Pediatric Nutrition in Chronic Diseases and Developmental Disorders

Pediatric Nutrition in Chronic Diseases and Developmental Disorders

Prevention, Assessment, and Treatment

Edited by

Shirley Walberg Ekvall, Ph.D., FAAMD, FACN, R.D.

New York   Oxford
OXFORD UNIVERSITY PRESS
1993

Oxford University Press

Oxford   New York   Toronto
Delhi   Bombay   Calcutta   Madras   Karachi
Kuala Lumpur   Singapore   Hong Kong   Tokyo
Nairobi   Dar es Salaam   Cape Town
Melbourne   Auckland   Madrid

and associated companies in
Berlin   Ibadan

Published by Oxford University Press, Inc.,
198 Madison Avenue, New York, New York 10016

Oxford is a registered trademark of Oxford University Press

Library of Congress Cataloging-in-Publication Data
Pediatric nutrition in chronic diseases and developmental disorders:
prevention, assessment, and treatment
edited by Shirley Walberg Ekvall.
p.   cm.   Includes indexes.   ISBN 0-19-507224-3
1. Developmentally disabled children—Nutrition.   2. Chronically
ill children—Nutrition.   I. Ekvall, Shirley.
[DNLM: 1. Child Development Disorders.   2. Child Nutrition.
3. Chronic Disease—in infancy & childhood.   4. Nutrition
Assessment.   5. Nutrition Disorders—in infancy & childhood.
WS   115 P3709]   RJ233.P43   1992   618.92—dc20   DNLM/DLC
for Library of Congress   91-45318

9 8 7 6 5

Printed in the United States of America
on acid-free paper

To all the children
with special health care needs
and to my husband, Ray,
for his understanding and support

Contributors

Linda Bandini, Ph.D.
Assistant Professor
Department of Pediatrics
Tufts University School of Medicine
Boston, Massachusetts

Mildred Bentler, M.A., R.D.
Pediatric Dietitian
Department of Nutrition Services
Newark Beth Israel Medical Center
Newark, New Jersey

Helen Berry, M.A.
Director, Metabolic Disease Center
Children's Hospital Medical Center
Professor of Pediatrics
University of Cincinnati College of Medicine
Cincinnati, Ohio

Eric Bonsall, M.D.
Assistant Professor, Department of Psychiatry
Director, Child Psychiatry In Patient Unit
Pennsylvania State University College of Medicine
Milton S. Hershey Medical Center
Hershey, Pennsylvania

Janet Borel, M.S., R.D.
Research Nutritionist
Department of Neurogenetics
Kennedy Institute for Handicapped Children
Baltimore, Maryland

Mariel Caldwell, M.P.H., M.S., R.D.
Regional Nutrition Consultant
Department of Maternal and Child Health
Public Health Service, U.S.D.H.H.S.
Chicago, Illinois

Harriet Cloud, M.S., R.D.
Director, Nutrition Division
Sparks Center Developmental and Learning Disorders
University of Alabama at Birmingham
Birmingham, Alabama

Shirley Walberg Ekvall, Ph.D., FAAMD, FACN, R.D., L.D.
Chief of Nutrition Services
University Affiliated Cincinnati Center for Developmental Disorders
Children's Hospital Medical Center and
Professor, Department of Health and Nutrition Sciences, University of Cincinnati
Cincinnati, Ohio

Valli Ekvall, L.P., R.D.
Nutrition/Psychology
Indiana University Medical Center
Indiana University and Purdue University
Indianapolis, Indiana

Sheila Farnan, M.P.H., R.D.
Nutrition Consultant
Minnesota Department of Health
Services for Children with Handicaps
Minneapolis, Minnesota

Michael Farrell, M.D., FACN
Associate Professor of Pediatrics
University of Cincinnati College of Medicine
Director of Nutritional Support Team
Children's Hospital Medical Center
Cincinnati, Ohio

Thomas Fischer, M.D., FAAP, FAAI
Associate Professor of Pediatrics
University of Cincinnati College of Medicine
Director, Division of Allergy/Immunology
Children's Hospital Medical Center
Cincinnati, Ohio

Deborah Gregg, R.D., L.D.
Research Dietitian
Clinical Research Center
Children's Hospital Medical Center
Cincinnati, Ohio

Shirley Hack, R.D.
Clinical Dietitian, Nutrition Support Team
Department of Gastroenterology and Nutrition
Children's Hospital of Los Angeles
Los Angeles, California

Carol Henderson, R.D., L.D.
Dietitian
Division of Pediatric Rheumatology
Children's Hospital Medical Center
Cincinnati, Ohio

James Heubi, A.B., M.D.
Assistant Program Director/Clinical Research Center
Children's Hospital Medical Center
Professor of Pediatrics
University of Cincinnati
Cincinnati, Ohio

R. Jean Hine, Ph.D., R.D.
Associate Professor
Department of Dietetics and Nutrition and
Arkansas Cancer Research Center
University of Arkansas Medical Center
Little Rock, Arkansas

Vanja Holm, M.D.
Associate Professor
Department of Pediatrics
University of Washington
Seattle, Washington

Lusia Hornstein, M.D.
Professor of Pediatrics
University of Cincinnati
Director of Pediatrics
University Affiliated Cincinnati Center for
*   Developmental Disorders*
Children's Hospital Medical Center
Cincinnati, Ohio

Agnes Huber, Ph.D., R.D., FAAMD
Professor of Nutrition
Simmons College
Boston, Massachusetts

Alison Hull, M.P.H., R.D.
Nutritionist
Pediatric Department
Georgetown University
Washington, D.C.

Melanie Hunt, M.Ed., R.D.
Nutritionist
The Metabolic Disease Center
Children's Hospital Medical Center
Assistant Professor of Clinical Pediatrics
University of Cincinnati
Cincinnati, Ohio

Kathleen Huntington, M.S., R.D.
Nutritionist
Metabolic Clinic and Nutrition Services
Oregon Health Sciences University
Child Development and Rehabilitation Center
Portland, Oregon

Susan Iannaccone, M.D.
Associate Professor
Director of Neuromuscular Clinic
Department of Neurology
Children's Hospital Medical Center
Cincinnati, Ohio

Ellen Gerber Illig, M.Ed., R.D., L.D.
Dietitian
The Cholesterol Center
The Jewish Hospital
Cincinnati, Ohio

Karen Kalinyak, M.D.
Assistant Professor of Pediatrics
Division of Hematology/Oncology
Children's Hospital Medical Center
Cincinnati, Ohio

Kristine Kelsey, M.S., R.D.
Nutrition/Public Health
Nutrition Department
School of Public Health
University of North Carolina
Chapel Hill, North Carolina

Marietta Llenado, M.Ed., R.D.
Nutrition Consultant
Private Practice
Wayne, New Jersey

Daniel Lovell, M.D., M.P.H.
Associate Professor of Pediatrics
Rowe Division of Pediatric Rheumatology
Children's Hospital Medical Center
Cincinnati, Ohio

Susan Dickerson Mayes, Ph.D.
Assistant Professor of Psychiatry
Pennsylvania State University College of Medicine
Milton S. Hershey Medical Center
Hershey, Pennsylvania

Barbara Niedbala, R.D., M.Ed.
Former Head Clinical Dietitian
St. Louis Regional Medical Center
Consultant/Instructor
Memphis State University
Memphis, Tennessee

Bonnie Patterson, M.D.
Assistant Professor of Pediatrics
University of Cincinnati College of Medicine
Department of Pediatrics

University Affiliated Cincinnati Center for
* Developmental Disorders*
Cincinnati, Ohio

Peggy Pipes, M.A., M.P.H.
Assistant Chief Nutritionist
Child Development and Mental Retardation Center
Lecturer, Parent/Child Nursing and
School of Nursing
University of Washington
Seattle, Washington

Barbara Mathis Prater, Ph.D., R.D., C.D.
Professor Emeritus
Utah State University
Salt Lake City, Utah

Ann Prendergast, M.P.H., R.D.
Chief Nutritionist
Department of Maternal and Child Health
United States Department of Health and Human
* Services*
Rockville, Maryland

Karyl Rickard, R.D., Ph.D.
Professor of Nutrition and Dietetics
Department of Nutrition and Dietetics
James Whitcomb Riley Hospital for Children
Indiana University School of Medicine
Indianapolis, Indiana

Cecilia Rokusek, Ed.D., R.D.
Executive Director
South Dakota University Affiliated Program
Center for Interdisciplinary Disabilities
Associate Professor of Family Medicine and Dental
* Hygiene*
University of South Dakota School of Medicine
Vermillion, South Dakota

Jack Rubinstein, M.D.
Director
University Affiliated Cincinnati Center for
* Developmental Disorders*
Professor of Pediatrics
University of Cincinnati
Cincinnati, Ohio

Donna Runyan, M.S., R.D.
Director of Nutrition Division
Child Development Center
Georgetown University
Washington, D.C.

Nina Scribanu, M.D.
Associate Professor
Department of Pediatrics, Georgetown University
Director, Center for Genetic Counseling and Birth
* Defects Evaluation*
Washington, D.C.

Marshal Shlafer, Ph.D.
Professor of Pharmacology
Medical School
University of Michigan
Ann Arbor, Michigan

Ninfa Saturnino Springer, Ph.D., R.D., FAAMD
Associate Professor
School of Nursing
University of Michigan
Ann Arbor, Michigan

Florence Stevens, M.S., R.D., L.D.
Nutritionist
Nutrition Department
University Affiliated Cincinnati Center for
* Developmental Disorders*
Cincinnati, Ohio

Reginald Tsang, B.B.S., M.D., FACN
Director of Perinatal Research Institute
Vice Chairman of Academic Affairs and Reseach
Children's Hospital Medical Center
Professor of Pediatrics, Obstetrics, and Gynecology
University of Cincinnati College of Medicine
Cincinnati, Ohio

Elizabeth Wenz, M.S., R.D.
Nutritionist
Phenylketonuria, Galactosemia, Medical Genetics
Children's Hospital of Los Angeles
Los Angeles, California

Illustrator
Bradley Ekvall
College of Design, Architecture, Art, and Planning
University of Cincinnati
Cincinnati, Ohio

Foreword

Interest in nutrition and its relation to health has waxed and waned during this century. Discovery and characterization of essential dietary factors in the early years led to recognition of disease states associated with deficiencies, and, by the 1940s, extraction and synthesis of vitamins brought hopes for a universal cure. The 1960s and 1970s broadened our knowledge of metabolic pathways by which food chemicals are converted to body chemicals and increased our understanding of the role of vitamins and trace minerals as catalysts for the enzymatic reactions involved. Only recently has nutrition taken its place beside drugs and surgical techniques as therapy for disease. Nutrition offers the added advantage of prevention of problems associated with many chronic diseases.

Nutrition intervention strategies for children with chronic diseases and developmental disorders must have both short- and long-term goals. The short-term goals, which are more obvious, involve support of growth and development while avoiding nutritional deficiencies both in calories and specific nutrients. Long-term goals are even more important. For example, many children for whom these strategies are developed have reduced physical activity. Of utmost importance, therefore, is the tailoring of diet to caloric expenditure to avoid the complicating factor of obesity. For children with such chronic disorders as myelomeningocele or hemophilia, obesity can be a devastating problem in management. As treatment for developmental disorders and chronic diseases has improved, so has longevity. Therefore, long-term goals must take into account the avoidance of nutritional risk factors for chronic adult diseases, such as coronary artery disease, hypertension, and cancer.

Health care professionals with varied experience and professional backgrounds should be assembled into a team to provide appropriate guidance and follow-up. Each child will need individualized programs depending on the severity of the disorder and his or her personal nature. The family must participate fully in the planning process and act as a full partner with health professionals in the implementation of the nutrition program if the above-mentioned goals are to be achieved and the child is to become as independent as possible.

Pediatric Nutrition in Chronic Diseases and Developmental Disorders, although directed toward children with special health care needs, provides a wealth of information on current issues in preventive nutrition and normal growth for all ages. As can be seen by a review of the Table of Contents, the diseases and disorders of children necessitating nutritional intervention are extremely varied. The diverse topics include acquired disorders, such as obesity, pica, and anorexia nervosa; inherited metabolic diseases; other genetic diseases, such as diabetes and cystic fibrosis; chromosomal defects; cancer; heart disease; the premature infant; and normal prenatal and postnatal growth.

The editor, Shirley Walberg Ekvall, is a nationally recognized expert in the field of pediatric nutrition with 25 years experience and numerous publications and national/international presentations. Since 1983, she has served as director of a national nutrition workshop for children with special health care needs, as well as a federal research grant reviewer and editorial consultant for the *Surgeon General's Report on Nutrition and Health*, several nutrition journals, and publishers. Dr. Ekvall has assembled a knowledgeable and experienced group of experts in the fields of nutrition, medicine, and biochemistry to bridge the gap from research to practice in nutrition for each of the topics in this book. The authors provide a careful analysis and clear guidelines to proper nutrition for children with special health needs. This volume offers to health professionals greater understanding of the nutritional implications of various disease states, how nutrition can affect brain development and learning behavior, and approaches to improving the health status of individuals.

Helen Berry, M.A.
Director, Metabolic Disease Center
Children's Hospital Medical Center
Professor of Research Pediatrics
University of Cincinnati
College of Medicine
Cincinnati, Ohio
National President, Society for
Inherited Metabolic Diseases

Alvin Mauer, M.D.
Chief, Division of Hematology
and Medical Oncology
Professor of Medicine and Pediatrics
University of Tennessee
Memphis, Tennessee
Former Chairman of the Nutrition
Committee American Academy of Pediatrics

Preface

The *Surgeon General's Report on Nutrition and Health*, 1988, and the *Surgeon General's Report: Chldren with Special Health Care Needs Campaign '87* both verified the need for better nutrition through early intervention, particularly for children with special health care needs. Public Law 99-457 underscores the importance of early intervention and identifies the need for family-centered care to reduce nutrition problems and their related cost in our society. In the last six years, several interdisciplinary national workshops/short courses have convened to make other disciplines aware of the impact of nutrition on chronic diseases and developmental disorders. These programs have been given under the auspices of the Maternal and Child Health Bureau (MCHB). As a follow up from the Surgeon General's Reports, *Healthy People 2000, National Health Promotion and Disease Prevention Objectives*, Institute of Medicine, 1990, and *Call to Action: Better Nutrition for Mothers, Children and Families*, MCHB, 1991, provide action strategies to improve nutrition for the nation. This growing recognition of the importance of nutrition has been enhanced by the ongoing federally sponsored health and examination studies (NHANES studies)—initiated in the United States in the early 1970's.

This book, a much-needed resource, spans the void between nutrition research and its practical application to children with chronic diseases and developmental disorders. It includes numerous recently diagnosed diseases and disorders such as Pediatric AIDS, Fragile-X, Williams Syndrome, Rett Syndrome, and Fetal Hydantoin Syndrome.

This volume reviews the current status of research in the role of nutrition in developmental disorders and chronic diseases of children and helps translate this research into clinical practice. Although the main thrust of the book is treatment, with the goal of enabling children who have special health care needs to develop their potential, techniques on assessment (including *behavior*) and prevention for all ages also are addressed. It should be a valuable reference for pediatricians, nutritionists, family practitioners, dietitians, pediatric residents, medical students, nutrition students, nursing students, and allied health personnel.

Each chapter focuses on Biochemical and/or Clinical Abnormalities, Techniques in Nutrition Evaluation or Diagnosis, Nutritional Treatment or Management, and Follow-Up Procedures. Section I deals with preventive techniques in assessing and averting disorders and other high risk problems. Resource materials and quality assurance standards in nutrition also are addressed. Section II contains topics related to nutrition in chronic diseases and developmental disorders. Section III describes hereditary in-born errors of metabolism and provides methods of diagnosis and treatment.

We hope that the use of this book will help improve the nutritional status of children with special health care needs and will stimulate and basic research in this field.

Cincinnati, Ohio   Shirley Walberg Ekvall
June 1992

Acknowledgments

I appreciate the editorial reviews by Helen Berry, Alvin Mauer, Kessey Keiselhorst, Susan Krug Wispe, and Grace Falciglia. I also extend thanks to the following people: current and former fellows at the University Affiliated Cincinnati Center for Developmental Disorders: Mariann Beutell, Jenny Heber, Betsy Bigley, Connie Arman, Cate Beck, Alison Rathke, Elizabeth Wheby, Becky Gruenwald, Gerri Leonti, Cynthia Vallo, Holly Murray, Tammy White, Lynnette Schwiegeraht, Stacey Johnston, Lisa Haven, and Staff Nutritionists, UACCDD, Elaine Howell, and Florence Stevens for their assistance with the book and Ramona Conley, Amy Merkley and Beverly York for typing manuscripts. I also appreciate the monetary contributions by Mr. and Mrs. James Rosenthal, Wyeth Pediatrics, Sandoz Nutrition, Gerber Products, Mead Johnson Nutritional Division, Miles Inc., The Upjohn Company, and Clintec Technologies in supporting publication of this book.

Contents

Pediatric Nutrition in Chronic Diseases and Developmental Disorders

Part I
Preventive Nutrition

Shirley Walberg Ekvall

This section focuses on preventive nutrition. Normal pre- and postnatal growth and development and prematurity are described. The behaviors and circumstances that might interfere with normal growth and the preventive measures and treatments for them are identified. Because the ability to measure nutritional status is key in identifying the possible need for intervention, nutritional status tools and training programs on how to provide nutrition services for children with special health care needs are reviewed. This section concludes with a discussion of the standards for delivering and evaluating the quality of these nutritional services.

Some effects of early malnutrition on growth reported by Myron Winick[1] are shown in the three figures below: cellular changes in various organs in malnourished rats after re-feeding (Fig. I-1), the reduction in human brain cells in infancy caused by malnutrition (Fig. I-2), and developmental quotients of 4-year-old children who had suffered early malnutrition and had not been rehabilitated until 4 months of age (Fig. I-3).

The severity, age of incidence, and duration of early nutritional deprivation determine the extent of its negative impact on growth and learning capability. The adverse effects of malnutrition on intellectual development are of interest, but need further investigation. The interplay of other environmental factors also cannot be ignored.

Proper maternal nutrients are essential for normal prenatal growth and for development during the first 3 years of life as 90% of the brain and 50% of the skeletal growth are developed by that age. High-risk factors affecting maternal nutrition and fetal outcome and associated corrective actions are discussed in Chapter 1 on prenatal growth. Some of the high-risk problems in infancy, such as iron-deficiency anemia, hypernatremia, obesity, and hyperlipidemia, are described, with their treatment, in Chapter 2. Because of the many assessment and treatment factors—enteral and parenteral nutrition, fluid balance, increased nutrient needs, and so forth—related to prematurity, Chapter 3 is devoted entirely to the premature infant.

Topics in this section relate to early intervention as mandated by Public Law (PL) 99-457 (102–119).[2] This law, passed originally in 1986 as an amendment to the Federal Education to the Handicapped Act, is earmarked for children from birth to 3 years of age who have developmental delays (children with special health care needs) or a high-risk problem that may result in a developmental delay. Preventive services have been extended to children ages 3 to 5 to strengthen the role of the family in their treatment. Children with these conditions are eligible for early intervention: mental retardation, speech and language impairment, hearing deficit, visual handicap, special learning disability, orthopedical impairment, emotional disturbance, and various other medical conditions categorized as health impairment. Early intervention encompasses a constellation of physical and cognitive services designed to prevent the need for later special education services. Disciplines involved in early intervention include nutrition, medicine, nursing, special education, speech/language pathology, audiology, psychology, occupational and physical therapy, and social work. These services may be transdisciplinary or interdisciplinary in nature. Dental referral may be appropriate as well.

The American Dietetic Association encourages and supports nutritional services that are coordinated, interdisciplinary, family centered, and community based for children with special health care needs and advocates that students be trained to provide such services.[3–7] The American Academy of Pediatrics and other health care associations also support PL 99-457 (102–119). Federal monies are provided to the states to fund the early intervention services for children who are developmentally delayed or at high risk from birth. At the state level, these services are administered either by the departments of health, education, or mental health and mental retardation. Nutrition education is a major component of PL 99-457 (102–119). Education related to nutrition may not only alleviate problems of these children with special health care needs so they may attain their full growth and development (e.g., feeding problems in children with cerebral palsy) but it may also prevent the delay from occurring.[8,9]

Techniques to screen, assess, diagnose, and correct high-risk nutrition problems in chronic diseases and developmental disorders such as those seen in children eligible for services mandated by PL 99-457 (102–119) are presented in the second part of this section. The five-point nutritional assessment includes dietary/nutrient intake and physical activity, biochemical values, anthropometric measurements, physical signs, and feeding. Several assessment methodologies are described comprehensively in Chapter 4, including anthropometric illustrations of measurement techniques for developmental disorders. Assessment forms, grids, tables, and illustrations covering infancy to adulthood are provided in the appendices. Three levels of nutritional status assessment—mini (community), midlevel (clinics), and in depth (physical examination)—are discussed throughout the chapter.

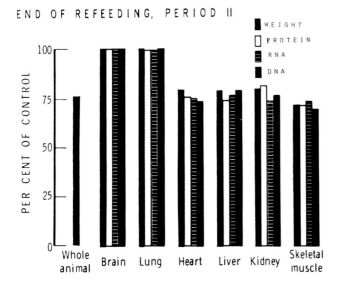

END OF REFEEDING, PERIOD II

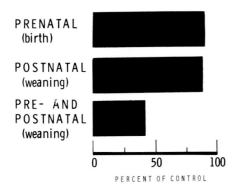

MALNUTRITION
TOTAL BRAIN CELL NUMBER

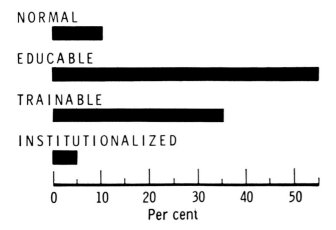

INFANTILE MARASMUS

Figs. I–1, I–2, and I–3 From Winick, M. *Cellular Changes During Early Malnutrition.* Currents in Maternal and Child Health. Columbus, OH: Ross Laboratories; 1971. Used with permission.

Of course, without the necessary nutritional resources and training materials at the clinics and other community-based programs, nutritional intervention would not be possible. Program planning tools for implementing community- and family-centered care are given in Chapter 5. One such resource is an interdisciplinary, short nutrition course for developmental disorders and chronic diseases sponsored annually by Maternal and Child Health in Cincinnati, Birmingham, and Los Angeles; this course includes training manuals and videotapes available from Cincinnati.[10] Long-term interdisciplinary nutrition training programs in other university-affiliated centers also are described.[11]

Quality assurance criteria and standards in nutrition are discussed in the last chapter of this section, Chapter 6. Detailed quality assurance standards of care for developmental disorders and for myelomeningocele are given in the appendices. Quality assurance standards for specific diseases or disorders are discussed throughout the book in the relevant chapters as well.

References

1. Winick, M. *Cellular Changes During Early Malnutrition.* Columbus, OH: Ross Laboratories; 1971. Currents in Maternal and Child Health.
2. Individuals with Disabilities Education Act. Early Intervention Program for Infants and Toddlers with Handicaps: Final Regulations. Public law #99-457 (102–119), *Federal Register.* June 22, 1989, 54(3)119:26306.
3. Lucas, B.L. Serving infants and children with special health care needs in the 1990s—are we ready? *J. Am. Diet. Assoc.* 1989;89:1599.
4. Kaufman, M. Are dietitians prepared to work with handicapped infants? P. L. 99-457 offers new opportunities. *J. Am. Diet. Assoc.* 1989;89:1602.
5. Hine, R.J., Cloud, H.H., Carithers, T., Hickey, C., Hinton, A. Early nutrition intervention services for children with special health care needs. *J. Am. Diet. Assoc.* 1989;89:1636.
6. Gooder, J.B., Ekvall, S.W. Extension of health and nutrition services via advanced telecommunications. *J. Am. Diet. Assoc.* 1989;89:821.
7. American Dietetic Association: Nutrition services for children with special health care needs. *J. Am. Diet. Assoc.* 1989;89:1133.
8. Sharbough, C., ed. *Call to Action: Better Nutrition for Mothers, Children and Family*, Washington, D.C., National Center for Education in Maternal and Child Health, 38 and R Streets, 1991.
9. Penziner, A.J., Amundson, J.A., Nelson, R.P. *Regional Nutrition Services for Children with Special Needs*, Child Health Specialty Clinics, The University of Iowa, Iowa City, Iowa, 52242, 1989.
10. Ekvall, S., Grace, E., Niemes, L., Wheby, E., Stevens, F. *Nutritional Needs of the Child with a Handicap or Chronic Illness (Child with Special Health Care Needs)*. Manuals I–III, Cincinnati University Affiliated Cincinnati Center for Developmental Disorders, 1987–1989.
11. Thompson, M.L., Smith, M.A., eds: 1987 Update: *Guidelines for Nutrition Training in University Affiliated Programs*. Memphis, University of Tennessee, Child Development Center, 1987.

Chapter 1
Prenatal Growth in Pregnancy

Shirley Walberg Ekvall

The causes of developmental disabilities in prenatal growth can be categorized into two major areas: (1) genetic inheritance, which includes single gene disorders (autosomal dominant, autosomal recessive, and X-linked), and chromosomal disorders (trisomy 21 and Down syndrome) and (2) the intrauterine environment, which includes maternal infection (herpes simplex type II), maternal diseases, and maternal lifestyles (use of toxic substances in the workplace or home, drug abuse, malnutrition, and smoking).

Maternal Nutrition and Fetal Outcome

Studies conducted during the past 40 to 50 years have demonstrated conclusively that improved nutrition during pregnancy (especially beginning in the first trimester) is associated with improved pregnancy outcomes. A study by Kennedy,[1] at the Harvard University School of Public Health, showed improved birth outcomes of 1303 women who had participated in the USDA Special Supplemental Food Program for Women, Infants, and Children (WIC). The subjects served as self-controls. They did not participate in the WIC food and nutrition education program for the first birth, but did participate for the second birth. There was a 23% decrease in low birth weight in those mothers who used the program for only one trimester and a 47% reduction in low birth weights for those who used the program for two trimesters. The WIC and Maternal and Infant Care Programs in general have produced a 42% increase in women's adherence to the prenatal care programs. These nutrition programs also have been cost effective: by reducing the incidence of low birth weight, each dollar spent on good nutrition has saved more than three dollars on subsequent treatment costs. With poverty reaching an all-time 17-year high, the impact of these nutrition programs can be critical.

Trends in Maternal and Infant Mortality

Maternal mortality rates in the United States declined 72% from 1960 to 1982.[2] The proportion of mothers beginning prenatal care in the first trimester has remained stable at 76% each year since 1979.[3]

Two-thirds of the deaths in the first month of life and 60% of all infant deaths occur in infants with low birth weight.[2] One-month survival increased from 36.5% to 89% from 24 to 29 weeks gestation.[4] The powerful effect of gestational age on survival highlights the need for an accurate

neonatal tool to assess gestational age of very low birth weight neonates.

The U.S. infant mortality rate of live births has decreased from 28/1000 in 1950 to 12.5/1000 in 1980 to 10.4/1000 in 1986,[5] to 9.7/1000 in 1989, and to 9.1/1000 in 1990 (preliminary estimates by the National Center for Health Statistics). However, the United States still ranked eighteenth in developed countries in 1985 (Table 1–1) and sixteenth in 1986 (Fig. 1–1). The mortality rate for black infants in 1986 in the United States was 6.3 compared to 3.1 for white infants per 1000 live births, and this disparity remained similar in 1989. Neonatal mortality risk and postneonatal mortality risk were 22% and 24% lower, respectively, among black foreign-born mothers than among black native-born mothers.[6] Only postneonatal mortality risk was 20% lower for white foreign-born mothers.[6] The baby born to an adolescent mother from a low socioeconomic background is most at risk for infant mortality.[5] Twin infant mortality rates are four to five times that of singletons.[7] Postneonatal mortality for selected countries and for selected causes of death from several countries are shown in Tables 1–2 and 1–3.[8].

Biochemical, Pathological, Clinical, and Nutrient Abnormalities

The effects of malnutrition are determined by its severity, timing, and duration (Fig. 1–2). When malnourished, the liver, heart, kidney, and skeletal muscle work harder and remain small to spare the brain and lung from damage. The last trimester of pregnancy and the first 6 months after birth are important for brain development. By age 3, 90% of the brain development has occurred, but the child has increased only 50% in height. The number of brain cells of infants in Chile dying from malnutrition were less than 40% of normal infants.[9] Studies in Mexico by Winick demonstrated that if infants were malnourished and then rehabilitated, 10% showed a total recovery in I.Q., 52% were educable, 33% were trainable and 5% were institutionalized.[10] (see Fig. I–3, Part I.) In the United States, problems caused by malnutrition may be revealed in more subtle changes in perceptual thinking, abstract thinking, verbalization, and maladaptive behavior. The incidence of fetal malnutrition is estimated to range from 3% to 10% of live births in developed countries and 15% to 20% in less developed countries.[11]

One of the major risk factors for developmental disabilities is the mother herself. Maternal high-risk indicators include:[12,13] smoking (20 cigarettes per day); adolescence (under

Table 1–1. Birth* and Infant Mortality† Rates for 25 Countries with Populations Greater Than 2,500,000, 1984 and 1985

Country	Birth Rate	Infant Mortality Rate 1985	Infant Mortality Rate 1984	% Births To Women Under 20
Japan	12.5		6.0	1.2
Sweden	11.8	6.7	6.4	3.8
Finland	13.3		6.5	4.3
Switzerland	11.5		7.1	3.2
Denmark	10.6		7.7	4.2
France	14.1	8.4	8.0	4.3 (1981)
Canada	14.9		8.1	7.8 (1982)
Norway	12.1		8.3	6.3
Netherlands	12.1	7.9	8.4	2.7
Hong Kong	14.4		8.8	3.0 (1982)
Singapore	16.6	9.3	8.8	3.2
Australia	15.0		9.2	6.9
German Fed. Rep.	9.6		9.6	4.4
United Kingdom	12.9		9.6	8.6
German Dem. Rep.	13.7	9.6	10.0	13.4
Ireland	18.2		10.1	4.4
Belgium	11.5	9.4	10.7	5.9 (1981)
U.S.A.	15.5	10.6	10.7	13.7
Austria	11.5	11.0	11.5	10.4
New Zealand	16.0	10.8	11.6	9.5
Italy	10.1	10.9	11.6	6.9 (1980)
Spain	12.5		12.3	6.9 (1979)
Israel	23.7	12.3	12.8	5.1
Greece	12.8	14.0	14.1	12.2 (1982)
Czechoslovakia	14.5		15.3	11.8 (1982)

*Infant mortality rate = number of deaths per 1000 live births.
†Birth rate = number of life births per 1000 population.
From Wegman, M.E. Annual summary of vital statistics, 1985. *Pediatrics.* 1986;78:983. Used with permission.

15 years); more than three pregnancies in 2 years (lower stores of iron, folate, B complex, and vitamin C); an inadequate diet (especially of protein, iron, folate, B_{12}, and vitamin A); food faddism (bizarre food habits or pica such as eating laundry starch or clay); economic deprivations and drug addiction or alcoholism (more than 5 ounces of whiskey or equivalent per day). Drugs, such as heroin and barbituates, can produce withdrawal in the infant. Heroin (causes hyperkalemia), morphine (results in calcium inhibition), and cocaine (depresses appetite)[14] are more damaging as their use results in lower birth weight than barbiturate addiction. Prescription drugs can also affect maternal nutrition. Oral contraceptives reduce serum B_6 and folate. Anticonvulsants—for example phenytoin—reduce folate as well. Abnormalities in fetal development can be caused by prescription drugs taken by the mother during pregnancy. Diuretics reduce oxygen to the fetal brain. Tetracycline produces abnormalities in bone development, including decalcification of dentition. Thalidomide, diethylstilbestrol, lysergic acid diethylamine, warfarin, antihistamines, cortisone, some antibiotics and tranquilizers, and Accutane® or isotretinoin, a vitamin A analog, have caused major problems in prenatal growth,[15,16] although other drugs have been accepted as nonteratogenic with customary use (Tables 1–4 and 1–5). Megavitamin usage, such as excessive ingestion of vitamins A, D, and C: calcium, and iodine, may result in prenatal damage to the infant (Table 1–6).

Other high-risk maternal indicators are chronic disease or a prior child with birth defects, 15% underweight or 20% overweight; poor obstetrical or fetal history; hemoglobin under 11 g/dL or hematocrit under 33% in the second trimester; inadequate weight gain (under 2 pounds per month or reduced growth of fetal skull by ultrasound); excessive weight gain (more than 2 pounds per week); breastfeeding; proteinuria; and glucosuria. Environmental substances suspected of causing congenital malformation in humans are shown in Table 1–4.

Maternal diseases can cause problems in prenatal growth. They include epilepsy, diabetes, heart disease, phenylketonuria, RH blood factor, hypertension (related to toxemia and pre-eclampsia), and anemia. Although folic acid is recommended prenatally to prevent neural tube defects, the intake of large quantities of folate during pregnancy should be evaluated during nutrition counseling to prevent possible deleterious interaction with other nutrients. A recent study in seven countries, however, has firmly concluded that women receiving 4 mg of folic acid supplementation had a significantly lower recurrence of fetal neural tube defects and has recommended increased folic acid for this population as well as for all pregnant women. The supplementation of 4 mg of folic acid, however, is much higher than the supplementation in some former studies.[18] (see Chapter 10.) Only a supplementation of 0.3 mg folic acid is given in vitamins in the United States.[19] Laboratory values in pregnant women for hemoglobin, hematocrit, serum transferrin, transferrin saturation, thiamine, riboflavin, and urinary n'methyl nicotinamide (mg/g of creatinine) differ from the acceptable adult values (see Appendix 10 for exact laboratory values).

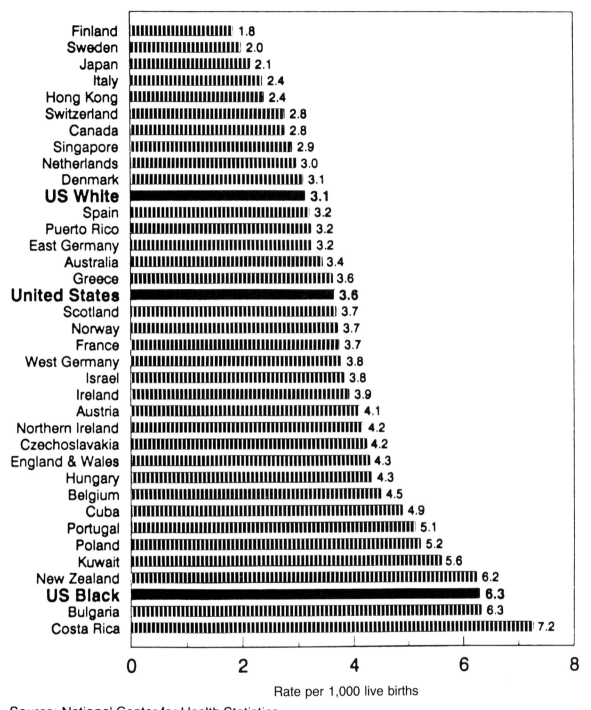

Fig. 1–1. Infant mortality rates. From Kleinman, J.C., Kiely, J.L. Postneonatal mortality in the United States: an international perspective: part 2. *Pediatrics.* 1990;86 (suppl). Used with permission.

Factors to be Considered in Nutritional Evaluation and Dietary Management

The suggested assessment of the mother includes her medical history as well as the physical screening of four parameters: dietary history and food frequency; anthropometric measures of mother's fatfold, height, and weight; physical activity of mother; and laboratory tests (see the WIC nutritional assessment form and computerized perinatal nutrition assessment form in Appendix 5).

In the dietary history, the mother should be asked about quantities of various foods eaten and any unusual food habits, such as pica during pregnancy. Women who are malnourished before pregnancy and during early pregnancy require additional nutrients and dietary counseling,[15] especially teenagers whose bodies are still growing. The recommended daily dietary intake for the pregnant adolescent and for the pregnant adult is shown in Table 1–7. Because this daily food plan may be low in some nutrients, such as folate and

Table 1–2. Postneonatal Mortality Rates per 1000 Live Births: Selected Countries, 1950 to 1987

	1950	1960	1970	1980	1985	1986
Canada	17.1	9.3	5.3	3.8	2.7	2.8
England and Wales	11.3	6.3	5.9	4.4	4.0	4.3
France	26.6	9.8	5.5	4.3	3.7	3.7
Netherlands	8.8	4.5	3.3	2.9	3.0	3.0
Norway	13.5	7.2	3.3	3.0	3.8	3.7
Sweden	5.7	2.8	1.9	2.0	2.6	2.0
United States	8.7	7.3	4.9	4.1	3.7	3.6
U.S. black	16.1	16.5	9.9	7.3	6.1	6.3
U.S. white	7.4	5.7	4.0	3.5	3.2	3.1

From Child Health in 1990: the United States compared to Canada, England and Wales, France, the Netherlands, Norway, and Sweden: part 2. *Pediatrics*. 1990;86(suppl). Used with permission.

Table 1–3. Postneonatal Mortality for Selected Causes of Death: Selected Countries, 1986

	Canada	England and Wales	France	Netherlands	Norway	United States	U.S. White	U.S. Black
All causes	276.3	427.2	373.2	296.4	369.4	364.1	313.4	628.9
Infectious and parasitic diseases	6.4	15.6	11.6	10.8	7.6	17.3	13.3	36.1
Nervous system diseases	14.0	20.1	14.0	14.6	15.2	14.9	13.7	23.5
Respiratory system diseases	17.2	47.0	15.0	28.2	19.0	28.4	22.6	57.1
Pneumonia and influenza	11.3	20.3	5.9	14.6	17.1	13.6	10.8	28.3
Congenital anomalies	69.5	74.0	62.7	76.4	83.8	55.6	53.1	69.9
Perinatal conditions	24.4	30.7	24.2	20.1	34.3	28.5	23.4	55.9
Symptoms and ill-defined conditions	102.6	197.4	181.3	111.1	194.2	146.5	127.5	248.7
Sudden infant death syndrome	92.9	195.4	158.3	99.7	190.4	130.9	115.1	215.1
Accidents	15.0	11.5	36.6	14.6	1.9	21.8	18.1	39.6
Residual	27.2	30.9	27.9	20.6	13.3	51.1	41.7	98.1

From Kleinman, J.C., Kiely, J.L. Postneonatal mortality in the United States: an international perspective: part 2. *Pediatrics*. 1990;86(suppl). Used with permission.

other B vitamins (depending on the foods selected) a prenatal vitamin supplement is frequently recommended by the physician for both pregnancy and lactation unless the client is nutrition knowledgeable. The daily diet during pregnancy should include at least *14 extra grams of protein, 300 extra calories*, and increased quantities of most vitamins and minerals, except for vitamins A and D, calcium, and phosphorus (Table 1–8 and 1989 recommended daily allowance (RDA) in Appendix 1). In the 1989 RDA table, recommendations for copper, manganese, fluoride, chromium, and molybdenum are listed as ranges for all age groups, but were not determined for pregnancy and lactation. A 1989 RDA value for selenium has been added for all age groups, including pregnancy and lactation.

Mineral deficiencies

Some mineral deficiencies may produce problems in pregnancy. Zinc deficiency results in impaired synthesis of nucleic acids.[20] Vitamin A is needed for the transport protein, a carrier of zinc into the blood. Low manganese levels, as measured in the mother's hair, which may be inaccurate, have been found in mothers of infants with congenital malformations.[21] Magnesium deficiency may be responsible for spasms of the umbilical and placental vasculature in preeclampsia; magnesium sulfate is effective therapy.[22] Because anemia due to iron deficiency or folic acid deficiency is common and the infant may also become anemic, food sources

with high iron and folic acid content are essential, as is supplementation of iron and folic acid in prenatal vitamin capsules. Without iron supplementation, most women exhaust their iron stores and are iron deficient as manifested by low ferritin levels. Iron supplementation appears to be needed until about 20 to 24 weeks gestation (Fig. 1–3). If no iron supplement is given, it takes about 2 years after pregnancy to attain prepregnancy ferritin levels. Ascorbic acid and meat, fish, or poultry may increase nonheme iron bioavailability fourfold.[23] Villar et al.[24] noted that individuals with high calcium intake have lower blood pressure and that rats with restricted calcium intake develop hypertension, which is reversible by calcium supplements. In addition, the eclampsia syndrome is similar to tetany caused by hypocalcemia, (a finding that requires more research).[25]

Age

A 30% increase in frequency of low birth weight was found in infants born to adolescent mothers.[26] Early prenatal care promoted better pregnancy outcome for younger teenagers than for older teens or adults.[27] Five percent of 10- to 14-year-old mothers had 2+ or greater acetonuria versus 2% of mothers between 17 to 32 years of age.[28] Neonatal and fetal deaths were 56% more frequent when mothers had 2+ or greater acetonuria.[28] "Encouraging young adolescents to gain larger amounts of weight during pregnancy may be one way to decrease the risk of low birth weight

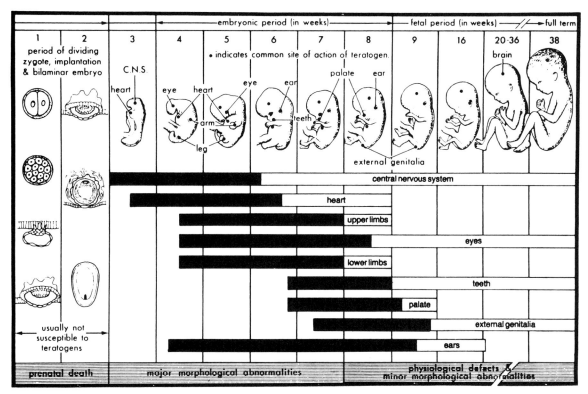

Fig. 1–2. Schematic illustration of the sensitive or critical periods in human development. The dark band denotes highly sensitive periods; the light band indicates stages that are less sensitive to teratogens. Note that each organ or structure has a critical period during which its development may be deranged and physiological defects, functional disturbances,and minor morphological changes are likely to result from disturbances during the fetal period. Severe mental retardation may result from exposure of the developing human to high levels of radiation during the 8- to 16-week period. From Moore, K.L. *Before We Are Born. Basic Embryology and Birth Defects.* 2nd Ed. Philadelphia: W.B. Saunders; 1974. Used with permission.

deliveries."[29] Infants born to mothers after age 35 have a higher incidence of Down syndrome (see Chapter 16).

Weight gain

Abrams and Russell[30] found that pregravid body mass and weight gain significantly influenced birth weight. For the underweight, ideal weight, and moderately overweight woman, each kilogram of maternal weight gain increased infant birth weight by 25.9, 28.3, and 17.8 grams, respectively.[30] When assessing the nutritional requirements of pregnant women, weight gain related to the changes due to the pregnancy itself must be considered (Table 1–9).

As shown in Table 1–9, a prenatal weight gain of 25 to 35 pounds produces an optimum pregnancy outcome for one infant (35 to 45 pounds for twins).[31] The caloric cost of pregnancy is about 70,000 calories.[15] The woman who does not gain sufficient weight must catabolize maternal tissue, which may produce ketosis and thus may impair the neurological development of the fetus.[32] Normal weight pregnant women should gain about one pound per week during the second and third trimesters. Brown et al.[33] found that more than 50% of underweight women failed to gain more than 9 kg in pregnancy and the infant weighed less than 2501 grams; thus weight gain is of critical importance to underweight women who become pregnant. Mitchell and Lerner[34] found similar results. Springer et al.[35] found a significant relationship between weight gain at 20 weeks gestation and

infant birth weight. Brown et al.[36] have developed a prenatal weight gain intervention program using social marketing methods to encourage early weight gain. Muscati et al.[37] and Springer et al.[35] also found that smoking was significantly associated with reduced prenatal weight gain, particularly for teenagers. Resting metabolic rate (RMR) increased more during pregnancy than previous estimates on well-nourished women would indicate, and the increase was significantly correlated with the birth weight of the baby.[38] Increased incidence of hypertension (43.6%), hyperglycemia (16.9%), and subnormal urinary estriol excretion (18.6%) were found in obese pregnant women.[38] The complications of labor also are much greater with obesity.[39] Figures 1–4 and 1–5 show recommended weight gain as related to pre-pregnancy weight and weight gain for selected subsets.

The fetus is fed first by the trophoblast (secretion of *uterine milk* from uterine glands), then by *syncytium* (formed between maternal and fetal tissues) when the blastocyst is implanted in the uterine epithelium, and finally by the *placenta* (through placental circulation). The velocity of weight gain peaks at 33–34 weeks at about 220 g/wt (Fig. 1–6 and see Fig. 2–1 in Chapter 2). Carbohydrates reach the fetus as glucose, which is used to synthesize fat. The essential lipids and phospholipids in the cell walls and nervous system are transferred to the fetus from the maternal circulation. The lipid content is 1% at 20 weeks, 2.8% at 34 weeks, and 15% at term. The nitrogen—as polypeptides, proteins, and

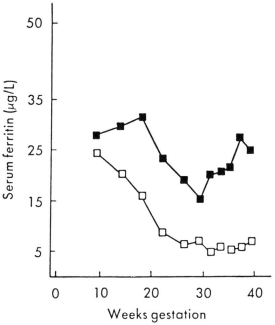

Fig. 1–3. Changes in serum ferritin during pregnancy in women treated with (■) or without (□) oral iron supplementation. Results are given as means + SD. From Romslo, I., et al. Iron requirement in normal pregnancy assessed by serum ferritin, serum transferrin saturation and erythrocyte protoporphyrin determinations. *Br J Obstet Gynecol* 1983;90:101. Used with permission.

immunoglobulins—required for the synthesis of many different proteins reaches the fetus mainly by the active transport of amino acids. The proportion of protein increases with gestational age and is greater than fat until 35 weeks of age[40] (Fig. 1–7). The rate of calcium increases from 0.3 g/wk at 18 weeks gestation to 1.3 g/wk at 40 weeks; phosphorus increases from 0.3 g/wk at 18 weeks to 2.6 g/wk at 40 weeks (Fig. 1–8). Trace elements enter the fetus early in gestation, probably in the plasma attached to specific proteins, whereas water-soluble vitamins cross the placenta by active transport since their concentration is higher in fetal than maternal blood. Fat-soluble vitamins are found in lower concentrations in the fetus than in maternal plasma, but the method of transfer is unknown. The oxygen consumption of the fetus is 30 kcal/kg/24 hr in utero, 32 kcal/kg/24 hr at birth, and 43 kcal/kg/24 hr by day.[40]

Colostrum only provides 18 kcal/kg/24 hr, but provides 12.5 g immunoglobulins (12% to 15% protein) on day one or 1% to 2% by day five, which limits bacterial and viral antigens in the intestinal tract. Colostrum also binds iron and makes it unavailable to *Escherichia coli* in the intestine, thereby inhibiting bacterial growth. Colostrum also has two times as much vitamin A, eight times as much carotenoids, and five times as much vitamin B_{12} per 100 mL as mature milk. Since nutrition after birth is less efficient, 120 kcal/kg/24 hr is needed during the first month and 100 kcal/kg/24 hr during the second month.[41] Breast milk provides about 100 kcal/kg/24 hr or less but some nutrients are better absorbed in breast milk.

Exercise

Engaging in moderate exercise of limited duration during pregnancy does not appear to produce fetal cardiovascular stress if the exercise was practiced before pregnancy.[41] It can strengthen the lower extremities, abdominal muscle, and pelvic floor and increase circulation to muscle fibers.[42] New or strenuous exercise programs should not be started during pregnancy because of a potential drop in blood flow in the body and reduced fetal oxygenation or fetal dissipation of heat through the placenta.[42] In one study, continued jogging throughout pregnancy did not increase the rate of abortion, prematurity, or fetal, maternal or neonatal deaths. However, the incidence of fetal anomalies did increase to 6% from the average of 2% to 3%.[43] These anomalies were not life threatening. Pregnant women should therefore ask their physician about the amount and type of exercise to pursue during pregnancy. More research is needed in this area.[43]

Diseases or disorders

Smokers have chronically decreased placental flow, and their infants weigh up to 200 grams less at birth.[44] *Alcohol* and *drugs* should be avoided during pregnancy (see Chapters 14 and 15). Data from human studies are inconsistent regarding caffeine usage. *Caffeine* should only be used minimally, or intake should be lower than 150 mg/day as late spontaneous abortions are more likely with higher levels.[25]

In the United States, geophagia, pagophagia, and anylophagia are the most commonly reported practices of *pica* during pregnancy. Anemia (iron deficiency) and zinc deficiency are common problems of pica (see Chapter 26). Clay and starch are the most commonly ingested substances. Pregnant women need to be questioned about food cravings and pica in particular, (particularly because of the harmful effects of lead toxicity).[45]

Mothers with *diabetes* have a higher incidence of congenital malformations. In rats these malformations were due to reduced arachidonic acid during organogenesis.[46] Women who are obese are more likely to develop gestational diabetes during pregnancy. In addition, women who are diabetic tend to deliver infants who weigh more than 9 lb. Frequently, these infants are delivered by cesarean section before they are full term. Eating a well-balanced diet and exercising regularly are particularly important for the mother with diabetes.

In recent years, *toxemia* in pregnancy has become less life threatening as blood pressure has come to be controlled more effectively, thereby reducing the incidence of intracranial hemorrhage. Prompt use of blood transfusion and broad-spectrum antibiotics for complications is needed.[47] The mean serum of placental isoferritin was found to be low in women with pre-eclamptic toxemia compared with women having a normal pregnancy. Thus, placental isoferritin may be a useful marker for pre-eclamptic toxemia of pregnancy.[48] It appears that the fetus whose mother has pre-clampsia-eclampsia is unlikely to be thrombcytopenic during labor and delivery; thus, scalp blood counts and cesarean delivery to avoid labor probably are not needed.[49] The Doppler ultrasound measurement of cardiac output in the pre-eclampsia patient has been validated.[50] Treating hypertension with medication during pregnancy may not be needed unless the pressure is above 170/100 mm Hg as diuretics may decrease the fetal oxygen supply.[51] A low 1 gm sodium and high 2 gm calcium diet possibly may be helpful, however.

Table 1–4. Environmental Substances Suspected of Causing Congenital Malformations in Human Beings (Teratogenic)

Contaminants and Additives

Cadmium
Cyclamates
Dioxin
Dichlorodiphenyl
 trichloroethane
Food colorings
Hair dyes
Lead
Mercury*
Monosodium glutamate
Nitrates
Nitrites
Polyhalogenated biphenyls
Saccharin
Sodium fluoride
2,4,5-T herbicide

Natural Substances

Blighted potatoes
Cyanide in cassava
Goitrogens in brassicae

Personal Habits

Alcohol
Cigarettes
Coffee
Gasoline sniffing
Lysergic acid diethylamide
Marijuana
Methadone
Phencyclidine
Tea
Tobacco chewing
Toluene sniffing

Occupational Exposure

Anesthetic gases
Fat solvents
Hairspray adhesives
Hexachlorophene
Hydrocarbons
Organic solvents
Printing trades
Smelter
University laboratories

*Of these substances, only mercury is today accepted to be a proven human teratogen.
From Kalter, H., Warkany, J. Congenital malformations. *N Eng J Med.* 1983;308:424.

Table 1–5. Possible Nonteratogenic Drugs or Drug Classes in Customary Use

Adrenocorticoids	Lithium*
Amphetamines	Meclizine
Nonquinine antimalarials	Nalidixic acid
Aspirin	Oral hypoglycemics
Bendectin	D-Penicillamine*
Captopril	Phenothiazines
Clomiphene	Podophyllum
Diazepam	Propoxyphene
Ergonovine	Sulfonamides
Imipramine	Tuberculostatics

*Since 1983, there is a question whether lithium and D-penicillamine may be teratogenic.
From: Kalter, H., Warhany, J. Congenital malformations. *N. Engl. J. Med.* 1983;308:491. (see Chapter 27.)

Proteinuria should be evaluated for its cause if at 1+, 2+, or 3+ levels.

Prevention management

A complete annotated resource list may be found in *Prevention Strategies For Developmental Disabilities, Module VI, The Importance of Optimum Nutrition at Conception, During Pregnancy, and in Early Childhood.*[52] Nutrition resources on prenatal growth are also readily available from the following sources: Food, Dairy and Nutrition Councils, selected federal information clearinghouses and national resource centers, Planned Parenthood affiliates, Maternal and Child Health projects, Women's, Infants, and Children's projects, March of Dimes chapters (*Maternal Nutrition Modules 1–10* and *Inside My Mom*), American Dietetic

Association (e.g., position papers related to chemical dependency.[53]) and dietary departments in hospitals. The Bureau of Maternal and Child Health Resources, Department of Health and Human Services asked the National Academy of Sciences to study maternal nutrition. Thus, the Committee on Nutritional Status During Pregnancy and Lactation, Food and Nutrition Board, Institute of Medicine, Na-

Table 1–6. Embryopathology Reported in Animal Models with Specific Nutritional Imbalances

Water	Deficiency	—
Food	Deficiency	—
Food and water	Deficiency	—
Vitamin A	Deficiency	Excess
Vitamin D	Deficiency	Excess
Vitamin K	Deficiency	—
Vitamin E	Deficiency	—
Vitamin C	Deficiency	Excess
Riboflavin	Deficiency	—
Thiamine	Deficiency	—
Niacin	Deficiency	—
Pyridoxine	Deficiency	—
Folic acid	Deficiency	—
Pantothenic acid	Deficiency	—
Vitamin B_{12}	Deficiency	—
Calcium	Deficiency	Excess
Magnesium	Deficiency	—
Iodine	Deficiency	Excess
Copper	Deficiency	—
Manganese	Deficiency	—
Zinc	Deficiency	—
Iron	Deficiency	—

From Brent[17] with permission.

Table 1–7. Daily Food Plan

Food Group	Adolescent Pregnancy	Adult Pregnancy	Lactation
Milk (milk products may be used)	5 c	4 c	6 c
Meat, liver, fish, poultry, eggs, or beans	2 servings (4 oz each)	2 servings (3 oz each)	4 servings (2½ oz each)
Fruit (vitamin C food source)	2 servings	2 servings	2 servings
Other	2 servings	2 servings	2 servings
Vegetables as source of			
Vitamin A	1 serving	1 serving	1 serving
Other, including raw vegetables	2 servings	2 servings	2 servings
Bread and cereal (whole grain preferred)	5–6 servings	4 servings	5 servings
Other foods	Foods to meet caloric needs may be selected from above groups, or fats and sweets may be added in moderation (about 200 cal).		
Liquids (cups per day)	8–12	8–12	12

Table 1–8. Recommended Dietary Allowances (RDA) for Pregnancy and Lactation for Ages 19 to 24, 1989

	RDA for Nonpregnant, Nonlactating Adults	Pregnant First Trimester	Lactation First 6 Months	Lactation Second 6 Months
Energy	2200	0*	+500†	+500†
Protein	46	60	65	62
Vitamin A (mcg RE)	800	800	1300	1200
Vitamin D (mcg)	10	10	10	10
Vitamin E (mg TE)	8	10	12	11
Vitamin K (mcg)	60	65	65	65
Vitamin C (mg)	60	70	95	90
Thiamin (mg)	1.1	1.5	1.6	1.6
Riboflavin (mg)	1.3	1.6	1.8	1.7
Niacin (mg NE)	15	17	20	20
Vitamin B$_6$ (mg)	1.6	2.2	2.1	2.1
Folate (mcg)	180	400	280	280
Vitamin B$_{12}$ (mcg)	2.0	2.2	2.6	2.6
Calcium (mg)	1200	1200	1200	1200
Phosphorus (mg)	1200	1200	1200	1200
Magnesium (mg)	280	320	355	340
Iron (mg)	15	30	15	15
Zinc (mg)	12	15	19	16
Iodine (mcg)	150	175	200	200
Selenium (mcg)	55	65	75	75

*Only need +300 cal/day if mother has depleted reserves or during second or third trimester.
†+500 cal/day is adequate, unless gestational weight gain is subnormal, then over 650 cal/day is needed.
Modified from The Food and Nutrition Board National Research Council: *Recommended Dietary Allowances.* 10th ed. Washington, DC: National Academy Press; 1989.

tional Academy of Sciences produced a valuable resource with information on weight gain and nutrient supplements during pregnancy and is entitled *Nutrition During Pregnancy*.[54] An annotated bibliography on *Nutrition and Adolescent Pregnancy, 1986* is available from the National Material Child Health Clearinghouse, 38 and R Streets, N.W., Washington, D.C. 20052.

Since the need to assess nutrition parameters in prenatal growth is so critical, dietitians and nutritionists should be employed in obstetric and pediatric offices. Likewise, since homeless women have higher pregnancy rates (11.4%) versus American women overall (5%) and lower birth weight infants (16.3%) to low income women (11.4%) and to overall births in New York City (7.4%),[55] dietitians and nutritionists should be consultants to homeless shelters. Doing

so is very cost effective, preventing the need for subsequent costly health care, in the United States. Third party reimbursement for nutrition services also is cost effective.

Preventive measures are important in reducing infant mortality.[55] Since lower net weight gains in pregnancy are associated with increased risk for the infant, young adolescent, Asian-American, and black mothers should strive for higher weight gains based on prepregnancy weight for height or body mass index (BMI) (weight/height^2)[56] (Fig. 1-5). The recommended weight gain is as follows:[57]

- Low (BMI < 19.8) = 28–40 lbs
- Normal (BMI 19.8 – 26.0) = 25–35 lbs
- High (BMI 26.0–29.0) = 15–25 lbs

Adolescents and underweight women tended to report prepregnancy weight and height more accurately than over-

Table 1–9. Weight Gain Related to Pregnancy

	Weight (lb)
Baby	7.0–8.5
Placenta	2.0–2.5
Increase in weight of uterus	2.0
Amniotic fluid	2.0
Increase in weight of breasts	1.0–4.0
Increase in blood volume and extracellular fluid	8.0–10
Mother's stores*	3.0–6.0
TOTAL	25.0–35.0

*Extra stores of fat and a little protein are required to support the energy required for pregnancy, labor, delivery, and milk production.

weight women.[58] Using pictures to show stages of growth and development of the fetus and plotting the weight change on a grid (Fig. 1–5) can reinforce the importance of weight gain, particularly for adolescents.[59]

A study in Guatemala examined women who became pregnant with a second child and continued to breast feed into the second trimester of pregnancy. The stress of lactation depleted the maternal nutrient stores, but did not affect fetal growth significantly.[60] These nutrients—iron, zinc, calcium, copper, magnesium, vitamins D and B[6], and folate—and caloric intake should be further studied to relate maternal and fetal nutritional status to pregnancy outcome.[56,61,62] If a daily multivitamin/mineral preparation is

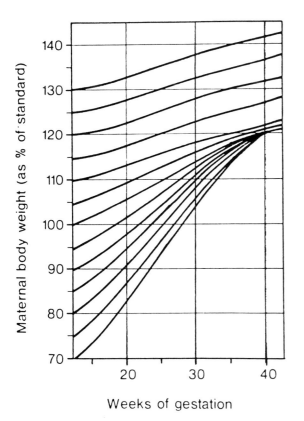

Fig. 1–4. Chart used to monitor weight gain during pregnancy considering prepregnancy weight and height. From Rosso, P. A new chart to monitor weight gain during pregnancy. *Am J Clin Nutr.* 1985;41:644. Used with permission.

recommended at the beginning of the second trimester it should contain: iron (30 mg), zinc (15 mg), copper (2 mg), calcium (250 mg), vitamin B[6] (2 mg), folate (300 mcg), vitamin C (50 mg), and vitamin D (5 mcg); it should be taken between meals or at bedtime.[56] In a study by Dubois et al.[63] results suggest that nutritional intervention can significantly improve twin-pregnancy outcome. Likewise Susser[64] found that to enhance infant birth weight, maternal diet appeared to deserve more attention than weight gain. Because many people patronize fast-food establishments, dietitians and nutritionists should encourage the reduction of sodium, sugar, and fat content in foods and the increased usage of whole-grain products and vegetables. Restaurants also would benefit from input by nutritionists and dietitians, particularly through the National Restaurant Association.

Lactation

The American Dietetic Association's position paper on breastfeeding states, "The American Dietetic Association advocates breastfeeding because of the nutritional and immunologic benefits of human milk and physiological, social, and hygienic benefits of the breastfeeding process for the mother and infant."[65] Breastfeeding has the advantage of reducing allergens if there is a history of allergies in the family and of increasing immunoglobulin. It may protect against clinical symptoms of some diseases (e.g., celiac and Crohn's disease) and bestow psychological benefits.[60] These advantages are particularly important for children with developmental disorders or chronic illness who are prone to upper respiratory infections. Benefits to the mother include more rapid loss of weight gained during pregnancy, enhanced maternal-infant bonding, amenorrhea, and more rapid uterine involution. However, the mother who does not choose to breastfeed should not be made to feel guilty because infant formulas are nutritious.

In 1988, 64% of white infants, 32% of black infants, and 54% of Hispanic infants were breastfed.[2] In 1991, Susser[59] reported that the Southeast Asian infants were the smallest minority group being breastfed. Some situations need special consideration. Breast milk provides less protein, calcium, phosphorus, and trace elements for the preterm infant than are available in the uterus, and thus a supplemental formula is needed as well[40] (see Table 3–6). Although most medications are excreted into breast milk at concentrations that are not harmful to the infant, some medications may be harmful and all should thus be investigated.[6] To breastfeed successfully, working mothers need extra support and guidance as are provided by part-time employment, flexible schedules, and partial breastfeeding.

During lactation at least *19 more grams of protein* and *500 calories* above the adult diet RDA should be consumed,[57] and the intake of vitamins and minerals, except for vitamin D, iron, calcium, and phosphorus, should be increased as well (Table 1–8). The 1989 RDA requirements for lactation have been separated into two time periods—the first 6 months and second 6 months of lactation—with the nutrient requirements being slightly higher during the first period. The daily food plan for lactation can be seen in Table 1–7. The study of maternal nutrition during lactation was undertaken (at the request of the Maternal and Child Health Program) by the Committee on Nutritional

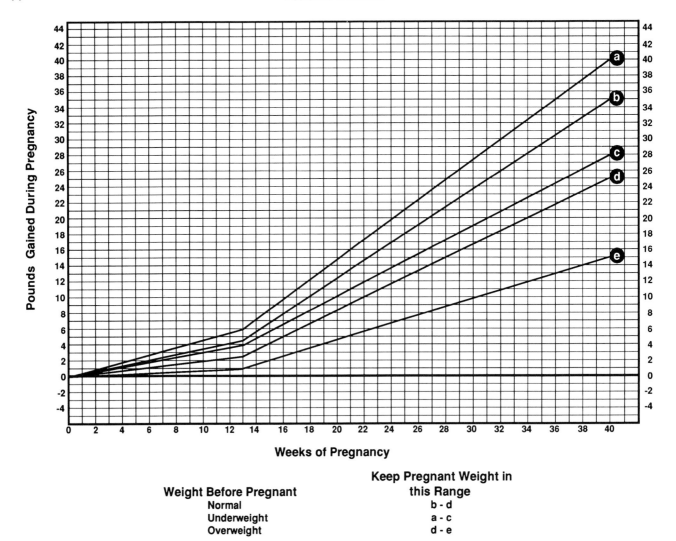

Weeks of Pregnancy

Weight Before Pregnant	Keep Pregnant Weight in this Range
Normal	b - d
Underweight	a - c
Overweight	d - e

Fig. 1–5. Adapted from the National Academy of Science's *Nutrition During Pregnancy*, National Dairy Council, Rosemont, Illinois, 1991. Used with permission.

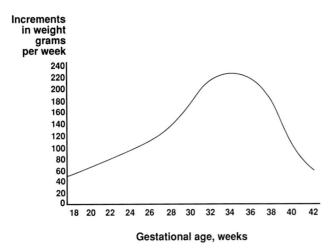

Fig. 1–6. Velocity of weekly gain in weight in utero. From Widdowson[40] with permission.

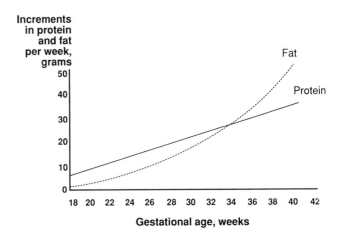

Fig. 1–7. Increments of fat and protein in fetal body per week. From Widdowson[40] with permission.

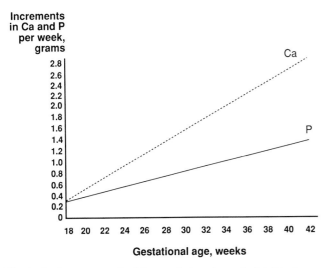

Fig. 1–8. Increments of calcium and phosphorus in fetal body per week. From Widdowson[40] with permission.

Status During Pregnancy and Lactation, Food Nutrition Board, Institute of Medicine, National Academy of Sciences.[66] For lactating women, the following nutrients should not be consumed above the recommended daily allowance for lactation by the mother as they are secreted into human milk:[66] iodine, vitamin B6, vitamin D, and selenium. Major minerals (calcium, phosphorous, sodium, and potassium) in human milk are not affected by the mother's diet.[66] The stores of vitamin C, thiamine, biotin, folate, vitamin B12, vitamin A, vitamin E and the composition of fatty acids in the mother's diet may influence nutrients in human milk; however, the influence of other vitamins and trace minerals is yet unknown.[66] Increased fluids as well as increased nutrients are recommended for the mother's diet during lactation. Problems appear to occur with the following: high risk mothers who consume less than 1800 calories per day (supplement daily with high nutrient dense foods and multivitamin-mineral supplement); complete vegetarian mothers who avoid animal foods (supplement daily with 2.6 mcg vitamins B12; mothers who have low calcium intake or lactose intolerance, although lactose tolerance may improve during pregnancy (supplement with 600 mg elemental calcium with meals); mothers who have limited exposure to sunlight and consume few vitamin D fortified foods (supplement daily with 10 mcg vitamin D).[66] Mothers should not breast feed if HIV positive or using drugs, alcohol, and large amounts of tobacco and caffeine (with abstinence after birth they may breastfeed).[67] Regional poison control centers or university pharmacies are excellent sources for information on drug nutrition information (see Chapter 27). The newborn infant should be given the following: 7.5 mcg of vitamin D daily if sunlight exposure is limited, fluoride supplement daily if less than 0.3 parts per million fluoride in the water, and 1 to 2 mg vitamin K immediately after birth only.[61] At six months of age, the infant should be given foods rich in bioavailable iron or a daily low dose iron supplement.[64] Research is needed on the relationship between maternal diet during lactation and nutritional status and milk volume. The use of the urinary lactose: creatinine ratio

is being investigated as a research and clinical tool for estimating lactation performance.[68]

Dietitians have the responsibility to provide education and training about breastfeeding and lactation to other health care professionals, as well as to the public. (Culture sensitivity, less formula distribution, supportive workplaces and reduced language barriers must be further developed to better coordinate services for minority groups.[69]) Lactation failure usually is preventable if the mammary gland is appropriately stimulated after the postpartum period.[70] Common problems, such as sore nipples and mastitis, usually can be alleviated and breastfeeding continued on the uninvolved breast.[70] The infant may lose 8–10% of birth weight initially when breast feeding, but it should be regained in two weeks. If the infant falls below the fifth percentile or gains less than 15 g daily a 24 hr tracking for problems is needed.[71] Best Start or LaLache League also may be helpful.

Follow-up

Prenatal care is essential, particularly in high-risk pregnancies. Dietary/physical, anthropometry, biochemical, and medical or clinical histories and measurements are needed at each health care visit.

References

1. Kennedy, E.T., Kotelchuck, M. The effect of WIC supplemental feeding on birth weight. A case-control analysis. *Am. J. Clin. Nutr.* 1984;40:579.
2. Office of Disease Prevention and Health Promotion. *Disease Prevention/Health Promotion—The Facts.* Washington, DC: U.S. Department of Health and Human Services; 1988.
3. National Center for Health Statistics. *Advance Report of Final Natality Statistics.* Hyattsville, MD: Public Health Service; 1990.
4. Phelps, D., Brown, D., Tung, B., Cassady, G., McClead, R., Purohit, D., Palmer, E. 28-day survival rates of 6676 neonates with birth weights of 1250 grams or less. *J. Pediatr.* 1991;87:7.
5. Wallace, H.M. Infant mortality. In: Wallace, H.M., Ryan, G., Oglesby, A., eds. *Maternal and Child Health Practices.* 3rd ed. Oakland, CA: Third Party; 1988.
6. Kleinman, J. Differences in infant mortality by race, nativity status, and other maternal characteristics. *Am. J. Dis. Child.* 1991;145:194.
7. Kleinman, J., Gowler, M., Kessel, S. Comparison of infant mortality among twins and singletons: United States 1960 and 1983. *Am. J. Epidemiol.* 1991;133:133.
8. Escobar, G., Littenberg, B., Petitti, D. Outcome among surviving very low birth weight infants: a meta-analysis. *Arch. Dis. Child.* 1991;66:204.
9. Winick, M., Rosso, P. Effects of severe early malnutrition on cellular growth of human brain. *Pediatr. Res.* 1969;3:181.
10. Winick, M. *Cellular Changes During Early Malnutrition.* Columbus, OH: Ross Laboratories; 1971. Currents in Maternal and Child Health.
11. Metcoff, J., Costiloe, J., Crosby, W., Bentle, L., Sechachalman, D., Sandstead, H., Bodwell, C., Weaver, F., McClain, P. Maternal nutrition and fetal outcome. *Am. J. Clin. Nutr.* 1981;34:708.
12. American College of Obstetrics and Gynecologists and the American Dietetic Association. *The Assessment of Maternal Nutrition.* Chicago: ACOG; 1978.
13. American Dietetic Association. *National nutrition consortium on vitamin-mineral safety, toxicity and misuse.* Chicago: ADA; 1978.
14. Mohs, M., Watson, R., Leonard-Green, G. Nutritional effects of marijuana, heroin, cocaine, and nicotine. *J. Am. Diet Assoc.* 1990;90:1261.
15. Worthington-Roberts, B., Williams, S. *Nutrition in Pregnancy and Lactation.* 4th ed. St. Louis: Times Mirror/Mosby; 1989.

16. Bigby, M., Stern, R.S. Adverse reactions to isotretinoin. *J. Am. Acad. Dermatol.* 1988;18:543.

17. Brent, R.L. Maternal nutrition and congenital malformations. Birth Defects: Original Article Series. *March of Dimes Birth Defects Fdtn.* 1985;21:1.

18. Huber, A.M., Wallins, L.L., DeRusso, P. Folate nutriture in pregnancy. *J. Am. Diet. Assoc.* 1988;88:791.

19. MRC Vitamin Research Group: Prevention of neural tube defects—results of the Medical Research Council study. *Lancet* 1991;338:131.

20. Hurley, L. Teratogenic aspects of manganese, zinc, and copper nutrition. *Physiol. Rev.* 1981;61:249.

21. Saner, G., Dagoglu, T., Ozden, T. Hair manganese concentrations in newborns and their mothers. *Am. J. Clin. Nutr.* 1985;41:1042.

22. Altura, B., Altura, B., Carella A. Magnesium deficiency-induced spasms of umbilical vessels: relation to preeclampsia, hypertension, growth retardation. *Science.* 1983;221:376.

23. Monsen, E. Iron nutrition and absorption: dietary factors which impact iron bioavailability. *J. Am. Diet. Assoc.* 1988;88:786.

24. Villar, J., Repke, J., Belizan, J.M. Calcium and blood pressure. *Clin. Nutr.* 1986;5:153.

25. Worthington-Roberts, B. Nutritional support of successful reproduction: an update. *J. Nutr. Ed.* 1987;19:1.

26. Graham, D. The obstetric and neonatal consequences of adolescent pregnancy. *Birth Defects.* 1981;17:49.

27. Elster, A. The effect of maternal age, parity, and prenatal care on perinatal outcome in adolescent mothers. *Am. J. Obstet. Gynecol.* 1984;149:845.

28. Naeye, R. Teenaged and pre-teenaged pregnancies: consequences of the fetal-maternal competition for nutrients. *Pediatrics.* 1981;67:146.

29. Stevens-Simon, C., McAnarney, E.R. Adolescent maternal weight gain and low birth weight: a multifactorial model. *Am. J. Clin. Nutr.* 1988;47:948.

30. Abrams, B., Russell, L. Prepregnancy weight, weight gain, and birth weight. *Am. J. Obstet. Gynecol.* 1986;154:503.

31. Pederson, A.L., Worthington-Roberts, B., Hickok, D.E. Weight gain patterns during twin gestation. *J. Am. Diet. Assoc.* 1989;89:642.

32. Berendez, H. Effect of maternal acetonuria on IQ of offspring. In: Cole, I., ed. *Early Diabetes in Early Life.* New York: Academic; 1975.

33. Brown, J.E., Jacobson, H.N., Askue, L.H., Peick, M.G. Influence of pregnancy weight gain on the size of infants born to underweight women. *Obstet. Gynecol.* 1981;57:13.

34. Mitchell, M.C., Lerner, E. Weight gain and pregnancy outcome in underweight and normal weight women. *J. Am. Diet. Assoc.* 1989;89:634.

35. Springer, N., Bischaping, K., Sampselle, C., Mayes, F., Petersen, B. Using weight gain and other nutrition-related risk factors to predict pregnancy outcomes. *J. Am. Diet Assoc.* 1992;92:217.

36. Brown, J., Tharp, T., McKay, C., Richardson, S., Hall, N., Finnegan, J., Splett, P. Development of prenatal weight gain intervention program using social marketing methods. *J. Nutr. Ed.* 1992;24:21.

37. Muscati, S.K., Mackey, M.A., Newsom, B. The influence of smoking and stress on prenatal weight gain and infant birth weight of teenage mothers. *J. Nutr. Ed.* 1988;20:299.

38. Forsum, E., Sadurskis, A., Wager, J. Resting metabolic rate and body composition of healthy Swedish women during pregnancy. *Am. J. Clin. Nutr.* 1988;47:942.

39. Calandra, C., Abell, D., Beischer, N. Maternal obesity in pregnancy. *Obstet. Gynecol.* 1981;57:8.

40. Widdowson, E.M. Fetal and neonatal nutrition. *Nutr. Today.* 1987;22:16.

41. Pijpers, L., Wladimiroff, J., McGhie, J. Effect of short-term maternal exercise on maternal and fetal cardiovascular dynamics. *Br. J. Obstet. Gynecol.* 1984;91:1081.

42. Hanzlink, J. Wellness and preventive medicine: the role of exercise. In: Ekvall, S., Wheby, E., eds. *Nutritional Needs of the Chronically Ill/Handicapped Child: Clinical Nutrition, Manual II.* Cincinnati, OH: University Affiliated Cincinnati Center for Developmental Disorders; 1987.

43. Jarett, J.C., Spellacy, W.N. Jogging during pregnancy: an improved outcome. *Obstet. Gynecol.* 1983;61:705.

44. Werler, M., Pober, B., Holmes, L. Smoking and pregnancy. *Teratology.* 1985;32:473.

45. Danford, D.E. Pica and nutrition. *Annu. Rev. Nutr.* 1982;2:303.

46. Goldman, A., Baker, L., Piddington, R., Marx, B., Herold, R., Egler, J. Hyperglycemia-induced teratogenesis is mediated by a functional deficiency of arachidonic acid. *Proc. Natl. Acad. Sci.* 1985;82:8227.

47. Sachs, B.P., Brown, D.A.J., Driscoll, S.G., Schulman, E., Acker, D., Ransil, B.J., Jewett, J.F. Hemorrhage, infection, toxemia, and cardiac disease, 1954–85: causes for their declining role in maternal mortality. *Am. J. Public Health.* 1988;78:671.

48. Maymon, R., Bahari, C., Moroz, C. Placental isoferritin: a new serum marker in toxemia of pregnancy. *Am. J. Obstet. Gynecol.* 1989;160:681.

49. Pritchard, J.A., Cunningham, F.G., Pritchard, S.A., Mason, R.A. How often does maternal preeclampsia-eclampsia incite thrombocytopenia in the fetus? *Obstet. Gynecol.* 1987;69:292.

50. Easterling, T.R., Watts, D.H., Schmucker, B.C., Benedetti, T.J. Measurement of cardiac output during pregnancy: validation of Doppler technique and clinical observations in preeclampsia. *Obstet. Gynecol.* 1987;69:845.

51. Redman, C.W.G. Therapy of non-preeclamptic hypertension in pregnancy. *Am. J. Kidn. Dis.* 1987;9:324.

52. Ekvall, S., Hedrick, B. The impact of nutritional status before conception, during pregnancy, and early childhood. Training module IV. Prevention Continuing Education in Rural Areas Project (84-1), Ohio Developmental Disabilities Council and Ohio Department of Mental Retardation and Developmental Disabilities (funded by PL. 50-602); August, 1985.

53. American Dietetic Association Position paper: Nutrition intervention and recovery from chemical dependency. *J. Am. Diet Assoc.* 1990;90:1274.

54. Dunn-Strohecker, M. Nutrition and health services needs among the homeless. *Public Health Reports.* 1991;106:364.

55. Luder, E., Cupens-Okado, E., Karen-Roth, A., Martinez-Weber, C. Health and nutrition survey in a group of urban homeless adults. *J. Am. Diet Assoc.* 1990;90:1387.

56. Food and Nutrition Board, Institute of Medicine, National Academy of Sciences: Effect of gestational weight gain on outcome in singleton pregnancies. In: *Nutrition During Pregnancy.* Washington, DC: National Academy Press; 1990.

57. King, J. (Chairman), Allen, L. (Chairman). Subcommittee on Nutritional Status and Weight Gain During Pregnancy and Subcommittee on Dietary Intake and Nutrient Supplements During Pregnancy: Nutrition during pregnancy. *Nutr. Today.* 1990;25:13.

58. Stevens-Simon, C., Roghmann, K., Mcanarney, E. Relationship of self reported prepregnant weight and weight gain during pregnancy to maternal body habitus and age. *J. Am. Diet Assoc.* 1992;92:85.

59. Gong, E. Weight issues and management. In: Story, M., ed. *Nutrition Management of the Pregnant Adolescent.* Washington, DC: National Clearing House; 1990.

60. Merchant, K., Martorell, R., Haas, J. Maternal and fetal responses to the stresses of lactation concurrent with pregnancy and of short recuperative intervals. *Am. J. Clin. Nutr.* 1990;52:280.

61. Hemminki, E., Rimpela, U. A randomized comparison of routine versus selective iron supplementation during pregnancy. *J. Am. Coll. Nutr.* 1991;10:3.

62. Brown, J.E. Improving pregnancy outcomes in the United States: the importance of preventive nutrition services. *J. Am. Diet. Assoc.* 1989;89:631.

63. Dubois, S., Dougherty, C., Suquette, M-P., Hanley, J., Moutquin, J-M. Twin pregnancy: the impact of Higgins Nutrition Intervention Program on maternal and neonatal outcomes. *Am. J. Clin. Nutr.* 1991;53:1397.

64. Susser. Maternal gain, infant birth weight, and diet: causal sequences. *Am. J. Clin. Nutr.* 1991;53:1384.

65. American Dietetic Association: Position paper on breast feeding. *J. Am. Diet. Assoc.* 1986;86:1580.

66. Food and Nutrition Board, Institute of Medicine, National Academy of Sciences, Maternal nutritional needs during lactation. *Nutrition During Lactation*. Washington, D.C., National Academy Press, 1991.

67. Frank, D., Bauchner, H., Zuckerman, B., Fried, L. Cocaine and marijuana use during pregnancy by women intending and not intending to breast-feed. *J. Am. Diet Assoc.* 1992;92:215.

68. Strand, F., Johnston, C. Urinary lactose as an index of lactation preformance. *J. Am. Diet Assoc.* 1992;92:83.

69. Ghaeni-Ahmadi, S. Attitudes toward breast-feeding and infant feeding among Iranian, Afghan, and Southeast Asian immigrant women in the United States: implications for health and nutrition education. *J. Am. Diet Assoc.* 1992;92:354.

70. Haphenson, J., Garza, C. Management of breastfeeding. In: Tsang, R.C., Nichols, B.L., eds. *Nutrition During Infancy*. Philadelphia: Hanley and Belfus; 1988.

71. Humphrey, N. Advances in perinatal and pediatric nutrition. *Conference Highlights Stanford University Carnation Nutritional Practices*. New York: Raven Press, 1991.

Chapter 2
Postnatal Growth in Infancy

Barbara Niedbala and Shirley Walberg Ekvall

Although controversies related to infant feeding practices still exist,[1] the American Academy of Pediatrics Committee on Nutrition (AAP-CON) is unequivocal in its recommendation of breastfeeding for all infants.[2] When breastfeeding is not possible, it recommends use of an iron-fortified formula from birth to 1 year of age. The introduction of solid foods is recommended when the infant is able to indicate hunger by leaning forward, has good head and neck control, and can indicate satiety by turning away from food. Usually this stage of development occurs between 4 to 6 months of age.[2] Infant weight gain averages 20–30 g/day. Controversies related to infant feeding practices still exist.[3]

Unconventional feeding practices include the barley water formula, nondairy creamer formula, Zen macrobiotic diet, megavitamin therapy, and a prolonged elimination diet, which can be dangerous (see Chapter 28).[4,5]

These simple guidelines for infant nutrition, which are of use both to professionals and to parents, are found in a 1989 brochure published by the Gerber Products Company.[6]

1. Build to a variety of foods.
2. Listen to your baby's appetite to avoid overfeeding or underfeeding.
3. Don't restrict fat and cholesterol too much.
4. Don't overdo high-fiber foods.
5. Sugar is okay, but in moderation.
6. Sodium is okay, but in moderation.
7. Babies need more iron, pound for pound than adults.

Problems in infant nutrition often center around birth weight and the baby's functional abilities. Growth charts in Figure 2–1 show sizes of infants who are small, appropriate, and large for gestational age. The infant should not deviate more than two channels from the normal growth pattern in weight or height for age and should fall between the 5th and 95th percentile (see Appendix 3 for infant growth charts). Infant weight gain should average 20–30 g/day. The Apgar score at birth is also an important index of the maturity and functional abilities of the infant (Fig. 2–2). Four of the major nutrition-related problems noted in infants in the United States are iron-deficiency anemia, obesity, hypernatremic dehydration, and hyperlipidemia. These problems, along with dietary management recommendations, are discussed below (hyperlipidemia is also presented separately in Chapter 54).

Iron Deficiency and Iron-Deficiency Anemia

The most prevalent nutritional disease in infants today is iron-deficiency anemia (see biochemical section in Chapter 4). Although simple methods of preventing this condition have existed for decades in the United States, it still remains a significant health problem. Evidence has accumulated showing the detrimental effects of iron deficiency without anemia and the possibility of irreversible damage caused by severe anemia has been documented.[7] A recent report indicates that the prevalence of iron-deficiency anemia is declining steadily—from 7.8% in 1975 to 2.9% in 1985—in children aged 6 months to 5 years.[7] However, this study may overstate the decline as it reports progress among high-risk children enrolled in a supplemental food program. Other recent studies report the incidence of iron-deficiency anemia to be approximately 9% to 10% in infants and young children,[8,9] which does represent a decline from those figures reported a decade earlier.

Common symptoms associated with iron-deficiency anemia are rather nonspecific and include fatigue, irritability, and restlessness. Adverse effects are decreased energy, a reduced tolerance to heat and cold stress, and cellular immunity incompetence. The decrease in hemoglobin level and the body's compensatory mechanisms for the decrease in oxygen transport are responsible in part for these adverse effects. More important, iron-dependent tissue enzymes are affected, causing health impairment even before anemia occurs.[11,12] In children, iron deficiency and iron-deficiency anemia affect mental and motor development. Developmental test scores of iron-deficient children are significantly lower than those of children with sufficient iron stores.[10] However, researchers suggest that the correction of iron deficiency may not necessarily result in improvement in test scores.[10,13,14]

Etiology

Healthy full-term infants are born with iron stores sufficient to provide for the first early growth spurt, that of birth weight doubling. Infants with intrauterine growth retardation and those born prematurely have smaller reserves of iron; yet, their postnatal growth may occur more rapidly. As a result, low birth weight infants deplete their iron reserves quickly, often in the first 2 to 3 months compared to 4 months for the full-term well-grown infant. Regardless of birth weight or gestational age, all infants eventually need an exogenous source of iron during the period of rapid growth in the first 2 years of life. Thus, the infant's diet becomes particularly important.

The food deemed most appropriate for the young infant, breast milk, contains a very small amount of iron in a highly absorbable form. An average of 49% of the iron in human milk is absorbed by the infant.[15] Although it is common practice to prescribe oral iron supplements for breastfed

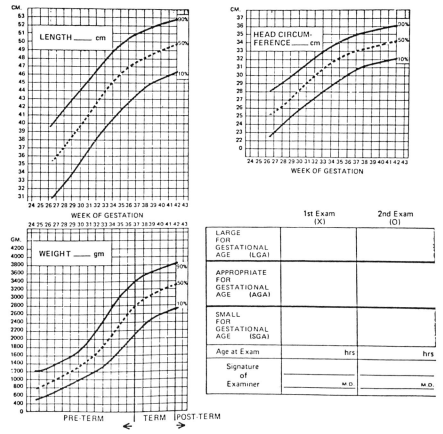

Fig. 2–1. Classification of newborns based on maturity and intrauterine growth. X = 1st exam, 0 = 2nd exam. Adapted from Lubchenco, L.C., Hansman, C., Boyd E. *Pediatrics.* 1966; 37:403; and Battaglia, F.C., Lubchenco, L.C. *J. Pediatr.* 1967;71:159.

infants, they are not necessary for healthy, full-term infants who are being breastfed exclusively. Several studies document that full-term infants breastfed for at least 6 months retain substantial iron stores and show no signs of deficiency.[16,17] However, infants fed breast milk alone until the age of 9 months begins to show lowered iron levels at that time.[17] In the United States, less than one-quarter of infants continue exclusive breastfeeding for 5 months.[18] The majority are fed a commercially prepared infant formula with a cow milk or soy protein base. Iron-fortified infant formula is the most appropriate choice for bottle-fed infants. Despite a low absorption rate of 3.4% to 5.4% of the iron in fortified milk- and soy-based formulas, infants fed a quantity of formula sufficient to provide for growth are well protected against iron deficiency.[19,20]

Iron-deficiency anemia and iron deficiency occurring in the first year of life are largely attributed to the introduction of whole cow milk too early into the infant's diet. The total dietary intake of iron and the absorption of iron are lower in infants fed whole cow milk during the first year.[21] The incidence of iron deficiency is significantly higher in infants fed whole cow milk before the age of 6 months than in those given whole cow milk after 6 months of age.[22] Weaning from breast milk to whole cow milk before 6 months is also associated with a significantly higher incidence of iron deficiency and its anemia.[10] In addition to the absorption of insufficient quantities of iron from whole cow milk, whole cow milk also predisposes the young infant to gastrointes-

tinal blood loss, a condition that contributes further to the development of anemia.[23]

The foods given in the first year as a supplement to breast or bottle feeding also play a significant role in the prevention of iron deficiency. The absorption of iron, rather than the total quantity ingested, is the most important measure, and certain food combinations enhance iron bioavailability. The iron present in foods commonly given to infants is primarily nonheme iron, a poorly absorbable form. Iron-fortified cereals, vegetables, and fruits contain iron in this form. Including a source of ascorbic acid or small amounts of heme iron—from meat, fish, or poultry—with the meals of starches, fruits, and vegetables can greatly increase the absorption of iron from these foods.

Biochemical abnormalities

The various laboratory indices used in the diagnosis of iron deficiency and its related anemia correspond to the overlapping stages of iron depletion. The first stage, loss of storage iron, is reflected by a fall in serum ferritin concentration. A decline in circulating iron occurs next and may be measured by serum iron or transferrin saturation. At this point, iron-dependent enzymes are impaired, and some of the deleterious effects of iron deficiency are seen, even before the circulating hemoglobin concentration drops. Free erythrocyte protoporphyrin also increases at this stage and is often used in the differential diagnosis. The final stage is

ESTIMATION OF GESTATIONAL AGE BY MATURITY RATING
Symbols: X - 1st Exam O - 2nd Exam

NEUROMUSCULAR MATURITY

	0	1	2	3	4	5
Posture						
Square Window (Wrist)	90°	60°	45°	30°	0°	
Arm Recoil	180°		100°-180°	90°-100°	< 90°	
Popliteal Angle	180°	160°	130°	110°	90°	< 90°
Scarf Sign						
Heel to Ear						

Gestation by Dates _____ wks

Birth Date _____ Hour _____ am / pm

APGAR _____ 1 min _____ 5 min

MATURITY RATING

Score	Wks
5	26
10	28
15	30
20	32
25	34
30	36
35	38
40	40
45	42
50	44

PHYSICAL MATURITY

	0	1	2	3	4	5
SKIN	gelatinous red, transparent	smooth pink, visible veins	superficial peeling &/or rash, few veins	cracking pale area, rare veins	parchment, deep cracking, no vessels	leathery, cracked, wrinkled
LANUGO	none	abundant	thinning	bald areas	mostly bald	
PLANTAR CREASES	no crease	faint red marks	anterior transverse crease only	creases ant. 2/3	creases cover entire sole	
BREAST	barely percept.	flat areola, no bud	stippled areola, 1–2 mm bud	raised areola, 3–4 mm bud	full areola, 5–10 mm bud	
EAR	pinna flat, stays folded	sl. curved pinna, soft with slow recoil	well-curv. pinna, soft but ready recoil	formed & firm with instant recoil	thick cartilage, ear stiff	
GENITALS Male	scrotum empty, no rugae		testes descending, few rugae	testes down, good rugae	testes pendulous, deep rugae	
GENITALS Female	prominent clitoris & labia minora		majora & minora equally prominent	majora large, minora small	clitoris & minora completely covered	

SCORING SECTION

	1st Exam = X	2nd Exam = O
Estimating Gest Age by Maturity Rating	_____ Weeks	_____ Weeks
Time of Exam	Date _____ Hour _____ am/pm	Date _____ Hour _____ am/pm
Age at Exam	_____ Hours	_____ Hours
Signature of Examiner	_____ M.D.	_____ M.D.

Fig. 2–2. Newborn maturity rating and classification. Scoring system from Ballard, J.L., et al. A simplified assessment of gestational age. *Pediatr. Res.* 1977;11:374. Figures adapted from Sweet, A.Y. Classification of the low birth weight infant. In: Klaus, M.H., Fararoff, A.A., eds. *Care of the High-Risk Infant*, Philadelphia: W.B. Saunders. 1977:47. Used with permission.

a decrease in hemoglobin concentration, indicating anemia. Iron-deficiency anemia is microcytic; therefore a decrease in the mean corpuscular volume is also seen.[11,12]

No single laboratory value definitively indicates the presence of iron deficiency or iron-deficiency anemia. Rather, diagnosis of these states depends on the results of three or more indices. Commonly accepted laboratory values for anemia are hemoglobin < 11 g/dL, hematocrit < 33%, transferrin saturation < 16%, and plasma ferritin < 7 mg/dL.[24] A typical acceptable hemoglobin level at 1 week is 13–20 g/dL; at 1 month, 14 g/dL; at 6–24 months, 10+ g/dL; at 2–5 years, 11+ g/dL; at 6–12 years, 11.5+ g/dL; at 13–16 males, 13+ g/dL; at 13–16 females, 11.5+ g/dL; at 16+ males, 14+ g/dL; and at 16+ females, 12+ g/dL (see Appendix 10). In cases of mild anemia, infection, or chronic disease, iron deficiency may be difficult to diagnose correctly. Often, a therapeutic trial of iron is given in those cases.

Factors to be considered in nutrition evaluation and dietary management

Treatment of established iron deficiency and iron-deficiency anemia consists of providing supplemental iron orally at a dosage of 2–3 mg/kg/day.[24,25] Treatment should continue for 3 to 4 months, with laboratory values verified at the end of treatment. The iron supplement is best absorbed when given between meals and with an ascorbic acid food source. A divided dose may be given if stomach upset occurs.

Iron deficiency can be prevented easily by a diet of appropriate foods and food combinations. From the time of birth, infants should be fed either breast milk or iron-fortified infant formula. Infants with a low birth weight should be given additional iron supplements starting between 2 and 8 weeks, with the dosage calculated according to birth weight (< 1000 mg, use 4 mg/kg; < 1500 g, use 3 mg/kg; and < 2500 g, use 2 mg/kg). Supplementary iron should continue until the age of 6 months.[25]

When the infant begins to consume solid foods, a food source of ascorbic acid should be provided with meals to enhance iron absorption. Iron-fortified infant cereal may be included in the diet as a reliable source of iron. This type of cereal should also be fed with ascorbic acid-rich food or given with small amounts of meat, fish, or poultry to allow for optimal absorption of the fortified iron. If the infant is being breastfed, strained meats and iron-rich cereals usually are added first because of the lower protein content of breast milk. If the infant is formula fed (especially by one fortified with iron), fruits and vegetables are usually added first. Infant fruits and vegetables should be purchased in glass jars or seamless cans or homemade, using frozen or thoroughly cleansed fresh fruits and vegetables.

The introduction of whole cow milk should be delayed until the infant is between 9 and 12 months of age. By this time, infants are usually consuming at least one-third of their calories as solid foods. As long as the supplemental foods include a balanced mixture of starches, vegetables, fruits, and protein sources, thereby providing adequate sources of iron and ascorbic acid, whole cow milk may be given.[22] However, to ensure adequate iron stores, breastfeeding or iron-fortified infant formula (at least 20 oz/day) should be continued throughout the first year of life.[26,27]

Obesity

Obesity in children is a significant health problem in modern industrialized society both because of its increasing prevalence and the accompanying morbidities of hypertension, diabetes, cardiovascular and respiratory diseases, orthopedic disorders, and psychosocial dysfunction.[27,28] Because it is difficult to treat obesity successfully, much research is currently being devoted to its prevention. Two questions—does the obese infant become an obese child and does the obese child become an obese adult—are under investigation, as well as the roles that heredity and environment play in the development of obesity.

The incidence of overweight children in the United States is estimated to be between 6% and 25% in the population aged birth through 5 years (as opposed to 5% as predicted by growth charts).[29–31] In children aged 6 to 11 years, the incidence is still higher—12% to 24%—and in adolescents the incidence is approximately 14% to 22%.[28,32] Severely obese children comprise a smaller part of the population: estimates of 8% to 12% of preschool children and 6% to 14% of older children and adolescents are reported in the literature.[31–33] Obesity is noted to be more prevalent among certain subgroups of the population: native Americans and Hispanics and, in general, groups with low socioeconomic status.[29] The greater incidence in certain cultural or racial groups may not actually exist, but may be an artifact of using one growth chart standard to define obesity in a heterogeneous population.

Evidence indicates that the already high incidence of obesity in the United States is increasing. Using the United States National Health Examination Survey and National Health and Nutrition Examination Survey data, Gortmaker and colleagues[28] in 1987 calculated a 54% increase in obesity in children 6 to 11 years of age and a 39% increase in those aged 12 to 17 years. Severe obesity has also increased dramatically, with 98% and 64% increases in the above-cited age groups over the 13 years of data collection. The researchers expect that the prevalence of related medical conditions will increase correspondingly as well.

Etiology

The primary function of adipose tissue is energy storage. The adipocytes have a seemingly limitless capacity to store fat, or energy, in contrast to the small storage capacity of the body for protein and carbohydrate. Fatness, or obesity, reflects an imbalance between energy intake and energy expenditure; the excess energy is stored for future use in the form of fat tissue.

Secondary functions of adipose tissue include thermoregulation, cushiony protection for organs, and storage of fat-soluble vitamins and essential fatty acids. The normal, nonoverweight, newborn infant body is approximately 16% fat by weight. From 1 to 12 months after birth an increase in fat cell size occurs, and from 12 to 18 months of age, an increase in fat cell number occurs, resulting in a gradual increase in percent body fat. The percent body fat of a normal-weight toddler is approximately 28% like that of an adult. However, the fat cell number and size are still far below that of an adult.[35] After the first postnatal 18 months of growth, the amount of adipose tissue normally remains stable as the child continues to gain in height. This change is reflected by the apparent slimming of the child. A second period of rapid growth in adipose tissue begins around 6 years of age. This stage is termed the "adiposity rebound" by Rolland-Cachera and her colleagues[36] and is a normal phase of fat cell proliferation and growth.

Abnormalities of the normal evolution of fat tissue have been observed, but as of yet are unexplained. Knittle et al.[37] observed that, in obese children, adipocyte size increased to adult values, whereas nonobese children displayed either a reduction or no change in lipid content. Adipocyte number also increased in the obese children at a time when no change was noted in the normal-weight children. Rolland-Cachera et al.[36] have observed that the age at which the adiposity rebound occurs is related to future obesity as an adolescent. Children who exhibited an early adiposity rebound (before 5.5 years) were significantly more likely to become obese than children who exhibited that phase at a later age (after 7 years). In the same study, it was found that groups of children with early and late adiposity rebounds had corresponding bone maturations. This result is consistent with other studies citing accelerated growth and skeletal maturation in obese children.[38,39] However, whether the high prevalence of obesity in children with advanced adiposity rebounds is due to overnutrition or solely to genetic or hormonal factors is currently unknown. The main predictors of adult obesity are also unknown, as some obese children do not become obese adults.[36]

The prevalence of obesity is higher in populations with documented higher caloric intake.[32] Obesity has become more prevalent as societies have reduced their activity levels and have adapted to energy-dense diets.[40] Although it is possible to document the direct relationship between increased caloric intake and obesity on the societal level, it has been difficult to do so on the individual level. The majority of studies report no correlation between individual caloric intake and degree of adiposity.[32,41] Nevertheless, the basic cause of obesity is energy imbalance: energy expenditure is too low for the amount of calories consumed. After an individual becomes overweight or obese, a steady state with little weight change may occur, explaining in part the average or below-average caloric intake of obese individuals.

Few research reports have linked obesity directly to decreased energy expenditure. Increased television viewing is positively correlated with obesity, but whether this effect is due to inactivity or increased snacking done while viewing is unclear.[42] An observation that obese female children playing tennis were stationary on the tennis court for 80% of the time supports the assumption that the energy imbalance may be caused by lower energy expenditure, rather than by a higher energy intake.[43] Other researchers theorize that obesity adversely affects motor activity.[33,44]

Some reports have attempted to link eating behaviors to the development of obesity. Drabman et al.[45] document that overweight children take fewer chews per bite and more bites per unit of time than do age-matched normal-weight children. Waxman and Stunkard[46] observed that mothers served their overweight children more food than they served their normal-weight children. It is commonly thought that bottle feeding and the early introduction of solid foods in infancy leads to infantile obesity because of the caregiver's tendency to encourage the infant to finish all of each feeding. Although early studies suggest that breastfeeding and the delayed introduction of solids help protect against obesity,[47,48] more recent studies find no difference in the incidence of obesity in either bottle-fed or breastfed infants or those with early versus late introduction of solid foods.[30,34,49,50] However, from the time solid foods are introduced to an infant, the infant learns valuable lessons about the role of food. Poor eating behaviors that are practiced by family members and that have led to their obesity are likely to be learned and practiced by the infant and toddler. These practices include eating past the point of satiety, "cleaning the plate," and using food as a method of showing affection or relieving emotional stress. Although children may have a genetic tendency toward obesity, as seen by an early adiposity rebound, the environment plays a great role in controlling the development of obesity.

Factors to be considered in nutritional evaluation

The definitions of the two terms "obesity" and "overweight" vary throughout the scientific literature. Despite controversy over strict definitions used to delineate statistically various population subgroups, obesity in the individual infant or child is quite apparent upon visual examination. Because the child or caregiver may dispute the presence of obesity, several anthropometric measurements may be obtained, as evidence.

Anthropometric and clinical assessment. Commonly employed methods of measuring fatness include triceps and subscapular skinfold measurements and various weight-height indices. Triceps skinfold measurements correlate highly with the percent of body weight as fat.[51] Using this measurement alone, obesity is defined as a triceps skinfold in excess of the 85th percentile for age and sex; a triceps skinfold in excess of the 95th percentile describes severe obesity.[28,52] Skinfold measurements are particularly helpful in differentiating the obese from the nonobese child, but these measures lack reproducibility in those identified as obese.[52]

Although body frame size may confound weight-for-height indices, the body mass index (BMI or Quetlet index) calculated by weight/height[2] correlates well with the percentage of body weight as fat.[51] The BMI is recommended as the most suitable index for ascertaining the degree of adiposity in children.[53] Percentile graphs shown in Figure 2–3 illus-

trate the evolution of adiposity during growth. The normal increase in fat tissue during the first 18 months and the second increase in adiposity around 6 years of age are depicted clearly on the BMI curves.

Another common method of estimating degree of obesity is to compare the infant's or child's actual weight with the "ideal" weight for height. The "ideal" weight is that weight corresponding to the 50th percentile when height is displaced to the 50th percentile. Using the results from the equation:

$$\frac{\text{actual weight}}{\text{ideal weight}} \times 100$$

percents $\geq$ 110 indicate overweight and those $\geq$ 120% indicate obesity. A problem inherent in this method is that the child may not be at the same stage of growth as the children measured to represent the 50th percentile for height on the growth chart.

In infants and young children, no single measurement is a good predictor of future obesity, as the individual's adiposity may be increasing or decreasing at any particular time.[36] Serial measurements of height, weight, and skinfold thickness are therefore most useful. Other methods taking into account fat-free mass should also be considered for accuracy, such as the formula proposed by Salas: resting energy expenditure = 54.4 LBM(kg) + 0.095 creatinine (mmol/Hg) = 4.7[54] (see Chapters 4 and 19 for other methodologies).

Dietary management

Treatment of obesity requires a two-pronged approach that increases energy expenditure and decreases caloric intake. A four-pronged approach is used as the child grows older. (see Chapter 19). In growing children, weight maintenance, rather than weight loss, is the goal as stature will continue to increase. Dietz[55] estimates that 1.5 years of weight maintenance is required for each 20% increment of weight over ideal weight to achieve ideal body weight in a growing child.

However simple the treatment for obesity, to a child or young adult results may seem slow to occur. Increasing activity level and decreasing the amount of food consumed are difficult changes in behavior that must be maintained for a lengthy period of time. Such behavioral changes are difficult to implement and sustain, particularly if the psychosocial environment, which may have encouraged the development of obesity, does not change. The most successful pediatric weight loss programs combine exercise, caloric control, behavior modification, and emotional support. When there is parental support as well, the success rate increases substantially.[55-57]

Before beginning a weight control regimen, a complete diet history should be obtained. It must include the behavioral antecedents to eating and information regarding the child's physical activity level. Caloric needs may be calculated either by decreasing 100–500 calories from the client's usual daily intake or by calculating the recommended energy intake[58] per kilogram of ideal body weight for height and adjusting it for age and physical maturity. A meal pattern of three meals per day, with one or two snacks, should be emphasized, and the types of food to be included in each meal and snack should be specified. Overeating and periods

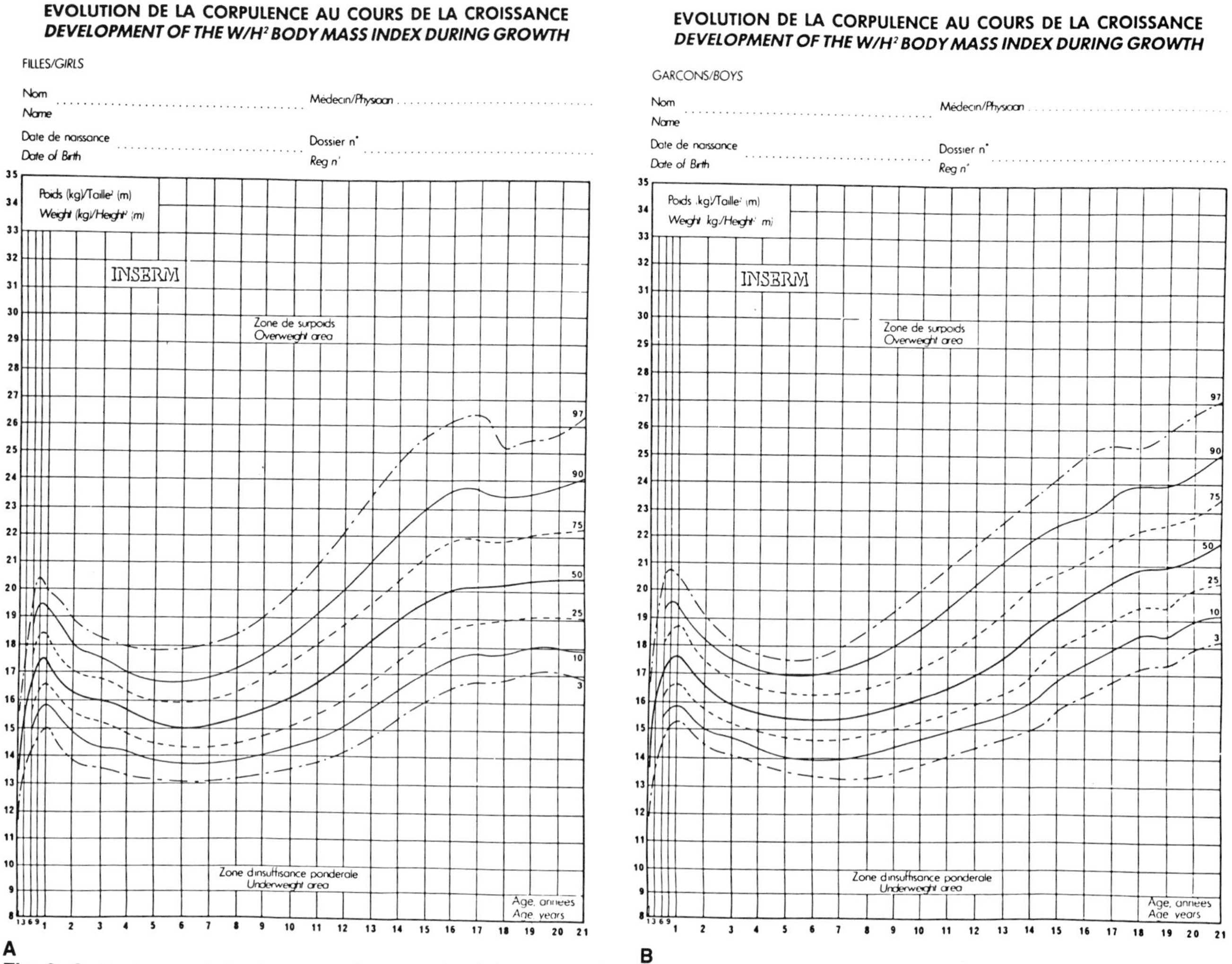

EVOLUTION DE LA CORPULENCE AU COURS DE LA CROISSANCE
DEVELOPMENT OF THE W/H² BODY MASS INDEX DURING GROWTH

FILLES/GIRLS

EVOLUTION DE LA CORPULENCE AU COURS DE LA CROISSANCE
DEVELOPMENT OF THE W/H² BODY MASS INDEX DURING GROWTH

GARCONS/BOYS

A   B

Fig. 2–3. Body mass index in percentile ranges for (A) girls and (B) boys. From Rolland-Cachera, M.F., Semp, M., Guilloud-Bataille, M., Patois, E., Peguignot-Guggenbuhl, F., Fautrad, V. Adiposity indices in children. *Am. J. Clin. Nutr.*, 1982;36:178. Used with permission.

of hunger are to be avoided. Caloric level is derived from the child's diet history. Yet, because caloric expenditure depends upon the child's activity level, frequent monitoring of his or her weight is needed to ensure that weight control is being maintained. Although a nutritionist's expertise is in foods and nutrition, the effect of physical exercise must not be overlooked or underemphasized. An exercise regimen should be developed and adhered to as closely as the dietary regimen.

Prevention. Prevention of future obesity remains the best method of management. Healthy eating patterns are developed early in life by trusting the infant's signals of hunger and satiety, rather than by feeding a certain amount of food according to a preset schedule. Following the infant's instinct can be done whether the infant is breast or bottle fed. The American Academy of Pediatrics Committee on Nutrition advises the support of both feeding methods while there is still doubt regarding the obesity-preventive effect of breastfeeding.[59] The years of solid food intake and the environmental mileu in which it is offered and consumed most likely have a greater effect than does the relatively

short time spent breast or bottle feeding. Current research concerning key times for the occurrence of adipocyte hyperplasia and hypertrophy and the effects of heredity and environment in the development of obesity will help delineate key times for nutrition education.

Hypernatremic Dehydration

Incidence

Hypernatremic dehydration most commonly occurs in infants and toddlers as the result of an infectious diarrheal disease in combination with inappropriate fluid therapy. This situation accounts for well over 90% of the cases of hypernatremic dehydration in children younger than 2 years of age.[60] Other cases occur in relation to disease states, such as diabetes insipidus, diabetes mellitus, or renal disease or to psychomotor retardation; a few cases are caused by dietary errors alone. For example, skim milk, with a high renal solute load, can overburden the infant kidney, especially if inadequate water is consumed.

Biochemical abnormalities

Hypernatremic dehydration is defined as dehydration associated with an elevated serum sodium concentration of 150 mEq/L or higher; the normal range is 136–145 mEq/L.[60] It reflects a body water deficit relative to sodium. Severe dehydration does not have to occur for the infant to become hypernatremic; one study documented that 50% of infants with hypernatremic dehydration were less than 10% dehydrated.[61] Infants presenting with hypernatremic dehydration may show few of the usual signs of dehydration—diminished skin turgor, dry shrunken tongue, and lack of tears. More often, signs of central nervous system dysfunction—lethargy, irritability, or seizures—are apparent. These signs may occur in as many as 70% of infants when serum sodium rises above 158 mEq/L.[62] Central nervous system dysfunction is probably caused by the maintenance of the intravascular volume through the influence of the sodium ion, which allows cellular dessication of the brain to occur. Severe brain damage, caused by the hypernatremia itself or by too-rapid replacement fluid therapy, is often irreversible.[63] The mortality rate in hypernatremic dehydration is high: in a review of eight studies, the combined mortality rate was 11.5%.[60]

Factors to be considered in nutrition evaluation

Hypernatremic dehydration occurs more frequently in infants and small children because of (1) their large ratio of body surface area to weight,[64] which causes more evaporative water losses; (2) a normally higher metabolic rate in children weighing less than 15 kg;[65] and (3) their susceptibility to metabolic water loss during febrile periods.[66] In a small child with diarrhea, increased gastrointestinal water and potassium losses induce further respiratory water loss and a release of nonextracellular sodium that may result in hypernatremia.[67] Inappropriate fluid therapy can aggravate the existing water deficit and sodium retention when a fluid that is too high in sodium is given. The excess sodium both increases the renal solute load and induces fever. Figure 2–4 depicts the mechanisms of hypernatremia.

Clinical management

Treatment of hypernatremic dehydration consists of slow correction of the serum osmolality. When given too rapidly, fluid replacement can cause cerebral edema or seizures from water movement into the cells.[68] A solution of one-quarter or half-normal saline in 5% dextrose water, with potassium added after adequate renal function is evidenced, is given intravenously over 48 to 72 hours to correct the fluid deficit and provide maintenance fluid. If the child is less than 10% dehydrated and alert, oral rehydration therapy may be given under medical supervision. Once the child is stable, fluids for maintenance of hydration are given, orally when possible.

Prevention of Hypernatremic Dehydration. Correct management of mild, moderate, or severe diarrheal dehydration is necessary to prevent the majority of cases of hypernatremic dehydration in the United States. Bouts of infectious diarrhea may be treated successfully at home, thereby avoiding the costs and complications associated with hospitalization. The usual symptoms of this acute illness are vomiting, increased frequency of loose or watery stools, and a decreased intake of food and fluid. Oral maintenance solutions (OMS), such as Pedialyte® and Lytren®, have been designed specifically for use in developed countries for treatment of these symptoms in otherwise healthy children.[68] These solutions contain 30–60 mEq/L sodium together with small amounts of glucose to facilitate sodium absorption; they also contain potassium, chloride, and an anionic base (Table 2–1). They are recommended for the home treatment of diarrhea, to prevent dehydration and maintain a physiological electrolyte balance. By using an OMS, the caregiver can provide the appropriate fluid, rather than choosing among the "clear liquids" that are typically available in the home. Table 2–2 shows the range in sodium content and osmolality of various clear liquids, some of which contain dangerously high levels of sodium or are hyperosmolar and may induce further gastrointestinal water losses.

When an OMS is recommended by the clinician, guidelines should be given as to the amount offered per day and whether any other fluids may be offered. In general, the amount of OMS should not exceed 150 mL/kg/day (100 mL/kg/day in children weighing greater than 10 kg). If additional fluid is needed to satisfy thirst, low-solute fluids may be used (sodium less than 8 mEq/L). To ensure the correct dilution and final electrolyte content, ready-to-feed OMS are preferred to powders that must be mixed with water. Vomiting is not a contraindication to the use of OMS. When fluid is administered by spooning rather than through a nipple or from a cup, successful retention is usually obtained even if small amounts are vomited.[68] If the caregiver must

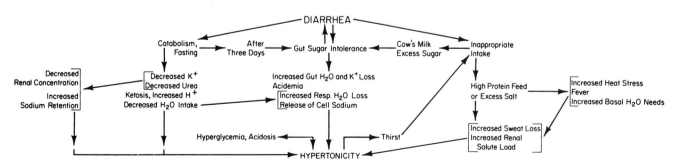

Fig. 2–4. Events leading to the development of hypernatremic dehydration following diarrheal losses. From Hirschorn, N. The treatment of acute diarrhea in children. A historical and physiological perspective. *Am. J. Clin. Nutr.* 1980;33:637. Used with permission.

Table 2-1. Composition of Oral Electrolyte

Solutions	Na + (mEq/L)	K + (mEq/L)	Cl − (mEq/L)	Base (mEq/L)	Glucose (g)
Oral maintenance solutions					
Pedialyte®	45	20	35	30	25
Lytren®	50	25	45	30	20
Oral rehydration solutions					
Rehydralyte®	75	20	65	30	25

give clear liquids available in the home, guidelines about the recommended types and amounts should be given.

Oral rehydration solutions (ORS), such as Rehydralyte®, differ from OMS in that they are intended for treatment rather than prevention of acute dehydration and are designed for use under medical supervision. Because the sodium content of ORS is greater than that of OMS, these solutions could be dangerous if given incorrectly. Normally, ORS are used for short periods of time—4 to 6 hours—and after rehydration is complete, an OMS is given to maintain hydration during ongoing diarrheal losses.

Although cases of hypernatremic dehydration caused by dietary errors alone do not constitute a large percentage nationwide and few reports of them appear in the current literature, it is important to address this problem and its prevention. All infants, as well as any small children who have severe psychomotor retardation or are comatose, are unable to communicate thirst and therefore are the most susceptible to hypernatremic dehydration caused by a faulty diet. A diet excessive in sodium together with inadequate free water is likely to cause hypernatremic dehydration in the absence of increased water loss.[69] When hyperosmolar feedings are given in addition to inadequate water and excessive sodium, vomiting and diarrhea may result, causing hypernatremia and dehydration to occur more rapidly. Cases of hypernatremic dehydration caused by improper mixing of powdered infant formulas, using undiluted concentrated liquid infant formula,[70-72] and feeding blenderized diets excessive in sodium[73] have been reported through the years. They have occurred both in the home setting and in institutions. Clinicians responsible for the direct preparation and provision of infant formulas and tube feedings in institutions must accurately calculate their nutrient contents, particularly water and sodium. Home caregivers must be given precautions concerning the mixture of infant formulas and

home blenderized diets; hands-on demonstration, when possible, of preparation methods is recommended.

Hyperlipidemia/Atherosclerosis

The AAP-CON recommendations for dietary practices in childhood that reduce the risks of atherosclerosis disease in adulthood suggest that greater efforts be made to detect potential cardiovascular disease problems by obtaining a family history and regular screening of weight, stature, and blood pressure on all children during well-baby visits to the pediatrician.[74,75] Follow-up counseling for appropriate body weight management and regular exercise are also recommended.[76] Children determined to be at risk because of their family history should be checked at least twice before school age for serum cholesterol levels. If total lipid levels for children are greater than the 75th to 90th percentile (170–185 mg/dL) for age and sex, high-density lipoprotein cholesterol screening is recommended (see Chapter 54, Hyperlipidemias in Children, for evaluation and treatment).

In infancy, reduced fat milks are not recommended as human milk is the base guideline for the infant diet. Calories for milk should consist of 50% fat and cholesterol as in human milk. The content of infant formulas is similar to human milk in fat and caloric content.[6] For those not at risk for atherosclerotic disease, the AAP-CON suggests that dietary fat for children 2 years of age or older should be restricted to 35% of total calories and should include the essential fatty acid, linoleic acid. (In fact the 1990 Canada nutrition recommendations include specific amounts of Omega-3 and Omega-6 fatty acids for pregnancy and lactation and various age groups.)[77] Fruits and all greens are encouraged, as well as reduced salt and refined sugar intake. The importance of exercise as a preventive factor in the development of atherosclerosis disease should be emphasized.[78]

The use of unusual or extreme diets, such as only plant (not animal) proteins or long-term parenteral nutrition in infancy, may result in taurine deficiency and retinol dysfunction as noted in animals. Taurine is important in cellular proliferation and membrane protection and is needed in the infant diet.[79]

Follow-up and Summary

Evaluation of family dietary practices and nutrition education are essential components of primary pediatric care; they are a worthwhile long-range investment for the child. Breastfeeding lowers infant mortality, particularly during

Table 2-2. Sodium Content and Osmolality of Clear Liquids

Product	Na (mEq/L)	Osmolality (mosm/kg H20)
Chicken broth	251–357	501
Beef broth	114–135	326
7-Up	5–7	548
Ginger ale	0.8–2.7	557
Cola drinks	1.3–6.5	601
Cranberry cocktail	1.1–4.2	1212
Kool-Aid®	0.9–1.1	251–509
Jello®	22–27	644
Popsicles	4.7–5.6	719
Gatorade®	21	NA

Adapted from Wendland, B.E., Arbus, G.S.[69]

the first few months of life when 20% of fetal infections occur in respiratory organs and 40% in the digestive organs, with one-half of affected infants dying during the first month.[80] In nutritional evaluation and counseling with families, the pediatrician, nurse, or dietitian should do the following:

- Ask about the diet and use of supplements (vitamins D and C, iron, and fluoride).
- Evaluate the diet and determine if it adequately meets the child's needs (at least 20 ounces of iron-fortified formula per day or human milk for 1 year and solid foods after 6 months from the four food groups and foods rich in iron.). If breast-feeding the newborn infant requires: 1 to 2 mg vitamin K immediately after birth, 7.5 mg vitamin D daily if sunlight is limited, and fluoride if less than 0.3 ppm in the water supply.[81]
- Be sensitive to cultural diversity in families (see references, Chapters 4 and 5) and be aware of high risk groups. For example, according to the *Hispanic* Health and Nutrition Survey, Mainland children of Puerto Rican heritage in the US seemed at greatest risk for poor health.[82]
- Determine the reason for an unusual dietary or feeding practice.
- Counsel the family regarding the nutritional adequacy and safety of the diet.[4,5]
- Evaluate anthropometry values continually with the normal growth chart.
- Check infant hemoglobin values (11 g/dL) or hematocrit (33%) and other biochemistries as needed to be sure they are normal (Table 4–13 and Appendix 10).
- Evaluate dental caries related to nursing bottle syndrome (see Infant Nutrition Form, Appendix 4).
- Determine that the infant does not lose more than 5% of body weight or remain on intravenous dextrose or clear liquids more than 2 days without nutritional support if hospitalized.

Treatment should be given by a qualified dietitian or nutritionist.

References

1. Beaton, G.H. Nutritional needs during the first year of life: some concepts and perspectives. *Pediatr. Clin. North Am.* 1985;32:275.
2. American Academy of Pediatrics. Policy statement based on Task Force Report. The promotion of breast-feeding. *Pediatrics.* 1982;69:654.
3. American Academy of Pediatrics Committee on Nutrition. On the feeding of supplemental foods to infants. *Pediatrics.* 1980;65:1178.
4. Hanning, R., Zlotkin, S. Unconventional eating practices and their health implications. *Pediatr. Clin. North Am.* 1985;32:429.
5. Sinatra, F. Food faddism in pediatrics. *J. Am. Coll. Nutr.* 1984;3:169.
6. Committee on Nutrition. *Dietary Guidelines for Infants (Consistent with American Academy of Pediatrics Policy Statements).* Fremont, MI: Gerber Products Company; 1989.
7. Lozoff, B., Brittenham, G.M., Wolf, A.W., McClish, D.K., Kuhnert, P.M., Jimenez, E., Jimenez, R., Mora, L.A., Gomez, I., Krauskoph, D. Iron deficiency anemia and iron therapy. Effects on infant development test performance. *Pediatrics.* 1987;79:981.
8. Yip, R., Binkin, N.J., Fleshood, L., Trowbridge, F.L. Declining prevalence of anemia among low-income children in the Unites States. *JAMA.* 1987;258:1619.
9. Expert Scientific Working Group. Summary of a report on assessment of the iron nutritional status of the United States population. *Am. J. Clin. Nutr.* 1985;42:1318.
10. Miller, V., Swaney, S., Deinard, A. Impact of the WIC program on the iron status of infants. *Pediatrics.* 1985;75:100.
11. Finch, C.A., Cook, J.D. Iron deficiency. *Am. J. Clin, Nutr.* 1984;39:471.
12. Scrimshaw, N.S. Iron deficiency and its functional consequences. *Compr. Ther.* 1985;40:40.
13. Oski, F.A., Honig, A., Helu, B., Howanitz, P. Effect of iron therapy on behavior performance in nonanemic, iron deficient infants. *Pediatrics.* 1983;71:877.
14. Deinard, A.S., List, A., Lindgren, B., Hunt, J.V. Chang, P.N. Cognitive defects in iron-deficient and iron-deficient anemic children. *J. Pediatr.* 1986;108:681.
15. Saarinen, U.M., Siimes, M.A., Dallman, P.R. Iron absorption in infants: high bio-availability of breast milk as indicated by the extrinsic tag method of iron absorption and by the concentration of serum ferritin. *J. Pediatr.* 1977;91:36.
16. Saarinen, U.M. Need for iron supplementation in infants on prolonged breast feeding. *J. Pediatr.* 1978;93:177.
17. Siimes, M.A., Salmenpera, L., Perheentupa, J. Exclusive breast-feeding for 9 months: risk of iron deficiency. *J. Pediatr.* 1984;104:196.
18. Martinez, G.A., Krieger, F.W. 1984 milk-feeding patterns in the United States. *Pediatrics.* 1985;76:1004.
19. Rios, E., Hunter, R.E., Cook, J.D., Smith, N.J., Finch, C.A. The absorption of iron as supplements in infant cereal and infant formulas. *Pediatrics.* 1975;55:686.
20. Hertrampf, E., Cayazzo, M., Pizzaro, F., Stekel, A. Bioavailability of iron in soy-based formula and its effect on iron nutriture in infancy. *Pediatrics.* 1986;78:640.
21. Martinez, G.A., Ryan, A.S., Malec, D.J. Nutrient intakes of American infants and children fed cow's milk or infant formula. *Am. J. Dis. Child.* 1985;139:1010.
22. Sadowitz, P.D., Oski, F.A. Iron status and infant feeding practices in an urban ambulatory center. *Pediatrics.* 1983;72:33.
23. Fomon, S.J., Ziegler, E.E., Nelson, S.E., Edwards, B.B. Cow milk feeding in infancy: gastrointestinal blood loss and iron nutritional status. *J. Pediatr.* 1981;98:540.
24. Koerper, M.A., Mentzer, W.C., Brecher, G., Dallman, P.R. Developmental change in red blood cell volume: implication in screening infants and children for iron deficiency and thalassemia trait. *J. Pediatr.* 1976;89:580.
25. Dallman, P.R. Iron deficiency in the weanling: a nutritional problem on the way to resolution. *Acta Paediatr. Scand.* 1986;323(suppl):59.
26. American Academy of Pediatrics, Committee on Nutrition. Iron-fortified formulas. *Pediatrics.* 1989;83:1114.
27. American Academy of Pediatrics, Committee on Nutrition. Follow-up weaning formulas. *Pediatrics.* 1989;83:1069.
28. Gortmaker, S.L., Dietz, W.H., Sobol, A.M., Wehler, C.A. Increasing pediatric obesity in the United States. *Am. J. Dis. Child.* 1987;151:535.
29. Trowbridge, F.L. Prevalence of growth stunting and obesity: pediatric nutrition surveillance system, 1982, *MMWR. CDC. Surveill. Summ.* 1983;32(4SS):23SS.
30. Wolman, P.G. Feeding practices in infancy and prevalence of obesity in preschool children. *J. Am. Diet. Assoc.* 1984;84:436.
31. Patterson, R.E., Typpo, J.T., Typpo, M.H., Krause, G.F. Factors related to obesity in preschool children. *J. Am. Diet. Assoc.* 1986;86:1376.
32. Rolland-Cachera, M.F., Bellisle, F. No correlation between adiposity and food intake: why are working class children fatter? *Am. J. Clin. Nutr.* 1986;44:779.
33. Jaffe, M., Kosakov, C. The motor development of fat babies. *Clin. Pediatr.* 1982;21:619.
34. Vobecky, J.S., Vobecky, J., Shapcott, D., Demers, P. Nutrient intake patterns and nutritional status with regard to relative weight in early infancy. *Am. J. Clin. Nutr.* 1983;38:730.
35. Hager, A., Sjostrom, L., Arvidsson, B., Bjorntrop, P., Smith, U. Body fat and adipose tissue cellularity in infants: a longitudinal study. *Metabolism.* 1977;26:607.
36. Rolland-Cachera, M.F., Deheeger, M., Belisle, F., Sempe, M., Guilloud-Bataille, M., Patois, E. Adiposity rebound in children: a simple indicator for predicting obesity. *Am. J. Clin. Nutr.* 1984;39:129.
37. Knittle, J.L., Timmers, K., Ginsberg-Fellner, F., Brown, R.E., Katz, D.P. The growth of adipose tissue in children and adolescents. Cross-sectional and longitudinal studies of adipose cell number and size. *J. Clin. Invest.* 1979;63:239.
38. Forbes, G.B. Nutrition and growth. *J. Pediatr.* 1977;91:40.
39. Bonnet, F.P., Recour-Brumioul, D. Normal growth of human adipose tissue. In: Fernand, P., Bonnet, M.D., eds. *Adipose Tissue in Childhood.* Boca Raton, FL: CRC; 1981.

40. Poskitt, E.M.E. Obesity in the young child: whither and whence? *Acta Paediatr. Scand.* 1986;323(suppl):24.
41. Rolland-Cachera, M.F., Deheeger, M., Peguignot, F., Guilloud-Batoille, M., Vinit, F. Adiposity and food intake in young children: the environmental challenge to individual susceptibility. *Br. Med. J.* 1988;296:1037.
42. Dietz, W.H. Gortmaker, S.L. Do we fatten our children at the TV set? Television viewing and obesity in children and adolescents. *Pediatrics.* 1985;75:807.
43. Mayer, J. Quoted by Passmore, R. IVth International Nutrition Congress. *Lancet.* 1963;2:327.
44. Wenzell, B.J., Stults, H., Mayer, J. Hypoferremia in obese adolescents. *Lancet.* 1962;2:457.
45. Drabman, R.S., Hammer, D., Jarvie, G.J. Eating styles of obese and nonobese black and white children in a naturalistic setting. *Addict. Behav.* 1977;2:83.
46. Waxman, M., Stunkard, A.J. Caloric intake and expenditure of obese boys. *J. Pediatr.* 1980;96:187.
47. Overfeeding in the first year of life. *Nutr. Rev.* 1973;31:116.
48. Crow, R.A., Fawcett, J.N., Wright, P. Maternal behavior during breast- and bottle-feeding. *J. Behav. Med.* 1980;3:259.
49. Dine, M.S., Gartside, P.S., Glueck, C.J., Rheines, L., Greene, G., Khoury, P. Where do the heaviest children come from? A prospective study of white children from birth to 5 years of age. *Pediatrics.* 1979;63:1.
50. Jung, E., Czajka-Narins, D.M. Birth weight doubling and tripling times: an updated look at the effects of birth weight, sex, race and type of feeding. *Am. J. Clin. Nutr.* 1985;42:182.
51. Roche, A.F., Siervogel, R.M., Chumlea, W.C., Webb, P. Grading fatness from limited anthropometric data. *Am. J. Clin. Nutr.* 1981;34:283.
52. Dietz, W.H. Childhood obesity. *Ann. NY. Acad. Sci.* 1987;499:47.
53. Rolland-Cachera, M.F., Sempe, M., Guilloud-Bataille, M., Patois, E., Peguignot-Guggenbuhl, F., Fautrad, V. Adiposity indices in children. *Am. J. Clin. Nutr.* 1982;36:178.
54. Sales, J., Mouharzel, E., Dozio, E., Goulet, O., Putet, G., Recoir, C. Estimating resting energy expenditure by simple lean body mass indicators on total parenteral nutrition. *Am. J. Clin. Nutr.* 1990;51:958.
55. Dietz, W.H. Childhood obesity. Susceptibility, cause and management. *J. Pediatr.* 1983;103:676.
56. Mellin, L.M., Slinkard, L.A., Irwin, C.E. Adolescent obesity intervention: validation of the SHAPEDOWN program. *J. Am. Diet. Assoc.* 1987;87:333.
57. Brownell, K.D., Kelman, J.H., Stunkard, A.J. Treatment of obese children with and without their mothers: changes in weight and blood pressure. *Pediatrics.* 1983;71:515.
58. Food and Nutrition Board, National Research Council. *Recommended Dietary Allowances.* 10th ed., Washington, DC: National Academy; 1989.
59. American Academy of Pediatrics Committee on Nutrition. Nutrition aspects of obesity in infancy and childhood. *Pediatrics.* 1981;68:880.
60. Paneth, N. Hypernatremic dehydration of infancy. *Am. J. Dis. Child.* 1980;134:785.
61. Habel, A.H., Simpson, H. Osmolar relation between cerebrospinal fluid and serum in hyperosmolar hypernatremic dehydration. *Arch. Dis. Child.* 1976;51:660.
62. Rosenbloom, L., Sills, J.A. Hypernatremic dehydration and infant mortality. *Arch. Dis. Child.* 1975;50:750.
63. Macaulay, D., Watson M. Hypernatremia in infants as a cause of brain damage. *Arch. Dis. Child.* 1967;42:485.
64. Finberg, L. Hypernatremic dehydration. *Adv. Pediatr.* 1969;16:325.
65. Holliday, M.A., Segar, W.E. The maintenance need for water in parenteral fluid therapy. *Pediatrics.* 1957;19:823.
66. McCauley, D., Blackhall, M.I. Hypernatremic dehydration in infantile gastroenteritis. *Arch. Dis. Child.* 1961;36:543.
67. Ahmed, I., Agusto-Odutola, T.B. Hypernatremia in diarrheal infants in Lagos. *Arch. Dis. Child.* 1970;45:97.
68. American Academy of Pediatrics Committee on Nutrition. Use of oral fluid therapy and posttreatment feeding following enteritis in children in a developed country. *Pediatrics.* 1985;75:358.
69. Wendland, B.E., Arbus, G.S. Oral fluid therapy: sodium and potassium content and osmolality of some commercial "clear" soups, juices, and beverages. *Can. Med. Assoc. J.* 1979;121:564.
70. Taitz, L.S., Byers, H.D. High calorie/osmolar feeding and hypertonic dehydration. *Arch. Dis. Child.* 1972;47:257.
71. Chambers, T.L., Steele, A.E. Concentrated milk feeds and their relation to hypernatremic dehydration in infants. *Arch. Dis. Child.* 1975;50:610.
72. Birenbaum, E., Shahar, E., Aladjem, M., Brish, M. Neonatal hypernatremic dehydration due to excessively concentrated prepared milk formula. *Clin. Pediatr.* 1981;20:627.
73. Listernick, R., Sidransky, E. Hypernatremic dehydration in children with severe psychomotor retardation. *Clin. Pediatr.* 1985;24:440.
74. American Academy of Pediatrics Committee on Nutrition. Toward a prudent diet for children. *Pediatrics.* 1983;71:78.
75. American Academy of Pediatrics Committee on Nutrition. Prudent lifestyle for children: dietary fat and cholesterol. *Pediatrics.* 1986;78:521.
76. Haust, M.D. The genesis of atherosclerosis in pediatric age-group. In: *Pediatric Diseases.* Ontario, Canada: Hemisphere Publishing Co; 1990.
77. Simpoulos, A. Omega-3 fatty acids in health and disease and in growth and development. *Am. J. Clin. Nutr.* 1991;54:438.
78. Roy, C., Galeano, N. Childhood antecedents of adult degenerative disease. *Pediatr. Clin. North Am.* 1985;32:517.
79. Kendler, B.S. Taurine: an overview of its role in preventive medicine. *Prevent. Med.* 1989;18:79.
80. Nichols, B.L. Infant feeding practice. In: Tsang, R.C., Nichols, B.L. eds. *Nutrition During Pregnancy.* Philadelphia: Hanley & Belfus; 1988.
81. Food and Nutrition Board, Institute of Medicine, National Academy of Sciences, Maternal nutrient needs during lactation. Nutrition During Lactation, Washington, D.C., 1991, National Academy Press.
82. Mendaza, F., Ventura, S., Valdez, B., Costello, R., Saldivar, L., Baisden, K., Martarell, R. Selected measures of health status for Mexican-American, Mainland Puerto Rican and Cuban-American children. *JAMA.* 1991;265(2):227.

Chapter 3
The Premature Infant

Barbara Niedbala and Reginald Tsang

A premature birth is defined as a birth occurring before 37 weeks of gestation. In the United States, premature births account for approximately 9% to 10% of all live births.[1] Causes include premature rupture of the membranes, maternal hypertension, preterm spontaneous labor, and antepartum hemorrhage.[2] Also associated with premature delivery are low maternal weight, poor socioeconomic status, diabetes, nephritis, anemia, fetal anomalies, and multiple pregnancy.

Premature infants, because they have an inadequate time to complete growth in utero, are born with low birth weights. Commonly used classifications of birth weight are as follows:

- low birth weight (LBW)   1500–2500 grams
- very low birth weight (VLBW)   1000–1499 grams
- extremely low birth weight (ELBW)   < 999 grams

Infants are further judged to be small, appropriate, or large for gestational age (SGA, AGA, or LGA) after plotting the birth weight against gestational age on a standard chart (Figure 12-1 in Chapter 12). Gestational age is determined by the clinician after calculation of maternal dates and from the results of clinical and neurological examinations of the newborn infant (see Chapter 2).

Mortality and morbidity are related to birth weight and gestational age. Survival rates over the past decade have increased from 13% to 21% at gestational ages < 26 weeks (ELBW), from 64% to 78% at gestational ages 27–29 weeks (VLBW), and from 88% to 100% at gestational ages 30–32 weeks (VLBW).[3] Morbidities in surviving infants include hyperbilirubinemia, respiratory distress syndrome, retinopathy of prematurity, patent ductus arteriosus, intraventricular hemorrhage, bronchopulmonary dysplasia, sepsis, and necrotizing enterocolitis.[4]

Premature infants have a higher incidence of neurodevelopmental sequelae than those born at term. Data collected from developed countries show the incidence of major handicaps (cerebral palsy, mental retardation, hearing or visual losses severe enough to necessitate special schooling, and hydrocephalus) to be 6% to 9% in VLBW infants.[4] The incidence increases with a lowered birth weight: 27% to 44% of ELBW may have major sequelae.[5]

Biochemical Abnormalities

Physiological, functional, and iatrogenic problems

To survive, the premature infant has to overcome the disadvantages of immature organ systems and adapt to extrauterine life. Nutrition plays a primary role as adequate substrate material must be present for growth and development to continue outside the uterus. Advanced medical technology enables infants with inefficiently functioning organs (such as the lungs by using exogenous surfactant) to survive, but often induces other clinical problems prohibitive to growth.[6] These problems and their nutritional implications are summarized in Table 3–1.

Although this type of assessment is controversial, adequate postnatal growth in the premature infant is assessed by comparison to intrauterine growth standards.[7] The most appropriate nutritional goal for the premature infant is not yet known. The Committee on Nutrition of the American Academy of Pediatrics recommends that the in utero growth of a normal fetus at the same postconceptional age be used as the standard for both postnatal growth and the determination of body accretion rates for macro- and micronutrients.[8,9]

Factors to be Considered in Nutritional Evaluation

Anthropometric

Baseline anthropometric measurements of the premature infant are obtained immediately after delivery. Birth weight, length, and head circumference are measured according to standard procedures.

In the first week of life, there occurs a physiological weight loss of 5% to 15% of the original birth weight. It is a naturally occurring diuresis caused by sodium and water loss from the extracellular space, and it occurs independently of the volume of fluid intake.[10] Thereafter, weight gain is dependent upon nutritional intake. Healthy, enterally fed premature infants usually regain birth weight by the second or third postnatal week.[11] During the hospital admission, weight should be obtained daily, and crown-heel length and head circumference should be obtained weekly. Both intra- and extrauterine growth charts are available for the assessment of postnatal growth. Pereira and Barbosa[12] discuss the controversies surrounding the use of various growth charts.

Assessment of the head circumference measurement in premature infants deserves special attention, as an increased velocity of growth may indicate developing hydrocephalus.[13] The clinician should scrutinize the weekly anthropometric measurements for increases in head growth that do not correspond to increases in weight, length, nutritional intake, and overall improved clinical status.

Biochemical assessment

Serum albumin and total protein concentrations may not be accurate measures of nutritional status in premature infants,

Table 3–1. Nutritional Implications of Postnatal Care of the Premature Infant

System	Problems	Nutritional Implications
Respiratory	Immature Lungs –Respiratory distress syndrome –Bronchopulmonary dysplasia	Fluid restriction and assisted ventilation may interfere with adequate enteral or parenteral feedings. Assisted ventilation may result in palatal groove formation, tooth enamel hypoplasia and acquired cleft palate.
Circulatory	Patent ductus arteriosus	Fluid restriction and/or surgical treatment may interfere with provision of adequate feedings.
	Frequent phlebotomy	Anemia
Renal	Immature excretory capacity	Limitations placed on nutrients in diet contributing to renal solute load (electrolytes, protein).
Gastrointestinal	Immature suck-swallow reflex	Tube feedings or parenteral feedings may be necessary.
	Small gastric capacity	Smaller feedings may be nutritionally inadequate.
	Immature digestion and absorption of carbohydrate, lipid	Modified milk feedings may be necessary. Absorption of fat-soluble vitamins may be impaired.
	Poorly developed nutrient stores of vitamin E, iron	Anemia
	Necrotizing enterocolitis	Bowel rest may be necessary, requiring parenteral feeding.
Endocrine	Need for high mineral accretion rate: calcium, phosphorus	Metabolic bone disease is likely when soy or human milk or parenteral nutrition is used.

particularly those of extremely low birth weight. These concentrations increase significantly with gestational age; there is also a postnatal rise in albumin concentration, regardless of gestational age at birth, of approximately 15% in the first 3 weeks.[14] Subcutaneous edema can be seen in the premature infant during the first few days of life, but it may be a normal finding and is not significantly linked to hypoalbuminemia.[14,15] Healthy premature infants often show lowered albumin and total protein concentrations, despite an adequate protein and energy intake and without clinical correlates of hypoproteinemia.[16] In contrast, other premature infants may develop clinical evidence of protein deficiency (hair depigmentation) without exhibiting significantly low serum albumin concentrations.[17] Prealbumin concentration appears to be a better marker of nutritional status in premature infants, most likely because of its shorter half-life. Significantly low prealbumin concentrations are documented in premature infants consuming inadequate protein and energy.[18]

Infants receiving parenteral nutrition should be monitored routinely for various laboratory measurements (Table 3–2). In enterally or parenterally fed infants, clinical signs of specific nutrient deficiencies and documentation of dietary inadequacy should be sought before laboratory assessment is made because of the risk and expense of having blood drawn from the infant and the infrequency of certain deficiencies. Zinc, folate, vitamin A, and essential fatty acid deficiencies may occur in individual infants with exceptionally low prenatal stores and/or dietary deficiencies. The acceptable hemoglobin and hematocrit values should be greater than 10 mg/dL and greater than 30%, respectively.

Clinical assessment

Clinical examination of the premature infant is a necessary part of ongoing nutritional monitoring. The infant should be routinely visually inspected for signs of edema, dermatitis, and changes in hair color and an overall evaluation of fat stores and musculature. Nursing records should be reviewed for notes on feeding intolerance. Late-occurring peripheral edema, noted upon visual inspection, and pulmonary edema, noted upon ascultation of the chest, may be

Table 3–2. Suggested Laboratory Monitoring Schedule during Parenteral Nutrition Therapy

	First Week	Thereafter
Electrolytes	Daily	3 times weekly to weekly
BUN	Daily	Weekly
Calcium	As needed*	Weekly
Phosphorus	As needed*	Weekly
Magnesium	As needed	Weekly
Alkaline phosphatase	Once	Weekly
Total protein/albumin	Once	Weekly to bi-weekly
Liver function tests	Once	Weekly to bi-weekly
CBC, platelets	As needed	Weekly
Triglycerides or lipid levels	With each incremental dose of intravenous lipid	Weekly
Urine specific gravity	2-3 times daily	2-3 times daily
Urine glucose	2-3 times daily	2-3 times daily

*Daily high infusion rates of calcium or phosphorus are given.

signs of overhydration, vitamin E deficiency, or hypoalbuminemia. The infant's skin should be observed for signs of dry, flaky dermatitis, which is indicative of essential fatty acid or zinc deficiency.

Feeding intolerance is manifested by the presence of an increased amount of residual matter withdrawn from the stomach just before the next enteral feeding. A small amount of gastric juice residual is normal. However, large amounts of residue, greater than one-third of the volume of the previous bolus feeding or greater than the amount delivered hourly by continuous drip, are indicative of bowel stasis. Abdominal distention—measured as an increase of more than 2 cm over the baseline measurement for the previous 24-hour period in a 2-kg infant—is also indicative of bowel stasis.[19]

Nutritional intake

Calorie, protein, vitamin, and mineral intakes from enteral and parenteral alimentary formulas are easily calculated from nursing records of the infant's intake and output and current formulary information. Additives to the enteral intake (glucose polymers, protein modulars, lipid supplements, human milk fortifier, etc.), intravenous solutions other than parenteral nutrition solutions (dextrose used for medication administration, calcium gluconate, etc.), and oral vitamin and mineral supplements should be duly recorded. Any excessive emesis or gastric residues not returned to the gastrointestinal tract should be subtracted from the enteral intake. Actual input and output records, rather than the physician's written orders, should always be used in intake calculations for assessment of nutrition and fluid intake. Totals of calculated nutrient intake data must be converted into meaningful units, such as kcal/kg/day, mg calcium/kg/day, g lipid/kg/hour, or percent of kcal provided by lipid. The results may then be compared with appropriately chosen reference standards based on current research.

When assessing nutritional intake in relation to the infant's gastrointestinal tolerance of an enteral formula, caloric density and osmolality must be considered. High caloric density is associated with inhibition of gastric emptying, although the degree of inhibition from any one nutrient is unknown. There is no significant difference in emptying time between 20 kcal/oz formula and 24 kcal/oz formula,

both of which are commonly utilized in feeding premature infants, but a density above 24 kcal/oz may be expected to cause delayed gastric emptying.[20]

Hyperosmolar formulas may also cause delayed gastric emptying, emesis, or diarrhea. An osmolality of less than 400 mO/sm/kg H_2O is recommended for infant feedings;[21] however, in the neonatal intensive care unit, various vitamin, mineral, and oral medication preparations are mixed together with infant formula, greatly increasing their osmolality. The osmolality of a drug-formula mixture may be calculated by the method of Ernst et al.[22]

Other drug-nutrient interactions should be considered when judging the adequacy of nutritional intake and the causes of formula intolerance. Diuretic therapy, specifically furosemide, causes hypercalciuria.[23] Long-term antibiotic treatment is a well-known causative factor in diarrhea because of its destruction of the gut flora necessary for carbohydrate digestion.

Feeding ability

The choice of feeding method—parenteral, enteral, gavage, bottle, or breast—is determined after evaluation of the infant's suck-swallow mechanism, gut maturity, and general clinical condition. The infant is first assessed for bowel sounds; if no ileus is present, enteral feedings may begin. When an oro- or endotracheal tube is in place for artificial respiration, the infant will require tube (gavage) feeding. The infant receiving bolus intermittent feedings by gavage is monitored for bradycardia during feeding and for signs of delayed gastric emptying, gastroesophageal reflux, and abdominal distention. If any of these signs occur repeatedly, continuous drip feedings into either the stomach or the jejunum (transpyloric) may need to be instituted. Parenteral nutrition is utilized when the gastrointestinal tract cannot be used or when enteral feedings are nutritionally insufficient.

The infant may be assessed for the ability to bottle or breast feed when artificial respiration is discontinued or when a permanent tracheostomy is in place. Coordination of the suck-swallow reflex is dependent upon postconception age and usually is not developed fully until 34–36 weeks of gestation.[24] Other developmental disorders affecting the central nervous system or muscular system may further delay development of suck-swallow coordination. Gagging, choking, spitting, apnea, severe bradycardia, and cyanosis are indications that the infant is not yet ready for nipple feeding.

Assessment of the infant's position during enteral feeding may be useful when delayed gastric emptying and reflux are seen. Gastric emptying occurs faster and reflux may be prevented by placing the infant in either the prone or right lateral position; a 30 degree elevated prone position is used in treating severe cases of gastroesophageal reflux.[24]

Factors to be Considered in Nutritional Evaluation and Dietary Management

Both enteral and parenteral modes of nutritional alimentation are used in feeding premature infants. Parenteral nutrition is used in up to 80% of premature infants in current nursery settings, almost a doubling of the usage 5 years ago.[25] The incidence of use is highest in infants of VLBW. The duration of intravenous alimentation is positively associated with lower gestational age and birth weight.[25] Although numerous problems are associated with the use of parenteral nutrition, sepsis and metabolic disorders being the largest, the advantages of this method of feeding cannot be disputed when its use is indicated clinically. Parenteral nutrition support in premature infants may be used for only a few days until enteral feedings can begin and are nutritionally sufficient; total parenteral nutrition may be used for weeks or months in premature infants with severe gastrointestinal impairment.

Enteral nutrition

Feeding methods. Various methods of gavage feeding may be employed as there is no general agreement about the ideal method to provide feedings to premature infants whose sucking and swallowing mechanisms are impaired.[12] Intermittent gavage feeding, in which a bolus of formula is passed to the stomach at timed intervals by gravity drip, syringe, or infusion pump, appears to be the most physiological feeding method.[26] The feeding tube may be passed through the nose or the mouth. Continuous gavage feeding, delivered by gravity drip or infusion pump, provides constant infusion of formula at a consistent rate. Continuous feedings may be used in those infants whose respiratory status is transiently compromised during bolus feedings[27] or who exhibit delayed gastric emptying without ileus. Feedings may be delivered to the stomach, or the feeding tube may be advanced through the pylorus to the duodenum or jejunum. Although transpyloric feedings decrease the incidence of pulmonary aspiration and abdominal distention, they may cause such complications as diarrhea and bacterial overgrowth and may decrease the absorption of potassium and fat.[28]

Nonnutritive sucking on a pacifier is recommended for infants fed by gavage. It is important for the infant to learn the association between pleasant oral stimulation and the cessation of hunger. Nonnutritive sucking in premature infants is associated with enhanced weight grain, earlier tolerance of nipple feeding, and earlier hospital discharge.[29-31] Increased weight gain is thought to be due to a decrease in motor activity during sucking periods. Respiratory status is also seen to stabilize during sucking periods.[32]

Gavage feedings are begun as soon after birth as possible, when the infant has stabilized and bowel sound are apparent. Feedings of formula or human milk may initially be diluted to one-quarter or half-strength. The rate, volume, and schedule of feedings are chosen based on the infant's size (Table 3–3). The rate and strength of feedings should not be advanced simultaneously; the infant must be monitored for tolerance to feeds before any increase is made. There is some evidence that advancing the volume of feedings before increasing the calorie density results in a significantly earlier attainment of adequate energy intake and decreases the need for concurrent intravenous fluids.[19] Different intensive care nurseries may use preset feeding protocols based on the preferences and experiences of the clinicians, but deviations from written protocols are often necessary for the individual infant (see Appendix 6 for University Hospital Protocol, Cincinnati).

Bottle feeding may be attempted in infants who have reached a postconception age of 32–36 weeks. Contraindications to bottle feeding include endo- or orotracheal intubation, an increased respiratory rate, and lack of suck-swallow coordination. Infants fed by continuous gavage are first gradually converted to an intermittent gavage schedule. When tolerance of gavaged bolus feedings is documented, gradual replacement of gavage feedings by bottle feedings may begin. Bottle-feeding sessions may last 20 to 40 minutes, depending on the amount to be consumed. Initially, a time limit may be set. Any unconsumed formula after the time allowed is gavage fed. Signs of respiratory distress, gagging, or choking may be present during some feedings but not others. Experimentation with nipple types and sizes may be helpful. The smaller, "premature" nipples are designed for infants with weaker sucking ability. Enlarging the hole in standard or premature nipples is not recommended as the infant will not then learn to integrate the muscle activity involved in oral control.

Indications and contraindications for breastfeeding are similar to those for bottle feeding. Clinically stable infants expected to show suck-swallow coordination may be put directly to the breast for feedings. However, it is often more convenient for nursery staff to evaluate the infant's feeding ability initially with an artificial nipple feeding. In addition, the frequency of scheduled feeding and the nutritional content of human milk (discussed below) may preclude breastfeeding at each feeding. Recent research has suggested that infants of 32 weeks gestation and a birth weight of 1200 grams may breastfeed successfully without disruption of ventilation.[33]

Individual nutrients

Fluid. Fluid needs range from 100 to 150 mL/kg/day after day 2 of life (Table 3–4). Water requirements are based on insensible water loss and on urine, sweat, and fecal losses. There is an inverse relationship between gestational age and insensible water loss because of the increased permeability of the premature infant's skin to water, a greater surface area per unit of body weight, and an increased skin vascularity. Insensible water losses are increased by the use of radiant warmers and phototherapy and by fever and increased activity. Mechanical ventilation and high humidity decrease insensible water loss. Hydration status is best meas-

Table 3–3. Guidelines for Initiating Oral Feedings

Birth Weight	≤1250 Grams*	1251–1500 Grams	1501–2000 Grams	>2000 Grams
Volume and type of first feeding	1 cc 5% glucose or sterile water	3 cc 5–10% glucose or sterile water	5 cc 5–10% glucose or sterile water	15 cc 5% glucose or sterile water
Number of glucose water feedings	1–2	1–2	1–2	1–2
Volume of first milk feeding	1–3 cc	5 cc	8 cc	15 cc
Schedule of feedings	Hourly	Every 2–3 hours	Every 2–3 hours	Every 3 hours
Volume and rate of milk increases	1 cc as tolerated	1 cc every other feeding	1 cc every other feeding	5 cc every other feeding

*After 24–48 hours of IV feeding.
From Ohio Neonatal Nutritionists. Feeding methodologies. In: Ohio Neonatal Nutritionists. eds. *Nutritional Care for High Risk Newborns*. Philadelphia: Stickley, 1985. Used with permission.

ured by urine osmolality and urine specific gravity. Normal urine osmolality is 150–400 mOsm/L; desirable urine specific gravity is 1.006–1.013.[34]

Energy. In the healthy, growing premature infant, energy needs are estimated to be 120–150 kcal/kg/day.[35–37] This amount usually allows for growth rates comparable to intrauterine growth rates at similar gestational ages, at least 20–30 g/day. Energy needs are partitioned among basal metabolic rate, growth, physical activity, protein synthesis, fecal and urinary losses, and cold stress.[35] Because sick premature infants are often unable to consume the recommended energy intake, the initial growth rate for these infants may be less than the expected intrauterine rate for gestational age.[38] One study suggested that a minimum intake of 85 kcal/kg/day still allows for head growth in sick premature infants, with concurrent suboptimal gains in weight and length.[39] A second phase of "catch-up" growth then occurs when adequate energy intake begins, and a third phase of growth along standard rates occurs last.

Protein. The desirable protein intake for premature infants is between 2.4–4.0 g/kg/day based on fetal accretion rates and metabolic balance studies.[40] Lower amounts may affect the overall growth rate, and higher amounts may cause metabolic acidosis, hyperammonemia, and azotemia. The relationship between protein and energy intake is important—10% to 15% of the calories should be provided by protein. The type of protein best tolerated and metabolized by the premature infant is thought to be whey-predominant and similar to that of human milk. Bovine milk may be modified to have a predominance of whey, although the ideal amino acid content for premature infants is still under study. Casein-predominant formula can cause more frequent, severe, and prolonged episodes of metabolic acidosis in premature infants.[40]

Carbohydrate. The carbohydrates most easily assimilated by the premature infant are sucrose, glucose, and glucose polymers. The use of sucrose or glucose is discouraged because of the resulting high osmolality of the feeding. Lactose, the only carbohydrate in "natural" milks, is usually well tolerated by premature infants despite low lactase activity in the immature intestine. Lactose is recommended as a partial or full carbohydrate source as it also enhances the absorption of calcium. Glucose polymers can be used in place of or to supplement lactose as the carbohydrate source. The osmotic load is low, and hence it is a useful means of measuring calorie density without unduly increasing osmotic load. Carbohydrate should comprise about 40% to 45% of the total caloric intake.

Fat. Fat provides the majority of energy intake—40% to 50% of total calories—and is also needed to prevent fatty acid deficiency. Polyunsaturated fats and medium-chain triglycerides are the most easily absorbed type of fat by the premature infant. At least 3% of the total caloric intake should be provided by linoleic acid to prevent fatty acid deficiency.[9]

Vitamins/Minerals. Recommendations for vitamin and mineral intakes for enterally fed premature infants are summarized in Table 3–5. The minimum, ideal, and maximum intakes of these nutrients remain under study, particularly for infants born at varying gestational ages. Current literature has been reviewed and compiled by Tsang[46] (see Appendix 6).

Table 3–4. Fluid Requirements (mL/kg/day)

Birthweight (g)	Days 1–2	Day 3	Days 15–30
<750–1,000	105	140	150
1,001–1,250	100	130	140
1,251–1,500	90	120	130
1,501–1,750	80	110	130
1,751–2,000	80	110	130

From Nash,[34] with permission.

Table 3–5. Intake Range Recommended for Growing, Stable 2-Week-Old, 29-Week Gestational Age Infant (Cow-Milk-Based Formula)

Nutrient	Intake Range
Vitamin B$_{12}$	0.15 μg/100 kcal
Folate	15 μg/kg per day
Vitamin C	30 mg/100 kcal
Niacin	4 mg preformed niacin/100 kcal
Thiamine	250 μg/100 kcal
Riboflavin	335 μg/100 kcal
Pyridoxine	250 μg/100 kcal
Vitamin A	1400 IU/day
Vitamin E	25 IU/day*
Vitamin K	5 μg/kg per day
Vitamin D	400 IU/day
Fe	2 mg/kg per day by doubled with birth weight[†]
Ca	Up to 200 mg/kg per day[‡]
P	Up to 113 mg/kg per day[‡]
Mg	5–6 mg/kg per day
Na	3–8 mEq/kg per day[§] up to 3 weeks, then 1–3 mEq/kg[§] per day[‖]
K	1–3 mEq/kg per day
Cl	3–8 mEq/kg per day (can reduce to 1.0 if HCO$_3^-$ given)
Zn	800–1,200 μg/kg per day[¶]
Cu	100–200 μg/kg per day
Se	1.5–2.5 μg/kg per day
Mn	10–20 μg/kg per day
Cr	2–4 μg/kg per day
Mo	2–3 μg/kg per day
Biotin	0.6–2.3 μg/kg per day
Pantothenic acid	1.0–1.4 mg/kg per day
Choline	5–9 mg/kg per day

*25 IU/day is recommended to establish tissue vitamin E stores in the first 2–4 weeks; beyond that 5 IU/day is satisfactory.

[†]1–2 mg/kg per day prior to this time, if blood loss not replaced.

[‡]Low calcium and phosphorus concentrations in human milk fed to preterm infants result in low bone mineral content, which may be prevented by using mineral supplements. Preterm infants receiving exclusively human milk for prolonged periods should be examined, at least at 2 months of age, for rickets and fractures using x-ray, serum phosphorus, and possibly alkaline phosphate measurements.

[§]Decrease to 2 mEq/kg per day if serum Na is greater than 144 mEq/L.

[‖]Increase again if serum sodium less than 132 mEq/L.

[¶]Infants appear to be generally in negative balance even at these levels of intake.

From Tsang,[41] with permission.

Use of commercial formula, human milk, and supplements

Human milk is clearly the food of choice for full-term infants; the nutrient content of human milk is used as a quality standard for the production of commercial formulas. For premature infants, human milk, particularly as the sole nourishment, can result in lowered growth rates and inadequate bone mineralization. However, the ease of digestion and the presence of host defense mechanisms and growth factors in human milk cannot be reproduced technologically by current manufacturing methods. Therefore, human milk, insofar as its metabolic and physiological effects are concerned, does remain a quality standard for the production of premature infant formulas. The goal of nutritional care for the premature infant is a well-grown infant with a body composition and chemical balance matching first the fetus in utero and then the term infant who is nourished postnatally by human milk. It appears therefore that, despite its limitations in this condition, human milk will always play a role in the nourishment of the premature infant.

Currently, three major brands of premature infant formula are available to hospitals for feeding premature infants. All are associated with adequate growth and metabolic stability when fed in amounts consistent with energy needs.[42,43,44] Although their macronutrient content is similar, the formulas vary in vitamin and mineral content. They have been developed specifically for the nourishment of premature infants with rapidly growing but immature systems and thus are used in most premature infants only until discharge from the neonatal nursery. In comparison to the standard formula, these formulas provide a higher protein content with a 60:40 whey:casein ratio, fat comprised of medium-chain triglycerides and polyunsaturated long-chain triglycerides, carbohydrate as part lactose and part glucose polymers, and significantly higher calcium and phosphorus content. Energy content may or may not be higher: both 67 kcal/dL and 81 kcal/dL formulas are available.

Standard milk- and soy-based formulas and low-mineral-containing formulas are not recommended for the rapidly growing ELBW or VLBW infant. These formulas do not provide sufficient calcium and phosphorus for bone mineralization[45]; the protein level may also be insufficient. In premature infants requiring highly specialized formula, such as those needed for the treatment of severe gastrointestinal, liver, or renal disease or inborn errors of metabolism, particularly close monitoring of growth, protein adequacy, and osteopenia is necessary, with individual supplementation of nutrients as indicated.

Still under investigation are cholesterol, taurine, carnitine, and omega-3 fatty acids (eicosapentaenoic and docosahexaenoic acids) in relation to the growth and development of the premature infant.

Preterm human milk contains higher concentrations of fat, protein, sodium, chloride, magnesium, and iron on a gram/liter basis in comparison to mature human milk.[45] The inadequacy of pooled and banked mature human milk for feeding premature infants is well known,[45] and most neonatal intensive care units currently do not use this milk. Despite the high concentration of some nutrients, deficiencies of protein, sodium, vitamin D, calcium, phosphorus, iron, zinc, and copper are possible in infants fed preterm human milk because of insufficient or highly variable concentrations relevant to preterm infant needs.[47] Adequate growth and nitrogen retention are possible in premature infants fed their own mother's milk,[48,49] but the majority of controlled studies report significantly higher gains in weight, length, and head circumference in formula-fed premature infants.[46]

Bone demineralization remains a problem in infants fed their own mother's preterm milk even when their growth rate is adequate.[50,51] Frequent monitoring of calcium and phosphorus laboratory values is warranted, but the optimal management of osteopenia while continuing to feed human milk is uncertain. Human milk fortifiers have been developed to increase the nutrient content of human milk; individual nurseries may also have their own formulations. Although the commercial human milk fortifiers may increase nutrients to a favorable level, few clinical studies report a positive effect on bone mineralization.[51,52] In addition, nutrient losses occur during gavage feeding of fortified human milk. Greater than 40% of the calcium and phosphorus may not be delivered to the infant; smaller losses of energy, zinc, copper, and magnesium may occur.[53] Lactoengineering, a process in which isolates of human milk protein and fat from banked donor milk, with or without supplementary minerals, are added to the infant's own mother's milk, is currently under investigation.[54]

Clinicians must decide together with the infant's mother whether expressed human milk or breastfeeding will be appropriate for the individual infant. Nursery personnel should be knowledgeable about collection, storage, and handling procedures for expressed human milk. The mother may need additional emotional support and encouragement.

Other supplements added to either formula or human milk consist of modified carbohydrate or lipid. These supplements are used to increase the energy content while making little change in the osmolality and volume of the feeding. Care must be taken when using these supplements to ensure that the nutritional content of the resulting formula remains balanced, with adequate protein, vitamin, and mineral content. The infant must also be monitored closely for gastrointestinal disturbances, particularly diarrhea and delayed gastric emptying.

Premature infants are born with lower stores of iron; yet, their postnatal iron needs are greater than those of a full-term infant because of the need to sustain a more rapid rate of growth. Typically premature infant formulas have not contained iron because of concerns of inducing vitamin E deficiency-related hemolysis. Early iron supplementation at 2 weeks of age may be begun in premature infants as long as plasma vitamin E is normal. Otherwise, supplementation of iron should begin at least by the eighth postnatal week. Supplements of 2–4 mg/kg/day[55] are given to both formula-fed and human-milk-fed infants, or the infant may be changed to an iron-containing premature formula. If birth weight is less than 1000 grams, 4 mg/kg/day iron is needed; if 1000–1500 grams, 3 mg/kg/day; and if 1501–2500 grams, 2 mg/kg/day.[55]

Vitamin E supplementation is necessary in many premature infants because of poor placental transfer, inadequate stores developed in utero, and postnatal malabsorption. Vitamin E requirements are increased by high intakes of both iron and polyunsaturated fatty acids. The recommended intake of vitamin E is 0.7 IU per 100 calories and at least 1.0 IU per gram of linoleic acid.[8] Infants receiving premature formula may not need any further vitamin E supplementation, as these amounts are provided by the formula, unless iron supplements are given concurrently.[56] Infants receiving human milk may benefit by vitamin E supplements of 5 IU/day when iron is also given.[56] Other researchers recommend vitamin E supplements of 25 IU/day for the first 2–3 postnatal weeks, regardless of formula or milk intake, with a subsequent decrease to 5 IU/day after the third week in healthy, growing neonates.[57]

Calcium, phosphorus, and vitamin D supplements may be necessary for either human milk-fed or formula-fed infants. Recommendations for calcium and phosphorus intakes are summarized in Table 3–6. Although the minimum requirement for these calcium and phosphorus is unknown, both minerals should be supplemented if hypophosphatemia is seen, keeping the calcium:phosphorus ratio between 1.4 and 2.0.[58] Osteopenia of prematurity has been shown generally to be related to calcium and phosphorus mineral insufficiency and to occur unrelated to vitamin deficiency. However, premature infants may still develop vitamin D-deficiency rickets if intake of this nutrient is inadequate. Therefore, a supplement providing 400 IU/day is recommended for human milk-fed infants.[59]

If preterm infant formulas are not used, a general pediatric multivitamin or "preemie" supplement is usually provided daily to premature infants. It contains 5 IU vitamin E/day and 400 IU vitamin D/day as recommended for most infants. It also provides supplements of vitamins A, B_6, and B_{12}; ascorbic acid; thiamin; riboflavin; folate; and niacin. Premature infants' requirements for these vitamins are unclear. The minimal needs are most likely provided by formula or human milk when used with the addition of a daily multivitamin supplement or when preterm infant formulas are used alone (except for vitamin E as described earlier).[59]

Table 3–6. Required Calcium and Phosphorus Intakes to Meet the Fetal Accretion Rate

Gestational Age (w)	Weight (g)	Fetal Accretion (mg/kg/day)		Required Intake From			
				Human Milk* (mg/kg/day)		Preterm Formula†	
		Ca	P	Ca	P	Ca	P
28	1150	120	71	240	79	185	100
32	1715	125	72	250	81	190	101
36	2710	130	80	260	90	200	113

*Retention of calcium is 50% of intake; retention of phosphorus is 89% of intake.
†Retention of calcium from U.S. commercial premature formulas is 65% of intake; retention of phosphorus from same is 71% of intake.
Adapted from Greer and Tsang.[58]

Parenteral nutrition

Clinical indications for instituting parenteral nutrition include intestinal ileus; severe gastrointestinal disease requiring bowel rest; extreme immaturity associated with intestinal hypomotility and decreased gastric capacity; and poorly tolerated, nutritionally insufficient enteral feedings. Fluid needs during parenteral nutrition therapy are based on birth weight and postnatal age (Table 3-4). In the first 2 to 3 postnatal days of life, the infant's fluid therapy is monitored carefully, to allow for slow diuresis and to keep sodium, glucose, and acid-base balances stable. Once stability is established, partial parenteral alimentation may begin with the addition of an amino acid solution and an increase in glucose administration. If enteral feedings are expected to be delayed even a few days, parenteral lipid administration will be required. When enteral feedings have begun but are slow to advance, parenteral alimentation may be manipulated such that energy and protein needs are met by both enteral and parenteral sources combined. Fluid balance requires careful monitoring during this time.

Energy needs during parenteral nutrition administration are slightly lower than those estimated for enteral feedings because the digestive system is bypassed. Glucose, lipid, and amino acids can all be used for energy. However, because acids should be provided for synthesis of new tissue rather than for energy, only the glucose and lipid sources are considered in energy intake calculations. Positive nitrogen balance has been documented in premature infants with an energy intake of 45 kcal/kg/day.[59] Nitrogen balance is dependent also on protein intake and rate of body growth. Consistent weight gain along intrauterine standards is generally not seen until nonprotein energy is supplied at 80–85 kcal/kg/day.[60,61] In adults, energy may be supplied by either glucose or lipid, but the sole use of either substrate poses problems for the premature infant. The amount of glucose infused is limited by the mode of administration, as well as by metabolic capacity. If given via a peripheral vein, the glucose concentration in solution should remain under 130 g/L ($D_{13}W$) to avoid vein thrombosis or local tissue irritation caused by a high osmolality (if fluids leak into the tissues). Greater concentrations may be given via a central vein. However, hyperglycemia frequently occurs if glucose administration is begun at a rate greater than 6 mg/kg/min.[62] If this amount is tolerated (blood sugar concentrations < 125 mg/dL), the infusion rate or solution concentration may be increased gradually over several days to provide a max-

imum of 11–12 mg/kg/min. In some cases, insulin may be administered concurrently to prevent hyperglycemia.

The use of intravenous lipid is required in premature infants receiving only parenteral nutrition for longer than 4 to 5 days. Lipid administration of 0.5 g/kg/day prevents fatty acid deficiency, which is quick to develop in premature infants because of their limited fat stores. Lipid also provides a concentrated source of energy while minimizing overall fluid intake and lowering total solution osmolality. The recommended administration is 0.5 g/kg/day initially, with an increase of 0.5 g/kg/day to a maximum of 3.0 g/kg/day.[63] The rate should not exceed 0.25 g/kg/hr. Complications of lipid infusion include hypertriglyceridemia and hyperglycemia, as the premature infant's ability to clear lipid from plasma is reduced.[64] The effects of lipid administration during infection, acute pulmonary disease, and in extreme prematurity are still under investigation. Reports of lipid deposition in the lungs,[65] impaired immunological function,[66] and interference with bilirubin binding sites and photometric measurement of bilirubin[67,68] are becoming more numerous in the literature. Particularly in view of the concerns regarding adverse pulmonary effects, many nurseries only use minimal amounts of lipid when infants have pulmonary disease. When lipid is administered, frequent laboratory monitoring of serum triglycerides is essential; the concentration should be kept below 150 mg/dL.

Protein needs are met by providing 2.0–3.5 g/kg/day through administration of a crystalline amino acid solution. Although commercial amino acid solutions developed for use in adults are most frequently used in neonatal intensive care units, pediatric formulations have been developed. The pediatric solutions provide a different amino acid content that allows the treated infants' plasma aminograms to appear similar to those of breastfed infants. The clinical benefit of these solutions in regard to protein status is still under investigation.

Electrolytes must be added to the parenteral fluid in amounts sufficient to maintain serum concentrations. With current formulations, it is difficult, but possible, to provide calcium and phosphorus in amounts large enough theoretically to prevent osteopenia. Precipitation may be reduced at low temperatures and low pH and in the presence of high amino acid and glucose concentrations. The calcium:phosphorus ratio in solution may also affect its solubility.[69] Amino acid solutions specifically designed for infants allow a lower pH through the addition of cysteine hydrochloride. This lower pH maximizes mineral stability, but the net retention of calcium and phosphorus may still be lower than the intrauterine accretion rate.[70] Under investigation are alternatives to the conventional calcium and phosphorus salts, which may allow greater concentrations to remain in solution.[71] Frequent monitoring of serum phosphorus and alkaline phosphatase concentrations and estimates of renal tubular reabsorption of phosphorus are helpful in following disease progression. Once enteral feeding can begin, oral supplements that provide a total intake of 220–250 mg calcium/kg/day and 110–125 mg phosphorus/kg/day may be given in cases of documented osteopenia.[72]

Vitamin and trace element requirements of premature infants during parenteral nutrition have been reviewed extensively by the Subcommittee on Pediatric Parenteral Nutrient Requirements of the Committee on Clinical Practice Issues of the American Society for Clinical Nutrition.[73] This subcommittee has published two sets of guidelines for vitamin dosage (Table 3–7). The first set is based on the amounts of vitamins provided when 40% of the MVI-Pediatric® (Armour) formulation per kilogram body weight per day is infused. This amount of the formulation does not maintain blood levels of all vitamins within an acceptable range, yet, it is the only pediatric parenteral vitamin formulation currently available in the United States. The second set of guidelines illustrate the best estimate for a new vitamin formulation. Provision of the trace elements—copper, selenium, chromium, manganese, and molybdenum—through the parenteral infusate is generally not required unless parenteral fluids is the sole source of nutrition for more than 4 weeks. When parenteral nutrition is only supplemental or is limited to less than 4 weeks, only zinc need be added.[73] Recommended intakes of the trace elements are summarized in Table 3–8.

Complications of parenteral nutrition are numerous and range from metabolic problems to sepsis and include problems stemming from catheter insertion and maintenance. Frequent laboratory monitoring to avoid metabolic complications and ensure nutritional intake is recommended highly. An oral stimulation program is needed if the infant is not feeding by mouth.

Follow-up

Continuing nutritional care

Slow growth and behavioral eating problems are common nutrition-related concerns in premature infants dismissed from the neonatal nursery. Preliminary data suggest a relationship between protein intake in the neonatal period and behavioral outcome at the end of the feeding period in the absence of differences in gross markers of protein nutritional status.[74] Before discharge, most infants are consuming all nutrients orally and are thriving on 20 kcal/oz formula or breast milk fed every 3 to 4 hours or "on demand." A caretaker demonstration session on feeding practice and on infant stimulation is essential.[75] Posthospitalization follow-up care in which nutrition recommendations are provided to the primary health provider is necessary to ensure that the intake is appropriate nutritionally and developmentally and that it is meeting the infant's needs for growth. Premature AGA infants generally follow the growth patterns of term AGA infants, when growth is plotted by corrected age rather than chronological age.[76,77] (Corrected age is postnatal age less the number of weeks the infant was premature; see Chapter 4, Table 4–18.) Correction for prematurity is only used when plotting growth on standard curves developed from the postnatal growth patterns of term infants. The use of corrected age is recommended during the first 1.5 years for measurements of heal circumference, 2 years for weight, and 3.5 years for stature; after these periods, the difference in curves plotted by corrected and chronological ages is no longer significant.[76] Other growth curves developed by following the postnatal growth of premature infants may also be used for posthospitalization assessment of growth (see Chapter 12) until the infant surpasses the last age on the chart.

Growth delay appears to be related to gestational age, with a large proportion of ELBW infants exhibiting stunting

Table 3–7. Suggested Intakes of Parenteral Vitamins in Premature Infants

Vitamin	Term Infants (dose/day)	Premature Infants (dose/kg Body Weight/day) (dose not to exceed term infant dose)	
		Current Guidelines*	Best Estimate for New Formulation
A, μg	700	280	500
E, mg	7	2.8	2.8
K, μg	200	80	80
D, IU	400	160	160
Ascorbic acid, mg	80	32	25
Thiamin, mg	1.2	0.48	0.35
Riboflavin, mg	1.4	0.56	0.15
Pyridoxine, mg	1.0	0.4	0.18
Niacin, mg	17	6.8	6.8
Pantothenate, mg	5	2	2
Biotin, μg	20	8	6
Folate, μg	140	56	56
Vitamin B_{12}, μg	1.0	0.4	0.3

*Provision of 40% of the MVI-Pediatric® formulation per kg body weight. Adapted from Greene et al.[73]

Table 3-8. Suggested Daily Intake of Trace Elements During Parenteral Nutrition

Nutrient	Intake (μg/kg)
Zinc	400
Copper	20
Chromium	0.2
Manganese	1.0
Selenium	2.0
Molybdenum	0.25

Adapted from Greene et al.[73]

Table 3-9. Percentage of Former Premature Infants with Anthropometric Measurements Falling Under the Third Percentile at Ages One and Two Years (Corrected Age).

	ELBW Infants	VLBW Infants
Weight		
1 year	66.7	25.7
2 years	37.1	17.8
Length		
1 year	32.5	11.6
2 years	20.0	7.8
Head circumference		
1 year	14.6	1.4
2 years	7.5	2.8

Adapted from Brothwood et al.[4]

and low weight for length at age 2 years. Table 3-9 depicts the percentage of children with anthropometric measurements under the third percentile (after correction for prematurity) at ages 1 and 2 years. Infants of ELBW are at a significant disadvantage relative to those of VLBW, but the difference lessens as age increases.[4] Unfortunately, in the majority of studies, nutritional intake before or after hospitalization is not described in relation to the growth data. In two studies that attempted to discern the nature of growth delay in infants with bronchopulmonary dysplasia, decreased nutritional intake in VLBW infants was not related to slow postnatal growth.[78,79] With bronchopulmonary dysplasia, the effect of gastrointestinal, pulmonary, renal, and neurological dysfunction, as well as of activity level, diet, and cultural practices, on growth must be evaluated continually. The role of antioxidants in bronchopulmonary dysplasia is being investigated.[80]

In contrast, there has been concern regarding reports of increased fat deposition in premature infants and the effect that it may have on future adiposity and predisposition to chronic diseases associated with obesity. Fat accretion occurs in premature infants at a faster rate than seen in utero, but this postnatal fat accretion appears to be similar to the changes occurring in a term infant during the first 4 months of life.[81,82] A study documenting postnatal growth of premature infants shows that by 6 months premature infants have a body mass index (BMI) 103% of standard; thereafter, BMI drops to 94% of standard at 36 months.[83] Therefore, it appears that premature infants exhibit a normal pattern of development of adipose tissue.

References

1. National Center for Health Statistics. Advance report of final natality statistics, 1985. *Monthly Vital Stat. Rep.* 1987;36(suppl).
2. Hewitt, B.G., Newnham, J.P. A review of the obstetric and medical complications leading to the delivery of infants of very low birthweight. *Med. J. Aust.* 1988;149:234.
3. Heinonen, K., Hakulinen, A., Jokela, V. Survival of the smallest. Time trend and determinants of mortality in a very preterm population during the 1980's. *Lancet.* 1988;2:204.
4. Brothwood, M., Wolke, D., Gamsu, H., Cooper, D. Mortality morbidity, growth, and development of babies weighing 501–1000 grams and 1001–1500 grams at birth. *Acta Paediatr. Scand.* 1988;77:10.
5. Skouteli, H.H., Dubowitz, L.M., Levene, M.I., Miller, G. Predictors for survival and normal developmental outcome of infants weighing less than 1001 grams at birth. *Dev. Med. Child. Neurol.* 1985;24:588.
6. Whitsett, J.A., Hull, W.M., Luse, S. Failure to detect surfactant protein-specific antibodies in sera of premature infants treated with Survanta, a modified bovine surfactant. *Pediatrics* 1991;87:505.
7. Stern, L. Early postnatal growth of low birthweight infants: what is optimal? *Acta Paediatr. Scand.* 1982;296(suppl):6.
8. American Academy of Pediatrics Committee on Nutrition. Nutritional needs of low-birth-weight infants. *Pediatrics.* 1977;60:519.
9. Mauer, M.A., Dweck, H.S., Finberg, L., Holmes, F. Reynolds, J.W., Suskind, R.M., Woodruff, C.W., Hellerstein, S. American Academy of Pediatrics Committee on Nutrition: Nutritional needs of low-birth-weight infants. *Pediatrics* 1985;75:976.
10. Lorenz, J.M., Kleinman, L.I., Kotagal, U.R., Reller, M.D. Water balance in very low-birth-weight infants: relationship to water and sodium intake and effect on outcome. *J. Pediatr.* 1982;101:423.
11. Brosius, K.K., Ritter, D.A., Kenny, J.D. Postnatal growth curve of the infant with extreme low birth weight who was fed enterally. *Pediatrics.* 1984;74:778.
12. Pereira, G.R., Barbosa, N.M.M. Controversies in neonatal nutrition. *Pediatr. Clin. North Am.* 1986;33:65.
13. Sher, P.K., Brown, S.B. A longitudinal study of head growth in preterm infants. II. Differentiation between "catch-up" head growth and early infantile hydrocephalus. *Dev. Med. Child. Neurol.* 1975;17:711.
14. Cartlidge, P.H.T., Rutter, N. Serum albumin concentrations and oedema in the newborn. *Arch. Dis. Child.* 1986;61:657.
15. Watkinson, M., Miller, P.W. Serum albumin concentrations and oedema in the newborn. *Arch. Dis. Child.* 1986;61:1244.
16. Zlotkin, S.H., Casselman, C.W. Percentile estimates of reference values for total protein and albumin in sera of premature infants (<37 weeks of gestation). *Clin. Chem.* 1987;33:411.
17. Shulman, R.J., DeStefano-Laine, L., Petitt, R., Rahman, S., Reed, T. Protein deficiency in premature infants receiving parenteral nutrition. *Am. J. Clin. Nutr.* 1986;44:610.
18. Moskowitz, S.R., Pereira, G., Spitzer, A. Prealbumin as a biochemical marker of nutritional adequacy in premature infants. *J. Pediatr.* 1983;102:749.
19. Currao, W.J., Cox, C. Shapiro, D.L. Diluted formula for beginning the feeding of premature infants. *Am. J. Dis. Child.* 1988;142:730.
20. Siegel, M., Lebenthal, E., Krantz, B. Effect of caloric density of gastric emptying in premature infants. *J. Pediatr.* 1984;104:118.
21. Rickard, K., Gresham, E.L. Nutritional considerations for the newborn requiring intensive care. *J. Am. Diet. Assoc.* 1975;66:592.
22. Ernst, J.A., Williams, J.M., Glick, M.R., Lemons, J.A. Osmolality of substances used in the intensive care nursery. *Pediatrics.* 1983;72:347.
23. Atkinson, S.A., Shah, J.K., McGee, C., Steele, B.T. Mineral excretion in premature infants receiving various diuretic therapies. *J. Pediatr.* 1988;113:540.
24. Myers, W.F., Herbst, J.J. Effectiveness of positioning therapy for gastroesophageal reflux. *Pediatrics.* 1982;69:768.

25. Beganovic, N., Verloove-Vanhorick, S.P., Brand, R., Ruys, J.H. Total parenteral nutrition and sepsis. *Arch. Dis. Child.* 1988;63:66.

26. Lebenthal, E., Leung, Y.K. Feeding the premature and compromised infant: gastrointestinal considerations. *Pediatr. Clin. North Am.* 1988;35:215.

27. Heldt, G.P. The effect of gavage feeding on the mechanics of the lung, chest wall, and diaphragm of preterm infants. *Pediatr. Res.* 1988;24:55.

28. Roy, R.N., Pollnitz, R.P., Hamilton, J.R., Chance, G.W. Impaired assimilation of nasojejunal feeds in healthy low-birth-weight newborn infants. *J. Pediatr.* 1977;90:431.

29. Bernbaum, J.C., Pereira, G.R., Watkins, J.B., Peckham, G.J. Nonnutritive sucking during gavage feeding enhances growth and maturation in premature infants. *Pediatrics.* 1983;71:41.

30. Field, T., Ignatoff, E., Stringer, S. Nonnutritive sucking during tubefeedings: effects on preterm neonates in an intensive care unit. *Pediatrics.* 1982;70:381.

31. Woodson, R., Hamilton, C. The effect of nonnutritive sucking on heart rate in preterm infants. *Dev. Psychobiol.* 1988;2:207.

32. Daniels, H., Devlieger, H., Casaer, D. Nutritive and nonnutritive sucking in preterm infants. *J. Dev. Physiol.* 1986;8:117.

33. Meier, P., Anderson, G.C. Responses of small preterm infants to bottle- and breast-feeding. *Matern. Child. Nurs.* 1987;12:97.

34. Nash, M.A. Nutrition, body fluids, and acid-base homeostasis. Part two. Provision of water and electrolytes. In: Fanaroff, A.A., Martin, R.J., eds. *Neonatal-Perinatal Medicine: Diseases of the Fetus and Infant.* 4th ed., St. Louis: CV Mosby Co; 1987.

35. Reichman, B.L., Chessex, P., Putet, G., Verellan, G.J.E., Smith, J.M., Heim, T., Swyer, P.R. Partition of energy metabolism and energy cost of growth in the very-low-birth-weight infant. *Pediatrics.* 1982;69:446.

36. Sauer, P.J.J., Dane, H.J., Visser, H.K.A. Longitudinal studies on metabolic rate, heat loss, and energy cost of growth in low-birth-weight infants. *Pediatr. Res.* 1984;18:254.

37. Catzeflis, C., Schutz, Y., Mitcheli, J.L., Welsch, C., Arnaud, M.J., Jequier, E. Whole body protein synthesis and energy expenditure in very low birth weight infants. *Pediatr. Res.* 1985;19:679.

38. Maisels, M.J., Marks, K.H. Growth chart for sick premature infants. *J. Pediatr.* 1981;98:663.

39. Georgieff, M.K., Hoffman, J.S., Pereira, G.R., Bernbaum, J., Hoffman-Williamson, M. Effect of neonatal caloric deprivation on head growth and 1-year developmental status in preterm infants. *J. Pediatr.* 1985;107:581.

40. Raiha, N.C.R., Heinonen, K., Rassin, D.K., Gaull, G.E. Milk protein quantity and quality in low-birthweight infants. I. Metabolic responses and effects on growth. *Pediatrics.* 1976;57:659.

41. Tsang, R.C., ed. *Vitamin and Mineral Requirements in Preterm Infants.* New York: Marcel Dekker; 1985.

42. Tyson, J.E., Lasky, R.E., Mize, C.E. Growth, metabolic response and development in very-low-birth-weight infants fed banked human milk or enriched formula. I. Neonatal findings. *J. Pediatr.* 1983;103:95.

43. Gross, S.J. Growth and biochemical response of preterm infants fed human milk or modified infant formula. *N. Engl. J. Med.* 1983;308:237.

44. Davies, D.P. Adequacy of expressed breast milk for early growth of preterm infants. *Arch. Dis. Child.* 1977;52:296.

45. Anderson, G.H. Human milk feeding. *Pediatr. Clin. North Am.* 1985;32:335.

46. Lucas, A., Morley, R., Cole, T.J., Gore, S.M., Davis, J.A., Bamford, M.F.M., Dossetor, J.F.B. Early diet in preterm babies and developmental status in infancy. *Arch. Dis. Child.* 1989;64:1570.

47. Mendelson, R.A., Bryan, M.H., Anderson, G.H. Trace mineral balance in preterm infants fed their own mother's milk. *J. Pediatr. Gastroenterol. Nutr.* 1983;2:256.

48. Svenningsen, N.W., Lindroth, M., Lindquist, B. A comparative study of varying protein intake in low birth weight infant feeding. *Acta Paediatr. Scand.* 1982;296(suppl):28.

49. Lewis, M.A., Smith, B.A.M. High volume milk feeds for preterm infants. *Arch. Dis. Child.* 1984;59:779.

50. Chan, G., Mileur, L.J. Post hospitalization growth and bone mineral status of normal preterm infants. *Am. J. Dis. Child.* 1985;139:896.

51. Abrams, S.A., Schanler, R.J., Garza, C. Bone mineralization in former very low birth weight infants fed either human milk or commercial formula. *J. Pediatr.* 1988;112:956.

52. Greer, F.R., McCormick, A. Improved bone mineralization and growth in premature infants fed fortified own mother's milk. *J. Pediatr.* 1988;112:961.

53. Bhatia, J., Rassin, D.K. Human milk supplementation. *Am. J. Dis. Child.* 1988;142:445.

54. Schanler, R.J., Garza, C., Nichols, B.L. Fortified mother's milk for very low birth weight infants: results of growth and nutrient balance studies. *J. Pediatr.* 1985;107:437.

55. Dallman, P.R. Iron deficiency in the weanling: a nutritional problem on the way to resolution. *Acta Paediatr. Scand.* 1986;323(suppl):59.

56. Gross, S.J., Gabriel, E. Vitamin E status in preterm infants fed human milk or infant formula. *J. Pediatr.* 1985;106:635.

57. Farrell, P.M., Zachman, R.D., Gutcher, G.R. Fat-soluble vitamins A, E, and K in the premature infant. In: Tsang, R.C., ed., *Vitamin and Mineral Requirements in Preterm Infants.* New York: Marcel Dekker; 1985.

58. Greer, F.R., Tsang, R.C. Calcium, phosphorus, magnesium, and vitamin D requirements for the preterm infant. In: Tsang, R.C., ed. *Vitamin and Mineral Requirements in Preterm Infants.* New York: Marcel Dekker; 1985.

59. Heird, W.C., Hay, W., Helms, R.A., Storm, M.C., Kashyap, S., Dell, R.B. Pediatric parenteral amino acid mixture in low birth weight infants. *Pediatrics.* 1988;81:41.

60. Zlotkin, S.H., Bryan, M.H., Anderson, G.H. Intravenous nitrogen and energy intakes required to duplicate in utero nitrogen accretion in prematurely born human infants. *J. Pediatr.* 1981;99:115.

61. Duffy, B., Gunn, T., Collinge, J., Pencharz, P. The effect of varying protein quality and energy intake on the nitrogen metabolism of parenterally fed very low birthweight (<1600 g) infants. *Pediatr. Res.* 1981;15:1040.

62. Dweck, H.S., Cassady, G. Glucose intolerance in infants of very low birth weight. I. Incidence of hyperglycemia in infants of birth weight, 1,110 grams or less. *Pediatrics.* 1974;53:189.

63. American Academy of Pediatrics. Use of intravenous fat emulsions in pediatrics. *Pediatrics.* 1981;68:738.

64. Cooke, R.J., Yeh, Y.Y., Gibson, D., Debo, D., Bell, G.L. Soybean oil emulsion administration during parenteral nutrition in the preterm infant: effect on essential fatty acid, lipid and glucose metabolism. *J. Pediatr.* 1987;111:767.

65. Dahms, B.B., Halpin, T.C., Jr. Pulmonary arterial lipid deposit on newborn infants receiving intravenous lipid infusion. *J. Pediatr.* 1980; 97:800.

66. Fischer, G.W., Wilson, S.R., Hunter, K.W., Mease, A.D. Diminished bacterial defenses with Intralipid. *Lancet.* 1980;2:819.

67. Burkhart, G.J., Whitington, P.F., Helms, R.A. The effect of two intravenous fat emulsions and their components on bilirubin binding to albumin. *Am. J. Clin. Nutr.* 1982;36:521.

68. Shennan, A.T., Cherian, A.G., Angel, A. Bryan, M.H. The effect of Intralipid on the estimation of serum bilirubin in the newborn infant. *J. Pediatr.* 1976;88:285.

69. Eggert, L.D., Rusho, W.J., MacKay, M.W., Chan, G.M. Calcium and phosphorus compatibility in parenteral nutrition solutions for neonates. *Am. J. Hosp. Pharm.* 1982;39:49.

70. Koo, W.W.K., Hollis, B.W., Horn, J., Steiner, P., Tsang, R.C., Steichen, J.J. Stability of vitamin D_2, calcium, magnesium, and phosphorus in parenteral nutrition solution: effect of in-line filter. *J. Pediatr.* 1986;108:478.

71. Whyte, R.K., Yuen, D.E., Draper, H.H. A soluble source of calcium and phosphate improves bone mineralization in piglets fed by total parenteral nutrition. *Pediatr. Res.* 1984;18:355A.

72. Shenai, J.P., Jhaveri, B.M., Reynolds, J.W., Huston, R.K., Babson, S.R. Nutritional balance studies in very low birth weight infants: role of soy formulas. *Pediatrics.* 1981;66:631.

73. Greene, H.L., Hambidge, K.M., Schanler, R., Tsang, R.C. Guidelines for the use of vitamins, trace elements, calcium, magnesium, and phosphorus in infants and children receiving total parenteral nutrition: report of the Subcommittee on Pe-

diatric Parenteral Nutrient Requirements from the Committee
on Clinical Practice Issues of the American Society for Clinical
Nutrition. *Am. J. Clin. Nutr.* 1988;48:1324.

74. Bhatia, J., Rassin, D., Cerreto, M., Bee, D. Effect of protein/
energy ratio on growth and behavior of premature infants:
Preliminary findings. *J. Pediatr.* 1991;119:103.

75. Lester, B., Tronick, E. Stimulation and the preterm infant:
the limits of plasticity. *Clin. Perinatol.* 1990;17:1.

76. Brandt, I. Growth dynamics of low-birth-weight infants with
emphasis on the perinatal period. In Falkner, F., Tanner, J.M.,
Eds. *Human Growth. vol. 2: Postnatal Growth.* New York:
Plenum Press; 1978.

77. Karniski, W., Blair, C., Vitucci, J.S. The illusion of catch-up
growth in premature infants. *Am. J. Dis. Child.* 1987;141:520.

78. Greer, F.A., McCormick, A. Bone mineral content and growth
in very-low-birth-weight premature infants: does bronchopulmonary dysplasia make a difference? *Am. J. Dis. Child.*
1987;141:179.

79. Sarue, R.S., Singhal, N. Long-term morbidity of infants with
bronchopulmonary dysplasia. *Pediatrics.* 1985;76:725.

80. Falciglia, H., Jinn-Pease, M., Falciglia, G., Lubin, H., Frank,
D., Chang, W. The role of vitamin E and selenium in the
development of bronchopulmonary dysplasia. *J. Pediatr. Perinatal. Nutr.* 1988;2:35.

81. Reichman, B., Chessex, P. Putet, G., Verellen, G., Smith,
J.M., Heim, T., Swyer, P.R. Diet, fat accretion, and growth
in premature infants. *N. Engl. J. Med.* 1981;305:1495.

82. Foman, S.J. Body composition of the male reference infant
during the first year of life. *Pediatrics.* 1967;40:863.

83. deGamarra, M.E., Schutz, Y., Catzeflis, C., Freymond, D.,
Calame, A., Micheli, J.L., Jequier, E. Composition of weight
gain during the neonatal period and longitudinal growth follow-
up in premature babies. *Int. J. Vit. Nutr. Res.* 1987;57:339.

Chapter 4
Nutritional Assessment and Early Intervention

Shirley Walberg Ekvall

Nutritional assessment, an essential task of the nutritionist and dietitian, is an important disease prevention measure that has been shown to reduce health care costs. Meyer,[1] in one of the early position papers of the American Dietetic Association on health care delivery, stated, "In terms of money as in terms of human suffering—one can well argue that every dollar spent on nutrition instruction may save tens of dollars in later medical care." Kennedy[2] reported that participation of prenatal patients in the USDA Special Supplemental Food Program for Women, Infants, and Children (WIC), which includes nutrition education, showed a positive effect on pregnancy outcome: A 107 gram increase in mean birth weight and a 4% decrease in the incidence of low birth weight. High-risk teenage, black and Hispanic women gained even stronger benefits, particularly when they were followed for two trimesters. In another study, malnourished patients were hospitalized 2 days longer than nonmalnourished patients, resulting in an additional cost of $2750 per patient. The malnourished surgical patients required an additional 5 days of hospitalization, with an additional cost of $5575 per patient.[3] Nutrition support teams helped reduce the incidence of malnutrition. However, only one-fifth of the patients received home counseling or other form of posthospitalization follow-up care.[4] Butterworth and Blackburn found that protein-calorie malnutrition affected one-fourth to one-half of medical and surgical patients whose hospitalization extended 2 weeks or longer.[5] Likewise, one-third of the patients showed hypoalbuminemia in laboratory tests.[5]

Nutritional status evaluation has five steps.

1. screening and/or referral
2. nutritional assessment
3. interpretation of assessment
4. intervention or treatment plan
5. follow-up plan

There are three different levels of nutritional assessment: an *in-depth assessment* performed as part of a complete physical examination; a *midlevel assessment* performed in a specialty clinic, such as a myelomeningocele, cerebral palsy, or high-risk infant clinic; and a *mini-assessment* performed in the community (Table 4–1). The choice of assessment depends on the expertise and amount of time available, the age of the child, and the problem. This chapter focuses primarily on the in-depth assessment.

In Depth Nutritional Assessment

Physical exam

The five key elements of any nutritional assessment are dietary and physical activity, biochemistry, anthropometry,

physical signs, and feeding (Table 4–1). A problem noted in the assessment of dietary intake will show up physiologically in the biochemical assessment, later in the anthropometry, and finally in the physical signs. (Clinically, anthropometry and physical signs are assessed before the biochemical assessment is performed.) Thus, the problem should be corrected at the dietary stage—the first level of assessment.

Malnutrition

Economically, socially, and educationally deprived populations are at nutritional risk for *primary malnutrition*, which occurs when there are inadequacies and imbalances in the quantity or quality of foods consumed. There are three states of primary malnutrition which are described below, with their International Classification Disease (IDC) codes[6]:

- *A visceral attrition state of kwashiorkor-like syndrome* (ICD 267): The patient may appear well nourished, but has depressed serum levels of albumin, transferrin, and other circulating proteins. Anthropometric measurements are maintained, but cellular immunity is comprised. The patient requires protein. Protein-sparing regimens are recommended along with the provision of more than adequate calories, fluid, electrolytes, and vitamins and minerals.
- *Marasmus-like syndrome* (ICD 268): The patient is visibly underweight with depleted muscle and fat stores. Serum proteins are maintained until late in the course. The patient requires high-calorie, high-protein foods that are generally augmented by oral supplements.
- *Acute state combining both kwashiorkor and marasmus* (ICD 269.9): This syndrome is often caused by severe trauma and stress in mildly undernourished individuals. The patient exhibits the signs of both visceral attrition and cachexia and requires vigorous nutritional support, oral feedings of high nutrient and caloric density, and, if indicated, peripheral or total parenteral nutrition.

In the human brain, early malnutrition in the cerebellum causes a reduction in the number of cells in the cerebrum and brainstem; the largest reduction is in the cerebrum.[7] Postnatal cell division also appears to occur most rapidly in the cerebrum;[7] In a study of malnutrition in an underdeveloped country, Chase and Martin[8] followed 19 children who were hospitalized for malnutrition in the first year of life for 4 years after rehabilitation. Only 10% achieved normal intelligence; 52% were educable, 33% were trainable, and 5% were institutionalized. In the United States, more subtle changes in development, such as delays in language or cognitive development, may be related to malnutrition, especially if it occurred before 6 months of age.[9]

Table 4–1. Guidelines for Nutritional Status Assessment

Dietary Assessment (Minimal)	Biochemical Assessment (Minimal)	Anthropometric Assessment (Minimal)	Physical or Clinical Signs (Minimal)	Feeding and Behavioral Assessment (Minimal)
Feeding history questionnaire Twenty-four hour recall Food frequency recall	Hemoglobin or CBC Hematocrit Routine urinalysis	Head circumference Weight 　–Beam Scale Height 　–Recumbent 　–Standing 　–Upper and lower ratio (if needed)	Medical and dental records Clinical signs of malnutrition Skin Lips–tongue–gums Teeth Eyes	Parental perception Professional perception
(Midlevel) Minimal	**(Midlevel)** Minimal	**(Midlevel)** Minimal plus	**(Midlevel)** Minimal plus	**(Midlevel)** Minimal plus
Parental knowledge: Nutrition-drug interaction Basic nutrition Fiber and fluid Caloric expenditure		Plot growth curve Special growth grids	Physical limitations score Allergies Infections	Gross motor Fine motor Reinforcers
(In-Depth) Midlevel plus	**(In-Depth)** Midlevel plus	**(In-Depth)** Midlevel plus	**(In-Depth)** Midlevel plus	**(In-Depth)** Midlevel plus
Three day diet diary Quantitative Supplements Special diet Physical activity record Caloric expenditure Mobility	Transferrin saturation Total serum protein and albumin Fasting glucose Serum urea nitrogen Quantitative urinary plasma amino acid screen Organic acids **(Special Conditions)**	Skinfold or fatfold 　–Triceps 　–Subscapular 　–Abdominal (obese) Arm circumference Waist circumference (obese) Bone age or density (as needed)	Clinical signs of malnutrition Hair Posture Abdomen Skeletal development General appearance– behavior, speech Prenatal history–maternal weight gain and diet Postnatal history of chronic illness or disease Blood pressure	Physical A. Oral reflexes (suck, swallow, chew) B. Neuromuscular development (fine and gross motor) Behavioral A. Parent-child interaction B. Reinforcers C. Environmental influences
	Anticonvulsant:　Folic acid and vitamin C 　　　　　　　　Vitamin D and calcium 　　　　　　　　Alkaline phosphates 　　　　　　　　Pyridoxine Prader Willi:　Glucose Tolerance Test Pica:　Lead, hemoglobin			

Adapted from Smith, M.A., ed. *Guides for Nutritional Assessment of the Mentally Retarded and Developmentally Disabled.* Memphis, TN: The Child Development Center for Health Services, 1976.

Secondary malnutrition is produced by disease and disability, such as fever, cardiovascular disease, diabetes mellitus, cystic fibrosis, and cerebral palsy. Some disease-related problems are malabsorption, anorexia, hypermetabolic and metabolic dysfunction, organ failure, and treatment-induced causes.[4] These and other conditions affecting nutritional status are shown in Table 4–2 and Appendix 8–12.

Obesity also may be a form of malnutrition—both primary and secondary—particularly with children who are immobile. Obesity is a pathological condition in which there is an accumulation of fat in excess of what is needed for body functioning (see Chapter 19)

For both primary and secondary malnutrition, the grade of malnutrition may be evaluated according to Waterlow's classification[10] (Table 4–3.)

An initial nutritional medical screening for clients at risk of malnutrition (Table 4–4) is often obtained before referral

is made for an in-depth nutritional assessment. Table 4–5 shows referral criteria of a specialty clinic and a hospital. Health care providers should be well informed about these criteria so they can make appropriate referrals for the in-depth assessment.

Dietary Physical Activity Assessment

In this part of the assessment, information on both the developmental and current dietary history is obtained (Appendix 4). Dietary intake is calculated, and conditioning factors, such as problems of malabsorption and medication, are evaluated (Table 4–2). For the child with a handicap or chronic illness, it is particularly important to know what is actually being consumed as a large amount of the food may be spilled. Socioeconomic information is also reviewed in the dietary assessment.

Table 4–2. Conditions That Affect Nutritional Status

Condition	Increased Nutrient Needs
Infections	Vit A, Vit C, Fe, N, calories, H_2O, Na, K
Drugs	Vit C, N, Na, K, B_{12}, folic acid
Emotion	Iodine, Vit C and B complex, Ca, N
Malnutrition	Vit C, Vit A, N, Chol, K, P
Obesity	Calories, macro- and micronutrients
Immobilization	Ca, Na, K, N, H_2O
Malabsorption	Vit C, B complex, A, D, E, B_{12}, fat, calories, H_2O, N, Ca, P, Na, K
Physical activity	Vit C, B complex, N
Pregnancy and Lactation	Ca, N, Fe, folic acid
Surgery	Vit C, B_{12}, K, N, H_2O
Burns or injury	Vit C, B complex, K, N,
Environment (heat)	Ca, Cu, Mn, P, K, Fe, N, Na

From Ekvall, S. UACCDD, and Bozian, R. College of Medicine, University of Cincinnati, Cincinnati, OH. Used with permission.

Three methods for collecting dietary data are available:

1. food list—quantity of food eaten over time
2. food record—inventory of food on hand at the beginning and end of a study or plate waste record
3. family food account—description of food purchased

The food list method that is used most frequently is a 1-, 3- or 7-day dietary list or diary (see UACCDD Nutrition Record for a 3-day food list in Appendix 4). Food lists are useful in obtaining presumptive evidence of dietary inadequacies, not the absolute values consumed. In general, a deficiency in one nutrient is a good indicator of other nutritional problems.

Dietary history

The dietary history is based on the 24-hour recall of foods eaten and the food summary, which is a frequency cross-check of the 24-hour recall (see Appendix 4–1). The food summary is evaluated according to a 15-point system. Points are subtracted for the intake of large quantities of sugar, salt, soft drinks, sweet desserts, and foods high in saturated fat and cholesterol; they are subtracted as well if the diet contains inadequate amounts of fiber and water. If the child scores below a 10, the parent is given a 3-day dietary intake list or diary to complete (Appendix 4),[11] and a follow-up visit with the family is usually planned. The nutrient content of the 3-day diet diary is then analyzed by computer or manually according to food composition tables that are based

Table 4–3. Assessment of Malnutrition: Waterlow Classification

Grade of Malnutrition	Weight/Height % of Standard	Height/Age % of Standard
0	>90	>95
1	81–90	90–95
2	70–80	85–89
3	<70	<85

From Waterlow,[10] with permission.

on the 1989 recommended dietary allowances (U.S. RDA Appendix 1–1). The controversial Recommended Dietary Intakes (Appendix 1–3) proposed by the Food and Drug Administration, mainly for labeling purposes, uses an average value for nutrients (lower than the U.S. RDA's) rather than separate values for sex and age. The Canadian Recommended Nutrient Intakes are listed in Appendix 1–4 and include polyunsaturated fatty acid recommended values. The Canadian nutrient values generally are lower than the U.S. RDA's (more like the WHO values); however the Japanese RDA's are even higher than those of the U.S. At UACCDD, 56 nutrients are calculated from the 3-day diet diary and 24-hour recall (Table 4–6). For children 1–10 kg, fluid requirements are 100 mL/kg; for those 10–20 kg, 1000 mL plus 50 mL/kg for each kilogram over 10 kg; and for those over 20 kg, 1500 mL plus 20 mL/kg for each kilogram over 20 kg.[12,13] By body surface area, daily fluid needs are 1500–1800 mL/m^2.[14,15]

Food intake patterns as based on the Basic Four Food Group are shown in Table 4–7. Other classifications, such as the Basic Five Food Groups with a separate fruit and vegetable group and more whole grains (particularly increasing the antioxidants, Vitamin A, C, E and selenium) is shown in Appendix 4–1. The Eating Right Pyramid for food groups accepted by the U.S. Department of Agriculture (similar to the Australian Pyramid) increases grains, fruits and vegetables (Appendix 4–1). The recommended method for the gradual introduction of solid foods is shown in Table 4–8.

Physical activity assessment

Information about the physical activity of the child is obtained either from the 24-hour recall of physical activity or the 3-day diet/activity diary (Appendix 4). It is necessary to evaluate the child's level of physical activity to determine his or her caloric and muscle mass needs. Caregivers also need to understand that the child's caloric requirements vary according to the level of activity (Quality Assurance Standards, Appendix 7).

Both the 1989 RDA[16] and the *Surgeon General's Report on Nutrition and Health*[17] cite the benefits of increased physical activity. To condition the cardiovascular system, one should engage in 20-minute periods of exercise for at least three times per week in which one's target heart rate is attained. The target heart rate (THR) for an individual in good physical condition is determined by subtracting age from 220 and then multiplying that figure by 70% or 85% (85% for those in excellent health). Swimming and fast walking are two excellent forms of aerobic exercise that involve large muscle groups and that children with special health needs can engage in to attain their THR. Other aerobic exercises are bicycling, aerobic dancing, rowing, hiking, skating, skiing, and jogging. Anaerobic exercises include sprinting, weightlifting, and calisthenics.

Parents of children with developmental disorders (DD) and chronic illnesses have developed innovative exercise games and equipment to meet their special needs, such as a body-sized skateboard that is moved by the arms. The benefits of increasing lean body mass through physical activity and thus increasing the caloric requirements for over-

Table 4–4. Initial Nutritional Screening Data

The presence of one or more of the following conditions should alert the health care professional that the patient has the potential of developing malnutrition or has had a condition in the past requiring

General

Does the patient have any conditions that cause nutrient loss, such as malabsorption syndromes, draining abscesses, wounds, fistulas, or protracted diarrhea?

Does the patient have any conditions that increase the need for nutrients, such as fever, burn, injury, sepsis, or antineoplastic therapies?

Has the patient been NPO for 3 days or more?

Is the patient receiving a modified diet or diet restricted in one or more nutrients?

Is the patient being enterally or parenterally fed?

Does the patient describe food allergies, lactose intolerance, or limited food preferences?

Has the patient experienced recent unexplained weight loss?

Gastrointestinal (GI)

Does the patient complain of nausea, indigestion, vomiting, diarrhea, or constipation?

Does the patient exhibit glossitis, stomatitis or esophagitis?

Does the patient have difficulty chewing or swallowing?

Does the patient have a partial or total GI obstruction?

What is the patient's state of dentition?

Cardiovascular

Does the patient have ascites or edema?

special nutritional care. Incorporation of the following questions and observations into a routine history and physical can facilitate identification of patients who are at risk for malnutrition.

Is the patient able to perform activities of daily living?

Does the patient have congestive heart failure?

Genitourinary

Does fluid input approximately equal fluid output?

Does the patient have an ostomy?

Is the patient hemodialyzed or peritoneally dialyzed?

Respiratory

Is the patient receiving mechanical ventilatory support?

Is the patient receiving oxygen via nasal prongs?

Does the patient have chronic obstructive pulmonary disease?

Skin

Does the patient describe nail or hair changes?

Does the patient have rashes or dermatitis?

Does the patient have dry or pale mucous membranes or decreased skin turgor?

Does the patient have pressure areas on the sacrum, hips, or ankles?

Extremities

Does the patient have pedal edema?

Does the patient exhibit cachexia?

Modified from *Nutritional Assessment: What is it? How is it used?* Columbus, OH: Ross Laboratories; G593 1988. Used with permission.

weight children with DD need further investigation. When calculating caloric needs of children with myelomeningocele, Down syndrome, cerebral palsy, and other disorders, one must remember to subtract the weight of limbs lost from amputation or atrophy (Fig. 4–1).

Energy expenditure

The *basal metabolic rate (BMR)*, also termed the resting metabolic rate (RMR), is measured in a postabsorptive state and at complete rest in a thermoneutral environment, which is an artificial condition. In practice, therefore, BMR is only reflective of a resting state and has been termed the *resting energy expenditure (REE)*. These terms are interchangeable.

The REE is the largest component of total energy expenditure (TEE) and is the preferred measure of energy needs unless the physical activity level is unusually high or if heavy work is performed at high (37°C) or low (below 14°C) temperatures.[16] REE correlates well with lean body mass (LBM) and differs from the BMR by less than 10%.

Methods for calculating REE are described in Table 4–9 and the energy expenditures of various activities are shown in Table 4–10. The thermic effect of food varies with its content and is only 5% to 10% of the energy ingested.

Differences in LBM account for about 80% of the variability when measuring the REE of individuals of similar sex, height, weight, and age.[16] Body composition changes at different ages and is also affected by disease; these changes in turn markedly affect energy needs. The LBM of infants (1.7–2.0 × REE) is higher than for adults (1.45–1.50 × REE).[16] Metabolic rates of organs and tissues vary with age, affecting the REE. For example, the brain is most active for the neonate, and the liver and muscle are most active for the adult. Except during the first year of life, growth is a very small component of energy needs (about 1%).[16] Sex differences in body composition are small until children reach adolescence, when young men have greater LBM and young women have greater fat.

Energy needs may be determined by actual weight or median weight according to sex, age, and height. Median heights and weights and recommended energy intake by age

Table 4–5. Referral Nutrition Criteria for an In-Depth Assessment

Specialty Clinic*

Under 3 years of age
Height or weight below the 10th or above the 75th percentile or a large discrepancy in weight for height
Mechanical feeding problems
Conditions such as allergies, chronic diarrhea, excessive use of vitamins, food faddism
Family income less than $25,808 for four people
Mother younger than age 20 at time of child's birth
Postmenarcheal adolescent girl

Hospital†

Height less than 85% of standard (stunted)
Weight/height less than 90% of standard (underweight) or greater than 120% of standard (obese)
Weight loss greater than or equal to 5% of usual body weight
Serum albumin less than 3 g/dL (infants less than 2.5 g/dL)
Lymphocyte count less than 1500 cells
Sustained fever, major organ failure, etc.
Nothing passed orally for at least 2 days without parenteral nutrition
On clear full-liquid diet for at least 2 days
Referred by other disciplines

*From the University Affiliated Cincinnati Center for Development Disorders.
†Modified from Queen & Gallagher.[21]

Table 4–6. Nutrients Used in Analysis of a Dietary History

Kilocalories	Tyrosine	Niacin	Magnesium
Carbohydrate	Histidine	Vitamin B6	Iron
Sugar	Trytophan	Folacin	Zinc
Fiber in diet	Fat	Vitamin B12	Iodine
Fiber–crude	Saturated fat	Biotin	Selenium
Protein	Poly fat	Pantothenic acid	Copper
Threonine	Cholesterol	Vitamin A	Manganese
Leucine	Lineoleic FA	Vitamin D	Fluoride
Methionine	Oleic FA	Vitamin E–total	Chromium
Phenylalanine	Mono fat	Vitamin E–AT	Molybdenum
Valine	Vitamin K	Calcium	Ash
Isoleucine	Vitamin C	Phosphorus	Alcohol
Lysine	Thiamin	Sodium	Caffeine
Cystine	Riboflavin	Potassium	Water

FA = fatty acid; AT = alpha tocophenol
Used at the University Affiliated Cincinnati Center for Developmental Disorders, Cincinnati, OH.

using multiples of the REE values are shown in Appendix 1. The weight of undernourished or obese individuals should be adjusted to the normal height and weight (Appendix 4). People with large body frames require more energy per unit of time than those with small frames. Yet, when individuals of the same weight vary in height and thus in body mass index, height or stature variations have little effect on energy needs, except for the elderly. Weight is thus the influencing factor in BMR, RMR, and REE. However, a predictive equation to calculate REE using LBM and creatinine showed more significance than one based on weight or height in children on total parenteral nutrition (see Chapter 3).

Appendix 1 shows caloric requirements based on energy needs. Pregnant and lactating women need additional ca-lories. For children under age 10, caloric needs are based on normal growth patterns; over age 10, the caloric needs of boys and girls differ. Appendix 1–2 uses the World Health Organization's energy allowances.

Physical activity is the second largest component of total energy expenditure (TEE). For sedentary people, increasing physical activity during their leisure time is essential to increase their LBM and ultimately their nutrient needs. The activity factors for a range of typical daily activities are found in Table 4–11. The activity factor is then multiplied by the REE to determine energy needs. The total energy factor for the digestion of food is small but may require an additional 7% for TEE in research versus clinical situations.

Another method of assessing energy needs is based on the *basal energy expenditure* (*BEE*), or basal energy requirements, which is the measure of energy needs when at complete rest. BEE does not include activity level, stress factors, temperature, specific dynamic action of food, or other conditioning factors. It can be estimated three ways.

1. Multiply the metabolic rate (kcal/hr) by 24 (see Chapter 19).[17]
2. For children weighing more than 15 kg and measuring greater than 85 cm in height and who are near ideal body weight (IBW), use the Mayo Clinic nomogram (Chapter 19) to determine surface area. Then use this equation:
   (m) × (kcal/m/hr × 24 hr/day = kcal/day)
3. For persons 18 years and older who are close to IBW, use the Harris-Benedict equations:
   BEE (men) = 66 + (13.75 × W) + (5.0 × H) − (6.8 × A)
   BEE (women) = 655 + (9.6 × W) + (1.70 × H) − (4.7 × A)
   where W = weight in kilograms (use IBW unless 30–40 lb under IBW, then use usual body weight; use actual weight unless 100% above IBW, then use IBW + 20% difference between actual and IBW), H = height in centimeters, and A = age in years.

However, a revised Harris-Benedict equation[18] is needed for the malnourished person due to increased resting oxygen consumption as follows:

Females

REE = 447.593 + 3.098 S + 9.247 W − 4.330 A

Males

REE = 88.362 + 4.799 S + 13.397 W − 5.677 A

Total energy expenditure (TEE) can be determined several ways, depending on the problem, age of the client, and expertise available. The most exact methods, described in Chapter 19 on obesity, are a doubly labeled water method[19] of indirect calorimetry and K_{40} in the whole body counter.[20] These methods were evaluated for developmental disorders as well. The doubly labeled water method combined with heart-rate monitoring also is being investigated in England and Ireland.[21] A less precise method is to multiply BEE by activity, stress, and fever factors (Table 4–12). The energy needs of those requiring parenteral and enteral feeding are shown in Tables 4–13 and 4–14.

Several procedures can be used to determine caloric needs based on energy expenditure. This following method is used by McCardle et al.[22]

1. BMR cal/24 hr × surface area.
2. BMR × 5 physical activity (sedentary 20%, light 30%, moderate 40%, and very active 50%) = physical activity calories.
3. BMR cal + physical activity cal × 10% = food digestion calories.

Table 4–7. Food Intake Patterns for Optimal Nutrition at Different Age Levels

Food Group*	Servings/day	Average size servings									
		0–2 months	3–4 months	5–7 months	8–12 months	1 year	2–3 years	4–5 years	6–9 years	10–12 years	13–16 years
Milk and Cheese	4										
1.5 oz Cheese = 1 C milk (or 8 oz)	**	~ 1 C** formula with iron	~ 1-1/4 C** formula with iron	~ 1 C** formula with iron	3/4 C formula with iron	3/4 C Whole Milk	1/2 C	1/2 C	3/4 C–1 C	1 C	1 C
Meat Group	2										
Lean meat, fish		–	–	–	1 T egg yolk	1 egg	1 egg	1 egg	1 egg	1 egg	
egg, poultry		–	–	1 T	3 T	3 T	3–4 T	4 T	4–6 T	6–8 T	8 T or more
Peanut butter		–	–	–	–	–	1 T	2 T	2–3 T	3 T	3 T
Dried beans, peas		–	–	–	–	1/4 C	1/4 C	1/2 C	1/2 C	3/4 C	3/4 C
Fruits and Vegetables	4† include:										
Vitamin C source (citrus fruits, berries, tomato, cabbage, cantaloupe)	1	–	–	1/4 C	1/4 C	1/2 C	1/2 C	1/2 C	1/2 C or 1 medium orange	1/2 C or 1 medium orange	1/2 C or 1 medium orange
Vitamin A source (green or yellow fruits and vegetables)	1	–	–	1 T	2 T	2 T	3 T	4 T	4 T	1/3 C	1/2 C
Other fruits and vegetables	2	–	–	1 T	2 T	2 T	3 T	4 T	4 T	1/3 C	1/2 C
Bread or Grains†	4										
Bread		–	–	–	1/2 sl	1/2 sl	1 sl	1–1 1/2 sl	1–2 sl	2 sl	2 sl
Cooked cereal		–	–	1 T	2 T	1/4 C	1/3 C	1/2 C	1/2 C	3/4 C	1 C or more
Dry cereal		–	–	–	–	6 T	1/2 C	3/4 C	3/4 C	1 C	1 C or more
Macaroni, spaghetti, rice		–	–	–	–	1/4 C	1/3 C	1/2 C	1/2 C	3/4 C	1 C or more

*Fats added only if needed to meet caloric needs after 1 year of age.
*Adapted by Marjorie Michell and Shirley Ekvall from: Bennet, M.J., and Hansen, A.J. *Four Groups of the Daily Food Guide.* Washington, DC: Institute of Home Economics, USDA publication no. 30.
**Breastfeeding or quantity of formula according to physician prescription.
†Add more if needed for calories or other nutrients (particularly antioxidants).

4. BMR cal + physical activity cal + food digestion cal = total energy needs.

A quick method to determine the caloric needs of adults, which can be useful in a mini-assessment, is adapted from the American Diabetes Association's *Guide for Professionals: The Effective Application of Exchange Lists for Meal Planning.*[23]

1. Determine the build according to this formula:

$$\frac{Ht\ (cm)}{Wrist\ (cm)}$$

Measure the wrist from the styloid process, which is above the radius (outer bone of forearm, thumb side) to the ulna (large inner bone of forearm, opposite thumb side. Determining the frame size by elbow breadth may be even more accurate (Appendix 10).

	Men	Women
Small build	10.4	11.1
Medium build	9.6–10.4	10.1–11.0
Large build	9.6	10.1

2. Calculate desirable body weight.

	Men	Women
Medium build	Allow 106 lb for first 5 ft of height, plus 6 lb for each additional inch	Allow 100 lb for first 5 ft of height, plus 5 lb for each additional inch
Small build	Subtract 10%	Subtract 10%
Large build	Add 10%	Add 10%

3. Determine caloric needs based on activity level. Basal level equals desirable body weight (DBW) in pounds × 10.
   Sedentary = DBW × 3
   Moderate = DBW × 5
   Strenuous = DBW × 10
4. Add calories for indicated weight gain, growth (pregnant women), and lactation.
   Pregnancy—add 300 cal/day to gain 22–27 lb in 9 months
   Lactation—add 500 cal/day
   To gain 1 lb/wk, add 500 cal/day
5. Subtract calories for indicated weight loss.
   To lose 1 lb/wk, subtract 500 cal/day

Another simple method of determining caloric needs is based on weight and activity level–sedentary, moderate,

Table 4–8. Introduction of Solids

Steps to Table Texture	Age	Food Types	Table Texture
Avoid items with added sugar and salt; encourage high-iron foods	5–6 mo.	Enriched cereal; strained fruits, juices, vegetables, and meats	Strained
Use teething biscuit; cooked or canned fruits and vegetables	6–7 mo.	By 7 months, cooked or canned fruits and vegetables, ripe banana	Mashed* (strained to Junior texture)
Begin finger foods	7–9 mo.	By 9 months, enriched bread, toast, potato, rice, macaroni	Minced fine (including meats)
Use varied finger foods	9–12 mo.	By 12 months, whole-grain bread, cereal breadsticks, crackers, hard cheese, whole egg, pieces of fruit and vegetables, whole milk	Chopped
Begin raw fruits and vegetables	12–15 mo.		Cut table food

*This is an important step—when increase in texture is delayed beyond this time, infant may resist change.
Adapted from Fomon, S.J., et al. Recommendations for feeding normal infants. *Pediatrics* 1979;63:52. Used with permission.

and active. For an overweight individual the range is from 20–30 cal/kg; for one of normal weight, 30–40 cal/kg; and for an underweight individual, 30–50 cal/kg.[24]

Biochemical Assessment

Biochemical or laboratory tests provide the most precise or quantitative method of evaluating nutritional status. Bio-chemical data are used to detect marginal deficiencies before any overt clinical or physical signs appear or to corroborate questionable dietary histories. The laboratory test is the most expensive method of evaluation, and the interpretation of the data is sometimes difficult since it may not correlate with dietary or other assessment parameters.

The intake of large quantities of some nutrients, such as fat, or an imbalance of nutrients can produce biochemical abnormalities.[25] Likewise a deficiency of one nutrient may

The following information may be used to estimate body weights for patients with amputations. For limbs, the averages for left and right are given.

Body Part	% Desirable Body Weight	Example (kg)
Entire body	100	55.70
Head and neck	7	3.93
Trunk without limbs	43	23.80
Entire upper extremity	6.5	3.62
Upper arm	3.5	1.98
Forearm without hand	2	1.27
Hand	1	0.47
Entire lower extremity	18.5	10.38
Thigh	11.5	6.45
Leg, without foot and thigh	5	2.94
Foot	2	1.00

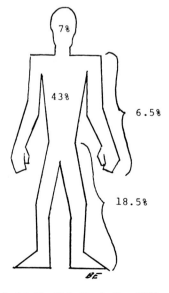

Fig. 4–1. Segmental weights for limbs. Modified from Brunnstrom, S. *Clinical Kinesiology.* Philadelphia: F.A. Davis Co.; 1972.

Table 4–9. Equations for Predicting Basal Metabolic Rate from Body Weight in Kilograms

Age Range (yr)	Kcal_th/Day	Correlation Coefficient	SD*	MJ/Day	Correlation Coefficient	SD*
Males						
0–3	60.9 W − 54	0.97	53	0.255 W − 0.226	0.97	0.222
3–10	22.7 W + 495	0.86	62	0.0949 W + 2.07	0.86	0.259
10–18	17.5 W + 651	0.90	100	0.0732 W + 2.72	0.90	0.418
18–30	15.3 W + 679	0.65	151	0.0640 W + 2.84	0.65	0.632
30–60	11.6 W + 879	0.60	164	0.0485 W + 3.67	0.60	0.686
>60	13.5 W + 487	0.79	148	0.0565 W + 2.04	0.79	0.619
Females						
0–3	61.0 W − 51	0.97	61	0.255 W − 0.214	0.97	0.255
3–10	22.5 W + 499	0.85	63	0.0941 W + 2.09	0.85	0.264
10–18	12.2 W + 746	0.75	117	0.0510 W + 3.12	0.75	0.489
18–30	14.7 W + 496	0.72	121	0.0615 W + 2.08	0.72	0.506
30–60	8.7 W + 829	0.70	108	0.0364 W + 3.47	0.70	0.452
>60	10.5 W + 596	0.74	108	0.0439 W + 2.49	0.74	0.452

*Standard deviation of differences between actual BMRs and predicted estimates.
From WHO (World Health Organization). *Energy and Protein Requirements. Report of a Joint FAO/WHO/UNU Expert Consultation.* Technical Report Series 724. Geneva: World Health Organization; 1985. Used with permission.

indicate other nutrient abnormalities. A nutrient deficiency may be caused not only by decreased intake but also by these *inhibiting factors: interference with ingestion, absorption, storage, or utilization; excessive excretion or loss; increased requirements for the nutrient; or the presence of analogs.* Progressive depletion of a nutrient results in these sequential changes in nutritional status: *lowered plasma concentration; lowered intercellular fluid concentration; lowered concentrations of red and white blood cells; lowered intra-cellular concentration; biochemical and physiological abnormalities in pyruvate, kynurenic acid, phosphatase, p-hydroxyphenyl acids, electrocardiogram, electroencephalogram, and dark adaptation; morphological change; and ultimately death of the cell.*

According to Steinbaugh and Sauls,[26] the four most important biochemical measures in nutritional assessment are urinary excretion of nitrogen and creatinine, serum protein level, skin testing of cellular immunity, and determination

Table 4–10. Approximate Energy Expenditure for Various Activities in Relation to Resting Needs for Men and Women of Average Size*

Activity Category†	Representative Value for Activity Factor per Unit Time of Activity
Resting	REE × 1.0
Sleeping, reclining	
Very light	REE × 1.5
Seated and standing activities, painting trades, driving, laboratory work, typing, sewing, ironing, cooking, playing cards, playing a musical instrument	
Light	REE × 2.5
Walking on a level surface at 2.5 to 3 mph, garage work, electrical trades, carpentry, restaurant trades, housecleaning, child care, golf, sailing, table tennis	
Moderate	REE × 5.0
Walking 3.5 to 4 mph, weeding and hoeing, carrying a load, cycling, skiing, tennis, dancing	
Heavy	REE × 7.0
Walking with load uphill, tree felling, heavy manual digging, basketball, climbing, football, soccer	

*Based on values reported by Durnin, J.V.G.A. *Energy requirements of pregnancy. An integration of the longitudinal data from the 5-country study.* Nestle Foundation Annual Report. Lausanne, Switzerland: Nestle Foundation; 1986 and WHO (World Health Organization). *Energy and Protein Requirements. Report of a Joint FAO/WHO/UNU Expert Consultation.* Technical Report Series 724. Geneva: World Health Organization; 1985.
†When repeated as multiples of basal needs, the expenditures of men and women are similar.
From National Research Council[16] with permission.

Table 4–11. Factors for Estimating Daily Energy Allowances at Various Levels of Physical Activity for Men and Women (Ages 19 to 50)

Level of Activity	Activity factor* (× REE)	Energy Expenditure† (kcal/kg per day)
Very light		
Men	1.3	31
Women	1.3	30
Light		
Men	1.6	38
Women	1.5	35
Moderate		
Men	1.7	41
Women	1.6	37
Heavy		
Men	2.1	50
Women	1.9	44
Exceptional		
Men	2.4	58
Women	2.2	51

*Based on examples presented by World Health Organization: *Energy and Protein Requirements. Report of a Joint FAO/WHO/UNU Expert Consultation*. Technical Report Series 724. Geneva: World Health Organization; 1985.
†REE was computed from formulas in Table 4–9 and is the average of values for median weights of persons ages 19 to 24 and 25 to 74 years: men 24.0 kcal/kg; women 23.2 kcal/kg.
From National Research Council[16] with permission.

Table 4–12. Factors Used in the Calculation of Total Energy Expenditure

Activity factors	
Bedridden	1.20
Ambulatory	1.30
Fever factors	
Per degree Fahrenheit deviation from	1.07
Injury factors	
Starvation	0.70
Minor surgery	1.00–1.20
Peritonitis	1.20–1.50
Soft tissue trauma	1.14–1.37
Skeletal trauma	1.35
Major sepsis	1.40–1.60
Thermal injury	2.00

From Long, C., Schaffel, N., Geiger, J., Schiller, W., Blackmore, W. Response to injury and illness: estimation of energy and protein needs from indirect colorimetric and nitrogen balance. *J.P.E.N.* 1979; 3:452. Used with permission.

of percent of lymphocytes. The choice of laboratory tests depends on the expertise required, cost of the tests, and the child's problem. Laboratory equipment is required for calorimetry, fluorometry, spectrophotometry, chromatography, and microbiological assay. Tests for various nutrients, their methods, and acceptable values are given in Table 4–15 and Appendix 8. Stages of depletion of iron and nitrogen can be seen in Appendix 8–12.

Parental and/or the child's consent is required to perform biochemical tests for research studies. To minimize the trauma and cost of repeated tests, one should always consult the child's chart to see if a recent blood chemistry value is available.

Creatinine

Somatic proteins are found in skeletal muscle, whereas visceral proteins are found in other body compartments (Table 4–16). The urinary excretion of creatinine correlates well with the status of skeletal muscle. However, it is difficult to collect a 24-hour urine sample from children, which is needed to calculate the creatinine height index (CHI)

$$CHI = \frac{measured\ urinary\ creatinine}{ideal\ urinary\ creatinine} \times 100$$

where ideal creatinine excretion is ideal body weight (IBW) × 23 mg for men and 18 mg for women. Moderate depletion is 60% to 80% of that level, and severe depletion is less than 60%.

Serum Protein Level

Albumin is a better measure of protein nutrition than the globulins as it has a shorter biologic half-life.[27,28] The visceral proteins in the liver, such as retinol-binding protein, prealbumin, and transferrin, have even shorter half-lives than albumin and thus are even more sensitive in detecting early nutritional changes. However, the serum transferrin assay is not routinely available in clinical laboratories.[25] Transferrin can be calculated from total iron-binding capacity (TIBC) using the equation, calculated transferrin = (0.68 × TIBC) + 21.[29] Ranges of serum transferrin and serum albumin levels give some indication of malnutrition severity[24] (Table 4–17).

Estimates of daily amino acid requirements are provided in Table 4–18.

Immune Competence

Immunological abnormalities, such as a reduction in lymphocyte count or changes in lymphocyte response to in vitro stimulation by phylohemogglutinins, are indicators of poor nutritional status. The *total lymphocyte count*, an indication of immune reserves, is calculated according to this equation:

$$\frac{\%\ lymphocyles \times WBC}{100}$$

where WBC = white blood cell count. Mild depletion is indicated by *1200–2000/mm³*, moderate by *800–1199/mm³*, and *severe* by less than *800/mm³*.

Cell-mediated immunity is determined by intradermal testing with such antigens as streptokinase, streptodornase, *Candida* and *Trichophyton* species, mumps, and the purified protein derivative of tuberculin. Intact immunity is indicated by one or more positive responses—a wheal measuring at least 5 mm × 5 mm. Anergy, a diminished reactivity to specific antigens, is frequently associated with increased sepsis and mortality rates.

Nutrients important in maintaining immunocompetence include nucleotides (mainly found in meat, poultry, fish, eggs, milk, nuts, legumes); a balance of omega 6 acid or linoleic acid (vegetable seed oils, meat, and milk), omega 3 fatty acids (fish oils, canola, walnut or soybean oils, plant leaves); zinc (meat, eggs, milk, poultry, whole grain, oysters); iron (liver, beef, poultry, eggs, raisins); and vitamin A (leafy green or dark yellow vegetables, liver, cheese). However, some of these nutrients—iron, zinc, fat, omega

Table 4–13. Energy Needs of Nutritional Therapy

Energy requirements	Kilocalories required/24 hr	
Parenteral anabolic therapy	$1.75 \times$ BEE	
Oral anabolic therapy	$1.50 \times$ BEE	
Oral maintenance therapy	$1.20 \times$ BEE	
Prescriptions for anabolism*	Protein (g/day)	Calories (kcal/day)
Oral protein-sparing therapy	$1.5 \times$ weight†	
Total parenteral nutrition	$(1.2$ to $1.5) \times$ weight†	$40 \times$ weight†
Oral hyperalimentation	$(1.2$ to $1.5) \times$ weight†	$35 \times$ weight†

*Levels of protein intake are to be adjusted according to blood urea nitrogen values and nitrogen balance.
†Weight = actual weight in kilograms.
From Blackburn, G.L., Bistrian, B.R., Maini, B.S., et al. Nutritional and metabolic assessment of the hospitalized patient. *J.P.E.N.* 1977;1:17. Used with permission.

6 fatty acids, and linoleic acid—can suppress immunity when administered in high amounts.[30]

A prognostic score index with four parameters, developed by Mullen et al., provides a quantitative estimate of risk for anergy, sepsis, and death.

$$PNI = 158\% - (16.6 \times ALB) + (0.78 \times TSF)$$
$$+ (0.2 \times TFN) + (5.8 \times DH)$$

where ALB = serum albumin concentration, g/dL; TSF = triceps skinfold, mm; TFN = transferrin, g/dL; DH = delayed hypersensitivity in interdermal cellular immunity testing—grade of reactivity to any of three antigens (*Candida*, mumps, or streptokinase/streptodornase): Nonreactive = 0 induration, 1 = <5 mm induration, and 2 = >5 mm induration

The higher the percentage, the greater the mortality rate. For example,

$$ALB = 3.0 \text{ g/dl} \times 16.6 = 49.8$$
$$TSF = 10.1 \text{ mm} \times 0.78 = 7.9$$
$$TFN = 155 \text{ g/dl} \times 0.2 = 31.0$$
$$DH = 1 \times 5.8 = 5.8$$
$$94.5$$
$$PNI = 158\% - 94.5 = 63.5\%$$

The 63.5% risk of anergy, sepsis, or death is high in this malnourished person: less than 30% indicates mild risk; 30% to 59%, moderate risk; and over 60%, high risk.

Bone mineralization

For the child under age 10 who is immobile, on anticonvulsants, or is growth retarded, a bone mineralization measurement using the left forearm is useful in determining the loss of minerals. The photon absorption method using a bone mineral analyzer is preferred.[32–40]

- The Cameron method[33] using direct in vivo photon absorptiometry should be used for measurement of bone mineral content (BMC). Precision and accuracy are 4% to 7% and 2%, respectively (greater than in other radiographic or photodensitometric techniques). Older methods had error rates as large as 20% or 30%. Methods used to diagnose early rickets include radiographs of the wrist, which show changes of cupping, fraying, and widening of the metaphysis at the distal end of the ulna or increasing space between the proximal metacarpal bones or the epiphysis and metaphysis caused by lack of mineralization of osteoid.
- Cameron's photon source is a well-collimated 27.3 Kay I source. The transmitted monochromatic photons are detected by a well-collimated scintillation detector. Transmission through the bone is a function of mineral content. The source and detector move simultaneously across the bone at the rate of 1 mm/sec.
- The BMC is proportional to the area under the curve.[30] The absorbance of the gamma ray is measured by comparing soft tissue to bone. Bone width (BW) is also measured by this method. BMC and BW are expressed in g/cm of longitudinal bone section. Even in cadaver soft tissue-covered bone, the BMC is measured accurately. Bone mass by the Cameron method[33] correlated at 0.96 with actual bone weight. The weight of standard sections of excised bone and total ulna weight correlated very highly with Cameron's method using scans of excised bone sections and at one site of the human ulna.[35,36] Scans on different

Table 4–14. Nutritional Needs of Children (Birth to Age 15) on Enteral Feeding

Energy needs	Protein needs (g/Kg)	
Basal = $(55 - 2 \times$ age$) \times$ kg	0–6 mo	2.2
Maintenance = $20\% \times$ basal	6 mo–1 yr	1.6
Growth = $50\% \times$ basal	1–3 yr	1.2
*Activity = $0 - 25\% \times$ basal	4–6 yr	1.1
Sepsis $- 13\%/1$ degree C $\times$ basal	7–14 yr	1.0
Simple trauma = $20\% \times$ basal		
Multiple injuries = $40\% \times$ basal		
Burns = $50 - 100\% \times$ basal		

*50% $\times$ basal in very active children.
Adapted from Seashore, J. Nutrition support of children. *Yale J. Biol. Med.* 1984;51:111.

Table 4-15. Biochemical Chart

Test	Specimen (Method)*	Normal Range or Mean Value Children†	Amount of Specimen‡ (mL)
Hemoglobin	Whole blood (cyanmethemoglobin)	12.5 g/dL (100 mL)	0.1
Hematocrit	Whole blood (micro centrifuge)	35–37%	0.1
Iron	Serum (chromogenic complex)	50–60 mcg/dL	2.0
Transferrin saturation	Serum (Fe saturation)	≥ 20%	2.0
Copper	Serum (chromogenic complex, atomic absorption)	70–140 mcg/dL	3.0
Magnesium	Serum (chromogenic complex, atomic absorption)	1.5–2.1 mEq/L	3.0
Zinc	Serum (atomic absorption)	80–120 mcg/dL	2.0
Calcium	Serum (chromogenic complex, atomic absorption)	9–10 mg/dL	0.5
Phosphorus	Serum (chromogenic complex)	3.5–5.5 mg/dL	0.5
Vitamin A	Serum (chromogenic complex, fluorometric)	30–65 mcg/dL	2.0
Carotene	Serum (optical density)	80–200 mcg/dL	1.0
Vitamin D	Serum (25-OH-C-cholecalciferol)	15–40 ng/mL	5.0
Ascorbic acid	Plasma (chromogenic complex, fluorometric)	0.5–1.5 mg/dL	1.0
Folic acid	Serum, erythrocytes (radio-immuno-assay (RIA) microbiological)	5–6 ng/mL	1.0
Vitamin B_{12}	Serum (RIA microbiological)	200–1000 pg/mL	1.0
Vitamin B_6	Erythrocytes (SGOT-SGPT index)	1.5	1.0
Pyridoxic acid	Urine (chromogenic complex)	≥ 0.8 mg/24 hr	5.0
Thiamine	Erythrocytes, serum, urine (transketolase, TPP effect, fluorometric)	0–14% TPP effect	2.0
Riboflavin	Erythrocytes, serum, urine (glutathione reductase fluorometric)	activation coefficient <1.20	2.0
Protein (total)	Serum (chromogenic complex, Biuret)	6–8 g/dL	0.2
Albumin	Serum (chromogenic complex, B.C. green)	3.5–5.0 g/dL	0.2
BUN	Serum (chromogenic complex, enzymatic)	10–20 mg/dL	0.5
Glucose	Serum (chromogenic, enzymatic)	70–90 mg/dL	0.5
Essential amino acids	Serum (amino acid analyzer)	Varies for amino acid (Table 4-16)	0.5–5.0
Alkaline phosphatase	Serum (chromogenic, enzymatic)	Infants, 100–150 mU/mL Children, 50–125 mU/mL	0.1

*Use of serum or plasma is adequate in most cases; however, the type of specimen is determined by the analytical method. Determinations of micronutrients in serum, plasma, or urine can be used to establish correlations among themselves and other metabolites and functional tests, i.e., TPP activation, to assist in the biochemical evaluation.
†Variability of values dependent on age. Values indicated are guidelines for the interpretation of results.
‡Volume of specimen is determined by the analytical method.
Modified from H. V. Nino, Ph.D., Christ Hospital, Cincinnati, OH, 1978

Table 4-16. Body Compartments and Common Methods of Assessment

Body Compartments	Assessed By	Interpretation Affected By
Adipose	Skinfold measurements, body weight.	Presence of clothing and dressings, technician error, patient age, hydration status, frame size.
Skeletal muscle— somatic proteins	Body weight, arm muscle circumference, Creatinine Height Index (CHI).	Same as above. Plus, completeness of sample collection, stress, injury, patient age, body build, renal function.
Visceral proteins	Serum albumin, serum transferrin.	Nephrotic syndrome, albumin infusion, stress, injury, blood products, patient hydration status, liver function.
Plasma proteins Extracellular Skeleton		

From *Nutritional Assessment: What Is It? How Is It Used?* Columbus, OH: Ross Laboratories; 1988.

Table 4-17. Visceral Proteins and Immune Competence Useful in Nutritional Assessment of Malnutrition

A			Malnutrition Values		
Protein	Half-Life	Normal	Mild	Moderate	Severe
Albumin	21 days	3.5–5.5 g/dL	3.0–3.5 g/dL	2.1–3.0 g/dL	<2.1 g/dL
Transferrin	10 days	200–400 mg/dL	150–175 mg/dL	100–150 mg/dL	<100 mg/dL
Thyroxine-binding protein	2 days	15.7–29.6 mg/dL			
Retinol-binding protein	12 hours	2.6–7.6 mg/dL			
Somatomedin C	2 hours	0.4–2 U/mL			
B					
Total lymphocyte count (% lymphocyte × *WBC*)*			1200–2000/m²	800–1199/m³	<800/m³

Cell-mediated immunity (immune function):
antigen analysis, including streptolinase,
streptodornase, *Candida* spp., mumps and PPD.*

*WBC = white blood count; PPD = purified protein derivative of tuberculin.
Modified from Long, C.R. Historic review of nutritional assessment techniques in applying new technology to nutritional assessment. *Report of the Ninth Ross Roundtable on Medical Issues*. Columbus, OH: Ross Laboratories, 1989. Used with permission.

Table 4-18. Estimates of Daily Amino Acid Requirements

	Requirements, by age group			
Amino acid	Infants 3–4 mo*	Children under 2 yr†	Children 10–12 yr‡	Adults§
	(mg/kg/day)			
Histidine	28	?	?	8-12
Isoleucine	70	31	28	10
Leucine	161	73	42	14
Lysine	103	64	44	12
Methionine plus cystine	58	27	22	13
Phenylalinine plus tyrosine	125	69	22	14
Threonine	87	37	28	7
Tryptophan	17	12.5	3.3	3.5
Valine	93	38	25	10
Total without histidine	714	352	214	84

*Based on amounts of amino acids in human milk or cow's milk formulas fed at levels that supported good growth. Data from Formon, S.J., Filer, L.J., Jr. Amino acid requirements for normal growth. In: Nyhan, W.L., ed. *Amino Acid Metabolism and Genetic Variation*. New York: McGraw-Hill; 1967.
†Based on achievement of nitrogen balance sufficient to support adequate lean tissue gain (16 mg N/kg per day). Data from Pineda, O., Torun, B., Viteri, F.E., Arroyave, G. Protein quality in relation to estimates of essential amino acids requirements. In: Bodwell, C.E., Adkins, J.S. Hopkins, D.T., eds. *Protein Quality in Humans: Assessment and In Vitro Estimation*. Westport, CT: AVI Publishing; 1981.
‡Based on upper range of requirement for positive nitrogen balance. Recalculated by Williams, H.H., Harper, A.E., Hegsted, D.M., Arroyave, G., Holt, I.E., Jr. Nitrogen and amino acid requirements. In: Food and Nutrition Board. *Improvement of Protein Nutriture. Report of the Committee on Amino Acids*. Washington, DC: National Academy of Sciences; 1974.
§Based on highest estimate of requirement to achieve nitrogen balance. Data from several investigators (reviewed by) FAO/WHO (Food and Agriculture Organization/World Health Organization). *Energy and Protein Requirements. Report of a Joint FAO/WHO Ad Hoc Expert Committee*. Technical Report Series No. 552; FAO Nutrition Meetings Report Series 52. Rome: World Health Organization; 1973.
From National Research Council[16] with permission.

bones (ulna, radius, femur) are highly intercorrelated (r = 0.80 to 0.90), correlated with weights of other bone (r = 0.90), and also with the weight of the total skeleton (r = 0.90).[37-39]

- The maximum exposure per photon absorption scan is about 0.08 rem limited to a small area of the forearm, and the maximal dose per child is about 0.32 rem (four scans per examination of 0.08 rem per scan) compared with the maximal allowable dose to forearms of children of 7.5 rem per year.[40]

Anthropometry Assessment

The Health and Nutrition Examination Survey (HANES II) provides the basis for anthropometric measurements. HANES was conducted by the National Center for Health Statistics according to a multistage stratified probability design.[41] Bishop et al[41] reviewed the accumulated data and developed age- and sex-specific percentile distributions for the various anthropometric measurements.

HANES III will be completed in 1994 with a portion of the data released in 1992. The survey includes: dietary interviews, body measurements, hematological tests, biochemical analysis of whole blood and serum, oral glucose tolerance tests, blood pressures, electrocardiograms, urine tests, bone densities, and dental examinations on 40,000 noninstitutionalized civilians 2 months of age and older.[42]

The measurements of most significance in children and adolescents include the following[43]:

- height (recumbent length if less than 2 years of age and under 1 meter in length; otherwise, stature/standing or upper and lower body ratio
- weight
- head circumference (up to 6 years of age)
- triceps (subscapular, thorax, and other) skinfolds or fatfolds
- arm circumference (after infancy)
- chest circumference (in infancy to age 5, particularly in underdeveloped countries)
- upper and lower arm length (atrophy of lower extremities)
- arm span (atrophy of lower extremities)
- other circumferential measurements
- bone or skeletal age.

To ensure accuracy, measurements should be recorded directly on the appropriate forms.

Bone or skeletal age

The anthropometry assessment for three different levels (minimal, mid-level, and in-depth) are shown in Table 1. Height and weight values for males and females ages 1 month to 18 years are shown in Appendix 3. Median heights and weights by age can be seen in Appendix 1 and weights for heights of adults in Appendix 10. Standing height using a flexible steel tape attached to the wall or door frame and a triangular block of wood with a leveler or an accurate measuring rod attached to birch wood (Figures 2 and 3) should be used only if the child is older than two years of age and is capable of standing as follows:

Height

Heights and weights of both biological or adoptive parents and siblings should be documented to determine the relationship of growth to the child's genetic potential and to identify growth retardation caused by nutritional and other factors. The impact of nutrition on anthropometric measures is illustrated in an interesting study of parent-child pairs. In that study, Garn[44] found the dimensions of adoptive parents and children to be similar. They were genetically unrelated, but after living together they began to resemble each other in growth and stature, fatness, and even urinary analysis and serum vitamin levels.

Height, weight, and head circumference should be plotted on standard growth grids developed from the HANES data to determine the child's height for age, weight for age, and weight for height ratios (Fig 4–2; Appendix 3). A deviation of 15% or one standard deviation above or below the mean is abnormal. Special grids have been developed for children with Down's syndrome, myelomeningocele, Prader-Willi syndrome, and sickle cell anemia (Appendix 3). The height:weight ratio should be used for children with other special health care needs.

At birth, length is related to maternal height, but by age 2, length correlates best with mean parental height. A 1-month-old infant gains 30 mm/day and grows 1.5 mm/day. A 3-year-old gains 5 g/day and grows 0.2 mm/day. Table 4–19 shows normal growth and development, and Table 4–20 can be used to adjust the infant's length in relation to parental stature.

Height or Stature and Length. (*Measure twice without shoes to nearest 0.5 cm*).

Standing

- Equipment: Dermographic pencil, flexible or plastic coated tape, a leveler, clipboard or block.
- Procedure: Height is measured by using a flexible steel or plastic measuring tape attached to wall or door frame.

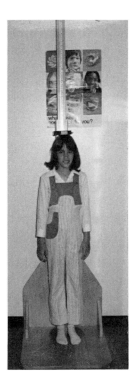

Fig. 4–2. Measuring stature. From the UACCDD Nutrition Department, Cincinnati, OH, with permission.

Table 4–19. Normal Growth and Development

Weight			
Birth weight		7.7 lb	(3.5 kg)
Six months	Doubles	15.4 lb	(7.0 kg)
One year	Triples	23.1 lb	(10.5 kg)
Two years	Quadruples	28.0 lb	(13.0 kg)
Two years to adolescence	about 5.0 lb/yr		
Adolescence	about 10.0 lb per year		
Length			
Birth length		19.5 in	(50.0 cm)
One year		30.0 in	(74.0 cm)
Four years	Doubles	41.0 in	(100.0 cm)
Thirteen years	Triples (girls)	60.0 in	(150.0 cm)
Thirteen years and greater—	Rapid linear growth (boys)		

From UACCDD Nutrition Department (extrapolated from HANES Growth Grids, Appendix 3).

- The child stands against the tape or stadiometer with shoes removed. Heels, lower back, and shoulders should be touching the wall or door frame.
- A block of wood or clipboard should be lowered to make firm contact with the child's scalp (Fig. 4–3).

Variability in measurements should be within *0.5 cm or repeated two times again in all stature and length measurements.* Otherwise, recumbent length using a standard headboard should be used:

Recumbent

- Equipment: A rigid measuring board or headboard and two people.
- Procedure: If the child is less than 2 years of age or under 1 meter in length, recumbent height should be taken using a headboard. Measurers should change position for each measurement.

Table 4–20. Adjustments (cm) for Parental Stature To Be Made to an Infant's Measured Length (Birth and 2 Years) or Stature (4 to 18 Years)

Age (yr)	Short Parents†		Tall Parents‡	
	Boys	Girls	Boys	Girls
Birth	+1	0	−1	−1
2	+3	+3	−4	−4
4	+4	+4	−6	−6
6	+6	+6	−7	−7
8	+7	+6	−9	−8
10	+8	+6	−10	−8
12	+8	+7	−10	−9
14	+8	+7	−10	−8
16	+11	+8	−15	−10
18	+13	+7	−17	−9

Himes JH, Roche AF, Thissen D, et al: Parent-specific adjustments for evaluation of recumbent length and stature. *Pediatrics.* 1985;75:304–313.
†Mother approximately 153 cm (5 ft) and father approximately 165 cm (5 ft 5 in.).
‡Mother approximately 176 cm (5 ft 9 in.) and father approximately 191 cm (6 ft 4 in.).
From Moore, W.M., Roche, A.F., Eds. *Pediatric Anthropometry.* 3rd ed., Columbus, OH: Ross Laboratories; 1987. Used with permission.

- The child lies on his back in the center of the measuring board (Fig. 4–4).
- One person holds the crown of his head against the headboard.

Recumbent height. Many studies have shown recumbent height to be longer than standing height by about 2 cm and thus to be a more accurate measure of length[45] (*1.8 cm* by age 2, gradually decreasing to *1.1 cm* by age 9 and then gradually increasing to *1.9 cm* to age 16 boys, and *1.9 cm* to age 14 girls. The *1.9 cm* remains until age 28 for both sexes[45]). One study found that this difference remained into

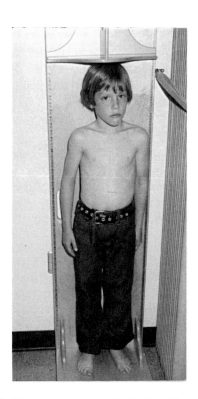

Fig. 4–3. Upright measurement with the head board. From the UACCDD Nutrition Department, Cincinnati, OH, with permission.

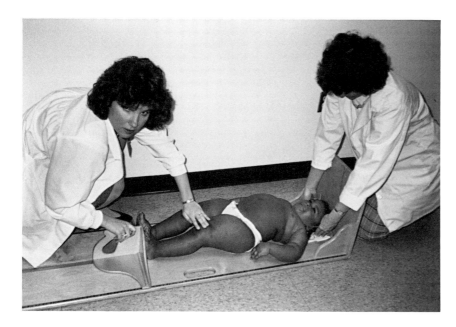

Fig. 4–4. Head board measurement in a supine or recumbent position. From the UACCDD Nutrition Department, Cincinnati, OH, with permission.

adulthood and was about 1 to 2 cm.[46] In adults, Gray et al.[46] determined that recumbent body length was significantly longer by an average of 3.68 cm than standing height as measured on a standard balance beam scale.

Recumbent height is measured as follows:

- Grip both ankles with one hand and place the child's heel firmly against the foot board, which is manipulated with the other hand. If the infant's knees are flexed, firmly but gently press them down on the table with the lateral edge of the hand.
- Turn the head board upright to measure an older child (Figs 4–3 and 4–4).

Sitting Height. Sitting height from crown to rump is used to determine the length of children whose legs are severely deformed or shorter than normal (Appendix 8).[47]

- Use an anthropometer
- Place child in erect, sitting position with head oriented.
- Measure the vertical distance from the sitting surface to the vertex (top of the head).

Weight

Weight should be measured using a beam scale with a capacity of 200–350 lb,[48] unless the child weighs less than 13.6 kg or 30 lb. The scale should be checked weekly with known weights.

Measurement of weight. *For a small child*

- Use an infant scale for children under 13.6 kg (30 lb)
- Remove all of the child's clothing.
- Balance the scale and place the child on it.
- Weigh twice to the nearest *30 g.*

For a child over 13.6 kg (30 lb)

- Use a beam scale with a capacity from 220–350 lb with a support pillar (Fig 4–5)
- Have the child remove shoes and all clothing but underwear.
- Balance the scale.
- Place the child in a standing position on the scale, facing the beam with hands on hip or support pillar.

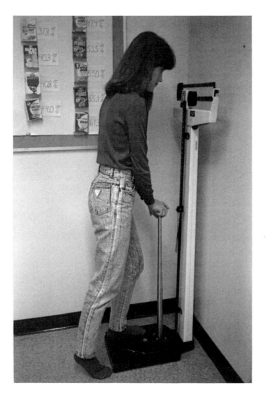

Fig. 4–5. Person being weighed using a support pillar. From the UACCDD Nutrition Department, Cincinnati, OH, with permission.

- Weigh twice to the nearest *100 g.* Have the child step off the platform after each weighing.

Head circumference

Head circumference is an important measure in young children because it reflects brain growth. The rate of brain growth is greatest during the last trimester of pregnancy and the first 6 months after birth. However, it is important to take head circumference measurements through age 6 for the child who is developmentally delayed. Head circumference should be measured with a nonstretchable tape (Fig 4–6). The standard growth grid for head circumference is shown in Appendix 3.

Measurement of head circumference

- Use a flexible narrow 7-mm width steel or platic-coated tape.
- Apply the tape firmly around the head above the supraorbital ridges or the most prominent part of the frontal bulge, anteriorly, and over that part of the occiput that gives maximum frontal-occipital circumference (Fig 4–6).
- Measure twice to nearest 0.1 cm.

Triceps Skinfolds

The distribution of subcutaneous fat varies from individual to individual and changes with aging, but alterations caused by dietary changes appear to occur proportionately throughout the body. Thus, changes in subcutaneous fat are assumed to reflect changes in total body fat. The triceps skinfold thickness provides an estimate of body fat, and the arm muscle circumference or area that is calculated from the triceps skinfold thickness and upper arm circumference provides an indication of body muscle, skeletal mass, lean body mass (LBM), or the somatic proteins.[49] Since caloric needs and perhaps nutrient needs are based on LBM or fat-free mass, which is active tissue (rather than the more inactive fat tissue), it is essential to determine LBM. A urinary creatinine measurement collected over 24 hours also provides an indication of skeletal muscle or somatic proteins (see section on biochemical assessment).

The most commonly measured skinfold thickness in nutritional assessment is the triceps. However, recent studies by Bray et al,[50] and Bradfield,[51] have suggested that other measurements might be more accurate indicators of body fat. Chumlea and Roche[52] found a good correlation between total body fat and the sum of multiple skinfold thickness measurements, including triceps, biceps, chin, subscapular,

midaxillary, paraumbilical, superiliac, thigh, and medial calf skinfolds (Appendix 10). In routine clinical practice, however, adequate accuracy and reproducibility can be obtained from measurement and summation of just the triceps and subscapular skinfolds thickness.[52] Triceps and subscapular skinfold grids have been developed for boys and girls from age 0 to 6 years, 6 to 12 years, and 12 to 18 years (Appendix 8). These grids correlate well with total fat and percent body fat in children. Standards for skinfold measurements are shown in Appendix 3. Skinfold and circumferential measurements are described in even more detail in the *Anthropometry Standardization Reference Manual*.[54]

Measurement Techniques for Skinfolds

Skinfold thickness

- Use Lange or Holtain calipers and tape measure.
- *Measure twice to the nearest .02 millimeter.*

Triceps skinfold thickness

- Place the child in sitting position with right arm relaxed and flexed 90 degrees at the elbow.
- Measure the distance between the olecranon and acromial processes of the relaxed, hanging right arm and mark the midpoint.
- After the midpoint is marked, grasp a full fatfold lifting it cleanly from the underlying muscle tissue, and apply the calipers below the fingers to the fatfold with the arm flexed 90 degrees at elbow (Fig 4–7).
- Read triceps skinfolds measurement with the arm hanging freely and not compressed about 3 sec after the caliper tension is released.

Biceps skinfold thickness

- Place child in sitting position with right arm relaxed and flexed 90 degrees at the elbow.
- Use midpoint mark as in the triceps skinfold measure.
- Grasp the skin and the subcutaneous tissue on the bicep of the relaxed arm, which is flexed 90 degrees at the elbow.
- Place the calipers 1 cm below the fingers to the fatfold.
- Read the biceps skinfold measurement with arm hanging freely and not compressed.

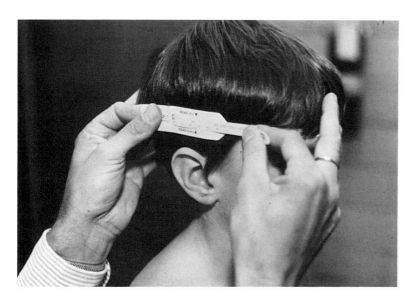

Fig. 4–6. Head circumference measurement. From Chumlea,[48] with permission.

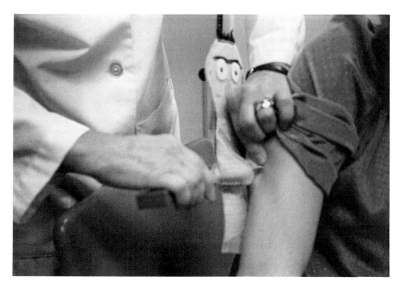

Fig. 4–7. Triceps skinfold measurement using a puppet. From the UACCDD Nutrition Department, Cincinnati, OH, with permission.

Subcapular skinfold thickness

- Place child in standing, erect position with shoulders and arms relaxed.
- Measure by grasping the skin and the subcutaneous tissues 1 cm below the tip of the right scapula with the forefinger at the lower tip of the scapula.[53] The skinfold forms a line about 45 degrees below the horizontal, extending diagonally toward the right elbow.
- Place the calipers perpendicular to the length of the fold about 1 cm over the inferior angle of the scapula directly lateral to the finger at the mark. (Fig 4–8).

Abdominal skinfold

- Place the child in standing position breathing quietly.
- Grasp skin and subcutaneous tissues 3 cm to the right and 1 cm below the umbical cord.
- Apply the calipers horizontally to the abdominal skinfold.

Thorax or midaxillary skinfold

- Place child in standing position with arms extended to shoulder line.
- Grasp skin and subcutaneous tissue parallel over the tenth rib or xiphi-sternal junction in the axillary line.
- Place the calipers on a horizontal fold adjacent to the grasping fingers.

Anterior thigh skinfold

- Extend the child's leg flat on the bed.
- Measure the anterior upper thigh with a flexible tape from the lower pelvis to the upper knee cap, and mark the midpoint as for measuring thigh circumference.
- Grasp the skin and subcutaneous fat at the mark, and apply the calipers 1 cm distal to the marked level.

Medial calf skinfold

- Place child in standing position.
- Measure the medial calf skinfold at the most prominent part of the lower leg. Measure calf circumference initially, and mark the point at that time.
- Grasp the skin and subcutaneous fat 1 cm above the marked point at the medial calf muscle, and apply the calipers at marked point for calf circumference.
- For lateral calf skinfold, use side instead of medial calf muscle.

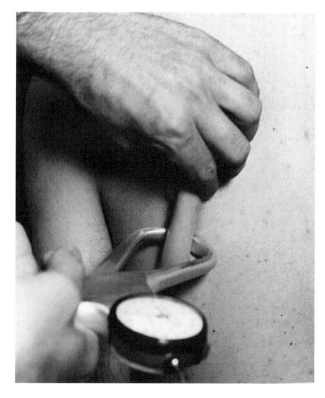

Fig. 4–8. Subscapular skinfold measurement. From Chumlea,[48] with permission.

Anterior chest skinfold

- Place the child in standing position with the arm hanging relaxed at the side.
- Grasp the anterior axillary skinfold as high as possible. The long axis of the fold should slant medially and inferior.
- Place the caliper perpendicular to the length of the fold about 1 cm below the fingers.

Superilliac skinfold

- Place the child in standing position.
- Select site in midaxillary line, superior to the illiac crest.
- Apply the calipers parallel to the cleavage line of the skin, not quite horizontal.

Thigh skinfold

- Use the thigh circumference marked area.
- Grasp a double fold of skin and subcutaneous tissue 1 cm distal to marked level.
- Apply calipers perpendicular to fold at marked level.

Circumferential Measurements

Midarm muscle circumference (MAMC) is derived from the following formula:

MAMC or AMC (cm) = Midarm circumference (cm)

$$- 3.14 \times \frac{\text{triceps skinfold (TSF) in mm}}{10}$$

MAMC estimates somatic protein, and TSF estimates subcutaneous fat but variability in size of the bone is not determined.

The midarm muscle area (MAMA or AMA) is calculated by the following equation:

$$\frac{\left[\text{midarm circumference (cm)} - \left(3.14 \times \frac{\text{TSF mm}}{10}\right)\right]^2}{12.56}$$

A combination of triceps skinfold and upper arm circumference to compute upper arm muscle area or muscularity in children using the nomogram developed by Gurney and Jelliffe.[55] (Fig 4–9) is a good general index of growth and nutritional status. The *corrected MAMA* (c MAMA or also called c AMA) by Heymsfield[56] which *subtracts for bone* (a 20% reduction) is using the *same equation but subtracting − 6.5 for females and − 10 for males*. A nomogram using the correction factor is not available, however. The MAMA or AMA prediction equations are not recommended for persons having a relative weight ≥ 125%[56] or a triceps skinfold thickness > 85 percentile. AMA appears to be a useful index for body muscle in young children as it significantly correlated with creatinine excretion in this population.[57] Techniques for many circumferences follow, all use plastic-coated nonstretchable tape and should be done *twice to the nearest 0.1 cm.*

Mid-upper arm circumference

- Place the child in a standing position.
- Encircle the upper arm at the midpoint mark, between the tip of the acromial process of the scapula and the tip of the elbow, as determined in measuring the triceps skinfold.
- Locate the level with the forearm flexed at 90 degrees, but the measurement is made with the arm hanging freely. The tape should be snug but not too tight to avoid compressing the tissue.[45]
- Use combination of skinfold and upper arm circumference measurements to compute arm muscle area or muscularity using the nomogram developed by Gurney and Jelliffte (Fig 4–9).

Chest circumference

- Place the child in a sitting position with arms at side.
- Apply the tape to the chest so as to encompass the areolae for boys and the axillae above the area of breast fullness for girls.

Medial calf circumference

- Place the child in a sitting position with feet flat on the floor.
- Apply tape to the most prominent area of the calf.

Waist, abdomen, and hip circumference

- Place the child in a standing position, with feet together, weight evenly distributed, and arms hanging at sides.
- Measure the horizontal circumference at the waist, abdomen (at the largest part of the abdomen) and hip (the largest part of buttocks area) during normal breathing.

Wrist circumference

- Place the child in a standing position, arm flexed at the elbow, palm side up (useful for frame size).
- Apply tape perpendicular to long axis of the forearm, just distal to the styloid processes of the radius and ulna.

Thigh circumference

- Place child in standing position and ask child to take one half step backwards with left foot (shifts weight to left foot).
- Mark the point ½ the distance from the proximal border of the patella to the inguinal crease and measure perpendicular to shaft of the thigh. (If unable to stand, place right knee at 90 degree angle on the bed and mark point ⅓ distance from the proximal border of the patella to the anterior superioriliac and measure).

Elbow breadth

- Elbow breadth is a good indicator of skeletal dimensions (frame size) because it is not affected by percent fat weight. See Appendix 10.
- Use sliding caliper on frameter (distributed by Health Products, 2126 Ridge, Ann Arbor, Michigan, 48104).
- Place the child in a sitting position facing the examiner.
- Extend the right arm and bend the forearm toward the shoulder at a 90 degree angle, turning the palm of the hand toward the body. Place the elbow on a table or board containing calipers.
- Slide the caliper jaws against the side the child's elbow.
- Measure the greatest bony width across the elbow.

Ankle breadth

- Place the child in an erect, standing position with feet apart and weight evenly distributed.
- Use a sliding caliper.
- With paddle blades of the sliding caliper, measure the minimum horizontal breadth of the right ankle (narrowest part) above the malleous (ankle bone).

Arm muscle area is a more physiological parameter than arm muscle circumference and skinfold or fatfold measures. Changes in the arm muscle area result in larger changes in the arm muscle area values as a function of the formula used to calculate it.[58] Mid-upper arm muscle area can be calculated from the triceps skinfolds and the upper arm circumference by using the arm anthropometry nomogram for the appropriate age[45] (see Fig 4–9 and Appendix 10).

Arm span and length

The arm span is measured as it should equal[59] height. Likewise, upper arm length multiplied by a factor can be used to determine height.[60]

Arm length

- Use a plastic-coated tape measure.
- Place child in erect standing position, with upper arms hanging at sides and arms flexed 90 degrees.
- For upper arm length, measure the distance from the acromion process to the radiale.
- *Measure twice to the nearest 0.1 cm.*

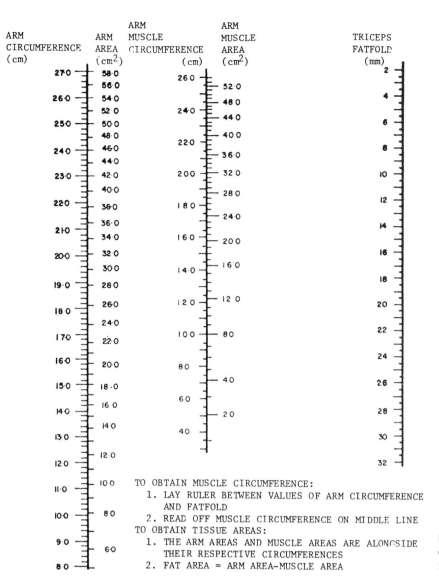

TO OBTAIN MUSCLE CIRCUMFERENCE:
1. LAY RULER BETWEEN VALUES OF ARM CIRCUMFERENCE
   AND FATFOLD
2. READ OFF MUSCLE CIRCUMFERENCE ON MIDDLE LINE
TO OBTAIN TISSUE AREAS:
1. THE ARM AREAS AND MUSCLE AREAS ARE ALONGSIDE
   THEIR RESPECTIVE CIRCUMFERENCES
2. FAT AREA = ARM AREA-MUSCLE AREA

Fig. 4–9. Arm anthropometry nomogram for children. From Gurney & Jelliffe,[55] with permission.

Arm span

- Have the child stretch both arms maximally with back against the wall.
- Measure from the tip of the middle finger to the tip of the other middle finger.
- *Measure twice to the nearest 0.1 cm.*

Knee height

- Use knee height caliper.
- Child should lie on his back and bend left knee and ankle to 90 degrees.
- Place caliper down against the thigh about 2 inches behind the patella (knee cap).
- *Measure twice to the nearest 0.1 cm. (see Appendix 8).*

Bone age

An x-ray of the hand and wrist is an accurate method to assess skeletal age with minimal skin dose radiation. The procedure described here is modified for children over 3 years of age.[61] It uses an x-ray machine and plastic paddle to obtain a left hand and wrist posteroanterior radiograph.

- Place the hand flat on table. Place plastic paddle on top of hand to retain posture. Use nonscreen film. Specify size of nonscreen film tube-to-film distances for x-ray and KVP and MaS so technician knows how to set dials.[62] X-ray skin dosage should be 0.005–0.01 rad and gonadal dosage a fraction of a millirad per view.
- Follow standards of Greulich and Pyle[63] to diagnose bone age of children 3 to 10 years of age.
- Use results of study by National Center for Health Statistics to compare group data in children 6 to 11 years until more data become available on developmentally disabled children.
- For research purposes and comparison, count the number of ossification centers and look at sequence of ossification centers (useful in certain syndromes).[63] According to Garn et al.,[63] the ten most consistent secondary centers in order of time of appearance are distal phalanx, third finger; distal phalanx, fourth finger; proximal phalanx, second finger; third metacarpal; distal phalanx, fifth finger; distal phalanx, second finger; middle phalanx, fourth finger; fifth metacarpal; proximal phalanx, fifth finger; and middle phalanx, second finger.

In the clinical estimate of maturation the skeletal age should be correlated with other findings, such as motor performance, mental age, race, height, weight, and nutritional status.

Application of Anthropometric Measures in a Nutritional Assessment

All anthropometric measurements are useful in completing a nutritional assessment. The more measurements one can obtain, the more precisely the client's body composition can be interpreted and therefore the more accurate the nutritional assessment. However, clinical measurements must be both reliable (two measurement samples), and accurate (using adequate equipment and proper technique), or wrong conclusions regarding nutritional status, growth and intervention may be drawn. If the limit for differences is excluded, a second set of measurements should be taken. Table 4–21 shows some applications of anthropometric measurements to nutritional status.

The National Center for Health Statistics growth grids or charts for children are found in Appendix 3.[64] Standardized growth grids for triceps and skinfold measurements and midarm circumference can be seen in Appendix 8. Incremental growth charts showing the velocity, slope of the curve, or rate of growth per unit of time demonstrate the rate of the child's growth against normal American children.[65] Thus, the amount of change or increment from one visit to the next can be quantified.

Body mass index (BMI) compares weight to height, but is not useful in children with unusual body composition, such as increased LBM. It is calculated according to this equation.

$$BMI = \frac{weight\ (kg)}{height^2\ (meters)}$$

BMI correlates better with body fat than body weight using the standard of Bray et al.[50] A BMI index of 24–27 for females and 25–27 for males is an indication of overweight, and a BMI greater than 27 indicates obesity in adults. However, this figure cannot be translated into recommendations of how much weight to lose[66] (see Chapters 2 and 19). The BMI in adolescence is correlated more closely with percent body fat in girls, whereas triceps skinfold (TSF) is correlated more closely with body fat in boys.[67] The BMI as well as the sum of two skinfolds for children 6 to 17 years by Lohman[68] is shown in Appendix 8–7). A TSF of 60% to 80% indicates a moderate deficit and less than 60% a severe deficit[69] (see Fig 4–9 for nomogram). The weight for height ratio is the most widely used index for adipose tissue, but it does not differentiate muscle and soft tissue from fat, especially with young children. An arm muscle circumference of 75% to 85% is a moderate to mild deficit and less than 75% a severe deficit (Table 4–20).

Skeletal muscle, like fat, can be used as an energy source if calories are not sufficient although it is not intended for that purpose. Muscle can be estimated by midarm circumference, midarm muscle circumference, and creatinine height index (see section on biochemical assessment).

The relationship of the head circumference to recumbent length is a useful indicator; length should not exceed head circumference by more than *40 percentile points*, or vice versa. For example, a 6-month-old boy who is 70 cm (80th percentile) and has a head circumference of 41.5 cm (5th percentile) should be evaluated further.[70]

Gestational age of the child must be assessed properly in the first 2 or 3 years of life. If the child is determined to be at 32 weeks gestation or later, correction must be made until

he or she reaches 24 months of age, whereas for an infant born 28 weeks gestation or earlier, correction must be made until 36 months of age. By age 4, generally, corrections for gestational age are no longer needed (Table 4–22).[48] Z-scores, which are used to categorize data, are calculated according to this formula:

$$\frac{standard\ mean\ value\text{-}value\ of\ subject}{standard\ deviation}$$

In normal distribution the Z-score and percentile equivalents are

- below 5th percentile—Z-score is less than -1.650
- 5.0 to 15th percentile—Z-score is between -1.654 and -1.040
- 15.1 to 85th percentile—Z-score is between -1.036 and $+1.030$
- 85.1 to 95th percentile—Z-score is between $+1.036$ and $+1.640$
- 95.1 to 100th percentile—Z-score is equal to or greater than $+1.645$.

See Appendix 8 for the usage of Z-scores for an 8-year-old boy.

Anthropometric Assessment of Children with Special Needs

An anthropometric assessment of children with special needs must use alternate measurement techniques and special growth grids or charts for certain disorders or diseases. The grid should be used to plot longitudinal data on the child to see if he or she is improving, deteriorating, or remaining the same.[48]

Short parental stature is rarely the cause of length or weight below the 5th percentile[71], nor is tall parental stature often the cause of weight or length above the 95th percentile. A 1987 study lists these other causes of abnormal growth.[72] Growth above the 95th percentile

- weight—tallness, obesity, edema
- length of stature—tall parents, accelerated maturation, Marfan syndrome, pituitary gigantism
- weight-for-length or weight-for-stature—obesity, edema, achondroplasia
- Head circumference—hydrocephaly
- Triceps skinfold thickness—obesity

Growth below the 5th percentile

- weight—shortness, malnutrition, chronic renal disease, psychosocial deprivation, infectious disease, iron-deficiency anemia
- length or stature—short parents; malnutrition; psychosocial deprivation; delayed maturation; endocrinopathies, especially hypothyroidism and hypopituitarism; chromosomal and genetic abnormalities, e.g., Turner syndrome; chronic renal disease
- weight-for-length or weight-for-stature—dehydration, recent febrile illness, recent malnutrition, Marfan syndrome
- head circumference—microcephaly, e.g., fetal alcohol syndrome; craniostenosis; genetic disorders
- triceps skinfold thickness—malnutrition; chronic illness, e.g., cystic fibrosis

Accurate measures of height and weight can still be obtained in children who cannot stand. Jensen et al[73] found that the TSF and arm circumference obtained in the upright position correlated significantly with those obtained in the supine position. Arm span[59] or arm length[60] multiplied by a factor, rather than recumbent length, can also be used to measure length. Belt et al found that upper arm length,

Table 4–21. Some Anthropometric Measurements Applied in Nutritional Assessment

Measurements	Age groups	Nutritional indication	Reproducibility	Advantages	Disadvantages	Observer error	Interpretation
Weight	All groups	Present nutritional status; under and over	Good	Common in use	Difficult in field, can't tell body composition, need accurate age, height related (insensitive)	<100 g in children <250 g in adults	<60% severe 60–80 moderate 80–90 mild 90–110 normal 110–120 over 120 and over obese
Height	All groups	Chronic nutritional status (under)	Good	Common in use Simple to do in field	Other factors play a role	<0.5 cm <3.0 cm in adults	<80% dwarf 80–93 short 93–105 normal >105 giant
	7 years child	Chronic under nutrition in early childhood	Good				
Head circumference	0–4 years	Intrauterine and childhood nutrition (chronic under-nutrition)	Good	Simple	Other factors play a role e.g. brain development	<0.5 cm	
Midarm circumference	All groups	Present under and over nutrition	Fair	Simple, age independent, child need not be stripped, suitable for rapid survey	No limits for over nutrition, No standard for adult	<0.5 cm	<75% severe 75–80 moderate 80–85 mild >85% normal
Skinfold thickness, subscapula or triceps	All groups	Present under and over nutrition	Fair	Measures body composition, detects obesity in adults	Needs expensive caliper, difficult with child and in the field, ? ethnic differences	1.0–1.5 mm	Similar to item (1)
Weight/height/ age ratio	All ages	Present under and over nutrition	Good	Index of body build, age independent 1–4 years and adults	Need proper scales, need trained personnel		<75% severe 75–85 moderate 85–90 mild 90–110 normal 110–120 over >120 obese
Midarm/head ratio	3 months– 48 months	Present under nutrition	Good	Simple, age independent, sex independent, any person can do it in field	No standard for adults		<0.25 severe 0.25–0.28 moderate 0.28–0.31 mild 0.31–0.35 normal >0.35 obese
Chest/head circs. ratio	1–2 years	Present under nutrition	Fair or poor	Simple, age. independent	For limited age No classification method		<1 malnourished >1 normal

From McLaren, D.S. Nutritional assessment. In: McLaren, D.S., Burman, D., eds., *Textbook of Pediatric Nutrition*. 2nd ed. New York: Churchill Livingstone; 1982. Used with permission.

Table 4–22. Adjusted Ages at Which Growth Measurements Should Be Plotted for Infants of Different Gestational Ages (GA) at Birth

Actual Age (mo)	Adjusted Age (mo) for Plotting		
	28 wk GA	32 wk GA	36 wk GA
3	0	1	2
6	3	4	5
9	6	7	8
12	9	10	11
15	12	13	14
18	15	16	17
21	18	19	20
24	21	22	23
27	24	25	26
30	27	28	29
33	30	31	32
36	33	34	35

From Moore & Roche[72] with permission.

rather than lower arm length or total arm length, multiplied by a factor, correlated most significantly when evaluating children with myeomeningocele (Chapter 10). Leg length plus a factor can be used to measure length or weight if the child has normal leg development and is over 6 years of age (Appendix 8). Weight can be measured by a moveable wheelchair beam scale or by weighing the caregiver and child and then subtracting the caregiver's weight.

Each recumbent position is taken in the same body location as the corresponding standing measurement.[52] Recumbent measurement techniques for triceps and subscapular skinfold and midarm circumference can be used with a few exceptions. The arm being measured for midarm circumference is placed alongside the body, palm upward, and raised slightly by placing a sandbag under the elbow (Fig 4–10). Measurement of triceps and subscapular skinfolds is made with the child lying on the side with one arm extending from the front of the body at a 45 degree angle, the trunk in a straight line, and the legs bent and tucked up slightly. The arm being measured rests along the trunk, palm down.

An imaginary line connecting the acromion processes should be perpendicular to the surface of the bed and the spine. The procedure for recumbent triceps skinfold measurement is shown in Figure 4–11.

Standards for the measurement of standing height (stature), recumbent length, head circumference, skinfold thickness, and arm circumference for chronically ill and handicapped children are adapted from Chumlea.[48] Age-related anthropometric trends are discussed by Bowen and Custer.[58]

Body Composition

Lean body mass (LBM) is mainly being measured by the doubly-labeled water method or whole body K_{40} count as discussed in Chapter 19. However, other advanced technologies are becoming available as well which evaluate the four compartments (water, protein, mineral, and fat) and are particularly useful in diseased states.[74–76] Most techniques measure the whole body average, such as the 24-hour excretion of creatinine as a measure of muscle mass, dilution of oxygen-labeled water as a measure of total body water, and potassium 40 as a measure of body cell mass. The distribution of fat and muscle at selected sites, which can predict risk for certain metabolic diseases, requires imaging techniques, such as magnetic resonance imaging (MRI) or computed tomography (CT).[77,78] These are expensive techniques and require better "phantoms" for standards and thus mainly are used for research. In one study that measured adipose tissue distribution by CT and MRI, average errors of the method were 5.4%, 10.6%, and 10.1% for total, visceral and subcutaneous fat areas, respectively.[79]

Bioelectric impedance (BIA) is a new method of determining total body water and fat and FFM or LBM composition in human subjects; however, better evaluation of laboratory variability and development equations are needed.[80] The method is based on the nature of electrical conduction, which is influenced by water and electrolyte distribution. Since FFM or LBM contains nearly all of the water and conducting electrolytes in the body, electrical

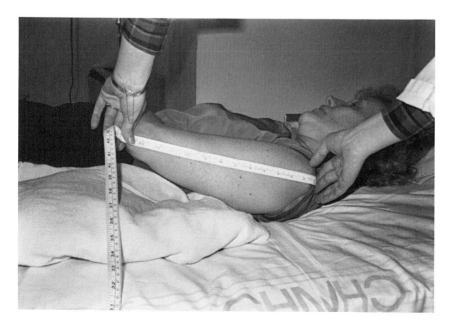

Fig. 4–10. Recumbent midpoint upper arm measurement technique. From the UACCDD Nutrition Department, Cincinnati, OH, with permission.

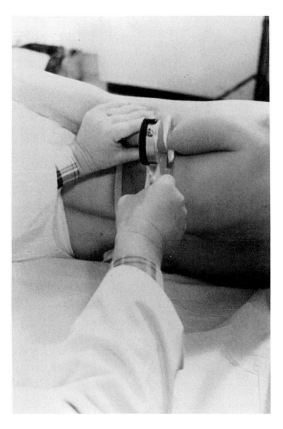

Fig. 4–11. Recumbent triceps skinfold measurement technique. From Chumlea,[48] with permission.

conductivity is far greater in FFM than in fat mass. The equation developed by Lukaski and Bolonchuk[81] to measure FFM follows:

$$FFM (LBM) = [(0.734 \ Ht^2)/R] \times 0.116 \ Wt$$
$$+ \ 0.096 \ X_c + 0.878 \times gender - 4.03$$

where Ht = height in cm, Wt = body weight in kg, R = low resistance, X_c = reactance, and gender = male (1), female (0).

Guo, et al.[82] predicted FFM in children 7–25 years using a multicomponent model of BIA and anthropometric variables—triceps, biceps, subscapular, midaxillary, and lateral skinfolds; arm muscle and calf muscle circumference; weight, and height—as well as age and percent body fat. The correlation between weight and FFM or LBM generally ranges from 0.4–0.7; for arm circumference and FFM, it is approximately 0.7 in men and 0.5 in women; and for skinfold thickness and FFM, it is a low 0.06–0.04. Five independent variables seemed adequate in predicting FFM in the study. For men, the selected variables were weight, lateral and midaxillary skinfold, arm circumference, and BIA; for women, they were weight, lateral calf and triceps skinfold, subscapular skinfold, and BIA.

The multicomponent model of Lohman[83] is based on this equation:

$$\% \ body \ fat = (\frac{2.74}{body \ density} - 0.71 \ body \ water)$$
$$+ \ 1.27 \ bone \ mineral - 2.045) \times 100$$

This model reflects the concentrations of water, protein,

and mineral and thus appears to be more accurate than the Siri two-component model, which only includes percent body fat and body density from underwater weight as follows:

$$\% \ body \ fat = (\frac{4.95}{body \ density} - 4.5) \times 100$$

Body density may be measured by K40, underwater weighing, skinfolds and bone mineral by photon absorption (see Biochemical Section). For example, body density for an adult female = 1.0994921 − 0.0009929 (sum of triceps, suprailiac and thigh skinfolds) + 0.0000023 (sum of same 3 skinfolds)^2 − 0.0001392 (age).[84,85] The most accurate prediction equation for children 8 years and older is based on a multicomponent system for determining percent body fat, including density, water, and bone, that uses a *sum of the triceps and calf skinfolds* as follows[73]:

$$Male \ \% \ body \ fat = 0.735 \ (triceps + calf) + 1.0$$

$$Female \ \% \ body \ fat = 0.610 \ (triceps + calf) + 5.1$$

See Appendix 8–9 for the conversion charts by Lohman and a grid to determine percent body fat. Equations and normal percent body fat for those age 18 and above and for athletes and nonathletes can be found in Appendix 10–7 thru 10–9.

The sum of triceps and subscapular skinfolds may also be used to determine percent body fat, but they must be calculated separately for various age groups and thus are much more complicated to use than the triceps and calf skinfolds.

Houtkooper et al.[86] recently developed a prediction equation to estimate the body composition of children (FFM) from 10–18 years of age and, indirectly, the percent body fat using only BIA, height, and, weight, without the need for any other anthropometric measures by cross validation.

$$FFM = 0.61 \times \left(\frac{h^2 \ cm}{resistance}\right) + 0.25 \ weight \ (kg) + 1.31$$

The percentage body fat may be determined by this equation:

$$Total \ weight - FFM = \frac{Fat \ weight \times 100}{Total \ weight} = \% \ body \ fat$$

Charts predicting percent body fat, such as those for the sum of the triceps and calf skinfolds, will soon be available using the BIA equations, which are now being cross-validated in other populations of children.[86] Methods to determine body fat based on BIA are useful, but require expensive BIA equipment ($4000–$5000) versus the caliper ($200) used in the triceps and calf skinfold equation by Lohman. Body composition can be as accurate using skinfolds as BIA (if skinfold measurements are taken accurately). Both are better predictors than BMI, particularly in men.[74] Hydration may affect BIA measurements.[68,87] However, skinfolds may not be as good a predictor as circumferential measures if body fat is above 35%. Fat patterning differences (age, ethnic group, fatness, physical activity, and areas of the body) will be evaluated by using skinfold equations in future research.[68] Likewise, basic equations are being modified for adult obesity (for example, see waist/hip nomogram Appendix 10). Other methods of determining human body composition and their limitations are shown in Table 4–23. Target weight for adults (Appendix 10–13) may be used to achieve a certain percent body

Table 4–23. Limitations of Methods of Determining Human Body Composition*

Method	Cost	Technical difficulty	Precision Fat-free mass	% Fat
Water				
Deuterium	2	3	3	3
Oxygen-18	5	5	4	4
Tritium	3	3	3	3
Potassium	4	4	4	3
Creatinine	2	3	2	1
Densitometry				
Immersion	3	4	5	5
Plethysmography	4	3	5	5
Skinfold thickness	1	2	2	2
Arm circumference	1	3	2	2
Neutron activation	5	5	5	5
Photon absorptiometry	4	4	4	4
3-Methylhistidine	2	3	3	?†
Electrical				
Conductivity	5	1	4	4
Impedance	2	1	4	4
Computed tomography	5	5	?	?
Ultrasound	3	3	3	3
Infrared interactance	4	3	3	3
Magnetic resonance	5	5	?	?

*Ranking system: ascending scale, 1 = least and 5 = greatest.
†Unknown at this time.
From Lukaski, H. Methods for assessment of human body composition: traditional and new. *Am. J. Clin. Nutr.* 1987;46:537. Used with permission.

fat and is accurate as long as the % body fat is determined correctly. The target weight formula follows:

Fat weight = total body weight × % body fat

FFM = total body weight − fat weight

Target weight = %FFM / (100 − desired body fat).[84]

Clinical Or Physical Signs Assessment

Clinical or physical signs are the last to appear, usually after a prolonged inadequate intake of nutrients. Therefore, dietary depletion should be evaluated carefully and corrected when it first appears so the potential for the child's growth is not reduced by inadequate nutrition.

Clinical findings caused by nutrient deficiency can be seen in Table 4–24. Many signs of malnutrition are subclinical, however. It is necessary to evaluate children frequently to become a good clinician and become knowledgeable in clinical or physical signs of malnutrition. Slides developed by Sandstead et al. are available from the *Nutrition Today*[88] journal office for identification and review of physical signs related to nutrient and other deficiencies.

According to the World Health Organization, the physical signs are classified as

- those associated with nutritional deficiency
- those that need further investigation (e.g., malnutrition related to chronic problems or poverty)
- those signs not related to malnutrition

A physical signs assessment should evaluate the oral musculature and its possible relationship to feeding problems; the use of drugs, such as anticonvulsants; general appear-

ance; and behavioral characteristics (see Appendices 4 and 5 for the physical signs assessment sections of the UACCDD and Boston Evaluation Center nutrition records). Blood pressure measurements should be taken on all children over 3 years of age (see Table 4–25 for standards). Physical signs of excessive weight change or loss need to be investigated thoroughly. Severe weight loss is greater than 2% in 1 week, 5% in 1 month, 7.5% in 3 months, and 10% in 6 months.

Psychosocial evaluation

Social and psychological components are increasingly important parts of the nutrition assessment and must be considered when planning the proper nutrition intervention (see Chapters 19 and 23). The parent-child psychosocial evaluation is particularly crucial if the child or family is in a stressful state. Calorie and protein needs may require adjustment during times of stress (Table 4–26).

The degree of stress is often related to the magnitude of change brought about by different life situations. Holmes' Social Readjustment Rating Scale[89] assigns numerical values to a number of stressful situations (Table 4–27). Ways to cope more effectively with stress are outlined in Table 4–28. The Prognostic Score Index[27] as related to stress and mortality is described in the section on biochemical assessment.

Standardized instruments are available to measure the following conditions[15]:

- anxiety state: 40-item STAI[90]
- depression: Beck Depression Inventory Index (Appendix 9)[91]
- functional status: Karnofsky Index of Performing Status[92]

Table 4–24. Clinical Nutrition Examination

Clinical findings	Possible deficiency	Possible excess
Hair, nails		
Flag sign (transverse dyspigmentation of hair)	Protein, copper	
Hair easily pluckable	Protein	
Hair thin, sparse	Protein, biotin, zinc	Vitamin A
Nails spoon-shaped	Iron	
Nails lackluster, transverse ridging	Protein calorie	
Skin		
Dry, scaling	Vitamin A, zinc, essential fatty acids	Vitamin A
Erythematous eruption (sunburnlike)		Vitamin A
"Flaky paint" dermatosis	Protein	
Follicular hyperkeratosis	Vitamins A, C; essential fatty acids	
Nasolabial seborrhea	Niacin, pyridoxine, riboflavin	
Petechiae, purpura	Ascorbic acid, vitamin K	
Pigmentation, desquamation (sun-exposed area)	Niacin (pellagra)	
Subcutaneous fat loss	Calorie	
Yellow pigmentation sparing sclerae (benign)		Carotene
Eyes		
Angular blepharitis	Riboflavin	
Band keratitis		Vitamin D
Corneal vascularization	Riboflavin	
Dull, dry conjunctiva	Vitamin A	
Fundal capillary microaneurysms	Ascorbic acid	
Papilledema		Vitamin A
Scleral icterus (mild)	Pyridoxine	
Perioral area		
Angular stomatitis	Riboflavin	
Cheilosis	Riboflavin	
Oral area		
Atrophic lingual papillae	Niacin, iron, riboflavin, folate, vitamin B_{12}	
Glossitis (scarlet, raw)	Niacin, pyridoxine, riboflavin, vitamin B_{12}, folate	
Hypogeusesthesia (also hyposmia)	Zinc, vitamin A	
Magenta tongue	Riboflavin	
Swollen, bleeding gums (if teeth present)	Ascorbic acid	
Tongue fissuring, edema	Niacin	
Glands		
Parotid enlargement	Protein	
Sjögren's syndrome	Ascorbic acid	
Thyroid enlargement	Iodine	
Heart		
Enlargement, tachycardia, high-output failure	Thiamine (wet beriberi)	
Small size, decreased output	Calorie	
Sudden failure, death	Ascorbic acid	
Abdomen		
Hepatomegaly	Protein	Vitamin A
Muscles, extremities		
Calf tenderness	Thiamine, ascorbic acid (hemorrhage into muscle)	
Edema	Protein, thiamine	
Muscle wastage (especially temporal area, dorsum of hand, spine)	Calorie	
Bones, joints		
Beading of ribs (child)	Vitamins C, D	
Bone and joint tenderness (child)	Ascorbic acid (subperiosteal hemorrhage)	Vitamin A
Bone tenderness (adult)	Vitamin D, calcium, phosphorus (osteomalacia)	
Bulging fontanelle (child)		Vitamin A
Craniotabes, bosselation (child)		Vitamin D
Neurologic considerations		
Confabulation, disorientation	Thiamine (Korsakoff's psychosis)	
Decreased position and vibratory senses, ataxia	Vitamin B_{12}, thiamine	
Decreased tendon reflexes, slowed relaxation phase	Thiamine	
Drowsiness, lethargy		Vitamins A, D
Opthalmoplegia	Thiamine, phosphorus	
Weakness, paresthesias, decreased fine tactile sensation	Vitamin B_{12}, pyridoxine, thiamine	
Other		
Delayed healing and tissue repair (e.g., wound, infarct, abscess)	Ascorbic acid, zinc, protein	
Fever (low-grade)		Vitamin A

From Weinsier, R.L., Butterworth, C.E., Jr., *Handbook of Clinical Nutrition*, St. Louis: C.V. Mosby, 1981, pp. 30–31. Used with permission.

Table 4–25. Normal Blood Pressure for Various Ages*

Ages	Mean systolic ± 2 S.D.	Mean diastolic ± 2 S.D.
Newborn	80 ± 16	46 ± 16
6 mo.–1 year	80 ± 29	60 ± 10*
1 year	96 ± 30	66 ± 25*
2 years	99 ± 25	64 ± 25*
3 years	100 ± 25	67 ± 23*
4 years	99 ± 20	65 ± 20*
5–6 years	94 ± 14	55 ± 9
6–7 years	100 ± 15	56 ± 8
7–8 years	102 ± 15	56 ± 8
8–9 years	105 ± 16	57 ± 9
9–10 years	107 ± 16	57 ± 9
10–11 years	111 ± 17	58 ± 10
11–12 years	113 ± 18	59 ± 10
12–13 years	115 ± 19	59 ± 10
13–14 years	118 ± 19	60 ± 10

*In this study the point of muffling was taken as the diastolic pressure. From Nadas, A.S., Fyler, D.C., eds. *Pediatric Cardiology*. 3rd ed. Philadelphia: W. B. Saunders, 1972. Used with permission.

• quality of life: Quality of Life Index (QOLI) designed by a sociologist[93] or the Spilzer Quality of Life (QL) index designed by a physician[94] (Table 4–29)
• mood states: Profile of Mood States measuring tension-anxiety; depression-dejection, anger-hostility, fatigue-inertia, and con-fusion-bewilderment[95] (see Appendix 9).

Adolescent stresses

In Western society, adolescence is a time of change and stress. There are three stages of adolescence, each involving significant psychosocial changes:

1. Age 10–14: early puberty, with changes in body image
2. Age 14–18: peer groups, with cognitive awakening and much risk taking
3. Age 18–21 or 36: separation from family, less peer involve-ment, and increased self-sufficiency

The changes taking place in adolescence are related to the need for autonomy, independence, assumption of adult sex-ual and work roles, and economic independence.[96,97] Adult-hood can be seen as a continuation of development that starts in childhood and passes into adolescence, eventually reaching various stages of adulthood (Fig 4–12).

In adolescence, stress is caused by changes in body image, sexuality conflicts, academic and athletic pressures, and re-lationships with peers and with others. David Elkind[86] writes that these stresses are manifested in 12 problem behaviors:

low self-image, inconsiderate of others and of self, authority problems, misleads others and is easily misled, aggravates others and is easily angered, stealing, alcohol or drug use, and fronting.

Adolescence can be much less stressful if the child has a good self-image and has been treated consistently well by parents. In adolescence, the basis of a good parent-child relationship shifts from power to companionship and from instructing to advising.[98] Parents can help their adolescent children cope better with stress by (1) developing skills in receiving and giving affection, limit setting, and discipline, (2) by providing opportunities for self-learning, decision making, self-responsibility and freedom; and (3) by being authoritative, not authoritarian. Adolescent girls whose pa-rental relationships do not change may have problems with separation, and adolescent boys may have difficulty devel-oping relationships with others.[99]

A peak period of growth occurs in adolescence, beginning at age 13.5 years for boys and 11.5 years for girls.[100] A boy may gain 9.5 cm and a girl 8.3 cm in height during this year. The nutritional status of a North American adolescent is assessed better by the Tanner and Davis maturational charts than standard growth grids (Appendix 9) since nutrient needs are related to maturity not age during adolescence. Boys tend to have a weight/fat gain early in puberty and then become leaner, whereas girls tend to have a constant rise in adipose tissue (see growth grids in Appendix 3 and Tanner grids for sexual maturity in Appendix 9). Men may not reach maximum adult height until the third decade of life.[101] The body composition of adolescents is shown in Appendix 9. Athletes, women on diets, ballet dancers, and others may have delayed menarche until 19 years due to reduced fatness (hormones are stored in fat tissue) (see Chapter 23). Hemo-globin values should be 13 g/dL or more for boys and 12 g/dL or more for girls.

Data from the Hanes II survey[102] indicated that adolescent boys and girls are at risk for iron-deficiency anemia, par-ticularly because of boys' increased muscle mass and menses for girls, and for marginal intakes of calcium, riboflavin, and vitamin A.[96] Teenage girls and boys often skip breakfast and snack frequently. Likewise, many teenagers eat meals away from home. In one study, 37% of the girls were on diets.[96] Pregnancy for the girl 15–17 years of age or younger is a high-risk problem in that increased nutrients are needed for the adolescent, as well as for the growing fetus (see Chapter 1).

Adolescents usually respond well to invitations to partic-ipate and do problem solving in nutrition planning. There-

Table 4–26. Calorie and Protein Needs in Stress

Stress level	Clinical setting	Estimated kcal need–total kcal/kg/day	NPC:N	AA g/kg/day	% total kcal AA	CHO	Fat
0	Simple starvation	28	150:1	1.0	15	60	25
1	Elective surgery	32	100:1	1.5	20	50	30
2	Polytrauma	40	100:1	2.0	25	40	35
3	Sepsis	50	80:1	2.5	30	70	0

From Cerra, F.B., ed. Open forum: Branched chain amino acids. Part I: stress nutrition. Cerra, F.B. *Nutr. Supp. Serv.*, January, 1985: 5. Used with permission.

Table 4–27. Stress Caused by Change in Life Situations

Life event	Mean value
Death of spouse	100
Divorce	73
Marital separation	65
Jail term	63
Death of close family member	63
Personal injury or illness	53
Marriage	50
Fired at work	47
Marital reconciliation	45
Retirement	45
Change in health of family member	44
Pregnancy	40
Sex difficulties	39
New family member	39
Business readjustment	39
Change in financial state	38
Death of close friend	37
Change to different line of work	36
Change in number of arguments with spouse	35
Mortgage over $10,000	31
Foreclosure of mortgage or loan	30
Change in responsibilities at work	29
Son or daughter leaving home	29
Trouble with in-laws	29
Outstanding personal achievement	28
Wife begin or stop work	26
Begin or end school	26
Change in living conditions	25
Revision of personal habits	24
Trouble with boss	23
Change in work hours or conditions	20
Change in residence	20
Change in schools	20
Change in recreation	19
Change in church activities	19
Change in social activities	18
Mortgage or loan less than $10,000	17
Change in sleeping habits	16
Change in number of family get-togethers	15
Change in eating habits	15
Vacation	13
Christmas	12
Minor violations of the law	11

Adapted from Holmes.[89]

fore, they should be interviewed separately from their parents or caregivers. The interview also must be nonjudgmental.

Dietitians and nutritionists working with adolescents need to be knowledgeable about sports nutrition; anorexia nervosa, bulimia, and obesity (eating disorders); alcohol and drug abuse (substance abuse); nutrient-drug interactions; affective mood disorders, psychiatric illnesses, and behavioral and psychotherapies, particularly with eating and mood disorders and handicapping conditions.[103,104] They also need extensive listening and counseling skills[91] and must be able to provide nutrition education both to the adolescent alone and to the family as a whole. Core areas of a nutritional assessment of an adolescent are weight history, height, sexual maturity, reproductive history, food beliefs, dietary behavior, fluid balance and hydration, iron status, medications, exercise patterns, and elimination patterns. Specialized training in working with this population is available at 8 adolescent health centers and 22 university-affiliated programs for developmental disorders in the United States.

The nutritionist should be aware of the special concerns of adolescents participating in athletic events. For example, a complex carbohydrate diet[70,71] and reduced exercise a few days prior to an athletic event may be useful for some long-endurance sports. Rather, a well-balanced diet with adequate protein, iron, and fluid that meets the RDA for age usually is recommended. Added calories, preferably supplied by complex carbohydrates, may be needed depending on the calories expended in competition, and increased fluids should be given to replace those lost in perspiration. Special psychic foods, such as concentrated sweets and unusual diets, are of no benefit and should be evaluated individually. Alcohol can lead to obesity; protein-energy malnutrition; deficiencies in thiamine, folate, and other vitamins; and depletion of magnesium and zinc.[102] The second most commonly used drug, cocaine, and other stimulants, such as amphetamines, result in weight loss, abnormal dietary patterns, and nutrient deficiencies.[105] Most patients with mood disorders show weight loss, but increased appetite, particularly in the winter, occurs in a few patients.[91] Schizophrenia may produce delusions relating to certain foods or fluids, which may result in nutrient deficiencies, protein-energy malnutrition, and dehydration.

The nutritionist must become knowledgeable about psychiatric illness and its treatment, reviewing its neuro-biochemistry and neurophysiology. Diet and psychotrophic medications can produce dry mouth, riboflavin deficiency, constipation, weight gain, nausea, and loose stools. When used in combination with alcohol, they can produce further sedation, whereas caffeine can reduce their effectiveness. Large amounts of ascorbic acid may decrease the absorption of antipsychotics, and exercise may eliminate the effect of antidepressants. Increased sodium can eliminate lithium's activity, but a low-sodium diet may cause lithium retention and toxicity. Chapter 27 describes drug-induced malnutrition in more detail. With chemical dependency the biological, psychological and social factors must be investigated.[92] It is essential for the dietitian to become a member of the treatment team for both assessment and rehabilitation.[106] Likewise, drug abuse, inadequate nutrition, and lack of prenatal care are problems among homeless pregnant girls which must be addressed by dietitians due to double the average infant mortality rate in this population (24.9/1000),[107] (see Chapter 1). Problems of anemia, diarrhea, nutritional deficiencies and lead poisoning are common among the homeless.[107,108]

Feeding Assessment

To perform a feeding assessment, one must know the normal milestones of feeding skill development, such as grasping the cup with both hands by age 15 months. One must also observe the child eating. The child must be able to chew before he or she is able to speak. Simulating this problem requires trying to speak without moving the tongue. Simulating swallowing problems requires tilting the neck toward the cervical spine and trying to swallow. A menu developed at UACCDD to help with the mechanics of feeding includes these foods:

Table 4–28. Ways to Cope More Effectively with Stress

Strengthen your body
  Learn to relax.
  Eat a nutritionally balanced diet.
  Get proper rest.
  Get regular exercise.
  Lose weight.

Develop self-understanding
  List your goals.
  Listen to the rhythm of your body.
  Write a diary or journal.
  Get feedback from others on how
    they perceive you.
  Analyze your strengths and
    weaknesses.

Improve your mind
  Read about stress and human growth.
  Be sensitive to all dimensions of life.
  Do light reading.

Develop healthy attitudes
  Think positively.
  Develop the attitude of gratitude.
  Learn to accept what you cannot
    change.

Control your emotions
  Admit to yourself how you feel.
  Practice self-expression.
  Work off your anger.

Improve your personal relationships
  Seek out friendships.
  Share yourself with significant others.
  Contact new people.
  Do something for others.
  Take charge of getting involved.

Control your job
  Focus on one thing at a time.
  Manage your time.
  Define the purpose of work.
  Don't try to be perfect.

Lift your spirit
  Keep things in proper perspective.
  Work toward deepening your life.
  Allot time for daily meditation.
  Learn to let go.

Improve your environment
  Spend time in a new environment.
  Find security.
  Change residences.

Live a healthy life-style
  Be yourself.
  Arrange to have variety in your life.
  Take one thing at a time.
  Don't let things drift.
  Learn to vary your pace.
  Plan for maximum comfort.

Control all your input.
Utilize medical check-ups.
Dress the way that feels right.
Practice good posture.

Keep track of your stress level.
Make use of the helping professions.
Be honest with yourself.
Find out what is controllable in your life
  and what isn't.

Clear your mind.
Take a course.
Go to the public library.
Think about great ideas.

Practice living in the present.
Don't be afraid of failure.
Get friendly with leisure.
Learn to love yourself.

Face your fears.
Experiment with new feelings.

Listen to others.
Don't criticize and blame others.
Give in occasionally.
Make clear choices.
Face painful questions directly.

Redefine your job.
Take some time off.
Be assertive.

Encourage your gentleness.
Engage in organized religious activity.
Laugh.
Learn to play.

Cut down excessive noise.
Rearrange and redecorate your home.
Control the TV set.

Set up desirable futures.
Take time to be alone.
Plan relaxed vacations.
Practice relaxed driving.
Develop your own list of coping devices.
Develop a hobby.

Adapted from Holmes.[89]

Table 4–29. Quality of Life Index Scoring Form

Score each heading 2, 1 or 0 according to your most recent assessment of the patient.

ACTIVITY — *During the last week, the patient*
- has been working or studying full-time, or nearly so, in usual occupation, or managing own household, or participating in unpaid or voluntary activities, whether retired or not 2
- has been working or studying in usual occupation or managing own household or participating in unpaid or voluntary activities; but requiring major assistance or a significant reduction in hours worked or a sheltered situation or was on sick leave 1
- has not been working or studying in any capacity and not managing own household 0

DAILY LIVING — *During the last week, the patient*
- has been self-reliant in eating, washing, toileting and dressing; using public transport or driving own car 2
- has been requiring assistance (another person or special equipment) for daily activities and transport but performing light tasks 1
- has not been managing personal care nor light tasks and/or not leaving own home or institution at all 0

HEALTH — *During the last week, the patient*
- has been appearing to feel well or reporting feeling "great" most of the time 2
- has been lacking energy or not feeling entirely "up to par" more than just occasionally.......................... 1
- has been feeling very ill or "lousy", seeming weak and washed out most of the time or was unconscious 0

SUPPORT — *During the last week,*
- the patient has been having good relationships with others and receiving strong support from *at least one* family member and/or friend 2
- support received or perceived has been limited from family and friends and/or by the patient's condition 1
- support from family and friends occurred infrequently or only when absolutely necessary or patient was unconscious...................... 0

OUTLOOK — *During the last week, the patient*
- has usually been appearing calm and positive in outlook, accepting and in control of personal circumstances, including surroundings 2
- has sometimes been troubled because not fully in control of personal circumstances or has been having periods of obvious anxiety or depression...................... 1
- has been seriously or very frightened or consistently anxious and depressed or unconscious...................... 0

QL INDEX TOTAL

How confident are you that your scoring of the preceding dimensions is accurate? Please ring the appropriate category.

Absolutely Confident	Very Confident	Quite Confident	Not Very Confident	Very Doubtful	Not at all Confident
1	2	3	4	5	6

Adapted from Spitzer et al.[94]

- thin, peeled apple slices or orange sections with tough membranes removed
- cereals cooked in milk with raisins or fruit added to increase texture; graham cracker bits or animal crackers sprinkled on pudding
- toast sticks, enriched animal crackers, and zwieback dry cereals (preferably not sugar coated which also may be used to encourage finger feeding)
- cooked vegetables and fruits, gradually advanced to raw, such as carrots
- cottage cheese in varying degrees of lumpiness, combined with fruits, such as applesauce, to encourage acceptance
- cheese of varying degrees of hardness used by itself or combined with whole-grain crackers
- hamburger, meat balls, tender chicken, meat cubes, and finally more chewy meats

Until feeding milestones are accomplished, a mixture of cottage cheese, yogurt, ice cream, pureed fruit, and citrotein jello, or formula (Appendix 6) may be used to increase protein and calories.

Other disciplines, particularly occupational therapy, dentistry;[109] and speech and hearing, also provide information related to feeding problems. A psychologist may assist in the area of motivation.

The feeding assessment section of the UACCDD and Boston Evaluation Center nutrition records is shown in Appendices 4 and 5, respectively. The feeding skill assessment chart can be used to observe changes over several visits. Likewise, the Mueller Prespeech and Feeding evaluation is an important inter-disciplinary assessment tool. The feeding assessment is described in more detail in Chapter 24.

Intervention and Follow-up

The treatment or intervention plan is designed to achieve a behavioral objective. It specifies the *goal, time frame* for completion, measurement for *accomplishment*, the *client* and the *nutritionist evaluator.*

The interpretation of the findings of the in-depth nutritional assessment includes a *summary of the pertinent nutritional history, current nutritional status, anthropometry data, biochemistry, clinical or physical signs, presenting nutritional problem, the impression or diagnosis*, and the *recommendations*. Evaluation points for the UACCDD summary are shown in Appendix 4–1.

In-Depth Nutritional Assessment of Adults and Older Adults. As the child with developmental disorders and chronic

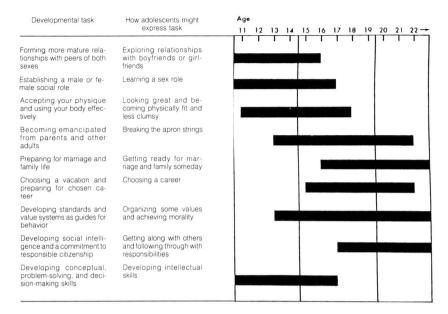

Fig. 4–12. Developmental tasks in adolescents. From: Eggert, L.L. Psychological development in adolescence In: Mahan, L.K., Rees, Z., eds. *Nutrition in Adolescence.* St. Louis: CV Mosby; 1984, with permission.

diseases passes through adolescence and into adulthood, other biochemical, dietary, anthropometric, and physical signs are manifested and aging may occur more rapidly than with the general population. The basal metabolic rate or basal energy expenditure decreases approximately 20% between 30 and 90 years of age, calcium content of the skeleton decreases, collagen and elastin become more polymerized, and connective tissue becomes brittle.[110,111] The female hormones, estrogen and progesterone, decline more than do male hormones, thus producing greater osteoporosis in women. Estrogen is found in most foods of plant or animal origin. It is particularly high in soybean oil, palm kernel oil, cabbage, wheat germ, clover, and eggs, but the estrogenic biological activity is only about 1% to 0.1%. Women with high calcium and high estrone levels have significantly greater bone density than women with less estrone and calcium levels.[111] High-density lipoproteins (HDL) and low-density lipoproteins (LDL) may change with age. The LDL is calculated as follows:

$$\text{Cholesterol} - \frac{\text{triglycerides}}{5} - \text{HDL} = \text{LDL}$$

Normal desirable adult values are:

- LDL: 62 to 130 mg/dL
- HDL: 32 to 72 mg/dL
- Cholesterol: 120 to 200 mg/dL
- Triglycerides: 15 to 200 mg/dL
- LDL/HDL: 1.0 to 4.0
- Cholesterol/HDL: 1.9 to 4.2

Values for children can be found in Chapter 54. (Body weight and saturated fat intake appear to be important indicators of cholesterol in children). The lipid and lipoprotein composition of the following is: HDL = 50% protein, 18% cholesterol, 30% phospholipids, and 2% triglycerides: LDL = 25% protein, 43% cholesterol, 23% phospholipids, and 9% triglycerides; VLDL = 13% protein, 15% cholesterol, 12% phospholipids, and 60% triglycerides.

Diets supplemented with eicosapentaenoic (EPA) and docosahexaenoic acid (DHA) from fish oil produce a significant lowering of systolic blood pressure (4.5 mm Hg), but a 4% increase in LDL cholesterol.[112] The stroke-reducing effect of the blood pressure reduction would be expected to outweigh the effect of the rise in cholesterol. Therefore, blood pressure levels should be checked frequently at this age and preferably by self-measurement using a home blood pressure kit (see Appendix 10 for normal adult blood pressure values pathophysiology diagram of obesity and coronary heart disease/stroke risk prediction). Dietary fat appears to be more obesity promoting than carbohydrate in an isocaloric diet.[113] Because obesity is a major problem in the U.S.A. recent research has focused on the use of drug therapy in treatment of obesity in adults. Anorectic drugs such as centrally acting (on opioid receptors, peptide antagonists), thermogenic (adrenergic antagonists) and gastrointestinal (enzyme inhibitors, absorption inhibitors and synthetic foods) are being developed.[114] For example, seritoninergic drugs such as Fluoxetine have been used for weight control and depression[115] while andrenergic agents such as amphetamine have been used to suppress appetite.[116] Gut peptides appear to increase satiety.[117] These drugs, however, should be *carefully studied before use for children* with morbid obesity.

For older persons of both sexes, the kidneys, liver, and pancreas function less efficiently. Overloading the body with sweets may result in insulin deficiency. Sodium intake needs to be reduced since it is 50 times the requirement in the U.S. diet (10,000–20,000 mg versus 200 mg). Chloride measurement may soon become available as a method to check the compliance of the patient on a low sodium diet.[118] Medications stay in the body longer because of less efficient kidney function. The need for protein and calcium is increased.[119] Likewise, folic acid and vitamin B_{12} frequently become deficient. The problems of adolescents, such as alcohol abuse, overmedication, depression or mood disorders, and anorexia, also plague the elderly. (see Appendix 8 for Depression Inventory.) In addition, lactose intolerance, hydration/constipation, and poor oral health may occur, particularly in the disabled older adult. The social ills or institutionalization, or the one fourth who live near poverty and the one third who live alone, compound the nutritional problems of the elderly. Likewise, arthritis and osteoporosis may bring about changes in physical activity and meal preparation. Inappropriate food intake (one third skip meals), reduced mid arm circumference and triceps skinfold, and multiple medications (taken by nearly one half of this population) must be evaluated. Adults with developmental disorders living in group homes need to obtain at least one third of the USRDA in the evening meal especially when working outside the group home. At least 64% of the meals only contained two food groups according to one study. Snacks mainly added calories rather than other nutrients.[120] Carbohydrate overeating has been reported among adults who were mentally retarded and depressed.[121]

Serum albumin appears to be the simplest and best single predictor of mortality and can provide early identification of increased risk of death for this population.[122] Serum albumin does not change, however, for 3–4 weeks. Serum transferrin is more sensitive and has a shorter half-life; but iron deficiency can elevate transferrin so the test must be interpreted carefully (prealbumin may also be used, see biochemical section). Serum transferrin should be repeated every 7–10 days and serum albumin every 3–4 weeks. Electrolytes, calcium, and phosphorus should be checked regularly.[110] If serum albumin and transferrin are normal it is assumed that there is no loss of organ mass or functional impairment.

If malnutrition is identified, protein and calorie assessment are essential. For the hospitalized patient, determining nitrogen balance may be important and should be repeated every 3–4 weeks. If nitrogen balance is positive, 1 gram means a gain of 1 ounce of protoplasm. A negative nitrogen balance of 16 grams means a loss of a pound of muscle, cardiac muscle, or organ tissue. A sample nitrogen balance calculation follows[110]:

Urinary area nitrogen (UUN)—7.8 g/24 hr
Nitrogen intake—70 g protein from TPN
Blood urea nitrogen (BUN)
   Initial—2 mg/dL
   End—9 mg/dL
Weight
   Initial—59 kg
   End—61.5 kg

1. TN_u = (UUN + 1.24) × 1.1
   = (7.8 + 1.24) × 1.1
   = 9.9 g total nitrogen excreted in urine
2. Patient receiving TPN (no oral intake)
   0.017 g nitrogen/kg × kg initial body wt = integumental losses
   0.017 g nitrogen/kg × 59 kg = 1 g nitrogen
3. Initial body water
   59 kg body wt × 0.50 = 29.5 kg water = 29.5 L water
4. Weight change during the 24-hour urine collection
   61.5 kg − 59 kg = 1.5 kg water = +1.5 L water
5. Body water at end of collection
   29.5 L + 1.5 L = 31 L water

6. Urea nitrogen content of the body (initial)
   2 ÷ 100 = 0.020 g/L water
   29.5 L water × 0.020 g UN/L = 0.59 g UN
7. Urea nitrogen content of the body (end)
   9 ÷ 100 = 0.090 g/L water
   31 L water × 0.090 g UN/L = 2.79 g UN
8. Change in urea nitrogen content of the body
   2.79 g UN (end) − 0.59 g UN (initial) = +2.2 g UN (change)
9. Add change in UN content to the nitrogen output
             TN_u = 9.9
     Integumental loss = 1.0
     UN content change = 2.2
                 13.1 g nitrogen output

10. Nitrogen intake = 70 g protein from TPN
   70 ÷ 6.34 = 11.0 g nitrogen
11. Nitrogen balance
   11 − 13.1 = −2.1 g nitrogen/d

where TPN = total parenteral nutrition, TN_u = total urinary nitrogen, and UN = urea nitrogen.

This calculation is explained in more detail below. Obtain blood urea nitrogen (BUN) and body weight at the beginning and end of the 24-hour urine collection. Determine kg of body water by multiplying initial body weight by 50%. Convert kg of water to liters of water (1 kg of weight gain = 1 kg of water = 1 liter of water). This value is the starting total body water. Determine weight gain in kg (ending body weight minus initial body weight) and convert to liters of water. Add this value to the initial body water to obtain the amount present at the end of the study. If body weight decreases during the 24-hour study period, assume this loss is due to loss of fluid. Convert kg of weight into liters of water, but subtract this value from the initial body water. To determine total urea content of the body at the beginning of the urine collection, convert initial BUN from mg/dL to g/L by dividing BUN by 100. Multiply liters of body water at the beginning of the collection by g urea nitrogen/L. To determine urea content of the body at the end of the urine collection, convert BUN at the end of the study from mg/dL to g/L as before. Multiple liters of body water at the end of the collection by g of urea nitrogen/L. Change in urea content of the body is computed by subtraction of the initial body urea from the end value. If the result is positive, add it to the nitrogen output. If the result is negative, assume that the urea nitrogen was excreted via the kidneys and collected during the 24-hour study period.

Energy expenditure is determined indirectly by measuring oxygen consumption. "By also determining carbon dioxide production, the substrate(s) being oxidized can be assessed and the respiratory quotient (RQ) calculated. A caloric equivalent for a liter of oxygen is assigned based on this RQ, resulting in a more accurate measure of energy requirements.[110]

Some of the anthropometric standards and nomograms for adults can be seen in Appendix 10. A loss of one-third of LBM is associated with death due to malnutrition.[110] The total lymphocyte count should be 20% to 40% of the white blood cells (WBC); however, an infection can elevate WBCs and result in a misdiagnosis of nutritional adequacy.[98]

A nutritional assessment for this population includes these five steps:

"*Step 1. Anthropometric evaluation*
   Height

Actual weight
Body frame size
Expected weight range—% expected body weight
Usual weight—% usual body weight
Body composition
    % body fat (sum of four skinfolds)—kg body fat and
      kg lean body mass
Midarm muscle circumference
Triceps skinfold
Upper arm muscle area
Upper arm fat area
Step 2. Biochemical evaluation
Visceral proteins
    Serum albumin
    Serum transferrin
Immunocompetence
    Total lymphocyte count
    Delayed cutaneous hypersensitivity
Step 3. Nutritional diagnosis
Adequate
Marasmus (starvation)
Visceral protein depletion (kwashiorkor)
Marasmus with visceral protein depletion (marasmus-
    kwashiorkor mix)
Step 4. Energy and protein requirements
Harris-Benedict equations basal energy expenditure
    (BEE)
Maintenance
    Oral: BEE × 1.2
    Parenteral: BEE × 1.5
    Anabolic
      Oral: BEE × 1.5
    Parenteral: BEE × 1.75
    Protein requirement = 1.0 to 1.4 g/kg body weight
      Use expected weight if normal weight or obese
      Use actual weight if underweight
Step 5. Evaluation of nutritional therapy
Daily weights
Anthropometric measurements
Laboratory tests
Indirect calorimetry
Nitrogen balance"

An Individual Nutrition Assessment form for this age group
is found in Appendix 10.

Anthropometry, biochemical, and dietary tests provide
information on body fat stores, muscle mass, visceral proteins, and immunocompetence.[123] Assigning the adult the
proper classification or nutritional diagnosis is important. If
visceral proteins, lymphocyte count, and cellular immunity
are moderate or severely depleted, a kwashiorkor state is
noted (*weight* may be normal). If *weight*, creatinine, and
cellular immunity are moderately depleted, a marasmus or
starvation state is noted (*albumin* may be normal). If both
are depleted, it is a mixed state. Since the nutritional status
at the time of admission in the elderly population correlates
with the risk of subsequent complications, even when selected nonnutritional factors are controlled,[123] protein and
caloric intake and weight must be determined when making
a diagnosis (*albumin* and *weight loss* are essential parameters). The nutritional diagnosis should be documented as
well.

Mid-Level Assessment

The midlevel nutritional assessment (Table 4–1) is performed in outpatient clinics, such as the high-risk infant
(Early Intervention), myelomeningocele, and cerebral palsy
clinics at UACCDD. The criteria for referral to these clinics
are shown in Table 4–30. The UACCDD nutritionist par-
ticipates in assessing the nutritional status of children referred for nutrition problems to the clinic. This evaluation
requires about 20 minutes per child as part of the interdisciplinary team assessment or as the nutrition discipline only.[13]
Nutrition record forms for midlevel assessment in the clinics
are shown in Appendix 4.

It is essential to determine calorie, protein, fluid, and
basic nutrient needs and the caregiver's knowledge of calorie
expenditure, nutrition, fiber and fluid needs. Developmental milestones, drug interactions, anthropometry, physical activity, biochemical, physical signs, and socioeconomic
condition should also be assessed. The interpretation or
summary is presented as a subjective-objective-assessment-
plan (SOAP) with recommendations and follow-up. Goals
with a time table and measurement methods are also noted.
A 3-day diet/physical activity diary is collected if the child
is determined to be at high nutritional risk, e.g., if food
summary score is below 10.

Mini-Level Assessment

The mini-level or minimal nutrition assessment is an interdisciplinary evaluation and frequently is performed in the

Table 4–30. Criteria for Nutrition Referral to Specialty Clinics

High-Risk Infant
  Seizure disorder
  Hydrocephalus
  Multiple congenital anomalies
  Chromosomal anomalies
  Condition requiring neurosurgical intervention
  Metabolic disorders
  Fetal drug and alcohol syndromes
  Congenital infectious diseases: STORCH—syphilis,
    toxoplasmosis, rubella, CMV, herpes
  Any question of developmental disorder
Myelomeningocele
  Under 5 years
  Weight above 50th or below 5th percentile or discrepancy in
    height and weight
  Mobility loss greater than 25%
  Mechanical feeding problems
  Premenarcheal adolescent girls
  Certain conditions, such as allergy, diarrhea, excessive use of
    vitamins or medications, or food faddism.
Cerebral Palsy
  Height below the 10th percentile and weight above the 75
    percentile.
  Mobility loss greater than 25%
  Sudden weight loss or gain
  Mechanical or behavioral feeding problems
  Gastrointestinal problems (especially diarrhea or constipation)
  Conditions that affect food intake, such as allergy,
    vegetarianism, low income, food faddism, excessive use of
    vitamins or medications, family problems
  Parents' request for nutrition consultation

community (Table 4–1). The nurse or teacher may evaluate the physical and behavioral condition of the child (see Screening/Mini-Evaluation in Appendix 4) which is often closely related to nutritional status. The nutritionist may obtain information on height and weight and some of the other physical signs noted in the mouth, eyes, hair, skin, and nails. A 100-point food frequency list based on the Basic Four Food Groups with emphasis on whole grains, increased fiber, and high-density nutrients may be used in the mini, midlevel, and in some instances in the in-depth assessment (Appendix 4). The social worker may seek information on food purchasing or preparation while making the home visit. The occupational therapist, dentist, or physician may obtain information on feeding problems. The mini-assessment may also function as a screening device for nutrition problems.

Family-centered care for children with special health care needs as mandated by PL 99-457 is of special importance in the interdisciplinary mini-level evaluation.[104] It is based on teamwork and early intervention. Due to this law which authorizes early intervention programs for infants and toddlers with potential developmental delays, dietitians and nutritionists need more education in pediatric nutrition with developmental disorders (particularly behavioral and feeding skills), cultural diversity, community nutrition, and interdisciplinary teams in order to develop the individualized family service plans.[125–136]

Likewise preschool children appear cognitively ready to learn about food, nutrition, and health and greater effort must be made to educate[137,138] them. (For example, at UACCDD preschool children in the CP classroom receive education on food and nutrition). Nutrition education programs for head start parents also have had a positive effect on the quality of diet for their children.[139] Reliable tools also have been developed to assess and thus prevent or alleviate hunger in children and women.[140] Universal reference standards being established by new research on energy metabolism at the cellular level should provide assistance in future nutritional assessment.[141]

Summary

The nutritional assessment of the child who has a developmental disability or chronic illness has five components: *dietary/physical activity, biochemical, anthropometry, physical signs*, and *feeding*. The level of assessment employed— *in-depth, midlevel, or mini*—depends on the problem, age of the child, and time and expertise available.

The interpretation of the assessment findings or *diagnosis* and the follow-up or *treatment* plan by the nutritionist/dietitian are essential. The nutritionist/dietitian is the key in reducing health care costs by *preventing* nutrition problems or *correcting* these problems early so that the person can develop to his or her full potential.

References

1. Meyer, J. The American Dietetic Association. Position paper on the nutrition component of health care services delivering systems. *J. Am. Diet. Assoc.*, 1971; 58:538.
2. Kennedy, E.T., Kotelchuck, M. The effect of WIC supplemental feeding on birth weight: a case-control analysis. *Am. J. Clin. Nutr.*, 1984; 40:579.
3. *Benefits of Nutrition Services: A Costing and Marketing Approach.* Columbus, OH: Ross Laboratories; 1987. Report of the Seventh Ross Roundtable on Medical Issues.
4. Gilbride, J.A., Cowell, C., Simko, M.D. Overview of nutrition assessment. The process of nutrition assessment. In: Simko, M.D., Cowell, C., Gilbride, J.A., eds.: *Nutrition Assessment: A Comprehensive Guide for Planning Intervention.* Rockville, MD: Aspen Publishers; 1989.
5. Butterworth, C.E., Blackburn, G.L. Hospital malnutrition and how to assess the nutritional status of a patient. *Nutr. Today.* 1975; 10:8.
6. Vazquez, R.M. *Manual of Nutritional Support.* Chicago: Northwestern Memorial Hospital; 1982.
7. Winick, M., Rosso, P., Waterlow, J. Cellular growth of cerebrum, cerebellum, and brain stem in normal and marasmic children. *Exp. Neurol.* 1970; 26:393.
8. Chase, P.H., Martin, H.P. Under-nutrition and child development. *N. Engl. J. Med.* 1970; 282:933.
9. Stock, M.G., Smythe, P.M. Does undernutrition during infancy inhibit brain growth and subsequent intellectual development? *Arch. Dis. Child.* 1963; 38:546.
10. Waterlow, J.C. Classification and definition of protein-energy malnutrition. In: Boston, G.H., Bengoa, J.M., eds. *Nutrition in Preventive Medicine: The Major Deficiency Syndromes, Epidemiology and Approaches to Control.* Geneva: WHO; 1976.
11. Ekvall, S. Nutritional assessment. In: Ekvall, S., Stevens, F.S., eds. *Nutritional Needs of the Handicapped/Chronically Ill Child, Nutrition Assessment, Manual 3.* Cincinnati, OH: University Affiliated Cincinnati Center for Developmental Disorders; 1989.
12. Kerner, J., ed. *Manual of Pediatric Parenteral Nutrition.* New York: Wiley; 1983.
13. Howard, R.B., Herbold, N.H., eds. *Nutrition in Clinical Care.* New York: McGraw-Hill; 1982.
14. Peterson, K., Washington, J.S., Rathburn, J. Team management of failure to thrive. *J. Am. Diet. Assoc.* 1984; 84:810.
15. MacLean, W., deRomana, G., Massa, E., Graham, G. Nutritional management of chronic diarrhea and malnutrition: primary reliance on oral feeding. *J. Pediatr.*, 1980; 97:316.
16. National Research Council. *Recommended Dietary Allowances. 10th ed.*, Washington, DC: National Academy Press; 1989.
17. Queen, P.M., Gallagher, L., eds. *Pediatric Nutrition Handbook.* Boston: Department of Nutrition and Food Service, The Children's Hospital; 1987.
18. Roza, A., Shizgal, H. The Harris-Benedict equation reevaluated: resting energy requirements and body cell mass. 1984; 40:168.
19. Bandini, L., Schoeller, D., Fukagawa, N., Wyhes, L., Dietz, W. Body composition and energy expenditure in adolescents with cerebral palsy and myelodysplasia. *Ped. Res.* 1991; 29:70.
20. Grogan, C., Ekvall, S. The body composition of spina bifida patients as determined by K_{40} urinary creatinine and anthropometric measures. In: *International Union of Nutritional Sciences* and *Publication Committee* of the *Tenth International Congress* of *Nutrition.* Kyoto, Japan: The Science Council of Japan; 1975.
21. Livingstone, B., Prentice, A., Coward, W., Ceesay, S., Strain, J., McKenna, G., Nevin, G., Barker, M., Hickey, R., Simultaneous measurement of free-living energy expenditure by the doubly labeled water method and heart-rate monitoring. *Am. J. Clin. Nutr.* 1990; 52:59.
22. McArdle, W., Katch, F., Katch, V. Nutrition, Diet, and Weight Control. 3rd ed. Philadelphia: Lea & Febiger; 1989.
23. American Diabetes Association. *A Guide for Professionals: The Effective Application of Exchange Lists for Meal Planning.* Chicago: ADA; 1977.
24. McArdle, W., Katch. F., Katch, V. *Energy, Nutrition and Human Performance: Exercise Physiology.* 2nd ed. Philadelphia: Lea & Febiger, 1986.
25. *Surgeon General's Report on Nutrition and Health.* Washington, DC: Government Printing Office; 1988. U.S. Department of Health and Human Services publication 88-50210.
26. Steinbaugh, M.L., Sauls, H.S. *Applying New Technology to Nutrition Assessment.* Ross Laboratories; Columbus, OH: 1989. Report of the Ninth Ross Round Table on Medical Issues.

27. American Academy of Pediatrics. *Pediatric Nutrition Handbook*. 2nd ed. Elk Grove, VIL: American Academy of Pediatrics; 1985.

28. Craig, R.M. Serum albumin as a nutritional marker. *Ann. Intern. Med.* 1987; 106:327.

29. Miller, S.F., Morath, M.A., Finley, R.K. Comparison of derived and actual transferrin: a potential source of error in clinical assessment. *J. Trauma.* 1981; 21:548.

30. Gottschlein, M. Nutritional immunoodeclation. *Dietitians Nutr. Supp. Newsl.* April, 1990; 12.

31. Mullen, J.L., Buzby, G.P., Waldman, M.T., et al. Prediction of operative morbidity and mortality by preoperative nutritional assessment. *Surg. Forum.* 1979; 30:80.

32. Steichen, J., Chen I.W., Disney, T., Minton, S.D., Tsang, R. Bone mineral content (BMC) and 25 hydroxyD in preterm (AGA) and small for gestational age (SGA) infants. *Pediatr. Res.* 1976; 10:415.

33. Cameron, J.R., Sorenson, J.A. Measurement of bone mineral in vivo. An improved method. *Science.* 1963; 142:230.

34. Smith, D.M., Johnston, C.C., Jr., Yu, P.L. In vivo measurement of bone mass. *JAMA* 1972; 219:325.

35. Mazess, R.B., Cameron, J.R., O'Connor, R., Knutsen, D. Accuracy of bone mineral measurements. *Science.* 1964; 145:388.

36. Cameron, J.R., Mazess, R.B., Sorenson, J.A. Precision and accuracy of bone mineral determination by direct photon absorptiometry. *Invest. Radiol.* 1968; 3:9.

37. Mazess, R.B. Estimation of bone and skeletal weight by direct photon absorptiometry. *Invest. Radiol.* 1971; 6:52.

38. Mazess, R.B. Estimation of bone and skeletal weight by direct photon absorptiometry. *Invest. Radiol.* 1971; 6:433.

39. Memma, H.E. Estimation of bone and skeletal weight by direct photon absorptiometry. *Invest. Radiol.* 1971; 6:432.

40. Rauschkolb, E.W., David, H.W., Finsmore, D.C., Black, H.S., Fabre, L.F. Identification of vitamin D_3 in human skin. *J. Invest. Dermatol.* 1969; 53:289.

41. Bishop, C.W., Bowen, P.E., Ritchey, S.J. Norms for nutritional assessment of American adults by upper arm anthropometry. *Am. J. Clin. Nutr.* 1981; 34:2530.

42. *Nutrition Monitoring in the United States*. Washington, DC: Government Printing Office; VSDHHS publication 89-1255-1.

43. Hooley, R. clinical nutritional assessment: a perspective. *J. Am. Diet. Assoc.* 1980; 77:682.

44. Garn, S. The anthropometric assessment of nutritional status. In: Smith, M.A., ed. *Guides for Nutritional Assessment of the Mentally Retarded and the Developmentally Disabled*. Proceedings of the Third National Nutrition Workshop for Nutritionists from University Affiliated Facilities, sponsored by the Bureau of Community Health Services; 1976. The Child Development Center, University of Tennessee Center for Health Sciences, Memphis.

45. Roche, A.F., Davila, G.H. Differences between recumbent length and stature within individuals. *Growth.* 1974; 38:313.

46. Gray, D.S., Crider, J.B., Kelley, C., Dickinson, L.C. Accuracy of recumbent height measurement. *JPEN.* 1985; 9:712.

47. Roche, A.F. Growth assessment of handicapped children. *Ross Diet. Curr.* 1979; 6:25.

48. Chumlea, W.C. Assessing growth and nutritional status of children who are chronically ill or handicapped. In: Ekvall, S., Stevens, F., eds. *Nutritional Needs of the Handicapped/ Chronically Ill Child, Manual III*, Cincinnati: UACCDD; 1989.

49. Burgert, S.L., Anderson, C.F. An evaluation of upper arm measurements used in nutritional assessment. *Am. J. Clin. Nutr.* 1979; 32:2136.

50. Bray, G.A., Greenway, F.L., Molitch, M.E., Dahms, W.T., Atkinson, R.L., Hamilton, K.E. Use of anthropometric measures to assess weight loss. *Am. J. Clin. Nutr.* 1978; 31:769.

51. Bradfield, R.B. Skinfold changes with weight loss. *Am. J. Clin. Nutr.* 1979; 32:1756.

52. Chumlea, W.C., Roche, A.F. Nutritional anthropometric assessment of non-ambulatory persons using recumbent techniques. *Am. J. Phys. Anthrop.* 1984; 63:1.

53. Grant, J.P., Custer, P.B., Thurlow, J. Current techniques of nutritional assessment. *Surg. Clin. North Am.* 1981; 61:437.

54. Lohman, T., Roche, A., Martorell, R. *Anthropometry Standardization Reference Manual*. Champaign, IL: Human Kinetics, Books, 1988.

55. Gurney, J.M., Jelliffe, D.B. Armanthropometry in nutritional assessment: nomogram for rapid calculation of muscle circumference and cross-sectional muscle and fat areas. *Am. J. Nutri.* 1973; 26:913.

56. Heymsfield, S., McManus, C., Smith, J., Stevens, V., Nikon, D. Anthropometric measurement of muscle mass: revised equations for calculating bone-free arm muscle area. *Am. J. Clin. Nutr.* 1982; 36:680.

57. Trowbridge, F., Hiner, C., Robertson, A. Arm muscle indicators and creatinine excretion in children. *A. J. Clin. Nutr.* 1982; 36:691.

58. Bowen, P.E., Custer, P.B. Reference values and age-related trends for arm muscle area, arm fat area, and sum of skinfolds for United States adults. *J. Am. Coll. Nutr.* 1984; 3:357.

59. Engstrom, F.M., Roche, A.F., Mukherjee, D. Differences between arm span and stature in white children. *J. Adolesc. Health.* 1981; 1:19.

60. Belt-Niedbala, B.J., Ekvall, S., Cook, C.M., Oppenheimer, S., Wessel, J. Linear growth measurement: a comparison of single arm-lengths and arm-span. *Develop. Med. Child. Neurol.* 1986; 28:319.

61. Palmer, S., Ekvall, S., eds. *Pediatric Nutrition in Developmental Disorders*. Springfield, IL: Charles Thomas; 1978.

62. Garn, S.M., Silverman, F.N., Rohmann, C.G. A rational approach to the assessment of skeletal maturation. *Ann. Radiol.* 1964; 7:297.

63. Greulich, W.W., Pyle, S.I. *Radiographic Atlas of Skeletal Development of the Hand and Wrist*. 2nd ed. Palo Alto, CA: Stanford University Press; 1959.

64. Hamill, P.V.V., Johnson, C.L., Reed, R.B., Roche, A.F., Moore, W. Physical growth: National Center for Health Statistics percentiles. *Am. J. Clin. Nutr.* 1979; 32:607.

65. Roche, A.F. Himes, H.J. Incremental growth charts. *Am. J. Clin. Nutr.* 1980; 33:2041.

66. Schulz, L.O. Obese, overweight, desirable, ideal. Where to draw the line in 1986. *Am. J. Diet. Assoc.* 1986; 86:1702.

67. Johnston, F.E. Validity of triceps skinfold and relative weight as measures of adolescent obesity. *J. Adoles. Health Care.* 1985; 6:185.

68. Lohman, T. Prediction equations and skinfolds, bioelectric impedance, and body mass index. In: Lohman, T. Advances in Body Composition Assessment. Champaign, IL: Human Kinetics, Books, 1992.

69. Cronk, C.E., Roche, A.F. Race and sex-specific reference data for triceps and subcapular skinfolds and weight/stature^2. *Am. J. Clin. Nutr.* 1982; 35:347.

70. Dine, M., Gartside, P., Glueck, C., Rheins, L., Greene, G., and Khoury, P.: Relationship of head circumference to length in the first 400 days of life. *Pediatrics*, 1981; 67:506.

71. Assessment of nutritional status. In: Forbes, G.B., Woodruff, C.W., eds. *Pediatric Nutrition Handbook* 2nd ed. Elk Grove Village, IL: American Academy of Pediatrics; 1985.

72. Moore, W.M., Roche, A.F., eds. *Pediatric Anthroporietry*, 3rd ed. Columbus, OH: Ross Laboratories; 1987.

73. Jensen, T., Dudrick, S., Johnston, D. A comparison of triceps skinfold and arm circumference values measured in standard supine positions. *JPEN.* 1979; 3:513. Abstract.

74. Heymsfield, S., Waki, M. Body composition in humans: advances in the development of multicompartment chemical models. *Am. J. Clin. Nutr.* 1991; 49:97.

75. Roubenoff, R., Kehayias, J. The meaning of measurement of lean body mass. *Nutr. Rev.* 1991; 49:163.

76. Heymsfield, S., Lickman, S., Baumgartner, R., Wang, J., Kamen, Y., Aliprantis, A., Pierson, R. Body composition of humans: comparison of two improved four compartment models that differ in expense, technical complexity, and radiation exposure. *Am. J. Clin. Nutr.* 1990; 52:52.

77. Hayes, P.A., Sowood, P.J., Belyavin, A., et al. Subcutaneous fat thickness measured by magnetic resonance imaging, ultrasound, and calipers. *Med. Sci. Sports Exerc.* 1988; 20:303.

78. Enzi, G., Gasparo, M., Biondetti, P.R., et al. Subcutaneous and visceral fat distribution according to sex, age, and over-

weight, evaluated by computed tomography. *Am. J. Clin. Nutr.* 1986; 44:739.

79. Seidell, J.C., Bakker, C.J.G., van der Kooy, K. Imaging techniques for measuring adipose-tissue distribution—a comparison between computed tomography and 1.5-T magnetic resonance. *Am. J. Clin. Nutr.* 1990; 51:953.

80. Segal K.R., Van Loan, M., Fitzgerald, P.I., Hodgdon, J.A., Van Itallie, T.B. Lean body mass estimation by bioelectrical impedance analysis: a four-site cross-validation study. *Am. J. Clin. Nutr.* 1988; 47:7.

81. Lukaski, H.C., Bolonchuk, W.W. Theory and validation of the tetrapolar bioelectrical impedance method to assess human body composition. In: Ellis, K.J., Wasumura, S., Morgan, W.D., eds. *In Vivo Body Composition Studies.* London: Institute of Physical Science and Medicine; 1987.

82. Guo, S., Roche, A.F., Houtkooper, L. Fat free mass in children and young adults predicted from bioelectric impedance and anthropometric variables. *Am. J. Clin. Nutr.* 1989; 50:435.

83. Slaughter, M.W., Lohman, T.G., Boileau, R.A., Horwill, C.A., Stillman, R.J., Van Loan, M.D., Bemben, D.A. Skinfold equations for estimations of body fatness in children and youth. *Human Biol.* 1988; 60:709.

84. Jackson, A., Pollock, M. Practical assessment of body composition. *Phys. and Sportsmed.* 1985; 13:76.

85. Golding, L., Meyers, C., Sinning, W. *The Y's Way to Physical Fitness* 3rd ed. Champaign, IL: Human Kinetics, Books; 1989.

86. Houtkooper, L. Cross-validation of prediction equations for children using bioelectric impedance height and weight only. *J. Appl. Physiol.* 1992; 72:366.

87. Houtkooper, L., Lohman, T., Going, S., Hall, M. Validity of bioelectric impedance for body composition assessment in children. *J. Appl. Physiol.* 1989; 66:814.

88. How to diagnose nutritional problems in daily practice. Teaching aid No. 5. *Nutr. Today.* 1969; 4:2.

89. Holmes, T.H. The social readjustment rating scale. *J. Psychosom. Res.* 1967; 11:213.

90. *STAI Manual.* Palo Alto, CA: Consulting Psychologists Press; 1970.

91. Beck, A.T., Ward, C.H., Mendelson, M., et al. An inventory for measuring depression. *Arch. Gen. Psychiatry.* 1961; 4:53.

92. Hutchinson, T.A., Boyd, N.F., Feinstein, A.R. Scientific problems in clinical scales as demonstrated in the Karnofsky index of performance status. *J. Chronic Dis.* 1979; 32:661.

93. Padilla, G.V., Present, C., Grant, M.M., et al Quality of life index for patients with cancer. *Res. Nurs. Health.* 1983; 6:117.

94. Spitzer, W.O., Dobson, A.J., Hall, J., et al. Measuring the quality of life of cancer patients: a concise QL-Index for use by physicians. *J. Chronic Dis.* 1981; 34:585.

95. McNair, D.M., Lorr, M., Droppleman, L.F. *EITS Manual for the Profile of Mood States.* San Diego: Educational and Industrial Testing Service; 1981.

96. Truswell, A.S., Dornton-Hill, I. Food habits of adolescents. *Nutr. Rev.* 1981; 39:73.

97. Elkind, D. *The Hurried Child.* 2nd ed. New York: Addison-Wesley; 1988.

98. Elkind, D. *All Grown Up and No Place To Go.* New York: Addison-Wesley; 1984.

99. Story, M., Blum, R.W. Adolescent nutrition: self-perceived deficiencies and needs of practitioners working with youth. *J. Am. Diet. Assoc.* 1988; 88:591.

100. Carruth, B.R. Nutritional assessment guide for nutrition educators. *J. Nutr. Ed.* 1988; 20:280.

101. Hulanecha, B., Korlarg, F. The final phase of growth in height. *Ann. Human Biol.* 1983; 10:429.

102. Carrol, M.D., Abraham, S., Dresser, C.M. *Vital and Health Statistics.* Series 11-NO. 231. Washington, DC: Government Printing Office; March, 1983. DHHS publication (PHS) 83-1681.

103. Gray, G.E., Gray, L.K. Nutritional aspects of psychiatric disorders. *J. Am. Diet. Assoc.* 1989; 89:1492.

104. Lehmann, H.E. Affective disorders: clinical features. In: Kaplan, H.J., Sadock, B.J., eds. *Comprehensive Textbooks of Psychiatry.* Baltimore: Williams & Wilkins Co.; 1985.

105. Mohs, M., Watson, R., Leonard-Green, T. Nutritional effects of marijuana, heroin, cocaine, and nicotine. *J. Am. Diet Assoc.* 1990; 90:1261.

106. American Dietetic Association Position paper. Nutrition intervention in treatment and recovery from chemical dependency. *J. Am. Diet Assoc.* 1990; 90:1274.

107. Wiecha, J., Dwyer, J., Dunn-Strohecker, M. Nutrition and health services needs among the homeless. *Public Health Reports* 1991; 106:364.

108. Luder, E., Cupens-Okado, E., Karen-Roth, A., Martinez-Weber, C. Health and nutrition survey in a group of urban homeless adults. *J. Am. Diet Assoc.* 1990; 90:1387.

109. McKinney, L. Palmer, C., Dwyer, J., Garcia, R. Managing dentally related nutrition concerns of children with special needs: Part 2. *Top. Clin. Nutr.* 1991; 6:76.

110. Shuran, M., Nelson, R. Updated nutritional assessment and support of the elderly. *Geriatrics.* 1986; 41:48.

111. Anderson, J.B. Dietary calcium and bone mass through the life cycle. *Nutr. Today.* 1990; 2:9.

112. Kestin, M., Clifton, P., Belling, G.B., Nestel, P.J. n-3 Fatty acids of marine origin lower systolic blood pressure and triglycerides but raise LDL cholesterol compared with n-3 and n-6 fatty acids from plants. *Am. J. Clin. Nutr.* 1990; 51:1028.

113. Datillo, A.M. Dietary fat and its relationship to body weight. *Nutrition Today* 1992; 27:13.

114. Bray, G. Drug treatment of obesity. *Am. J. Clin. Nutr.* 1992; 55:538S.

115. Wise, S., Clinical studies with fluoxetine in obesity. *Am. J. Clin. Nutr.* 1992; 55:181S.

116. Wellman, P. Overview of adrenergic anorectic agents. *Am. J. Clin. Nutr.* 1992; 55:1935.

117. Bray, G. Peptides affect the intake of specific nutrients and the sympathetic nervous system. 1992; 55:265S.

118. Dubbert, P., Rowland, A., Maury, P., Liggert, V., Terre, L., Krug, L. Estimation of sodium intake by analyzing food records with augmented nutrition software and by overnight urine collections. *J. Am. Diet Assoc.* 1992; 92:87.

119. Cauley, J.A., Gutai, J.P., Kuller, L.H., LeDonne, P., Sandler, R.B., Sashnin, D., Powell, J.G. Endogenous estrogen levels and calcium intakes in postmenopausal women. Relationships with cortical bone measures. *JAMA* 1988; 260:3150.

120. Mercer, K., Ekvall, S. Comparing the diets of adults with mental retardation in intermediate care facilities and in group homes. *J. Am. Diet Assoc.* 1992; 92:356.

121. O'Brien, G., Whitehouse, A. A psychiatric study of deviant eating behavior among multiply handicapped adults. *Br. J. Psychiatry* 1990; 157:281.

122. Agarval, W., Acevedo, F., Leighton, L.S., Coyten, G.D., Pitchumoni, C.S. Predictive ability of various nutritional variables for mortality in elderly people. *Am. J. Clin. Nutr.* 1988; 48:1173.

123. Sullivan, D.H., Patch, G.A., Walls, R.C., Lipschitz, P.A. Impact of nutrition status on morbidity and mortality in a select population of geriatric rehabilitation patients. *Am. J. Clin. Nutr.* 1990; 51:749.

124. Gooder, J.B., Ekvall, S. Extension of health and nutrition services via advanced telecommunications. *J. Am. Diet. Assoc.* 1989; 89:821.

125. Wodarski, L.A. Nutrition intervention in developmental disabilities: an interdisciplinary approach. *J. Am. Diet. Assoc.* 1985; 85:218.

126. U.S. Department of Health and Human Services, *Healthy People 2000* National Health Promotion and Disease Prevention Objectives, DHHS Publication No. (PHS) 91-50212, Superintendent of Documents, U.S. Government Printing Office, Washington D.C., 1990.

127. Maternal and Child Health Bureau *Call to Action: Better Nutrition for Mothers, Children and Families*, Washington D.C., National Center for Education in Maternal and Child Health, 38 and R Streets, 1991.

128. Maternal and Child Health Bureau. *Development of Community-Based Service Systems By State CSHCN Programs Guidance Material with Comments.* Washington, D.C., National Center for Education in Maternal and Child Health, 1991.

129. Randall, D.E. *Strategies for Working with Culturally Diverse Communities and Clients.* Bowman Gray School of Medicine and Comprehensive Hemophilia Program, Washington, D.C.,

National Center for Education in Maternal and Child Health, 1991.

130. Kaufman, M. Are dietitians prepared to work with handicapped infants? P.L. 99-457 offers new opportunities. *J. Am. Diet Assoc.* 1989; 89:1604.

131. Hine, R.J., Cloud, H.H., Carithers, T., Hickey, C., and Hinton, A.W. Early nutrition intervention services for children with special health care needs. *J. Am. Diet Assoc.* 1989; 89:1636.

132. American Dietetic Association: Nutrition services for children with special health care needs. *J. Am. Diet Assoc.* 1989; 89:1133.

133. Lucas, B.L. Interdisciplinary nutrition training: Children with special health care needs. *Top. Clin. Nutr.* 1990; 5:24.

134. Thompson, M.L., and Smith, M.A., eds. 1987 Update: *Guidelines for Nutrition Training in University Affiliated Programs.* Memphis, University of Tennessee, Child Development Center, 1987.

135. Palmer, C., Dwyer, J., Clark, E. Planning for continuing education: perceived training needs of public health nutritionists in management of children with special health care needs. *J. Nutr. Ed.* 1991; 23(6):291.

136. Position of the American Dietetic Association: Nutrition in comprehensive program planning for persons with developmental disabilities. *J. Am. Diet. Assoc.* 1992; 92:613.

137. Singleton, J., Achterberg, C., Shannon, B. Role of nutrition in the health perceptions of young children. *J. Am. Diet Assoc.* 1992; 92:67.

138. Conclusions, guidelines and recommendations from the IUNS/WHO workshop: nutrition in the pediatric age group and later cardiovascular disease. *J. Am. Col. Nutr.* 1992; 11:1S.

139. Koblinsky, S., Guthrie, J., Lynch, L. Evaluation of a nutrition education program for head start parents. *J. Nutr. Ed.* 1992; 24:4.

140. Rodimer, K., Olson, C., Green, J., Campbell, C., Habicht, J. Understanding hunger and developing indicators to assess it in women and children. *J. Nutr. Ed.* 1992; 24:365.

141. Kinney, J.M., Tucker, H.N. *Energy Metabolism. Tissue Determinants and Cellular Correlaries.* New York: Raven Press, 1992.

Chapter 5
Nutrition in Community-Based Programs and Nutrition Resources

Cecilia Rokusek, Ann Prendergast, and Shirley Walberg Ekvall

Nutrition in Community-Based Programs

Within the last 25 years the field of developmental disabilities has changed significantly. According to PL 98-52, the Developmental Disabilities Act of 1984, a developmental disability is a severe, chronic disability of a person which: (1) is attributable to a mental or physical impairment or combination of mental or physical impairments; (2) manifests before age 22; (3) is likely to continue indefinitely; (4) results in substantial functional limitations in three or more of the following areas of major life activity—self-care, reception and expressive language, learning, mobility, self-direction, capacity for independent living and economic self sufficiency; and (5) reflects the need for a combination and sequence of special interdisciplinary or generic care, treatment, or other services which are lifelong or of extended duration, and are individually planned and coordinated. Deinstitutionalization, integrated community living programs, supported employment options, and least restrictive learning environments have been the new directions employed to reach the overarching goals of independence, productivity, and integration of persons with developmental disabilities. These new directions have placed an additional challenge on the nutrition professional, who now must work not only in the traditional clinical and institutional settings but also in the community environment, serving all age groups from those in preschool programs to those living in independent elderly apartment dwellings. In addition, the qualified nutritionist must become a key player in interdisciplinary healthcare delivery, planning for the ongoing nutritional needs of the person with developmental disabilities who is being served within the community setting. This chapter (1) presents an overview of nutrition services in the community, (2) identifies potential resources to use within the community, (3) presents financing options for nutrition services, and (4) provides an overview of quality assurance programs and standards established to monitor nutrition services within the community setting.

Because nutritional needs of the person with developmental disabilities vary and the skills required to meet those nutrition needs are also different, there is an increased significance to the interdisciplinary role of the nutrition professional. It is essential that the nutritionist in developmental disabilities work with the (1) parents or primary caregivers; (2) physicians; (3) allied health professionals (i.e., nurses, occupational therapists, speech clinicians, or physical therapists); (4) food service personnel (in a school setting); (5) teachers; and (6) health care financing agencies (i.e., insurance companies and federal and state entitlement programs).

For the population with developmental disabilities, nutrition can serve both a preventive and restorative role. The community setting provides challenges in meeting this dual goal, particularly when health professionals, such as registered dietitians, are not available on a daily basis. Most community-based programs depend upon nutrition consultants to provide the direction and clinical expertise for the nutrition services provided. The consultant must assure that the ongoing nutritional needs are identified and met through his or her leadership. Private accreditation agencies, as well as state and federal standards, have developed quality assurance guides for community programs, including schools.

Funding for nutrition services in community agencies is a complex issue. The need for third party reimbursement and adequate funding for nutrition services must be addressed. The resources available for nutrition services, both in personnel and materials, such as feeding equipment and special formula diets, must also be considered. These resources must be readily available for registered dietitians working in the community. Ongoing training must be provided at the preservice and inservice levels for these nutrition professionals. Appropriate consultation models and additional resources for dietitians in community settings still need to be developed. With these needs met, nutritionists can make a significant contribution to the success and overall productivity, independence, and integration of persons with developmental disabilities within the community setting.

Resources

The impact of nutrition services for persons with developmental disabilities is ongoing and lifelong. Nutrition services for the special needs infant, child, adolescent, or adult should be integrated fully throughout the individual education and/or habilitation plan. Within the school system, this mandate is outlined clearly in Public Law 99-142, the Education for the Handicapped Children's Act enacted in 1975. It mandates that all public schools provide education in the least restrictive setting based on an interdisciplinary evaluation for all handicapped children. Nutrition services, when needed, must be provided through the school system by trained and qualified professionals. Because of the increasing number of medically fragile and technology-dependent children who are being fully integrated into the public schools, the role of the registered dietitian in the school system must be expanded. Unfortunately, many schools do not employ a qualified nutrition professional, despite the need for the services and the implied mandate to service through PL 94-142.

Public Law 99-457 (102–119 in 1992), enacted in 1986, provides another opportunity for the early involvement of registered dietitians in meeting the challenging nutrition needs of the population aged birth through 5 years in a family-centered team approach.[1-3] Parents and caregivers must be informed of all the interdisciplinary services available as a result of PL 99-457 (102–119). The purposes of PL 99-457 (102–119) are to

- ensure that children with disabilities and chronic illness are identified as early as possible
- make referral to an appropriate services agency or treatment facility
- ensure that individual children are not "lost" to the service system
- determine future personnel needs
- understand developmental outcomes of children who have risk factors
- understand developmental outcomes of children who were differently managed in different care systems
- identify personnel training needs

This legislation provides a basis for early nutrition intervention and transitional planning as follows:

In meeting the purposes of PL 99-457 (102–119), nutrition professionals may be called upon to work in schools; hospitals; Head Start programs, child care settings; early periodic screening, diagnosis, and treatment programs (EPSDT), and state interagency councils. These councils provide the direction and coordinated plan for the state's future work with the preschool population.[4] While working in these community settings, nutritionists need to use such programs as the Special Supplemental Food Program for Women, Infants, and Children (WIC), Maternal and Child Health Specialty Clinics, and University-Affiliated Programs (UAP).[5]

More interdisciplinary training is needed to inform health care administrators about the impact of good nutrition on children with developmental disorders or a chronic illness (children with special health care needs). Three university-affiliated programs (Cincinnati, Los Angeles, and Birmingham) have been funded to provide interdisciplinary training in nutrition awareness for this population annually at each program site for 5 years. Manuals on program planning,[6] clinical nutrition,[7] and nutritional assessment[8] and 35 video- or audiotapes from an earlier 5-year program for children with special needs have been developed at the University Affiliated Program at the Cincinnati Center for Developmental Disorders (UAPCCDD). These training materials can be disseminated widely through advanced telecommunications technology using a personal computer or terminal. Two-way, interactive television created by a microwave telecommunications system and videoimaging by telephone, as well as by computer, will also be available in the near future.[9]

School-aged children and adolescents with special needs may also require specialized nutrition services. PL 99-142 mandates that public schools provide free and appropriate education in the least restrictive environment for all handicapped children. As a result of this 1976 legislation and with the emphasis on the "least restrictive environment" during the late 1980's, many, and ultimately all, handicapped and chronically ill children can enroll in public schools and participate in the National School Lunch and School Breakfast Programs. Therefore, school lunch programs must provide special needs children and adolescents with the assistance they need to meet their dietary needs so they can participate fully in the educational process.

In 1984, South Dakota conducted a survey of school lunch directors to assess their attitudes, knowledge, and needs regarding the preparation of meals to meet the special feeding and nutrition needs of handicapped children as mandated by PL 94-142. Attitudes of school lunch directors were favorable toward meeting the nutrition and feeding needs of handicapped children, but knowledge of how to do so was limited. This lack of knowledge was substantiated by the directors' failure to identify the actual nutritional needs of the handicapped children.[10] As a result of this survey, the South Dakota Department of Education worked with the nutrition staff of the South Dakota University Affiliated Program (SD UAP) to develop a *Nutrition and Feeding for the Developmentally Disabled How-To Manual.*[11]

In 1986 the Virginia Division of Children's Specialty Services in the Department of Health surveyed special education directors in the state to investigate the number of children requiring special feeding procedures or diets during the school day and the availability of nutrition services for these children. The Virginia survey identified the need for increased training and support for school personnel so nutrition services for students with special health care needs could be integrated more fully into the school curriculum.[12] As a result of this study, Virginia developed an interagency teaching and staff development program of the state health and education departments to develop nutrition services for handicapped children within the school system. The Virginia project was developed with a three-fold purpose:

1. to increase awareness and knowledge of the nutritional needs of handicapped and chronically ill children
2. to create networks among families of handicapped children
3. to initiate ongoing nutrition programs for school-aged handicapped children.

Its ultimate goal is to improve the health of handicapped and chronically ill school children by identifying, controlling, and resolving their nutrition problems.

Achievement of this goal in any school must be dependent on interagency collaboration and family involvement at the preschool, elementary, and secondary levels. Nutrition professionals must be advocates for their services in the educational setting.

A myriad of community-focused nutrition resources for all age groups, although primarily for children, have developed over the last 10 years (Table 5–1). Nutrition services for adults with developmental disabilities are provided through the Medicaid legislation by federal and state funds. Effective resources have been those that could be integrated into an agency's total plan for education and health services. Appropriate preparation for registered dietitians to work in community settings with the special needs population remains a problem at both the preservice and inservice level. Interdisciplinary nutrition training programs at several University Affiliated Programs, such as those at Cincinnati, Los Angeles, and Birmingham, have provided valuable training in the 1980's for nutrition and other professionals to work more effectively with this special needs population.

Table 5-1. Nutrition Services for Children with Special Needs

The competencies listed in this document describe assessment, intervention and follow-up service provided by nutritionists skilled in the delivery of nutrition services to high-risk children. Such individuals will have been credentialed by the Commission on Dietetic Registration of the American Dietetic Association and be a registered dietitian (RD). They will have received specialized training and be involved in continuing education addressing the needs of children "at risk."

DIRECT CARE SERVICE

I. Assessment
  A. Nutritional Status
    1. Collect and interpret anthropometric and growth data.
    2. Assess clinical status with special attention to problems affecting nutritional status; define the need to refer.
    3. Assess dietary intake.
    4. If appropriate, collect feeding history which may affect current food intake.
    5. Collect and/or assess the need to collect biochemical data.
    6. Collect medication information which may affect nutrient needs.
    7. Collect data regarding mobility status and physical activity.
  B. Feeding Skills
    1. Assess feeding skill development considering present level of function to determine normal vs. delayed feeding skills.
    2. Assess oral motor development to determine normal, delayed, or pathological development and the need for referral to appropriate therapy.
    3. Evaluate appropriateness of food textures offered, based on feeding development.
  C. Feeding Behavior
    1. Collect caregiver-child interaction information; if appropriate, observe feeding.
    2. Define noneating behaviors (throwing food, refusing to eat, gagging, etc.) which affect nutrient intake.
    3. Define eating behaviors (pica, using fingers/utensils appropriately, stuffing food in mouth, etc.) which affect feeding skill development.
  D. Feeding Environment
    1. Evaluate feeding environment, i.e., equipment, timing of meals and snacks, sanitation and safety.
    2. Assess caregiver's knowledge of food sources/appropriate foods for child.
    3. Assess caregiver's economic ability to provide food for child and use of available resources.
  E. Caregiver's Expectations
    1. Evaluate the appropriateness of caregiver's expectations for feeding skills.
    2. Evaluate appropriateness of caregiver's expectations for quantity of food the child should consume.
II. Develop Nutrition Care Plan
III. Counseling and Consultation
  A. Counsel caregiver regarding:
    1. Improving nutrient deficiencies/excesses through food sources and/or supplements;
    2. Feeding skills and appropriate foods to support developmental progress;
    3. Management of feeding behaviors;
    4. Improvement of feeding environment within framework of individual's need, socio-economic status, and lifestyle.
  B. Provide consultation to health care professionals (therapists, M.D., public health nurse, etc.) in methods of improving the child's nutrient and energy intake as in "A" above.
  C. Make referrals to appropriate health professionals and health care agencies.
  D. Participate in interagency and interdisciplinary team conferences to determine priorities for therapy, follow-up and referral.
IV. Monitor effectiveness of nutrition care plan and counseling; follow-up as needed.

AGENCY AND CONSULTATIVE SERVICES

I. Nutrition Education
  A. Collect and evaluate materials on nutrition and feeding for use by families, caregivers and other health professionals.
  B. Develop, arrange, conduct and evaluate nutrition education programs for health professionals and the public.
II. Policy Making and Program Planning
  A. Identify individuals at nutritional risk by soliciting consumer and professional input.
  B. Assess nutrition and diet related health problems in the community.
  C. Plan or participate in planning, developing, implementing and evaluating the nutrition components of community programs.
  D. Consult with Group centers or health agencies regarding nutrition standards and nutrition care criteria.

This document was prepared by the participants of the first short-term Nutrition and Handicapped Children Training Program of the Child Development and Mental Retardation Center, University of Washington. These activities were supported by the State of Washington Department of Social and Health Services, Bureau of Parent-Child Health Services (sponsoring number 1640-67510).

The model for the provision of services at the community level—in Head Start Programs, schools, and adult service agencies—is primarily the consultation model. However, the increased role of nutrition services in the community delivery system may require more full-time registered dietitians in the future. In general, nutrition professionals within community settings should strive to

- be an *advocate* for nutrition services and strive for their incorporation throughout the interdisciplinary planning process for an individual requiring special nutrition and feeding intervention
- provide the leadership in the development, implementation, and ongoing evaluation of an integrated nutrition services component
- work to develop an agency-specific nutrition program and manual outlining program requirements and policy standards.
- provide ongoing technical assistance and in-service training in nutrition to other interdisciplinary staff
- work closely with state and private accreditation agencies on quality assurance

In addition to providing direct services via consultation or full-time delivery, nutrition professionals in community settings must continually plan and provide education programs for other health care professionals within their community environment, such as teachers, administrators, physicians, nurses, and occupational and physical therapists. These individuals can promote nutrition services and can facilitate the successful delivery of nutrition services by their understanding of it.

Community nutrition programs at all levels must include the following components:

- screening
- complete assessment
- development of nutrition care plans through an individual education plan (IEP) or individual habilitation plan (IHP)
- implementation of a nutrition care plan by an interdisciplinary team, including parents/guardians when appropriate
- nutrition counseling focusing on the individual with special needs and his or her ability to follow through on the recommendations made
- follow-up and referral to other community agencies when appropriate

Referral to other community resources presents a real challenge. For example, overweight adults with Down syndrome most appropriately should join local weight loss groups, rather than be put in a segregated one-on-one weight loss program or a group program only for persons with developmental disabilities. All community resources should be identified carefully so that a comprehensive and fully integrated nutrition program can be delivered by the most appropriate agency or school.

Community resources for nutrition services, training, and technical assistance are found on the local, state, regional, and federal levels. Specific federal programs that can assist agencies and nutrition professionals in meeting the nutrition challenges of persons with handicaps and special health needs—the medically fragile or chronically ill—include the following:

- The National School Lunch Program helps child care centers (including Head Start preschool programs), school systems, and community-based programs for adults provide nutritious and well-balanced meals. Governmental food commodities provided through the U.S. Department of Agriculture, reduce the costs of overall meal preparation to the schools. Other programs included in the umbrella school lunch program include the School Breakfast Program, Child Care Food Program, Summer Feeding Program, and the Special Milk Program.
- The Women, Infants, and Children (WIC) program is a federally funded food program initiated in 1974 and designed to improve the nutrition status of low-income pregnant and post partum women and preschool children up to age 5 who are at nutritional risk. Nutrition education, health care referral, and supplemental food items are provided through this program.
- Food stamps, as is WIC, is an entitlement program designed to aid low-income individuals by enabling them to purchase supplemental food items through food coupons. Both WIC and food stamps are resources for families or individuals in need because of a lack of money resulting from an ongoing disabling and/or medical condition that is not totally covered by a financing or reimbursement system. In addition, adults with special needs who live independently may need one of the supplemental programs until they are fully employed.
- The Expanded Food and Nutrition Education Program (EFNEP) provides grants to land-grant universities to assist counties in developing programs to improve the nutrition status of special needs families. This program is not used often by eligible familes with a handicapped child. It may provide nutrition education and special meal planning ideas.
- The Head Start program provides special nutrition services through a qualified nutrition professional. Approximately 10% of the children in Head Start Programs have handicaps.
- Maternal and Child Health Services, funded under Title V of the Social Security Act, provides intervention and prevention nutrition services through clinics, education programs, and research. An early childhood intervention program established in 1991 (Parent-Child Centers) provides comprehensive services (health, social, and education) for children under 3 years of age.
- University Affiliated Programs (UAPs), with core federal support from Maternal and Child Health and/or the Administration on Developmental Disabilities, provide state-of-the-art training for nutrition professionals at the preservice (undergraduate and graduate) and in-service (working professionals) levels to work with children and adults who have developmental disabilities and/or chronic health problems. In addition, UAPs with a nutrition component provide ongoing service, technical assistance, state-of-the-art information, and research to professionals, parents, and consumers.
- Through the Title VII Nutrition Program, elderly individuals, especially those in need, can receive low-cost, nutritious meals in community settings where they can also receive social and rehabilitative services. This program, often referred to as the Congregate Meal Program, provides an excellent opportunity for elderly persons with developmental disabilities to be integrated more fully into the community with other elderly persons.

Funding

Nutrition services have always been considered an important component of health care dating to ancient Greece, when physicians identified food as a source of good health and healing ability. Nutrition services were initiated in public health programs in the 1920s with the passage of the Maternity and Infant Act. The Social Security Act in 1935 further expanded nutrition services in state health agecies. In the 1950s and 1960s federal funding for specialized programs for chronic disease, maternal and infant care, child health, and mental retardation resulted in a significant increase in the direct provision of nutrition services by nutrition personnel. Federal initiatives in comprehensive state and federal health planning and primary health care further increased the scope and coverage of nutrition services during the 1970s.[13]

These programs placed an emphasis on improving the nutritional status of pregnant women, infants, children, and adults through nutritional screening and assessment, dietary counseling and treatment, nutrition education, follow-up, referral, and, in some cases, the direct provision of food. For the past two decades, Maternal and Child Health (Title V) programs have focused on the role of nutrition in contributing not only to the overall health of a person with developmental disabilities but also in preventing other health problems and developmental disabilities in future generations.

Appropriate and ongoing nutrition services within the community setting for persons with developmental disabilities can not only enhance the quality of life for individuals but can also save money by bringing about overall health improvement.[14,15] Nutrition services are a cost-effective strategy for health maintenance.[16]

To support all nutrition service activities and to provide a full complement of nutrition professionals and the necessary support staff requires that nutrition services be adequately and fairly reimbursed. Obtaining funding for nutrition services in the community setting is a complex and challenging task. To provide an adequate funding base, agencies must obtain resources from multiple funding sources, including education, medicine, social services, human services, and insurance carriers. Table 5–2 provides an overview of the primary funding or resource options available to community agencies.

For many of these funding sources, states can determine, with federal approval, the eligibility requirements and the funding service options. Therefore, nutrition professionals must be advocates for the inclusion of nutrition services throughout the special needs delivery system. Funding for children is closely tied to Maternal and Child Health resources and education programs. Funding for adults comes primarily from the Medicaid system. Children with special needs may also use Medicaid funds if they meet the individual state guidelines.

Dollars appropriated for Intermediate Care Facilities for the Mentally Retarded (ICF-MR) have been the usual reimbursement source for most community and institutional settings. All health care needs, including nutrition,[17] as identified by the interdisciplinary team, are reimbursable through ICF-MR. The Home and Community Based Services (HCBS) waiver replaces the ICF-MR and focuses on the needs of an individual within a community. Usually individuals on the HCBS waiver are not as medically fragile or in need of ongoing and daily medical attention as those in institutions. The system is moving more in the direction of providing a waiver for each individual in need. Food cannot be purchased with waiver dollars, but needed nutrition and feeding services may be reimbursable. Special care during a period of hospitalization is covered by Medicaid when an individual is on a waiver.

In addition to the established reimbursement sources, nutrition professionals should be aware of other funding sources as well. On the state level, there are state block grants, such as those in social services and health. In addition, state general funds to specific departments can be allocated for

special needs, such as nutrition training programs for handicapped children and adults; advocacy again becomes critical in obtaining these funds. In community settings, such as clinics or special weight loss groups, a sliding fee may be established for persons with developmental disabilities, with the subsidy provided by state agencies or insurance companies. If a fee for services is established, third party reimbursement is a viable option when a registered dietitian is providing the nutritional services ordered by a physician. Third party reimbursement provided by insurance carriers represents a significant financing option for the future. State departments will need to use third party carriers for funding their services, including nutrition, to supplement federal and state financing programs.

The implementation of reimbursement based on diagnosis-related groupings (DRGs) together with rising medical costs, requires that such services as nutrition be planned and implemented carefully to ensure adequate reimbursement in hospital, institutional, and community settings. Although DRGs are not yet used in pediatric care, the registered dietitian should examine closely the fees for nutrition services. Those working with persons who have developmental disabilities and/or handicapping conditions need to maintain records of their actual time spent in assessment, counseling, follow-up, and planning. These time records provide justification for salaries as well as the need for additional professional staff.

Medicaid funding is the most direct avenue for reimbursement of nutrition services. Each state designs its own system to allow for reimbursement of specific health-related areas, such as nutrition. Recent changes in the legislation mandate Medicaid coverage for children under age 6 whose families have incomes below 133% of the poverty level, with the option to cover children up to age 19 in families with incomes below 100% of poverty.[12] The expansion of Medicaid-covered services for pregnant women and children, which includes more services for Early and Periodic Screening, Diagnosis, and Treatment, increases the need for nutrition services.

The WIC Reauthorization Act of 1989 (PL 101-147) enhances WIC services for the homeless, increases coordination with Medicaid and Maternal and Child Health, strengthens the emphasis on breastfeeding, and modifies the WIC food package to reflect current U.S. dietary Guidelines. It also provided a $223 million increase in funding for Fiscal year 1992.[18,19]

An example of a state-run Medicaid-funded project, in which nutrition services play a key role, is the High-Risk Channeling Project (HRCP) of South Carolina. HRCP provides risk assessment, high-risk perinatal care, social work services, nutrition services, and case management to pregnant women and their infants up to 1 year after birth.[12,20] To qualify for this project, the woman or infant must meet the high-risk criteria and be Medicaid eligible. The Health and Human Services Finance Commission, as the state Medicaid agency, is responsible for developing Medicaid policies and for administering financial components of this program.

A comprehensive nutrition assessment must be completed on all HRCP patients. It must be performed by a registered dietitian or by a nutritionist who is eligible to be registered by the American Dietetic Association. The nutritional assessment process and follow-up encounters must be indi-

Table 5–2. Financing Structure for Nutrition Services

I.

TITLE XIX-Medicaid
(Authorized through Social Security Act)
Administered by
Health Care Financing Administration (HCFA)

All Ages

Intermediate Care Facilities for the Mentally Retarded (ICF-MR) (may or may not be institution based)	Home and Community Based Waiver (HCBS) Must be noninstitutional; (food cannot be purchased with this money)

Eligibility includes all those who are eligible and receiving SSI (aged, blind, and disabled). Also can include others as determined by individual states with approval of federal governmental regulation agency (HCFA).

II.

Education Dollars

1) Through PL 99-457 (Education of the Handicapped, Amendment, 1986) nutrition services may be identified as a needed reimbursable service. 2) Head Start programs provide nutrition services.	Through PL 94-142 (Education for all Handicapped Students Act, 1976) the provision of a free and appropriate education for all students may include nutrition services when needed.

School lunch should be provided to all students, including those with special needs.

III

Social Services Block Grant Money

All Ages

Individual states can determine what services can be purchased for special needs (nutrition may not be included; only "non-institutional types of services)

IV

Maternal and Child Health*
(Funded through Title V of the Social Security Act)

Through the provision of nutrition services at the state level and through specialty clinics such as PKU, spina bifida, Down's syndrome, etc. persons gain access to specialized nutrition services and resources.

V.

Entitlement Programs*
(income dependent)

Women-Infant, and Children Supplemental Feeding Program (Both programs should contain nutrition education provided by a qualified nutrition professional.	Food Stamp program

*These programs are administered through various agencies from state to state.
From C. Rokusek, 1989, South Dakota University Affiliate Program, USD School of Medicine, Vermillion, SD.

vidual, face-to-face encounters with the patient and be documented by completing the nutrition assessment form in the patient's record. The number of follow-up visits are dictated by the identified nutritional problems and planned interventions as noted on the initial assessment. Medicaid reimbursement for nutrition services is completed by documenting staff time to the agency personnel cost-accounting system and by the chart recording activities.

In summary, financing for nutrition services can come from (1) federal funding, such as special appropriation dollars or grants; (2) state and local funding; (3) medicaid funding; (4) insurance companies; (5) individual consumer payment on a sliding fee schedule; and (6) entitlement support programs, such as WIC or food stamps.

Quality Assurance Programs and Standards

The term "quality assurance" came into widespread use after the Professional Standards Review Organization (PSRO) legislation (PL 92-603) was passed in 1972. This legislation required that the Maternal and Child Health (MCH), Medicare, and Medicaid programs evaluate the quality and cost of health care services provided through their funds. The PSRO regulations are as equally concerned with the cost of care, as with its quality. However, after passage of the legislation, health care professionals began writing criteria measuring the quality of care that reflected their concerns not only about the delivery of services as professional judgment and the "state-of-the-art" required but also that patients improved as a result.

The American Dietetic Association defines quality assurance (QA) as "the certification of continuous, optimal, effective, and efficient health and nutrition care."[13,21] Within a health care system, QA is an ongoing problem-solving vehicle that is "a system organized and administered by health practitioners and consumers designed to certify continuous, optimal, effective, and efficient health and nutrition care with appropriate corrective action whenever a performance deficiency or discrepancy is identified."[22]

In the field of developmental disabilities, QA measures for nutrition programs and services come primarily from state health, social service, and human service agencies; state developmental disabilities and mental retardation programs; private nonprofit agencies. Components of state QA programs vary from state to state. For example, New Hampshire, New York, Tennessee, and Texas have developed state-specific standards, QA measures and ongoing program monitoring. In addition, the Head Start program has developed a set of performance standards and QA measures that can be used in program monitoring of nutrition services.

Two private nonprofit organizations have established standards for a national QA program for agencies—both institutional and community-based—serving persons with developmental disabilities. The Accreditation Council for Services for People with Developmental Disabilities (ACDD), with its early roots in the American Association of Mental Deficiency (AAMD) Review Standards developed in 1952, has developed and published standards for professionals, including nutritionists, and lay people who represent both providers and recipients of services in MR/DD programs.[23] These standards, which are revised every 2 years, reflect services for the individual focusing on individual empowerment and control. Standards emphasize the development of a nutrition plan ensuring that individual needs and preferences are met. There are approximately 150 ACDD-accredited agencies in the United States. Full accreditation is for a 2-year period. The review is conducted by an outside professional team.

The Commission on Accreditation of Rehabilitation Facilities (CARF) reviews and accredits rehabilitation/habilitation organizations and programs.[24] CARF was organized in 1966 and presently has accredited more than 2480 agencies that include infant and childhood development, vocational, respite community mental health, and psychosocial programs; drug abuse centers; and rehabilitation facilities, among its standards review for 19 individual programs or services. Reviews of individual agencies are conducted by peers. The CARF standards manual is revised and published yearly. Standards focus on the provision of comprehensive assessment, planning, intervention, training, and follow-up when needed by qualified nutrition professionals.

Although many states have developed individual standards for various service classifications—health, social services, mental retardation, developmental disabilities, etc.—some have adopted QA components from federal nonprofit accrediting bodies, such as ACDD and CARF, and these agencies have in turn adopted components from state agencies. The key aspect of this shared influence is the input of professionals from individual discipline areas into the ongoing review and development of standards.

Qualified nutrition professionals must be knowledgeable of these standards and their ongoing revision. They can play a critically important role as advocates in the standards development process.

Summary

Schools, communities, local, state, and federal programs, and private agencies serving persons with developmental disabilities must develop appropriate, comprehensive, and effective nutrition programs that are responsive to the diverse needs of that population. Services must be designed to be both restorative and preventive. Challenges for the qualified nutritionist lie in (1) advocacy for appropriate nutrition services in the community, (2) the development of interdisciplinary team leadership in family-centered care, (3) the incorporation of new models of service delivery—in the home, in the school, etc.—by use of teleconferencing and fiberoptic communications,[9] and (4) the development of creative financing structures to provide long-term nutrition services for the uninsured and/or underinsured.

A variety of resources inside and outside an agency need to be used not only to strengthen community linkages but also to promote a more efficient service delivery system that maximizes community service and use of experts and, at the same time, allows financial savings.[25,26] A delivery system is needed for children with special health care needs that includes comprehensive services which are coordinated, culturally competent/sensitive, family centered and community based.[27–37] A definition of some of these terms from the Ohio Department of Health follows: *culturally competent/sensitive* recognizes and respects the fact that different cultures may have different concepts and practices; *family-centered community-based* and *coordinated care* means diagnosis and treatment and primary, tertiary, and specialty care are available in the community, the child's family and their needs are considered, the child has a written plan, resources and financing services are identified and provided, communication is available among the family and providers, a non-physician care coordinator is provided as well as a mechanism for the family to report problems, quality is assured through examination of the process and outcome, support systems are identified, sufficient flexibility is provided for individual and family needs, and continuity of coordination exists regardless of ability to pay; *health care needs* means the physical, mental and social well-being, not merely absence of disease. Identification of these resources will ultimately promote continuity of care, efficient delivery of services without duplication, maximum use of community nutrition services, and thereby an even greater community integration.

References

1. Lucas, B.L. Serving infants and children with special health care needs in the 1990s—are we ready? *J. Am. Diet. Assoc.* 1989; *89:* 1599.
2. Kaufman, M. Are dietitians prepared to work with handicapped infants? P.L. 99-457 offers new opportunities. *J. Am. Diet. Assoc.* 1989; *89:* 1602.
3. Hine, R.J., Cloud, H.H., Carithers, T., Hickey, C., Hinton, A. Early nutrition intervention services for children with special health care needs. *J. Am. Diet. Assoc.* 1989; *89:* 1636.

4. Smith, B., ed. *Mapping the Future for Children with Special Needs*, Iowa City: University of Iowa; 1988.

5. Smoyer, D., Pappas, V. *UAPs: Making a Difference*, Silver Spring, MD: American Association of University Affiliated Programs; 1989.

6. Ekvall, S., Grace, E., Niemes, L. Nutritional needs of the child with a handicap or chronic illness. In: *Nutrition Program Planning, Manual I*. Cincinnati: University Affiliated Cincinnati Center for Developmental Disorders; 1987.

7. Ekvall, S., Wheby, E. Nutritioal needs of the child with a handicap or chronic illness. In: *Clinical Nutrition Manual II*. Cincinnati: University Affiliated Cincinnati Center for Developmental Disorders; 1988.

8. Ekvall, S., Stevens, F.: Nutritional needs of the child with a handicap or chronic illness (child with special health needs). In: *Nutritional Assessment, Manual III*. Cincinnati: University Affiliated Cincinnati Center for Developmental Disorders; 1989.

9. Gooder, J.B., Ekvall, S.W. Extension of health and nutrition services via advanced telecommunications. *J. Am. Diet. Assoc.* 1989; *89:* 821.

10. Axtman, C.D., Davis, J., Rokusek, C. *A Survey on Nutrition Attitudes, Knowledge, and Needs of School Lunch Directors in Relation to Special Needs Populations*, Pierre, SD: South Dakota Department of Education; 1983.

11. Rokusek, C., Heinrichs, E., eds. *Nutrition and Feeding for the Developmentally Disabled*, Pierre, SD: State Publishing; 1985/6.

12. Horsley, J., Allen, E. Expanding nutrition services for handicapped children. *School Food Serv. J.* 1989; August, 44.

13. Egan, M.C. Public health nutrition services: issues today and tomorrow. *J. Am. Diet. Assoc.* 1980; *77:* 423.

14. Gordon, T., Kannel, W.B. The effects of overweight on cardiovascular disease. *Geriatrics.* 1973; *28:* 80.

15. Davidson, J.K., Delcher, J.K., Englund, A. Spinoff costs/benefits of expanded nutritional care. *J. Am. Diet. Assoc.* 1979; *75:* 250.

16. American Dietetic Association. *Costs and Benefits of Nutritional Care.* Chicago: American Dietetic Association; 1979.

17. Mercer-Clark, K., Ekvall-Walberg, S. Comparing the diets of adults with mental retardation who live in intermediate care facilities and in group homes. *J. Am. Diet Assoc.* 1992; *92:* 356.

18. *Supplement to a Compendium of Program Ideas for Serving Low-Income Women.* U.S. Department of Health and Human Services. Washington, D.C.: Government Printing Office; 1990.

19. *USDA Budget Summary, FFY, 1992.* Alexandria, VA: Food and Nutrition Services, U.S. Department of Agriculture; 1991.

20. Nutrition services reimbursement by Medicaid. *Neonat. Nutr. News. 1(1):* 6.

21. Caldwell, M., ed. Quality assurance. In: Ekvall, S. Grace, E., Niemes, L., eds. Nutritional needs of the handicapped/chronically ill child. *Program Planning, Manual I* Cincinnati: University Affiliated Cincinnati Center for Developmental Disorders, 1987.

22. Kaufman, M. ed. *Guide to Quality Assurance in Ambulatory Nutrition Care*, Chicago: American Dietetic Association; 1983.

23. ACDD. *Accreditation Council on Services for People with Developmental Disabilities (ACDD) Standards.* 1987 ed.

24. *Commission on Accreditation of Rehabilitative Facilities (CARF) Standards Manual for Organizations Serving People with Developmental Disabilities.* Tucson, 1989.

25. Hohenbrink, K. Nutrition resources. In: Ekvall, S., Grace, E., Niemes, L., eds. Nutritional needs of the handicapped/chronically ill child. *Program Planning, Manual I.* Cincinnati: University Affiliated Cincinnati Center for Developmental Disorders; 1987.

26. Thompson, E., Bellamy, M., Kaufman, M., and Jacka, E. Capacity of state health agencies to meet nutrition objectives in maternal and child health. *J. Am. Diet. Assoc.* 1990; *90:* 1423.

27. U.S. Department of Health and Human Services: *Surgeon General's Report: Children With Special Health Care Needs.* Compaign '87: Commitment to family-centered coordinated care for children with special health care needs (DHHS Publ. No. HRS/D/MC 87-2). Washington, D.C., 1987.

28. Sharbaugh, C., (Ed.) *Call to Action: Better Nutrition for Toddlers, Children and Families*, Washington D.C., National Center for Nutrition in Maternal and Child Health, 38 and R Streets, 1991.

29. U.S. Department of Health and Human Services, *Healthy People 2000* National Promotion and Disease Prevention Objectives, DHHS Publication (PHS) 91-50212, Superintendent of Documents, U.S. Government Printing Office, Washington D.C., 1990.

30. Dwyer, J. and Egan, M.C., Eds.: *The Right to Grow: Putting Nutrition Services for Children with Special Long-Term Development and Health Needs into Action.* Boston: Frances Stern Nutrition Center, New England Medical Center Hospital, 1986.

31. American Dietetic Association: Child nutrition services. *J Am Diet Assoc.* 1989; *87:* 217.

32. American Dietetic Association: Nutrition services for children with special health care needs. *J Am Diet Assoc.* 1989; *89:* 1133.

33. Thompson, M.L., and Smith, M.A., Eds.: 1987 Update: *Guidelines for Nutrition Training in Univesity Affiliated Programs.* Memphis, University of Tennessee, Child Development Center, 1987.

34. Maternal Child and Health Bureau: *Nutrition Services for Children With Special Health Care Needs.* Abstracts of active and completed projects, Washington D.C. National Center for Education in Maternal and Child Health, 1991.

35. Penziner, A.J., Amundson, J.A., and Nelson, R.P. *Regional Nutrition Services for Children with Special Needs*, Child Health Specialty Clinics, The University of Iowa, Iowa City, Iowa, 52242, 1989.

36. Maternal and Child Health Bureau: *Needs Assessment and the Development of Community Based Service Systems.* An Annotated Bibliography of Resources, Washington D.C., National Center for Education in Maternal and Child Health, 1991.

37. University Child Development Center: *Developing Cultural Competent Programs for Families of Children with Special Needs.* National Center for Education in Maternal and Child Health, 3800 Reservoir Rd., Washington, D.C. 20007, 1991.

Chapter 6
Quality Assurance Standards

Mariel Caldwell

Quality assurance (QA) has been defined as the "certification of continuous, optimal, effective and efficient health and nutrition care."[1] It uses a problem-solving approach to measure and monitor health care to assure that it is both effective and efficient.[2] A QA program can determine the effectiveness of care, provide direction for improving the quality of care, document the types of problems and needs often found in a particular population, be used to advocate for health services, and help providers of good care achieve some measure of job satisfaction.

Assuring quality of care should be a concern of every health care provider, just as it is a concern of clients or patients and those who are paying for care. The Joint Commission on Accreditation of Healthcare Organizations has identified many factors that influence the quality of health care: practitioner, health care team, organizational or institutional, clinical care, health care policy, and patient variables.[3] These variables should be taken into consideration in any QA program. Fortunately they can be considered within the traditional measures of quality care: structure, process, and outcome.[4-7]

Structural criteria are the organizational elements and resources that contribute to the quality and quantity of health care. They include staff qualifications and ratios, staffing patterns, physical facilities and equipment, accreditation status, organizational arrangements, and financial resources and their management.[1,4,6] They also include the organization's mission statement, program plan, and policies.

Process criteria are "pre-determined elements of care selected to identify key activities or procedures by health professionals in a course of management for a defined health condition in the delivery of patient care."[1] They involve what is done to or for a patient.[6] Process criteria may incorporate the care protocol of the organization or institution, which describes how care is provided in that institution.[8]

Outcome criteria are "pre-determined elements demonstrating measurable and observable end results of change in health status of the patient or client.[1] Changes in knowledge and in behavior of clients are useful and valid indicators of care, along with the more traditional end result indicators based on anthropometric, biochemical, and clinical data.[1,5] Similarly, patient satisfaction with care has become accepted as a valid indicator of quality care.[4,9]

To some extent, consumers, practitioners, and purchasers of health care have varying conceptions of quality health care. For example, consumers may be more concerned about the courtesy and responsiveness of the care providers, purchasers about the efficiency and related costs of care, and practitioners about their own technical skills and professional judgment. Although the specific elements of quality health care that take priority may vary among consumer, practitioner, and purchaser of care, all are concerned with the outcomes of health care.[3]

Traditionally, the health care profession directed much of its QA efforts to meeting and assuring structure criteria. However, in the 1970s outcome criteria began to receive greater emphasis, partly because of the Professional Standards Review Organization legislation, Public Law 92-603, of 1972. This law required that several federal programs—Medicare, Medicaid, and Maternal and Child Health—evaluate the quality and cost of health care services provided through them.

In the late 1970s public health nutritionists and dietitians developed a QA manual to help health care providers assure that the nutrition services they provided were based on the most recent findings of nutrition science and were demonstrated to have positive impacts on health status. Another purpose of the manual was to provide guidance on the development and use of QA in ambulatory nutrition care.[1]

The manual—*Guide to Quality Assurance in Ambulatory Nutrition Care*[1]—was published in 1983 by the American Dietetic Association. It delineated a process for developing QA criteria sets to be used in measuring the quality of nutrition care. (Fig. 6-1).

Steps in Developing Quality Assurance Criteria

Step I: Select the Target Population

Step I involves selecting the target population for whom the criteria will be written. Characteristics to consider in selecting the population include that the population is at high risk for nutrition-related health problems, the problems occur frequently and are responsive to nutrition intervention, and nutrition management methods are generally not controversial.[1] The population may be a particular age group or have a particular medical condition or both; for example, children from 0–18 years of age or individuals with diabetes mellitus or children from 1 to 8 years of age with Type I diabetes mellitus.

Step II: Select Specific Condition(s)

In Step II, the specific condition of the population is defined clearly. The problem is often delineated in terms of being a healthy population with no complications or a population with additional medical complications or chronic conditions: children from 0–18 years of age with Type I diabetes mellitus and no additional complications versus children from

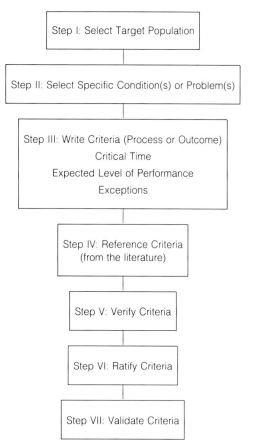

Fig. 6-1. Steps in developing quality assurance criteria. From *Guide to Quality Assurance in Ambulatory Nutrition*, with permission.

0–18 years of age with Type I diabetes mellitus and retinopathy or cardiovascular disease. Clear delineation of the population and the conditions is essential for writing the criteria and identifying the sample to be selected for study or monitoring.

Step III: Write the Criteria

In Step III, criteria are written, usually by individuals with expertise in nutritional care of the particular target population. The nominal group process, a structured group method, is often used in this step.[8] The decision must be made as to the type of criteria to be written: process or outcome or both. Criteria are written to embody the characteristics described by the acronym *RUMBA*: *r*elevant, *u*nderstandable, *m*easurable, *b*ehavioral, and *a*chievable. These characteristics are similar to those of the clinical indicators being developed by task forces of the Joint Commission on Accreditation of Healthcare Organizations (JCAHO), as part of its Agenda for Change. This project is a research and development activity to develop an outcome-oriented monitoring, continuous quality improvement, and evaluation process that will assist health care organizations to improve the quality of the care they provide.[3,4] By definition, clinical indicators are defined, measurable dimensions of the quality or appropriateness of important aspects of patient care. Health professional organizations, including the American Dietetic Association,

are cooperating with the JCAHO on the development of indicators by establishing clinical indicators relevant to their field of practice. The process of developing clinical indicators is similar to that for developing QA criteria.[10] Many nutrition criteria developed to date could be adapted for use as clinical indicators.[3]

In addition to the criteria themselves, the critical time by which each criterion should be met if good care is provided must be stipulated, as well as any exceptions that describe those instances or circumstances that prevent the criterion from being met because of conditions beyond the control of the practitioner or client. The expected level of performance indicates how often this criterion could be expected to be met with good nutritional care and is usually indicated as a percent of time. At present, the level of performance must be determined by each institution or health care organization as there are no national standards or norms and the research literature is inadequate to provide guidance to practitioners. The term threshold is also used to differentiate between good and poor care.

Step IV: Reference the Criteria

References from the research literature substantiate the scientific basis, as well as the efficiency and safety of the criteria. Referencing also provides partial validation for the criteria.

Step V: Verify the Criteria

After writing and referencing, the criteria are verified by determining the source of documentation, generally the patient's health care record, and the type of data to be used to determine if the criteria are met. The task of verification assists in determining whether the criteria are measurable.

Step VI: Ratify the Criteria

In the ratification process, the draft criteria are submitted to other nutrition care providers, often experts in the care of the target population, who review them for clarity and appropriateness and check them against the RUMBA characteristics. When criteria do not meet those characteristics, they are rewritten. After any revision, the criteria must be accepted by the group before proceeding to the step of validation or field testing.

Step VIII: Validate the Criteria

In a field test, the criteria are audited in a manner similar to an actual quality assessment or review, however, it is the criteria, rather than the quality of care, that are being assessed. Generally, the criteria sets are field tested in settings considered to provide good care. At each site a statistically valid sample of charts is selected based on members in the population for which the criteria were written.[1,11] Two or more auditors review the same charts to determine if each criterion is met. The use of more than one auditor helps ensure the reliability or reproducibility of the criteria. Field test results are summarized by site and then compiled. If field test results indicate the criteria are not substantially met, they are rewritten and again submitted for field testing.

Quality Assurance in Nutrition Care

Using the process described in the *Guide to Quality Assurance in Ambulatory Nutrition Care*,[1] public health nutritionists and dietitians concerned with services for children with special health care needs established QA criteria to monitor nutrition services for children with myelomeningocele and developmental disabilities. (see Chapter 10 and the Appendix for two samples)

In 1980, the Pediatric Nutrition Practice Group (PNPG), formerly the Dietitians in Pediatric Practice of the American Dietetic Association, established a QA committee to develop guidelines to determine the level of nutrition care provided to children in hospitals. This group focused its efforts on developing outcome and process criteria. Populations first selected for writing criteria sets were the normal infant of 0–6 months and 6–12 months of age and children with phenylketonuria (PKU), cystic fibrosis, and renal disease. Following the established procedure, small groups of pediatric dietitians with expertise in providing care to the target populations wrote the criteria, which were then submitted to other pediatric nutrition experts for review and ratification. The criteria were then field tested in two or three sites across the country by at least two auditors at each site. The field test results were summarized and reviewed by the original committee to determine whether the criteria were valid and reliable. If they were not, they were then rewritten and once again field tested.

Because some of the criteria referred to patient care protocols, examples of such protocols were included with the criteria sets. As a protocol defines the specific process of providing care in a specific institution, it may vary from institution to institution.

Additional criteria sets were developed by PNPG task forces in a similar fashion for the following populations: normal adolescents, pregnant adolescents, normal healthy premature infants, pediatric intensive care patients, patients with insulin-dependent diabetes mellitus, and oncology patients. The criteria sets were published by the American Dietetic Association in 1988 in *Quality Assurance Criteria for Pediatric Nutrition Conditions: A Model*.[12] Additional criteria sets are being developed by the PNPG for the following conditions: bronchopulmonary dysplasia, cardiac disease, home TPN/enteral nutrition, vegetarianism, inborn errors other than PKU, failure to thrive, craniofacial anomalies, obesity, burns, gastrointestinal disease, anorexia-bulimia, AIDS, renal transplant, chronic liver disease, hyperlipidemia, and inflammatory bowel disease. It is expected that these will also be published by the American Dietetic Association.

QA criteria sets are not intended for use as national standards. Rather, they are guidelines for care that can be adapted by health care institutions for use in monitoring care in their own setting, as noted in Manual I on *Nutrition Program Planning*.[13] The complete criteria sets may be used to conduct in-depth studies of nutritional care, or portions of the sets may be used in monitoring total patient care. When used to monitor total patient care, the criteria considered to be the most important indicators of care in that setting can be selected for use as part of a multidisciplinary review or audit.[1,12,13] The level of performance that constitutes good care must be determined by the institution before conducting the care review as there are no nationally accepted standards.

Although the review or audit process described above relates to field testing QA criteria, a similar process is used in actual monitoring of patient care. The monitoring process requires that there be appropriate documentation of care in the data sources used to verify that care, usually the health care records. Recording important aspects of care is a valuable tool for communication among all health care providers and is essential for assuring and being able to "prove" the type and quantity of care provided to a patient.

QA should focus on identifying and solving problems that adversely affect patient care.[6] If patient care audits show significant findings indicating inadequate or inappropriate care, a plan must be developed for improving care. The plan may involve such activities as in-service education, individual counseling of care providers, adjustments in staffing, or revised policies or procedures to correct the identified deficiencies. Once the plan for improving care has been implemented, a re-audit is essential to assure that the plan is effective in improving patient outcomes.[1,6,13,14]

It is important to remember that QA criteria are indicative of good care at the time the criteria are written. As new research describes better methods of providing care or care resulting in better patient outcomes, criteria sets must be updated to take this new knowledge into consideration.

The emphasis on process and outcome criteria does not mean that structure criteria are not important. Assuring that health care providers have adequate training and experience to allow them to provide the level of care required in the setting in which they work and to provide the quality of care to achieve the best possible patient outcomes is still a major component of a QA program.[5–7,9,13,14] Similarly, the mission statement, program plan, and policies of the health care organization or institution; the equipment; facilities; laboratory services; space; staffing patterns; and budget are all important determinants of the provision of quality health care.[9,14,15] The QA system for each Maternal and Child Health program includes nutrition program guidelines, screening/assessment protocols, intake recommendations, intervention policies, referral policies, health education guidelines, and provider credentials.[10] The Study Committee, Institute of Medicine, also recently reported a strategy for promoting quality assurance in Medicare through ten major recommendations.[16]

References

1. Kaufman, M., ed. *Guide to Quality Assurance in Ambulatory Nutrition Care*. Chicago: American Dietetic Association; 1983.
2. Michnich, M. E., Harris, J. L., Willis, R. A., Williams, J. E. *Ambulatory Care Evaluation: A Primer for Quality Review*. Los Angeles: CA, A.C.E. Project, School of Public Health, University of California, 1976.
3. *Overview of the Joint Commission's Agenda for Change*. Chicago: Joint Commission on Accreditation of Healthcare Organizations; 1987.
4. *The Joint Commission Guide to Quality Assurance*. Chicago: JCAHO; 1988.
5. Donabedian, A. Criteria and standards for quality assurance and monitoring. *Qual. Rev. Bull.* 1986; 12:99.
6. Batalden, P. B., O'Connor, J. C. *Quality Assurance in Ambulatory Care*. Rockville, MD: Aspen Systems Corp.; 1980.
7. *Nutrition Services for Children with Handicaps: A Manual for State Title V Programs*. Los Angeles: University Affiliated Pro-

gram Center for Child Development and Developmental Disorders; 1982.

8. Delbecq, A. L., Van de Ven, A. H., Gustafson, D. H. *Group Techniques for Program Planning: A Guide to Nominal Group and Delphi Process.* Glenview, IL: Foresman, 1975.

9. Benson, D. S., Miller, J. A. *Quality Assurance for Primary Care Centers.* Indianapolis: Methodist Hospital of Indiana, Inc.; 1988.

10. *Primer on Indicator Development and Application. Measuring Quality in Health Care.* Oakbrook Terrace, IL: Joint Commission on Accreditation of Healthcare Organizations, 1990.

11. Slonim, M. J. *Sampling.* New York: Simon and Schuster; 1960.

12. Wooldridge, N. H., ed. *Quality Assurance Criteria for Pediatric Nutrition Conditions: A Model.* Chicago: American Dietetic Association; 1988.

13. Caldwell, M. Quality Assurance. In: Ekvall, S., Grace, E., Niemes, L., eds. *Nutrition Program Planning, Nutritional Needs of the Handicapped/Chronically Ill Child,* Manual I. Cincinnati, OH: University Affiliated Cincinnati Center for Developmental Disorders; 1987.

14. *Quality Assurance in Obstetrics and Gynecology.* Washington, DC; American College of Obstetricians and Gynecologists; 1989.

15. Owens, J., Geibig, C., Mirtello, J. Concurred quality assurance for a nutrition support service. *Am. J. Hosp. Pharm.* 1989; 46:2469.

16. Lohr, K.N., Harris-Wehling, J. Medicare: A strategy for quality assurance, I: A recapitulation of the study and definition of quality of care. *Qual. Rev. Bull.* 1991; 17:6.

Part II
Chronic Diseases and Developmental Disorders

Shirley Walberg Ekvall

This section describes nutritional and biochemical abnormalities in chronic diseases and developmental disorders. It examines multiple factors to be considered in nutritional diagnosis or evaluation and management of these diseases and/or disorders. Nutrition intervention on both a long- or short-term basis and resources are presented as well. Moving from general preventive nutrition, which was presented in Part I, more specific nutrition management related to diseases/disorders is addressed in this part. The knowledge from Part I on normal growth and development and assessment is essential in order to understand nutritional intervention in the diseased states discussed in Parts II and III. The topics in this part cover children of all ages.

Although based on a relatively small survey of 83 children, the distribution of nutritional disorders found among children referred to the University Affiliated Cincinnati Center for Developmental Disabilities (UACCDD) nutrition department for in-depth assessment in 1990 provides some perspective on the global experience with nutrition for children with special health care needs. The disorders were overweight, underweight, feeding, nutrient deficiency, bizarre food habits, and metabolic disorders (Fig II–1). Although only 13% of the children were referred because of major nutrient deficiencies, significant nutrient deficiencies in diets (less than 77% of the recommended daily allowance or RDA) were found in children in most other referral categories. The 1982 survey by Smith et al.[1] corroborates some of the experience at UACCDD; of 1230 children who were

retarded, 65% were short stature, with 10% overweight and 17% underweight.

The sample of 83 children in the in-depth UACCDD nutrition assessment survey had these demographic characteristics: mean age—5.4 years; sex—31% girls and 69% boys; race—65.1% Caucasian, 32.5% African-American, and 2.4% other. The survey sample did not include children seen by nutrition in midlevel (special clinics) or mini-level (community setting) assessments.

Earlier dietary assessment studies reported a deficiency of iron, calories, calcium, niacin, and vitamins A, C, and D,[1] and iron and vitamin C deficiency correlated with feeding problems.[2] These nutrient deficiencies, as well as others, were found in 8%–45% of the children in the UACCDD 1990 survey (Fig II–2). Children in the general population suffer from some of the same deficiencies. According to a 1986 survey of the Nutritional Monitoring Division of the United States Department of Agriculture (USDA), diets for children ages 1 to 5 were deficient in calcium, zinc,

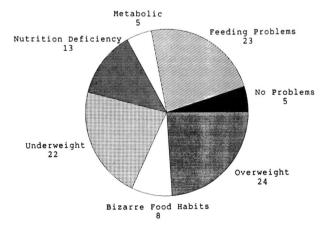

Fig. II–1. Distribution of nutritional disorders among children referred to the UACCDD nutrition department for in-depth assessment in 1990.

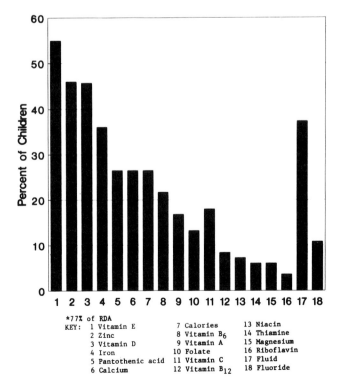

Fig. II–2. Nutrient deficiencies found in 1990 UACCDD survey.

magnesium, vitamin E, iron, and vitamin B₆, in descending order. In addition, adolescents in their late teens (USDA and UACCDD surveys) and women (USDA survey) were deficient in folate. In fact, folate was the most deficient nutrient (52% of RDA consumed) and was of greatest concern for pregnant females in their late teens or older because of the increased need for this nutrient during pregnancy (see Chapter 10). Folate status of adolescents can improve significantly with supplementation according to a 1990 study by Tsui and Nordstrom.[3]

The UACCDD survey also revealed evidence of excessive intake of some nutrients. Vitamin and mineral supplements were consumed by 36% of the children in the survey. The very high percentage of children with more than 100% of the RDA of specific nutrients considered to be harmful to the body is shown in Figure II–3. Most remarkable is the fact that 94% of the children had an excessive sodium intake of 621% of RDA. Daily or more frequent consumption of soft drinks and candy or sugar items was found in 34% and 30% of the children, respectively. Fat and sodium excess has been shown in other studies of children.[4]

A Food Summary Score based on the Basic Four Food Groups (see in-depth nutrition record in Appendix 4) of less than 10 points was found in 40% of the children. This low score reflected an intake of low nutrient-dense foods—for example, soft drinks—and means that 40% of the children evaluated required more treatment sessions to improve nutrition. The percentage of children with a low number of servings in each of the Basic Four Food Groups ranged from a low of 45% for the meat group to a high of 63% with deficient servings for the fruit and vegetable group; the milk and bread group were deficient 59% and 52%, respectively. For the fruit and vegetable group, which provides the protective action of antidioxidants such as retinoids and beta-carotene, vitamin E and vitamin A were found to be low in

55% and 17% of the children, respectively (see Fig II–2). The UACCDD is changing to the Five Food Groups classification because it separates the fruit and vegetable group and increases the number of servings, and expands the grain group.

A great deal of nutrition education is needed to encourage intake of more nutrient-dense foods, especially for children on restricted diets or limited calories. The reduction of sugar and sodium for all age groups and of calories and fat for children over 2 years of age is essential. For example, milk or milk products should replace excessive usage of soft drinks to increase calcium and vitamin D intakes, both of which were deficient in 27% (40% of adolescents) and 46% (60% of adolescents), respectively, of the 83 children surveyed. The low dietary calcium (27%) and low physical activity (59%) can result in reduced bone mass for children who are developmentally delayed or chronically ill. The need for calcium to enhance bone mass is particularly acute during adolescence.[5] Those children using anticonvulsant medication and who are dark skinned have a superimposed problem of reduced vitamin D absorption. Yet, the use of calcium supplements without adequate fluid (low in 37% of the children) or little physical activity can be harmful to the kidneys. Thus, calcium intake from the diet is preferred. This problem illustrates the complexities of nutritional diagnosis and treatment of children with special health care needs.

Many nutrients also may be deficient because of the effect of medications, such as anticonvulsants, taken by children with chronic diseases and developmental disorders. For example, in a 1987 study, lower thyroxine and higher retinol-binding protein were found among children who received diphenylhydantoin, phenobarbital, or anticonvulsant combinations; however, vitamin A was higher in those on diphenylhydantoin.[6] The effect of medication on nutrition is addressed in Chapter 27. Feeding (both behavioral and neuromotor) was a problem in 23% of children in our survey (Fig II–1). This topic is presented in Chapter 24, as well as in other chapters on cerebral palsy, cleft palate, craniofacial anomalies, and gastrointestinal disorders. At UACCDD underweight occurred in 24% of the children (Fig II–1) with many of the above conditions being related to feeding. Overweight occurred in 23% of the children with developmental disorders—myelomeningocele, Down syndrome, Prader-Willi syndrome, and so forth. In a study in Norway of children who were disabled the prevalence of feeding disorders was: 23 to 43% for mentally retarded, 26 to 52% for cerebral palsy and 10 to 49% for congenital heart disease.[7] Height was subnormal in 50% and weight subnormal in 25% of the children with feeding problems. Height for age was most deficient in children with cerebral palsy and mental retardation and least for children with epilepsy. Dyphagia or difficulty in swallowing results in one of the greatest risks for malnutrition and severe feeding problems.[8]

Interestingly, in the UACCDD 1990 survey, 20% of the children were below the 5th percentile for height; 23% of these children had a weight:height ratio above the 95% percentile and 11% below the 5th percentile. Likewise, 10% of the children had a midarm muscle circumference above the 95th and below the 5th percentiles. Physical activity was low in 59% and high in 20% of the 83 children surveyed. This indicates a critical need to address low physical activity, especially for children who have developmental disorders

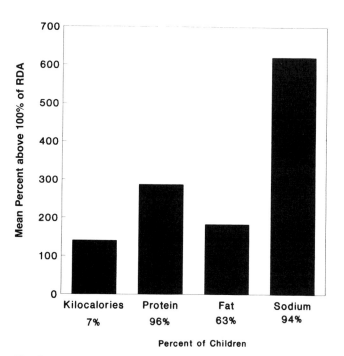

Fig. II–3. Percent of children with excess nutrients (mean percent above 100% of RDA), UACCDD 1990 survey.

(see Chapter 4). A special weight and height growth grid for myelomeningocele is being developed at UACCDD using national data (preliminary growth grids are shown in Appendix 2). Other special growth grids for Down syndrome, sickle-cell anemia, Prader-Willi syndrome, and Turner's syndrome have been developed and are shown in Appendix 2. The assessment of energy needs is difficult for this population and must be performed on an individual basis. It should always include the physical activity level, as well as caloric intake computation due to the effect of physical activity in increasing lean body mass. The chapters on obesity, failure to thrive and other specific diseases in this part and on nutritional assessment in Part I address this problem.

Eating and other psychological and behavioral disorders, such as failure to thrive, anorexia nervosa, and obesity, are receiving widespread attention today. Bizzare food habits were noted in 8% of the children at UACCDD. Some of these problems may be neurological in nature, such as attention deficit hyperactivity disorder. Children with neurological disorders—epilepsy, muscular dystrophy, autism, etc.—have nutrition and other related problems that require interdisciplinary intervention. For example, the effect of nutrients and neurotransmitters on brain dysfunction is a promising new research frontier. Some of these topics have been addressed in collaboration by a nutritionist, psychologist, gastroenterologist, and/or psychiatrist.

Children with diseases, such as cancer, congenital heart disease, and renal disease, require special nutritional management with specific standards of care. In many instances, developmental disorders and chronic diseases overlap; both require long-term, consistent, and preventive care.

Nutrition is the key to open the door to better health. During the last decade several position papers of the American Academy of Pediatrics Committee on Nutrition addressed the nutritional health of children in the general population[9,10] (see Chapter 2) and of children with disabilities.[11,12] Likewise, position papers for children in the general population (referenced throughout the book) and children with developmental disorders have been developed by the American Dietetic Association.[13,14] The American Dietetic Association Pediatric Nutrition Practice Group (PNPG), with input from the Developmental and Psychiatric Disorders Practice Group, have published quality assurance criteria for several diseases and disorders.[15] Children from low-income families are in particular need of adequate nutrients for proper growth and development. Proper nutrition is cost effective by reducing the incidence of infections, anemia, stunted growth, and hospitalization, thereby providing these children with enough energy to develop and learn to their potential (see Chapter 4). The interdisciplinary team approach based on coordination of services and family-centered input provides the best means for improving the health and potential of children with special health care needs (developmental disorders and chronic diseases).

References

1. Smith, M., Connolly, B., McFadden, S., Nicrosi, C., Nuckolls, L., Russell, F., Wilson, W. *Feeding Management of a Child with a Handicap: A Guide for Professionals.* Memphis, TN: University of Tennessee Center for the Health Sciences, Child Development Center; 1982.
2. Gouge, A.L., Ekvall, S.W. Diets of handicapped children: physical, psychological and socioeconomic correlations. *Am. J. Ment. Def.* 1975; 80:149.
3. Tsui, J., Nordstrom, J. Folate status of adolescents: effects of folic acid supplementation. *J. Am. Diet. Assoc.* 1990; 90:1551.
4. Simons-Morton, B.G., Baranowski, T., Parcel, G.S., O'Hara, N.M., Matteson, R.C. Children's frequency of consumption of foods high in fat and sodium. *Am. J. Prev. Med.* 1990; 6:218.
5. Anderson, J. Dietary calcium and bone mass through the life cycle. *Nutr. Today.* 1990; 25:9.
6. Kozlowski, B.W., Taylor, M.L., Baer, M.T., Blyler, E.M., Trahms, C. Anticonvulsant medication use and circulating levels of total thyroxine, retinol binding protein, and vitamin A in children with delayed cognitive development. *Am. J. Clin. Nutr.* 1987; 46:360.
7. Thommessen, M., Heiberg, A., Kase, B.F., Larsen, S., Riis, G. Feeding problems, height and weight in different groups of disabled children. *Acta Pediatr. Scan.* 1991; 80:527.
8. Gines, D.J., ed. *Nutrition Management in Rehabilitation.* Rockville, MD: Aspen Publication, 1990.
9. American Academy of Pediatrics Committee on Nutrition. Iron-fortified formulas. *Pediatrics.* 1989; 83:1114.
10. American Academy of Pediatrics Committee on Nutrition. Follow-up on weaning formulas. *Pediatrics.* 1989; 83:1069.
11. American Academy of Pediatrics Committee on Children with Disabilities and Committee on School Health. Children with health impairments in schools. *Pediatrics.* 1990; 86:636.
12. American Academy of Pediatrics Committee on Sports Medicine and Committee on Children with Disabilities. Exercise for mentally retarded children. *Pediatrics.* 1987; 80:447.
13. American Dietetic Association. Infant and child nutrition concerns regarding the developmentally disabled. *J. Am. Diet. Assoc.* 1981; 78:443.
14. American Dietetic Association. Nutrition in comprehensive program planning for persons with developmental disabilities. *J. Am. Diet. Assoc.* 1987; 87:1068.
15. Woolridge, N.H., and Quality Assurance Committee, Dietitians in Pediatric Practice, eds. *Quality Assurance Criteria for Pediatric Nutrition Conditions: A Model.* Chicago: American Dietetic Association; 1988.

Chapter 7
Cerebral Palsy

Linda Bandini, Bonnie Patterson, and Shirley Walberg Ekvall

Cerebral palsy (CP) is a group of chronic, nonprogressive disorders of the brain in infants and young children that produce abnormalities of posture, muscle tone, and motor coordination. The prevalence of CP among children at school entry is consistently 2 per 1000 live births.[1] There is no firm evidence that this figure is on the decline. The two major risk factors for cerebral palsy are low birth weight and birth asphyxia. Other causes include congenital infections and brain anomalies and perinatal metabolic conditions—hyperbilirubinemia, hypoglycemia, and amino acid disorders.

Types of Cerebral Palsy. CP is classified according to the predominant neurological sign, specifically abnormalities in muscle tone and extrapyramidal functioning.[2] Muscle tone can be either increased (hypertonicity, spasticity) or decreased (hypotonic, floppy). In some cases, children present with variable tone or tone that changes from infancy to childhood. Many hypotonic infants develop spasticity at about 1 or 2 years of age. Extrapyramidal signs include choreoathetosis, ataxia, and dystonia.

Failure to achieve normal maturation of, or injury to, the central nervous system may produce disorganization of movement and abnormal postures. These postures represent early developmental reflexes that are present in all infants up to a certain age (3 to 4 months), at which time they are replaced by voluntary motion. Examples of these early reflexes include the atonic neck reflex, grasp reflex, tongue thrust, and rooting reflexes. These early or primitive reflexes often persist in children with cerebral palsy. Voluntary motion is decreased, absent, or erratic while abnormal posturing persists. Presenting symptoms of CP can include the following:

- excessive fussiness
- poor feeding
- stiffness when diapering, feeding, handling, or bathing
- low threshold to sensory stimuli with easily evoked and pronounced startle reflex
- early abnormal rolling or standing
- disassociated development with gross motor skills lagging far behind language, adaptive, and social skills

Different types of CP are usually diagnosed at different ages and at different rates of occurrence. *Spastic CP* involves increased muscle tone of the "clasp knife" variety, persistent primitive reflexes, and increased deep tendon reflexes in the involved extremities found in one of the three characteristic patterns: hemiplegia, involving the arm and leg on one side of the body; diplegia, involving predominantly the lower extremities, although upper extremities may have associated minor deficits of fine motor function; and quadriplegia, involving all four extremities and may include significant trunk

pseudobulbar movement (Table 7–1). Various combinations of these patterns also may occur.[3] Spastic hemiplegia is often difficult to diagnose in the first few months of life, and it may not be until 9 to 12 months that the asymmetry is first noted by the parent or physician. In spastic diplegia, the gait is often more affected than hand skills, and the diagnosis is often not made until the child should begin to ambulate at about 1 year of age. Children with spastic quadriplegia frequently are very severely involved, and the diagnosis may be made early in infancy. These children present with difficulties in positioning, handling, and feeding due to diffusely increased tone, tongue thrusting, and swallowing problems.

In *athetoid CP* the child has uncontrolled and continuous involuntary movements. It is characterized by slow, wormlike, writhing movements, usually involving all four extremities, neck, face, and trunk. The most common cause of athetoid forms has been kernicterus, but the ability to prevent Rh sensitization has brought a significant decline in

Table 7–1. Classification of Cerebral Palsy and Frequency of Various Forms of Cerebral Palsy

Classification		
Physiological		
Abnormalities of tone		
Spastic		
Hypotonic or atonic		
Rigid		
Dystonic		
Abnormalities of movement		
Athetoid		
Choreiform		
Ataxic		
Topographic		
Monoparesis: involvement of one limb only		
Hemiparesis: involvement of one side, arm more than leg		
Quadriparesis: significant involvement of all limbs		
Diparesis: significant involvement of legs with little or no involvement of arms		

	Frequency (%)	
Spastic		75
Hemiparesis	30	
Diparesis	25	
Quadriparesis	20	
Athetoid		5
Dystonic athetoid		10
Mixed and other		10

From Erenberg, G. Cerebral palsy: current understanding of a complex problem *Postgrad. Med.* 1984, 75:87. Used with permission.

kernicterus and thus in athetoid CP. This has resulted in a corresponding increase in the percentage of cases classified as spastic.[4] *Mixed CP* refers to the condition when both athetosis and spasticity may be present.

CP, as noted above, is primarily a motor disability. However, frequently there are associated developmental problems that are seen in higher incidence in children with CP. These include mental retardation, learning disabilities, attention deficit disorder, speech and language problems, hearing problems, seizure disorder, and growth retardation. The most common associated problem in cerebral palsy is a decrease in intellectual and cognitive function. More than 50% of persons with CP show signs of mental retardation (MR) or a learning disability.[3,5] The degree of mental retardation can vary from mild to severe. Perceptual problems can reduce learning ability in persons whose overall intelligence is normal.

Behavioral problems, such as hyperactivity and decreased attention span, also are common in persons with CP. An attention deficit disorder with or without hyperactivity involves decreased attention span, fidgeting and restlessness, poor ability to concentrate, distractibility, poor peer relationships, fearlessness, low frustration tolerance, need for instant gratification, and general immaturity.[5] When these behaviors occur in children with CP, the disorder is often complicated by retardation or learning disability.

A frequent neurological problem is the occurrence of seizures, which affect about 30% of persons with CP. Nearly all seizure types can occur, including grand mal, psychomotor, focal, and petit mal.[5] Ocular motor problems are much more frequent in children with CP than in the general population.[5] Blindness in children with CP is not common except when the disorder is a result of intrauterine infection such as rubella, but visual field deficits may occur. Speech and language impairment often are associated with CP due to dyspraxia of the oral musculature (tongue, lips, cheeks, and palate), which can result in poor chewing, swallowing, and excessive drooling.[5]

Biochemical and Functional Abnormalities

The use of medications to treat spasticity has not been particularly successful. Medications that have been used include Dantrium[R], Valium[R], Lioresal[R], and occasionally Cogentin[R] and Clonopin[R].[6] The first three drugs result in relaxation of muscle tension, but most studies to date have shown a very poor effect on functional ability. In addition, the sedative side effects of the medication may have a detrimental effect on development. Cogentin and Clonopin have been used to produce relaxation in children who primarily show rigidity. These drugs have been somewhat more effective, although sedation may be difficult to avoid.

Many educational and therapeutic programs are now available to serve children with cerebral palsy. The rehabilitation is aimed not only at improving the child's physical status but also at maximizing the child's potential for achieving independence in all functional areas, including mobility, fine motor skills, self-care, and communication.[6] Appropriate timing of intervention strategies is very important. The therapeutic system most commonly used today is that developed by the Bobaths in the early 1960s called neuro-developmental therapy (NDT). This treatment program emphasizes positioning and handling of the child in such a way as to promote as near-normal movement patterns as possible. An important aspect of this therapy involves inhibition of abnormal primitive reflex patterns. Early infant stimulation programs are frequently seen as complementing the individual therapy and are often started when a child is diagnosed as being at risk.

A vital adjunct to therapy and medication is the use of adaptive equipment that can enhance mobility, hand function, and communication skills.[6] The use of computer-assisted and electronically powered devices has become prevalent with the advent of today's technology. Adaptive seating provides support for children with poor control of their trunk, through the use of lateral head, trunk, and hip supports; abduction pommel; foot straps or stirrups; seatbelts; and trunk harness when needed. These adaptive forms can fit into most strollers or travel chairs. Sport wheelchairs, which are light weight and more cosmetically acceptable, are now available for the child with good trunk and upper extremity control. Electric wheelchairs with adaptive seating can provide much independence for children with severe physical involvement, but with good cognitive and visual-perceptual skills.

Such devices as holders and cuffs, which are strapped to the child's hand, can be used to fit utensils, crayons, and the like to assist with fine motor activities. Environmental control units, which can be used to operate the television, telephone, and page turners, provide considerable functional independence for even profoundly physically impaired people. Augmentative communication devices are also now available that can provide a means of communication for the nonverbal child.

Factors to be Considered in Nutritional Evaluation

Growth

Children with CP are often shorter than children without CP of the same age. It is not clear whether CP children are congenitally short or whether their short stature is a result of chronic undernutrition. Several studies[7,8] have observed a correlation between the severity of motor involvement in handicapped children and the degree of impairment in growth. Tobias et al.[8] found that a severe deviation in stature was associated with dependency in feeding and ambulation. Sixteen of 21 dependent feeders had heights below two standard deviations, in contrast to 29 of 65 independent feeders ($P < 0.02$). Studies by Krick and Duyn[9] suggest that oral motor impairment, when superimposed on a central nervous system insult, may exacerbate the growth retardation observed in CP.

There are limited data on the body composition of children with CP. Berg and Isaksson[10] measured total body water (TBW) and body cell mass (BCM) in a group of children with CP and compared their findings to those predicted for age. They concluded that TBW was increased and BCM decreased in subjects with CP. The decrease in BCM would be expected since children with CP are less active. However, calculations from their data suggest that some children had a fat-free mass that was greater than their body weight. Further studies on the body composition of CP individuals, including measures of extracellular water, are needed to verify these alterations in body composition.

Because of deviations in growth patterns in CP, anthropometric measures of height and weight are often of limited use in the nutritional assessment. In children without CP, weight for age,[11] height for age,[12] and weight for height[13] are useful indices for determining the prevalence of undernutrition. In the CP child, comparisons based on weight for age and height for age provide only a rough estimate of the degree of undernutrition. Skinfold thickness may overestimate body fatness because fatfolds have been shown to increase over paralyzed limbs.[14] Many children with CP are often below the 3rd percentile of height for age; thus, weight for height may be a more reliable indicator of current nutritional status. Johnson and Maeda[15] used the weight:height ratio as an index of nutritional status in 94 children with CP seen in an outpatient clinic. In 14 patients, height was difficult to obtain because of severe joint contractures. In these patients arm span was measured, and a conversion factor of arm span divided by 1.03 for nondeformed height (8) was used. They found 20% of the population to be at nutritional risk (5th–10th% or 90th–95th% of weight for height). Thirty-four percent had poor nutritional status—either below the 5th percentile or above the 95th percentile.

In a survey of 33 children and adolescents at a residential facility in Massachusetts, Dietz[16] reported that the prevalence of malnutrition was dependent on the criteria used. When weight for age was the standard, 47% of the children were considered malnourished, when height for age was used—38%, and when weight for height was the criteria—12%. Twenty-four percent had a triceps skinfold in excess of the 85th percentile, and 21% had skinfolds equal to or less than the 3rd percentile.

An accurate index of linear growth is difficult to obtain in children with joint contractures. Thus, several studies have investigated the reliability of upper arm length (and possibly lower leg length in some children) as an index of linear growth in children. Belt et al.[17] found that upper arm length was more reliable than either lower arm length, total arm length, or arm span—using a reliable plastic-coated tape measure—when measuring linear growth in the normal population. Because of the high correlation between linear growth and upper arm length,[18,19] Spender et al. have recommended that this measure be used to assess linear growth if height or length cannot be measured reliably. Spender et al. also noted that black children appeared to have longer legs than white children, suggesting that growth grids may overestimate their growth measurement.[19]

Anthropometric measures are useful in determining changes in nutritional status. The National Center for Health Statistics (NCHS) growth charts may be used to evaluate changes in weight with increasing age where ideal weight is the weight at the 50th percentile of weight for height. However, children with CP, especially those who are nonambulatory, may have decreased muscle mass. Therefore, clinical judgment must be used to determine individual ideal body weight, which may be more appropriate at the 25th–50th percentiles. Height:age ratio can be used to compare the child to NCHS reference data.

When assessing individual nutritional status in children with CP, it is helpful to take several anthropometric measurements, including height, weight, circumferences, arm and leg length, and skinfold thickness. Although absolute values may be difficult to interpret in this population, repeated measures are useful in determining the effectiveness of the dietary treatment. These measurements should be repeated frequently and used as the child's own standard to assess changes in growth and fatness.

Energy Requirements

Energy requirements specific for children with CP are not available. Although it has been frequently documented that children with CP have caloric intakes less than 90% of the RDA,[20–22] many children with spastic CP appear overweight.[17]

Only a few studies of energy expenditure of CP children have been reported in the literature. Wakoh et al.[23] studied the metabolic rate of 11 boys with CP and concluded that 9 had decreased caloric requirements for age. However, they failed to present any details on the methodology of their study or the standards they used for comparison. Berg and Olsson[24] measured 24-hour energy expenditure in four subjects with heart rate monitoring in conjunction with indirect calorimetry. In six other subjects they measured oxygen consumption at one point and extrapolated from the data of the other subjects to determine energy expenditure. Comparison with normal subjects is not given. Nonetheless, the use of heart rate monitoring for the determination of energy expenditure in sedentary individuals is associated with significant error. Eddy et al.[25] measured basal metabolic rate (BMR) and the energy expended in various activities in three CP children. The two athetoid children had metabolic rates that were normal and slightly below normal according to standards of Robertson and Reid. The spastic child weighed 65 kg and had a BMR that was equivalent to a normal child weighing 30–35 kg. During activity, the subjects with CP had higher energy expenditures per activity than normal subjects when the activity approached their physical limitations.

Bandini et al.[26] found that resting metabolic rate (RMR) and fat-free mass in a group of nine adolescents with cerebral palsy (six spastic, one athetoid, and two mixed) were significantly lower than in a group of normal adolescents. However, RMR predicted from body weight was not significantly different from that observed. Total energy expenditure (TEE) measured by the doubly-labeled water method was also significantly lower than in normal adolescents of the same age. The ratio of total energy expenditure:resting metabolic rate (TEE/RMR) was reduced in the subjects with CP who were nonambulatory. These results suggest that the decreases in TEE in the CP subjects were caused by decreases in both fat-free mass and physical activity.

Cully and Middleton[27] found no significant differences in energy intake expressed per centimeter of body height in ambulatory children with or without a motor deficit. However, they found a significantly lower caloric intake per centimeter of height in children with motor dysfunction. They have recommended that caloric requirements be based on stature and severity of the dysfunction, rather than age. For children 5 to 11 years of age, they recommended a caloric intake of 13.9 cal/cm height for the mild to moderate cases of motor dysfunction and 11.1 kcal/cm height in cases of severe motor dysfunction.

Because of the lack of data regarding energy requirements in persons with CP, energy needs must be determined on an individual basis. Children with athetoid CP exhibit exaggerated involuntary movements of the arms and legs that result in extra energy expenditure, thereby increasing caloric needs. Children with spastic CP and with very limited physical activity may have lower energy needs. Whether energy needs are determined from dietary intake, estimate of BMR and an activity factor,[26] or body height,[27] careful monitoring of body weight is necessary to adjust the caloric intake to meet individual energy needs. Bandini et al.[26] found measured energy expenditure to be the following in a small study of CP. 9.0–12.5 kcal/cm height in girls with spastic quadriparesis, 10.6 kcal/cm height in one male primarily athetoid, nonambulatory, and 16.1 kcal/cm height in one female primarily athetoid, ambulatory.

Protein

There are no reported studies of the protein requirements of severely physically handicapped children. Studies have reported intakes of protein below the RDA for age.[21,22] Whether requirements are altered because of a decreased muscle mass is not clear.

Vitamins and minerals

Specific recommended daily allowances for vitamins and minerals have not been determined for persons with handicaps. It is assumed that, in handicapped children without other complicating factors, vitamin and trace element requirements appear comparable to those observed in normal children. However, children receiving chronic anticonvulsant therapy are at risk for vitamin D deficiency and pathological fractures. Approximately 30% of children with CP receive long-term anticonvulsant therapy. Anticonvulsants are thought to increase the activity of the hepatic microsomal enzymes that metabolize vitamin D, thus making less available for use.[28] Limited mobility, lack of exposure to sunshine, and inadequate intakes of milk, fish, or eggs contribute to the susceptibility for vitamin D deficiency. The dose of vitamin D required to prevent rickets or osteomalacia remains unclear. Care should be taken to ensure that the child is receiving the amounts of vitamin D recommended for the general population. If a child is receiving chronic anticonvulsant therapy, serum calcium, phosphorus, and alkaline phosphatase should be measured at least annually to assess vitamin D status. Biochemical signs of deficiency should be treated (see Chapter 8).

Folate, biotin and vitamin B_{12} deficiency may also occur among patients receiving diphenylhydantoin therapy, although the mechanisms remain unclear. Monitoring of the patient is indicated to detect any signs of megaloblastic anemia. Other medications should be evaluated for any possible drug-nutrient interactions.

The physical impairments and feeding difficulties associated with CP often result in decreased food intake. Low serum iron, reduced transferrin, decreased hemoglobin, and hypochromic anemia, as well as deficiencies in calcium, protein, thiamine, and vitamins A and C,[10,20,25,29] have all been reported in children with CP. Careful assessment of the individual's diet will alert the nutritionist to any potential nutrient deficiencies.

Constipation

Due to weak abdominal muscles, insufficient roughage, dehydration associated with excessive vomiting, sweating, hypertonia, and hypotonia, constipation may be a problem (see Chapter 15).

Feeding

Poor motor skills contribute to the feeding problems of the child with CP. Lack of sitting balance; lack of head, mouth, and trunk control; the inability to bend hips sufficiently to enable stretching of the arms forward to grasp and to maintain that grasp, and finally the lack of eye-hand coordination enabling food to be brought from hand to mouth,[30] are all factors that make the feeding process more difficult for the child with CP. The child's degree of impairment can be evaluated using the Mueller prespeech evaluation and feeding skill assessment chart (UACCDD In-depth Nutritional Record, Appendix 4).

Oral motor impairment often results in reduced nutrient intake, reduced growth, and poor nutritional status. Some common feeding problems include difficulties in sucking; incoordination of swallowing or chewing; abnormal reflexes, such as tongue thrust; and poor lip and tongue control.[9] Children with CP have difficulty manipulating food in their mouth, placing them at risk for unsafe feeding.[9] They may become exhausted before finishing their meal placing them at risk for inadequate nutrient intake, growth retardation, and safety in feeding. A study of feeding efficiency in children with severe CP and growth failure found that these children required 2 to 12 times longer to chew and swallow a standard amount of pureed food and 1 to 15 times longer for solid food than did their weight-matched controls.[31] The authors concluded that, in some children with CP, feeding time in excess of the waking hours would be needed to meet their nutritional needs (see Chapter 24).

Gastroesophageal reflux (GER), the re-entry of acidic stomach contents into the esophagus, is a serious feeding problem that is characterized initially by eager food consumption followed shortly by pain. Children who cry persistently during and after feeding, make gurgling sounds when eating, or have frequent respiratory problems or aspiration should be evaluated by a physician. The recurrent pain and aspiration that accompany persistent GER should be viewed as aversive stimuli that may prompt food avoidance (see Chapter 34).

For some children with CP, feeding difficulties may be so severe as to prevent an adequate intake of nutrients. In these cases, a gastrostomy tube may be indicated to safely achieve good nutritional status.

Dental problems are common in children with CP and may contribute to feeding difficulties. Poor oral hygiene, and dentition, dental caries, enamel hypoplasia, bruxism, and malocclusion are encountered frequently. Hyperplasia of the gums may occur with long-term usage of phenytoin (Dilantin®), an anticonvulsant drug. This problem may be exacerbated by poor dental hygiene, contributing to poor chewing, hyperplasia of gums, or hypersensitivity in the mouth.[29]

Dietary Management

Nutrients

The major objectives of dietary treatment in CP include prenatal nutritional counseling and nutritional rehabilitation in undernourished children, intervention for treatment of specific feeding problems, and prevention of overweight in children with spastic CP. Regular monitoring of anthropometric measurements is needed to ensure that energy needs are adequate but not excessive. Signs of malnutrition must be evaluated in children with severe dysfunction due to CP. An albumin measurement less than 3.5 g/dL or transferrin less than 200 mg/dL must be investigated (see Chapter 4). Other physical signs of malnutrition, such as dehydration and skeletal muscle wasting, should be evaluated. Multivitamin and mineral supplements may be necessary if caloric intake is limited.

The nutritionist must consider several factors when treating the child with CP. The diet must be evaluated to determine if it is well balanced. Many caregivers are often involved in the care of the severely handicapped child; thus, it is important that the information gathered be consistent among them. Because of feeding difficulties, the child may not swallow the foods and liquids offered to him or her. Thus, it is important for the nutritionist to determine that the diet record or recall reflects actual intake. Energy and protein requirements must be determined on an individual basis. The foods and liquids in an oral diet should be the appropriate texture and consistency for the child to swallow easily.

Feeding

Because feeding is often a very long and tiresome process for the handicapped child, mealtimes, the quantities consumed, and the endurance of the child are important factors to consider. Although it is important to promote the child's independence in self-feeding, care must be taken so as not to compromise the child's nutritional status. Finally, the influence of the environment must also be considered. Too much stimulation from the environment during mealtime may be distracting for the child who has to work hard to eat.

The management of feeding problems often requires the expertise of an occupational, physical, or speech therapist (see Chapter 24). The normalization of the feeding pattern should lead to both improvements in oral motor behavior and an increase in body weight.[32] A study by Hulme et al.[33] found that adaptive seating devices (ASDs) had a positive effect on eating and drinking behaviors. Head alignment was improved, less liquid was lost, food consistency was advanced from pureed to blended or chopped, and the bottle was replaced by a cup.[33] The use of ASDs has been described in several studies in which control of the head and trunk and maintenance of symmetrical alignment were considered important precursors to oral-motor intervention and feeding.[33–35] It has been proposed that positioning is the most important consideration in preparing the child for a meal and that special adaptations are usually needed for optimal results.[34,36] Banerdt and Brecker[37] reported that positioning in an adaptive highchair improved a child's hand-to-mouth coordination enough to begin self-feeding with minimal as-

sistance. Hulme et al.[33] also concluded that self-feeding behavior improved after ASDs were introduced. Sitting posture, maintaining head control alignment, self-finger feeding, and drinking have all been reported to improve with ASDs.[33,34]

Drooling is a problem in many children with CP and is caused by oral motor dysfunction. Excessive drooling may place the child at risk for infection or dehydration.[38] Mouth closure, jaw stability, and swallowing techniques are important in controlling drooling.[39] Neuromuscular stimulation techniques, together with ASDs, can play a significant role in improving feeding problems in children with CP. It is important, however, that treatment be started early before poor feeding patterns are established (see Chapter 24).

Nutrition therapy

Recently, there has been an increase in the use of feeding gastrostomies in children with neurological impairment. Patrick et al.[39] have reported improvements in nutritional status with supplementary nasogastric feedings. Rampel et al.[40] studied the growth characteristics of 57 children with feeding gastrostomies and found that gastrostomy feeding in children severely affected by CP can improve nutritional status, but does not eliminate growth retardation. They suggested that the greatest benefit may lie in the facilitation of patient care. Therefore, when a gastrostomy feeding is being considered, the complication rate, occasional lack of improvement in nutritional status, and the risk of obesity should be weighed against patient comfort and facilitation of care (see Chapter 34).

Sanders et al.[41] studied the use of enteral feedings providing 1 cal/mL in three groups of children with CP (within 1 year, 8 years, and more than 8 years since their CNS insult). Caloric intake for 6 months was 11 cal/cm, 10 cal/cm, and 9.5 cal/cm for the three groups, respectively. A weight gain of 3.3, 2.8, and 1.5 g/kg/day was found.[41] These results support early aggressive use of enteral feedings if weight for age is reduced (before growth reduction occurs), although some benefits in weight and height were noted in the older age groups as well.

Constipation

High-roughage foods, such as fresh fruits and vegetables, whole-grain breads and cereals, and prune juice, often alleviate constipation. Plenty of fluids should be offered in addition to high-fiber foods. Laxatives containing mineral oil should be avoided because of their interference with the absorption of fat-soluble vitamins (see Chapter 35).

Dental

Parents and caregivers should be educated on appropriate methods of preventing dental problems. They should frequently offer fresh fruits and vegetables when appropriate, encourage frequent brushing, and discourage sweet snacks that promote dental decay. A pediatric dentist should be consulted for problems of dentition in CP.

Follow-up

Nutritional management of a child with CP should include short- and long-term goals or behavioral objectives. Follow-up should include repeat anthropometric measures and nutrient analysis, as well as an assessment of feeding skills and progress with any nutrition-related problems (see quality assurance guidelines for developmental disorders in Appendix 7).

Health professionals working with parents must recognize the significant role that the parents and caregivers play in the development of the child's character and behavior, particularly in the functional development of the child with CP. The challenging goal is to help parents to promote independence in the management of the child with CP. Helping the child function independently appears to increase longevity and provide a better quality of life for persons with CP.

References

1. Paneth, N. Etiologic factors in cerebral palsy. *Pediatr. Ann.* 1986; 15:191.
2. Barabas, G., Taft, L.T. The early signs and differential diagnosis of cerebral palsy. *Pediatr. Ann.* 1986; 15:203.
3. Lord, J. Cerebral palsy: a clinical approach. *Arch. Phys. Med. Rehabil.* 1984; 65:542.
4. Levine, M.I. Cerebral palsy—a permanent disability. *Pediatr. Ann.* 1986; 1593:183.
5. Erenberg, G. Cerebral palsy: current understanding of a complex problem. *Postgrad. Med.* 1984; 75:87.
6. Diamond, M. Rehabilitation strategies for the child with cerebral palsy. *Pediatr. Ann.* 1986; 15:230.
7. Cully, W.J., Jolly, D.H., Mertz, E.T. Heights and weights of mentally retarded children. *Am. J. Ment. Def.* 1963; 68:203.
8. Tobias, J.S., Saturen, P., Larios, G., Posniak, A.O. Study of growth patterns in cerebral palsy. *Arch. Phys. Med. Rehabil.* 1961; 42:475.
9. Krick, J., Duyn, M.A. The relationship between oral-motor involvement and growth: a pilot study in a pediatric population with cerebral palsy. *J. Am. Diet. Assoc.* 1984; 84:555.
10. Berg, K., Isaksson, B. Body composition and nutrition of school age children with cerebral palsy. *Acta Pediatr. Scand.* 1970; 205:41.
11. Gomez, F., Galvan, R.R. Mortality in second and third degree malnutrition. *J. Trop. Pediatr.* 1956; 2:77.
12. Waterlow, J.C. Note on the assessment and classification of protein-energy malnutrition in children. *Lancet.* 1973; 2:87.
13. McTaron, D.S., Reed, W.W.C. Weight/length classification of nutritional status. *Lancet.* 1975; 2:219.
14. Lee, M.M.C. Thickening of the subcutaneous tissues in paralyzed limbs in chronic hemiplegia. *Hum. Biol.* 1959; 31:187.
15. Johnson, R.K., Maeda, M. Establishing outpatient nutrition services for children with cerebral palsy. *J. Am. Diet. Assoc.* 1989; 89:1504.
16. Dietz, W.H. Nutritional requirements and feeding of the handicapped child. In: Grand, R.J., Stuphen, J.L., Dietz, W.H., eds. *Pediatric Nutrition, Theory and Practice.* Boston: Butterworths; 1987.
17. Belt, B., Ekvall, S., Cook, C., Oppenheimer, S., Wessel, J. Linear growth measurement: a comparison of single arm-length and arm-span. *Dev. Med. Child. Neurol.* 1986; 28:319.
18. Snyder, R.G., Schneider, L.W., Owings, C.L., Reynolds, H.M., Golomb, D.H., Schork, M.A. *Anthropometry of Infants, Children, and Youths to Age 18 for Product Safety Design*, Bethesda, MD; Consumer Product Safety Commission; (Report No. UM-HSRI-77-17), 1977.
19. Spender, Q.W., Cronk, C.E., Charney, E.B., Stallings, V.A. Assessment of linear growth of children with cerebral palsy: use of alternative measures to height or length. *Dev. Med. Child. Neurol.* 1989; 31:206.
20. Leamy, C.M. A study of the food intake of a group of children with cerebral palsy in the Lakewood Sanatorium. *Am. J. Public Health.* 1953; 43:1310.
21. Peeks, S., Lamb, M.W. Comments on the dietary practices of cerebral palsied children. *J. Am. Diet. Assoc.* 1951; 27:870.
22. Hammond, M.I., Lewis, M.N., Johnson, E.W. A nutritional study of cerebral palsied children. *J. Am. Diet. Assoc.* 1966; 49:196.
23. Wakoh, T., Hillman, J.C., Reiss, M. Energy metabolism of spastic children. *Int. J. Neuropsych.* 1965; 1:185.
24. Berg, K., Olsson, T. Energy requirements of school children with cerebral palsy as determined from indirect calorimetry. *Acta Pediatr. Scand.* 1970; 24:71.
25. Eddy, T.P., Nickolson, A.L., Wheeler, E.F. Energy expenditure and dietary intakes in cerebral palsy. *Dev. Med. Child. Neurol.* 1965; 7:377.
26. Bandini, L.G., Schoeller, D.A., Fukagana, N.K., Wykes, L., Dietz, W.H. Body composition and energy expenditure in adolescents with cerebral palsy or myelodysplasia. *Pediatr. Res.* 1991; 29:70.
27. Cully, W.J., Middleton, T.O. Caloric requirements of mentally retarded children with and without motor dysfunction. *J. Pediatr.* 1969; 75:380.
28. Mimaki, T., Walson, P.D., Haussler, M.R. Anticonvulsant therapy vitamin D metabolism: evidence of different mechanisms for phenytoin and phenobarbital. *Pediatr. Pharmacol.* 1980; 1:105.
29. Karle, I.P., Brieler, R.E., Ohlson, M.A. Nutritional status of cerebral palsied children. *J. Am. Diet. Assoc.* 1961; 38:22.
30. Finnie, N.R., ed. *Handling the Young Cerebral Palsied Child at Home.* 2nd ed. New York: Dutton; 1975.
31. Gisel, E.G., Patrick, J. Identification of children with cerebral palsy unable to maintain a normal nutritional status. *Lancet.* 1988; 1:283.
32. Ottenbacher, K., Hicks, J., Roarke, A., Swinea, J. Oral sensorimotor therapy in the developmentally disabled: a multiple baseline study. *Am. J. Occup. Ther.* 1983; 37:541.
33. Hulme, J.B., Shaver, J., Archer, S., Mullette, L., Eggert, C. Effects of adaptive seating devices on the eating and drinking of children with multiple handicaps. *Am. J. Occup. Ther.* 1987; 41:81.
34. Hulme, J.B., Poor, R., Schulein, M. Perceived behavioral changes observed with adaptive seating devices and training programs for multihandicapped developmentally disabled individuals. *Phys. Ther.* 1983; 62:204.
35. Moore, S., Bergman, J.S., Edwards, G., Cowsar, D., Echols, S.D., Forbes, J. The DESEMO customized seating device support-custom molded seating for severely disabled persons. *Phys. Ther.* 1982; 62:460.
36. Roberts, D.W. Positioning device for individuals with neuromuscular disabilities. *Phys. Ther.* 1982; 62:33.
37. Banerdt, B., Brecker, D. A training program for the motorically impaired. *AAESPH Rev.* 1980; 3:222.
38. Ray, S.A. Decreasing drooling through techniques to facilitate mouth closure. *Am. J. Occup. Ther.* 1983; 31:749.
39. Patrick, J., Boland, M., Staski, D., Murray, G.E. Rapid correction of wasting in children with cerebral palsy. *Dev. Med. Child. Neurol.* 1986; 28:734.
40. Rempel, G.R., Colwell, S.O., Nelson, R.P. Growth in children with cerebral palsy fed via gastrostomy. *Pediatrics.* 1988; 82:857.
41. Sanders, K.D., Cox, K., Cannon, R., Blanchard, D., Pitcher, J., Papathakis, P., Varella, L., Maughan, R. Growth response to enteral feeding by children with cerebral palsy. *JPEN.* 1990; 14:23.

Chapter 8
Epilepsy

Shirley Walberg Ekvall and Susan Iannaccone

Epilepsy affects 1.5% to 2% of the population with an incidence of 40 new cases per 100,000 persons per year or approximately 100,000 new cases in the United States annually. There is a bimodal distribution according to age, with the highest incidence occurring at the extremes of life: the neonatal period and old age.[1] A small increase in incidence occurs at adolescence as well, but is less significant. Epilepsy cases may account for 80% of the clinical practice of some pediatric neurologists.

Epilepsy is a symptom of brain dysfunction characterized by excessive fluctuations in electromechanical balance that may be expressed in spontaneous recurring seizures—sudden electrical discharges in the central nervous system (CNS) that alter behavior or function.[2,3] The abnormal discharge may be limited to a region of the brain or may spread throughout the CNS. Thus, seizures may produce a variety of clinical symptoms ranging from a mild alteration in level of consciousness to the dramatic "grand mal" seizure. The clinician relies greatly on eyewitness accounts of the seizure pattern for accurate diagnosis and classification of the epilepsy. Some clues that paroxysmal behavior may represent a form of epilepsy include abrupt onset, stereotypic behavior, abnormal mental status, and brevity and sudden cessation of the episodes.[4]

Several years ago, a system for the International Classification of Epileptic Seizures (ICES)[5] was established. This system enables the use of a common language among clinicians, researchers, and pharmacologists when discussing either evaluation or management of epilepsy. The ICES (Table 8–1) has facilitated more accurate assessment of diagnostic methods and treatment protocols for the various types of epilepsy. Most epileptic patients enjoy a significant decrease in number or complete control of their seizures when treated with the appropriate antiepileptic drug (AED) in an appropriate dose. Commonly used AEDs today include phenytoin, carbamezepine, valproic acid, and nitrazepam. Phenobarbital is very useful for infants and small children.[1,6] The anticonvulsant carbamazepene has a relatively low teritogenicity risk for use during pregnancy. A single anticonvulsant administered at the lowest dosage to achieve seizure control is recommended.[7]

The causes of epilepsy are as various as the clinical manifestations. The search for etiology is an important part of the diagnostic work-up, since knowledge of etiology is the only way to ensure specific treatment.[8] Most cases of epilepsy in childhood are idiopathic (no known cause) or familial (genetic cause).[4] However, many are caused by structural abnormalities of the brain, such as tumors, that can be corrected by surgery. If surgical intervention or correction of electrolyte imbalance cannot cure the epilepsy, then

Table 8-1. Classification of Epileptic Seizures

Partial Seizures	Generalized Seizures
Simple partial (conscious)	Absence (petit mal)
Motor: focal, adversive, jacksonian	Tonic-clonic (grand mal)
Sensory: tingling, light flashes,	Tonic or clonic
buzzing, smell, vertigo	Myoclonic
Autonomic: pallor, flushing	Atonic
Psyche: déjà vu, fear, macropsia,	Infantile spasms
music, scenes, forced thinking	
Complex partial (consciousnesss impaired)	
Impairment of consciousness at onset	
Without impairment of consciousness at onset (simple partial onset)	
Partial seizures evolving to generalized tonic-clonic seizures	

From Wright.[4] Used with permission.

treatment with AEDs is indicated. Selection of the appropriate AED depends almost entirely on accurate classification of the patient's epilepsy.[3]

Biochemical Abnormalities

Diphenylhydantoin (DPH), a hydantoin, may be useful for treatment of certain generalized epilepsies, as well as partial complex seizures. It usually does not produce sedation or respiratory depression and can be given intravenously for treatment of status epilepticus.[9] However, long-term therapy with DPH may cause hirsutism, gingival hypertrophy, and coarse facial features.[1] Higher retino 1 binding protein and lower T_4 were found in children receiving phenobarbitol, diphenylhydantoin, or anticonvulsant combinations, but vitamin A was higher among those who received diphenylhadantoin.[10] Its use during pregnancy has been associated with an embryopathy, the "fetal hydantoin syndrome," which carries a high risk of mental retardation in the exposed fetus[11] (see Chapter 15). Folic acid may be depleted by prolonged use of DPH, but anemia rarely occurs. Supplementation with high doses of folic acid may cause an increase in seizure frequency and even seizure status in some patients.[4] Higher retinol-binding protein and lower T_4 levels were found in children receiving phenobarbitol, DPH, or anticonvulsant combinations, but vitamin A was higher among those who received DPH.[12] Frank rickets has been reported in DPH-treated children from northern climates in which sun exposure may be restricted for part of the year.[13] DPH may interfere with absorption of calcium from the diet and accelerate the metabolism of vitamin D. In a study on dogs treated with phenytoin for 54 weeks, the RBC folate content decreased significantly, but hepatic folate did not decrease.[14] DPH may induce the liver to metabolize several drugs, or it may inhibit drug metabolism, such as when given with phenobarbital.[15] The availability of new, more effective AEDs, such as valproic acid, has enabled clinicians to manage many more patients with monotherapy,[16] thereby avoiding such complicating drug interactions.

DPH, phenobarbital, and other AEDs may raise triglyceride (TG) and cholesterol levels by altering the metabolism of fatty acids. This effect has been found to be temporary, disappearing after 2 years of continuous therapy.[1] Treatment with AEDs should be initiated only after careful consideration by the patient and the physician of the risk of recurrent seizures compared to the risk of long-term therapy.[17]

Factors to be Considered in Nutritional Evaluation

Prolonged anticonvulsant drug therapy can cause many nutritional disturbances (see Chapter 27). Young children with neurologic disabilities taking multiple antiepileptic drugs may have the greatest risk for carnitine deficiency; thus, carnitine levels should be measured.[18] Hypoglycemia has been found to be associated with seizure disorders, and early treatment is imperative to prevent brain damage caused by low blood glucose. A variety of inborn errors of protein metabolism, such as phenylketonuria, Hartnup's disease, alkaptonuria, cystinuria, maple syrup urine disease, and Fanconi's syndrome, are associated with convulsions.

Complete blood counts should be evaluated periodically to review signs of megaloblastic anemia from folic acid or vitamin B_{12} deficiency. Children on anticonvulsant medication also should be evaluated for vitamin D (1,25 dihydroxy cholecalciferol) and calcium levels. Over 40% of persons undergoing therapy may have decreased levels of calcium and phosphorus and elevated alkaline phosphate levels.[1] This decrease in calcium and phosphorus is thought to be due to vitamin D deficiency, which is produced by a drug-induced increase in hepatic microsomal catabolism of vitamin D and its biologically active metabolites. If not treated with vitamin D, osteomalacia or rickets may occur.[1,13] Exposure to sunlight of at least 15 to 20 minutes per day (and longer for darkly pigmented skin) and weight-bearing activity, such as walking or standing each day, are needed to reduce osteomalacia as well.

After a prolonged seizure-free period, the question arises for every patient with epilepsy of whether to discontinue the AED treatment. The relapse rate has been shown to range from 20% to 63% in children with epilepsy.[19] In a prospective study by Hirtz et al.,[20] the risk of recurrence after a first postneonatal nonfebrile seizure was 61% by 7 years of age. They demonstrated that focal seizures were more likely to recur than generalized motor seizures. Nearly 90% of the recurrences took place within 1 year and 96% within 2 years.[20]

Because of the risk of developing a variety of nutritional disturbances, a child with epilepsy who has been receiving anticonvulsant therapy should be monitored closely for these conditions: feeding problems caused by sore and swollen gums (gum hypertrophy is caused by phenytoin medication), loss of appetite associated with the use of drugs, and vitamin and mineral deficiencies.[21] Decreased calorie or nutrient intake may occur because of drowsiness associated with anticonvulsant usage or feeding problems at mealtimes (see Chapter 24).

Anthropometric measurements of height and weight, triceps skinfolds, and arm circumference (for arm muscle area) are needed to assess the adequacy of protein and energy intake.[22] A study by Uden et al.[23] supports the use of antioxidant supplements—selenium, vitamin C, and methionine—to help control painful exacerbations of chronic pancreatitis, especially when the person is taking anticonvulsant therapy and is producing increasing cytochromes P450 by using cigarettes or alcohol.

Dietary Management

A person with epilepsy should eat a normal, healthy diet, with adequate protein, calories, vitamins, and minerals as recommended by a physician or nutritionist. The diet should be particularly high in vitamin D, riboflavin, folic acid, and calcium. Correction of malnutrition during pregnancy can help prevent seizures.

The ketogenic diet (high-fat intake) was developed in 1921.[1] It initiates ketosis or the metabolic circumstances associated with starvation. Evidence suggests that ketosis is the major factor correlated with improved brain wave recordings and with clinical seizure control in the person with epilepsy. It was believed that ketonuria was the variable that controlled seizures. The ketogenic diet was particularly effective in children, but due to its unpalatability, it was very difficult to maintain over prolonged periods. With the discovery of effective anticonvulsant medications, the diet was gradually discarded. Today, the ketogenic diet is often used for those persons for whom medications induce toxic side effects.[1]

The breakdown of nutrients in the ketogenic diet is shown in this formula:

$$\frac{\text{ketogenic}}{\text{antiketogenic}} = \frac{0.90 \text{ F } 0.46 \text{ P } 0.0 \text{ C}}{0.10 \text{ F } 0.58 \text{ P } 1.00 \text{ C}}$$

where F = calories provided from fat, P = calories provided from protein, and C = calories provided from carbohydrate. The ratio of three or four acetoacetic acid (ketogenic) to one molecule of glucose (antiketogenic) is needed to obtain adequate results.[24]

Fortunately, a more palatable version of the diet—the medium-chain triglyceride (MCT) diet—has been developed.[25,26] A variation of the ketogenic diet, it is easier to adhere to because many of the fats are given in the form of special MCT oil. This oil can be used for cooking or mixed with other foods so that its taste is not noticeable. The use of MCT oil makes the diet more ketogenic and less hypercholesterolemic than the standard diet.[27] Drinking mixtures of MCT is small amounts also alleviates the troublesome side effects of nausea, vomiting, abdominal cramps, and diarrhea.[27] However, because of reduced carbohydrate and protein intake, vitamin and mineral deficiencies need to be evaluated carefully. Table 8–2 outlines the procedure for calculating the MCT diet. In one study, 50 children with drug-resistant epilepsy were treated with the MCT diet. Eight achieved complete control of seizures, four had seizures reduced by 90%, and ten by 50% to 90%.[25] Results using the MCT diet were best in children with astatic myoclonic and absence seizures versus those with tonic-clonic and complex partial seizures. An extra dose of MCT given before bedtime reduced nocturnal seizures.[22] Recent research showed that a corn oil ketogenic diet was effective in reducing the number and frequency of intractable seizures.[28]

In some patients, epileptic seizures sometimes coincide with migraine headaches and at other times occur independently. Opioid peptides have been implicated in the pathophysiology of epileptic seizures and in the induction of mast cells, suggesting a possible association among food hypersensitivity, migraine, and epilepsy. Egger et al.,[29] in a double-blind study, produced a 55% reduction in seizures in children with epilepsy, headaches, abdominal symptoms, or hyperkinetic behavior. Foods that provoked symptoms were identified and systematically reintroduced into the diet (see Chapters 28 and 20). Children with epilepsy alone did not benefit from the diet.

Other management

Growth between the 10th and 90th percentile in height and weight, daily exposure to sunshine to enhance vitamin D utilization, and daily weight-bearing activities should be monitored. Daily dental and oral hygiene is needed.

Table 8-2. Calculation of the Medium-Chain Triglyceride Diet

1. Establish caloric needs according to the RDA: 1900 kcal
2. Determine the amount of MCT oil to be given: 50% to 70% of total kcals
   60% of 1900 = 1140 kcal from MCT
   1 g MCT = 8.3 kcal
   1140/8.3 = 137 g MCT
   137 × 8.3 = 1137 kcal
   15 mL (1 tbsp) MCT = 14 g
   137/14 = 9.8 tbsp (tbsp + 1 tsp) MCT
3. Determine kcal to be provided by foods exclusive of MCT: 1900–1140 = 760 kcal
4. Establish protein intake according to RDA: at least 36 g protein for 5- to 7-year-old child weighing 28 kg.
   41 × 4 = 164 kcal protein
5. Estimate maximum kcal to be given in form of carbohydrate:
   19% of 1900 = no more than 361 kcal
   361 kcal/4 = no more than 90 g of CHO
   89 × 4 = 356 kcal
6. Estimate maximum kcal to be given in form of protein and carbohydrate:
   29% of 1900 = no more than 551 kcal from PRO + CHO 164 + 356 = 520 kcal from CHO + PRO
7. Estimate minimum kcal to be given in form of fats exclusive of MCT
   11% of 1900 = at least 209 kcal from other fats
   20 × 9 = 180 kcal exclusive from MCT
8. After determining above dietary requirements, calculate the dietary pattern using exchange lists (see Chapter 44).

Follow-up

Daily urine analysis for ketones, continual reassessment of anticonvulsant drug therapy, and monthly monitoring of nutritional status as described in this chapter are recommended.

References

1. Sugarman, G. *Epilepsy Handbook.* St. Louis: C.V. Mosby Co.; 1984.
2. Rodin, E. An assessment of current views on epilepsy. *Epilepsia.* 1987; 28:267.
3. Freeman, J.M. A clinical approach to the child with seizures and epilepsy. *Epilepsia.* 1987; 28:103.
4. Wright, E.S. Epilepsy in childhood. *Pediatr. Clin. North Am.* 1984; 31:177.
5. Commission on Classification and Terminology of the International League Against Epilepsy. Proposal for the classification of epilepsies and epileptic syndromes. *Epilepsia.* 1985; 26:268.
6. Delgado-Escuela, A.V., Treiman, D.M., Walsh, G.O. The treatable epilepsies. *N. Engl. J. Med.* 1983; 308:1508.
7. Kilpatrick, C.J., Moulds, R.F.W. Anticonvulsants in pregnancy. *Med. J. Aust.* 1991; 154:199.
8. Gomez, M.R., Klass, D.W. Epilepsies of infancy and childhood. *Ann. Neurol.* 1983; 13:113.
9. Lockman, L.A. Status epilepticus. In: Morselli, P.L., Pippenger, C.E., eds. *Antiepileptic Drug Therapy in Pediatrics.* New York: Raven Press; 1983.
10. Kozlowski, B.W., Taylor, M.L., Baer, M.T., Blyler, E.M., Trahms, C. Anticonvulsant medication use and circulating levels of total thyroxine, retinol binding protein, and vitamin A in children with delayed cognitive development. *Am. J. Clin. Nutr.* 1987; 46:360.
11. Majewski, R., Steger, M. Fetal head growth retardation associated with maternal phenobarbitone/primidone and/or phenytoin therapy. *Eur. J. Pediatr.* 1984; 141:188.
12. Kozlowski, B.W., Taylor, M.L., Baer, M.T., Blyler, E.M., Trahms, C. Anticonvulsant medication use and circulating levels of total thyroxine, retinol binding protein, and vitamin A in children with delayed cognitive development. *Am. J. Clin. Nutr.* 1987; 46:360.
13. Hunt, P.A., Wu-chen, M.L., Handal, N.J., Chang, C.T., Gomez, M., Howell, T.R., Hartenberg, M.A., Chan, J.C.M. Bone disease induced by anticonvulsant therapy and treatment with calcitriol (1,25-dihydroxyvitamin D_3). *Am. J. Dis. Child.* 1986; 140:715.
14. Bunch, S., Easley, J., Cullen, J. Hematologic values and plasma and tissue folate concentrations in dogs given phenytoin on a long term basis. *Am. J. Vet. Res.* 1990; 51:1865.
15. Levy, R., Moreland, T.A., Farwell, J.R. Drug interactions in epileptic children. In: Morselli, P.L., Pippenger, C.E., eds. *Antiepileptic Drug Therapy in Pediatrics.* New York: Raven Press; 1983.
16. Shakir, R., Johnson, R., Lambie, D. Comparison of sodium valproate and phenytoin as single drug treatment in epilepsy. In: Morselli, P.L., Pippenger, C.E., eds. *Antiepileptic Drug Therapy in Pediatrics.* New York: Raven Press; 1983.
17. Tharp, B.R. An overview of pediatric seizure disorders and epileptic syndromes. *Epilepsia.* 1987; 28:36.
18. Coulter, D. Carnitine, valproate and toxicity. *J. Child. Neurol.* 1991; 6:7.
19. Todt, H. The late prognosis of epilepsy in childhood: results of a prospective follow-up study. *Epilepsia.* 1984; 25:137.
20. Hirtz, D.G., Ellenberg, J., Nelson, K.B. The risk of recurrence of nonfebrile seizures in children. *Neurology.* 1984; 34:637.
21. Palmer, S., Kalisz, K. Epilepsy. In: Palmer, S., Ekvall, S., eds. *Pediatric Nutrition in Developmental Disorders.* Springfield, IL: Charles C Thomas; 1978.
22. Beran, R., Vajda, F. Weight reduction and epilepsy. *Am. Med. J. Aust.* 1991; 154:71.
23. Uden, S., Acheson, D.W.K., Reeves, J., Worthington, H.V., Hunt, L.P., Brown, S., Braganza, J.M. Antioxidants, enzyme induction, and chronic pancreatitis: a reappraisal following

studies in patients on anticonvulsants. *Eur. J. Clin. Nutr.* 1988; 42:561.

24. Wilder, R.M., Winter, M.D. The threshold of ketogenesis. *J. Biol. Chem.* 1922; 52:401.

25. Sills, M.A., Forsythe, W.I., Haidukewych, D., Macdonald, Robinson, M. The medium chain triglyceride diet and intractable epilepsy. *Arch. Dis. Child.* 1986; 61:1168.

26. Gasch, A. Use of the traditional hetogenic diet for treatment of intractable epilepsy. *J. Am. Diet. Assoc.* 1990; 90:1433.

27. Huttenlocher, P.R., Wilbourn, A.J., Signore, J.M. Medium chain triglycerides as a therapy for intractable childhood epilepsy. *Neurology.* 1971; 21:1097.

28. Woody, R.C., Brodie, M., Hampton, D.K., Fiser, R.H. Corn oil ketogenic diet for children with intractable seizures. *J. Child. Neurol.* 1988; 3:21.

29. Egger, J., Carter, C.M., Soothill, J.F., Wilson, J. Oligoantigenic diet treatment of children with epilepsy and migraine. *J. Pediatr.* 1989; 114:51.

Chapter 9
Muscular Dystrophy

Susan Iannaccone

Muscular dystrophy is a progressive, hereditary disorder of muscle that causes deterioration of strength in voluntary muscle. The most common form of muscular dystrophy is Duchenne, which is caused by a deletion of a large gene on the X chromosome at the Xp21 locus.[1] Deletion of this gene results in the absence of a protein, dystrophin, from the intracellular surface of the muscle membrane. The function of this protein is not yet understood, but it has been shown to occur in tissues other than skeletal muscle. This fact may explain why many patients also suffer from involvement of heart muscle (cardiomyopathy) and of the brain, resulting in mental retardation.[2] Duchenne dystrophy affects one male infant in 18,000.

The term "neuromuscular diseases" refers to all disease of muscle and nerve, including muscular dystrophy and other myopathies. The most common neuromuscular diseases of childhood are Duchenne muscular dystrophy (DMD); spinal muscular atrophy (SMA), a disorder of the motor neuron also known as Werdnig-Hoffmann disease; myasthenia gravis; myotonic dystrophy; and the congenital myopathies, such as nemaline myopathy (Table 9-1). As a group, such diseases account for a significant proportion of physical handicaps in childhood.[3] Up to 30% of hospitalized patients may have a neuromuscular complication. Most neuromuscular disease, as is Duchenne, is caused by a genetic defect. However, some, such as dermatomyositis or myasthenia gravis, are acquired and may be cured with specific therapy. A few may be either acquired or congenital, such as carnitine deficiency. Neuromuscular disorders that are caused by dietary

deficiency, such as vitamin E, are extremely rare. This chapter focuses only on nutritional problems resulting from diseases associated with weakness of skeletal muscle and not on any diseases caused by nutritional deficiencies.

Nutritional problems are most likely to be caused by weakness of the bulbar musculature resulting in inadequate caloric intake (Table 9-2). Thus, patients may present as failures to thrive. Conversely, some patients develop morbid obesity secondary to immobility.

Biochemical and Pathological Abnormalities

Accurate diagnosis of the neuromuscular disease[4,5] is essential before embarking on evaluation and management of the nutritional complications. Diagnosis is based on blood and urine tests, occasionally x-rays, electrodiagnostic study (EMG), and muscle biopsy. The single most important blood chemistry—the creatine kinase level—is helpful for diagnosing muscular dystrophy. It is generally elevated in cases of muscular dystrophy—up to 6×10^3 times normal in Duchenne dystrophy.

Specific diagnosis rests on the morphological examination of tissue. In certain cases, both muscle and nerve biopsies may be necessary. Frequently, the muscle biopsy can be done as a percutaneous procedure using a special needle. Occasionally, it must be done under general anesthesia as an "open" biopsy; in those cases the surgeon uses a longer incision, about 1–2 inches, allowing visualization of the mus-

Table 9-1. Neuromuscular Diseases and Nutritional Disorders Secondary to Weakness

Diagnosis	Growth Failure	Feeding Difficulty	Weakness Facial	Weakness Nasopharyngeal	Weakness Respiratory	Comments
Genetic Disorders						
Duchenne muscular dystrophy	—	Late	Late	Late	Late	Obesity
Spinal muscular atrophy	+	Early	Early	Late	Late	Obesity
Congenital myopathy*	+	Early	Early	Late	Late	—
Congenital myotonic dystrophy	+/−	Early	Early	Early	Possible	Mental retardation
Acquired (Reversible) Disorders						
Guillain-Barré syndrome	—	Possible	Possible	Possible	+	Good prognosis
Myasthenia gravis	—	Possible	Rare	+	+	Fatiguability prominent
Polymyositis/ dermatomyositis	—	Possible	Rare	Rare	Rare	—

*Nemaline myopathy, central core myopathy, centronuclear myopathy, myotubular myopathy.

Table 9-2. Neuromuscular Disease and Nutrition Problems

Disorder	Area of Weakness
Inadequate caloric intake caused by weakness*	
Duchenne muscular dystrophy	Trunk, arms
Spinal muscular atrophy	Trunk, arms, face
Myasthenia gravis	Face, tongue, nasopharynx
Myotonic dystrophy	Face, tongue, nasopharynx esophagus
Congenital myopathy	Face, tongue
Weakness caused by nutritional disorders	
Vitamin E deficiency	Limbs, trunk
Vitamin B deficiency (B$_1$, B$_6$, B$_{12}$)	Limbs
Carnitine deficiency	Trunk, limbs, heart

*Other causes of inadequate caloric intake are abnormal swallowing mechanism, poor positioning (against gravity), pulmonary congestion (weak cough), and dependency (lack of self-feeding).

cle at the time of biopsy. In either case, the biopsy is a short procedure, lasting no more than 30 minutes. The patient may resume normal activity immediately. Although these procedures may be available at most hospitals, they should be performed by specialists in neuromuscular diseases, since the diagnosis depends on appropriate technique and expert interpretation of the findings.

Factors to be Considered in Nutritional Evaluation

When nutritional problems occur secondary to inadequate caloric intake, strength and function of the bulbar musculature should be evaluated. A careful examination of the cranial nerves, both efferent and afferent pathways, is most important. Further evaluation of the swallowing mechanism should be done using radiological techniques (see Chapter 24).

The mechanics of normal eating involves four phases of swallowing. The *pre-swallow or oral phase* is the period of time during which the food is in the mouth. During this phase, solid food is chewed, and both solid and liquid are formed into a bolus in preparation for swallowing. Skeletal muscles are used for biting, chewing, and, in the case of infants, for sucking. If any of these muscle groups are weak, the oral phase of swallowing will be abnormal. The *second or pharyngeal phase* is the swallow reflex. During this phase, the bolus is propelled from the mouth into the pharynx and then to the esophagus. This propulsion requires that the tongue and nasopharynx, both of which are skeletal muscles, function normally so that the food is moved rapidly while the airway is protected by closure of the glottis. Weakness during this phase not only prevents entrance of food or liquid into the esophagus but also puts the patient at risk for aspiration into the lungs causing pneumonia or apnea. Pooling of oral secretions and an inability to swallow may provoke choking. This is the phase of swallowing that is most commonly affected in patients with neuromuscular disorders. During the *esophageal or third phase* of swallowing, the bolus moves through the esophagus by contraction of its wall. The upper one-third of the esophagus is lined with skeletal muscle, and the lower two-thirds are lined by smooth muscle. Some diseases, such as myotonic dystrophy, affect

both types of muscle, whereas other disorders, such as central core myopathy, only affect skeletal muscle. Therefore, this phase of swallowing may be fairly normal in some neuromuscular diseases and abnormal in others. Finally, in the *fourth or postswallow phase*, the food has entered the stomach. This phase is generally normal in neuromuscular disorders, but reflux may occur in children for other reasons. Obviously, if reflux does occur, then it will complicate the patient's management.

Nutrient and caloric intake, physical activity, anthropometry measurements (body weight, triceps skinfold, midarm muscle circumference), and biochemical values (hemoglobin, prealbumin, and serum transferrin) should be evaluated by the nutritionist.

Dietary Management and Treatment

Ideally, management of such patients is based on the team approach. The leader of the team is the primary care physician who is most often the pediatric neurologist, but may be a pediatric physiatrist or the pediatrician. The team leader is the primary communicator with the patient and the parents and their liaison with other specialists and members of the team. Team members include a nutritionist who specializes in the care of children, physical therapist, occupational therapist, physiatrist, respiratory therapist, nurse, and social worker. The participation of all members of the team may not be required at every stage of the disease, but the role of each should be considered carefully by the primary physician who calls on each as needed. Each member should be introduced to the patient and family early in the course of the disease, soon after diagnosis. Doing so provides continuity of care and allows the patient and family to become comfortable with the team effort.

Management depends on determination of the nature and scope of the swallowing problem, since it is important to know whether the child is at risk for aspiration, whether his or her nutritional needs are being met, and whether the problem can be explained in the context of the disease. Thus, accurate diagnosis of the neuromuscular disorder is essential before evaluation of the eating process.

The child should be observed while taking both liquids and solids (Table 9-3). Laryngoscopy and bronchoscopy may be indicated to evaluate the function of the glottis and vocal

Table 9-3. Evaluation of Swallowing Problems

	Physical Signs	Special Tests
Liquids	Poor coordination, delayed swallow, nasal regurgitation	Barium swallow with video
Solids (labeled food)	Delayed peristalsis, fatigue on chewing	Barium swallow with video
	Gag reflex, movement of palate, tongue motility	Laryngobronchoscopy

cords. If an abnormality is identified at any phase of swallowing, several options for management may be considered in the context of the patient's age, nutritional status, and degree of weakness (Table 9-4). The occupational therapist and the nutritionist play important roles in evaluating and managing the patient's swallowing function during phases 1 and 2 of swallowing and his or her feeding skills.

When the mechanics of swallowing are normal, weakness in other muscle groups may still interfere with attaining adequate nutrition. Supporting the infant or child in an upright position engages the help of gravity in the swallowing mechanism.[6] Chest physiotherapy should be done just before feedings to ensure optimal respiratory function and to clear the nasopharynx of all secretions.[7] Weak patients fatigue easily, and adequate rest periods should be allowed during the meal.[8,9] This may necessitate several small meals during the day, rather than the conventional three. The meal schedule should be adjusted to accommodate the child's school program. For older children with Duchenne muscular dystrophy or spinal muscular atrophy, table height, position of arms, and adaptive utensils may make the difference between complete dependency and self-feeding. Such devices should be provided at school, as well as at home (see Chapter 24).

Although the most common nutritional problem in infants with neuromuscular disease is failure to thrive, patients in midchildhood with muscular dystrophy are usually able to swallow normally. However, severe weakness of all other voluntary muscles renders the children hypomobile or completely immobile. In this situation, they frequently consume more calories than they can burn and become obese. Such obesity is difficult to reverse and poses a health threat not only for the patients but also for their mothers or other caregivers who must transfer them from bed to wheelchair to commode.[10] The early introduction of the nutritionist as part of the patient's management team may be helpful in preventing the development of obesity. The nutritionist assesses the diet and physical activity level and performs anthropometric measurements before prescribing a specific diet (see Chapter 19). In a recent study, however, six children with Duchenne muscular dystrophy, when given a nightly tube feeding by drip of 100 mL/0 $\times$ 10^0 of Osmolite® (supplies 1000 calories and 37.2 g of protein daily) for 3 months, showed a significant increase in body weight and 14% increase in midarm muscle circumference with only a small change in triceps skinfold, indicating an increase in muscle mass.[11] No changes occurred in these measures: urinary 3-methylhistidine excretion, suggesting improved muscle protein synthesis with no change in muscle protein degradation; hematological and biochemical parameters; liver or pulmonary function tests; or general activity index. No change was shown in body weight or anthropometric measures on three congenital muscular dystrophy patients following the same procedure.

Follow-up and Summary

In conclusion, an accurate diagnosis of the specific neuromuscular disorder affecting the child is essential. The nutritionist is part of the management team and should be consulted soon after the diagnosis has been established. At each clinic or hospital visit, the nutritionist should take a dietary and physical activity history and make anthropometric measurements. Evaluation of the swallowing mechanism will determine how best to achieve adequate nutrition. Gastric tube placement, temporary or permanent, may be indicated in certain cases where oral intake is inadequate to achieve or maintain normal growth. The team approach is most important, and for pediatric patients, the parents are an integral part of the team.

References

1. Arahata, K. Dystrophin and Duchenne's muscular dystrophy. *N. Engl. J. Med.* 1989; 320:138.
2. Rowland, L. Clinical concepts of Duchenne muscular dystrophy. The impact of molecular genetics. *Brain.* 1988; 111:479.
3. Dubowitz, V. *Color Atlas of Muscle Disorders in Childhood.* Chicago: Year Book Medical; 1989.
4. Brooke, M.H. *A Clinician's View of Neuromuscular Diseases.* Baltimore: Williams & Wilkins; 1977.
5. Szer, I. Congenital and metabolic abnormalities of the musculoskeletal system. *Curr. Opin. Rheumatol.* 1990; 2:832.
6. Berger, A.F., Colangelo, C. *Positioning the Client with Central Nervous System Deficits: The Wheelchair and Other Adapted Equipment.* Valhalla: Valhalla Rehabilitation; 1982.
7. Heckmatt, J.Z. Leading articles: respiratory care in muscular dystrophy. *Br. Med. J.* 1987; 295:1014.
8. Smith, P.E.M., Calverley, P.M.A., Edwards, R.H.T., Evand, G.A., Campbell, E.J.M. Medical progress: practical problems in the respiratory care of patients with muscular dystrophy. *N. Engl. J. Med.* 1987; 316:1197.
9. Jaffee, K., McDonald, C., Ingman, E., Haas, J. Symptoms of upper gastrointestinal dysfunction in Duchenne muscular dystrophy: case control study. *Arch. Phys. Med. Rehab.* 1990; 71:742.
10. Edwards, R.H., Round, J.M., Griffiths, R.D., Lilburn, M.F. Weight reduction in boys with muscular dystrophy. *Dev. Med. Child. Neurol.* 1984; 26:384.
11. Goldstein, M., Meyer, S., Freund, H. Effects of overfeeding in children with muscle dystrophies. *JPEN.* 1989; 13:603.

Table 9-4. Treatment of Swallowing Problems

Swallowing Phase	Remedy
Phase 1	Increase or decrease consistency
	Increase caloric concentration
	Retrain for sucking or chewing
	Use adapted nipples
Phase 2	Adjust consistency
	Bypass with nasogastric tube or gastrostomy/jejunostomy
Phase 3	Bypass
Phase 4	Use proper positioning
	Do Nissan procedure

Chapter 10
Myelomeningocele

Shirley Walberg Ekvall

Myelomeningocele (MM), a type of spina bifida and the most common malformation resulting from a disturbance in neurotation, occurs when a child is born with a protruding sac or lesion along the midline of the spinal cord, which results in no closure of the neural tube (Fig 10-1). This nonclosure occurs when the neuroectoderm is transformed into a neural tube and becomes detached from the cutaneous ectoderm. The defect occurs between 26–30 days gestation; the later the occurrence, the lower the lesion.[1] Removal of the sac and closure of the neural defect usually are performed within 24 hours of birth to avoid infection. The sac contains meninges, dura, cerebral spinal fluid, and other neural elements. Depending on the level of the sac or lesion, the higher the sac, the greater the extent of paralysis manifestations of range from weakness in the lower extremity to complete paralysis and loss of sensation and thereby incontinence of bladder. Upper extremity fine motor problems are also usually present, although to a lesser degree than lower extremity involvement. Approximately 90% of the children with MM have hydrocephalus,[2] which is not fatal if treated promptly before brain tissue is destroyed. A ventriculoatrial or ventriculoperitoneal shunt is used to relieve the pressure (Fig 10-2). The median IQ for children with MM is 88.[3] Even with normal intelligence, many children with MM have a learning disability.

Trophic ulcers, spontaneous fractures, and deformities of lower extremities occur because of reduced ambulation. Obesity follows and is also related to the level of lesion, with higher lesions producing the greatest obesity.[4]

In 1980 myolomeningocele occurred in 5 per 10,000 births in the United States and in 6.7 per 10,000 births in Ireland.[5] It is found 2.5 times more frequently in whites than in blacks or Asians[6] and more frequently in girls than boys in a ratio of 1.25:1.00.[7] Recurrence in families with one child with spina bifida is 2.5 times greater than in the general population; however, its etiology is still unknown.[6] The first-born child is at greatest risk of developing MM.[8]

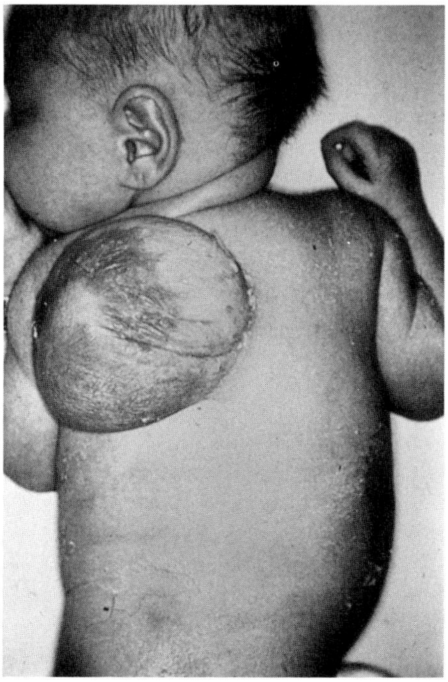

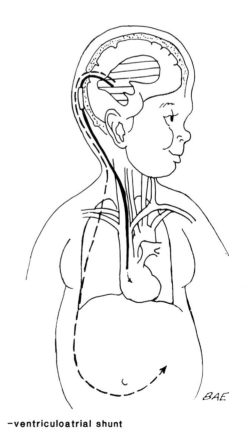

−ventriculoatrial shunt

---ventriculoperitonial shunt

Fig. 10-2. A ventriculoatrial shunt or ventriculoperitoneal shunt is used to relieve pressure.

Fig. 10-1. Protruding sac along the midline of the spinal cord which produces nonclosure of the neural tube. From the UACCDD, Cincinnati.

With surgical correction of hydrocephalus, removal of the lesion, prevention of renal damage, and the provision of aggressive nutrition, orthopedic, and other multidisciplinary therapy, survival may reach 80% to 95%, rather than the earlier levels of 50% to 70%.[2]

Biochemical Abnormalities

Biochemical factors that have been proposed to produce MM, a form of neural tube defect (NTD), are amphetamines, oral contraceptives, potato glycoalkaloids, nitrites, and salicylates; environmental factors, such as geography, maternal age (especially over 35 years) and illness, migration, socioeconomic status, ethnicity, and hyperthermia have also been implicated.[9] Drugs, such as valproic acid, also have been investigated, but currently the most promising area is nutritional deficiencies.[9] Several studies have shown that insulin-dependent diabetic women produce more infants with congenital abnormalities, including neural defects; aminopterin, a powerful folic acid antagonist, has produced neural tube defects in humans.[10] Maternal alcohol ingestion during neurotation also may produce NTD.[11] The etiology is unknown, but prenatal screening is available that can detect raised alphafetoprotein levels in amniotic fluid.[12] Ultrasound monitoring also is frequently performed prenatally for women and can show head malformations before 20 weeks gestation.

High levels of urinary excretion of p-hydroxyphenylacetic acid (pHPAA), 4-hydroxy-3-methoxymandelic acid (HMMA), and homovanillic acid (HVA) found in children with MM may be due to a disorder in the metabolism of ascorbic acid.[13] Ekvall et al.[14] also reported low levels of ascorbic acid and zinc in children with MM; however, the children with MM were able to become ascorbic acid saturated with ascorbic acid supplementation. In this study 40 children with MM were divided evenly into a group receiving ascorbic acid supplementation and a control group. Both groups were matched for age, sex, race, and physical activity. No evidence of vitamin B_{12} deficiency was noted in the 20 children receiving a mean dose of 1.65 g ascorbic acid by the urologist over an average period of 3.2 years when measured against the control group. The dietary intake of ascorbic acid was measured to rule out any influence on serum levels. Results demonstrated that the experimental group with supplementary ascorbic acid had significantly higher ascorbic acid and B_{12} levels than the control group and did not show a deficiency in serum vitamin B_{12} levels, anemia, or an elevated mean corpuscular volume.[14]

Factors to be Considered in Nutritional Evaluation

Nutritional deficiency

Research studies have focused on deficiencies of folic acid, zinc, and multivitamin supplements. In a small study, Laurence et al.[15] recommended that 4 mg of folic acid be administered 28 days before conception to produce less NTD. In a double-blind study Laurence and co-workers[16] investigated the effect of folic acid in early pregnancy and before conception on women who had previous births of children

with NTD. There was no recurrence in 10 who received folic acid, but six recurrences in 17 who had no folate supplement. Also, a good diet produced less recurrence in larger group studies (no recurrence with good diet and six recurrence in 27 women on a poor diet).[17] Laurence et al. concluded that a good diet and folate supplements were beneficial.[17]

Smithells et al.,[8] in England, compared 234 mothers who took a supplemental Pregnavite Forte F® vitamin preparation 28 days before conception to 219 mothers in the United States not receiving that vitamin preparation. The supplemented mothers had only 0.9% recurrence of NTD in England compared to 5.1% in the United States. This vitamin preparation contained slightly less vitamins and minerals than the current U.S. RDA, except for increased iron sulfate. The study's choice of controls was questionable, but called for further research in this area. Malloy et al.[18] suggested the value of better maternal nutritional status evaluation, particularly for folic acid and vitamin B_{12}, early in pregnancy.

A study showing the relation of NTD risk to multivitamin intake in general and to folic acid in particular involved 23,491 women who had alphafetaprotein screening or amniocentesis around 16 weeks gestation. Forty-nine of these women (3.5 per 1000) evaluated at delivery, gave birth to infants with NTD.[19] The prevalence of NTD in women who used folic acid with multivitamins during the first 6 weeks of pregnancy was only 0.09 per 1000, compared to 0.12 to 0.59 per 1000 for those women who used multivitamins without folic acid. The inclusion of folic acid in the multivitamin during the first 6 weeks of pregnancy was most significant in reducing NTD.[19] A recent study in seven countries firmly concluded that a 4 mg supplementation of folic acid (ten times the U.S. RDA of 0.4 mg) significantly lowered recurrence of fetal neural tube defects and recommended increased folic acid for this population as well as for all pregnant women. (The quantity of supplementation for all pregnant women was not given.[20])

Bergmann et al.[21] found increased zinc in hair concentrations during pregnancy in mothers who had produced one child with NTD. The plasma zinc level in maternal blood was significantly lower in 54 women delivering infants with congenital abnormalities. Nevin[22] found significantly higher amounts of zinc and copper in amniotic fluid of mothers in the NTD group. Smithells'[8] supplementation did not include zinc and copper, but zinc as a catalyst could have been spared by increased iron supplementation. Ekvall[14] also showed a reduction in serum zinc, as well as ascorbic acid, in children with MM. The synergistic effect of ascorbic acid and folic acid must be considered.

Avenues for future research include testing multivitamin preparations; examining the effect of other environmental factors, folic acid, and zinc; identifying women and siblings at risk with one affected child; and improving the diets of women during childbearing ages.

Height

Mean birth weight and length in children with NTD were significantly lower than in normal infants.[21] Reduced length and atrophy of the lower extremities seem to produce the reduced height of children with NTD, although other problems, such as hydrocephalus, renal disease, and malnutri-

Table 10-1. Nutritional Assessment for Myelomeningocele: UACCDD Clinic*

I. Dietary intake (based on 3-day annual food record or 24-hour recall with food frequency)
   A. Nutrients (calories, vitamins, minerals, protein)
   B. Fluids, fiber/bulk with bowel function
   C. Energy expenditure/ambulation
   D. Dietary modifications and compliance
   E. Client caregiver understanding
      1. Solid food after 6 months
      2. Increased texture
      3. Good feeding skills
      4. Low-calorie, high nutrient-dense foods and high-calorie, low nutrient-dense foods
      5. Demonstrate 1-day meal plan
         a. Number and size of servings
         b. Weight control/calorie expenditure
         c. Fluid and fiber
         d. Reward nonfood items
         e. Drug and nutrient interactions
         f. Diet modification, if needed

II. Anthropometry
   A. Weight for height
      1. 2 to 10 years of age, keep weight for height 10th to 75th percentile†
      2. 10 to 17 years of age, keep weight for height 10th to 90th percentile†
   B. Fatfold thickness (children over 1 year of age, keep 10th to 90th percentile for age and sex)
      1. Triceps
      2. Abdominal
      3. Waist circumference
   C. Upper arm length

III. Biochemical
   A. Iron status
   B. Nutrient supplementation
   C. Drugs affecting nutrient use/need

IV. Physical signs—clinical and dental
V. Feeding—feeding skills and behaviors

Care Plan

I. Behavioral objective
   A. Problem
   B. Goal
   C. Timetable and how measured
   D. Subject-object assessment plan (SOAP) notes

II. Intervention—within 2 weeks of assessment

*Follows quality assurance guidelines.
†Keep in 25th percentile for age if possible.
From Ekvall, S. Myelomeningocele: nutrition implications. *Top. Clin. Nutr.* 1988:3:41. Used with permission.

tion, may contribute to it. Little data exist on anthropometric measures or the stages of puberty in children with MM.[23] In a study by Rosenblum et al.,[24] children with MM who had a lower lesion showed no reduction in stature, whereas 43% with midlesions and 80% with high lesions were less than the 3rd percentile in height. LaFollette[25] determined that lesions as a collective group resulted in a significant reduction in stature, but no specificity occurred with the level of lesion.

However, in several studies ambulation was significantly affected by the level of the lesion.[25,26] Asher and Olson[26] also found the most important variable affecting ambulation was level of the lesion. LaFollette[25] showed that the linear growth rate of children with a high lesion who were wheelchair bound began to decline and increased weight ensued, whereas those with high lesions who were ambulatory showed more normal growth curves in both height and weight.

Keeping the child walking or physically active and out of the wheelchair is essential to avoid weight gain, regardless of the level of lesion.

Alternate methods of determining stature use arm span or single arm length multiplied by a factor.[26–29] An arm span to height ratio has been developed: arm span × 1.0 if no leg muscle mass loss (sacral lesion), arm span × 0.95 if partial leg muscle loss (mid- and lower lumbar lesion), and arm span × 0.9 if complete leg muscle loss (high lumbar or thoracic lesion). However, children with a high lesion or who are bedridden or wheelchair bound cannot be measured in this manner, and the procedure does require two observers. Belt et al.[30] found that upper arm length was not as affected by a high lesion in MM as the arm span in 48 children with MM (Fig 10-3). For example, in the 9.5 to 10.5 year age group, multiplying the upper arm length by 5.3 could determine stature thereby allowing the identifi-

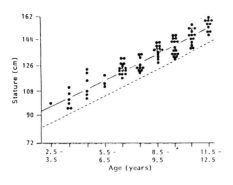

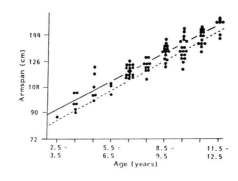

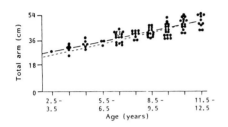

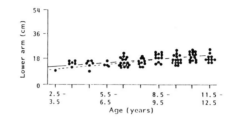

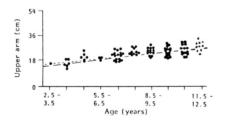

Fig. 10–3. Linear regressions relating stature and arm length measurements with age of control children (*solid lines*) and children with myelomeningocele (*broken lines*). From Belt et al.[30] Used with permission.

cation of pathological factors affecting growth. This procedure only requires one observer. The ratio of arm span to weight has also been examined.[31]

Weight

LaFollette[25] noted that by age 4, children with MM started to gain weight when bracing or walking began. In this study of 100 children with MM, the weight/height index was above the 95th percentile for girls and above the 95th percentile for boys, suggesting obesity. Further investigations with more children are now being conducted by the University Affiliated Cincinnati Center for Developmental Disorders (UACCDD). In a preliminary growth chart with data from several different centers, children with MM tended to follow their own growth curve from 4 to 10, with girls reaching their peak growth at 8 to 9 years and boys at 10 to 12 years (Appendix 2–5 and 2–6).

Skinfolds

Grogan et al.[32] found that the abdominal and thorax skinfolds and waist and abdominal circumferences were correlated significantly with percentage of body fat when measured in the whole body counter. Fat appeared to accumulate

around the hip and lower areas of the body below the neurological lesion. Hayes-Allen[4] found a significant correlation between weight and subscapular skinfold thickness in children with MM. Physical maturation[33] occurs earlier in children with MM (11.4 years versus 12.5–12.7 for children without MM), which may be due to increased adipose tissue (AT) or obesity. Shepherd et al.[34] found decreased body cell mass and total body water (increased extra cellular fluid and decreased intercellular fluid) and increased percentage body fat after ages 3–4 years, particularly in children with high lesions.

Caloric Needs

Since children with MM do not appear overweight on growth grids for age, weight for height or calories per centimeter of height must be used to determine caloric needs. In minimally active children with MM over 8 years old, caloric level was only 7 cal/cm of height, yet weight loss was slight, only 9–11 kcal/cm height was needed to maintain weight.[25,32] Physical activity increased the LBM (thereby calorie needs) better than diet restriction.[32] Braune and Fischer[35] determined that the loss of one limb in children without MM resulted in a 15% reduction in calories. Perhaps a reduction of weight and caloric needs due to limb reduction or atrophy should be considered in MM (see Chapters 4 and 19). Should a 30% or greater reduction in calories occur with atrophy of both limbs? Since there are decreased lean body mass (LBM) and increased adipose tissue (AT) in the paralyzed lower extremities, fat comprises a higher proportion of body mass, and available standards tend to underestimate the extent of obesity. In a small study of 8 adolescent girls with MM using the doubly labeled water method, Bandini et al. measured the following energy needs: 4 nonambulatory 10.2 (8.4–12.8) kcal/cm height and 4 ambulatory 12.6 (11.9–13.2) kcal/cm height. All subjects had developed their upper torso LBM however.[36]

Physical Activity

Obesity can impair ambulation potential to such a degree that children must spend their lifetime in a wheelchair if physical activity is not started early in life. In a study of 14 children with MM, increasing physical activity had more effect than reducing calorie intake in increasing LBM and reducing adipose tissue (AT).[32] Because increasing LBM increases calorie needs, physical activity, such as swimming, is crucial and should begin in infancy. Since the waist circumference test measurement correlates well with adipose tissue, a reduced measurement can be used as a measure of less AT or increased LBM. School-aged children with MM should be able to monitor their weight independently.

Physical Signs, Constipation, and Feeding Skills

Any physical signs of malnutrition or dental problems should be noted during each clinic visit. Poor skin condition due to pressure sores, increased weight, and lack of sensation in the lower extremities must be evaluated at each clinic visit by the nurse and nutritionist and then corrected. Constipation may be caused by the neurogenic bowel (without adequate system control), inactivity, a diet low in fiber and fluid, and the usage of anticholinergenic drugs to treat the neurogenic bladder. Feeding skills should be reviewed as needed due to bulsar palsy produced by the Arnold-Chiari brain malformation.

The study of Grogan et al.[32] found that the mean caloric intake to maintain growth for children over 8 years of age was approximately 50% of that for children without MM. The K_{40} content as a measure of protoplasmic muscle or LBM (indirect measure of AT) in the whole body counter of children with MM was 50% of that for children without MM. Since caloric needs are directly related to lean body mass, a much lower caloric intake is needed for children with MM. It may be as low as 7–9 kcal/cm height in some minimally active children with MM and decreased lean body mass. Caloric restrictions may need to begin between 3 or 4 years when the child should be walking. By this age the limbs fail to grow adequately, and stature is starting to fall off on the growth grid.[25,37,38]

Urinary tract infection (UTI)

Frequent urinary tract infections produce significant health problems.[14,37] Acidification of the urine by dietary means helps decrease bacterial growth. Thus, the acid-ash diet, which is high in meats, poultry, seafood, eggs, fats, and cereals and low in vegetable and fruits, has been promoted. The acid-ash foods include all foods from the meat and bread groups; a few from the vegetable (corn, hominy, and lentils) and fruit group (cranberries, plums, prunes); cakes; cookies; and plain gelatin. Most fats are neutral, except for bacon and brazil nuts, filberts, peanuts, and walnuts. Candy, coffee, and tea also are neutral. Milk and milk products (except for cheese) are alkaline-ash, as well as all fruits and vegetables except those few mentioned above, all salty items, carbonated beverages, chocolate, and items prepared with baking powder or soda. However, the lack of adequate fruits and vegetable, especially for a long period of time, makes this diet controversial. Synthetic vitamin C may also be used to acidify the urine to maintain a pH between 5.5 and 6.

Drug-nutrient interaction

Epilepsy may occur in approximately 20% of patients with MM. The following medications are used frequently: anticonvulsants for seizures, anticholinergics for bladder control, and antibiotics for frequent upper urinary infections (see Chapter 27).

Dietary Management

The criteria for nutrition referral by the Myelomeningocele Clinic at UACCDD are under 5 years; weight above 50th or below 5th percentile or discrepancy in height and weight; mobility loss greater than 25%; mechanical feeding problems; premenarcheal adolescent girls; and certain conditions, such as allergy, diarrhea, excessive use of vitamins, or food faddism. Prevention of health problems through the use of low-calorie, high-nutrient dense foods is emphasized when the child is very young as it is hard to change eating patterns after age 3. It is important to emphasize the introduction of solid foods after 6 months of age and the use of only 1 tbsp initially. Parents or caregivers must understand how much food is enough, to limit the intake to just the amount adequate for growth, and not to use food as a reward or substitute for love. They must be models to their children, eating low-calorie, nutrient-dense foods themselves, to help the child establish good food patterns.

At the UACCDD Preschool, children with MM are educated in the use of low-calorie, high-nutrient dense foods while the caregiver watches through a one-way mirror. This nutrition education is as important as teaching the diabetic exchange system to parents whose children have diabetes. Foods with high-fiber content (see Chapter 35) and plenty of water (8 c/day) help relieve constipation and facilitate weight control. Adequate nutrients—especially zinc, ascorbic acid, and folic acid—must be maintained in the diet of the mother, as well as of the child, since she is at risk for producing a second child with MM. The child with MM already may have low serum levels of ascorbic acid and zinc.

School-aged children should be allowed to select and determine their physical activity and to measure their own waist circumference (having been prepared for this independence during preschool years). The parents or siblings and the child with MM should plan, prepare, and shop for food together. By this time the child should have good dental care practices and be able to plan a 1-day menu as the caregiver has demonstrated to the nutritionist earlier.[39,40]

By the preteen age, children with MM should be in charge of their weight control and exercise programs by setting appropriate goals, keeping food records, taking their own measurements, and making decisions about follow-up care (see Chapter 19). Since weight affects self-image, parents or siblings and the interdisciplinary team—physician, nutritionist, social worker, nurse, physical therapist, psychologist—need to teach self-motivation techniques and the importance of the diet to the young child with MM. Dietary restrictions are imposed when weight is above the 25th percentile for age or 10th percentile for height on standard NCHS growth charts. The multidisciplinary approach to weight control also is described by Hanson and Graves.[41] Killiam et al.[42] Searff and Fronczak[43] and Parent et al.[44] discuss other rehabilitation measures related to weight for the child with MM. A wheelchair, bed, or chair scale can be used to measure weight; infants can be held by their mother. A gross measurement of weight can be obtained by using a tape measure to measure the change in waist circumference over time if no other method is available. Using this method has the advantage of giving children a feeling of control over their weight. Obesity[44] produces significant health problems.

Since exercise increases LBM, it should be started in infancy. Because the child should be kept below the 25th percentile of weight for age, increased exercise should be stressed by all members of the interdisciplinary team. The physical therapist and nutritionist must plan exercise goals together beginning in infancy. Since all children may not be seen by the nutritionist, a criteria for screening or referral should be developed as shown in Chapter 4 *Nutritional Assessment* and the Complete Quality Assurance Standards for MM and Developmental Disorders in Appendix 7. Nutrients related to drug interaction must be evaluated (see Chapter 27).

Follow-up

Caloric intake, physical activity, anthropometrics, and biochemical factors must be monitored and measurable goals specified in the follow-up care plan. The 3-day diet and physical activity diary or a 24-hour dietary recall and frequency cross-check must be obtained weekly in infancy, monthly after 1 month of age, and every 3 months after one year or age until the child reaches school age when it is obtained approximately every 6 months. The diet diaries may extend to the high-risk mother as preconceptual diet counseling is essential for her also.[45] The 24-hour dietary recall (including high-fiber foods, fluids, and nutrient-dense snacks)[46] a food frequency, and a physical activity score should be performed on all MM children who are immobilized or taking anticonvulsant medications. Anthropometric measures (weight, height, skinfold) should be performed each time the child is seen by the Nutrition Department (see Appendix 2 for preliminary growth grids on MM). At that time, biochemical information, physical signs and any feeding problems are also evaluated. Occasionally, bone mineralization measurements are taken (see Chapter 4 for more specific procedures).

References

1. McLaurin, R., Workony, J. Management of spina bifida and associated anomalies. *Comp. Ther.* 1986; 12:60.
2. Oppenheimer, S. Twenty year review: Cincinnati experience. In: McLaurin, R., Oppenheimer, S., Dias, L., Kaplan, W.E., eds. *Spina Bifida (A Multidisciplinary Approach).* New York: Praeger; 1986.
3. Raimondi, A.J. Intellectual development in shunted hydrocephalic children. *Am. J. Dis. Child.* 1974; 127:664.
4. Hayes-Allen, M.C. Obesity and short stature in children with myelomeningocele, *Dev. Med. Child. Neurol.,* 1972; 27(S):14.
5. Lorber, J. Spina bifida—a vanishing nightmare? In: Voth, D., Glees, P., eds. *Spina Bifida-Neural Tube Defects.* Berlin: Walther de Gruyter; 1986.
6. Leck, I. Epidemiological clues to the causation of neural tube defects. In: Dobbing, J., ed. *Prevention of Spina Bifida and Other Neural Tube Defects,* New York: Academic Press; 1983.
7. Laurence, K.M. The natural history of spina bifida cystica: detailed analysis of 407 cases. *Arch. Dis. Child.* 1964; 39:41.
8. Smithells, R.W., Nevin, N.C., Seller, M.J., Sheppard, S., Harris, R., Read, A.P., Fielding, D.W., Schorah, C.J., Wild, J. Further experience of vitamin supplementation for prevention of neural tube defect recurrences. *Lancet.* 1983; 1:1027.
9. Lemire, R.J. Causes of neural tube defects. In: McLaurin, R.L., Oppenheimer, S., Dias, L., Kaplan W.E., eds. *Spina Bifida (A Multidisciplinary Approach),* New York: Praeger; 1986.
10. Seller, M.J., Norman, C.N. Periconceptual vitamin supplementation and the prevention of neural tube defects in Southeast England and Northern Ireland. *J. Med. Genet.* 1984; 21:325.
11. Friedman, J.M. Can maternal alcohol ingestion cause neural tube defects? *J. Pediatr.* 1982; 101:232.
12. Brock, D.J.H., Bolton, A.E., Scrimgeour, J.B. Prenatal diagnosis of spina bifida and anecephaly through maternal plasma-alpha-fetoprotein measurement. *Lancet.* 1974; 1:767.
13. McKiben, B., Toseland, P.A., Duckworth, T. Abnormalities in vitamin C in spina bifida. *Dev. Med. Child. Neurol.* 1968; 15(S):55.
14. Ekvall, S., Chen, I.W., Bozian, R. The effect of supplemental ascorbic acid on serum vitamin B_{12} levels in myelomeningocele patients. *Am. J. Clin. Nutr.* 1981; 34:1356.
15. Laurence, K.M., James, N., Campbell, H. Blood folate levels and quality of the maternal diet. *Br. Med. J.* 1980; 285:216.
16. Laurence, K.M., James, N., Miller, M.H., Tennant, G.B., Campbell, H. Double-blind randomized controlled trial of folate treatment before conception to prevent recurrence of neural tube defects. *Br. Med. J.* 1981; 281:1509.
17. Laurence, K.M., Nanci, J., Miller, M., Campbell, H. Increased risk of recurrence of pregnancies complicated by fetal neural tube defects in mothers receiving poor diets, and possible benefit of dietary counseling. *Br. Med. J.* 1980; 281:1592.
18. Molloy, A.M., Kirke, P., Hillary, I., Weir, D.G., Scott, J.M. Maternal serum folate and vitamin B_{12} concentrations in pregnancies associated with neural tube defects. *Arch. Dis. Child.* 1985; 60:660.
19. Milursky, A., Jick, H., Jick, S.S., Bruell, C.L., MacLaughlin, D.S., Rothman, K.J., Willett, W. Multivitamin/folic acid supplementation in early pregnancy reduces the prevalence of neural tube defects, *JAMA.* 1989; 262:2847.
20. MRC Vitamin Study Research Group. Prevention of neural tube defects: results of the medical research council vitamin study. *Lancet* 1991; 33:131.
21. Bergmann, K.E., Makosh, G., Tews, K.H. Abnormalities of hair zinc concentration in mothers of newborn infants with spina bifida. *Am. J. Clin. Nutr.* 1980; 33:2145.
22. Nevin, N. Prevention of neural tube defects in an area of high incidence. In: Dobbing, J., ed. *Prevention of Spina Bifida and other Neural Tube Defects.* New York: Academic Press; 1983.
23. Green, S., Frank, M., Zackmann, M., Prader, A. Growth and sexual development in children with myelomeningocele. *Eur. Pediatr.* 1985; 144:146.
24. Rosenblum, M.F., Finegold, D.N., Charney, E.B. Assessment of stature of children with myelomeningocele, and usefulness of arm-span measurement. *Dev. Med. Child. Neurol.* 1983; 25:338.

25. Atencio-LaFollette, P., Ekvall Walberg, S., Oppenheimer, S., Grace, E. The effect of level of lesion and ambulation on growth chart measurements in children with myelomeningocele—A Pilot Study, *J. Am. Dietet. Assoc.* 1992, in press.

26. Asher, M., Olson, J. Factors affecting the ambulatory status of patients with spina bifida cystica, *J. Bone Joint Surg.* 1983; 65:350.

27. Engstrom, F.M., Roche, A.F., Mukherjee, D. Differences between arm-span and stature in white children. *J. Adolesc. Health Care.* 1981; 2:19.

28. Engelbach, W. *Endocrine Medicine*, Vol. I. Springfield, IL: Charles C Thomas; 1932.

29. Mitchell, C.O., Lipschitz, D.A. Arm length measurement as an alternative to height in nutritional assessment of the elderly. *JPEN.* 1982; 6:226.

30. Belt, B., Ekvall, S., Cook, C., Oppenheimer, S., Wessel, J. Linear growth measurement: a comparison of single arm-lengths and arm span. *Dev. Med. Child. Neurol.* 1986; 28:319.

31. Shurtleff, D., Lamers, J., Goiney, T., Gordon, L. Are myelodysplastic children fat? Anthropometric measures: A preliminary report. *Spina Bifida Ther.* 1982; 4:1.

32. Grogan, C., Ekvall, S., Bozan, R. The effect of nutrient intake and physical activity on the body composition of myelomeningocele patients as determined by K_{40} anthropometric measures and urinary creatinine. *Fed. Proc.* 1977; 36:1165.

33. Blum, R.W. The adolescent with spina bifida. *Clin. Pediatr.* 1983; 22:332.

34. Shepherd, K., Roberts, D., Golding, L., Thomas, B., Shepherd, R. Body composition in myelomingocele. *Am. J. Clin. Nutr.* 1991; 53:1.

35. Braune, Fisher, In: Brunnstrom, S., ed. *Clinical Kinesiology*, Philadelphia: F.A. Davis; 1972.

36. Bandini, L.G., Schoeller, D.A., Fukogawa, N.K., Wyhes, L., Dietz, W.H. Body composition and energy expenditure in adolescents with cerebral palsy and myelodysplasia. *Ped. Res.* 1991; 29:70.

37. Graves, M., Graves, M., Barron, M. The primary care physician's role in management of child with myelomeningocele. *J. Miss. State Med. Assoc.* 1988; 28:75.

38. Duval-Beupere, G., Kaci, M., Lougovoy, J., Caponi, M., Touzeau, C. Growth of trunk and legs of children with myelomeningocele. *Dev. Med. Child. Neurol.* 1987; 29:225.

39. Ekvall, S., Wheby, E., eds. *Quality Assurance Standards for Myelodysplasia. Manual II. Clinical Nutrition, Nutritional Needs of the Child with a Handicap or Chronic Illness.* Cincinnati: The University of Cincinnati Publications; 1987 (Sponsored by SPRANS Special Project Federal Grant).

40. Pediatric Practice Group. *Quality Assurance Standards.* Chicago: American Dietetic Association; 1988.

41. Hanson, R., Graves, M. Current concepts: care and habilitation of children with myelomeningocele—a multidisciplinary approach. *J. Miss. State Med. Assoc.* 1987; 28:145.

42. Killiam, P.E., Apida, L., Manilla, K.J., Varni, J.S. Behavioral pediatric weight rehabilitation for children with myelomeningocele. *Matr. Child Nurs.* 1983; 8:280.

43. Scarff, T.B., Fronczak, S. Myelomeningocele: a review and update. *Rehabilitation.* 1981; 42:143.

44. Parent, A., Miller, J., Graves, M. Current concepts: care and habilitation of the child with myelomeningocele—a multidisciplinary approach. *J. Miss. State Med. Assoc.* 1987; 28:173.

45. Ekvall, S., Hedrick, B. The impact of nutritional status before conception, during pregnancy, and early childhood. Training module VI. Prevention Continuing Education in Rural Areas Project (84-1). Columbus: Ohio Developmental Disabilities Council and Ohio Department of Mental Retardation and Developmental Disabilities; 1985.

46. Distrude, A., Prince, A. Provision of optimal nutrition care in myelomeningocele, *Top. Clin. Nutr.* 1990; 5:34.

Chapter 11
Nutrients, Neurotransmitters, and Brain Dysfunction

Valli Ekvall, Shirley Walberg Ekvall, and Eric Bonsall

The central nervous system (CNS) is a dynamic, complex, and fully integrated biological network that determines mood, cognition, and behavior and controls physiological homeostasis. The organizing center of this network is the brain, which comprises only 2% of the adult body weight but requires 15% of the total cardiac output and remarkably consumes 20% to 30% of the body's resting metabolic energy.[1] The brain does not have large energy stores and thus is dependent on a continuous supply of oxygen, glucose, and other nutrients for optimal development and function. This chapter reviews the current research linking nutritional state with CNS activity. Its focal point is the role of nutrients in the modulation of neurotransmitter synthesis and action, with reference to the impact of such modulation on more global CNS functions involving mood, cognition, behavior, and the maintenance of homeostasis. Initially, a brief overview of neurotransmitter biochemistry and physiology is presented, followed by a more comprehensive discussion of the relationships between nutrients and some specific neurotransmitter systems. The chapter concludes with some suggestions for further research in this important area.

Biochemistry and Physiology

Neurotransmitters are broadly defined as compounds "localized in specific neuronal systems and released on cell depolarization which produce changes in neuronal activity."[2] The inside of a nerve cell, or neuron, is maintained approximately 70 millivolts negative with respect to the outside of the cell by a system of ion pumps and channels involving primarily sodium, potassium, calcium, and chloride. A nerve impulse is propagated down an individual neuron by a decrease in this transmembrane potential, termed depolarization, which physically travels down the neuron to the terminal bouton. A small space, the synaptic cleft, separates the presynaptic terminal bouton from the postsynaptic neuron. Upon depolarization of the terminal portion of the presynaptic neuron, a neurotransmitter is secreted into the synapse and subsequently is recognized and bound by a postsynaptic receptor. The further propagation of an impulse down the postsynaptic neuron is a function of the balance between the concentration of the neurotransmitter in the synapse, the affinity and number of postsynaptic receptors, and whether the particular neurotransmitter is excitatory (leads to transmembrane depolarization) or inhibitory (leads to transmembrane hyperpolarization).

Currently, up to 40 putative neurotransmitters have been identified. These substances can be divided broadly into two major classes: (1) the traditional neurotransmitters synthe-sized in the nerve terminal and (2) the neuropeptide neurotransmitters, which are generally small proteins synthesized in the neuron cell body.[3] Traditional neurotransmitters include the catecholamines (norepinephrine, epinephrine, and dopamine), the biogenic amines (serotonin and histamine), amino acids (aspartic acid, glutamic acid, glycine, gamma-aminobutyric acid, homocysteine, and taurine), and acetylcholine. The list of putative neuropeptide neurotransmitters is lengthy and growing. A partial list of neuropeptides is found in Table 11-1. In addition to neurons, these compounds are found in tissues of the gastrointestinal tract, pancreas, pituitary, and even cells of the immune system.[4] These peptides may act as neurohormones to modulate distant biological processes, or they may act locally within the synaptic cleft.

Classically, neurons were thought to be committed to a single neurotransmitter, but more recent work has shown that the traditional neurotransmitters frequently exist together with neuropeptides in a single neuron, a concept known as co-localization.[3] Thus, each postsynaptic neuron is regulated by the interplay of excitatory and inhibitory forces from multiple, presynaptic neurons and possibly even from single, presynaptic neurons in which two types of neurons are co-localized.

Table 11-1. Neuropeptides

Gut-brain peptides
  Vasoactive intestinal polypeptide (VIP)
  Cholecystokinin octapeptide (CCK–8)
  Substance P
  Neurotensin
  Methionine enkephalin
  Leucine enkephalin
  Insulin
  Glucagon
Hypothalamic-releasing hormones
  Thyrotropin-releasing hormone (TRH)
  Luteinizing hormone-releasing hormone (LHRH)
  Somatostatin (growth hormone release-inhibiting factor, SRIF)
Pituitary peptides
  Adrenocorticotropin (ACTH)
  Beta-endorphin-melanocyte-stimulating
    hormone (Alpha-MSH)
Others
  Angiotensin II
  Bradykinin
  Vasopressin
  Oxytocin
  Carnosine
  Bombesin

From Snyder[2] with permission.

Factors to be Considered in Nutrients and Specific Neurotransmitter Synthesis and Function

Substantial evidence suggests that specific neurotransmitters are sensitive to relatively mild, physiological fluctuations in the quality of foods eaten even at a single meal.[5-7] It appears that brain neurotransmitter synthesis is affected by specific dietary precursors[8,9] and by more global nutritional status[10,11] (Table 11-2). Dietary precursors and their companion neurotransmitters are found in Table 11-3 and high food sources of dietary precursors in Table 11-4. The steps in the conversion of these nutrients into neurotransmitters and the regulatory enzymes involved are illustrated in Figure 11-1. Since the brain is separated from the peripheral circulation, these nutrients must pass through the blood-brain barrier either by diffusion through the capillary endothelial cell membrane or by active transport mechanisms (Fig 11-2).

Amino acid concentration in plasma is affected in two ways; one way is through the exogenous rhythm, which is controlled by the food that is consumed. A high protein meal increases the level of amino acids in the plasma. An internally set, endogenous circadian rhythm also controls amino acid concentration. In humans, the plasma amino acid levels are lowest between 2:00 A.M. and 4:00 A.M., but eating continuously or at night can affect these natural, internal rhythms.[12]

In addition to the intake of specific dietary precursors, the more global nutritional status of an individual affects neurotransmitter synthesis and function.[10,11] Foods ingested by malnourished individuals have less competition and thus can have a more pronounced effect. It seems that the rate of synthesis and the amount of neurotransmitter released vary in malnourished individuals, depending on what foods are eaten. These changes in neurotransmitter release can result in affective, cognitive, and behavioral changes, therefore directly linking nutrient intake with the global functioning of an individual[13] (Table 11-2). Specific neurotransmitters and their relationships to nutrient intake are reviewed in more detail below.

Serotonin

The amino acid tryptophan is the primary substrate for the synthesis of serotonin, 5-hydroxytryptamine. Tryptophan is first hydroxylated and then decarboxylated to form serotonin (Fig 11-1). Serotonin is found in platelets, mast cells, and enterochromaffin cells of the gastrointestinal tract. Only 1% to 2% of the serotonin in the body is synthesized in the brain.[14] As serotonin does not cross the blood-brain barrier, neuronal synthesis of this neurotransmitter is dependent upon an adequate supply of tryptophan from the periphery.

Of the neurotransmitter systems affected by precursor availability, the relationships among food composition, plasma, and brain tryptophan and brain serotonin are best understood.[15] Tryptophan cannot be synthesized in the blood as a result of protein ingestion or body protein breakdown and thus is truly an essential amino acid. Along with tyrosine, it is transported across the blood-brain barrier via a carrier mechanism specific for the large neutral amino acids.[6,7] The pathway of nutrient molecules crossing the blood-brain

Table 11-2. Some Physiological and Potentially Therapeutic Effects of Nutrients on Brain

Nutrient	Food Constituent that Increases Brain Levels	Effects
Tryptophan	Carbohydrates	Physiological: Decrease appetite for carbohydrates; drowsiness; calmness; modulate sensitivity to pain
		Therapeutic: Depression; insomnia
Tyrosine	Tyrosine	Physiological: Subjective vigor
		Therapeutic: Hypertension; shock; hyperprolactinemia; depression; Parkinson's disease
Choline	Lecithin (phosphatidylcholine)	Therapeutic: Tardive dyskinesia; memory disorders; mania, ataxias

Assessment of the Possible Effects on Brain of Food Additives Normally Present in the Blood Stream

1. Does its consumption in reasonable doses raise its plasma concentration (or that of a metabolite) beyond the normal range? (For a large neutral amino acid, is its plasma ratio raised beyond its normal range?)

2. Does an increase in its plasma level (or ratio) bring about a corresponding increase in its brain level?

3. Does its consumption affect the synthesis, release, levels, metabolism, or receptor effects of a neurotransmitter?

4. Does its consumption modify behavior, autonomic functions, neuroendocrine secretion, or subjective phenomena? Are such modifications consistent with its effects on neurotransmitters?

5. Are its functional or behavioral effects altered by drugs known to enhance or suppress transmission mediated by the neurotransmitter that it affects?

From Wurtman, R.J., Maher, T.J. Strategies for assessing the effects of food additives on the brain and behavior. *Fundam. Appl. Toxicol.* 1984; 4(S):318. Used with permission.

Table 11-3. Dietary Precursors Affecting Neurotransmitter Function

Food Source	Blood	Brain Neuron		
		Substrate	Regulatory Enzyme	Neurotransmitter
Protein	Tyrosine	Tyrosine	Hydroxylase	Dopamine or norepinephrine
	Tryptophan	Tryptophan	Hydroxylase	Serotonin
	Histidine	Histidine	Decarboxylase	Histamine
	Threonine	Threonine	Serinetranshydroxy-methylase	Glycine
Lecithin	Choline	Choline	Cholineacetyl-transferase	Acetylcholine

Modified from Anderson & Johnston.[6]

Table 11-4. High Food Sources of Dietary Precursors

Dietary Precursor (Amino Acids)	Food Source	Serving Size	Amount of Amino Acid (mg)
Tryptophan	Beef (round, lean + marbled, top, broiled)	3.5 oz	504
	Skim milk (dry, instant 3.2-oz envelope with water)	reconstit.	451
	Veal (round, lean + fat, cutlet/breaded, cooked)	3.5 oz	435
	Cottage cheese (2% fat)	1c	346
	Chicken (fryer/broiler, skinless, roasted)	3.5 oz	338
	Tuna fish (canned, oil or water packed)	3 oz	294
Tyrosine	Cottage cheese (2% fat)	1 c	1655
	Skim milk (dry, instant 3.2-oz envelope)	8 oz reconstit.	1542
	Chicken (fryer/broiler, skinless, roasted)	3.5 oz	977
	Cheddar cheese (shredded)	1/2 c	679
	Turkey ham luncheon meat	2 oz	424
	Evaporated milk (whole, canned)	1/2 c	414
Choline	Chicken egg (yolk)	1 large egg	253
	Wheat (whole, dry, cooked)	1 c	230
	Rice (white, enriched, long grain, cooked)	1 c	147
	Lamb (leg, raw)	3.5 oz	84
	Beef (rib, choice, lean, cooked)	3.5 oz	82
	Milk (whole)	1 c	49
Histadine	Cottage cheese (2% fat)	1 c	1032
	Chicken (fryer/broiler, skinless, roasted)	3.5 oz	898
	Skim milk (dry, instant 3.2-oz envelope)	8 oz reconstit.	866
	Cheddar cheese (shredded)	1/2 c	494
	Smoked link sausage (pork and beef)	1 link	475
	Tuna fish (canned, oil or water packed)	1 oz	453
Threonine	Beef (round, lean + marbled, top, broiled)	3 oz	1904
	Skim milk (dry, instant 3.2-oz envelope)	8 oz reconstit.	1442
	Veal (round, lean + fat, cutlet/breaded, cooked)	3.5 oz	1438
	Cottage cheese (2% fat)	1 c	1377
	Fish—halibut (broiled/baked)	1 serving (125 g)	1354
	Chicken (fryer/broiler, skinless, roasted)	3.5 oz	1222
Phenylalanine	Cottage cheese (2% fat)	1 c	1674
	Beef (round, lean + marbled, bottom, broiled)	3 oz	1666
	Skim milk (dry, instant 3.2-oz envelope)	8 oz reconstit.	1542
	Veal (round, lean + fat, cutlet/breaded, cooked)	3.5 oz	1346
	Chicken (fryer/broiler, skinless, roasted)	3.5 oz	1226
	Fish—halibut (broiled/baked)	1 serving (125 g)	1166

Modified from Pennington, J.A.T., Church, H.N. *Food Values of Portions Commonly Used.* 14th ed. New York: Harper & Row Publishers; 1985.

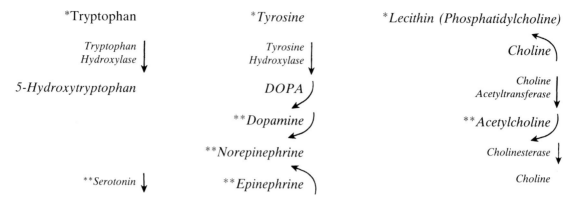

*Tryptophan   *Tyrosine   *Lecithin (Phosphatidylcholine)

Tryptophan $\downarrow$ Tyrosine $\downarrow$ Choline
Hydroxylase   Hydroxylase

5-Hydroxytryptophan   DOPA   Choline
                                                                    Acetyltransferase $\downarrow$

                              **Dopamine   **Acetylcholine

                          **Norepinephrine   Cholinesterase $\downarrow$

      **Serotonin $\downarrow$ **Epinephrine   Choline

Fig. 11–1. Steps in the conversion of nutrients into neurotransmitters. *-Dietary precursor; **-neurotransmitter.

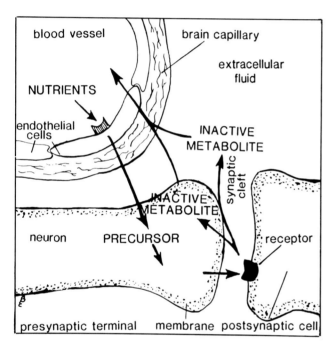

Fig. 11–2. The pathway of nutrient molecules crossing the blood-brain barrier. Modified from Wurtman, R.J. Nutrients that modify brain function. *Sci. Am.* 1982; 246:50.

barrier can be seen in Figure 11-2. Due to the competitive nature of amino acid transport, the effect of food ingestion on brain tryptophan is not simply related to tryptophan content alone. Because there is competition for available carrier sites,[16] the uptake of an individual amino acid is proportional to the ratio of its concentration to that of its competition.[12] For example, protein ingestion causes a greater increase in plasma branched-chain amino acids relative to tryptophan, decreasing the plasma tryptophan:neutral amino acid ratio (TRP/NAA) and therefore brain tryptophan uptake. Conversely, carbohydrate ingestion increases the plasma TRP:NAA ratio, thus increasing tryptophan availability to the brain.[6,7] This increase is caused by the carbohydrate-induced insulin release that increases the uptake of all amino acids into tissue, but has a lesser effect on tryptophan, which is carried in plasma both free and bound to albumin.[6] Tryptophan is released as albumin moves through the brain capillaries, and because of its competitive advantage in the

blood, more tryptophan enters the brain than other amino acids. Thus, protein ingestion decreases brain serotonin level, whereas tryptophan administration and carbohydrate ingestion increase the concentration of brain tryptophan and serotonin.[6,7] Also, supplementation of tryptophan in a low-protein diet can produce higher levels of serotonin in the brain.[17]

The neurobehavioral effects of serotonin are far ranging and include important effects on mood.[18] Young and colleagues[19] reported on the effects of tryptophan-free, balanced, and tryptophan-loaded diets on mood in normal volunteers. The tryptophan-free diet produced a mildly depressed mood, which correlated with low plasma tryptophan concentrations.[19] Tryptophan loading has been reported to elevate mood in normal volunteers.[20] Serotonin also has been reported to affect sexual behavior,[21] impulsiveness and suicide,[22] and the sensation of pain.[23] Serotonin is implicated in obsessive-compulsive disorder and other anxiety disorders.[24]

Tryptophan has been reported to improve sleep, presumably through serotonergic mechanisms,[25] and parachlorophenylalanine-induced suppression of serotonin synthesis causes insomnia.[26] Hepatic coma may in part be caused by increased serotonin synthesis in the brain.[27] A comatose state may be promoted further by the increased uptake of phenylalanine (as a result of increased plasma levels of this amino acid) into the brain. High levels of phenylalanine in the brain inhibit tyrosine hydroxylase and thus decrease the synthesis of the neurotransmitters, dopamine and norepinephrine.[28] These catecholamines are thought to be important for normal alertness. Other factors that may influence hepatic encephalopathy include elevated ammonia levels and the accumulation of false neurotransmitters in the brain. Dogs with hepatic encephalopathy can be aroused by the administration of branched-chain amino acids.[29] This arousal probably occurs because increased competition diminishes tryptophan entry into the brain. Patients with hepatic encephalopathy have been treated by using parenteral formulas with increased amounts of branched-chain amino acids.[30]

The influence of serotonin on carbohydrate appetite has been reviewed.[31] Increased serotonergic activity selectively decreases carbohydrate intake.[32] Conversely, low brain levels of tryptophan and serotonin have been linked with increased carbohydrate intake.[33] The use of tryptophan also reduced carbohydrate-rich snacking in subjects who were obese.[34] Dietary protein consumption affects the sympathetic nervous system and may have implications for energy efficiency in obese persons.[35] The digestion of gliadine and casein produces opiate-like activity or "exorphine" and thus may cross the intestinal mucosa.[36] Seasonal affective disorder, a specific form of recurrent depression, has been associated with carbohydrate craving,[37] and some investigations suggest that this excess carbohydrate intake is an attempt at self-medicating through modulation of the serotonergic system.[31]

Catecholamines

The catecholamines include dihydroxyphenylethylamine— dopamine—and its metabolic products, norepinephrine and epinephrine. Norepinephrine and epinephrine have been linked to arousal and the fight-or-flight respond, whereas the dopaminergic system is involved in involuntary movement disorders and hallucinations. The rate-limiting step in the synthesis of all of the catecholamines is the conversion of tyrosine to 3,4 dihyroxyphenylalanine (DOPA) (Fig 11-1). Tyrosine hyroxylase, the enzyme controlling this rate-limiting step, is activated whenever nerves are firing rapidly. At these times, the enzyme can handle much more tyrosine than is normally present in the brain. Thus, whenever tyrosine levels in brain increase, more catecholamines are synthesized within active neurons and are available for sending messages.[38]

Dietary precursors that may influence the neurotransmitter catecholamines were examined using radioenzymatic assays in 30 varieties of fruits and vegetables. The dopamine concentration differed with the variety of banana (red banana having a higher and plantains a lower dopamine concentration).[39] Also, the concentration varied by location within the banana; dopamine was highest near the skin and serotonin near the center of the fruit. No studies have shown that the ingestion of bananas, which are high in dopamine or serotonin, produces problems in healthy people. However, patients with carcinoid tumors, which typically synthesize serotonin but also can synthesize bradykinin and histamine, reported flushing attacks after consuming bananas. Fruits with a high and moderate dopamine concentration are shown in Table 11-5.

The relationship between diet composition, brain catecholamine, and brain tyrosine metabolism is not yet well defined. Tyrosine is formed in the liver and, to a limited extent in the brain, from phenylalanine; however, phenylalanine itself is an essential amino acid, and its conversion to tyrosine is probably insufficient to satisfy the body's need for tyrosine.[6,7] In a study using kittens,[40] the dietary requirement for phenylalanine was reduced by half when tyrosine was substituted for it. Although single meals containing both carbohydrate and protein increase brain tyrosine, with protein having the greater effect, chronic high-protein feeding decreases brain tyrosine concentration.[6,7] A large dose of tyrosine raises brain tyrosine levels and lowers tryptophan. Likewise, a large tryptophan or carbohydrate dose can lower brain tyrosine and may thereby compromise central catecholaminergic transmission.[6,7] This compromising effect is shown with a 50 mg/kg dose of tryptophan, which produces increased fatigue and decreased pain sensitivity without impairing sensorimotor activity.[41] Protein-containing meals that raise serum tyrosine levels also increase dopamine synthesis in the retina.[42] Large doses of tyrosine have been reported to make humans less depressed.[43] Tyrosine also can reduce high blood pressure and raise low blood pressure by its effect on norepinephrine-releasing neurons[44–46]; it can also modify the ventricular fibrillation threshold in dogs.[47] Tyrosine, however, had no effect on sympathetic nervous system activity in young mice. A decarboxylated product of tyrosine—tyramine—can cause norepinephrine release from neurons and also may decrease catecholamine synthesis.[48] Thus, patients with depression who are treated with monoamine oxidase inhibitors can be affected by foods high in tyramine, such as aged cheese, undistilled spirits, and mushrooms (see Chapter 27).

Vitamins and minerals appear to have a wide range of effects on catecholamine neurotransmitters in a manner similar to dietary precursors.[6] Marginal intakes of vitamin B_{12} and folate affect transmethylation. Folate is the precursor of tetrohydro-biopterin, a necessary co-factor in tyrosine hydroxylase activity. A high percentage of depressed patients have poor folate status.[49] Vitamin B_6 deficiency has been linked to a decrease in dopaminergic neuron function in the rat corpus striatum.[50] Vitamin A is involved in the physiology of the retina, and vitamin E acts as an antioxidant in brain tissue. Both ascorbic acid and copper affect the conversion of dopamine to norepinephrine. Magnesium has been shown to influence aggressive behavior in mice while altering the potency of catecholamine-stimulating drugs,[51] and magnesium levels have been studied in conduct-disordered youth.[52] Iron, a co-factor of tyrosine hydroxylase activity, also is linked to impaired phenylalanine conversion to tyrosine when it is deficient.[53] Iron-deficient rats have shown inhibition of serotonin and dopamine and a reduction in selective attention and vigilance. Zinc deficiency has caused lethergy and apathy in children and reduced cognition in all age groups.[54–56]. Essential fatty acid intake has been reported to modulate dopamine activity.[57] The effect of marginal deficiencies of these vitamins and minerals needs further exploration.

Acetylcholine

Acetylcholine was the first neurotransmitter to be identified.[58] It is the neurotransmitter at the neuromuscular junction that controls all voluntary movement and is also the neurotransmitter of the parasympathetic nervous system. Within the CNS, acetylcholine has been linked to aggression, depression, the stress response, and dreaming.[59] Research supports a strong role for this neurotransmitter in memory and the cognitive dysfunction associated with aging.[60]

Acetylcholine is synthesized by the action of choline ace-

Table 11-5. Fruits with a High and Moderate Dopamine Concentration

Fruit	High Concentration (mcg/g)	Moderate Concentration (mcg/g)	
Red banana	51.4	Smooth avocado	1.0
Yellow banana	42.0	Cocoa bean powder	1.0
Plaintain	5.5	Broccoli	1.0
Fuerte avocado	4.0	Brussels sprouts	1.0

tyltransferase on choline (Fig 11-1). Dietary intake of choline lecithin or choline-containing compounds elevates blood choline concentration.[61] Choline is transported across the blood-brain barrier by a specific carrier, which is capable of handling much more choline than is normally present.[62] Thus, when blood choline concentration rises, more choline enters the brain. Within neurons, the enzyme that produces the neurotransmitter acetylcholine from choline also can handle much more choline than is normally available. So, when brain choline levels rise, the synthesis of the neurotransmitter acetylcholine increases.[63] This brain messenger is then available for release. This enhancing effect of choline has also been observed in neurons outside the brain, such as in the nerves that innervate the heart[64] and the diaphragm muscles.[65]

Choline has been used with some success in the treatment of tardive dyskinesia, an involuntary motor movement disorder associated with long-term neuroleptic use.[66,67] Its use in Alzheimer's disease has been reviewed extensively.[60] Interestingly, though the usefulness of supplemental choline in the treatment of Alzheimer's disease is questionable, several studies suggest possible preventive effects.[68-70] Manic persons may benefit from therapy with choline-containing compounds,[71] whereas depressed individuals may become more depressed after such treatment.[72]

Histamine

Histamine cannot be produced totally from histidine. Histidine taken intraperitoneally or by dietary alteration can increase brain histidine and histamine.[6] Glycine, a neurotransmitter and nonessential amino acid, can be synthesized in the brain by threonine and serine. In turn, 1-threonine administered intraperitoneally increases glycine in rats. The effect of dietary variations on threonine levels needs investigation.[6]

Directions for Further Research and Applications Related to Nutrient and Drug Management

Clearly, investigations to date have documented the potential role of nutrition in modulating affect, cognition, and behavior. Future research involves determining the factors that control the rate by which precursor amino acids are resynthesized into polyproteins and the formation of active peptides,[73] which in turn affect behavior.[74] An interesting and rapidly developing area of cellular research is the identification of growth factors that keep nerve cells from dying by preventing the cells from producing killer proteins.[75]

Several peptides produced in the hypothalamus have been isolated from foods. Thyrotropin-releasing hormone has been found in alfalfa and luteinizing hormone-releasing hormone in oat leaves.[36] The clinical utility of these findings deserves further study. Monosodium glutamate has caused damage to hypothalamic neurons in young, immature rats. Likewise, erythrosine (red dye FD&C #3) appears to inhibit the uptake of neurotransmitters in rats, but more research is needed to determine the extent to which this food additive crosses the blood-brain barrier.[48] The potential for tryptophan to relieve pain and the effects of food on mood merit more research.[76,77] Investigations into the genetic control of differential responses to dietary manipulation may lead to treatment strategies targeted to more specific subtypes of patients with brain dysfunction.

The nutritionist, as an integral part of the multidisciplinary team working with psychiatrically ill patients, is required to have a broad knowledge base encompassing the basic signs and symptoms of a range of psychiatric disorders, as well as some knowledge of the standard psychopharmacological and psychotherapeutic treatment modalities used to treat these disorders.[78,79] Many psychiatric illnesses present with eating disturbances as part of their core symptomatology. Major depression, unipolar type, is an illness that afflicts approximately 10% of women and 5% of men during their lifetime.[80] Recent work documents that this illness can have its onset in early latency and perhaps even in the preschool period.[81] The core feature of this disorder is recurrent episodes of depressed mood that are frequently accompanied by appetite disturbances, as well as sleep disruption, fatigue, feelings of guilt, and suicidal ideation. The etiology is multifactorial, involving the interaction of an inherited vulnerability with environmental stressors. Current treatments include psychotherapy, antidepressant medications, and electroconvulsive therapy. The potential adjunctive role of dietary manipulation in the treatment of depressed patients and in the maintenance of normal mood in vulnerable individuals is an area in need of investigation.

Similarly, bipolar disorder, a cyclical illness presenting with alternating periods of depressed and elevated mood, warrants more research on the effects of nutritional status. This illness has a lifetime prevalence of 0.5% to 1.0% in both sexes[81] and may be linked to a defect on the short arm of chromosome 11 at a site near the gene that codes for tyrosine hydroxylase,[82] although further investigations have failed to confirm this linkage.[83]

In one study L-tryptophan did not appear to effect food intake[84] but when reduced in the brain correlated with anxiety, depersonalization, diurnal variation, obsessions, and paranoid symptoms.[85] Depressed mood, feelings of guilt, suicidal ideation and loss of interest were not related to biological data.[85] However, the degree of weight change appears to be a potential marker in depression.[86] Sertraline and fluoxetine serotonin-uptake inhibitors were found to inhibit food intake in animals and thus are being studied for human obesity.[87-91]

The eating disorders, anorexia nervosa and bulimia nervosa, clearly require the input of a skilled nutritionist in their comprehensive management. Estimates for the prevalence of bulimia nervosa, a disorder involving alternative binging and purging, range from 1.0% to 10.0% among women.[92] Anorexia nervosa, a life-threatening illness of extreme weight loss and distorted body image, affects approximately 1% of women.[92] Gastrin secretions were significantly decreased in anorexia nervosa. The effect of peptides and appetite control was noted (pancreatic polypeptides increased in anorexia nervosa and decreased in obesity).[93,94] Schizophrenia can involve delusions that may result in greatly increased intake of certain foods or can produce a catatonic state that results in almost no solid or liquid intake. Homeless people with schizophrenia, a group presumed at high risk for malnutrition, have not yet been studied systematically.[95]

More well-designed studies involving nutrients as part of the treatment of psychiatric illnesses are warranted. Perhaps more important, the possible preventive role produced by good nutritional status needs further research. For additional information, see the chapters on anorexia nervosa and bulimia (23), autism (13), fetal alcohol syndrome (14), attention-deficit hyperactivity disorder (20), and drug-induced malnutrition (27).

References

1. Bray, G., York, D. Neurotransmitters and consummatory behaviors. *Phsiol. Rev.* 1979; 59:719.
2. Snyder, S. Brain peptides as neurotransmitters. *Science.* 1980; 209:976.
3. Coyle, J.T. Neuroscience and psychiatry. In Talbott, Hales, Yeidofsky, eds. *The American Psychiatric Press Textbook of Psychiatry.* Washington, DC: American Psychiatric Press Inc.; 1989.
4. Solomon, G.F. Psychoneuroimmunology: interactions between central nervous system and immune system. *J. Neuroscience Res.* 1987; 18:1.
5. Wurtman, R.J. Effects of dietary amino acids, carbohydrates, and choline on neurotransmitter synthesis. *Mt. Sinai. J. Med.* 1988; 55:75.
6. Anderson, G., Johnston, J. Nutrient control of brain neurotransmitter synthesis and function. *Can. J. Physiol. Pharmacol.* 1983; 61:271.
7. Wurtman, R. Behavioral effects of nutrients. *Lancet.* 1983; 1:1145.
8. Gietzen, D.W., Leung, P.M.B., Rogers, Q.R. Dietary amino acid imbalance and neurochemical changes in three hypothalamic areas. *Physiol. Behav.* 1989; 46:503.
9. Yogman, M.W., Zeisel, S.H. Nutrients, neurotransmitters and infant behavior. *Am. J. Clin. Nut.* 1985; 42:352.
10. Goodwin, G.M., Fraser, S., Stump, K., Fairburn, C.G., Elliott, J.M., Cowen, P.J. Dietary and weight loss in volunteers increases the number of alpha-2-adrenoreceptors and 5-HT receptors on blood platelets without effect on [³H] imipramine binding. *J. Affect. Dis.* 1987; 12:267.
11. Goodwin, G.M., Fairburn, C.G., Cowen, P.J. The effects of dieting and weight loss on neuroendocrine responses to tryptophan, clonidine and apomorphine in volunteers. *Arch. Gen. Psychiatr.* 1987; 44:962.
12. Zeisel, S.H., Sheard, N.F. Nutrition and neurotransmitters—clinical implications. In: Ekvall, S.M., Wheby, E.A., eds., *Manual II: Clinical Nutrition, Nutritional Needs of the Child with a Handicap or Chronic Illness.* Cincinnati: UACCDD; 1987.
13. Wurtman, R.J. Ways that foods can affect the brain. *Nutr. Rev.* 1986; 5(S):2.
14. Cooper, J.R., Bloom, F.E., Roth, R.H. Catecholamines. II: CNS aspects. In: Cooper, J.R., Bloom, F.E., Roth, R.H., eds. *The Biochemical Basis of Neuropharmacology.* New York: Oxford University Press; 1986.
15. Li, E., Anderson, H. Self-selected meal composition, circadian rhythms and meal responses in plasma and brain tryptophan and 5-Hydroxytryptamine in rats. *J. Nutr.* 1982; 112:2001.
16. Pardridge, W.M. Regulation of amino acid availability to the brain. In: Wurtman, R.J., Wurtman, J.J., eds. *Nutrition and the Brain.* New York: Raven Press; 1977.
17. Yokogoshi, H., Iwata, T., Ishida, K., Yoshida, A. Effect of amino acid supplementation to low protein diet on brain and plasma levels of tryptophan and brain 5-hydroxyindoles in rats. *Am. Inst. Nutr.* 1986; 18:42.
18. Blier, P., Montigny, C., Chaput, Y. A role for the serotonin system in the mechanism of action of antidepressant treatments: preclinical evidence. *J. Clin. Psychiatr.* 1990; 51:14.
19. Young, S.N., Smith, S.E., Pihl, R.O., Ervin, F.R. Tryptophan depletion causes a rapid lowering of mood in normal males. *Psychopharmacology.* 1985; 87:173.
20. Charney, D.S., Heninger, G.R., Reinhard, J.F. The effect of intravenous L-tryptophan on prolactin and growth hormone and mood in healthy subjects. *Psychopharmacology.* 1982; 77:217.
21. McEwen, B.S., Parsons, B. Gonadal steroid action on the brain: neurochemistry and neuropharmacology. *Annu. Rev. Pharmacol. Toxicity.* 1982; 22:555.
22. Brown, G., Linnoila, M.I. CSF serotonin metabolite (5-HIAA) studies in depression, impulsivity and violence. *J. Clin. Psychiatr.* 1990; 51:31.
23. Von Knorring, L., Perris, C., Oreland, L., Eisemann, M., Eriksson, U., Perris, H. Pain as a symptom in depressive disorders and its relationship to platelet monamine oxidase activity. *J. Neural Transmission.* 1984; 60:1.
24. Murphy, D.L., Pigott, T.A. A comparative examination of a role for serotonin in obsessive compulsive disorder, panic disorder and anxiety. *J. Clin. Psychiatr.* 1990; 51:53.
25. Hartmann, E. Effects of L-tryptophan on sleepiness and on sleep. *J. Psychiatr. Res.* 1983; 17:107.
26. Sallanon, M., Janin, M., Buda, C., Jouvet, M. Serotonergic mechanisms and sleep rebound. *Brain Res.* 1983; 268:95.
27. Munro, H.N., Fernstrom, J.D. Insulin, plasma amino acid imbalance, and hepatic coma. *Lancet.* 1975; 1:722.
28. Dodsworth, J.M., James, J.H. Depletion of brain norepinephrine in acute hepatic coma. *Surgery.* 1974; 75:811.
29. Bernardini, P., Fischer, J.E. Amino acid imbalance and hepatic encephalopathy. *Annu. Rev. Nutr.* 1982; 2:419.
30. Fischer, J.E., Rosen, H.M. The effect of normalization of plasma amino acids on hepatic encephalopathy in man. *Surgery.* 1976; 80:77.
31. Wurtman, J.J. Carbohydrate craving, mood changes and obesity. *J. Clin. Psychiatry.* 1988; 49:37.
32. Garrattini, S., Mennini, T., Samanin, R. From fenfluramine racemate to d-fenfluramine: specificity and potency of the effects on the serotonergic system and food intake. *Ann. NY. Acad. Sci.* 1987; 499:156.
33. Wurtman, J.I., Moses, P.L., Wurtman, R.J. Prior carbohydrate consumption affects the amount of carbohydrate that rats choose to eat. *J. Nutr.* 1983; 113:70.
34. Wurtman, R.J., Wurtman, J.J. Carbohydrates and depression. *Sci. Am.* 1989; 1:68.
35. Johnston, J.L., Balachandran, A.U. Effects of dietary protein, energy and tyrosine on central and peripheral norepinephrine turnover in mice. *J. Nutr.* 1987; 117:2046.
36. Morley, J.E. Food peptides: a new class of hormones? *JAMA.* 1982; 247:2379.
37. Rosenthal, N.E., Sack, D.A., Gillin, C. Seasonal affective disorder, *Arch. Gen. Psychiatr.* 1984; 41:72.
38. Growdon, J.H. Neurotransmitters and the diet: their use in the treatment of brain disorders. In: Wurtman, R.J., Wurtman, J.J., eds. *Nutrition and the Brain.* Vol. 3. New York: Raven Press; 1979; 117.
39. Feldman, J.M., Lee, E.M., Castleberry, C.A. Catecholamine and serotonin content of foods: effect on urinary excretion of homovanillic and 5-hydroxyindoleacetic acid. *J. Am. Diet. Assoc.* 1987; 87:1031.
40. Williams, J.M., Morris, J.G., Rogers, Q.R. Phenylalanine requirement of kittens and the sparing effect of tyrosine. *J. Nutr.* 1987; 117:1102.
41. Lieberman, H.R., Corkin, S., Spring, B.J., Growdon, J.H., Wurtman, R.J. Mood, performance, and pain sensitivity: changes induced by food constituents. *J. Psychiatr. Res.* 1982/83; 17:135.
42. Gibson, C.J. Dietary control of retinal dopamine synthesis. *Brain Res.* 1986; 382:195.
43. Gelenberg, A.J., Wojick, J.D. Tyrosine for the treatment of depression. *Am. J. Psychiatr.* 1980; 137:622.
44. Sved, A.F., Fernstrom, J.D. Tyrosine administration reduces blood pressure and enhances brain norepinephrinie release in spontaneously hypertensive rats. *Proc. Natl. Acad. Sci. USA.* 1979; 76:3511.
45. Wurtman, R.J. Nutrients that modify brain function. *Sci. Am.* 1982; 246:50.
46. Wurtman, R.J., Hefti, F., Melamed, E. Precursor control of neurotransmitter synthesis. *Pharmacol. Rev.* 1980; 32:315.
47. Scott, N.A., DeSilva, R.A. Tyrosine administration decreases vulnerability to ventricular fibrillation in the normal canine heart. *Science.* 1981; 211:727.

Chapter 12
The Small for Gestational Age Infant

Barbara Niedbala and Reginald Tsang

Fetal growth retardation results in reduced overall weight gain of the fetus compared to an appropriately grown fetus of the same gestational age. The term "small for gestational age" (SGA) is used for such infants. SGA may be defined as birth weight less than two standard deviations below the mean[1] or as birth weight less than the 10th percentile[2] when plotted against gestational age on an intrauterine growth chart (see Chapter 2 and Fig 12–1).

SGA infants constitute a heterogenous group, and the different conditions resulting in growth retardation in the fetus affect weight, length, and head circumference to varying degrees. Intrauterine growth retardation (IUGR) occurring early in gestation is thought to result in a symmetrically small infant. Later growth retardation, occurring in the third trimester of pregnancy, is believed to affect weight more than length and head circumference, resulting in an asymmetrically grown infant.[3,4] SGA infants are often categorized as both symmetrical and asymmetrical types, and clear distinctions among preterm SGA, term SGA, and normally grown preterm infants, all described as low birth weight (LBW) infants, are seen with increasing frequency in the literature.

Worldwide, the majority of instances of IUGR are related to poor maternal nutrition and health. In developed countries the etiology is often unclear.[5] IUGR may be of fetal origin, with malformations and dysmorphic syndromes constituting 5% to 15% of cases and chromosomal abnormalities another 2%.[6,7] Viral infections acquired in utero account for another 3% of cases.[8] Maternal origins of IUGR— pre-eclampsia, hypertension, renal disease, sickle-cell disease, cyanotic heart disease, substance abuse (alcohol, drug, cigarette), and malnutrition—account for most other cases of IUGR, although in at least 30% the cause is unknown. In these idiopathic cases, uteroplacental vascular insufficiency is thought to play a role.[9]

Approximately 10% of all liveborn infants and 30% of low birth weight infants (birth weight <2500 g) are SGA.[9] The incidence in specific populations varies from 4% to 45%. Developing areas have an incidence of LBW infants four times higher than developed countries; of these births, IUGR is 6.6 times more prevalent, whereas prematurity is only twice as high compared with developed countries.[10] Villar and Belizan[10] theorize that in any population, when the incidence of LBW infants is greater than 10% of live births, it is almost all due to an increase in IUGR infants. It must be noted, however, that these counts still underestimate the incidence of IUGR, as infants born at term or postterm and weighing more than 2500 grams may also be SGA.

The prognosis for an infant with IUGR is difficult to predict, as it is related both to the etiology of the growth retardation and to certain perinatal events, such as asphyxia. Various research studies reporting growth, developmental, and neurological outcomes are conflicting, owing to different testing methods; failure to control for perinatal events, socioeconomic status, and familial factors; and lack of clarity regarding the cause of LBW or the type of IUGR. Several studies report catch-up growth in term, asymmetrical SGA infants[11–14]; other studies report that infants born SGA tend to remain smaller throughout childhood and adolescence than appropriate for gestational age (AGA) cohorts.[15–17] Developmental scores have been reported to be lower in some SGA infants and are correlated with a decreased head circumference.[14,18,19] Other studies have found no significant difference in developmental scores[15,17] and a comparable rate of neurological sequelae in SGA and AGA infants.[13]

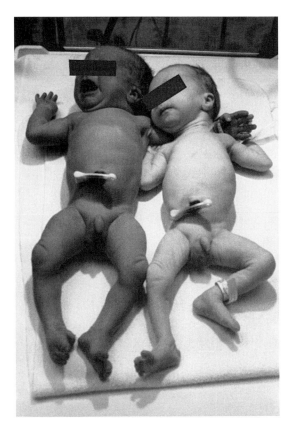

Fig. 12–1. Comparative size of a normal infant and small-for-gestational age infant, both born at full term. Courtesy of F. Hall, D.O., Section of Neonatal/Perinatal Medicine. The Children's Mercy Hospital of Kansas City. Used with permission.

Low socioeconomic status and a history of birth asphyxia appear to have a larger influence on developmental outcome than the presence of IUGR alone.

Biochemical and Clinical Abnormalities

Despite the varying causes of IUGR and differing body proportions of SGA infants, there are striking similarities in physical appearance and functional problems among these neonates. At birth, the term SGA infant resembles the normally grown term infant in behaviors, such as feeding eagerness, spontaneous activity, and the characteristic flexion into a fetal position. However, in contrast to normally grown term infants, the SGA infant has noticeable wasting of adipose and muscle tissues. This wasting causes the face to take on a wizened appearance, and the hands, feet, and head may appear unusually large for the body (Figs 12–1 and 12–2). The skin hangs loosely, is rough and dry, and desquamates easily. Cranial sutures are sometimes widened, and the fontanel may be larger than expected for the infant's size.

Birth asphyxia occurs frequently in SGA infants, but can be anticipated and potentially prevented when placental insufficiency is diagnosed before birth. Asphyxia causes hypoxia and hypercapnia in the newborn; anaerobic glycolysis follows and predisposes the infant to hypoglycemia. The hypocalcemia often seen in SGA infants is also thought to be a result of asphyxia, rather than an inherent defect in calcium metabolism.[20]

The sequelae of birth asphyxia may further affect the SGA infant's already poor nutritional status. Meconium aspiration and the resultant respiratory distress will delay feedings or affect the method of feeding the infant. Ischemia of the bowel wall may lead to necrotizing entercolitis. Renal hypoxia and hypoperfusion can result in acute renal failure. These problems are usually corrected soon after their occurrence, but central nervous system damage resulting from

birth asphyxia is lifelong. The infant with resultant cerebral palsy or severe mental retardation may need specialized feeding help (see Chapters 7 and 24).

Hypoglycemia in SGA newborns is a frequent metabolic complication and occurs unrelated to asphyxia in many infants. The incidence of prefeeding hypoglycemia (serum glucose less than 30 mg/dL) is between 18% to 67% in infants born SGA, with the highest incidence seen in preterm SGA infants. In contrast, approximately 10% of term AGA infants exhibit hypoglycemia.[21] The hypoglycemia is transient, but often symptomatic. The newborn appears jittery at first and then becomes lethargic, with tremors and apneic spells when the blood glucose drops below 20 mg/dL. Lower cardiac, hepatic, and muscle glycogen stores in SGA infants play an important role, particularly in asymmetrical SGA infants who have a larger than normal brain-to-body weight ratio.[22,23] Symptomatic hypoglycemia is seen less in premature SGA infants who are maintained on intravenous fluids immediately after birth. However, all infants with IUGR must be considered at high risk for hypoglycemia in the first few days of life.

In addition to the imbalance between glycogen stores and glucose-requiring stresses in SGA neonates, defects in the gluconeogenic pathway, fatty acid oxidation, and endocrine control of these mechanisms have been documented in hypoglycemic SGA infants. The absence of a normal glycemic effect of gluconeogenic precursors is indicated by high serum concentrations of lactate, alanine, and other gluconeogenic amino acids.[24-27] The high serum concentrations correlate inversely with the degree of hypoglycemia. In AGA hypoglycemic newborns, alanine feeding raises plasma glucagon and glucose concentrations,[28] whereas in SGA hypoglycemic newborns it does not. High serum concentrations of gluconeogenic precursors in SGA infants suggest that the hypoglycemia is caused by dysfunctioning gluconeogenic enzymes, specifically pyruvate carboxylase and phosphoenol pyruvate carboxykinase (PEPCK). Serum free fatty acid (FFA) concentrations are lower in hypoglycemic SGA in-

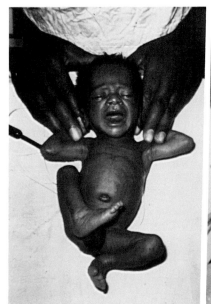
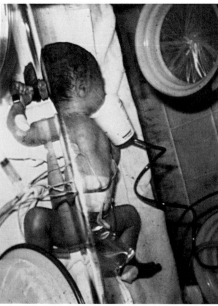

Fig. 12–2. Comparative size and posturing behavior of a term SGA infant and a preterm AGA infant. From the Perinatal Research Institute in Cincinnati. Used with permission.

fants when compared to normoglycemic SGA and AGA control groups.[29-32] The low FFA concentrations correspond to low serum β-hydroxybutarate levels, indicating that the low FFA levels are caused by a disturbance in fat mobilization, rather than a higher oxidation rate of fat.[33] Exogenous lipid injection (0.5 g lipid/kg) is known to raise triglyceride concentrations in SGA infants, but it also serves to stimulate gluconeogenesis, possibly by producing acetyl-CoA, a byproduct of β-oxidation, which is necessary to stimulate PEPCK.[34] The exact pathophysiology of the hypoglycemia is still unknown, however.

Reduced concentrations of serum nitrogenous products in SGA infants resemble those found in older infants with protein-calorie malnutrition, but whether this alteration is caused by impaired placental transport of amino acids or defective fetal production is unknown. Serum total protein, albumin, prealbumin, branched-chain amino acids, and retinol-binding protein concentrations are lower in term and preterm SGA infants soon after birth, but levels become normal after enteral feeding.[35-37] There is also evidence of lowered absorption and deranged metabolism of protein in preterm SGA infants. The significance of this finding is not fully understood, as it does not affect weight gain adversely.[38-40]

The immune system is adversely affected in adults with protein-calorie malnutrition, and similar changes occur in the growth-retarded infant. Decreased concentrations of serum thymic hormone, T lymphocytes, and IgG and impaired cutaneous delayed hypersensitivity have been documented in SGA infants.[41] The higher incidence of infections in infants with IUGR is thought to be the result of impaired immunocompetence caused by malnutrition.[41]

Hypothermia may occur in term SGA infants, despite the ability to decrease body surface area by flexion into the curled fetal position. Underdeveloped stores of subcutaneous adipose tissue and the presence of hypoxia hamper the thermoregulatory function of brown fat tissue.[42] Brown fat stores may also have been atrophied during growth retardation in utero, presumably related to reduced nutrient supply.[43] The SGA infant can compensate for heat losses by increasing the basal metabolic rate (BMR), but if heat losses are not reduced by artificial thermogenic control, poor growth will result. SGA infants are also believed to have an intrinsically higher BMR due to the large brain relative to body weight and to the faster accretion of body tissue during rapid growth phases.[38,44,45]

There is a paucity of information regarding vitamin and mineral stores of the SGA newborn. Overt vitamin or mineral deficiencies are not commonly seen. Most vitamins cross the placenta and accumulate in the fetus at greater blood concentrations than in the mother, even when maternal hypovitaminemia exists. Exceptions to this are vitamins A, B_6, E, and β-carotene.[46] Lower cord serum vitamin A is found in infants with IUGR born of poorly nourished mothers exhibiting low serum vitamin A concentrations.[47] Lower serum concentrations of retinol-binding protein in SGA infants may further restrict the amount of vitamin A available to these newborns.[36]

In a study in the United States, significant risk factors for SGA were: Black and Asian ethnicity, cigarette smoking, short stature (<152 cm), low pregravid weight for height (<90% ideal), low rate of maternal gain (<0.27 kg/week), primiparity, and maternal hypertensive disorder; whereas Preterm delivery risk factors were Black ethnicity, age <16 years, illicit drug abuse, low rate of maternal weight gain (<0.27 kg/week), short interpregnancy interval (<2 year), incompetent cervix and trauma, or anesthesia during pregnancy.[48] In England a low initial maternal weight in pregnancy (<51 kg) was the most effective maternal weight measurement for antinatal detection of SGA infants.[49]

Factors to be Considered in Nutritional Evaluation

History

A detailed prenatal history should be gathered from the mother and her prenatal medical records. It should include the amount and rate of weight gain, presence of hyperemesis, dietary intake (particularly during the third trimester), vitamin-mineral supplements, drug, cigarette and alcohol usage, and any significant medical conditions of the mother. The prenatal history may help elucidate the cause of IUGR, but will be used to a greater extent when counseling for prevention of IUGR in future pregnancies.

Birth events should be noted from the birth attendant's medical notes when examination of nutritional status is delayed for days or weeks. Apgar scores, hypoglycemia, intubation, and early feeding behaviors are important in later nutritional evaluation.

Anthropometric data

Birth weight, length, and head circumference should be measured as accurately as possible immediately after birth. Length may need to be repeated later on a standard neonatal length board, as measurement after delivery is often hurried and should not be relied upon as accurate. These measurements are then plotted on a growth chart appropriate for the infant's gestational age. Other measurements, such as midarm circumference, chest circumference, crown-rump length, and triceps or subscapular skinfold, may also be recorded.

Although weight for gestational age is the traditional method of diagnosing IUGR, further judgments concerning the degree of growth retardation and malnutrition, its possible etiology, and prognostic indicators for metabolic complications and future growth and development may be derived from manipulation of various anthropometric measurements into mathematical ratios. The most widely used is the ponderal index (PI) by Rohrer.[50]

$$\frac{\text{wt in g}}{\text{length}^3 \text{ in cm}} \times 100$$

The PI shows how heavy the infant is for its length and increases with the accumulation of muscle and adipose tissue. It has been used by various researchers to describe subgroups of SGA infants based on their body proportions. Type I SGA infants have a normal PI, defined as a PI greater than the 10th percentile on Miller's curve (Fig 12–3), have a head circumference less than the 10th percentile for gestational age, and thus are somewhat symmetrical. Type II SGA infants are disproportionately growth retarded, as evidenced by a PI less than the 10th percentile and a head

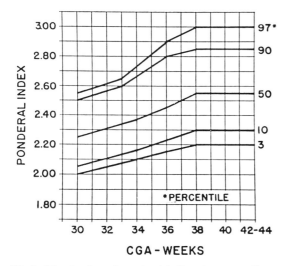

Fig. 12-3. Distribution of ponderal indices by percentile groups in a control group of newborn infants according to their fetal ages. From Miller, H.C., Hassanein, K. Diagnosis of impaired fetal growth in newborn infants. *Pediatrics.* 1971; 48:511. Used with permission.

circumference greater than the 10th percentile.[51] Studies using the ponderal index to classify infants support the theory that asymmetrical SGA infants have better catch-up growth and developmental outcomes than symmetrical SGA infants.[11,14]

The ponderal index has also been suggested for use in classifying infants at risk for hypoglycemia.[21] However, Georgieff and colleagues[52-54] have studied the use of the midarm circumference/head circumference ratio (MAC/HC) extensively and have demonstrated that it is a more discriminative measure for diagnosing IUGR and predicting metabolic complications. The MAC/HC ratio is based on the belief that malnutrition in a growing infant causes head circumference growth to be spared at the expense of length and weight and that midarm circumference, which reflects fat and muscle stores, will be the first measurement to decrease. Therefore, a ratio between the most affected (MAC) and least affected (HC) measurements should define IUGR more accurately. In contrast, the ponderal index combines weight and length measurements; both weight and length can be affected by IUGR, and length is often an inaccurate measurement.

In Georgieff's studies, the MAC/HC ratio identified significantly higher percentages of infants who had metabolic disturbances (glucose < 30 mg/dL, calcium < 7 mg/dL, and hematocrit > 65%) among infants who had physical signs of suspected growth retardation (subcutaneous muscle wasting, peeling skin, and metabolic symptoms) but were not SGA as defined by weight alone. A standard curve for MAC:HC has been developed, based on healthy preterm and term infant measurements (Fig. 12-4). IUGR infants who have metabolic disturbances tend to have ratios below the 5th percentile on the standard curve, whether they are AGA or SGA.[53]

Ounsted et al.[55] have attempted to divide SGA neonates into subgroups based on head circumference:chest circumference ratio and head circumference:crown-rump length ratio, but found that gestational age and gender have more

of an influence on these anthropometric measures than etiological factors. Skinfold thickness, in the triceps, subscapular, and abdominal areas, is decreased in infants who are SGA at birth,[56] as are midarm circumference and arm-fat area.[57] The usefulness of these measurements has yet to be determined.

When recorded serially, anthropometric measurements are particularly valuable in assessing growth. Continued documentation of head circumference, length, and weight measurements on the appropriate growth chart will illustrate whether nutritional intake has been adequate. The phenomenon of catch-up growth may be observed, particularly in SGA infants who were asymmetrical at birth. Symmetrical SGA infants tend to follow an individual growth curve below the standard percentiles.

In sick neonates, a triphasic growth pattern may be seen: an initial phase of suboptimal growth, a second phase of catch-up growth, and a third phase of growth along standard rates.[58] It is important in these infants to watch growth velocity, as catch-up growth measured by head circumference or weight gain may actually reflect the development of hydrocephalus or edema.[59] Any improvement of growth rate should correlate with improvements in nutritional intake and general medical condition.

Nutritional intake and feeding ability

The evaluation of the infant's suck-swallow mechanism should be done at the first feeding soon after birth. The feeding behavior of the term SGA infant is often aggressive, but severe asphyxia or premature birth may affect the oral reflexes. The infant in these instances may be sluggish to feed or may suck ineffectively. Depending on the circumstances, different nipples may be tried, or nasogastric or intravenous feedings may be initiated. The older infant with a history of IUGR, when receiving solid foods, should be evaluated for feeding abilities as described in Chapter 24.

A detailed and sequential historical record of the infant's nutritional intake should be constructed. It should include the type and amount of formula or human milk actually ingested, gastrointestinal tolerance of the feedings, and the use of vitamin or mineral preparations. If the infant has been hospitalized for a length of time after birth, it will be helpful to note when the infant was advanced to full, ad libitum oral feedings and whether any parenteral nutrition was provided. Average daily or weekly calorie, protein, and mineral intakes can then be calculated. Records should also be made of any other dietary supplements provided (carbohydrate, fat, protein modulars; human milk fortifier) and medications known to have interactions with nutrients.

When infants begin eating solid foods or when feedings are erratic in the home setting, a 3-day written record that the caregiver completes at home may provide more specific information.

After the nutritional intake information is analyzed, it is used in conjunction with the growth record, laboratory data, and clinical assessments to determine what further nutritional therapy is needed.

Laboratory and Clinical Assessments

Clinical signs of malnutrition in the SGA infant include thin, dry skin; prominence of bony skeleton; a scaphoid abdo-

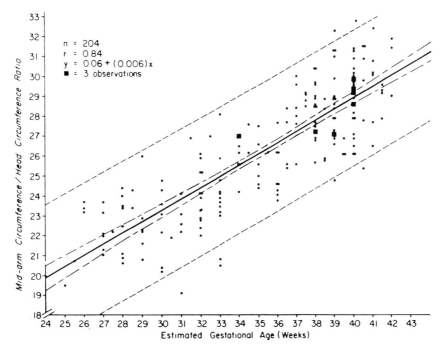

Fig. 12–4. Midarm circumference:head circumference ratio standard curve. ——— mean MAC:HC; — · — 95% limits on predicted mean MAC:HC for regression line; — — — 95% confidence limits for one observation. From Sasanow, S.P., Georgieff, M.K., Pereira, G.R. Mid-arm circumference and mid-arm/head circumference ratios: standard curves for anthropometric assessment of neonatal nutritional status. *J. Pediatr.* 1986; 109:311. Used with permission.

men; and absence of fatty tissue over the buttocks, cheeks, and extremities. Simple visual inspection and palpation can lead to a diagnosis of IUGR in term infants; these methods are less reliable in preterm infants. The degree of growth impairment is subjective, but largely based on anthropometric measurements.

Laboratory tests should be used thoughtfully as a method of nutritional assessment in SGA newborns due to their risk, invasiveness, expense, and lack of diagnostic ability. Lowered serum concentrations of albumin, total protein, and prealbumin have been documented in some, but not all, SGA neonates born at term.[35] Normal values of serum proteins for preterm infants are still unknown. When a confident judgment of protein-calorie malnutrition can be made from anthropometric measurements and the infant's physical appearance, biochemical measurements to corroborate malnutrition are usually unnecessary.

In sick SGA neonates or those with subsequent failure to thrive, indices of protein and iron stores are measured as part of the complete medical and nutritional evaluations. Other specific serum nutrient concentrations to be evaluated, such as zinc, vitamins A and D, and folate, should be determined based on the diet history, clinical signs, and growth status of the infant. In addition to having diagnostic value, the laboratory data are used as a baseline reference from which to measure the efficacy of nutritional therapy.

Dietary Management

As soon as feasible after birth, feedings are begun to prevent the occurrence of hypoglycemia in the SGA newborn. In-

fants with prefeeding hypoglycemia or respiratory distress who are otherwise unable to feed are maintained on intravenous glucose until oral feedings can begin and blood sugar is stabilized. Frequent feedings (every 2 to 3 hours) at the breast or of bottled formula should be given for several days thereafter. Blood glucose concentrations should be monitored closely for the first few days to be certain they remain in the normal range.

SGA infants who require intubation or those who have oral feeding dysfunction need to be fed by tube. The infant's condition will determine the feeding type, amount, and delivery method. Peripheral or total parenteral nutrition is limited to situations where the gastrointestinal tract is not functioning. Occasionally, pharmacotherapy, such as glucagon, may be needed.

The SGA infant who feeds well orally may be allowed to feed ad libitum at the breast or by bottle with standard iron-fortified infant formula. Intake and growth rate should be monitored closely. In more severe cases of IUGR, the formula concentration may be increased over the standard 67 cal/dL to 74 or 81 cal/dL by decreasing the water added to powder mix or liquid concentrate. Doing so has the advantage of concentrating all nutrients proportionately; carbohydrate or fat modulars increase the caloric value while decreasing the nutrient density, but they are valuable in certain cases.

There is some evidence that higher energy feedings in SGA infants are beneficial only up until 2 months of age; after this time, appetite control becomes more precise, and the infant compensates for the higher energy density by reducing intake.[40] Mothers who wish to continue breastfeeding should be encouraged to nurse frequently in the first few months. Eight to ten nursing periods per day, offering both breasts at each feeding, will establish an adequate milk supply. Poorly growing breastfed infants should not be given supplementary formula feedings before a careful evaluation of the mother-infant feeding relationship is made, as doing so will actually decrease the mother's milk supply.

The desired caloric intake is one that will support rapid growth of the infant. At least 56–76 kcal/kg/day are needed to support resting energy expenditure[38,44]; intakes above this level begin to provide for growth. The minimum needed for postnatal head growth is thought to be 85 kcal/kg/day.[58] In term SGA infants, adequate growth (15–30 g/day) has been documented on oral, ad libitum intakes of formula ranging from 129–163 kcal/kg/day.[25,40] Premature SGA infants show comparable weight gains on oral, and libitum intakes of 108–144 kcal/kg/day.[38,45,59] Very low birth weight (BW < 1500 g) premature SGA infants appear to need higher caloric intakes—154–158 kcal/kg/day—to reach growth rates of 30 g/day due to their poorer absorption of protein and fat.[44]

There is no evidence that SGA infants require a higher protein intake than that provided by the standard infant formulas (2.22–2.71 g protein/100 kcal). Protein intake of SGA infants from the above studies ranged from 2.0–3.4 g/kg/day.[25,38,44,59] In Boehm's study[39] using human milk feedings for very low birth weight infants, the authors suggest that even low protein intakes (1.98–2.41 g protein/kg/day) may not be tolerated well by preterm SGA infants. From these preliminary data they suggest that for this subgroup of SGA infants metabolic capacity for protein is initially lowered, but returns to normal after the third postnatal week.

A general multivitamin preparation is usually prescribed for term infants demonstrating IUGR. Iron should be provided in the form of drops or iron-fortified formula, and fluoride should be prescribed according to standard guidelines (see Chapter 2). Individual nutrient deficiencies in SGA infants, as determined by laboratory data, need to be corrected through appropriate supplementation.

Unfortunately, long-term studies of growth in SGA infants have not reported on nutritional intake and its effects. One study, by Ernst et al.,[60] did find that adverse nutritional practices were prevalent in a group of 122 very low birth weight infants followed for 12 months postnatally. Feeding solids earlier than developmentally appropriate (via bottle or infant feeder) and feeding cow's milk, particularly low fat and skim, during the first year of life were the identified practices that may have resulted in less favorable growth outcome. However, SGA and AGA infants were grouped together with regard to nutritional intake data.

Compared to AGA cohort groups, SGA infants tend to remain shorter and lighter, despite the occurrence of catch-up growth. Differences seem to exist between symmetrical and asymmetrical SGA infants, and between preterm and term SGA infants. As stated previously, contradictory results of growth are reported in the literature due to uncontrolled variables and differences in the categorization of SGA subgroups. Catch-up growth appears to occur at a greater rate in asymmetrical SGA infants than in symmetrical SGA infants,[11,14] suggesting that protein-calorie malnutrition with origin late in gestation is more amenable to correction. However, some studies still report significant differences in weight, length, and skinfold measurements up to 2 and 3 years of age between asymmetrical SGA infants and AGA infants.[11,12] Preterm SGA infants show extraordinary catch-up growth, resulting in no significant differences in length and weight at 12 and 24 months of age when compared to preterm AGA infants,[11,13] but differences have been documented later at 5 years of age in the same study group[13] and others.[16] Although socioeconomic status plays a greater role than IUGR in determining later developmental scores,[13,15] in Westwood's study[17] there were still significant differences in height, weight, head circumference, and triceps skinfold measurements between SGA and AGA subjects at adolescence when socioeconomic status was held constant. Westwood's study group comprised adolescents with a history of term birth without asphyxiation. Bone age and sexual development were not found to be delayed in the SGA adolescents, indicating that the growth deficits were permanent. Although poor nutritional status is often found in populations with low socioeconomic status, it is not possible to extrapolate from the above studies that differences in growth of SGA infants are due to poor postnatal nutrition.

Follow-up and Summary

Nutritional management of the SGA infant should focus on the provision of adequate nutrients to provide for catch-up growth and prevent deficiencies. The clinical condition and gestational age of the individual infant determine the mode and manner of nutrient delivery. Dietary intake in conjunction with growth records should be monitored closely to ensure the optimal chance for recovery after IUGR.

References

1. Gruenwald, P. Growth of the human fetus. I. Normal growth and its variation. *Am. J. Obstet. Gynecol.* 1966; 94:1112.
2. Lubchenco, L.O., Hansman, C., Dressler, M., Boyd, E. Intrauterine growth as estimated from live-born birth-weight data at 24 to 42 weeks of gestation. *Pediatrics.* 1963; 32:793.
3. Villar, J., Belizan, J.M. The timing factor in the pathophysiology of the intrauterine growth retardation syndrome. *Obstet. Gynecol. Surv.* 1982; 37:499.
4. Walther, F.J., Ramaekers, L. The ponderal index as a measure of the nutritional status at birth and its relation to some aspects of neonatal morbidity. *J. Perinat. Med.* 1982; 10:42.
5. Wennergren, M. Perinatal risk factors. With special reference to intrauterine growth retardation and neonatal respiratory adaptation. *Acta. Obstet. Gynecol. Scand.* 1986; 135(suppl):8.
6. Chen, A.T., Falek, A. Chromosome aberrations in full-term low birthweight neonates. *Hum. Genet.* 1974; 21:13.
7. Anderson, N.G. A five year survey of small for dates infants for chromosome abnormalities. *Aust. Paediatr. J.* 1976; 12:19.
8. Andreasson, B., Svenningsen, N.W., Nordenfelt, E. Screening for viral infections in infants with poor intrauterine growth. *Acta Paediatr. Scand.* 1981; 70:673.
9. Chiswick, M. Intrauterine growth retardation. *Br. Med. J.* 1985; 291:845.
10. Villar, J., Belizan, J.M. The relative contribution of prematurity and fetal growth retardation to low birthweight in developing and developed societies. *Am. J. Obstet. Gynecol.* 1982; 143:793.
11. Tenuvou, A., Kero, P., Piekkala, P., Korvenranta, H., Sillanpaa, M., Erkkola, R. Growth of 519 small-for-gestational age infants during the first two years of life. *Acta Paediatr. Scand.* 1987; 76:636.

12. Walther, F.J., Ramaekeers, L.H. Growth in early childhood of newborns affected by disproportionate intrauterine growth retardation. *Acta Paediatr. Scand.* 1982; 71:651.
13. Vohr, B.R., Oh, W. Growth and development in preterm infants small for gestational age. *J. Pediatr.* 1983; 103:941.
14. Villar, J., Smeriglio, V., Martorell, R., Brown, C.H., Klein, R.E. Heterogeneous growth and mental development of intrauterine growth-retarded infants during the first 3 years of life. *Pediatrics.* 1984; 74:783.
15. Low, J.A., Galbraith, R.S., Muir, D., Killen, H., Pater, B., Karchmar, J. Intrauterine growth retardation: a study of long-term morbidity. *Am. J. Obstet. Gynecol.* 1982; 142:670.
16. Sann, L., Darre, E., Lasne, Y., Bourgeois, J., Bethanod, M. Effects of prematurity and dysmaturity on growth at age 5 years. *J. Pediatr.* 1986; 109:681.
17. Westwood, M., Kramer, M.S., Munz, D., Lovett, J.M., Watters, G.V. Growth and development of full-term nonasphyxiated small-for-gestational age newborns: follow-up through adolescence. *Pediatrics.* 1983; 71:376.
18. Ounsted, M., Moar, V.A., Scott, A. Head circumference and developmental ability at the age of seven years. *Acta Paediatr. Scand.* 1988; 77:374.
19. Tenuvou, A., Kero, P., Korvenranta, H., Pickkala, P., Sillanpaa, M., Erkkola, R. Developmental outcome of 519 small-for-gestational age children at the age of two years. *Neuropediatrics.* 1988; 19:41.
20. Tsang, R.C., Gigger, M., Oh, W., Brown, D.R. Studies in calcium metabolism in infants with intrauterine growth retardation. *J. Pediatr.* 1975; 86:936.
21. Lubchenco, L.O., Bard, H. Incidence of hypoglycemia in newborn infants classified by birth weight and gestational age. *Pediatrics.* 1971; 47:831.
22. Hay, W.W. Fetal and neonatal glucose homeostasis and their relation to the small for gestational age infant. *Sem. Perinatol.* 1984; 8:101.
23. Pildes, R.S. Pyati, S.P. Hypoglycemia and hyperglycemia in tiny infants. *Clin. Perinatol.* 1986; 13:351.
24. Haymond, M.W., Karl, I.E., Pagliara, A.S. Increased gluconeogenic substrates in the small-for-gestational-age infant. *N. Engl. J. Med.* 1974; 291:322.
25. Robles, R., Gil, A., Faus, M.J., Periago, J.L., Sanchez-Pozo, A., Pita, M.L., Sanchez-Medina, F. Serum and urine amino acids patterns during the first month of life in small-for-date infants. *Biol. Neonate.* 1984; 45:209.
26. Lindblad, B.S. The venous plasma free amino acid levels during the first hours of life. I. After normal and short gestation and gestation complicated by hypertension. With special reference to the "small-for-dates" syndrome. *Acta Paediatr. Scand.* 1970; 59:1.
27. Mestyan, J., Soltesz, G., Schultz, K., Horvath, M. Hyperaminoacidemia due to the accumulation of gluconeogenic amino acid precursors in hypoglycemic small-for-gestational-age infants. *J. Pediatr.* 1975; 87:409.
28. Vileisis, R.A., Oh, W. Metabolic consequences of intrauterine growth retardation. *J. Pediatr. Gastroenterol. Nutr.* 1983; 2(suppl 1):S59.
29. Harris, R.J. Plasma nonesterified fatty acid and blood glucose levels in healthy and hypoxemic newborn infants. *J. Pediatr.* 1974; 84:578.
30. Keele, D.K., Kay, J.L. Plasma free fatty acid and blood sugar levels in newborn infants and their mothers. *Pediatrics.* 1966; 37:597.
31. deLeeuw, R., deVries, I.J. Hypoglycemia in small-for-dates newborn infants. *Pediatrics.* 1976; 58:18.
32. Schultz, K., Mestyan, J., Soltesz, G., Horvath, M. The metabolic effects of glucagon infusion in normoglycemic and hypoglycemic small-for-gestational-age infants. I. Changes in blood glucose, blood lactate and plasma free fatty acids. *Acta Paediatr. Hung.* 1976; 17:237.
33. Sabel, K.G., Olegard, R., Mellander, M., Hildingsson, K. Interrelation between fatty acid oxidation and control of gluconeogenic subtrates in small-for-gestational-age (SGA) infants with hypoglycemia and with normoglycemia. *Acta Paediatr. Scand.* 1982; 71:53.
34. Sabel, K.G., Olegard, R., Hildingsson, K., Karlberg, P. Effects of injected lipid emulsion on oxygen consumption, RQ,

35. Faus, M.J., Gil, A., Robles, R., Sanchez-Pozo, A., Pita, M.L., Sanchez-Medina, F. Changes in serum albumin, transferrin, and amino acid indices during the first month of life in small-for-dates infants. *Ann. Nutr. Metab.* 1984; 28:70.
36. Howells, D.W., Levin, G.E., Brown, I.R., Brooke, O.G.: Plasma retinol and retinol-binding protein in preterm infants born small for gestational age or of appropriate weight for age. *Hum. Nutr. Clin. Nutr.* 1984; 38:107.
37. Thomas, M.R., Massoudi, M., Chan, G.M., Wells, B.S. Eggert, L.D. Comparison of maternal energy and protein intake to cord blood and infant protein—energy assessment measures. *J. Am. Coll. Nutr.* 1984; 3:263.
38. Cauderay, M., Schutz, Y., Micheli, J.L., Calame, A., Jequier, E. Energy-nitrogen balances and protein turnover in small and appropriate for gestational age low birthweight infants. *Int. J. Vitam. Nutr. Res.* 1987; 57:338.
39. Boehm, G., Senger, H., Braun, W., Beyreiss, K., Raiha, N.C. Metabolic differences between AGA- and SGA-infants of very low birthweight. I. Relationship to intrauterine growth retardation. *Acta Paediatr. Scand.* 1988; 77:19.
40. Brooke, O.G., Kinsey, J.M. High energy feeding in small for gestation infants. *Arch. Dis. Child.* 1985; 60:42.
41. Xanthou, M. Immunologic deficiencies in small-for-dates neonates. *Acta Paediatr. Scand.* 1985; 319(suppl):143.
42. Hull, D. The structure and function of brown adipose tissue. *Br. Med. Bull.* 1966; 22:92.
43. Sinclair, J.C. Heat production and thermoregulation in the small-for-date infant. *Pediatr. Clin. North Am.* 1970; 17:147.
44. Chessex, P., Reichman, B., Verellen, G., Putet, G., Smith, J.M., Heim, T., Swyer, P.R. Metabolic consequences of intrauterine growth retardation in very low birthweight infants. *Pediatr. Res.* 1984; 18:709.
45. Brooke, O.G. Energy requirements and utilization of the low birthweight infant. *Acta Paediatr. Scand.* 1982; 296(suppl):67.
46. Baker, H., Frank, O., Thomson, A.D., Langer, A., Munves, E.D., DeAngelis, B., Kaminetzky, H.A. Vitamin profile of 174 mothers and newborns at parturition. *Am. J. Clin. Nutr.* 1975; 28:59.
47. Shah, R.S., Rajalakshmi, R. Vitamin A status of the newborn in relation to gestational age, body weight, and maternal nutritional status. *Am. J. Clin. Nutr.* 1984; 40:794.
48. Abrams, B., Newman, V. Small-for-gestational-age birth: Maternal predictors and comparisons with risk factors of spontaneous preterm delivery in the same cohort. *Am. J. Obstet. Gynecol.* 1991; 164:785.
49. Dawes, M.G., Grudzinskas, J.G. Repeated measurement of maternal weight during pregnancy. Is this a useful practice? *Br. J. Obstet. Gynaecol.* 1991; 98:189.
50. Rohrer, R. Der index der korperfulle als mass des ernahrungszustandes. *Munchener. Medizinische. Wochenschrift.* 1921; 68:580.
51. Walther, F.J., Ramaekers, L. The ponderal index as a measure of the nutritional status at birth and its relation to some aspects of neonatal morbidity. *J. Perinat. Med.* 1982; 10:42.
52. Georgieff, M.K., Sasanow, S., Pereira, G.R., Watkins, J.B. Mid arm circumference/head circumference ratio (MAC/HC) for identification of intrauterine growth disorders in neonates. *J. Am. Coll. Nutr.* 1984; 3:263.
53. Georgieff, M.K., Sasanow, S.R., Mammel, M.C., Pereira, G.R. Mid-arm circumference/head circumference ratios for identification of symptomatic LGA, AGA, and SGA newborn infants. *J. Pediatr.* 1986; 109:316.
54. Georgieff, M.K., Sasanow, S.R., Choekalingam, U.M., Pereira, G.R. A comparison of the mid-arm circumference/head circumference ratio and ponderal index for the evaluation of newborn infants after abnormal intrauterine growth. *Acta Paediatr. Scand.* 1988; 77:214.
55. Ounsted, M., Moar, V.A., Scott, A. Proportionality of small-for-gestational age babies at birth; perinatal associations and postnatal sequelae. *Early Hum. Dev.* 1986; 14:77.
56. Usher, R.H., McLean, F. Intrauterine growth of live-born Caucasian infants at sea level: standard obtained from meas-

urements in 7 dimensions of infants born between 25 and 44 weeks of gestation. *J. Pediatr.* 1969; 74:901.

57. Excler, J.L., Sann, L., Lasne, Y., Picard, J. Anthropometric assessment of nutritional status in newborn infants. Discriminative value of mid arm circumference and of skinfold thickness. *Early Hum. Dev.* 1985; 11:169.

58. Georgieff, M.K., Hoffman, J.S., Pereira, G.R., Bernbaum, J., Hoffman-Williamson, M. Effect of neonatal caloric deprivation on head growth and 1-year developmental status in pre-

term infants. *J. Pediatr.* 1985; 107:581.

59. Stanley, O.H., Speidel, B.D. "Catch-up" following severe intrauterine retardation of head growth. *J. Perinat. Med.* 1985; 13:253.

60. Ernst, J.A., Bull, M.J., Richard, K.A., Gray, S. Lemons, J.A. Growth outcome and feeding practices of very low birth weight infants (less than 1500 grams) within the first year of life. *J. Pediatr.* 1990; 117:5156.

Chapter 13
Autism

Bonnie Patterson, Shirley Walberg Ekvall, and Susan Dickerson Mayes

Autistic disorder is one of two forms of pervasive developmental disorder and was first identified by Leo Kanner in 1943. It is characterized by a pervasive disorder of affect, language, cognitive skills, and social development.[1] The diagnostic criteria for autistic disorder have been well established and are listed in Table 13–1.[2] When less than 8 of the 16 criteria for autistic disorder are met and there is a qualitative impairment in the development of reciprocal social interaction and communication skills, a diagnosis of pervasive developmental disorder not otherwise specified (PDDNOS) is made.

The etiology of autism is unclear, but it is felt to have a neurobiological basis. Like many other neurodevelopmental disorders, autism may have multiple causes. For example, structural abnormalities of the brain, viruses (rubella and cytomegalovirus), genetic disorders (e.g., Cornelia de Lange syndrome), chromosomal abnormalities (fragile X syndrome), metabolic disorders (phenylketonuria), and a specific seizure disorder (infantile spasms) have all been associated with autism. Children with autism have an increased incidence of congenital anomalies, persistence of primitive reflexes, unusual posturing and motor movements, nonspecific EEG abnormalities, increased incidence of seizures in adolescence, and delayed development of hand dominance.[1] Recent magnetic resonance imaging (MRI) studies have shown developmental hypoplasia of portions of the cerebellum in some children with autism.[3] This hypoplasia appears to be specific for neocerebellar vermal lobules six and seven. These abnormalities may be related to impaired cognitive functioning, which is seen in the majority of children with autism. Bioclinical markers—behavior, electrophysiological, and biochemical—can be analyzed.[4]

The prevalence of autism has been reported as four to five children in every 10,000.[1] Prevalence of pervasive developmental disorder (autistic disorder and pervasive developmental disorder not otherwise specified) has been estimated at 10 to 15 children in every 10,000.[5] Autism appears to be more common among boys than girls, with a ratio of three or four to one. It can be diagnosed readily in children between 1 to 3 years of age.[6]

Some girls diagnosed as autistic in reality have Rett's syndrome. This syndrome is characterized by regression in communication and social development, which is frequently thought to resemble autism. In addition, the girls have microcephaly, ataxia, repetitive hand washing or hand-wringing movements, severe to profound retardation, hyperventilation, decreased body fat and muscle mass, seizure disorder, and increasing spasticity with age. The autistic features often decrease as the girls become older. The etiology of Rett's syndrome is unknown at this time, but affects only girls (see Chapter 18).

Biochemical Abnormalities

Studies by Schain and Freedman[7] have revealed increased serotonin levels in people with autism. Dysfunction in the pineal-hypothalmic-adrenal axis may produce increased opiods, peptides, and serotonin.[8] This apparent hyperserotoninemia has led to attempts to treat autistic children with fenfluramine, which decreases both peripheral and central levels of serotonin. In a double-blind placebo-controlled cross-over study of 14 autistic individuals, fenfluramine resulted in significant improvement of many autistic symptoms, including social and affective dysfunction, sensory disturbance, and abnormal motor behavior, as well as an increase in developmental test scores.[9] However, in another study, fenfluramine did not produce significant positive results in relation to placebo.[10] Hashimoto et al., found significantly lower thyroid stimulating hormone (basal and peak values) and enhanced dopamingeric *or* reduced serotonergic activity in the central nervous system in boys with autism.[11]

Histamine, calcium, and uric acid levels have been measured in urine and whole blood or plasma in some individuals with autism. Only minor, generally insignificant changes were seen in histamine levels. Serum calcium levels were reported to be within normal ranges in one study, but Launay et al.[11] found that 50% of the children diagnosed with autism had low serum calcium levels and high amounts of urinary calcium. Furthermore, decreased serum calcium levels have been found in children with major depressed states. Uric acid levels in serum and urine also are decreased.[12] This might correspond to subgroups of the population labeled "autistic" in whom defects in purine metabolism might be related to immunological deficiencies affecting autism and in whom folate metabolism may interact with bioamine metabolism, particularly at the hydroxylase levels. These types of disturbances have been reported in various types of psychoses.[9] Adenylosuccinase deficiency—measured by succinyl-adenosine levels in urine—has been found in children with autistic behavior.[13] The formation of carbolines related to reduced folic acid levels is an area of investigation for autism research.[12] However, in most of the studies identifying possible biochemical abnormalities, dietary intake was not controlled; therefore, all of the findings may be secondary to dietary differences, rather than the metabolic parameters.[12]

Another area of biochemical investigation involves hair analysis for mineral concentrations (although hair analysis

Table 13-1. Diagnostic Criteria for Autistic Disorder

At least 8 of the following 16 items are present, these to include at least two items from A, one from B, and one from C.

Note: Consider a criterion to be met *only* if the behavior is abnormal for the person's developmental level.

A. Qualitative impairment in reciprocal social interaction as manifested by the following:

(The examples within parentheses are arranged so that those first mentioned are more likely to apply to younger or more handicapped, and the later ones, to older or less handicapped, persons with this disorder.)

(1) marked lack of awareness of the existence or feelings of others (e.g., treats a person as if he or she were a piece of furniture; does not notice another person's distress; apparently has no concept of the need of others for privacy)

(2) no or abnormal seeking of comfort at times of distress (e.g., does not come for comfort even when ill, hurt, or tired; seeks comfort in a stereotyped way, e.g., says "cheese, cheese, cheese" whenever hurt)

(3) no or impaired imitation (e.g., does not wave bye-bye; does not copy mother's domestic activities; mechanical imitation of others' actions out of context)

(4) no or abnormal social play (e.g., does not actively participate in simple games; prefers solitary play activities; involves other children in play only as "mechanical aids")

(5) gross impairment in ability to make peer friendships (e.g., no interest in making peer friendships; despite interest in making friends, demonstrates lack of understanding of conventions of social interaction, for example, reads phone book to uninterested peer)

B. Qualitative impairment in verbal and nonverbal communication, and in imaginative activity, as manifested by the following:

(The numbered items are arranged so that those first listed are more likely to apply to younger or more handicapped, and the later ones, to older or less handicapped, persons with this disorder.)

(1) no mode of communication, such as communicative babbling, facial expression, gesture, mime, or spoken language

(2) markedly abnormal nonverbal communication, as in the use of eye-to-eye gaze, facial expression, body posture, or gestures to initiate or modulate social interaction (e.g., does not anticipate being held, stiffens when held, does not look at the person or smile when making a social approach, does not greet parents or visitors, has a fixed stare in social situations)

(3) absence of imaginative activity, such as playacting of adult roles, fantasy characters, or animals; lack of interest in stories about imaginary events

(4) marked abnormalities in the production of speech, including volume, pitch, stress, rate, rhythm, and intonation (e.g., monotonous tone, questionlike melody, or high pitch)

(5) marked abnormalities in the form or content of speech, including stereotyped and repetitive use of speech (e.g., immediate echolalia or mechanical repetition of television commercial); use of "you" when "I" is meant (e.g., using "You want cookie?" to mean "I want a cookie"); idiosyncratic use of words or phrases (e.g., "Go on green riding" to mean "I want to go on the swing"); or frequent irrelevant remarks (e.g., starts talking about train schedules during a conversation about sports)

(6) marked impairment in the ability to initiate or sustain a conversation with others, despite adequate speech (e.g., indulging in lengthy monologues on one subject regardless of interjections from others)

C. Markedly restricted repertoire of activities and interests, as manifested by the following:

(1) stereotyped body movements, e.g., hand-flicking or twisting movements, spinning, head-banging, complex whole-body movements

(2) persistent preoccupation with parts of objects (e.g., sniffing or smelling objects, repetitive feeling of texture of materials, spinning wheels of toy cars) or attachment to unusual objects (e.g., insists on carrying around a piece of string)

(3) marked distress over changes in trivial aspects of environment, e.g., when a vase is moved from usual position

(4) unreasonable insistence on following routines in precise detail, e.g., insisting that exactly the same route always be followed when shopping

(5) markedly restricted range of interests and a preoccupation with one narrow interest, e.g., interested only in lining up objects, in amassing facts about meteorology, or in pretending to be a fantasy character

D. Onset during infancy or childhood.

Specify if childhood onset (after 36 months of age).

From American Psychiatric Association[2] with permission.

can be unreliable). In a study of 12 children diagnosed with infantile autism and 12 control children, scalp hair samples were analyzed for concentrations of calcium, magnesium, zinc, copper, lead, and cadmium.[14] The only statistically significant difference ($P < 0.05$) found between the two groups was a 62% lower cadmium concentration in the hair of the children with autism. No explanation for this difference was offered by the authors. It was noted that the study was limited by a small number of participants, as well as the variable reliability of hair analysis as a diagnostic tool in assessing mineral status of individuals.[14]

Factors to be Considered in Nutritional Evaluation

Behavioral problems affecting dietary intake

Behavioral problems associated with food acceptance or rejection are commonly recognized problems of children with developmental disabilities, particularly autism.[14-16] Often, such behaviors contribute to poor dietary intake and bizarre feeding patterns. These children may be indulged by caregivers who may tend to tolerate such behaviors in these children more readily than in unaffected children.[16] Additionally, caregivers may not know how to manage the unusual feeding problems of autistic children.

The atypical feeding patterns of autistic children are usually a reflection of their underlying, neurologically based disorder. Autistic children characteristically present with a variety of somatosensory disturbances, including feeding disorders. An increased frequency of physical anomalies and the persistence of primitive reflexes in children with autism may contribute to feeding problems as well. Other characteristics that may affect the development of feeding skills include delayed development of hand dominance, unusual postures, and unusual movements.[1] Feeding behaviors often associated with infantile autism include pica, food craving, specific food or food preparation preferences, idiosyncracies, and perceived eating problems according to parental report and clinical observation.[14,15,17] For example, there may be aversion to the swallowing of substances other than own secretions in extreme cases, and milder cases may exhibit oral tactile defensiveness (e.g., hypersensitivity to some textures), retention of bits of food in the mouth for prolonged periods of time, and idiosyncratic and rigid food preferences.

In one study, parents of children with autism were surveyed for their nutrition knowledge and attitudes related to the diet of the children. Their responses were compared to parents of control children who also participated in the study.[15] It was found that, as a group, parents of children with autism appear to have a more positive attitude toward nutrition and a higher nutrition knowledge score than did parents of the control children. Food-related idiosyncracies reported for children with autism included food cravings (53% versus 18% in controls) and pica (33% versus 3% in controls). In 38% of cases of food cravings in children with autism, the parents noted an association between the consumption of craved food and disturbed behavior. However, statistical analysis of these children's diets failed to reveal any significant relationship between the food item frequency of consumption and reported behavior. It revealed that children with autism generally consume more variety within each

food group each day than control children.[15] This finding is unusual as most children with autism like only a few foods and may eat large quantities of these foods; for example, one cup of butter at a time.

The three types of food habits most often seen are (1) the need for sameness and ritual; (2) specific eating behaviors, such as messy eating; and (3) limited and rigid food preferences; for example, a preference for high-carbohydrate foods. Whenever food aversions exist, there is the potential for nutritional deficiency.[18] Vitamin deficiencies are not as prevalent as mineral deficiencies because so many foods are fortified and/or enriched.[18]

Research in dietary intake

Because of the frequently described unusual food behaviors in children with autism, it is often assumed that the children will consume inadequate diets. Written dietary records kept by caregivers were analyzed for 12 children diagnosed with autism and 12 control children of normal behavior and intelligence.[14] All children were between 7 and 9 years of age, with the mean age for the autistic group at $8.0 \pm .8$ years and for the control children at $8.4 \pm .6$ years. Both groups were from middle-class, urban families, and none of the children was institutionalized. Caregivers kept 3-day food records for the children; vitamin and mineral supplements were not included in the dietary analysis. Eleven nutrients, in addition to energy or calories, were determined by computer analysis of the written diet records and compared to the 1980 Recommended Dietary Allowances (RDA) of the National Research Council for the children's age group. Intakes of both groups of children were found to be satisfactory as compared to the RDA. The lowest percentages of the RDA in the group of children with autism were for energy at $92 \pm 6\%$ and for calcium at $92 \pm 10\%$. Compared to the control children, the children with autism had intakes that were significantly lower ($P < 0.05$) in calcium and riboflavin, but this lower intake appears to be due to the greater consumption of milk by the control children than the children with autism. As compared to the RDA, the riboflavin intake of the children with autism was $116 \pm 9\%$, whereas the control children's intake was $147 \pm 14\%$.[14]

In comparing food intakes of children with autism to the Four Basic Food Groups, this study revealed that children with autism consumed, on the average, 1.9 ± 0.3 servings per day from the milk group as compared to the control children at 3.3 ± 0.4 servings per day. Although there was a statistically significant difference ($P < 0.05$) between the two groups on this item, there was not a statistical difference between the recommended three servings per day for the children's age group and the intake of the children with autism. No other statistically significant differences were reported. These other daily food group intakes were reported for the children with autism: meat, 2.0 ± 0.2 servings; fruits and vegetables, 4.1 ± 0.6 servings, which included foods rich in vitamins C (0.7 ± 0.2) and A (0.3 ± 0.1); and grain products 6.2 ± 0.5 servings. There was also no significant difference between the groups of children in sugar intake. Simple sugar intakes were approximately 17% and 19% of total calories for the autistic and control children, respectively. It was noted that sugar-based foods are often used as teaching prompters for children with autism, and therefore the sugar consumption of these children may be underestimated.[14]

Therefore, despite unusual food behaviors reported in this study, intakes of children with autism were overall not statistically different from those of the control children. This may be the result of greater attention paid to the diets of the children with autism and an increased awareness of their parents of the importance of nutrition to the health of their children. Because these results were interpreted from the dietary means of the groups, individual children with extreme food idiosyncracies and behaviors should continue to be monitored closely for dietary adequacy.[14,15] During adolescence, obesity may become a problem due to medications, such as phenothiazine, or the use of food reinforcers for behavior.[12] Anorexia nervosa may be a problem with some children with autism, particularly with hysterical, obsessional, or schizoid characteristics.[19] Food allergies may go unnoticed due to subnormal communication skills of autistic individuals.[1]

Dietary Management and Other Treatments

Megavitamin therapy

Various vitamin and dietary treatments have been investigated as possible management programs for children with infantile autism and other developmental disorders.[20] This dietary approach stems from the theory of genetotrophic disease, which holds that, because of genetic predisposition to a disease, the individual requires nutrients in megadoses to prevent or delay symptoms of the disease state.[21] Few well-controlled studies have been completed, and of those completed it is difficult to interpret their results as being beneficial for all children with the diagnosis of autism.[15] Much of the early work was completed on children who exhibited autistic-like characteristics, but who may not have met the diagnostic criteria for autism. A study by Harrell et al.,[21] which is widely cited in the literature concerning autism and vitamin supplementation, investigated the influence of daily doses of supplementary vitamins and minerals on 16 children diagnosed with mental retardation. None of these children appeared to have a diagnosis of autism. Results of this study were extremely varied, and areas of improvement, if present, differed widely among the children. Two later studies,[17,22] inspired by the work of Harrell et al.[21] provided vitamin and mineral supplements to young adults who had been diagnosed with mental retardation. Neither of these studies found any significant effects on intelligence testing after supplementation for a minimum of 5 months. The studies, although completed using older subjects, did not provide support for the earlier work. Generally, vitamin therapy is discouraged for children with autism. Care should be taken so that this type of therapy is not instituted in the place of more effective treatment approaches and at the expense of the child's education.[1]

One study that does support the earlier theory of genetotrophic disease was completed using a 2-week, cross-over, double-blind trial. Rather than supplementing diets with multivitamins and minerals for subjects who may or may not have been autistic, this study treated 44 children who were diagnosed with autistic symptoms with megadoses of vitamin B_6 and magnesium. Although this study did not

evaluate differences in intelligence before and after treatment, it did find improvement in the behavior of the children during the treatment phase and a worsening after discontinuing the supplements in 34% of the participants.[23] Magnesium is added to the vitamin therapy to prevent side effects of megavitamin doses of vitamin B_6, such as irritability, sound sensitivity, and enuresis; however, the regimen has not been fully investigated.[24]

Folate supplementation has been used in boys with autism and fragile X syndrome with variable results.[25] Calcium, when administered to children with low serum levels, has increased the antagonistic ability of the calcium channels, which may be associated with improvement in some autistic symptoms.[12]

The Feingold diet, or a no additive type diet, has been found to be ineffective for hyperactivity, except in a few young children; however, it has begun to be used for children with autism.[24] Although no extensive studies have been carried out to determine the effectiveness of the Feingold diet for children with autism, testimonials support its use and reflect the enthusiasm of the parents who enrolled children in programs utilizing the diet. Unproven treatment methods, such as the use of magnesium, vitamin B_6, folate, calcium, or the Feingold diet, are not recommended at this time (see Chapter 20).

Behavioral management

Several approaches to behavioral management of children and young adults diagnosed with autism have been proposed in recent years. These management concepts have implications for the development of feeding skills in the individual with autism. Behavior modification is based on the principles of reinforcement and punishment. Reinforcement is the procedure by which the frequency of a behavior increases because it is followed by a reinforcing consequence, either the presentation of a positive stimulus (which is called positive reinforcement) or the removal of a negative stimulus (referred to as negative reinforcement). There are several types of reinforcers, including tangible and activity reinforcers (e.g., food, toys, or access to a favorite activity, such as blowing bubbles or frolic play), social reinforcers (attention, praise, smiles, hugs), and for higher-functioning children, tokens or points (which can be exchanged for back-up reinforcers). Also, the removal of a negative stimulus can be reinforcing (e.g., doing one's work is reinforced by the cessation of adult scolding). In contrast to reinforcement, punishment occurs when a consequence decreases the behavior. The consequence can be the delivery of a negative stimulus or the withdrawal of a positive stimulus contingent on the target behavior.

Several behavioral techniques can be used to decrease undesired behaviors. These include time-out from reinforcement (i.e., the removal of all reinforcing stimuli in response to the inappropriate behavior), response cost (a reinforcer is lost or a penalty is imposed contingent on misbehavior), satiation (providing an excessive amount of something that is reinforcing so that it loses its reinforcing value), overcorrection (the consequences of the misbehavior are corrected to an exaggerated degree with the individual making restitution or extensively rehearsing the appropriate behavior), and aversive conditioning (using an aversive stimulus contingent on misbehavior). Aversive conditioning can range from a reprimand to a noxious stimulus, such as water mist to decrease self-injurious behavior. Effective behavior modification programs often integrate both reinforcing and punishing consequences.

One longitudinal study[26] attempted to provide constant behavioral management treatment during all waking hours to children with autism. Trained student therapists and the children's parents were involved in the treatment program. Its basic concept was positive reinforcement theory, with treatment focusing on the child's ability to discriminate an appropriate response to a stimulus from several possible responses. Ignoring undesirable behavior, employing time-out, and shaping alternative behaviors were used to discourage inappropriate actions. The behavioral intervention approach provides the caregiver with a well-designed program of consistent actions to take and responses to employ when presented with an action by the child. This approach to developing the child's functional abilities can be readily adapted for feeding activities. Since many parents spend a great deal of time attempting to feed these children, a program of consistent stimuli and reinforcement can be useful in shaping the child's eating behaviors and developing feeding skills.

Another management approach that also has implications in feeding is based on the concept of maternal bonding. Welch[27] proposes a program of holding therapy primarily involving the mother and child. The author theorizes that intense physical contact might break through the barrier between the caregiver and child that is manifested as apparent disinterest and rejection of physical contact by the child. Once a bond of trust is established, it can carry over into other aspects of the relationship, including feeding.

Feeding and dietary approaches

A third approach[28] employed with autistic adults also has implications for use with children in developing feeding skills. Life-skill tasks are analyzed for their component steps and then matched with prompting sequences. Once the adult or child completes a step of the sequence, a cue is given for the next step. Upon completion of the task sequence, the selected goal would be accomplished. This clearly has implications for the development of food preparation skills for adults or self-feeding skills for children. It should be noted that, although self-help skills, such as self-feeding, in a child may not be a true indication of mental development, it is critical in improving future adaptability of young children with autism.[29]

The desire for little food or fluid must be monitored closely to avoid deficiencies and dehydration, particularly if schizoid tendencies are present. An outpatient treatment center, as well as a residential treatment program, may be clinically effective and economical in some instances.[30]

Follow-up and Experimental Considerations

The future research into nutrition for children with autism should focus on three major areas. First, more must be learned through research about the nutritional needs of these children: actual energy and nutrient intakes, types and fre-

quency of foods consumed, feeding behaviors, energy expenditures, and parental response to the children's eating patterns and behaviors. A nutritious diet with iron-rich foods and complex carbohydrates, that is perhaps low in gas formers should be the goal. If the child if obese, low-calorie foods should be given with personalized plans for adequate physical activity (see Chapter 19). Hospitalization may be required if the child with autism shows severe food aversion or signs of undernutrition or anorexia nervosa (see Chapter 23). Parents of children with autism appear to be eager recipients of nutrition education information. Second, a greater understanding of the possible role of neurotransmitters and dietary influences on the symptoms, not cause, of autism must be investigated (see Chapter 11). Third, development and use of appropriate behaviral techniques in the acquisition and maintenance of appropriate oral intake and feeding skills for children with autism (and related skills for adults with autism) must become available to caregivers of these individuals. A multidisciplinary team may help provide this intervention and prevent parental stress.[31]

References

1. Volkmar, F.R., Cohen, D.J. Current concepts: infantile autism and the pervasive developmental disorders. *J. Dev. Behav. Pediatr.* 1986; 7:324.
2. American Psychiatric Association, *Diagnostic and Statistical Manual of Mental Disorders*, 3rd ed. rev. Washington, DC: APA; 1987.
3. Courchesne, E., Yeung-Courchesne, R., Press, G.A., Hesselink, J.R., Jernejan, T.L. Hypoplasia of cerebellar vermal lobules VI and VII in autism. *N. Engl. J. Med.* 1988; 318:1349.
4. Adrien, J.L., Barthelemy, C., Lelord, G., Muh, J.P. Use of bioclinical markers for the assessment and treatment of children with pervasive developmental disorders. *Neuropsychobiology.* 1989; 22:117.
5. Volkmar, F.R., Cohen, D.J. Neurobiologic aspects of autism. *N. Engl. J. Med.* 1988; 318:1390.
6. Gillberg, C., Ehlers, S., Schaumann, H., Jakobsson, G., Dahlgren, S.O., Lindblom, R., Bagenholm, A., Tjuus, T., Blidner, E. Autism under age 3 years: a clinical study of 28 cases referred for autistic symptoms in infancy. *J. Child. Psychol. Psychiatr.* 1990; 31:921.
7. Schain, R.J., Freedman, D.X. Studies on 5-hydroxyindole metabolism in autistic and other mentally retarded children. *J. Pediatr.* 1961; 58:315.
8. Chamberlain, R.S., Herman, B. A novel biochemical model linking dysfunctions in brain melatonin, propiomelanocortin peptides, and serotonin in autism. *Biol. Psychiatr.* 1990; 28:773.
9. Ritvo, E.R., Freeman, B.J., Geller, E., Yuwiler, A. Effects of fenfluramine on 14 outpatients with the syndrome of autism. *J. Am. Acad. Child Psychiatr.* 1983; 22:549.
10. Campbell, M., Small, A.M., Palij, M., Perry, R., Polonsky, B.B., Lukashok, D., Anderson, L.T. The efficacy and safety of fenfluramine in autistic children: preliminary analysis of a double-blind study. *Psychopharmacol. Bull.* 1987; 23:123.
11. Hashimoto, T., Aihara, R., Tayama, M., Miyazaki, M., Shirakawa, Y., Kuroda, Y. Reduced thyroid-response to thyrotropin-releasing hormone in autistic boys. *Dev. Med Child. Neuro.* 1991; 33:313.
12. Launay, J.M., Ferrari, P., Haimart, M., Bursztejn, C., Tabuteau, F., Braconnier, A., Pasques-Bondoux, D., Luong, C., Dreux, C. Serotonin metabolism and other biochemical parameters in infantile autism. *Neuropsychobiology.* 1988; 20:1.
13. Maddocks, J., Reed, T. Urine test for adenylosuccinase deficiency in autistic children. *Lancet.* 1989; 1:158.
14. Shearer, T.R., Larson, K., Neuschwander, J., Gedney, B. Minerals in the hair and nutrient intake of autistic children. *J. Autism Dev. Disord.* 1982; 12:25.
15. Raiten, D., Massaro, T. Perspectives on the nutritional ecology of autistic children. *J. Autism Dev. Disord.* 1986; 16:133.

16. Rice, B.L. Nutritional problems of developmentally disabled children. *Pediatr. Nurs.* 1981; September/October:15.
17. Ellman, G., Silverstein, C., Zingarelli, G., Schafer, E., Silverstein, L. Vitamin-mineral supplement fails to improve IQ of mentally retarded young adults. *Am. J. Ment. Defic.* 1984; 88:688.
18. Raiten, D.J. Nutrition and developmental disabilities. In: Schopler, E., Mesibov, G.B., eds., *Neurobiological Issues In Autism.* New York: Plenum; 1985.
19. Daldorf, J.S. Medical needs of the autistic adolescent. In: Schopler, E., Mesibov, G.B., eds., *Autism in Adolescents and Adults.* New York: Plenum; 1983.
20. Zeisel, S.H. Dietary influences on neurotransmission. *Adv. Pediatr.* 1986; 33:23.
21. Harrell, R.F., Capp, R.H., Davis, D., Peerless, J., Ravitz, L. Can nutritional supplements help mentally retarded children? An exploratory study. *Proc. Natl. Acad. Sci. USA.* 1981; 78:574.
22. Coburn, S., Schaltenbrand, W., Mahren, J.D., Clausman, R., Townsend, D. Effect of megavitamin treatment on mental performance and plasma vitamin B_6 concentrations in mentally retarded young adults. *Am. J. Clin. Nutr.* 1983; 38:352.
23. Lelord, G., Muh, J.P., Barthelemy, C., Martineau, J., Garreau, B. Effects of pyridoxine and magnesium on autistic symptoms—initial observations. *J. Autism Dev. Disord.* 1981; 11:219.
24. Martineau, J., Barthelemy, C., Cheliakine, C., Lelord, G. Brief report: an open middle-term study of combined vitamin B_6-magnesium in a subgroup of autistic children selected on their sensitivity to this treatment. *J. Autism Dev. Disord.* 1988; 18:435.
25. Dawson, G., ed. *Autism: Nature, Diagnosis and Treatment.* New York: Guilford; 1989.
26. Lovaas, O.I. Behavioral treatment and normal educational and intellectual functioning in young autistic children. *J. Consult. Clin. Psychol.* 1987; 55:3.
27. Welch, M.G. Toward prevention of developmental disorders. *Penn. Med.* 1987; 90:47.
28. Smith, M.D., Belcher, R. Teaching life skills to adults disabled by autism. *J. Autism Dev. Disord.* 1985; 15:163.
29. Kurita, H. Variables relating to the mental development of children with infantile autism. *Jpn. J. Psychiatr. Neurol.* 1986; 40:161.
30. Sherman, J., Barker, P., Lorimer, P., Swinson, R., Factor, D.C. Treatment of autistic children: relative effectiveness of residential, out-patient and home-based interventions. *Child Psychiatr. Hum. Dev.* 1988; 19:109.
31. Milgram, N.A., Atzil, M. Parenting stress in raising autistic children. *J. Autism Dev. Disord.* 1988; 18:415.

Chapter 14
The Fetal Alcohol Syndrome

Agnes Huber and Shirley Walberg Ekvall

Reference to the deleterious effects of alcohol on the developing human fetus have been made throughout history[1]; however, only in recent years have these effects been documented systematically. The observations of Lemoine[2] in France in 1968 and of Ulleland in Seattle in 1970[3] and 1972[4] gave the impetus to the recent interest in the effects of alcohol on fetal development. The growth retardation, malformations, and central nervous system (CNS) effects in infants related to alcohol exposure in utero were subsequently termed the "fetal alcohol syndrome" (FAS) by Jones et al. 1973.[5] Children who do not show the full spectrum of the fetal alcohol syndrome but have some abnormalities related to maternal alcohol consumption are considered to suffer from fetal alcohol effects (FAE).

Incidence

Estimates of the incidence of FAS vary from study to study. One publication cites a frequency of 1.1 affected children per 1000 live births.[6] In a national survey in which 46 states were contacted, only 4 stated an incidence ranging from 0.9 to 1.4 FAS cases per 1000 live births.[7] However, there is still some doubt about the reliability of these figures since underreporting does occur. In a review published in 1987 on the worldwide incidence of FAS, Abel and Sokol[8] give a figure of 1.9 per 1000 live births for the United States. This is a higher incidence than for cerebral palsy and Down's syndrome, making FAS the most common known cause of mental retardation. Among alcoholic pregnant women, the incidence of FAS has been estimated as 24 to 42 cases per 1000 live births, with the highest figures for alcohol-abusing women of the southwestern Apache and Ute tribes. Much higher incidence figures for FAS among alcohol-abusing women have been published in Ireland (209 per 1000) and Germany (259 per 1000),[8] suggesting that incidence figures may be influenced by diagnosis, reporting, and other factors. The partial expression of alcohol-related effects (FAE) is considered more common than FAS and can be expected in three to five cases for every 1000 live births.[9]

Features of FAS

FAS is characterized by the following triad of abnormalities[10]:

1. prenatal and/or postnatal growth retardation with weight, length, and/or head circumference below the 10 percentile
2. CNS involvement with neurological abnormality, developmental delay, or intellectual impairment
3. facial dysmorphology (birth defects) with at least two of the following signs:

a. microcephaly
b. microphthalmia and/or short palpebral fissures
c. poorly developed philtrum, thin upper lip, and/or flattening of the maxillary area

The principal and associated features of FAS are summarized in Tables 14-1 and 14-2 based on data from Clarren and Smith.[11] In Figure 14-1 the characteristic dysmorphic facial features are shown. Microcephaly, and abnormal length and weight are recognized at birth, as are the facial dysmorphies.

The dose-effect of ethanol on birth weight depends to some degree on the amount and timing of alcohol intake by the mother during pregnancy.[12] Birth weight seems least affected when mothers decrease their alcohol intake early during pregnancy.[13] However, a report by Little and coworkers[14] researching pregnancy outcomes of alcoholic mothers who abstained from alcohol throughout pregnancy indicates that birth weight for these infants is still decreased.

The teratological effect of alcohol abuse by pregnant women is thought to be most damaging during the first 8 weeks of gestation when organogenesis takes place. This is the period when many women are not aware of their pregnancy, and even a single binge drinking episode is capable of causing damage. Damage to the embryo and fetus during a critical period of development is not reversible.

Biochemical Abnormalities

Alcohol is water soluble and is taken up by the embryo and the fetus. Since the fetus has a higher water content than

Table 14-1. Principal Features of the Fetal Alcohol Syndrome

Mild to moderate mental retardation*
Microcephaly*
Poor coordination, hypotonia†
Irritability in infancy*
Hyperactivity in childhood†
Less than 2 SD for length and weight at birth*
Less than 2 SD for length and weight postnatally*
Disproportionately diminished adipose tissue†
Eyes—short palpebral fissures*
Short upturned nose†
Hypoplastic philtrum*
Hypoplastic maxilla†
Mouth—thin upper vermillion, retrognathia*
Micrognathia or relative prognathia in adolescence*

* In more than 80% of patients.
† In more than 50% of patients.
From Clarren & Smith[11] with permission.

Table 14-2. Associated Features of the Fetal Alcohol Syndrome

Area	Frequent*	Occasional†
Eyes	Ptosis, strabismus, epicanthal folds	Myopia, clinical microphthalmia, blepharophimosis
Ears	Posterior rotation	Poorly formed concha
Mouth	Prominent lateral palatine ridges	Cleft lip or cleft palate, small teeth with faulty enamel
Cardiac	Murmurs	Ventricular septal defect, great-vessel anomalies, tetralogy of Fallot
Renogenital	Labial hypoplasia	Hypospadias, small rotated kidneys, hydronephrosis
Cutaneous	Hemangiomas	Hirsutism in infancy
Skeletal	Aberrant palmar creases, pectus excavatum	Limited joint movements, nail hypoplasia, polydactyly, radioulnar synostosis, pectus carinatum, bifid xiphoid, Klippel-Feil anomaly, scoliosis
Muscular		Hernias of diaphragm, umbilicus, or groin distal recti

*Reported in 26% to 50% of patients.
†Reported in 1% to 25% of patients.
From Clarren & Smith[11] with permission.

the mother, alcohol concentrations are usually higher in the fetus than in the mother. Furthermore, the activity of liver alcohol dehydrogenase, the major alcohol-metabolizing enzyme, develops slowly and by birth is still lower in the fetus than in the mother. This results in longer exposure of the fetus to higher concentrations of alcohol and its effects.[15] The high and extended alcohol exposure can cause a wide array of effects. Alcohol can have a direct cytotoxic effect, may interfere with hormones or specific metabolic pathways, or act via drug-nutrient interaction.[16,17]

Alcohol effects on smooth muscle cells can produce especially damaging consequences in the fetus. It has been known for some time that ethanol in the fetus results in hypoxia, acidosis, and hypoglycemia. Studies have demonstrated that intravenous ethanol given to pregnant animals causes a transient collapse of the fetal vasculature and interruption of oxygen and nutrient supply.[18] Similarly, in vitro studies have shown that human umbilical blood vessels contract at a comparatively low ethanol exposure (equivalent to the intake of 1½ drinks by the pregnant women).[19]

The implications of these studies are that the fetus exposed to ethanol may experience intermittent collapse of the vasculature and thus reduced transfer of essential nutrients. The placenta also may oxidize ethanol and produce acetaldehyde, which may be harmful to the fetus and placenta as well.[20] The hypoglycemia may be aggravated further by decreased liver glycogen storage during fetal life, which has been demonstrated to result in hypoglycemia in the neonatal period.[21]

The mechanism of alcohol teratogenicity is at present not explained, although many studies, most of which involve animal models, have been published. Among cellular effects, the depression of ATP-activated sodium transport systems, abnormal mitochondrial action, and interference with protein synthesis have been proposed.[22] However, whether the congenital abnormalities relate to these actions is not known. In addition to reduced cellular multiplication,[23] which is caused by the direct toxicity of alcohol, actions, such as hormonal changes,[24] an autoimmune response,[25] and potential teratogenic effects of prostaglandins,[26] have been implied.

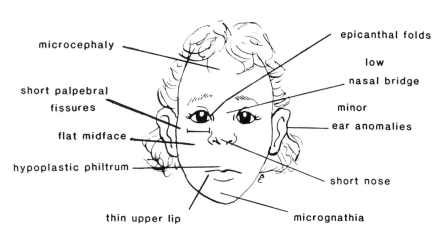

Fig. 14–1. Characteristic dysmorphic facial features of fetal alcohol syndrome.

Maternal alcohol consumption and undernutrition in rats altered proportions of the individual ganglioside fractions, decreased the production of ganglioside-catabolizing enzymes in the brain and spinal cord, and reduced the content of DNA and protein in the CNS of in utero pups. Maternal calorie and fluid intake of the rats did not decrease due to the alcohol consumption.[27]

Of special interest are the drug-nutrient interactions with alcohol, among which zinc has received the most attention. In a study by Lillien et al.,[28] 48% of a large population of pregnant women had suboptimal zinc intakes, and low plasma zinc levels have been reported in alcoholic pregnant women by Flynn and co-workers.[29] Zinc deficiency in animals[30,31] and in women[32] has been associated with a variety of congenital malformations. In a controlled animal study, Keppen et al.[33] showed that zinc deficiency acted as a co-teratogen with alcohol. When both were present at the same time, malformations and growth depression were much more pronounced than those caused by alcohol or zinc deficiency alone. Low zinc states in alcoholic mothers are not only due to low dietary zinc intakes, but also to decreased retention of zinc because of liver damage, which results in excessive urinary zinc loss. FAS children exposed to intrauterine alcohol similarly have decreased plasma zinc and elevated urinary zinc excretion, probably due to liver damage caused by the alcohol exposure.[34] Other nutrient interactions with alcohol can have contributive effects, but these are less well studied during pregnancy.

Factors to be Considered in Nutritional and Other Evaluation

In contrast to Down's syndrome, in which laboratory tests provide a definitive diagnosis, FAS is diagnosed by clinical symptoms.[35] Checklists have been developed to facilitate diagnosis of FAS in early childhood. Knowledge of the mother's drinking history during pregnancy is an important part of the diagnosis since some of the features characteristic of FAS apply to other diagnoses. Some researchers suggest that with a standardized method of morphometric analysis, FAS can be identified with high accuracy.[36] The phenotype of FAS in adolescents and older adults is more difficult to recognize.[35]

Fetal alcohol effects (FAE) can include one or several of the abnormalities seen in FAS. Some children function in the normal range, and others appear to be normal until they enter school. Learning disabilities related to speech or low attention span may become evident in a more formal learning situation. Some children may exhibit maladaptive behaviors. Because of the variety of abnormalities, it is difficult to diagnose the defects related to alcohol even when the mother's drinking history is known.

It also has been difficult to establish a dose-effect relationship between alcohol intake during pregnancy and the severity of alcohol-induced manifestations because the timing of drinking, the amount of alcohol ingested, nutritional status, and individual differences in sensitivity of the mother and fetus all affect the type and severity of abnormality (see Nutritional Assessment, Chapter 4). Vohees[37] described four types of teratogenic outcomes of alcohol: a dose-response for functional abnormalities, growth deficiency, malfor-

mations, and embryolethal effects. This means that a lower dose is required to produce growth abnormalities than malformations, and an even lower dose would produce abnormal functional outcomes. Therefore, although FAS is related to heavy drinking throughout pregnancy, the amount and timing of social or binge drinking by the pregnant women may determine the severity of effects in the offspring.

Dietary and Other Management

According to Streissguth and LaDue,[35] the developmental work-up should include a thorough physical examination, a family history in view of support services, a psychological/educational evaluation, and, at an appropriate age, a vocational training and developmental disabilities evaluation.

The prenatal growth retardation of FAS infants persists postnatally, and many FAS infants exhibit failure to thrive (see Chapter 21). They often have a poor suck, and thus are a challenge to feed. They are hypotonic and many exhibit irregular wake-sleep patterns. The characteristic craniofacial features identified in the FAS infant at birth persist throughout life. Organ and skeletal abnormalities may be identified at birth or when the child is older.

Early diagnosis of FAS and definition of the child's problems are beneficial in preventing secondary problems. It is also important to set realistic goals and expectations for the child and parents or caregivers. Mastropieri et al.[38] describe the assessment process as follows:

1. Age-appropriate testing of the child should be done to assess the child's developmental level and to identify the specific problem the child may have. The outcome of this assessment will be the basis for planning by parents, teachers, physician, etc.
2. Services helpful to the child and parents should be identified. This can help to diffuse crisis situations, soften and deal with guilt feelings, and identify peer groups for parents, the child, and siblings.
3. Realistic growth expectations that are consistent with the growth progress one can expect from FAS children should be established. Meal plans should be consistent with these patterns and with acceptable dietary practices. Early intervention often can prevent the development of behavior problems around meals.
4. Active follow-up should be provided to monitor progress and re-evaluate the child, preferably by a team of providers. Family issues, such as guilt, drinking relapse, marital stress, and child abuse, must be addressed.
5. There should be intellectual testing and the development of an educational plan for educating the child. The parents/caregivers' understanding and support of this plan is important.
6. Parents should be supported as advocates to gain or improve services for their infants.

Growth and development of FAS children should be assessed throughout childhood and the teens. Instruments for developmental assessments from birth to adulthood have been summarized.[38] Because children with FAS or FAE are highly variable in their development, behavioral, nutritional, and other problems must be assessed individually (see Chapter 4). Day et al. found that at three years of age, children who were prenatally exposed to alcohol did not exhibit catch-up growth and had slower rates of growth in weight, length and head circumference as well as minor physical abnormalities.[39] In this way the children's capabilities and potential for growth, development, and functioning can be maximized. In severe cases where oral intake is low, a gastrostomy tube may be needed to improve growth (see Chapters 24 and 34).

Implications for Prevention of FAS/FAE

Evidence is overwhelming that heavy drinking during pregnancy interferes with normal fetal growth and development. However, whether lower intakes of alcohol and/or occasional binge drinking are harmful is still debated.[12,40,41] Although effects of low intakes of alcohol are extremely difficult to separate from nutritional, smoking, and other factors, alcohol at any level poses a risk for the fetus.[42,43] Because alcohol exerts a potentially damaging effect on the fetus, the Surgeon General's *Advisory on Alcohol and Pregnancy* suggests that women should not drink at any time during pregnancy.[44]

Screening methods have been developed to elucidate the drinking habits of pregnant women, so that women whose alcohol intake puts them at risk for offspring with FAS can be referred for treatment.[45,46] A ten-step plan for identifying and treating drinking during pregnancy has been outlined by Dwyer.[47] This plan includes a systematic assessment of alcohol intake from beer, wine, and liquor, education of the mother about the alcohol effects on the fetus, suggestions for strategies to stop drinking, and planning for optimum pregnancy and aftercare. FAS and FAE are increasingly being recognized by local, state, and federal agencies as public health problems that can be prevented. According to the latest incidence figures, FAS is the leading identifiable cause of mental retardation. Eleven percent of the 11.7 billion dollars spent per year for residential facilities goes toward the care of people with FAS,[8] yet preventive efforts are sporadic and slow.

A 1986 survey[7] of state-sponsored programs to prevent FAS found that 50 states are conducting public awareness programs, 7% had sponsored public awareness campaigns in the past, 19% have initiated some type of professional education activity, and 17% have initiated awareness campaigns aimed at both professionals and the general public. In some states, FAS prevention efforts are included among other public health activities. The monies spent by the involved states ranged from $2,000 to $200,000 per year. States with a strong commitment to the prevention of FAS have established interagency task forces with the purpose of developing state prevention plans. Such plans have three objectives:

1. to establish the incidence of FAS and FAE cases by better diagnosis
2. to provide professional training in screening of and intervention with women at risk
3. to provide public education with attention toward reaching specific target populations.

FAS has been recognized as a national problem at the federal level, and the week of January 15–21, 1984 was proclaimed National Fetal Alcohol Syndrome week. Senate bill 2047, which requires a health warning on the labels of all alcoholic beverages of the detrimental effects of alcoholism in general and during pregnancy in particular, was passed in February 1988. A position paper on nutrition intervention in treatment and recovery from chemical dependency was published by the American Dietetic Association in 1990.[48]

Follow-up and Resources

Case histories and follow-up of FAS children can be found in publications by Barnett and Shusterman,[49] Lindor et al.[50] and Streissguth et al.[51] An in-depth nutritional assessment (see Chapter 4) and family history are required at each visit. An extensive bibliography with references up to September 1986 and an *FAS Resource Manual* can be obtained from the Shriver Center Fetal Alcohol Program, The Eunice Kennedy Shriver Center for Mental Retardation, 200 Trapelo Road, Waltham, MA 02254. Other resources are "Pregnancy and Health Program," University of Washington, School of Medicine, GI-80, Seattle, WA 98105; The National Clearinghouse for Alcohol Information, P.O. Box 2345, Rockville, MD 20852; and "Healthy Mothers, Healthy Babies," 600 Maryland Avenue, S.W., Suite 300, Washington, DC 20024.

References

1. Warner, R.H., Rosett, H.L. The effects of drinking on offspring: an historical survey of the American and British literature. *J. Stud. Alcohol.* 1975; 36:1395.
2. Lemoine, P., Harrousseau, H., Borteyru, J.P., Menuet, J. Les enfant de parents alcooliques. *Quest. Med.* 1968; 25:476.
3. Ulleland, C., Wenneberg, R.P., Igo, R.P., Smith, N.J. The offspring of alcoholic mothers. *Pediatr. Res.* 1970; 4:474.
4. Ulleland, C.N. The offspring of alcoholic mothers. *Ann. NY. Acad. Sci.* 1972; 197:167.
5. Jones, K.L., Smith, D.W., Ulleland, C.N., Streissguth, A.P. Pattern of malformations in offspring of chronic alcoholic mothers. *Lancet.* 1973; 1:1267.
6. Abel, E.L. *Fetal Alcohol Syndrome and Fetal Alcohol Effects.* New York: Plenum; 1984.
7. Baumeister, A.A., Hamlett, C.L. A national survey of state sponsored programs to prevent fetal alcohol syndrome. *Ment. Retard.* 1986; 24:169.
8. Abel, E.L., Sokol, R.J. Incidence of FAS and economic impact of FAS-related anomalies. *Drug Alcohol Depend.* 1987; 19:51.
9. Smith, D.W., Jones, K.L., Hansen, J.W. Perspectives on the cause and frequency of the fetal alcohol syndrome. *Ann. NY. Acad. Sci.* 1976; 273:138.
10. Ouellette, E.M. The fetal alcohol syndrome. *J. Dent. Child.* 1984; 51:222.
11. Clarren, S.K., Smith, D.W. The fetal alcohol syndrome. *N. Engl. J. Med.* 1978; 298:1063.
12. Mills, J.L., Graubard, B.I., Harley, E.E., Rhoads, G.G., Berendes, H.W. Maternal alcohol consumption and birth weight: how much drinking during pregnancy is safe? *JAMA.* 1984; 252:1875.
13. Rosett, H.L., Weiner, L., Edelin, K.C. Strategies for prevention of fetal alcohol effects. *Obstet. Gynecol.* 1981; 57:1.
14. Little, R.E., Streissguth, A.P., Barr, H.M., Herman, C.S. Decreased birth weight in infants of alcoholic women who abstained during pregnancy. *J. Pediatr.* 1980; 96:974.
15. Pikkarainen, P.H., Räiha, N.C.R. Development of alcohol dehydrogenase activity in the human liver. *Pediatr. Res.* 1967; 1:165.
16. Lieber, C.S. *Metabolic Aspects of Alcoholism.* Baltimore: University Park Press; 1977.
17. Roe, A.D. *Alcohol and the Diet.* Westport, CT: AVI Publishing; 1979.
18. Mukherjee, S.P., Hodgen, J.P.J. Maternal ethanol exposure induces transient impairment of umbilical circulation and fetal hypoxia in monkeys. *Science.* 1982; 218:700.

19. Altura, B.M., Altura, B.T., Carella, A., Chatterjee, M., Halevy, S., Tejani, N. Alcohol produces spasms of human umbilical blood vessels: relationship to fetal alcohol syndrome. *Eur. J. Pharmacol.* 1982; 86:311.

20. Fisher, S.E. Selective fetal malnutrition: the fetal alcohol syndrome. *J. Am. Coll. Nutr.* 1988; 7:101.

21. Witek-Januseke, L. Maternal ethanol ingestion: effect on maternal and neonatal glucose balance. *Am. J. Physiol.* 1986; 251:E178.

22. Abel, E.L. Prenatal effects of alcohol on growth: a brief overview. *Fed. Proc.* 1985; 44:2318.

23. Brown, N.A., Goulding, E.H., Fabro, S. Ethanol embryotoxicity: direct effects on mammalian embryos in vitro. *Science.* 1979; 206:573.

24. Root, A.W., Reiter, E.O., Andriola, M., Duckett, G. Hypothalamic-pituitary function in the fetal alcohol syndrome. *J. Pediatr.* 1975; 87:585.

25. Foster, J.W. Possible maternal autoimmune component in the etiology of the fetal alcohol syndrome. *Dev. Med. Child. Neurol.* 1986; 5:654.

26. Randall, C.L., Anton, R.F., Becker, H.C. Alcohol, pregnancy, and prostaglandins. *Alcoholism.* 1987; 11:32.

27. Prasad, V.V. Maternal alcohol consumption and undernutrition in the rat: effects on gangliosides and their catabolizing enzymes in the CNS of the newborn. *Neurochem. Res.* 1989; 14:1081.

28. Lillien, L.J., Huber, A.M., Rajala, M.M. Diet and ethanol intake during pregnancy. *J. Am. Diet. Assoc.* 1982; 81:252.

29. Flynn, A., Martier, S.S., Sokol, R.J., Miller, S.I., Golden, N.L., Del Villano, B.C. Zinc status of pregnant alcoholic women: a determinant of fetal outcome. *Lancet.* 1981; 1:572.

30. Hurley, L.S. *Developmental Nutrition.* Englewood Cliffs, NJ: Prentice-Hall; 1979.

31. Keppen, L., Moore, D., Cannon, D. Zinc nutrition in fetal alcohol syndrome. *Neurotoxicology.* 1990; 11:375.

32. Hambidge, K.M., Nelder, K.H., Walravens, P.A. Zinc, acrodermatitis enteropathica and congenital malformations. *Lancet.* 1975; 1:577.

33. Keppen, L.D., Pysher, T., Rennert, O.M. Zinc deficiency acts as co-teratogen with alcohol in fetal alcohol syndrome. *Pediatr. Res.* 1985; 19:944.

34. Assadi, F.K., Ziai, M. Zinc status of infants with fetal alcohol syndrome. *Pediatr. Res.* 1986; 20:551.

35. Streissguth, A.P., LaDue, R.A. Fetal alcohol, teratogenic causes of developmental disabilities. In: Begab, M.E. *Toxic Substances and Mental Retardation.* 1987. Washington, D.C.: AAMD Monograph Series.

36. Clarren, S.K., Sampson, P.D., Larsen, J., Donnell, D.J., Bar, H.M., Brookstein, F.L., Martin, D.C., Streissguth, A.P. Effects of fetal alcohol exposure assessment by photographs and morphometric analysis. *Am. J. Med. Genet.* 1987; 26:651.

37. Vohees, C.V. Principles of behavioral teratology. In: Riley, E.P., Vorhees, C.V., eds. *Handbook of Behavioral Teratology.* New York: Plenum; 1986.

38. Mastropieri, L., Boisvert, C.M., Smeallie, M.L. *Fetal Alcohol Resource Manual.* Waltham, MA: Shriver Program; 1986.

39. Day, N.L., Robles, N., Richardson, G., Geva, D., Taylor, P., Scher, M., Stoffer, D., Cornelius, M., Goldschmidt, L. The effects of prenatal alcohol use on the growth of children at three years of age. *Alcohol Clin. Exp. Res.* 1991; 15:67.

40. Alcohol and the fetus-is zero the only option. *Lancet.* 1983; 1:682.

41. Rosett, H.L., Weiner, L. Maternal alcohol consumption and birth weight. *JAMA.* 1985; 253:3550.

42. Forbes, R.E. Alcohol-related birth defects. *Pub. Health.* 1984; 98:238.

43. Lillien, L.J. *Diet, Ethanol Intake and Pregnancy Outcome.* Cambridge, MA: Harvard School of Public Health; 1981. Doctoral thesis.

44. *Surgeon General's Advisory on Alcohol and Pregnancy. FDA Drug Bull.* 1981; 11:9.

45. Russell, M., Bigler, L. Screening for alcohol-related problems in an outpatient obstetric-gynecological clinic. *Am. J. Obstet. Gynecol.* 1979; 134:4.

46. Bodendorfer, T.W., Broggs, G.G., Gunning, J.E. Obtaining drug histories during pregnancy. *Am. J. Obstet. Gynecol.* 1979; 135:490.

47. Dwyer, J. Substance abuse in pregnancy. *Pub. Health Curr.* 1986; 26:1.

48. American Dietetic Association. Nutrition intervention in treatment and recovery from chemical dependency. *J. Am. Diet. Assoc.* 1990; 90:1274.

49. Barnett, R., Shusterman, S. Fetal alcohol syndrome: a review of literature and report of cases. *J. Am. Dent. Assoc.* 1985; 111:591.

50. Lindor, E., McCarthy, A., McRae, M.G. Fetal alcohol syndrome: a review and case presentation. *J. Obstet. Gynecol. Neonatal. Nurs.* 1980; 2:222.

51. Streissguth, A.P., Clarren, S.K., Jones, K.L. Natural history of the fetal alcohol syndrome: a ten-year follow up of eleven patients. *Lancet.* 1985; 2:85.

Chapter 15
Fetal Hydantoin Syndrome

Shirley Walberg Ekvall and Agnes Huber

In the general population approximately 1 in 200 people has a seizure disorder.[1] The discovery in the late 1930s of anticonvulsant drugs led to the successful treatment of the majority of cases. Phenytoin (PHT) has been the drug of choice, although other types, such as phenobarbitone or valproic acid, have been used concomitantly or singly. In adults, minimal side effects from the long-time use of PHT may occur; however, a large number of clinical and epidemiological studies suggest an increased frequency of malformations in children exposed to PHT in utero.[2] For example, a 1981 study found that in one year 1384 children with major congenital malformations were born to 18,960 treated women with epilepsy.[1]

The common features shared by children exposed to PHT in utero form a pattern of associated characteristics described as fetal hydantoin syndrome (FHS), a term that was coined by Hanson and Smith in 1975.[3] FHS is defined as "a complex of birth defects associated with prenatal maternal ingestion of hydantoin derivatives."[4] The full features of FHS, as described by Hanson and Smith are shown in Figures 15-1 and 15-2 and, according to their estimates, may be seen in 1 in 5000 births. However, as many as 33% of hydantoin-exposed infants might have some stigmata related to FHS.[3]

Diagnosis

The diagnosis must be considered in any infant exposed prenatally to anticonvulsants—diphenylhydantoin, mephenytoin, ethotoin. The main features include abnormalities of pre- and postnatal growth, microcephaly, and small size; developmental delays to frank mental deficiency; dysmorphic craniofacial features including cleft lip and/or palate; limb anomalies, such as hypoplasia of nails and distal phalanges; and anomalies of the genitourinary, cardiac, and central nervous system (CNS), including a variety of ocular manifestations.[5-7] Table 15-1 summarizes the patterns of anomalies originally studied by Hanson and Smith[3] in five children who were severely affected by FHS.

Clinical features noted in first-born children affected by phenytoin versus those first-born children unaffected by phenytoin are shown in Table 15-2.[8] Mothers who had one affected child appeared to be at a much higher risk for having subsequent affected children (90%) if phenytoin was continued. The majority of infants born to mothers treated with hydantoin during pregnancy manifest less severe involvement. Up to 40% of the offspring of epileptic treated mothers are reported to have some features of the syndrome, such as orofacial clefts or congenital heart disease, which occur in perhaps 10% of children—a two- to threefold increase in risk compared with the general population.[3] Most

affected children present with milder craniofacial or limb abnormalities. Mild dysmorphic features, such as short nose with broad bridge, ocular hypertelorism, ptosis, or short neck, are subject to substantial variation in observer interpretation in clinical settings.[7] As a consequence, although more recent studies have confirmed the presence of such abnormalities, the diagnosis of fetal hydantoin effects is frequently overlooked.[9] Furthermore, these manifestations may be readily confused with the findings of other birth defect patterns. Included among such conditions are Coffin-Siris, Noonan, Williams, and Aarskog-Scott syndromes; neurofibromatosis; and other teratogenic effects, such as alcohol and maternal phenylketonuria. The craniofacial effects of other anticonvulsant drugs, such as barbiturates, primidone, and valproic acid, may be at least superficially similar.[10] In many cases, exposure to one or more of these agents may have occurred concomitantly. In such instances it is often difficult or impossible to ascribe observed effects to a single agent. In addition, certain genetic conditions may be responsible for abnormalities in the hydantoin-exposed infant.[9]

Some evidence suggests that epilepsy in the mother with and without anticonvulsants may increase the risk of abortions, stillbirths, and toxemia; may complicate delivery; and may place the newborn infant at greater risk for epilepsy.[11] A higher prevalence of malformations in children of treated epileptic fathers as compared to untreated fathers was also observed; this could be due either to a mutagenic effect of antiepileptic drugs or to differences in other uncontrolled risk factors between the two patient groups.[12] An increased malformation rate in children of epileptic fathers may support the hypothesis of a major role for genetic factors.[13] A number of authors have reported affected siblings; however, in some instances the effects among siblings have been dissimilar.[14] Of particular interest is the observation of heteropaternal twins born to an epileptic mother treated with phenytoin during pregnancy, only one of whom displayed features of FHS.[15]

Biochemical Abnormalities

At the present time, the pathogenetic mechanism responsible for the fetal hydantoin effects remains uncertain, although all of the teratogenic or embryopathic observations are found in offspring exposed to chronic anticonvulsant therapy. However, few, if any, of these observations can be the basis for determining the risk of short-term or acute exposure to these agents in pregnancy. A role has been postulated for arene oxide metabolites of phenytoin.[16] However, other metabolic factors may be important as well since animal studies reveal not only differences in susceptibilities

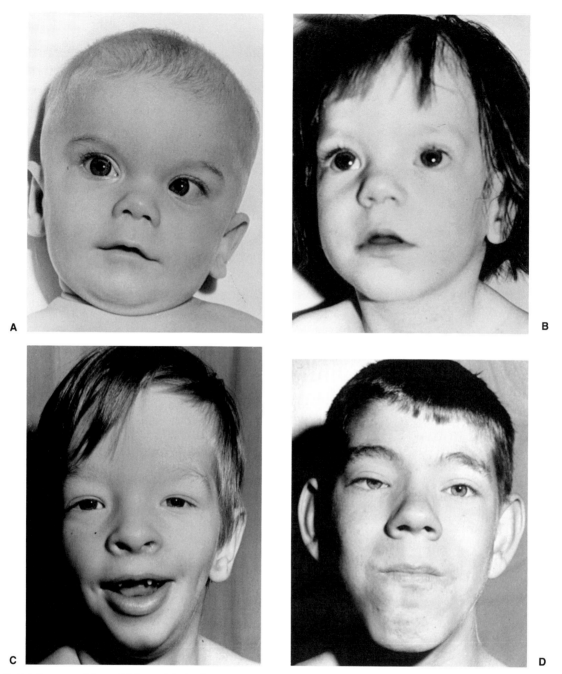

Fig. 15-1. Facial features of four children with the fetal hydantoin syndrome. A, Patient 1 at 5 months, B, Patient 3 at 15 months, C, Patient 4 at 4 years, D, Patient 5 at 5 years. A, courtesy of Weiswasser, W.H., Hall, B.D., Delevan, G.W., Smith, D.W. Coffin-Siris syndrome, *Am. J. Dis. Child.* 1973; 125:383. Used with permission.

among different species but also the existence of substantial strain differences.[17] A wide variety of teratopathogenic laboratory testing systems, as well as animal models, have been identified for further investigation for fetal hydantoin effects.

Factors to be Considered in Nutritional and Other Evaluation

Pregnant women with epilepsy can be divided into two categories: those identified as having epilepsy before their child was conceived and in whom a level of seizure control has been established and those who experience a seizure disorder not related to toxemia for the first time during pregnancy.[19] Fewer than one-quarter of the women in the latter group, to which the term "gestational epilepsy" has been applied, will have seizures only during pregnancy. The occurrence of gestational epilepsy in one pregnancy does not mean that it will recur in subsequent pregnancies.[19]

Antiepilepsy therapy is usually continued throughout pregnancy to ensure adequate seizure control. Most studies suggest that approximately 50% of women with epilepsy will have no change in their seizure activity, 40% will have

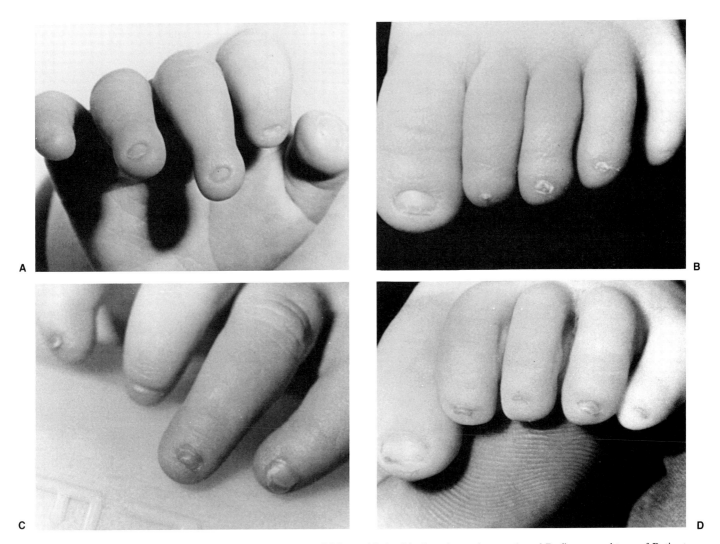

Fig. 15-2. Hypoplasia of distal phalanges and nails in two children with fetal hydantoin syndrome: A and B, fingers and toes of Patient 1; C, fingers of Patient 3; and D, toes of Patient 2. A, courtesy of Weiswasser, W.H., Hall, B.D., Delevan, G.W., Smith, D.W. Coffin-Siris syndrome. *Am. J. Dis. Child.*, 1973; 125:838. Used with permission.

more seizures, and 10% will have fewer seizures.[19] Factors that inhibit seizure control during pregnancy are lower serum concentration of anticonvulsants, maternal age, number of pregnancies, type and duration of epilepsy, prepregnant number of seizures, fluid retention, and stress.[18,19] It is felt that any changes in seizure activity occurring during pregnancy will return to the prepregnant state after delivery.

The woman with epilepsy who is pregnant or is planning to become pregnant should be counseled about the risks of congenital malformations associated with antiepileptic drugs, the risk that the child might develop epilepsy owing to genetic transmission, and the risk of injury to the fetus or infant if the mother should have a seizure.[20] Careful attention to patient compliance with drug regimens is essential. Problems of sleep deprivation ought to be sought and corrected. If seizures occur despite these measures, dosages of the anticonvulsant drugs should be increased, with plasma concentrations used as a guide to therapy.[20]

Nutritional concerns

Excessive weight gain and fluid retention should be prevented because these factors may increase the frequency of seizures during pregnancy.[21] Chronic administration of anticonvulsants may result in low plasma folic acid levels. Folic acid is required for the synthesis of DNA and is essential for the normal development of the human fetus; low folate status in the early weeks of pregnancy has been suspected of causing damage to the fetus. Folic acid deficiency has also been correlated with third trimester bleeding and neonatal hemorrhage.[2] Serum folate concentration decreases progressively during normal pregnancy if no folate supplement is taken. This decrease may be more pronounced in the presence of phenytoin. It is therefore suggested that women receiving this drug should take folate supplements of 400 mcg (the RDA) during and preferably before pregnancy to ensure an adequate supply for the fetus.[2,21] A low dosage of supplemental folate (100–1000 μg folate/day) throughout pregnancy is sufficient to prevent folate deficiency even in epileptic women, despite the folate-antagonizing properties of antiepileptic drugs.

Neonatal hemorrhage

Bleeding at delivery may be increased in the epileptic women because of the vitamin K deficiency produced by phenytoin.

Table 15-1. Pattern of Anomalies in the Fetal Hydantoin Syndrome

Abnormalities	1	2	3	4	5	Total
Growth and performance						
Motor or mental deficiency	+	−	+	+	+	4/5
Microcephaly	+	+	+	±	+	5/5
Prenatal growth deficiency	±	−	±	+	?	3/4
Postnatal growth deficiency	+	+	+	+	+	5/5
Craniofacial						
Short nose with low nasal bridge	+	+	+	+	+	5/5
Hypertelorism	+	+	+	+	+	5/5
Epicanthic folds	−	−	+	+	−	2/5
Ptosis of eyelid	−	−	+	−	+	2/5
Strabismus	+	−	−	−	+	2/5
Low-set and/or abnormal ears	±	+	±	±	+	5/5
Wide mouth	−	+	+	+	−	3/5
Prominent lips	−	−	+	+	+	3/5
Cleft palate	−	−	−	−	+	1/5
Metopic sutural ridging	−	−	+	−	−	1/5
Wide fontanels	+	−	+	?	?	2/3
Limb						
Hypoplasia of nails and distal phalanges	+	+	+	±	+	5/5
Fingerlike thumb	+	+	±	+	−	4/5
Abnormal palmar creases	−	−	+	+	+	3/5
Five or more digital arches	+	+	+	?	−	3/4
Other						
Short or webbed neck ± low hairline	±	+	+	±	+	5/5
Coarse hair	−	−	+	−	+	2/5
Widely spaced, hypoplastic nipples	+	−	+	−	+	3/5
Rib, sternal, or spinal anomalies	+	−	−	−	+	2/5
Hernias	−	−	−	+	−	1/5
Undescended testes	−	−	−	+	−	1/5

(Patient No. columns: 1 2 3 4 5)

+ = Present, ± = mild degree, − = absent, ? = unknown
From Hansen & Smith[3] with permission.

Table 15-2. Clinical Features in Affected and Unaffected Children.

	Affected (n = 24)		Unaffected (n = 115)		Probability (P)
	n	%*	n	%	
Physical abnormalities					
Nail hypoplasia	24	100	0		ND
Growth failure	13	54	0		< 0.001
Hypertelorism	10	42	0		< 0.001
Microcephaly	4	17	1	< 1	< 0.005
Cleft lip/palate	3	13	3	3	NS
Depressed nasal bridge	3	13	1	< 1	< 0.05
Midfacial hypoplasia	3	13	1	1	< 0.05
Ocular ptosis	3	13	0		< 0.005
Strabismus	2	8	2	< 2	NS
Radial/ulnar synostosis	2	8	0		0.05
Broad alveolar ridge	2	8	0		< 0.05
Ridging of metopic suture	1	4	0		NS
Developmental problems					
Developmental delay/mental retardation	10	42	1	< 1	< 0.001
School/learning problems	8	33	8	7	< 0.001
Speech/language problems	2	8	4	3	NS
Behavior problems	2	8	1	< 1	NS

*Some children fall into more than one category, so percentages add up to more than 100.
ND = comparison not done; NS = not significant.
From Van Dyke et al.,[8] with permission.

In newborns exposed to phenytoin in utero, bleeding tendencies may develop during the first day of life that are related to decreased levels of vitamin K-dependent clotting factors. Therefore, an injection of vitamin K should be given routinely to all newborns after delivery.[19] Because of the depression of vitamin K-dependent clotting factors, the following steps should be taken:

- Avoid drugs in the third trimester with adverse effects on hemostatic mechanisms—aspirin, promethazine, thiazides.
- Administer phytonadione to the mother before delivery and to the infant (intravenously) immediately after birth.
- Consider cesarean section if a difficult or traumatic delivery is expected.
- Submit cord blood for immediate clotting studies and fresh-frozen plasma for diminished vitamin K-dependent factors.
- Watch the neonate carefully and provide an exchange transfusion at the first sign of development of a hemorrhage.[19]

Lactation and breastfeeding

The ability to lactate is not impaired by epilepsy or antiepileptic drugs. Breast milk is essentially an ultrafiltrate of plasma, and the concentration of an antiepileptic in breast milk is similar to the concentration of unbound drug in plasma.[22] The risk to the infant from the epileptic drugs is controversial. Therefore, breastfeeding is best avoided in mothers taking antiepileptic drugs because of the risk of sedation, poor feeding and idiosyncratic reactions to drugs, the slow and unpredictable metabolism of antiepileptic drugs by the neonate, and the possibility that antiepileptic drugs may interfere with brain maturation.[22,23]

Treatment

At present the only known treatments of FHS are primary prevention and, later the secondary prevention of life-threatening and/or disfiguring abnormalities. Prevention measures rely on the exclusion of the teratogen from the prenatal environment. Unfortunately, the safety of alternative drugs remains poorly defined. Barbiturates, primidone, and, most recently, valproic acid, have all been implicated as potential teratogenic agents. Well-designed studies or dose-dependent dysfunctions and exposure-period-dependent agents[24] are needed. Combinations of medications may be particularly hazardous; thus, monotherapy is a desirable objective whenever possible. The relative contributions of possible genetic and other factors affecting hydantoin metabolism continue to be unclear at the present time. Women with seizure disorders should be informed of the nature and magnitude of risks to the fetus arising from hydantoin therapy before becoming pregnant. Although accurate prenatal diagnostic tests currently are not available for the abnormalities likely to occur, the epoxy hydrolase activity biomarker may prove useful in fetuses at high risk for FHS.[25] Perhaps with better understanding of the psychiatric manifestations of this syndrome, earlier diagnosis

and establishment of training and/or educational programs can help these patients reach their maximal potential.

References

1. Kalter, H., Warkany, J. Congenital malformations: etiological factors and their role in prevention. *N. Engl. J. Med.*, 1983; 308:424.
2. Janz, D., Dam, M., Richens, A., Bossi, L., Helge, H., Schmidt, D., eds. *Epilepsy, Pregnancy, and the Child.* New York: Raven Press; 1982.
3. Hansen, J.W., Smith D.W. The fetal hydantoin syndrome. *J. Pediatr.*, 1975; 87:285.
4. Glanze, W.D. ed. *Medical and Nursing Dictionary.* St. Louis: C.V. Mosby; 1986.
5. Kogutt, M.S. Fetal hydantoin syndrome. *South. Med. J.* 1984; 77:657.
6. Hampton, G. Ocular manifestations of the fetal hydantoin syndrome. *Clin. Pediatr.* 1981; 20:470.
7. Kelly, T.E. Teratogenicity of anticonvulsant drugs. *Am. J. Med. Genet.* 1984; 19:413.
8. Van Dyke, D.C., Hodge, S.E., Heide, F., Hill, H. Family studies in fetal phenytoin exposure. *J. Pediatr.* 1988; 113:301.
9. VanLang, Q., Tassinari, M.S., Keith, D.A., Holmes, L.B. Effects of in utero exposure to anticonvulsants on craniofacial development and growth. *J. Craniofacial Genet. Dev. Biol.* 1984; 4:115.
10. DiLiberti, J.H., Farndon, P.A., Dennis, N.R., Curry, T.R. The fetal valproate syndrome. *Am. J. Genet.* 1984; 19:473.
11. Nelson, K.B., Ellenberg, J.H. Maternal seizure disorder, outcome of pregnancy, and neurological abnormalities in the children. *Neurology.* 1982; 32:1247.
12. Moriselli, P., Pippinger, C., Penry, J. *Antiepileptic Drug Therapy in Pediatrics.* New York: Raven Press; 1983.
13. Karpathios, T., Zervoudakis, A., Venieris, F., Parchas, S., Youroukos, S. Genetics and fetal hydantoin syndrome. *Acta Paediatr. Scand.* 1989; 78:125.
14. Krauss, C.M., Holmes, L.B., VanLang, Q., Keith, D.A. Four siblings with similar malformations after exposure to phenytoin and primidone. *J. Pediatr.* 1984; 105:750.
15. Phelan, M.C., Pellock, J.M., Nance, W.E. Discordant expression of fetal hydantoin syndrome in heteropaternal dizygotic twins. *N. Engl. J. Med.* 1982; 307:99.
16. Strickler, S.M., Miller, M.A., Andermann, E., Dansky, L.V., Seni, M., Spielberg, S.P. Genetic predisposition to phenytoin-induced birth defects. *Lancet.* 1985; 2:746.
17. Finnell, R., Chernoff, G. Mouse fetal hydantoin syndrome: effects of maternal seizures. *Epilepsia.* 1982; 23:423.
18. Philbert, A., Dam, M. The epileptic mother and her child. *Epilepsia.* 1982; 23:85.
19. Clifford, D.B. Seizures and pregnancy. *Am. Fam. Physician.* 1984; 29:271.
20. Committee on Drugs. Anticonvulsants and pregnancy. *Am. Acad. Pediatr.* 1981; 63:331.
21. Ek, J., Mangnus, E. Plasma and red blood cell folate during normal pregnancy. *Acta Obstet. Gynecol. Scand.* 1981; 60:247.
22. Kaneko, S., Suzuki, K., Sato, T., Ogawa, Y., Nomura, Y. The problem of antiepileptic medication in the neonatal period: is breastfeeding advisable? In: Janz, D., Dam, M., Richens, A., Bossi, L., Helge, H., Schmidt, D., eds. *Epilepsy, Pregnancy, and the Child.* New York: Raven Press; 1982.
23. Bossi, L. Neonatal period including drug deposition in newborns, review of the literature. In: Janz, D., Dam, M., Richens, A., Bossi, L., Helge, H., Schmidt, D., eds. *Epilepsy, Pregnancy, and the Child.* New York: Raven Press; 1982.
24. Adams, J., Vorhees, C., Middaugh, L. Developmental neurotoxicity of anticonvulsants: human and animal evidence on phenytoin. *Neurotoxicol. Teratol.*, 1990; 12:203.
25. Buchler, B., Delmont, D., van Waes, M., Finnell, R. Prenatal prediction of risk of the fetal hydantoin syndrome. *N. Engl. J. Med.* 1990; 322:1567.

Chapter 16
Down Syndrome

Bonnie Patterson and Shirley Walberg Ekvall

Down syndrome (DS), first described by John Langdon Down in 1866,[1] is the most common chromosomal abnormality associated with mental retardation. Incidence, which is reported to be 1 in 800–1000 live births, increases significantly with increasing maternal age. Therefore, prenatal screening is recommended for women after age 35. The chromosomal abnormality in approximately 96% of people with DS is an extra 21 chromosome (trisomy 21). In the remainder of the cases, there is a translocation abnormality by which the extra 21 chromosome is attached to another autosomal chromosome, usually another 21 or 14. In these cases of translocation, it is important that chromosomal studies be done on the parents, as well as the child, since one of the parents may have a balanced translocation and be a carrier of the abnormality. Mosaic DS occurs when only some of the cell lines contain the extra 21 chromosome.

Features of Down Syndrome

Children with DS resemble their parents, but in addition, have many common features described in the syndrome. These features can change with age, such as the epicanthal folds and abundant neck tissue that are often seen in early childhood, but decrease as the person becomes older (Fig. 16-1). Fissure tongue anomalies often become more apparent with increasing age. Physical features that are often associated with DS but are not pathognomonic include the following[2]:

- flattened nasal bridge
- oblique palpebral fissures
- eipcanthal folds
- brachycephaly
- higher arched narrow palate
- gap between the first and second toe
- short, broad hands
- transverse crease on the palm of the hand
- hyperflexibility
- hypotonia
- Brushfield spots in the iris
- abnormal teeth
- furrowed tongue

In addition to the characteristic physical features, many people with DS have congenital anomalies of major organ systems. Approximately 40% of children with DS are born with significant congenital heart defects (endocardial cushion defect, ventricular septal defect, atrial septal defect), and 15% are born with gastrointestinal malformations, including duodenal atresia, annular pancreas, and malrotations.

People with DS are at risk for medical complications that can have a dramatic effect on their overall development. A Preventive Medicine Checklist was developed in the early 1980s by Dr. Mary Coleman and is used to guide physicians and families in monitoring the health status of children and

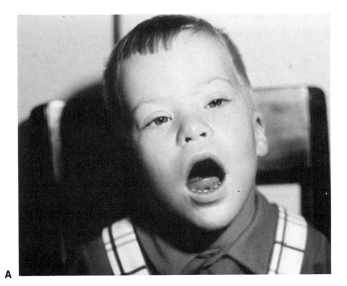
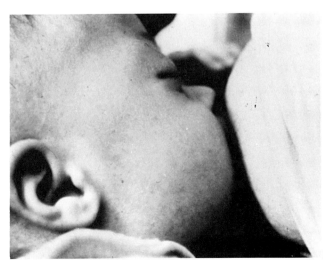

Fig. 16-1. A, Boy with Down syndrome. B, Child with Down syndrome: breastfeeding. Used with permission.

adults with DS.[3] There appears to be a higher incidence of infections, particularly of the upper respiratory tract and middle ear in DS. Because middle ear infections can result in hearing loss, it is recommended that people with DS have yearly audiologic evaluations. Visual problems are commonly seen in DS, including strabismus, blepharitis, and myopia. Yearly eye examinations are also recommended. Other areas of medical concern include endocrine problems (diabetes, hypothyroidism), orthopedic problems (atlantoaxial instability, hip dislocation, patellar instability), leukemias, and skin problems (psoriasis, alopecia).

Variability in development is seen in DS, with the majority of people functioning in the mentally retarded range. The intellectual abilities of people with DS range from low normal to severe and profound retardation. With the advent of infant stimulation programs and greatly improved special education services, many children with DS are now functioning in the mild to high moderate range of retardation. It is strongly recommended that infants with DS be referred to infant stimulation programs within the first few months of life.

The prognosis for children with DS has improved greatly with the advent of better medical care and educational and vocational services. In the 1950s, the life expectancy of a person with DS was approximately 9 years. At this time, many people with DS are living well into their fifties and sixties. Improved life expectancy is related to the advent of antibiotics and cardiac surgery. With the passage of PL 94-142, educational and vocational services are now available for all people with DS. Individual education programs can be developed, and many children are doing quite well in a combination of special education and mainstreamed programs. Many people with DS are developing academic skills in such areas as reading and mathematics and are able to work in the community. Institutionalization is no longer necessary or recommended for people with DS. Most children live at home with their parents and family, and as adults, many live in residential group home settings within the community.

Growth

Linear growth in children with DS is retarded beginning in prenatal life and extending to the end of the growing years. A study done by Cronk et al.[4] found that the growth rate was reduced by about 20% during infancy (3–36 months) in each sex, but only by about 5% between 3 and 10 years in girls and about 10% between 3 and 12 years in boys. Earlier, Cronk[5] had found the length velocity to be most deficient between 6 and 24 months. During the remainder of the growing period (10 to 17 years in girls and 12 to 17 years in boys) reduction in growth rate was 27% and 50% for girls and boys, respectively. This study supported earlier observations that the adolescent growth spurt in children with DS is less vigorous than in children without DS. Rarick and Seefeldt[6] measured sitting height and found that the reduction in stature was largely due to the reduction in lower segment length throughout the period of their study (8–18 years). Ratcliffe[7] noted reductions in birth weight by approximately 400 g and birth length by approximately 2 cm; a reduction in the rate of height growth, with the final height being approximately 151–156 cm in men and 141 cm in women; the occurrence of an adolescent growth spurt; height attainment independent of midparent stature; and bone age consistent with chronological age.

Children and adolescents with DS also have a tendency to be overweight beginning in infancy.[4] The percentage of children with DS who are overweight appears to increase from the expected value of about 15% during early infancy to nearly 50% in girls by the third year of life and in boys by early childhood. Cronk[5] found that weight velocity was most deficient between 6 and 18 months. It is likely that differences in environment—for example, the increased opportunity for physical activity, greater emotional support, improved nutritional adequacy—have a substantial influence on growth during childhood and adolescence. Moderate to severe congenital heart disease can affect stature and weight beginning in infancy and extending through the entire growing period. On the average the girls may be 1 cm shorter and 1 kg lighter and the boys 2 cm shorter and 1–2 kg lighter with cardiac disease and DS during infancy and childhood. (see Chapter 31).

Cronk et al.[4] have devised growth charts for children with DS from ages 1 month to 18 years. These charts give values for five centiles of stature and weight for each sex and two age intervals (Appendix 2). Deficiencies in growth velocity occur at varying times in children with DS and are of widely different magnitude, particularly in infancy. Compared with a child without DS, a child with DS may not remain at the same centile level on these charts. Weight gain for children with DS is more rapid than growth in stature, often resulting in overweight (50% above the 85th percentile for age) by 36 months of age. Cronk et al.[8] found mean weights of children with DS to be significantly higher than those of a reference group at 4 to 6 years of age. Differences in weight for stature were greater when children with DS were institutionalized, rather than reared at home, and were also greater for girls than boys.[9] Because these new growth charts reflect this tendency, they should always be used in conjunction with the NCHS charts for nonhandicapped children when assessing body weight. In addition, it is strongly recommended that the NCHS weight for length chart also be used for assessment of body fatness. Greater than expected percentage of children with DS also are overweight by the W/S^2 measurement.

Dental problems

Abnormalities in tooth shape and size are common in DS. The incidence of microdontia has been reported to range from 35% to 55%[10] Dental agenesis of both deciduous and permanent teeth is reported to be four to five times greater in DS.[2] The most frequently missing teeth are the lateral incisors.[11]

Periodontal disease appears to be very prevalent among patients with DS. Decreased resistance to the bacteria that accumulate in the gingival margins may be a contributing factor. Other factors, such as malocclusions, tooth morphology (including short roots), lack of normal masticatory function, and bruxism, have also been suggested as contributing to periodontal disease. The incidence of periodontal problems appears to be lower in individuals with DS who live at home.

The incidence of dental caries has frequently been reported to be lower in DS; however, Kroll et al.[12] used radiographs of the dentition and reported that the incidence of dental caries in DS was not significantly lower than in non-DS subjects. Since the eruption of both deciduous and permanent dentition is delayed in Down's syndrome, the difference may be due to the shorter time period that the teeth were exposed to the oral environment, rather than any innate protection against caries seen in DS.

Many people with DS have malocclusions, malalignment of the teeth, and abnormal jaw relationships. The major contributing factor to the malocclusions appears to be underdevelopment of the maxilla. The tongue also plays a primary role in the development of malocclusions. Dental abnormalities can certainly have an effect on the nutritional status of the child, particularly those abnormalities that affect chewing and mastication.

Biochemical Abnormalities

Numerous reports in the literature since the early 1940s have described biochemical abnormalities in DS that are attributable to the extra chromosome. However, for every study that showed some specific abnormality in protein, carbohydrate, or fat metabolism, another study found no abnormalities. These studies have not been highly specific and have been very difficult to interpret. The link between elevated levels of certain enzymes and the extra dose of genes located on the trisomic chromosome 21 is invoked as the explanation for some of the deviations, but further studies are indicated.[13,14]

An increased incidence of hypothyroidism has been documented in people with DS. Yearly thyroid studies—thyroxine (T_4) and thyroid-stimulating hormone (TSH) levels—are recommended.[15] A high incidence of leukemia has also been noted with this syndrome.[16]

Protein metabolism

Since the early 1950s many studies have assessed protein metabolism in people with DS. These reports present much conflicting information and are open to various interpretations. Serum albumin levels in DS are often reported to be decreased, whereas globulin concentrations are increased. Many studies have reported higher than normal gammaglobulin levels for people with DS. A study done by Donner[17] in 1954 found increased gammaglobulin concentrations in long-term institutionalized individuals with DS. However, new patients in the institution did not show these increases levels. This data suggested that environmental circumstances, such as current infections and dietary or other factors specific to residential facilities, may be responsible for the increase in gammaglobulin levels, rather than a direct association with DS. In 1967, Appleton and Pritham[18] found no significant difference between people with DS or control groups for any of the protein fraction studies. With advancing age, they did note a tendency for the concentration of albumin to decrease and gammaglobulin to increase. These authors felt that the increase in quantity of gammaglobulin in DS represented an attempt to compensate for the poor quality of antibody production.

Alpha-1-antitrypsin phenotypes were studied in 40 patients with DS by Arnaud and co-workers in 1976.[19] Thirty-six of the patients were found to have normal M phenotypes, whereas two deficient phenotypes of the MS variety were observed. The authors concluded that a deficiency in alpha-1-antitrypsin does not play a role in the respiratory problems exhibited by some individuals with DS.

Carbohydrate metabolism

Milunsky and Neurath in 1968[20] examined the frequency of carbohydrate metabolic disturbances in DS compared to control populations. Raiti and co-workers[21] studied eight children with DS during adolescence and found three of the eight patients had inadequate plasma insulin response to glucose or to arginine infusion. The glucose disappearance was suggestive of possible diabetic tendencies. There does appear to be a higher incidence of diabetes in people with DS; however, most studies have shown that the majority of patients with DS are asymptomatic with regard to carbohydrate metabolism.

Fat metabolism

There have been many conflicting studies regarding cholesterol levels in people with DS. Nishida and co-workers in 1977[22] found no significant difference between subjects with DS and those in control groups with regard to serum total cholesterol, phospholipids, or free fatty acids. However, the patients with DS did have significantly increased plasma triglyceride levels (224 mg/dL versus 173 mg/dL).

In 1984, Dorner et al.[23] looked at 186 patients with DS, ages 1 year to 68 years, and determined total cholesterol and triglycerides levels. A control group of 51 mentally handicapped adults without DS, who were living in the same institution was used. The DS patients total cholesterol, beta cholesterol, and triglyceride levels did not differ from those of controls. However, alpha cholesterol levels were significantly lower and beta/alpha lipoprotein ratios were significantly higher in patients with DS. In the general population, these findings are linked with a high risk of premature atherosclerosis. Yet, mortality cause data and pathological findings in DS show no increased frequency of cardiovascular disease. The discrepancy between the low incidence of cardiovascular disease in people with DS and the high risk factor of a strongly elevated beta/alpha lipoprotein ratio is obvious and leads to the conclusion that either in these patients a high ratio is not a risk factor or other risks not studied are considerably lower.

Minerals

Many studies, beginning in the late 1930s, have attempted to determine whether there are mineral abnormalities in people with DS. In 1981, Barlow et al.[24] using atomic absorption spectroscopy, estimated the trace elements content of suboccipital hair in 69 male and 67 female patients with DS and compared the results with 69 control patients in the same environment. Multiple deficiencies were noted, particularly in calcium, copper, and manganese. Some striking differences were noted in manganese levels in women with DS, which were significantly lower than those in women without DS. There were no comparative differences between men with DS and other men. Copper was more significantly reduced in males than in females with DS. Ceruloplasmin levels were found to be normal. Studies performed on 10 children with DS, aged 14 to 17, who were living at home revealed that they too were low in hair calcium, copper, and manganese. However, it is important to note that hair analysis of nutrient deficiencies is currently of limited use because of the lack of standardized collection techniques and normative values.

In 1986, Anneren[25] in Sweden compared a group of 22 children with DS (ages 2 to 15 years) to a control group of 22 healthy children from the same age group. Concentrations of iron, copper, and zinc in serum were determined by atomic absorption spectrophotometry, and serum proteins were quantitated by using the radial immunodefusion technique. Patients with DS had significantly lower mean serum iron and zinc levels. In more than 60% of the DS patients, the zinc concentration fell below normal range. Children with DS had significantly higher mean serum copper but lower serum iron and zinc levels than their healthy siblings living in the same family at the same time. Bjorksten[26] was able to double the serum levels of zinc and improve the immunological status through zinc supplementation. However, the serum copper was reduced.[27] Thus, a double-blind study using a placebo versus zinc is needed.

In 1983 and 1984 Neve et al.[28] and Sinet et al.[29] found low plasma levels of selenium in children with DS in comparison to the control group, but levels in the red cells did not differ. Further research is needed on selenium status.

Vitamins

Vitamin deficiencies, malabsorption of specific vitamins, and abnormalities of vitamin metabolism in DS have all been described in the literature. Interest in absorption and utilization of vitamin A was encouraged by the fact that people with DS often exhibited symptoms characteristic of vitamin A metabolic disturbances. These included hyperkeratotic skin lesions, increased incidence of upper respiratory infection, and poor dark adaptation ability.[30] In 1958, Sobol et al.[31] found that children with DS had a lower absorption of vitamin A. However, another study in 1976 by Cutress et al.[32] did not find significant differences of vitamin A absorption after oral vitamin A tolerance tests. This study included a control group of patients without DS. Matin et al.[33] in 1981 investigated the relationship of hypovitamin A to hyperkeratosis and also vitamin E, thiamin, nicotinic acid, and ascorbic acid status in children with DS. Six patients with hyperkeratosis were matched with six unrelated patients with DS but without hyperkeratosis. A group of non-DS patients acted as control. There were no significant differences between the mean values of the groups for vitamin A. A study by Barden[34] in 1977 determined vitamin A and carotene values of 44 patients with DS, 56 retarded patients without DS, and 40 normal subjects. The subjects with DS had significantly higher vitamin A values than those of the non-DS retarded population; these values were similar to those of the normal patients. Carotene values were similar in the DS and non-DS retarded groups, but were significantly higher than those of normal subjects.

In 1976, Schmid[35] examined the relationship of vitamin B metabolism in persons with DS to clinical symptoms. He proposed that the apathy and lethargy often described in DS might be due to vitamin B_1 deficiency and that the cheilosis, gingivitis, conjunctivitis, and changes of the taste buds on the tongue may be due to lack of vitamin B_2. Several studies have reviewed vitamin B_6 availability in patients with DS, citing abnormal tryptophan-loading tests as evidence of decreased vitamin B_6. However, Hansson[36] in 1969 questioned the value of this test as a predictor of vitamin B_6 deficiency. In 1985, Coleman et al.[37] conducted a double-blind study of the clinical effects of pharmacological doses of vitamin B_6 administered to 19 patients with DS. The administration of the vitamin began at less than 8 weeks of age and continued until 3 years of age. Ten patients received the vitamin and nine a placebo. No statistically significant differences were found between the two groups in mental age, height, weight, cranial circumference, or tongue protrusion. A study of side effects conducted on a larger open population (not double-blind) found vitamin B_6 to be relatively safe when administered over long periods of time, with photosensitive blisters as the major complication.[37]

Recently, there have been many claims that large, nonspecific doses of vitamins and minerals can improve the physical appearance and intellectual performance of children with DS. These reports have appeared both in the scientific and lay literature. A double-blind case control study was performed by Bennett et al.[38] in 1983. This study involved 20 home-reared children with DS between the ages of 5 and 13 years. The children were randomly assigned by matched pairs to either a vitamin/mineral group or placebo group for an 8-month period. There were no significant group differences or trends in any test area of development or behavior, including intelligence, school achievement, speech and language, and neuromotor function. Neither were any group differences in appearance, growth, or health seen. The results of this study indicated that there was no apparent support for the orthomolecular hypothesis of vitamin/mineral supplementation in school-aged children with DS.

Orthomolecular therapy is just one of many controversial unproven interventions, including vitamin B_6 administration, fetal animal brain cell injections, and plastic surgery, advocated for children with DS. Critics have pointed out that dessicated thyroid preparation has not been administered to subjects in the studies reported subsequent to that of Harrell et al.[39] and have suggested that the "Harrell regime" therefore has not been replicated by the other investigators. However, the idea of dietary supplementation for a child with DS is not without some precedent. Specific nutrient deficiencies—for example, vitamin A, vitamin B_6, and zinc—have been suggested by previous studies, but have never been consistently documented. Biochemical differences have not yet been associated with reproducible clinical signs or symptoms.

Uric acid

Reports have appeared in the literature concerning uric acid concentration in tissues of persons with DS. The majority of these studies have reported a markedly increased uric acid level.[40] The pathogenic mechanism leading to a high uric acid concentration in persons with DS is not well understood. There is no evidence to date to support the hypothesis that the increased uric acid serum concentrations damage the kidneys or interfere with other vital functions in the body. Much more investigation is needed to assess these and other aspects of hyperuricemia in DS.

Factors to be Considered in Nutritional Evaluation

There is no evidence at the present time that nutrition plays a specific role in the etiology of DS; however, due to the high incidence of growth problems, endocrine abnormalities, and feeding difficulties, nutritional assessment plays an important role in the total care of this patient population. The following nutritional parameters are significant in the overall evaluation and care of the patient.

Feeding Problems and Feeding Skills

Many infants with DS have feeding difficulties soon after birth.[41] They may be secondary to hypotonia, placidity, and/or weak sucking and rooting reflexes. However, the majority of children with DS eventually establish breast or bottle feeding skills without undue difficulty. For the slower-feeding child with DS, the usual procedures, such as experimenting with the size and type of nipple, are often sufficient to establish good feeding skills. It is vital to persevere for longer than usual before deciding a certain method of feeding is not working, particularly in attempts at breast-feeding. Typically, infants with DS maintain the tongue thrusting action required for rooting and sucking longer than normally expected. Often the mother interprets this action as a sign of food rejection. Persistence of the protrusion reflex well past the first or second year often results in the delayed progression to solid foods. Infants with DS often choke when drinking from a cup either because liquid fills the mouth too quickly or the baby is continually thrusting out the cup's spout. The development of self-feeding skills in infants with DS is often delayed.

Lack of feeding skills or mobility may be predictors of life expectancy.[42] Feeding difficulties are often seen in older children with DS as well. Slow physical growth and inactivity due to hypotonia are common characteristics of young children with DS and may limit caloric needs.[43] The importance of developmental readiness for feeding skills is sometimes not recognized in children with delayed development, and the parents' emotional response to having a handicapped child further interferes with feeding and eating. Feeding problems recognized by parents and/or professional staff members include the following[43]:

- inappropriate, excessive, or low intake of calories
- poor eating habits; that is, retention of infantile feeding habits, food refusal, and unacceptable behavior around food
- inappropriate parental feeding practices and delays in self-feeding skills in the children beyond an age when they are developmentally ready to acquire this skill

Nutrients

Pipes in 1980[43] completed a retrospective chart review of 49 children with DS between the ages of 6 months and 6-1/2 years. Eighty percent of the children had problems related to food or feeding, including excessive calorie intake and low intakes of calcium, iron, ascorbic acid, and fluid. These problems of nutrient intake were similar to those in non-handicapped children, but occurred with a higher frequency. Excessive calorie intake appeared to be related to the high intake of carbohydrates resulting, in part, from consumption of large quantities of easy-to-chew starches and the use of sweets as rewards for good behavior. Physical factors related to DS also were found to contribute to some nutritional inadequacies. For example, excessive nasal discharge is common in children with DS. Some children are on a low milk intake in an effort to decrease mucous production, but this technique has not been proven helpful and these children should receive the basic four serving requirement for milk or milk products. Occasionally, children with DS have difficulties in chewing stemming from the delayed appearance of the chewing reflex, late appearance of teeth, and other dental problems. Some children have a tendency to store food in their high arched palate and/or to thrust particular foods out of their mouths with their tongues. These problems often occur at about 2 years of age.

Cullen et al.[44] in 1981 reviewed the mastery of social development and feeding skills in 89 children with DS. The sex, cardiac status, and muscle tones of the subjects and parental follow-through data were examined for their potential influence on Vineland Social Maturity Scale (VSMS) scores and on a selected subset of feeding milestones. Young children with DS who obtained significantly higher scores on the VSMS achieved most feeding milestones earlier, if they had no or only mild congenital heart disease, if their parents followed through appropriately with furnished guidelines, and if they had good muscle tone.

Laboratory and clinical data

The DS Preventive Medicine Checklist was developed by Dr. Mary Coleman in the early 1980s. This checklist is a guideline for medical evaluations and laboratory studies that should be obtained for people with DS at various ages. The laboratory and dietary recommendations[3] are summarized below.

- *Neonatal period*—laboratory studies should include chromosomes, CBC, thyroid-stimulating hormone (TSH), and thyroxine (T$_4$) levels
- *Two- to 12-month examination*—laboratory studies should include thyroid-stimulating hormone (TSH), thyroxine (T$_4$), and CBC. Diet should maintain good carotene intake—that is, deep green, orange-yellow vegetables and fruits—as foods are added.
- *One year to puberty*—laboratory studies should include annual TSH and T$_4$. Energy (caloric) intake should be based on height (rather than age) and be related to activity level. Total calorie recommendations probably should be below the recommended daily allowance (RDA) for children of similar age and height.
- *Adolescence and adulthood*—laboratory studies should include serum thyroid tests, including antiglobulin factor and hepatitis screening. The diet should be well balanced and low calorie. Total caloric requirements should probably be below the RDA due to decreased activity level.

The incidence of thyroid disease, as noted above, is significantly increased among individuals with DS. The absorption of vitamin A from the gastrointestinal tract may be diminished, although this has not been clearly documented. Normal levels of thyroid and vitamin A are needed for growth, resistance to infection, and cognitive functioning. Monitoring is best achieved by obtaining blood levels on a yearly basis.

Some medical problems are seen more commonly in people with DS. Their appearance dictates certain laboratory studies.

- *Alopecia areata*—vitamin A and thyroid functioning, look for other autoimmune conditions
- *Constipation*—discontinue iron in infant formula; if no physical reason (such as Hirschsprung's disease), add magnesium
- *Obesity*—check for thyroid malfunction and steatorrhea, obtain a calorie count, encourage exercise
- *Paleness or petechiae on skin*—hematological evaluation and serum carotene levels
- *Peripheral neuropathy*—check niacin metabolites in the urine; check folate and vitamin B_{12} levels in serum
- *Roughness and cracking of the skin*—check thyroid tests, serum vitamin A, vitamin E, and riboflavin levels
- *Tremors*—obtain serum and 24-hour urine for magnesium and calcium
- *Unusually poor growth*—check for cardiac lesion, thyroid malfunction, steatorrhea, and vitamin A

Constipation

Constipation occurs with relatively high frequency in people with DS and may be related to several factors. In many cases it can be caused by a lack of physical activity or roughage in the diet. The generalized hypotonia observed in most people with DS may also play some role. Particularly in the neonatal period, the differential diagnosis would also include GI malformations—in particular, Hirschsprung's disease—which can often present with a history of constipation. Another medical complication often seen in DS is hypothyroidism, which can also present with the symptom of constipation.

Anthropometry, energy expenditure, and nutrients

Chad et al.[45] recently found that body height had the strongest and body fat the weakest correlation with resting metabolic rate in 11 male and seven female noninstitutionalized children with DS. Energy expenditure was significantly lower $(39.93 \text{ m}^2/\text{hr}^{-1})$ than in children without DS $(44 \text{ m}^2/\text{hr}^{-1})$. Daily caloric intake was 1,433.84 calories (16.0% protein, 42.2% fat), and 40.6% carbohydrate), and iron and thiamine intakes were below the recommended daily allowance. Nutrition counseling recommended: increased complex carbohydrates, decreased protein and fat, and increased exercise.[45] DS growth charts (Appendix 2) are needed to determine appropriate growth and thereby calorie levels. The NCHS height weight ratio charts are recommended for weight goals. Exercise is particularly important to increase lean body mass and decrease fat tissue (see Chapter 19). Skinfold measurements should be assessed.

Dietary Management

The major objectives of dietary management in DS are promotion of the development of self-feeding skills, prevention of obesity and the prevention and/or correction of nutritional deficiencies that might develop in association with the above-mentioned biochemical abnormalities.

Feeding Problems and Skills

The majority of children with DS establish breast or bottle feeding without undue difficulty. However, it is often necessary for the mother to persevere for longer than usual before deciding that a particular feeding method is not working. It is important to remember that considerable repetition and patience are required when teaching skills to a child who is developmentally delayed. Some of the feeding problems (food throwing and refusal of specific groups of foods) often are more of a behavior problem than a true feeding problem. Professional guidance in helping the family of the child with DS progress in feeding patterns is often recommended. A child's developmental readiness to progress in feeding is not always easy to recognize. Children with DS are often susceptible to being infantilized by their parents due to their inability to recognize when the child is ready for the next step toward independent feeding.

Dental problems

It is strongly recommended that children with DS begin routine dental care at 2 years of age. Follow-up examinations should be at 6- to 12-month intervals. Foods with a high concentration of sucrose, especially sweet, chewy snacks, should be avoided. Desserts with high sucrose content should be eaten with meals, rather than as snacks throughout the day, to reduce the opportunities for bacterial action. Fresh fruits and vegetables should be an integral part of the child's diet.

Anthropometry and nutrient intake

Caloric intake should be based on height rather than age and related to the activity level of the individual child using DS Growth Charts (Table 16–1). Approximately 16.1 calories per cm of height for boys and 14.3 calories per cm of height for girls was determined from reduced height in a study by Culley et al.[46] and is noted on the special grids (Appendix 2). In many cases, the total calorie recommendation should be below the recommended daily allowance (RDA) for children of similar age and height. Because of the restricted intake of calories, the intake of vitamins, minerals, and proteins should be evaluated and additional supplements given when necessary. Megadoses of vitamins, either B_6 or others, should be used cautiously because of the possibility of adverse affects. One study found hypercarotenemia, rather than a deficiency of carotene or vitamin A, in DS.[47] Milk or milk products should not be severely limited due to the needed riboflavin, protein, calcium, and vitamin D content. Good food sources of zinc and iron (such as meat), magnesium and vitamin E (such as whole grains), folate (such as spinach), vitamin B_{12} (as in meat or milk), calcium (in milk products), vitamin A (as in dark green or orange vegetables), and vitamin C (in citrus fruits) should be evaluated in the diet.

Constipation

A diet high in fiber and fluids is recommended for treatment of atonic constipation. Foods high in roughage include fresh fruits, particularly prunes, fresh vegetables, and foods made

Table 16–1. Estimations for Caloric Requirements for Down Syndrome (B and D, Down Syndrome; A and C, General Population)

Age in Years	Weight (kg)	Weight (lb)	Height (cm)	Height (in)	Calories (per kg)	Calories (per cm)	Calories Per Person Per Day	RDA Calories
				Boys				
(A) 1–3	13	29	90	35	100	14.4	1300	(1000–1400)
4–6	20	44	112	44	80	14.5	1600	(1500–1800)
7–10	28	62	132	52	85	18.2	2400	(2100–2500)
11–14	45	99	157	62	57	17.2		(2500–2800)
(B) 1–3	11	24	81	32	109	16.1	1200	(1100–1300)
4–6	15	34	99	39	100	16.1	1500	(1400–1600)
7–10	20	43	112	45	90	16.1	1800	(1700–2000)
11–14	26	58	130	52	80	16.1	2100	(2100–2300)
				Girls				
(C) 1–3	13	29	90	35	100	14.4	1300	(1000–1400)
4–6	20	44	112	44	80	14.5	1600	(1500–1800)
7–10	28	62	132	52	85	18.2	2400	(2100–2500)
11–14	46	101	157	62	48	14.0	2200	(2000–2200)
(D) 1–3	9	20	81	32	122	14.3	1100	(1000–1200)
4–6	15	32	104	41	93	14.3	1400	(1300–1500)
7–10	21	46	119	47	80.9	14.3	1700	(1500–1800)
11–14	31	69	134	54	61	14.3	1900	(1800–2000)

*Estimations based on Down syndrome growth curves taken from Springer, N. S. *Nutrition Casebook on Developmental Disabilities*. Syracuse, NY: 1982 and Cronk et al.[4]; agrees with original data from Culley et al.[46] and Recommended Dietary Allowances, 10th ed. Washington, D.C.: National Academy Press, 1989.

from whole-grains and cereals. Fruit juices and water with meals also are recommended (see Chapter 35).

Follow-up

An important aspect of nutritional management in people with DS is regular monitoring of progress in various areas of growth and development, as well as nutritional assessment (laboratory, feeding, dietary, and anthropometry). Providing behavioral and professional support to parents following a recommended home program is essential.

References

1. Down, J.L.H. Observations on an ethnic classification of idiots. *Clin. Lect. Rep.* (London Hosp) 1866; 3:259.
2. Pueschel, S.M., Rynders, J.E., eds. *Down Syndrome—Advances in Biomedicine and the Behavioral Sciences*. Cambridge, MA: Academic Guild; 1982.
3. Lentz, G. Down Syndrome preventive medicine checklist. Papers and Abstracts for Professionals, 1987; 10:2.
4. Cronk, C., Crocker, A.C., Pueschel, S.M., Shea, A.M., Zachai, E., Pickens, G., Reed, R.B. Growth charts for children with Down Syndrome—1 month to 18 years of age. *Pediatrics*. 1988; 81:102.
5. Cronk, C.E. Growth of children with Down's syndrome: Birth to age 3 years. *Pediatrics*. 1978; 61:564.
6. Rarick, G.L., Seefeldt, V. Observations from longitudinal data on growth in stature and sitting height of children with Down's syndrome. *J. Ment. Defic. Res.* 1974; 18:63.
7. Ratcliffe, S.G. The effect of chromosome abnormalities on human growth. *Br. Med. J.* 1981; 37:291.
8. Cronk, C.E., Chumlea, W.C., Roche, A.F. Assessment of overweight children with trisomy 21. *Am. J. Ment. Defic.* 1985; 89:433.
9. Chumlea, W.C., Cronk, C.E. Overweight among children with trisomy 21. *J. Ment. Defic. Res.* 1982; 25:275.
10. Spitzer, R., Mann, I. Congenital malformations in the teeth and eyes in mental defectives. *Br. J. Psychol.* 1950; 96:681.
11. Lane, D., Stratford, B., eds. *Current Approaches to Down's Syndrome*, New York: Praeger; 1985.
12. Kroll, R.G., Budnick, J., Kobren, A. Incidence of dental caries and periodontal disease in Down's syndrome. *NY State Dent. J.* 1970; 36:151.
13. Stocchi, V., Magnani, M., Cucchiarini, L., Novelli, G., Dallapiccola, B. Red blood cell adenine nucleotides abnormalities in Down syndrome. *Am. J. Med. Genet.* 1985; 20:131.
14. Crosti, N., Serra, A., Rigo, A., Viglino, P. Dosage effect of SOD-A gene in 21 trisomic cells. *Hum. Genet.* 1976; 23:197.
15. Pueschel, S., Pezzulo, J.C. Thyroid dysfunction in Down syndrome. *Am. J. Dis. Child.* 1985; 139:636.
16. Hsia, D.Y., Justice, P., Smith, G.F., Dowben, R.M. Down's syndrome: a critical review of the biochemical and immunological data. *Am. J. Dis. Child.* 1971; 121:153.
17. Donner, M. An investigation into immunological reactions and antibody production in mongolism. *Ann. Med. Exp. Biol. Fenn.* 1954; 32(S):9.
18. Appleton, M.D., Pritham, G.H. Biochemical studies in mongolism. II. The influences of age and sex on the plasma proteins. *Am. J. Ment. Defic.* 1967; 67:521.
19. Arnaud, P., Burdach, N.M., Wilson, G.B., Fundenberg, H.H. Alpha-1-antitrypsin (Pi) types in Down's syndrome. *Clin. Genet.* 1976; 10:239.
20. Milunsky, A., Neurath, P.W. Diabetes mellitus in Down's syndrome. *Arch. Environ. Health.* 1968; 17:372.
21. Raiti, S., Lifshitz, F., Trias, E., Sigman, B. Down's syndrome. Study of carbohydrate metabolism. *Acta Endocrinol.* 1974; 76:506.
22. Nishida, Y., Akaoka, I., Nishizawa, T., Maruki, M. Synthesis and concentration of 5-phosphorilosyl-1-pyrophosphate in erythrocytes from patients with Down's syndrome. *Ann. Rheum. Dis.* 1977; 36:361.
23. Dorner, K., Gaethke, A., Tolksdorf, M., Schumann, K.P., Gustmann, H. Cholesterol fractions and triglycerides in children and adults with Down syndrome. *Clin. Chim. Acta*, 1984.
24. Barlow, P.J., Sylvester, P.E., Dickerson, J.W. Hair trace metal levels in Down's syndrome patients. *J. Ment. Defic. Res.* 1981; 25:161.

25. Anneren, G., Gebre-Medkin, M. Tract elements and transport proteins in serum of children with Down's syndrome and healthy siblings living in the same environment. *Hum. Nutr. Clin. Nutr.* 1987; 41:291.

26. Bjorksten, B., Back, O., Hagglof, B., Tarnviks, A. Immune function in Down's syndrome, In: Guttle, F., Seakins, J.W.T., Harkness, R.A., eds. *Inborn Errors of Immunity and Phagocytosis.* Baltimore: University Park; 1979.

27. Correction of impaired immunity in Down's syndrome by zinc. *Nutr. Rev.* 1980; 38:365.

28. Neve, J., Sinet, P.M., Molle, L., Nicole, A. Selenium, zinc and copper in Down's syndrome (trisomy 21): blood levels and relations with glutathione peroxidase and superoxide dismutase. *Clin. Chim. Acta,* 1983; 133:209.

29. Sinet, P.M., Neve, J., Nicole. A., Molle, L. Low plasma selenium in Down's syndrome (trisomy 21). *Acta Pediatr. Scand.* 1984; 73:275.

30. Palmer, S. Influence of vitamin A nutritive on the immune system: findings in children with Down syndrome. *Int. J. Vitam. Nutr. Res.* 1977; 48:188.

31. Sobel, A.E., Strazzulla, M., Sherman, B.S., Elhan, B. Vitamin A absorption and other blood composition studies in mongolism. *Am. J. Ment. Defic.* 1958; 62:642.

32. Cutress, T.W., Mickleson, K.N., Brown, R.N. Vitamin A absorption and periodontal disease in trisomy G. *J. Ment. Defic. Res.* 1976; 20:17.

33. Matin, M.A., Sylvester, P.E., Edwards, P., Dickerson, J.W.T. Vitamin and zinc status in Down's syndrome. *J. Ment. Defic. Res.* 1981; 25:121.

34. Barden, H.S. Vitamin A and carotene values of institutionalized mentally retarded subjects with and without Down's syndrome. *J. Ment. Defic. Res.* 1977; 21:63.

35. Schmid, F. Das mongolismus—Syndrom. Deutsch. *Habammen. Z.* 1976; 28:169.

36. Hansson, O. Tryptophan loading and pyridoxine treatment in children with epilepsy. *Ann. N. Y. Acad. Sci.* 1969; 166:306.

37. Coleman, M., Sobel, S., Bhagavan, H.N., Coursin, D., Marquardt, A., Guay, M., Hunt, C. A double-blind study of vitamin B6 in Down's syndrome infants. Part 1—Clinical and biochemical results. *J. Ment. Defic. Res.* 1985; 29:233.

38. Bennett, F.C., McClelland, S., Kriegsmann, E.A., Andrus, L., Sells, C.J. Vitamin and mineral supplementation in Down's syndrome. *Pediatrics.* 1983; 72:707.

39. Harrell, R.F., Capp, R.H., Davis, D.R., Peerless, J., Ravitz, R. Can nutritional supplements help mentally retarded children? An exploratory study. *Proc. Natl. Acad. Sci.* 1981; 78:574.

40. Hestnes, A., Stovner, L.J., Husøy, Ø., Folling, I., Fougner, K.J., Sjaastad, O. Hormonal and biochemical disturbances in Down's syndrome. *J. Ment. Def. Res.* 1991; 35:179.

41. Eyman, R.K., Call, T.I., White, J.F. Life expectancy of persons with Down syndrome. *Am. J. Ment. Retard.* 1991; 95:603.

42. Aumonier, M., Cunningham, C. Health and medical problems in infants with Down's syndrome. *Health Visitor.* 1984; 57:137.

43. Pipes, P.L., Holm, V.A. Feeding children with Down's syndrome. *J. Am. Diet. Assoc.* 1980; 77:277.

44. Cullen, S.M., Cronk, C.E., Pueschel, S.M., Schnell, R.R., Reed, R.B. Social development and feeding milestones of young Down syndrome children. *Am. J. Ment. Defic.* 1981; 85:410.

45. Chad, K., Jobling, A., Frail, H. Metabolic rate: a factor in developing obesity in children with Down syndrome? *Am. J. Ment. Retard.* 1990; 95(2):228.

46. Culley, W.J., Goyal, K., Jolly, D.H., Mertz, E.T. Caloric intake of children with Down's syndrome (mongolism). *J. Pediatr.* 1965;66:772.

47. Storm, W. Hypercarotenaemia in children with Down syndrome. *J. Ment. Def. Res.* 1990;34:283.

Chapter 17
Prader-Willi Syndrome

Peggy Pipes

Prader-Willi syndrome evidenced at birth is characterized by hypotonia, genital hypoplasia, developmental delays, hyperphagia, and obesity which begins between 1 and 4 years. It is estimated to occur in 1 of 10,000 to 25,000 live births in all populations.[1] A small deletion of the proximal part of the long arm of the 15th chromosome is found in some but not all affected individuals. Lately, it has become evident that some individuals with this chromosomal deletion do not have the syndrome. Therefore, diagnosis is made on the basis of clinical symptomatology (personal communication, V.A. Holm, 1990). Symptoms that occur in more than 50% of individuals are shown in Table 17-1.

Linear growth charts specific to Prader-Willi syndrome have been prepared by V. Holm.[2] These, as well as the NCHS growth charts (Appendix 2), should be utilized when plotting growth data.

Factors to be Considered in Nutritional Evaluation

Changes in nutrition problems during growth

Infants with the Prader-Willi syndrome are hypotonic at birth. Most have a weak suck, and many require tube feeding initially. Failure to thrive is a common problem during the first year.

Between 1 and 4 years of age a rapid rate of weight gain occurs, which results in obesity unless restrictions are placed on the child's energy intake. Individuals with the Prader-Willi syndrome have less fat-free mass and therefore have lower energy expenditures than the average person of their age and height.[3] In addition, rates of linear growth are less than indicated by family expectations. Food behaviors, such as sneaking, foraging, and gorging, become manifest. Behavior management approaches to controlling this behavior are not successful. Although children with the Prader-Willi syndrome have been shown to be deficient in pancreatic polypeptide, infusion of this appetite-regulating factor makes no difference in the eating behavior of affected children[4] Environmental controls that make food inaccessible are important. Refrigerators, cupboards, and garbage cans need to be locked. Siblings, relatives, school personnel, and others in the child's food environment need to understand and develop procedures to control food availability in other settings.

As children grow older, other behaviors become a problem. Temper tantrums must be controlled. Stealing money to buy food and sack lunches from classmates and eating garbage from the school cafeteria may be observed. Shoplifting food sometimes occurs. It becomes apparent that independent living is not possible for individuals with the Prader-Willi syndrome, and plans for future placement need to be investigated.

During late adolescence or early adulthood, group home placement is generally considered. The most successful placements are in group homes designed specifically for individuals with the Prader-Willi syndrome. These homes have strict control of food available to residents. Most are designed so the kitchen and its contents, as well as garbage cans, are locked.

Dietary and Other Treatment

The multiplicity of conditions requiring intervention, the changes in clinical symptomatology as children grow older, and family adjustments required to rear children with the Prader-Willi syndrome make an interdisciplinary team the best approach to treatment. Children require ongoing intervention from a pediatrician, nutritionist, educator, and/or behaviorist and social worker. Physical and/or occupational therapy may be needed during infancy and early childhood. Psychological evaluations will be needed during the

Table 17–1. Symptoms of the Prader-Willi Syndrome

Percentage of Affected Individuals	
100%	50% to 90%
Central hypotonia	Small hands and feet
Abnormal delivery	
Poor suck	Skin problems
Delayed motor landmarks	Skin picking
	Easily bruised
Genital hypoplasia/	
cryptorchidism	Oral pathology
	Unusual sticky,
Hyperphagia and obesity	foamy saliva
	Abnormal bite
Dysfunctional CNS performance	
	Scoliosis
Dysmorphic facial features	
Narrow bifrontal diameter	Strabismus
Almond-shaped eyes	
Triangular mouth	Inability to vomit
Short stature	Behavior problems
	Violent outburst
	Temper tantrums

From Holm, V. A. The diagnosis of Prader-Willi syndrome. In: Holm, V. A., Sulzbacher, S., Pipes, P., eds. *The Prader-Willi Syndrome*. Baltimore: University Park Press; 1981.

school years. Speech therapy is often indicated. The use of anorexiant medications has been tried with mixed results.

At all ages nutrition and feeding intervention must be individualized to the needs of the child. Ranges of oral skills occur at birth, while ranges of appropriate energy intakes occur at any age. During infancy, hypotonia may make oral-motor intervention necessary to achieve a suck adequate for nippling. The caloric density of the formula may need to be increased to support adequate growth. Weight gain should be monitored carefully.

During the preschool years, prevention of obesity is the optimal approach. Usual anthropometric measures, such as triceps and subscapular fatfold measurements, are not reliable in estimating total body fat of these individuals.[3] Precise food intake data and calculation of the child's weight response to energy intake will indicate energy needs. In one protocol for establishing energy needs, the parents record as precisely as possible, in household measures, all food that the child consumes.[5] Any food stolen is estimated and recorded. The energy value of food consumed is calculated from these records. To this value the energy cost of weight lost or gained is added or subtracted, using a conversion figure of 7.7 kcal/g of weight change. The child's energy need per centimeter of height is estimated from these data, and a diet plan is designed to effect a weight loss or weight maintenance in growth channel, depending on the child's needs. The diet uses exchange lists (see Chapter 44). An exercise program should be planned and initiated as a part of the daily routine.

If parents are unable or unwilling to measure and record the food intake, reductions in the child's current food intake are based on weight gained during a certain time period. For example, parents of a child who gained an unwanted 500 grams during 30 days would be requested to reduce the child's energy intake by 130 kcal/day (7.7 × 500/30 = 128), which is necessary to prevent further weight gain. An additional reduction in caloric intake is added if it becomes necessary to effect weight loss.

Data collected on preschool and school-aged children with the Prader-Willi syndrome indicate that 8.5 kcal/cm is a reasonable energy intake to effect a slow weight loss and that 10 to 11 kcal/cm of height will maintain appropriate weight in the growth channel. Collected data indicate that energy needs are 37% to 77% of individuals of the same age and sex.[6]

For the obese child, the degree of obesity must be considered when calculating the appropriate food intake. In some cases a diet to maintain current weight may be appropriate. For the grossly obese child, a very slow rate of weight reduction may be attempted; however, linear growth should be monitored frequently. Experience of the author has shown that a weight reduction of 2 lb/month in grossly obese preschool and school-aged handicapped children has not affected their linear growth. Others, however, have reported that restricted calorie intakes did modify linear growth. Wolff[7] noted that children who lost 2% or more their weight per month grew in length at a less than expected rate. Children who either lost less than 2% of their body weight, did

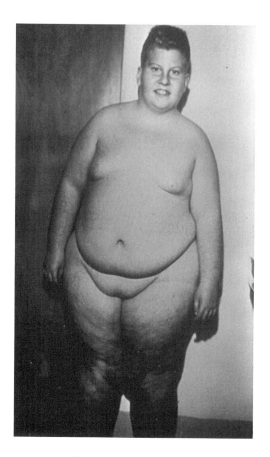
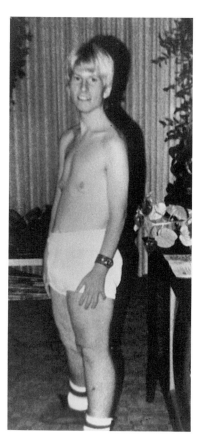

Fig. 17-1. Patient before and after nutrition intervention. Used with permission.

not lose, or gained weight grew at a rate faster than expected. Knittle[8] reported that children on a protein-sparing modified fast diet may experience a transient slowed rate of growth but that height percentile 6 months after weight reduction will return to previous channel.

During the later school and adolescent years, an appropriate placement will need to be considered. The placement should have a restricted food environment and nutrition support to design menus and establish appropriate intakes for Prader-Willi residents.

Follow-up

Successful programs of weight management use an interdisciplinary team and include not only the immediate but also the extended family, school personnel, and others in the food environment. Early intervention can prevent or delay the onset of obesity. Parents and children need continued guidance and support as the children grow older (see Figure 17-1 for the results of nutrition intervention). Behavior management and counseling for families are impor-

tant components of treatment programs for children with the Prader-Willi syndrome.

References

1. Cassidy, S.B. Prader-Willi syndrome characteristics, management and etiology. *Alabama J. Med. Ser.* 1987; 24:170.
2. Holm, V.A. Appendix A: Growth charts for Prader-Willi syndrome In: Greensway, L.R., Alexander, P.C., eds., *Management of Prader Willi Syndrome.* New York: Springer-Verlag; 1988.
3. Schoeller, D.A., et al. Energy expenditure and body composition in Prader-Willi syndrome. *Metabolism.* 1988; 37:115.
4. Zipf, W.B., Thomas, M.O., Bernston, G.G. Short-term infusion of pancreatic polypeptide: effect on children with Prader-Willi syndrome. *Am. J. Clin. Nutr.* 1990; 51:162.
5. Pipes, P.L. Nutrition management of children with Prader-Willi syndrome, In: Holm, V.A., Sulzbacher, S., Pipes, P. *The Prader-Willi Syndrome.* Baltimore: University Park Press; 1981.
6. Bray, G.A., Dahms, R.S., Swerdlaff, R.N., Fischer, R.H., Atkinson, R.L., Carrel, R.E. The Prader-Willi syndrome: a study of 40 patients and a review of the literature. *Medicine.* 1983; 62:59.
7. Wolff, O.H., Lloyd, J.K. Obesity in childhood. *Proc. Nutr. Soc.* 1973; 32:195.
8. Knittle, J.L., McLaren, D.S., Burman, B. Childhood obesity, In: Suskind, R.M., ed. *Textbook of Pediatric Nutrition.* New York: Raven Press; 1981.

Chapter 18
Rett Syndrome

Peggy Pipes and Vanja Holm

Rett syndrome is a disorder in which infant girls grow and develop normally until 6 to 18 months when developmental stagnation begins and previously acquired skills are lost. Deceleration of head growth begins between 6 and 12 months, and microcephaly becomes evident. Stereotypic hand movements characterized by hand wringing, clapping, tapping, and mouthing appear after purposeful hand movements are lost[1] (Fig. 18-1). Seizures often, though not always, are a problem. Some seizures are resistant to anticonvulsant medication.[2,3] It is estimated that Rett syndrome affects a minimum of 1 in 10,000–12,000 girls.[4] It has never been diagnosed in boys.[5]

Necessary criteria for the diagnosis of Rett syndrome are shown in Table 18-1. Clinical characteristics are divided into four stages (Table 18-2). Girls with Rett syndrome have been described as undernourished, despite good appetites and high-calorie diets.[6] However, obesity has been seen in two adolescents (Pipes & Holm, unpublished data, 1984).

Table 18–1. Diagnostic Criteria for Rett Syndrome

Apparently normal prenatal and perinatal period
Apparently normal psychomotor development through the first 6 months
Normal head circumference at birth
Deceleration of head growth between ages 5 months and 4 years
Loss of acquired purposeful hand skills between ages 6 and 30 months, temporarily associated with communication dysfunction and social withdrawal
Development of severely impaired expressive and receptive language and presence of apparent severe psychomotor retardation
Stereotypic hand movements, such as hand wringing/squeezing, clapping/tapping, mouthing, and "washing"/rubbing automatisms, appearing after purposeful hand skills are lost
Appearance of gait apraxia and truncal apraxia-ataxia between ages 1 and 4 years
Diagnosis tentative until 2 to 5 years of age

From Trevathan & Naidu,[3] with permission.

All individuals with Rett syndrome derive pleasure from food and have strong food preferences.[6]

Biochemical Abnormalities

The etiology of the syndrome remains unknown.[7] An inborn error of metabolism has been hypothesized to be the cause, and ultrasound investigation of the muscle has confirmed the presence of dumbbell-shaped mitochondria.[8] There is some speculation that carbohydrate metabolism may be involved. Haas and others[9] reported elevations of blood pyruvate in six of seven girls aged 5–10 years. Blood lactate levels were marginally elevated. Two had elevated blood glucose levels. Minimally elevated ammonia levels were found in three of five tested, two of whom were on valproic acid.[9]

Factors to be Considered in Nutritional Evaluation

Factors that need to be considered when planning for nutrition intervention change with age and must be individualized to the child. As with other children, physical growth, oral motor patterns, self-help skills, and current weight status are important.

Physical growth

Growth retardation defined as linear growth below the 5th percentile is often but not always a characteristic of the

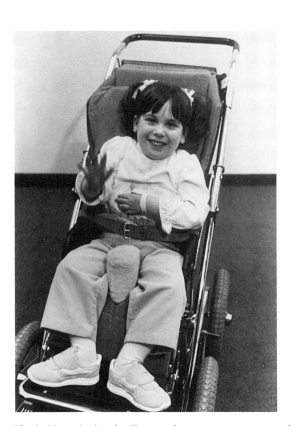

Fig. 18–1. Note the hand splints used to prevent movement in a 3-year-old girl with Rett syndrome. Used with permission.

Table 18–2. Rett Syndrome: Clinical Characteristics and Differential Diagnosis by Stage

Stages	Clinical Characteristics
Stage 1 Onset: 6–18 mo Duration: months	Developmental stagnation Deceleration of head/brain growth Disinterest in play activity and environment Hypotonia EEG background: normal or minimal slowing of posterior rhythm
Stage II Onset: 1–3 yr Duration: weeks to months	Rapid developmental regression with irritability Loss of hand use Seizures Hand stereotypies: wringing, clapping, tapping, mouthing Autistic manifestations Loss of expressive language Insomnia Self-abusive behavior (chewing fingers, slapping face) EEG: background slowing and gradual loss of normal sleep activity; focal or multifocal spike and wave
Stage III Onset: 2–10 yr Duration: months to years	Severe mental retardation, apparent dementia Amelioration of autistic features Seizures Typical hand stereotypies: wringing, tapping, mouthing Prominent ataxia and apraxia Hyperreflexia and progressive rigidity Hyperventilation, breath-holding, aerophagia during waking Weight loss with excellent appetite Early scoliosis Bruxism EEG: gradual disappearance of posterior rhythm, generalized slowing, absent vertex and spindle activity, epileptiform abnormalities activated during sleep
Stage IV Onset: 10+ yr Duration: years	Progressive scoliosis, muscle wasting, and rigidity Decreasing mobility, wheelchair-bound Growth retardation Improved eye contact Virtual absence of expressive and receptive language Trophic disturbance of feet Reduced seizure frequency EEG: poor background organization with marked slowing and multifocal spikes and slow spike and wave pattern activated by sleep

From: Trevathan & Naidu,[3] with permission.

syndrome. Holm[10] found only 10 of 21 girls ages 2 years and 3 months to 26½ years with linear growth that plotted below the 5th percentile. Eight of the remaining girls had measurements that had shifted downward in percentile on the growth charts. One was above average, and two were at the 50th percentile.[10] In another study, the mean age of menarche of six girls was 11 years, two months, an appropriate age for sexual development.[9]

Scoliosis appears to be present in about 50% of girls and occurs most frequently in the second decade.[11]

Oral motor dysfunction

Oral motor dysfunction is present in many girls with Rett syndrome. A survey of ten girls ages 2 years and three months to 16 years found that 70% drooled, 40% had poor lip closure, 10% had a bite reflex, and 10% had no gag reflex. Difficulty in consuming liquids was a problem of 80% of the girls. Thick liquids were easier to consume than thin liquids (Pipes & Holm, unpublished data, 1984).

Self-feeding

Most girls with Rett syndrome learn to feed themselves. Some girls lose self-feeding skills,[12] but then relearn them. Finger feeding is often the method of choice. Adapted utensils may be necessary (see Chapter 24).

Nutrition concerns

Nutrition concerns range from wasting and emaciation to overweight and obesity. Constipation requiring dietary intervention, which may affect appetite, is a problem of all girls with Rett syndrome. A ketogenic diet may be prescribed to control seizures.

Adaptations in food texture may be necessary. Soft chopped foods are often consumed in stage 3 of the syndrome. Pureed foods are offered to approximately 10% of girls with Rett syndrome.[6]

Dietary Management

The range of nutrition concerns mandate that intervention must be individualized. Therapy is most likely to focus on increasing weight of the undernourished, resolving constipation, and in some instances, controlling seizures with a ketogenic diet.

Increases in energy intake to effect weight gain for the undernourished child may require increasing the caloric density of the food offered by adding fat and sugar; using high-calorie, nutrient-dense beverages and/or supplements; and providing carefully planned snacks and bedtime feedings.

Constipation, which affects every girl with Rett syndrome, may respond to a high fiber intake. Parents report positive effects from bran, prunes and prune juice, and increased fruits and vegetables. Liquid intakes should be maintained or increased. Thickening the liquids may make them more acceptable. (Pipes & Holm, unpublished data, 1984).

A ketogenic diet may be prescribed for control of intractable seizures that do not respond to anticonvulsant therapy. Rice[6] describes a diet using medium-chain triglyceride (MCT) oil with a calorie distribution of 60% MCT oil, 10% other fats, 10% carbohydrate, and 20% protein. The diet, which was initiated in a three-step process, began with a fast to achieve ketosis; followed by feeding one-half of the prescribed calories, carbohydrate, and MCT oil for 24 hours;

and finally advancing the diet to the full prescription as tolerated. Monitoring patients for side effects, which included hypoglycemia, gas, vomiting, and diarrhea, determined how quickly the diet could be advanced to full prescription. Adjustments were then made dependent on weight gain, appetite tolerance of the fat, and seizure control. (For more detailed explanation of the MCT diet, see Chapter 8). Four patients who remained on the diet for 2 years demonstrated dramatic increases in weight; one patient actually doubled her weight.[6]

Nutrient supplements are appropriate for most girls with Rett syndrome. Those on anticonvulsants should be monitored biochemically and appropriate supplements prescribed. For other girls, supplements should complement the nutrients already consumed in food.

Follow-up

Until the etiology of Rett syndrome is determined, nutrition intervention is designed to respond to the symptoms presented. Individuals consuming a ketogenic diet should be monitored carefully for side effects of the MCT oil. The effect of anticonvulsants on vitamin D and folate metabolism should be determined periodically.

Physical growth and weight gain of all girls with the syndrome need to be followed. Adjustments in energy intake and food textures may need to be made as growth and development proceed. Some individuals may profit from oral motor therapy; others may benefit from learning self-feeding. An interdisciplinary team consisting of a pediatrician, nutritionist, behaviorist, occupational therapist, and social worker, remains the optimal approach to the nutrition care of these girls.

References

1. Rett, A. Cerebral atrophy associated with hyperammonaemia. In: Vinken, P.J., Bruyn, G.W., eds. *Handbook of Clinical Neurology*, Vol. 29. Amsterdam: North-Holland, 1977.
2. Hagberg, B., Aicardi, J., Dias, K., Ramos, O. A progressive syndrome of autism, dementia, ataxia and loss of purposeful hand use in girls: Rett syndrome: report of 35 cases. *Ann. Neurol.* 1983; 14:471.
3. Trevathan, E., Naidu, S. The clinical recognition and differential diagnosis of Rett syndrome. *J. Child. Neurol.* 1988; 3:S6.
4. Engerstrom, I. Rett syndrome in Sweden. Neurodevelopment-disability-pathophysiology. *Acta Paediatr. Scand.* 1990; 369(suppl):1.
5. Trevathan, E., Adams, M.J. The epidemiology and public health significance of Rett syndrome. *J. Child. Neurol.* 1988; 3:S17.
6. Rice, A., Haas, R.H. The nutritional aspects of Rett syndrome. *J. Child. Neurol.* 1988; 3:S35.
7. Hagberg, B. Rett syndrome: clinical peculiarities diagnostic approach, and possible cause. *Pediatr. Neurol.* 1989; 5:75.
8. Wahai, S., Vameda, K., Ishihowa, Y., Miyamoto, S., Nagaoka, M., Okabe, M., Minami, R., Tachi, N. Rett syndrome: findings suggesting axonopathy and mitochondrial abnormalities. *Pediatr. Neurol.* 1990; 6:339.
9. Haas, R.H., Rice, M.A., Trauner, D.A., Merritt, T.A. Therapeutic effects of a ketogenic diet in Rett syndrome. *Am. J. Med. Genet.* 1986; 24:225.
10. Holm. V.A. Physical growth and development in patients with Rett syndrome. *Am. J. Med. Genet.* 1986; 24:119.
11. Bassett, G., Tolo, V. The incidence and natural history of scoliosis in Rett syndrome. *Dev. Med. Child. Neurol.* 1990; 21:963.
12. Perry, A. Rett syndrome. A comprehensive review of the literature. *Am. J. Ment. Retard.* 1991; 96:275.

Chapter 19
Obesity

Shirley Walberg Ekvall, Linda Bandini, and Valli Ekvall

Obesity is the result of an excess accumulation of body fat. Increases in body fat are caused by an energy imbalance that occurs when energy intake exceeds energy expenditure. The causes of this energy imbalance are multifactorial and may include genetic, metabolic, psychological, and environmental factors.

Obesity is a serious nutritional disease in the United States, affecting an estimated 5% to 25% of children and adolescents.[1] It is estimated that 80% of obese adolescents will remain obese into childhood.[2] Approximately one-half to three-quarters of adults who were in excess of 160% of ideal body weight (IBW) were reportedly obese as children.[3] Obesity occurs in 50% of children with myelodysplasia[4] and is a characteristic of Prader-Willi syndrome.[5] Our clinical experience suggests that the prevalence of obesity in children and adolescents with spastic quadriparesis may be significant. Children with Down syndrome also are at risk for the development of obesity.

The pathophysiology of obestiy[6] can be found in Appendix 10. Childhood obesity is associated with an increased prevalence of hypertension[7] and can also lead to orthopedic problems and impaired glucose tolerance.[5] In addition to medical complications, obesity is also accompanied by negative social and psychological factors.

In the child who is physically disabled, obesity may further impair mobility and the development of progress in gross motor skills. It may reduce the child's ability to ambulate, thus decreasing the energy spent in activity and increasing the likelihoood that the child will remain obese. A child who is obese and physically disabled may cause increased burdens for parents and caregivers who provide assistance with activities of daily living. Obesity in the child with a handicap may make him appear even more different from the general population of children.

Identification of obesity in the child and adolescent will depend upon the criteria used. Because laboratory measures of body composition, such as underwater weighing, K^{40} counting, and measures of total body water, are too expensive and laborious to be used in clinical settings, anthropometric measures have been used to assess obesity in children and adolescents.[8] Measures of weight for height and triceps skinfold (TSF) are the most commonly used anthropometric indices. Roche et al.[9] have shown that both relative weight and the TSF are highly correlated to body fatness in both children and adolescents.

Obesity is characterized by an increase in adipose mass; thus, the development of this tissue is of great significance. Increases in adipose tissue occur as both an increase in fat cell size (hypertrophy) and fat cell number (hyperplasia). In normal-weight children the pattern of adipose tissue development consists of increases of both fat cell size and number up to 2 years of age. From age 2 through the onset of puberty there is little change in fat cell number. At puberty another increase in the number of fat cells occurs. This suggests that before age 2 and during adolescence a child is susceptible to hyperplastic obesity. Although fat cell size can be reduced, fat cell number cannot.

Although infancy through age 2 and the onset of puberty are critical periods in the susceptibility to obesity, increases in fat cell size can occur with increases in body weight at any time. Therefore, it is important that children at high risk for obesity be followed closely throughout childhood and adolescence.

Biochemical and Clinical Abnormalities

Biochemical assessment

Biochemical tests rarely provide answers to the etiology of obesity. Hypothyroidism is not a common cause of obesity in children or adolescents. However, thyroid function, fasting blood sugar, cholesterol, triglycerides, and liver function tests may be of some benefit in determining the etiology in some children.

Energy balance

An individual is in energy balance when energy intake equals energy expenditure. When energy intake exceeds energy expenditure, the excess calories are stored as adipose tissue. Relatively small excesses in energy intake that are maintained for long periods of time produce significant increases in body fat.

Clearly, children and adolescents become obese because energy intake exceeds energy expenditure. However, it is not clear whether obesity is the result of an excessive intake or a reduced energy expenditure. Studies reported in the literature do not suggest that obese children, adolescents, or adults eat more than their nonobese peers.[10-15] Nonetheless, the problems associated with obtaining accurate data from dietary intakes have been well documented.[13]

In a study in which energy intake and energy expenditure were measured simultaneously in obese and nonobese adolescents, both groups were found to report intakes that were significantly lower than energy expenditure.[16] Furthermore, reported energy intake as a percentage of daily energy expenditure was found to be significantly lower in the obese than nonobese. These findings are similar to those reported by Prentice et al.[17] who found reported energy intake as a percentage of daily energy expenditure to be significantly lower in obese than in nonobese women.

There have been several explanations for the inaccuracies in dietary intakes. It has been speculated that dietary behaviors may be changed from the usual pattern when keeping a diet record. Furthermore, the obese person may be ashamed or embarrassed about the amounts of food consumed and thus may underreport them. Errors in portion size may also contribute to the inaccuracies in reporting.

Because of the numerous problems with dietary intake methodology, recent research has focused on the role of energy expenditure in the development of obesity. Daily energy expenditure includes the basal metabolic rate, the thermic effect of food, the energy required for growth, and the energy spent in physical activity.

Basal metabolic rate. The basal metabolic rate (BMR) is the amount of energy required to maintain life processes and comprises 50% to 75% of the total energy expenditure (TEE). BMR can be measured by indirect calorimetry (Fig 19–1) or can be predicted on the basis of body size, body weight, and body height. A nomogram[18] (Fig 19–2) may be used to estimate body surface area. BMR can be calculated using standards for calories expended per square meter (Table 19–1; See Chapter 24 for BMR for children under 6 years of age). The FAO/WHO/UNU equations can be used to predict BMR from body weight or from body weight and height[19] (see Chapter 4).

Studies in both children[20,21] and adults[22,23] have shown that BMR is higher in the obese than nonobese when expressed in absolute terms (kcal/day), but is lower when expressed per kilogram of body weight. These findings can be attributed to the greater body size in the obese person. Because BMR is highly correlated with fat-free mass (FFM), recent studies have compared the relationship of BMR and FFM in obese and nonobese individuals. In adolescents, Bandini et al.[24] found that BMR adjusted for differences in FFM was higher in the obese than nonobese.

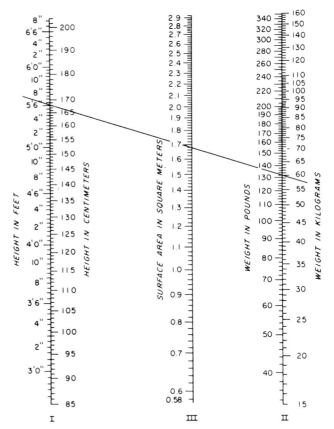

Fig. 19–2. Nomogram for calculating surface area. From Pike & Brown,[18] with permission.

These findings suggest that a reduction in BMR cannot be responsible for the maintenance of obesity in normal adolescents. Studies of metabolic rate in individuals with developmental disabilities and physical handicaps are limited. The only study reported on resting metabolic rate (RMR) of adolescents with myelomeningocele or myelodysplasia found metabolic rate to be significantly lower than in adolescents of normal weight.[25] The authors attributed the reduction in metabolic rate to the decrease in FFM observed in adolescents with myelodysplasia. Similar findings were apparent in individuals with the Prader-Willi syndrome, suggesting that metabolic rate is not altered but that decreases are due to a change in body composition.[26]

Thermic effect of food. The thermic effect of food (TEF) is the increase in energy expenditure observed after a meal. This increase is thought to be the result of the energy costs of digestion, transport, and storage of nutrients. Some studies in adults have suggested that adults who are obese have a decrease in the TEF.[27,28] In the two studies in children and adolescents in which the thermic effect of food was measured, no differences were found between obese and nonobese groups.[29,30]

Physical activity. The energy cost of physical activity is the third major component of TEE. Studies of activity among obese and nonobese children and adolescents have yielded conflicting results. In a study that used motion picture sampling to assess activity, the level of activity of obese girls at

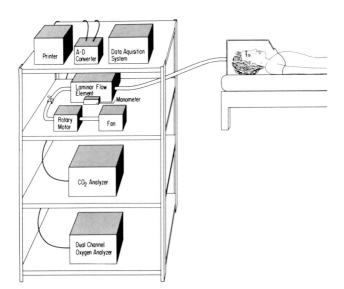

Fig. 19–1. Schematic drawing of an indirect calorimeter used for the measurement of metabolic rate. From L. Bandini, Massachusetts Institute of Technology. Used with permission.

Table 19–1. The Mayo Clinic Normal Standards (cal/sq m/hour)

Males		Females	
Age at Last Birthday	Mean (cal/m²/hr)	Age at Last Birthday	Mean (cal/m²/hr)
6	53.00	6	50.62
7	52.45	6½	50.23
8	51.78	7	49.12
8½	51.20	7½	47.84
9	50.54	8	47.00
9½	49.42	8½	46.50
10	48.50	9–10	45.90
10½	47.71	11	45.26
11	47.18	11½	44.80
12	46.75	12	44.28
13–15	46.35	12½	43.58
16	45.72	13	42.90
16½	45.30	13½	42.10
17	44.80	14	41.45
17½	44.03	14½	40.74
18	43.25	15	40.10
18½	42.70	15½	39.40
19	42.32	16	38.85
19½	42.00	16½	38.30
20–21	41.43	17	37.82
22–23	40.82	17½	37.40
24–27	40.24	18–19	36.74
28–29	39.81	20–24	36.18
30–34	39.34	25–44	35.70
35–39	38.68	45–49	34.94
40–44	38.00	50–54	33.96
45–49	37.37	55–59	33.18
50–54	36.73	60–64	32.61
55–59	36.10	65–69	32.30
60–64	35.48	*	
65–69	34.80		

*Obtain numbers beyond 69 by extrapolation. From Pike & Brown,[18] with permission.

summer camp was found to be less than that of nonobese girls.[31] Other investigators, however, found no differences in the activity levels of obese and nonobese adolescents determined from activity diaries.[10,11] Waxman and Stunkard found obese boys to be far less active than their controls at home, slightly less active outside the home, and equally active at the playground. However, the obese boys expended more calories in moving than the nonobese boys. Thus, the authors concluded that energy expenditure outside the home and at the playground was greater in obese than in the nonobese boys (see the section on physical activity in Chapter 4).

Daily energy expenditure. There is little information on the daily energy expenditure of children and adolescents. With the recent development of the doubly-labeled water method for the measurement of TEE in humans, daily energy expenditure can now be measured in free-living individuals.

The doubly-labeled water method is a type of indirect calorimetry that measures the rate of CO_2 production.[32] With the knowledge of the food quotient of the diet and CO_2 production,[33] daily energy expenditure can be determined. The method is noninvasive and nonrestrictive, requiring only periodic measurement of body fluids. It has been used for the measurement of TEE in several pediatric

populations, including obese and nonobese adolescents,[24] adolescents with myelodysplasia[25] and children and adolescents with Prader-Willi syndrome.[26] TEE was higher in obese than nonobese adolescents. Prader-Willi subjects were found to have a lower TEE than either obese or nonobese subjects.[26] These differences were attributed to a decrease in both FFM and activity. These findings are supported by those of Pipes and Holm[34] who found it necessary to reduce caloric consumption to 8.5 kcal/cm of height to produce effective weight loss and to 10–11 kcal/cm for weight maintenance in four boys with Prader-Willi syndrome[34] (see Chapter 17).

Similar findings were found in subjects with myelodysplasia. FFM was significantly reduced in adolescents with myelodysplasia.[25] TEE and the ratio of TEE/RMR (Fig. 19–3), which is a measure of the energy expended over resting, were significantly lower in the myelodysplasia subjects than in normal adolescents. Furthermore, the ratio of TEE/RMR was significantly lower in paraplegics than in those who could ambulate. These findings suggest that adolescents with myelodysplasia have a reduced energy expenditure due both to a decrease in FFM and a decrease in physical activity. These findings are supported by those of Grogan and Ekvall[35] who found a significant correlation between lean body mass or FFM determined by K[40] counting and physical activity determined by the physical activity score[35] (see Chapters 4 and 10). In this group of children 8–14 years of age with myelodysplasia and minimal physical activity FFM was reduced and weight loss was minimal when caloric

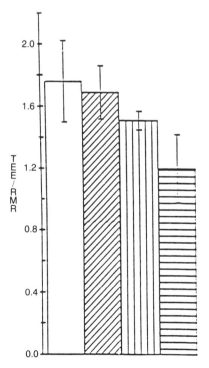

Fig. 19–3. Bandini et al.[24,25] Comparison of energy expenditure above resting in normal obese and adolescents with myelodysplacia. Group: ▢ normal; ▨ obese; ▥ myelodysplasia ambulatory; ▤ myelodysplasia nonambulatory.

intake was only 7 cal/cm and maintenance requirements were only 9–11 kcal/cm ht.[35] Ambulation also related to obesity in this population[36] (further suggesting that energy needs are related to active FFM rather than the less vascular adipose tissue).

Several investigators have estimated energy needs in physically handicapped children on the basis of body height. Berg and Isaksson[37] found that cerebral palsy subjects with normal physical activity needed 15 kcal/cm, whereas those with decreased physical activity required 10 kcal/cm per day. Culley and Middleton[38] did not measure energy expenditure directly in children with cerebral palsy, but categorized energy needs based on caloric intake in 5- to 11-year-old children according to the degree of motor dysfunction. Children with CP with mild to moderate motor dysfunction needed 13.9 kcal/cm, whereas those with severe impairment needed 11.1 kcal/cm.[38] For children with Down's syndrome, caloric intakes of boys and girls were estimated to be 16.1 kcal/cm for boys and 14.3 kcal/cm for girls (Table 19–2). Bandini et al., measured energy expenditure in adolescent children with CP. Energy expenditure was: 9.0–12.5 kcal/cm ht for those with spastic quadriparesis and 10.6–16.1 kcal/cm ht for two adolescents with athetosis.[25]

Factors to be Considered in Nutritional Evaluation

Family variables have been shown to be related to childhood obesity. The fatness level of children with two heavy parents has been reported to be three times the fatness level of children with two lean parents.[39] Obesity has been shown to be higher in children whose parents are divorced[40] and in families where the father has died.[41] Whether these factors are as significant for children with developmental disorders is not clear.

Clinical assessment

Obesity has been defined clinically as weight 20% above the standard desirable weight; *overweight* is body weight 10% to 20% above the standard desirable weight. A plot of weight for height on a growth chart allows for a rough approximation of the severity of obesity. In general, a child's ideal weight should correspond to his or her height percentile. Weight for height, or percent of ideal body weight, is calculated by dividing actual weight by the child's weight for height.[5]

Two important determinants of the natural history of childhood obesity are severity and age of onset.[42] Although the incidence rate remains stable throughout childhood and adolescence, the remission rate appears to decrease with advancing age.[42] Thus, obesity of later onset is more likely to persist. It is estimated that approximately 1½ years of weight maintenance is required to achieve IBW for each 20% increment in excess of ideal.[1] Thus, it is clearly evident that both the risk of after-effects and persistence rise with increasing severity.[42] Therefore, weight reduction before or during adolescence may help prevent adult obesity.

Measures of relative weight are limited by the fact that they do not take body composition into consideration. For example, some athletes, such as college football linemen, may be overweight because of an increase in muscle mass,

Table 19–2. Estimated Calorie Requirements for Specific Developmental Disabilities (according to individual heights)*

Developmental Disability	Guide for Caloric Intake
Down syndrome[38] Results from an extra 21 chromosome causing developmental problems, such as congenital heart disease, mental retardation, small stature, and decreased tone	Boys 16.1 kcal/cm (40.9 kcal/in) Girls 14.3 kcal/cm (36.3 kcal/in)
Prader-Willi syndrome[34] A disorder characterized by uncontrollable eating habits, inability to distinguish hunger from appetite, severe obesity, poorly developed genitalia, and moderate to severe mental retardation	10–11 kcal/cm (26.7 kcal/in) for maintenance 8.5 kcal/cm (21.6 kcal/in) for weight loss
Spina bifida (myelomeningocele)[35,36] Results from a midline defect of the skin, spinal column, and spinal cord; characterized by hydrocephalus, mental retardation, and lack of muscular control	9–11 kcal/cm (25.0 kcal/in) for maintenance or estimate LBM or AT 7 kcal/cm (17.78 kcal/in) for weight loss (or about 50% of kcal level of child without myelomeningocele) if weight is above the 50th percentile, has minimal physical activity, and > 3 years of age. After age 6 may be determined by AT or LBM. Keep < 25th percentile weight for age.
Cerebral palsy[38] A disorder of muscle control or coordination resulting from injury to the brain during its early (fetal, perinatal, and early childhood) stages of development. There may be associated problems with intellectual, visual, or other functions.	13.9 kcal/cm (35.3 kcal/in) 5–11 years; mild-moderate activity level 11.1 kcal/cm (28.2 kcal/in) 5–11 years; severe restrictions

*Guide for caloric intake references can be found in chapters on that disorder.
Modified from: Rokusek, C., Heinrichs, E., eds. *Nutrition and feeding for the Developmentally Disabled. A How To Manual.* Vermillion, SD: South Dakota University Affiliated Facility Center for the Developmentally Disabled; 1985. Used with permission.

not body fat. Body fat assessment in the normal obese adolescent may be complicated by the fact that excess weight is due to both fat and fat-free mass. Therefore, ideal body weight may be underestimated if the excess fat-free tissue is not taken into consideration.

Skinfold thickness is a measure of subcutaneous fat. When the diagnosis of obesity is questionable, a measure of skinfold thickness should be made. Sex- and age-specific standards for skinfold thickness are available.[43] Obesity may be diagnosed by a triceps skinfold thickness greater than the 85th percentile or by a weight for height greater than 120% of the ideal controlled for age and sex.[1] (see Chapter 4 and midarm circumference and triceps skinfold standards and grids in Appendix 8.) Obesity has been defined as body fat > 30% for prepubertal children, > 25% for pubertal boys, and > 30% for pubertal girls.[44] A method of calculating body fat percentage from the sum of biceps, triceps, subscapular, and suprailiac skinfold thicknesses is presented in Table 19–3 by using prediction equations based on measures of body density.[44] In extremely fat children—sum of four skinfold thicknesses > 120-140 mm—skinfold thickness cannot be used to estimate body fat percentage.

The diagnosis of obesity in the child with a handicap is complicated by the fact that growth often differs significantly from the norm. Children with myelodysplasia and Prader-Willi syndrome are of short stature and often below the 5th percentile of height for age. Thus, the growth charts are inadequate to determine IBW and the degree of obesity. The triceps skinfold (TSF) may not be an accurate assessment of body fatness in paraplegic children because there may be an alteration in fat distribution. In adolescents with myelodysplasia, TSF significantly underestimates the prevalence of obesity determined from measurements of total body water.[45] Furthermore, it has been shown that fatness increases over paralyzed limbs.[46] In a small sample of subjects with Prader-Willi syndrome, body fatness measured directly by the isotope dilution technique was considerably different from that calculated from skinfold thickness.[26]

These preliminary data suggest that specific anthropometric indices need to be developed to assess accurately body fatness in children who are developmentally disabled. Data by Grogan and Ekvall[35] on children with myelomeningocele or myelodysplasia found that the abdominal skinfold correlated best with the child's fatness as determined from K[40] counting. Each developmental disability should be considered with reference to current research on growth, body composition, and caloric requirements.

Criteria for selecting patients for a weight control program vary with each facility. The guidelines of the Nutrition Department at the University Affiliated Cincinnati Center for Developmental Disorders for identifying children at high risk for obesity are as follows:

- children with a family history of heart disease
- children with one or both parents and/or siblings who are obese
- children who show a tendency toward a discrepancy of weight for height (> 10% overweight for height or weight above 75th percentile), especially those from birth to 4 years of age and those entering adolescence (9–13 years of age).
- children with greater than 25% immobility determined from physical activity score (see Chapter 4) and above 50th percentile in weight for age
- children with Down syndrome, Prader-Willi syndrome, cretinism, myelomeningocele, spastic cerebral palsy, or Rubinstein-Taybi or Klinefelter's syndrome.

Management

The most successful treatment of this disease is *prevention*. However, obesity is a complex problem and is best treated using an interdisciplinary approach. The four-pronged treatment program has been found to be successful. This approach combines nutritional counseling, exercise, behavior modification, and emotional or family support.

Nutritional counseling

Diet remains the cornerstone of effective weight reduction. Although caloric restriction is necessary to promote a negative energy balance, it should be initiated with caution in the obese child. Growing children require energy to support adequate growth. Thus, the key is to provide the right amount of calories that will allow for weight maintenance and at the same time support growth. Recommended amounts of nutrients are also vital for proper physical maturation. Any prescribed diet must contain adequate amounts of carbohydrate, fat, protein, vitamins, and minerals to promote good health. A suggested easy scheme to follow is the familiar Basic Four Food Groups.[47] If an adequate number of servings are consumed from each food group, most of the recommended dietary allowances will be met.

Table 19–3. Skinfold Thicknesses* at Different Body Fat Percentages in Children Aged 0–18 Years

Age	Percent Body Fat, Male					Percent Body Fat, Female				
	15%	20%	25%	30%	35%	15%	20%	25%	30%	35%
					(mm)					
0+	17	22	30	40	52	17	22	30	40	52
1+	18	24	32	43	58	18	24	32	43	58
2	18	25	34	45	60	18	25	34	45	60
4	20	27	37	51	68	18	25	34	46	62
6	22	30	41	57	78	19	25	35	47	63
8	23	33	46	64	88	19	26	35	47	65
10	25	36	51	72	101	19	27	37	51	69
12	27	40	57	81	115	21	30	42	58	80
14	27	44	63	92	132	23	33	47	66	92
16	32	48	71	104	152	25	37	53	75	106
18	34	52	79	117	175	27	40	58	85	122

*Sum of bicipital, tricipital, suprailiac, and subscapular skinfold thicknesses.
†Mean age was used (6 mo).
‡Mean age was used (18 mo).
Modified from Weststrate & Deurenberg,[44] with permission.

The child and family should also be aware of the energy content of foods. The diet counselor should explain to the family and child that a calorie is a measure of energy contained in all foods and that the body requires energy to function properly. The child and family should be informed that those foods that are high in fat and sugar are generally high in calories. Although no food should be forbidden, the child who is obese should learn to eat foods that supply essential nutrients without excess calories. By being made aware of low-calorie alternatives, the child thereby should be able to make wise food choices.

Weight and calorie goals for children who are obese should be determined according to the age and body composition (FFM or adipose tissue) of the child. The initial goal for all overweight children is to stop gaining weight. The weight for height ratio can be determined and the caloric needs based on this ratio. The weight change should be a behavioral objective, with the goal, method, and timetable determined. Unusual eating behaviors in association with obesity also must be addressed.[48-52]

Because physicians often feel unprepared to provide dietary counseling, it is essential for the nutritionist/dietitian to do so.[53]

Exercise

Another important factor required to promote weight loss is an increase in energy expenditure, which can be accomplished through an increase in physical activity. During childhood increases in daily lifestyle activity, such as climbing stairs and walking, may be easier to comply with than a programmed exercise activity. Comparison between programmed activity versus lifestyle activity showed equivalent short-term effects, but long-term advantages were greater in the lifestyle approach because of a higher rate of compliance.[54] Nevertheless, either behavior will increase energy output and loss of body fat.[55-57] In the child with a handicap, achieving increases in physical activity may be difficult. The assistance of a physical therapist may be useful in designing an activity appropriate for specific individual needs.

Behavior modification

A successful weight loss program may include techniques to change behavior (see Appendix 9, Eating Attitudes Test Multidimensional Inventory, and Depression Inventory). Both changes in diet and in activity involve difficult alterations in behavior; thus, counseling of techniques by which to modify these behaviors is necessary. The patient should initially be instructed to keep a detailed record of eating habits, noting the time, types and quantities of foods eaten and the emotional state surrounding mealtimes. This record will identify undesirable behaviors.

Weight control is more successful when achieved by a series of steps within a long-term process. Each step involves the alteration of an undesirable behavior. Every step should be reinforced through rewards to promote adoption and retention of the new behavior. The most common types of reinforcement include: verbal praise delivered immediately after the desired behavior and tangible rewards, such as toys or increases in allowance. Children respond both to social reinforcement and to tangible rewards from parents, sib-

lings, peers, and teachers. These rewards can be used effectively in a weight control program when channeled directly to the child to encourage eating well and exercise.[58] In the UACCDD Nutrition Department, the reward of a watch produced weight loss (Fig. 19–4). Other behavioral approaches such as signed contracts and group programs which provide peer support have also reported positive outcomes.[51,59]

Two critical components of successful behavior modification programs are individualization and an emphasis on the role others play in the social control of the patient.

Emotional or family support

Parents exert a powerful influence on the eating activity and attitude patterns of their children. They can help control a child's weight by determining the type and amount of food that enters the house. Family attitudes toward food also influence the child's eating habits as the child readily adopts the family's value system concerning food. For example, if the family equates large portions and a full refrigerator with generosity and hospitality, the child is more apt to become an overeater. If all of the family's recreational activities are centered around food, the child is likely to have a large appetite.

Family support is very important in the promotion of healthful eating. There are several advantages to a family-oriented approach to treatment.

- Obesity is redefined as a family problem, rather than the problem of the child only.
- Blame is not placed exclusively on the child.
- Strategies for increasing effectiveness are developed.

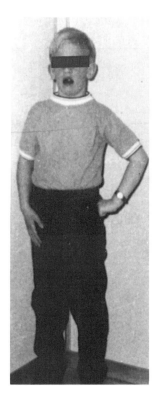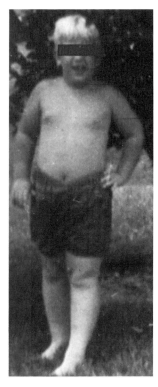

Fig. 19–4. Picture of child with watch after weight loss and before weight loss.

If the adolescent who is obese feels isolated and has little family involvement, efforts need to be focused on increased family interactional skills and behavioral education.[60] Brownell et al.[61] have shown that the nature of parental involvement is a significant determinant of the weight loss success rate. The results of this study indicated that a weight loss program administered separately to the child and mother produced the most successful short- and long-term results. This method of treatment (1) provided training for both parents and children, (2) allowed free discussion by both parents and children, and (3) gave the children more responsibility and better control than when the parents did not participate. Epstein et al. also found parental involvement to be a key factor in the maintenance of weight loss. However, in contrast to Brownell, Epstein et al. found the most effective program was one in which parents and children were both the targets of weight loss (the eight week session included diet, exercise, behavior, and education).[62]

In the child who is handicapped, energy requirements are often reduced markedly. Parents need to be educated about the nutritional needs of their child, given suggestions for low-calorie snacks, and instructed on portion sizes. Parents often feel guilty about restricting food intake, especially since eating may be one of the few pleasures they can provide. Because care is often shared by several individuals, consistency, plus compassion[63] must be enforced among caregivers. Long term treatment may be necessary.[64]

Follow-up and Research

For a weight reduction program to be successful, it is necessary to provide continued supportive therapy after the program has been completed. The components of this follow-up are similar to those used in the actual treatment—exercise, nutrition counseling, behavioral and emotional support—and are individualized to promote compliance. Many successful weight reductions are short term. Thus, to improve the overall long-term effectiveness of a weight loss program, a follow-up program is required. Working in groups may be an effective method for weight control. The most successful method of treatment is prevention or seeing the child at the early onset of overweight, particularly before age 7 years.[65] Prevention also is more cost effective than treatment of obesity.[66]

Future research is being conducted on energy metabolism at the cellular level which may provide new insights into understanding energy needs in various clinical populations.[67]

References

1. Dietz, W.H. Childhood obesity: susceptibility, cause and management. *J. Pediatr.* 1983; 5:676.
2. Lloyd, J.K., Wolff, O.H., Whelan, W.S. Childhood obesity. *Br. Med. J.* 1961; 2:145.
3. Rimm, I.J., Rimm, A.A. Association between juvenile onset obesity and severe adult obesity in 73,532 women. *Am. J. Pub. Health.* 1976; 66:479.
4. Hayes-Allen, M.C., Tring, F.C. Obesity: another hazard for spina bifida children. *Br. J. Prev. Soc. Med.* 1973; 27:192.
5. Dietz, W.H. Nutrition and obesity. In: Grand, R.J., Stephen, J.L., Dietz, W.H., eds. *Pediatric Nutrition, Theory and Practice.* Boston: Butterworth; 1987.
6. Bray, G. Pathophysiology of obesity. *Am. J. Clin. Nutr.* 1992; 55:488S.
7. Rames, L.K., Clarke, W.R., Connor, W.E., Reiter, M.A., Lauer, R.M. Normal blood pressures and the evaluation of sustained blood pressure evaluation in childhood: the muscatine study. *Pediatrics.* 1978; 61:245.
8. Bandini, L.G., Dietz, W.H. Assessment of body fatness in childhood obesity: evaluation of laboratory and anthropometric techniques. *J. Am. Diet. Assoc.* 1987; 87:1344.
9. Roche, A.F., Siervogel, R.M., Chumlea, W.C., Webb, P. Grading body fatness from limited anthropometric data. *Am. J. Clin. Nutr.* 1981; 34:2831.
10. Bradfield, R.B., Paulos, J., Grossman, L. Energy expenditure and heart rate of obese high school girls. *Am. J. Clin. Nutr.* 1971; 24:1482.
11. Stefaniak, P.A., Heald, F.P., Mayer, J. Caloric intake in relation to energy output of obese and non-obese adolescent girls. *Am. J. Clin. Nutr.* 1959; 7:55.
12. Johnson, M.L., Burke, B.S., Mayer, J. Relative importance of inactivity and overeating in the energy balance of obese high school girls. *Am. J. Clin. Nutr.* 1956; 4:37.
13. James, W.P.T., Bingham, S.A., Cole, T.J. Epidemiological assessment of dietary intake. *Nutr. Cancer.* 1981; 2:203.
14. Beaudoin, R., Mayer, J. Food intake of obese and non-obese women. *J. Am. Diet. Assoc.* 1953; 29:29.
15. Waxman, M., Stunkard, A.J. Caloric intake and expenditure of obese boys. *J. Pediatr.* 1980; 96:187.
16. Bandini, L.G., Schoeller, D.A., Cyr, H., Dietz, W.H. Comparison of energy intake and energy expenditure in obese and non-obese adolescents. *Am. J. Clin. Nutr.* 1990; 52:421.
17. Prentice, A.M., Black, A.E., Coward, W.A., Davies, H.L., Goldberg, G.R., Murgatroyd, P.R., Ashford, J., Sawyer, M., Whitehead, R.G. High levels of energy expenditure in obese women. *Br. Med. J.* 1986; 292:983.
18. Pike, R., Brown, M. *Nutrition: An Integrated Approach.* 2nd ed. New York: Wiley and Sons; 1975.
19. WHO: *Energy and Protein Requirements.* Report of a joint FAO/WHO/UNU Expert Committee. Geneva: World Health Organization; 1985.
20. Bruch, H. Obesity in childhood. II. Basal metabolism and serum cholesterol of obese children. *Am. J. Dis. Child.* 1939; 58:1001.
21. Talbot, N.B., Worcester, J. The basal metabolism of obese children. *J. Pediatr.* 1940; 16:146.
22. James, W.P.T., Davies, H.W., Bailes, J., Dauncey, M.J. Elevated metabolic rates in obesity. *Lancet.* 1978; 1:1122.
23. Ravussin, E., Burnand, B., Schutz, Y., Jequier, E. Twenty-four hour energy expenditure and resting metabolic rate in obese, moderately obese, and control subjects. *Am. J. Clin. Nutr.* 1982; 35:566.
24. Bandini, L.G., Schoeller, D.A., Dietz, W.H. Energy expenditure in obese and non-obese adolescents. *Pediatr. Res.* 1990; 2:197.
25. Bandini, L.G., Schoeller, D.A., Fukagawa, N.K., Wykes, L., Dietz, W.H. Body composition and energy expenditure in adolescents with cerebral palsy or myelodysplasia. *Pediatr. Res.* 1991; 29:70–77.
26. Schoeller, D.A., Levitsky, L.L., Bandini, L.G., Dietz, W.H., Walczak, A. Energy expenditure and body composition in Prader-Willi syndrome. *Metabolism.* 1988; 27:115.
27. Bessard, T., Schutz, Y., Jequier, E. Energy expenditure and postprandial thermogenesis in obese women before and after weight loss. *Am. J. Clin. Nutr.* 1983; 38:680.
28. Segal, K.R., Gutin, B., Nyman, A.M., Pi-Singer, F.X. Thermic effect of food at rest, during exercise and after exercise in lean and obese men of similar body weight. *J. Clin. Invest.* 1985; 76:1107.
29. Molnar, P., Varga, P., Rubecz, I., Hamer, A., Mestyan, J. Food-induced thermogenesis in obese children. *Eur. J. Ped.* 1985; 144:27.
30. Bandini, L.G., Schoeller, D.A., Edwards, J., Young, V.R., Oh, S.H., Dietz, W.H. Energy expenditure during carbohydrate overfeeding in obese and non-obese adolescents. *Am. J. Physiol.* 1989; 256:E357.
31. Bullen, B.A., Reed, R.B., Mayer, J. Physical activity of obese and non-obese adolescent girls appraised by motion picture sampling. *Am. J. Clin. Nutr.* 1964; 14:211.

32. Schoeller, D.A. Measurement of energy expenditure in free-living humans by using doubly labeled water. *J. Nutr.* 1988; 118:1278.

33. Elia, M. Energy equivalents of CO_2 and their importance in assessing energy expenditure when using tracer techniques. *Am. J. Physiol.* 1991; 260(1 Pt. 1):E75.

34. Pipes, P.L., Holm, V.A. Weight control of children with Prader-Willi syndrome. *J. Am. Diet. Assoc.* 1973; 62:520.

35. Grogan, C.B., Ekvall, S. The body composition of spina bifida patients as determined by K40, urinary creatinine, and anthropometric measures. In: *International Union of Nutritional Sciences and Publication Committee of the Tenth International Congress of Nutrition.* Kyoto, Japan: The Science Council of Japan; 1975.

36. Atencio-La Follette, P., Ekvall-Walberg, S., Oppenheimer, S., Grace, E. The effect of lesion level and ambulation on growth measurements in children with myelomeningocele. *J. Am. Diet Assoc.* 1992, in press.

37. Berg, K., Isaksson, B. Body composition and nutrition of school children with cerebral palsy. *Acta Paediatr. Scand.* 1970; 205(suppl):41.

38. Culley, W.J., Middleton, T.O. Caloric requirements of mentally retarded children with and without motor dysfunction. *J. Pediatr.* 1969; 75:380.

39. Garn, S.M., Clark, D.C. Trends in fatness and the origins of obesity. *Pediatrics.* 1976; 57:443.

40. Crisp, A.H., Douglas, J.W.B., Ross, J.M., Stonehill, E. Some developmental aspects of weight disorders. *J. Psychosom. Res.* 1970; 14:313.

41. Kahn, E.J. Obesity in children: identification of a group at risk in a New York ghetto. *J. Pediatr.* 1970; 77:771.

42. Dietz, W.H. Obesity in infants, children, and adolescents in the United States: identification, natural history, and after effects. *Nutr. Res.* 1981; 1:117.

43. Frisancho, A.R. New norms of upper limb fat and muscle areas for assessment of nutritional status. *Am. J. Clin. Nutr.* 1981; 34:2540.

44. Weststrate, J.A., Deurenberg, P. Body composition in children: proposal for a method for calculating body fat percentage from total body density or skinfold-thickness measurements. *Am. J. Clin. Nutr.* 1989; 50:1104.

45. Bandini, L.G., Schoeller, D.A., Fukagawa, N.K., Wyles, L., Dietz, W.H. Body composition and basal metabolic rate (BMR) in children and adolescents with myelodysplasia. *Am. J. Clin. Nutr.* 1988; 47:776A.

46. Lee, M.M.C., et al. Thickening of the subcutaneous tissues in paralyzed limbs in chronic hemiplegia. *Hem. Biol.* 1959; 31:187.

47. Cusack, R. Dietary management of obese children and adolescents. *Pediatr. Ann.* 1984; 13:455.

48. Brewerton, T.D., Heffernan, M.M., Rosenthal, N.E. Psychiatric aspects of the relationship between eating and mood. *Nutr. Rev.* 1986; 44(suppl):78.

49. Jacobsen, F.M., Wehr, T.A., Sack, D.A., James, S.P., Rosenthal, N.E. Seasonal affective disorder: a review of the syndrome and its public health significance. *Am. J. Pub. Health.* 1987; 77:57.

50. O'Brien, G., Whitehouse A. A psychiatric study of deviant eating behavior among mentally handicapped adults. *Br. J. Psychiatr.* 1990; 157:281.

51. Moss, N., Dadds, R.M. Body weight attributions and eating self-effiacy in adolescent obesity. *Addictive Behav.* 1991; 16:71.

52. Mills, L.K. Differences in locus of control between obese adult and adolescent females undergoing weight reduction. *J. Psychol.* 1991; 125:195.

53. Kimm, S.Y., Payne, G., Lahatos, E., Darby, C., Sparrow, A. Childhood screening and treatment practice of physicians. *Am. J. Dis. Child.* 1991; 144:967.

54. Epstein, L.H., Wing, R.R., Koeske, R., Ossip, D., Beck, S. A comparison of lifestyle change and programmed aerobic exercise on weight and fitness changes in obese children. *Behav. Ther.* 1982; 13:651.

55. Berdanier, C., McIntosh, M. Weight loss—weight regain a viscious cycle. *Nutr. Today* 1991; 26:6.

56. Brownell, K.D., Wadden, T.A. Confronting obesity in children: behavioral and psychological factors. *Pediatr. Ann.* 1984; 13:474.

57. Dattilo, A. Dietary fat, and its relationship to body weight. *Nutr. Today* 1992; 22:13.

58. Calleo-Escandon, J., Horion, E. The thermogenic role of exercise in the treatment of morbid obesity: a critical evaluation. *Am. J. Clin. Nutr.* 1992; 55:533S.

59. Devlin, C.L. Twelve step intervention in compulsive eating. *J. Am. Diet. Assoc.* 1991; 91:A136.

60. Goodrick, G.K., Foreyt, J.P. Why treatments for obesity don't last. *Am. Diet. Assoc.* 1991; 91:A151.

61. Brownell, K.D., Kelman, J.H., Stunkard, A.J. Treatment of obese children with and without their mothers: changes in weight and blood pressure. *Pediatrics.* 1983; 71:45.

62. Epstein, L.H., Wing, R.P., McCurley, J. Follow up of behavioral family based treatment for obese children. *JAMA* 1990; 264:2519.

63. Stunhard, A., Wadden, T. Psychological aspects of severe obesity. *Am. J. Clin. Nutr.* 1992; 55:524S.

64. Wing, R. Behavioral treatment of severe obesity. *Am. J. Clin. Nutr.* 1992; 55:545S.

65. Unger, R., Kreeger, L., Christoffel, K. Childhood obesity. Medical and familial correlates and age of onset. *Clin. Pediatr.* 1990; 29:368.

66. Spielman, A., Kandera, B., Kienholtz, M., Blackburn, G. The cost of losing: an analysis of commercial weight loss programs in a metropolitan area. *J. Am. Coll. Nutr.* 1992; 11:36.

67. Kinney, J.M., Tucker, H.N. *Energy Metabolism. Tissue Determinants and Cellular Correlaries.* New York: Raven Press, 1992.

Chapter 20
Attention Deficit Hyperactivity Disorder

Shirley Walberg Ekvall, Valli Ekvall, and Susan Dickerson Mayes

The term "hyperactivity" has been replaced by attention deficit hyperactivity disorder (ADHD) in the revised third edition of the American Psychiatric Association's *Diagnostic and Statistical Manual of Mental Disorders*.[1] The diagnostic criteria for ADHD are shown in Table 20-1. ADHD is one of the most common neurobehavioral problems seen in children today. The symptoms are not singular, but rather are a cluster of symptoms, which makes the etiology difficult to define. However, the general consensus is that ADHD is neurologically based.

Incidence

The prevalence rate is between 1.2% and 20%,[2] with the most commonly reported prevalence rate being 3% of all

Table 20–1. Diagnostic Criteria for Attention Deficit Hyperactivity Disorder

Note: Consider a criterion met only if the behavior is considerably more frequent than that of most people of the same mental age.

A. A disturbance of at least 6 months during which at least eight of the following are present:

   (1) often fidgets with hands or feet or squirms in seat (in adolescents, may be limited to subjective feelings of restlessness)
   (2) has difficulty remaining seated when required to do so
   (3) is easily distracted by extraneous stimuli
   (4) has difficulty awaiting turn in games or group situations
   (5) often blurts out answers to questions before they have been completed
   (6) has difficulty following through on instructions from others (not due to oppositional behavior or failure of comprehension), e.g., fails to finish chores
   (7) has difficulty sustaining attention in tasks or play activities
   (8) often shifts from one uncompleted activity to another
   (9) has difficulty playing quietly
   (10) often talks excessively
   (11) often interrupts or intrudes on others, e.g., butts into other children's games
   (12) often does not seem to listen to what is being said to him or her
   (13) often loses things necessary for tasks or activities at schools or at home (e.g., toys, pencils, books, assignments)
   (14) often engages in physically dangerous activities without considering possible consequences (not for the purpose of thrill-seeking), e.g., runs into street without looking

   Note: The above items are listed in descending order of discriminating power based on data from a national field trial of the DSM-III-R criteria for Disruptive Behavior Disorders.

B. Onset before the age of 7.

C. Does not meet the criteria for a Pervasive Developmental Disorder.

Criteria for severity of Attention Deficit Hyperactivity Disorder:

Mild: Few, if any, symptoms in excess of those required to make the diagnosis **and** only minimal or no impairment in school and social functioning.

Moderate: Symptoms or functional impairment intermediate between "mild" and "severe."

Severe: Many symptoms in excess of those required to make the diagnosis **and** significant and pervasive impairment in functioning at home and school and with peers.

From American Psychiatric Association,[1] with permission.

children.[1] This rate would translate into approximately one hyperactive child per classroom in school. The ratio of boys to girls receiving medication for ADHD in elementary school is 7:1 and in the middle or junior high school is 12:1.[3] The symptoms are usually apparent in the early preschool years, but the disorder is sometimes not recognized or diagnosed until the child reaches school age.[1] Although known as a childhood disease, ADHD may be present through adolescence and adulthood. ADHD predisposes the individual to antisocial disorders, such as substance abuse, oppositional defiant disorder, conduct disorder, or antisocial personality disorder.[2] Unfortunately, in many cases the ADHD etiology for these behaviors goes unrecognized. ADHD is more common in biological relatives with the disorder.[1] Approximately 20% to 30% of children with ADHD had one parent with ADHD in childhood. School failure is a major complication.

Clinical Abnormalities

The essential features of the disorder are inappropriate degrees of impulsiveness, hyperactivity, and inattention (Table 20-1). Some children may have behavior problems because of their impulsivity, and secondary emotional repercussions, such as low self-esteem, may ensue. Manifestations of the disorder appear in the school, home, and social situations. At school, the person may give the impression that he or she is not listening or makes comments out of turn. At home the person may fail to follow through with requests or interrupt other family members. With peers, excessive talking or failure to follow through on rules of the game is common (Table 20-1). Signs of the disorder may be reduced if the person is receiving appropriate psychotropic medication and consistent behavior management techniques.

Behavior rating scales offer a practical, quick, and inexpensive means of screening for ADHD and for augmenting a clinical evaluation. Many behavior rating scales have significant validity, reliability, and normative and factor analytic data. However, the scales are subjective and therefore susceptible to rater bias. Also, ADHD cannot be diagnosed or ruled out based on scale scores alone. A clinical evaluation by a professional, such as a psychologist, child psychiatrist, developmental pediatrician, or pediatric neurologist, is essential.[4]

Two types of rating scales are available. One focuses only on ADHD symptomatology, and the other evaluates multiple areas of psychopathology, including ADHD. The latter type assists in making a differential diagnosis and provides a comprehensive overview of the child's psychological functioning in several areas. One of the most researched and empirically sound instruments that evaluates psychopathology is the *Child Behavior Checklist* (CBCL; by T.M. Achenbach, 1981 from the University of Vermont, Burlington). The CBCL assesses multiple mood and behavior disorders and provides scores in such categories as hyperactive, depressed, anxious, and aggressive. There are several versions, including two parent scales (2 to 3 years and 4 to 16 years), a teacher scale for 6- to 16-year-olds, and a self-report scale for 11- to 18-year-olds. Depending on the version, there are between 100 and 113 items (e.g., "impulsive or acts without thinking") rated on a 3-point scale.

Each version is self-administered and takes approximately 15 minutes to complete. The factor scores are totaled separately and plotted on a graph with standard scores. Computer software is available that calculates the factor scores and generates a profile graph for each child.

The *Conners Teacher Rating Scale* (by C.K. Conners, 1989, 1990 from Western Psychological Services, Los Angeles) is a 39-item measure assessing multiple areas of psychopathology in children ages 4 through 12. Combined research publications provide empirical data on over 15,000 children and reveal a hyperactivity factor, with the item composition changing somewhat from study to study. The Conners Abbreviated Teaching Rating Scale comprised of 10 items from the full scale is one of the most frequently used instruments to assess ADHD. Each item (e.g., "restless or overactive") is assigned a weight of 0, 1, 2, or 3. The item scores are totaled, and a score of 15 or greater is generally considered to be in the hyperactive range. The Conners scales have recently been reissued with a new manual (incorporating prior studies) and with computer software.

The *Pediatric Behavior Scale* (PBS; by S.D. Lindgren, 1985 from Linden Press, Solon, Iowa) is a new and promising instrument for 6- to 16-year-olds especially designed for use in a medical setting (Table 20-2). The PBS comprises 165 items rated by an adult on a 4-point scale and requires about 20 minutes to complete. It yields scores in six categories: conduct, attention deficits, depression-anxiety, deviation, health, and cognition. Each of these six subscales is divided further, e.g., attention, impulsivity, and hyperactivity for the attention deficits subscale. Item scores are totaled and compared with the norms for the child's age and gender. A preschool version for 3- to 4-year-olds is being developed.

The most recent hyperactivity rating scale to become commercially available is the *Attention Deficit Disorders Evaluation Scale* (ÁDDES; by C.B. McCarney, 1989, from Hawthorn Educational Services, Columbia, Missouri). The ADDES has two versions—a 47-item parent scale and a 60-item teacher scale—both of which are rated on a 5-point continuum. The scales each take about 12 to 15 minutes to complete. ADDES has excellent empirical support and was standardized on 4876 children. Norms are available for children 4.5 to 18 years of age. For each child, scores are reported on three subscales (inattentive, impulsive, and hyperactive), which are plotted on a profile graph and converted into standard scores. The ADDES School Version has an accompanying 204-page manual providing intervention strategies for regular and special education teachers. Computerized versions are available for scoring and to generate a printout of intervention recommendations individualized for each student.

Differential diagnosis

Children with disorders other than ADHD may present with similar features. For example, children with an anxiety disorder or depression may show motor restlessness and problems with concentration, but they are a manifestation of their mood disorder and not ADHD. Some children may have multiple diagnoses. ADHD is more common in children with multiple handicaps than in nondisabled children, with prevalence rates as high as 25% to 50%.[5] Iron-deficiency anemia in young children has been linked to decreased cognitive and psychomotor performance and should be ruled out when evaluating for ADHD.[6] Also, school-aged children who are malnourished or who skip breakfast may perform less well on academic tests and should be evaluated if showing ADHD symptoms.[7]

Neurological and Biochemical Abnormalities

Central nervous system (CNS) abnormalities are often predisposing factors for ADHD. These conditions include cerebral palsy, epilepsy, neurological disorders caused by neurotoxins, and other difficulties that may affect the transmission of neurotransmitters, such as serotonin and catecholamines.[2] The brain is divided into different regions and organized into a system.[8,9] Since the attention system is widespread within the brain, it can be vulnerable to various insults, such as malnutrition. The effects of prolonged protein and calorie restrictions on the developing CNS are of particular concern. The amino acid transmitter is the predominant substance needed in transmission in the CNS, whereas monoamines and peptides function as neuromodulators.[10] Each of these classes of neurochemical messages has been implicated in the regulation of food intake[11,12] (see Chapter 11). Malnutrition at an early age is associated with cognitive and behavioral deficits, such as impaired language and motor skills, interpersonal relationships, and adaptive and motivational behavior. However, it is difficult to separate nutrition from other environmental and socioeconomic problems.[13]

Factors to be Considered in Nutritional and Other Evaluations

Medication

A comprehensive clinical evaluation of ADHD is essential using standardized measures and diagnostic criteria (Table 20-1) and can be done most effectively by an interdisciplinary team of a psychologist, physician, nutritionist, and educator. Pharmacological therapy, particularly stimulant medications, is a major component of treatment. The most widely used stimulants are methylphenidate, dextroamphetamine (Dexedrine®), and pemoline (Cylert®), with methylphenidate (Ritalin®) used most frequently. Dextroamphetamine is less frequently used because of its ability to suppress growth.[3] In 14 studies of school-aged ADHD children reviewed by Barkley, the average response rate to stimulant medication was 77%.[14,15] A methylphenidate response rate of 60% has been reported for multiply handicapped and mentally retarded preschool ADHD children.[16] Children who do not respond to stimulant therapy may benefit from tricyclic antidepressants and monoamine oxidase inhibitors.[2] The use of stimulant medication in public and parochial elementary, middle, and junior high schools has nearly doubled in the past decade.[3]

The primary action of stimulant drugs may be to restrict or lessen the variability of behavioral patterns or responses to environment stimuli, thereby attempting to bring about homeostasis of the monoamine-related neurotransmission process.[17,18] These medications generally are well tolerated, although there are a few adverse reactions, which usually subside within a week or two; irritability, decreased appetite, and insomnia are the most common side effects. If they do not subside, an alteration of the dosage may be needed. Stimulant medications may also act as growth suppressants in children receiving long-term treatment. Weight loss usually occurs first, with a later decrease in height (especially after 2–4 years of treatment).[19,20] Roche et al.[21] noted a temporary retardation in the rate of weight increase, suggesting a temporary slowing in growth and stature; yet, this slowing did not affect adult stature or weight. The temporary effect on growth was present in the first few years of treatment during the prepubertal period and appeared to be related to drug dosage and the absence of drug holidays, such as the cessation of medication during the summer vacation. In one study, Safer and Allen[22] discontinued stimulant medication during the summer in one group of children. These children grew in height and weight at a significantly greater rate than those who did not discontinue medication during the summer. This growth rebound was 15% to 68% above the age-expected increment. Satterfield et al.[23] found adverse effects on height and weight in the first year of treatment but not in the second year. Total dosage for summer holidays affected weight deficits more than growth deficits.[23]

Since ADHD is not a benign disorder that is outgrown automatically, it is important to combine drug therapy—treatment of choice for most prepubescent children—with counseling, education, behavior management strategies, and close communication among home, school, and professionals; this is a multimodal approach.

Lead

Hyperactivity may also be associated with increased lead levels. Physicians should be aware of potential increased lead levels in children with hyperactivity and test for lead levels (see Chapter 26).

Megavitamins

The use of megavitamins has been shown to produce no significant effect in lessening ADHD and may produce toxic effects in the child.[24,25] Haslam et al.[24] studied 41 subjects with ADHD using a double-blind repeated cross-over design. Initially, 12 or 29% of the children using megavitamins—3 g niacinamide, 3 g ascorbic acid, 1.2 g calcium pantothenate, and 0.6 g pyridoxine as advocated by Cott[26]—showed significant behavioral improvement during stage 1. However only 7% of these same subjects (all boys) elected to participate in a double-blind cross-over state stage 2. The subjects actually showed more disruptive classroom behavior when treated with vitamins versus the placebo during stage 2. There was no significant difference in serum pyridoxine and ascorbic acid levels between the 12 positive and 29 negative responders in stage 1, but both groups showed a significant increase (42%) in serum transaminase levels. The results showed that megavitamins were ineffective in the management of ADHD and should not be used because of the potential for gastrointestinal complaints and hepatotoxicity. Mothers felt that hyperactivity and learning prob-

Table 20–2. Pediatric Behavior Scale

This checklist asks you to provide some information about your child's behavior. Below is a list of items that describe common behavior problems in children. Some of the items may be true of your child and some may not. Similar items are listed together. Please read each statement and decide how well it describes your child during the past two months.

1. Disobedient; won't mind or follow rules
2. Argues or quarrels
3. Uncooperative; won't help or work together with others
4. Defies authority or talks back
5. Mean or cruel to others
6. Threatens, bullies, or picks on other children
7. Starts fights
8. Hits, bites, or throws things at people
9. Destructive; breaks or smashes things on purpose
10. Lies or cheats
11. Steals
12. Hangs around with "bad" friends who often get into trouble
13. Explosive, unpredictable, or violent outbursts
14. Irritable; gets angry or annoyed easily
15. Overreacts to minor problems; "flies off the handle"
16. Loses temper; has temper tantrums
17. Shouts or screams a lot
18. Excitable; gets "wound up" easily
19. Can't concentrate or pay attention for long; short attention span
20. Easily distracted
21. Shifts frequently from one activity to another
22. Doesn't listen to directions
23. Fails to finish things he or she starts
24. Impulsive; acts without stopping to think
25. Can't stand waiting, wants things right away
26. Interrupts, talks out of turn, or blurts things out
27. Grabs for things; gets "into" everything
28. Rushes into danger without thinking about getting hurt
29. Hyperactive; always "on the go"
30. Restless; can't sit still
31. Squirms or fidgets
32. Constantly in motion; rarely slows down
33. Always running about or climbing on things
34. Tense, can't seem to relax
35. Nervous, "jumpy," or jittery; seems "on edge"
36. Nervous movements, shaking, or twitching
37. Picks at things (such as skin, clothes, or hair)
38. Fearful, anxious, or worried
39. Shy or timid
40. Self-conscious or easily embarrassed
41. Afraid to try new things for fear of making mistakes
42. Makes self "sick" with worry

43. Clings to adults or is too dependent on others
44. Panic attacks, gets so worried or upset that he/she can't be easily comforted
45. Feelings are easily hurt; sensitive to criticism
46. Lacks self-confidence; has low self-esteem
47. Feels worthless or inferior
48. Blames self for problems; feels guilty
49. Feels lonely, unwanted, or unloved; complains that no one loves him/her
50. Lacks motivation; gives up easily or doesn't try
51. Sad, unhappy, or depressed
52. Cries a lot; cries easily for no good reason
53. Show little interest or pleasure in activities; apathetic, doesn't seem to care about anything
54. Thinks too much about death or dying; preoccupied with death
55. Talks about harming or killing self
56. Deliberately harms self or attempts suicide
57. Doesn't get along with other children
58. Has a hard time making friends
59. Ignored or rejected by others
60. Gets teased or picked on by other children
61. Withdrawn, doesn't get involved with others; spends a lot of time alone
62. Doesn't take part in normal social activities
63. Acts too young for his or her age, "childish" or immature
64. Acts silly or giggles too much
65. Pesters or nags, is demanding, won't take "no" for an answer
66. Asks personal or embarrassing questions
67. Loud
68. Talks too much
69. Hums or makes odd noises in public
70. Poor social judgment; not sensitive to other people's feelings or reactions
71. Careless about how he/she looks or dresses
72. Talks or thinks about sex too much
73. Plays with own sex parts too much
74. Bites or hits self, bangs head, or repeats other acts causing self-injury
75. Odd movements or unusual posturing (such as hand-flapping or toe-walking)
76. Needs close or constant supervision
77. Talks or thinks about the same things over and over
78. Repeats certain actions over and over (please explain)
79. Once he/she gets an idea, it's hard to get it out of his/her mind

80. Repeats or "echoes" words or phrases said by others
81. Upset by changes in routine; insists on doing things the same way every time
82. Sudden changes in mood or feelings; moody
83. Rapid shifts between sadness and excitement
84. Inconsistent; behavior or learning varies greatly from day to day
85. Shows changes in personality; is not always his/her "same old self"
86. Sees or hears things that aren't really there
87. Confuses reality and fantasy; unable to tell the difference between real and imaginary things
88. Says strange things that don't make sense; has odd or peculiar ideas (please explain)
89. Strange, unusual, or bizarre behavior (please explain)
90. Very suspicious of others; thinks people are out to get him or her
91. Drowsy or sleepy; not alert or wide awake
92. Sluggish or slow-moving; lacks energy
93. Stares into space; seems preoccupied or "in a world of his/her own"
94. Confused or disoriented; seems to be in a fog
95. Unresponsive; doesn't show feelings or emotions
96. Clumsy, awkward, or poorly coordinated
97. Bumps into things or falls a lot
98. Speech is slurred or hard to understand
99. Shaky movements or tremor; hands tremble or shake
100. Draws or writes poorly
101. Has trouble hitting, kicking, or throwing a ball
102. Eats too much
103. Overweight or gains too much weight
104. Poor appetite; doesn't eat much
105. Underweight or loses too much weight
106. Eats things that are not food (please explain)
107. Goes on eating binges; eats large amounts of food all at once
108. Vomits after eating (not due to illness or medication)
109. Sleeps more than most other children
110. Sleeps less than most other children
111. Has trouble falling asleep
112. Sleep is restless or disturbed; often tosses and turns in sleep
113. Wakes up often in the night
114. Has nightmares or bad dreams
115. Talks, walks, or cries out in sleep

Table 20–2. (*Continued*)

116. Wakes up too early in the morning	137. Wets self during the day	152. Has trouble remembering names for things or thinking of the right words to say
117. Headaches	138. Accident-prone; gets frequent cuts, scrapes, or bruises	
118. Stomach aches		153. Makes up words or substitutes words with similar meanings (such as "door" for "window")
119. Aches or pains in muscles, limbs, chest, or back	139. Illness requiring emergency room treatment or a stay in the hospital (please explain)	
120. Complains of feeling "sick"		154. Thinks and works slowly
121. Complains of dizziness of feeling faint	140. Other physical problems (please explain)	155. Unable to think clearly and logically; has trouble figuring out how to solve problems
122. Nausea or vomiting when nervous or emotionally upset	141. Doesn't follow doctor's orders for health problems	
123. Nausea or vomiting due to illness or medication	142. Refuses or "forgets" to take pills or medicine he/she is supposed to take	156. Comprehension problems; difficulty in understanding directions or discussions
124. Diarrhea or loose bowels	143. Refuses or "forgets" to complete special exercises or physical activities he/she is supposed to do	
125. Fever or high temperatures		157. Has trouble remembering things; forgets easily
126. Complains of hot or cold spells (without having a fever)	144. If on a restricted diet, he/she sneaks food or eats foods he/she is not supposed to eat	158. Thoughts are rambling or disorganized
127. Hearing problems (please explain)		159. Has difficulty learning, even when he or she tries hard
128. Problems with eyes or vision (other than needing eyeglasses) (please explain)	145. Worries about or is fearful of medical procedures (shots, blood tests, etc.)	160. Underachieving; not working up to potential
129. Rashes or other skin problems	146. Physically resists or combats medical procedures (shots, blood tests, etc.)	161. Has trouble with reading, writing, or arithmetic
130. Asthma, wheezing, or trouble breathing	147. Careless or irresponsible about his/her health	
131. Seizures that cause falling and loss of consciousness		162. Fails to complete schoolwork or homework
132. Seizures that are brief and do not cause complete loss of consciousness	148. Has trouble expressing self; "can't get the words out"	163. Schoolwork is sloppy, careless, or disorganized
133. Tires easily; lacks stamina or physical endurance	149. Quiet; doesn't talk very much	164. Gets low grades on school papers or tests
134. Constipated; doesn't have regular bowel movements	150. Speech or articulation problems (please explain)	165. Does not like school; doesn't want to go to school
135. Has bowel movements outside of the toilet; soils pants	151. Gets mixed up when telling a story or explaining how something happened	
136. Wets the bed at night		

From Lindgren, S. D. *Pediatric Behavior Scale.* Solon, IA: Linden Press; 1985.
Used with Permission. Note: Items 19–33 comprise the attention deficits subscale.

lems worsened during the vitamin treatment, but psychosomatic complaints were worse with the placebo. Fathers also found that the children were more hyperactive during the vitamin treatment. Teachers found no difference in hyperactivity with either treatment. In a review article in *Nutrition Reviews*,[25] it was stated that Haslam et al.[24] presented a carefully designed model to be used in future studies when evaluating responses under double-blind conditions.

Food allergies

Food allergies may be considered a potential cause of hyperactivity in children with ADHD. Some children do show allergic reactions, such as gastrointestinal upset or skin eruptions, to certain foods; however, food allergies seldom are the sole cause of hyperactivity. Feingold proposed that certain food additives, synthetic food colors and flavorings, and naturally occurring salicylates could cause hyperactivity.[8] The Feingold diet eliminated two groups of foods: those with naturally occurring salicylates and foods known to contain artificial colors and flavors (Table 20-3). Foods were placed in the latter category according to their ingredient labeling. However, *controlled double-blind experimental investigations have failed to show that Feingold's low-salicylate diet dramatically improves behavior.* On occasion, a few,

particularly very young children (3% of children with ADHD) responded positively on Feingold's low-salicylate diet.[27] Because of the Feingold theory and the studies related to it, a National Advisory Committee on Hyperkinesis and Food Additives was formed in 1975 to study food allergies and to report to the Nutrition Foundation.

Defined diet

Crook[28] stated that some children with dyslexia or ADHD improved with added B vitamins (especially B_6 and folic acid), and other children may be deficient in zinc, calcium, and magnesium, as well as essential fatty acids from the Omega 3 and Omega 6 series. *Candida albicans* also may cause health problems related to a depressed immune system. According to Crook,[28] several children with ADHD responded well to the following comprehensive approach.[28] However, the relative effectiveness of each of these components is not known:

- "avoidance of food allergens
- appropriate nutritional supplements
- antifungal therapy with nystatin and/or Nizoral®
- avoidance of environmental toxins, including lead, petrochemicals, and formaldehyde
- psychological support
- appropriate educational measures"

Table 20–3. The Salicylate-Free "Diet"*: Foods and Products that Should Be Avoided

Foods Containing Natural Salicylates

Almonds	Nectarines
Apples	Oranges
Apricots	Peaches
Blackberries	Plums or prunes
Cherries	Raspberries
Currants	Strawberries
Gooseberries	Cucumbers and pickles
Grapes or raisins	Tomatoes

Other Sources of Salicylates

Foods and products containing artificial flavors and colors

Ice cream	Oil of wintergreen
Oleomargarine	Toothpaste and toothpowder
Cake mixes	Mint flavors
Bakery goods (except plain bread)	Lozenges
Jello	Mouthwash
Candies	Jam or jelly
Gum	Luncheon meats (salami bologna, etc.)
Cloves	Frankfurters

Beverages

Cider (and cider vinegars)	Gin and all distilled drinks (except vodka)
Wine (and wine vinegars)	All tea
Kool-Aid and similar beverages	Beer
Soda pop (all soft drinks)	Diet drinks and supplements

Drugs and Miscellaneous

All medicines containing aspirin, such as Bufferin, Anacin, Excedrin, Alka-Seltzer, Empirin, Darvon Compound, etc.

Perfumes

Toothpaste and toothpower (a mixture of salt and soda can be used as a substitute or Neutregena soap, unscented)

*Check all labels of prepared foods or drugs for artificial flavoring and artificial coloring.
From Feingold B. Food additives and hyperactivity. *Hosp. Pract.* 1973;8:11. Used with permission.

The defined diet includes several dietary modifications, such as the low-salicylate diet of Feingold (Table 20-3). The low salicylate diet is not harmful but does limit the food sources of vitamin C (which should be supplemented). Other modifications included in the defined diet may be the exclusion of items, such as milk, corn, wheat, and sucrose. These may be eliminated and then added back into the diet individually. The defined diet, although not yet proven, has been useful to some families possibly because of a placebo effect. Yet, *diets and other treatment approaches that have not been empirically proven should not be used as a substitute for techniques that have scientific and unequivocal support, such as stimulant medication and behavior modification.*

In one study, food dyes were found to cause significantly impaired learning for some children with ADHD.[29] Other studies involving food dye point to some interaction with ADHD, especially if the child is of preschool age.[30] Perhaps the reaction to food dyes at this age is due to developmental immaturity, the sensitivity of specific areas of the brain, or the lack of certain enzymes.[31]

More conclusive research is needed on the effect of nutrition on hyperactivity. Food flavors and preservatives have not been studied in children. Placebo effects may account for some benefits of the defined diet. Approximately 35% to 39% of ADHD children respond to placebo,[32] which is a very high rate and must be taken into consideration when evaluating interventions. In general, in studies by Harley et al.[33] testing food colors on children with ADHD, parental ratings reveal more positive behavior changes for the experimental diet than do the school ratings. Hyperactive children generally do not eat differently from nonhyperactive children[34]; however, some children within both groups have individual sensitivities or reactions to some food substances. Kaplan et al.[34] concluded that nutrition-induced behavior changes were more a function of sensitivity to the product than ADHD.

Nitrogen metabolism in a substantial number of boys with ADHD appears to differ from that in boys without this syndrome, particularly daytime nitrogen excretion and flux[35] (Table 20-4). Perhaps protein turnover in stressed states is accompanied by increased urinary nitrogen excretion.[35] Results from this study suggest that hyperactive children differ from normal children in their amino acid and protein metabolism, which may provide a noninvasive biochemical means for categorizing children with hyperactivity into subgroups for later investigation.[35]

Table 20–4. Nitrogen Metabolism and ADHD

	Controls		Hyperkinetic	
No of boys	15		15	
Test score (%)	32	(3)	58	(3.4)†
Age (yr)	8.9	(0.2)	8.9	(0.2)
Ht (cm)	136.	(2)	136.	(2)
Wt (kg)	32.7	(1.5)	33.1	(1.7)
MAMC (cm)	16.4	(0.3)	17.5	(0.4)‡
Triceps skinfold (cm)	14.9	(1.7)	13.6	(1.4)
Nitrogen intake (g N/day)	12.5	(1.0)	12.3	(0.5)
Fat intake (g/day)	101	(6)	88	(4)
Carbohydrate intake (g/day)	320	(16)	273	(14)‡
Caloric intake (kcal/day)	2507	(129)	2188	(91)
Calorie/N ratio	208	(10)	179	(6)‡
Urine N excretion (g N/10 hr)	3.1	(0.2)	5.4	(0.5)†,§
Urine volume (ml/10 h)	306	(36)	489	(49)‡
Creatinine (mg/10h)	266	(20)	194	(16)†
N flux (g N/kg/day)	1.0	(0.1)	1.7	(0.4)§
PSR (g protein/kg/day)	4.8	(0.5)	8.2	(2.5)§

*MAMC, midarm muscle circumference; PSR, protein synthesis rate. Two hyperkinetic boys were excluded from the statistical analysis of the urine data. Data are mean ± S.E.M.
†$P < 0.01$ by AOV.
‡$P < 0.05$.
§Variances unequal by Bartlett's test, $P < 0.01$.
From Stein & Sammaritano,[35] with permission.

Dietary and Other Management

A complete nutritional assessment should be performed, taking into consideration medication, weight gain, and dietary habits. The dietary calculation is essential to understand the nutrient intake of the individual. A 24-hour food recall with the food frequency cross-check should be completed first and followed by a 3-day diet diary to ensure the nutritional assessment is as complete as possible (see Chapter 4). Information should be obtained about behavior at mealtimes, food habits, food allergies, and food likes and dislikes. The best dietary treatment may be to discuss with the family the lack of proven usefulness of a defined diet or unconventional diet therapy, but to be willing to evaluate the effects of the diet if the family insists on its use. For example, one should advise the family not to give too much attention to a special diet at the cost of neglecting scientifically proven treatments. Although no harmful physical effects may occur from the Feingold diet, it may be difficult to maintain.[27]

The National Institute of Health (NIH) Consensus Development panel[36] believes that defined diets should not be universally used in the treatment of childhood hyperactivity at this time. However, it recognizes that initiation of a trial of dietary treatment or continuation of a diet in patients whose families and physicians perceive benefits may be warranted. A defined diet should not be initiated until thorough and appropriate evaluation of the children and their families and full consideration of all traditional therapeutic options have taken place.[36] "The panel understands that existing *law* does not require identifying on the label, completely and accurately, all ingredients in food. The panel, therefore, recommends changes in the law to require the listing on labels of all ingredients of food and food products, and that this label include substances that may migrate from wrappers and containers that come in contact with foods."[36]

Asking the family about the basic five food groups consumed may produce the changes that are needed to achieve good nutrition management. Although sugar has not been linked to ADHD,[37] following the food groups will result in the reduction in consumption of sweets and an increase in more complex carbohydrates, which will enhance dental health. Reducing sugar by one-half in recipes is also feasible. Better food labeling is essential and is being requested by the American Dietetic Association.

Drug/medication

The use of methylphenidate during the school year, with reduced dosage in the summer, is a frequent component of treatment. However, many children may need medication throughout the entire day and year because their behavior is poorly controlled, interferes with functioning and learning in and outside school, and is a major problem to themselves and others. Of course, weight and height measurements should be taken monthly to be sure that growth parameters are being met.[38,39] ADHD children and families also need education about the disorder, behavioral and emotional counseling, and close communication between home, school, and clinic. ADHD tends to run in families and families must be told that it may continue into adolescence and adulthood. The adult ADHD residual type must be considered if the following symptoms are present and schizophrenia or major mood disorders are not diagnosed: impulsivity, depression, disorganization, low stress tolerance and short temper. Stimulant drugs and monoamine oxidase inhibitors appear to be of some benefit in adulthood; however, when using the monoamine oxidase inhibitors, red wines, aged cheese and other foods need to be limited (see Chapter 27).[40,41]

Research Directions

The NIH panel[36] determined that future research needs to take three different steps. The first step is to provide optimal measurements by using animal research to generate relative biological data for use in existing epidemiological studies. The second step is to determine defined populations of afflicted children through biological and neurophysiological diagnosis markers. The third step is to study the defined populations through longitudinal studies that address developmental, genetic, and environmental factors.

Animal studies

Animal studies that show the specific relationship of dosage to absorption, metabolism, distribution, and mechanism of action are needed. Various agents should be tested and made relevant to the human population.[36]

Diet, nutrients, and neurotransmitters

Improved study designs using random, double-blind trials to evaluate empirically the effectiveness of proposed treatments should be conducted, as has already been done in assessing the impact of stimulant medication on ADHD symptoms. The adverse effects of dietary interchange should be evaluated as it affects the family psychologically and biologically.[42,43]

New research is needed on the synthesis of brain neurotransmitters that respond to dietary fluctuations and fat in relation to neuronal function. Further studies linking diet, brain transmission, and brain dysfunction should be pursued[44] (see Chapter 11).

It has been speculated, but not proven, that high sugar intake relates to hyperglycemia or antisocial behavior.[45] Milich, et al.[46] reviewed 11 sugar challenge studies involving normal, hyperactive, and psychiatrically disordered children. In some of the studies, children were selected because parents reported they were sugar-reactive, whereas in other studies, this was not a criterion for inclusion. The review showed an overall lack of impact of sugar on ADHD symptoms. Following the sugar challenge, ADHD symptoms increased in two studies, decreased in two studies, and remained unchanged in seven studies.

The trace minerals—iron, copper, and zinc—influence neurotransmitter metabolism. For example, iron is a cofactor for tyrosine hydroxolase and serum zinc, i.e., copper-deficient rats have shown decreased brain tyrosine hydroxolase activity.[47] Benner[47] noted that children who responded to the Feingold diet had an elevated serum copper concentration. The reason for this is unclear. Zinc status also has an impact on catecholamine and hypothalamic pituitary activity. Calcium is known to be involved in nerve conduction. Effects of vitamin B_{12} and folate in transmethylation reactions and ascorbic acid in hydroxylation reactions continue to be of interest.[47] Thiamine plays a role in nerve conduction, and pyridoxal phosphate serves as a co-enzyme for amino acid decarboxylase. Serotonin, histamine, and glycine use dietary precursors from the amino acids—tryptophan, histidine, and threonine—whereas catecholamines use the dietary precursor tyrosine.[48] The behavioral effects of tryptophan, tyrosine, carbohydrate, protein, and caffeine are currently being studied[48] (see Chapter 11).

Behavioral research

New treatment strategies should be evaluated according to the following questions, as proposed by Golden[49]:

"1. Is theory consistent with modern scientific knowledge?
2. Are the claims for usefulness broad or highly specific?
3. What is the potential for biological harm?
4. What are the hidden time, financial, psychological and intrafamilial costs?
5. Based on the above, what is the final cost-benefit analysis?"

Schwab and Conners[50] developed standards for nutrient behavioral research with children. Research studies should fulfill these criteria:

• Study the hypothesis for the rationale (biochemical basis).
• Review subject description with appropriate recruitment methods, demographic characteristics, concurrent medication, and proper control group.
• Determine food challenge dosage level for subjects and its behavioral and psychological effects using double-blind, administration controlled, randomly assigned conditions.
• Evaluate dependent measures that relate to the hypothesis. Is it reliable, age appropriate, sensitive, replicable? Does it coincide with anticipated effects of the food, interrater reliabilities, and baseline scores?

Observation techniques for evaluating the effects of nutrients on mood are suggested.[51]

Follow-up

If the family insists on following a defined diet, the child should be evaluated monthly, if possible, with a complete nutritional assessment, including dietary, biochemical, anthropometry, and physical signs (see Quality Assurance Guidelines for Developmental Disorders in Appendix 7). If medication is administered, a complete nutritional assessment should be done periodically, with special attention given to growth parameters. Reducing or eliminating medication during weekends or summer holidays should be considered if the child is in the prepubertal period.

References

1. American Psychiatric Association. *Diagnostic and Statistical Manual of Mental Disorders, (DSM-III-R)*. 3rd ed. rev. Washington, DC: APA; 1987.
2. Bond, W. Recognition and treatment of attention deficit disorder. *Clin. Pharmacol.* 1987; 6:617.
3. Safer, D., Krager, J. Trends in medication of hyperactive school children. *Clin. Pediatr.* 1985; 22:500.
4. Bagnato, S.J., Mattison, R.E., Mayes, S.D. Diagnostic assessment of affective and behavioral disorders in children. *School Psychol. Int.* 1986; 7:40.
5. Fisher, W., Burd, L., Kuna, D.P., Berg, D. Attention deficit disorders and the hyperactivities in multiply disabled children. *Rehabil. Lit.* 1985; 46:250.
6. Pollitt, E., Saco-Pollitt, C., Leibel, R.L., Viteri, F.E. Iron deficiency and behavioral development in infants and preschool children. *Am. J. Clin. Nutr.* 1986; 43:555.
7. Meyers, A.F., Sampson, A.E., Weitzman, M., Rogers, B.L., Kayne, H. School breakfast program and school performance. *Am. J. Dis. Child.* 1989; 143:1234.
8. Feingold, B. *Why Your Child is Hyperactive*. New York: Random House; 1975.
9. Mirskey, A. Behavioral and psychophysiological markers of disordered attention. *Environ. Health Perspect.* 1987; 74:191.
10. Iverson, L. Amino acids and peptides: fast and slow chemical signals in the nervous system? *Proc. Roy. Soc. Lond. B.* 1984; 221:245.
11. Morley, J. The neuroendocrine control of appetite: the role of the endogenous opiates, cholecystokinin, TRH, gamma-amino-butyric-acid and the diasepam receptor. *Life Sci.* 1980;27:355.
12. Morley, J., Levine, A. Pharmacology of eating behavior. *Annu. Rev. Pharmacol. Toxicol.* 1985; 25:127.
13. Crnic, L. Nutrition and mental development. *Am. J. Ment. Defic.* 1984; 88:526.
14. Barkley, R.A. A review of stimulant drug research with hyperactive children. *J. Child Psychol. Psychiatr.* 1977; 18:137.
15. Barkley, R.A. *Hyperactive Children: A Handbook for Diagnosis and Treatment*. New York: Guilford; 1981.
16. Mayes, S.D., Bixler, E.O., Mattison, R.E., Humphrey, E.J. *Empirical Evaluation of Stimulant Medication Effects in Individual Hyperactive Children*. Annual Meeting of the American Academy of Child and Adolescent Psychiatry, Washington, DC; 1987.
17. Varley, C. A review of studies of drug treatment efficacy for attention deficit disorder with hyperactivity in adolescents. *Psychopharmacol. Bull.* 1985; 21:216.
18. Hechtman, L. Adolescent outcome of hyperactive children treated with stimulants in childhood: a review. *Psychopharmocol. Bull.* 1985; 21:178.
19. Mattes, J., Gittleman, R. Growth of hyperactive children on maintenance regimen of methylphenidate. *Arch. Gen. Psychiatr.* 1983; 40:319.
20. Friedmann, N., Thomas, J., Carr, R., et al. Effect on growth in pemoline-treated children with attention deficit disorder. *Am. J. Dis. Child.* 1981; 135:329.
21. Roche, A.F., Lipman, R.S., Overall, J.E., Hung, W. The effects of stimulant medication on the growth of hyperkinetic children. *Pediatrics.* 1979; 63:847.
22. Safer, D.J., Allen, R.P. Factors influencing the suppressant effects of two stimulant drugs on the growth of hyperactive children. *Pediatrics.* 1973; 51:660.
23. Satterfield, J.H., Cantwell, D.P., Schell, A., Blaschke, T. Growth of hyperactive children treated with methylphenidate. *Arch. Gen. Psychiatr.* 1979; 36:212.
24. Haslam, R.H.A., Dalby, J.T., Rademaker, A.W. Effects of megavitamin therapy on children with attention deficit disorders. *Pediatrics.* 1984; 74:103.
25. Megavitamins and the hyperactive child. *Nutr. Rev.* 1985; 43:105.
26. Cott, A. *The Orthomolecular Approach to Learning Disabilities*. San Rafael, CA: Academic Therapy Publications; 1977: 26–29.
27. Varley, C. Diet and the behavior of children with attention deficit disorder. *J. Am. Acad. Child Psychiatr.* 1984; 23:182.
28. Crook, W.G. Nutrition, food allergies, and environmental toxins. Letter to the Editor. *J. Learn. Dis.* 1987; 20:260.
29. Swanson, J.M., Kinsbourne, M. Food dyes impair performance of hyperactive children on a laboratory learning test. *Science.* 1980; 207:1485.
30. Weiss, B., Williams, J.H., Margen, S., Abrams, B., Caan, B., Citron, L.J., Cox, C., McKibben, J., Ogar, D., Schultz, S. Behavioral responses to artificial food colors. *Science.* 1980; 207:1487.
31. Conners, C.K. Nutritional therapy in children. In: Galler, J.R., ed. *Nutrition and Behavior*. New York: Plenum Publishing Corp; 1984.
32. Sroufe, L.A. Drug treatment of children with behavior problems. In: Horowitz, F.D., ed. *Review of Child Development Research*. Chicago: University of Chicago Press; 1975.

33. Harley, J.P., Matthews, C.G., Eichman, P. Synthetic food colors and hyperactivity in children: a double-blind challenge experiment. *Pediatrics.* 1978; 62:975.
34. Kaplan, B.J., McNicol, J., Conte, R.A., Moghadam, H.K. Overall nutrient intake of preschool hyperactive and normal boys. *J. Abnorm. Child Psychol.* 1989; 17:127.
35. Stein, T.P., Sammaritano, A.M. Nitrogen metabolism in normal and hyperkinetic boys. *Am. J. Clin. Nutr.* 1984; 39:520.
36. National Institute of Health Consensus Development Panel. Defined diets and childhood hyperactivity. *JAMA.* 1982; 248:290.
37. Lucas, B. Diet and behavior. In: Pipes, P., ed. St. Louis: Times Mirror/Mosby; 1989.
38. American Academy of Pediatrics Committee on Children with Disabilities and Committee on Drugs. Medication for children with an attention deficit disorder. *Pediatrics.* 1987; 80:758.
39. Calis, K., Grothe, D., Elia, J. Attention-deficit hyperactivity disorder. *Clin. Pharmacol.* 1990; 9:632.
40. Wender, P.H. *The Hyperactive Child, Adolescent, and Adult.* New York, Oxford University Press, 1987.
41. Wender, P.H., Reimherr, F.W., Wood, D., Ward, M. A controlled study of methylphenidate in the treatment of attention deficit disorder, residual type, in adults. *Am. J. Psychiatry* 1985; 142:5.
42. Lipton, M., Mayo, J. Diet and hyperkinesis: an update. *J. Am. Diet. Assoc.* 1983; 83:132.
43. Lipton, M.A., Golden, R.N. Nutritional therapies. In: Karasu, T.B., ed. *The Psychiatric Therapies.* Washington, DC: American Psychiatric Association; 1984.
44. Greenwood, C.E.L., Anderson, G.H. An overview of the mechanism by which diet affects brain function. *Food Tech.* 1986; 50:132.
45. Harper, A.E., Gans, D.A. Claims of antisocial behavior from consumption of sugar: an assessment. *Food Tech.* 1986; 50:142.
46. Milich, R., Wolraich, M., Lindgren, S. Sugar and hyperactivity: a critical review of empirical findings. *Clin. Psychol. Rev.* 1986; 6:493.
47. Benner, A. Trace mineral levels in hyperactive children responding to the Feingold diet. *J. Pediatr.* 1979; 94:944.
48. Lieberman, H.R., Corkin, S., Spring, B.J., Wurtman, R.J., Growdon, J.H. The effects of dietary neurotransmitter precursors on human behavior. *Am. J. Clin. Nutr.* 1985; 42:366.
49. Golden, G. Controversial therapies. *Pediatr. Clin. North Am.* 1984; 31:459.
50. Schwab, E.K., Conners, C.K. Nutrient-behavior research with children: methods, considerations, and evaluation. *J. Am. Diet. Assoc.* 1986; 86:319.
51. Barrett, D.E. An approach to the conceptualization and assessment of social-emotional functioning in studying nutrition-behavior relationships. *Am. J. Clin. Nutr.* 1982; 35:1222.

Chapter 21
Failure to Thrive

Kristine Kelsey

The term "failure to thrive" (FTT) is applied to infants and young children who do not achieve a reasonable rate of growth. The diagnostic criteria for FTT are variable, but the growth parameters usually used are weight and/or height consistently below the 3rd percentile for age based on standardized growth charts, weight for height below the 5th percentile, or a fall-off of growth velocity of two major percentiles.[1,2] FTT or growth delay accounts for between 1% to 5% of hospital pediatric admissions, and the long-term effects of this problem can include growth deficits through the school-aged years, disorders in personality, and cognitive defects.[3,4] Significant health problems have also been found to plague children with FTT upon follow-up after 3 years.[5]

Organic and Nonorganic FTT

The disorder is usually classified as either organic or nonorganic FTT depending on whether a diagnosable physical condition is present to cause the growth retardation. Only about 20% of the cases of FTT are found to be of the organic type.[1] The most common medical conditions causing organic FTT are gastrointestinal disorders (gastroesophageal reflux, chronic diarrhea, malabsorption, bowel malformations), central nervous system (CNS) problems (cerebral palsy, microcephaly, and asphyxia), cardiac lesions, pulmonary disease, and endocrinopathies.[1,3]

Often, the diagnosis of nonorganic FTT is made by exclusion after an initial evaluation fails to reveal any underlying physical disorder. The diagnosis is confirmed if there is in-hospital weight gain. Historically, nonorganic FTT was felt to be caused by a deprived environment, and because of the special role of the mother in caring for children, the problem was called "maternal deprivation syndrome."[6,7] It was considered to result from failure of the mother to provide a nurturing environment for the infant to develop normally. Currently, a broader view of the syndrome, labeled transactional or interactional, takes into account many aspects of the problem, including the parents (their childhood experiences, health, emotional status), the child (neurological status, temperament), the interaction between the child and the family, and the environment (level of stress, support in the family situation).[8–10] Recent views of the two types of FTT—organic and nonorganic—suggest that it may no longer be useful to consider these two types separately, but as concomitant causes of growth delay.[3,11,12] This view takes into account the emotional risks for the child failing to thrive secondary to an organic cause, as well as the medical risks that confront the child with nonorganic FTT who is also suffering from malnutrition.

Possible Etiology

In an attempt to discover the precursors of the syndrome, Vietze[7] and co-workers used a transactional approach in a prospective study of mothers and infants who were later diagnosed with nonorganic FTT and a comparison group of mothers and infants who did not develop nonorganic FTT. Their study differed from many of the other studies looking at characteristics of mothers and infants with FTT in that it was prospective and longitudinal and had an adequate comparison group. They collected data about maternal history, including social situation, developmental history, and attitudes regarding childrearing. The infant's biological and temperamental constitution was measured, as well as the various ways the infant and mother interacted during their earliest encounters while still in the hospital.

The results of this study were surprising in that there were no statistically significant differences in maternal characteristics, infant behavior, or biographical data of the mother between the two groups. However, infants later diagnosed with nonorganic FTT had significantly lower birth weights and shorter gestational ages. It was also found that mothers of infants with growth failure spent a significantly shorter time gazing at their infants than the comparison group of mothers. The authors concluded that it is possible that prematurity or a small baby, in the context of other adverse environmental conditions, such as poverty, absence of the father, and lack of support, could be the factor predisposing to an inadequate psychological bond between mother and infant that leads, ultimately, to the poor growth evidenced in nonorganic FTT.

In another study examining possible precursors of nonorganic FTT with a similar design, the inadequate childhood nurturing of the mother, overly stressful relationship with the father, and medical problems related to the pregnancy and birth of the child, including a shorter gestation time, were found to be predictive of later nonorganic FTT.[9] Hergenroeder et al.,[13] in a retrospective study of 40 children who were either abused and neglected or who failed to thrive, found a significantly higher percentage of these children with low birth weight than in the control group.

Biochemical Abnormalities and Nutritional Manifestations

Regardless of the underlying cause of FTT, whether organic or nonorganic, the syndrome presents as a purely medical disease—malnutrition.[12] Indeed, malnutrition can of itself cause irritability, disturbances in temperament, and difficulty in feeding. These characteristics are often noted in FTT.[10,12] An inadequate diet and problems with the feeding situation are important in the development of this disorder. Approaching the syndrome from a nutritional standpoint, the various nutritional inadequacies can be divided into several types[14]: adequate amounts of food to support normal growth in normal infants are offered, but are not accepted by the infant; large amounts of food are lost through vomiting or regurgitation; excessive fecal losses of nutrients and unusually high energy requirements occur; or an insufficient amount of food is offered to the infant. It is possible for infants to suffer from more than one of these nutritional problems.[14]

An infant may refuse food because of an immature sucking and swallowing mechanism, which can occur in young infants, especially if premature. Other causes are nasal obstruction, a small jaw, cleft palate or lip, or a large tongue. A disturbed mother-child interaction may also contribute to the refusal of food.[15] Vomiting or regurgitation of food can be secondary to abnormalities of the gastrointestinal tract. Excessive fecal losses resulting from malabsorption can produce diarrhea or steatorrhea. Specific examples include disaccharidase deficiency, milk allergy, and necrotizing enterocolitis. Increased caloric requirements are common in low birth weight infants and those with severe respiratory distress.[15]

An insufficient amount or inappropriate types of food may be offered when the family is following a fad or special diet such as vegetarianism, or because of erroneous parental beliefs concerning the elements of a healthy diet for infants.[16] Inappropriate test diets,[17] incorrect preparation of formula, and lack of success with breastfeeding can also result in insufficient intake of nutrients and growth failure. Sometimes, parents are not aware of the correct amount of food, how often to offer it, or when to introduce solid foods.[18] Rudolph[15] has listed many of the causes of inadequate intake of nutrients (Table 21-1). Calories, protein, and minerals affecting growth (phosphorus, calcium, magnesium, and zinc) need to be assessed.

Factors to be Considered in Nutritional Evaluation

A thorough nutritional evaluation of the infant suspected of FTT is necessary. The following information should prove very helpful: complete medical history, family and prenatal history, developmental assessment, clinical evaluation, anthropometric measurements, nutritional history, social situation, behavioral and interactional qualities, and biochemical tests.[3]

Medical, family, and prenatal history

The medical history should include any hospitalizations, medications, frequent illnesses, accidents, and any history of pica or lead ingestion.

Social data to be collected include information regarding the primary caregiver; number of family members living in the home; any disruptions in the family, such as separation or divorce; size of the home; level of concern of the parents

Table 21–1. Postnatal Nutritional Difficulties

Qualitative or Quantitative Inadequacy of Food Intake
Insufficiency of diet
  Incorrect preparation of formula
    Quality
    Quantity
  Unsuitable feeding habits
    Due to food fads
    Due to ignorance on the part of the mother
  Disturbed mother-child relationship
    Environmental deprivation
    Sensory deprivation
    Maternal deprivation
  Economic deprivation
Feeding difficulties due to mechanical or organic factors
  Congenital anomalies of nose, mouth, and jaw
    Choanal atresia
    Micrognathia and glossoptosis
    Harelip and cleft palate
  Congenital anomalies of the upper gastrointestinal tract
    Esophageal atresia or tracheo-esophageal fistula
    Diaphragmatic hernia
    Pyloric stenosis
  Dyspnea due to any cause
    Congenital heart disease
    Respiratory distress
  Neurological
    Immature sucking and swallowing mechanism
    Pharyngeal incoordination
    Generalized muscle weakness (hypotonia)
      Werdnig-Hoffman disease
      Myasthenia gravis
      Congenital hypotonia
    CNS damage due to birth injury or kernicterus
    Subdural hematoma
    Developmental retardation-infants may feed poorly and
      therefore gain slowly

Defects in Assimilation of Food (Malabsorption)
Immaturity
Congenital or acquired disaccharidase deficiency

Monosaccharide malabsorption	Congenital immunological deficiency
Milk allergy	Hirschsprung's disease
Cystic fibrosis	Acrodermatitis enteropathica
Celiac disease	Necrotizing enterocolitis
Protein-calorie malnutrition	Biliary atresia, neonatal hepatitis

Following neonatal surgery (gastroschisis, omphalocele, volvulus, etc.)

Increased metabolism	Storage diseases
chronic infection	glycogen-storage disease
hyperthyroidism	galactosemia
	mucopolysaccharidoses
	Aminoacidopathies
	Hyperammonemia
	Maple syrup urine disease, etc.
	Hypoxemia
	Cardiac
	Pulmonary insufficiency
	Hypothyroidism
	Congenital adrenogenital syndrome

Defective Utilization
Intrauterine infections
Chromosomal abnormalities
Mental retardation
Metabolic disorders

From Rudolph,[15] with permission.

over the child's slow growth; and amount of time the child spends outside the home.[19]

Information on the growth patterns of the parents and other siblings; inherited or familial diseases, such as Down's syndrome; thyroid insufficiency; microcephaly; or slow development in any other family member make up the family history. Prenatal and perinatal data of interest include any infections during the pregnancy; use of drugs, alcohol, and cigarettes; difficult pregnancy and/or labor; full-term or premature birth, gestational age and Apgar scores; medical problems; and problems with feeding during the perinatal period.[19]

Developmental and clinical assessment

The developmental assessment includes a record of developmental milestones as obtained from the parent, how the parent feels the child compares with others of his or her age developmentally, and a current rating of development using the Denver Developmental Screening test or a similar tool.[19]

Obvious signs of malnutrition should be noted, such as muscle wasting, very thin arms and legs, protuberant abdomen, thin skin with decreased subcutaneous fat, or a hollow look to the face. Indicators of possible neglect, such as untreated diaper rash, dirty clothes, or poor hygiene, should also be noted.[20]

Anthropometric assessment

Any previous height (or length if under 2 years), weight, and head circumference measurements should be obtained (see Chapter 4). It is also necessary to measure the present height, weight, head circumference, triceps skinfold, and arm circumference. Height and weight and weight for height, when compared with standards compiled by the National Center for Health Statistics (NCHS), enables the infant to be plotted on the growth grids (see Appendix 3). Serial height, weight, and head circumference measurements plotted on NCHS growth charts are of much greater use in determining growth retardation than are single measurements.[3,6] When weight or height is found to be below the 10th percentile, growth retardation is suspected, and these children should be monitored carefully.[3,14] Arm circumference and triceps skinfold measurements are used to determine midarm muscle circumference and arm fat area according to standards developed by Frisancho.[21] When these measurements are below the 5th percentile, depletion of fat stores and muscle protein is indicated.

Premature birth by 4 or more weeks should be age-adjusted until catch-up-growth occurs or until 2 years of age. The weight centile of a child between 4 and 8 weeks of age was found to be a better predictor of the centile at 12 months than the birth centile.[22]

Nutrition history and feeding pattern

It is necessary to question the parents carefully concerning the child's intake. One should ask specific questions about present intake, changes in intake, food likes and dislikes, and any problems surrounding the feeding situation. To determine nutritional adequacy, the parents should be instructed by a dietitian to complete a 7-day food record,

including only the amounts of foods actually eaten by the child. If formula is used, an exact description of the way the formula is prepared is important. Other factors to consider are the position of the infant during feeding, who usually feeds the infant, an estimation of any losses of nutrients due to diarrhea and vomiting, and urinary pattern.[19] For breastfed children, FTT is often caused by a failure to obtain enough food at the breast, and in some instances, this situation may be corrected by support and practical suggestions.[6]

To learn more about the feeding situation, one should ask about the length of time of a normal feeding, the emotional context (whether relaxed or tense), and whether the primary caregiver seems to respond appropriately and play with the infant. It is beneficial to observe the caregiver and child during a feeding session. At this time, the appropriateness of developmental feeding milestones, such as using the bottle, cup, or utensils, could be noted. Maladaptive feeding behaviors that may manifest during the feeding situation are gagging, choking, holding of the breath, pica, vomiting at the sight of food, rumination, and refusal of food.[18]

Behavioral and interactional qualities

Infants diagnosed with FTT have been described as jittery, irritable, and fussy[20]; older infants appear apathetic, withdrawn, and apprehensive, and do not vocalize very much.[6] Powell's group[23] compared specific behaviors among infants diagnosed with FTT and those with no signs of FTT. Behaviors that occurred significantly more frequently in the FTT group were flexed hips and knees, expressionless face, abnormal gaze, general inactivity, and lack of physical response to a stimulus.[23] Mothers of infants diagnosed with FTT also display behaviors that differ from those of mothers of infants with normal growth. Mothers of FTT infants were found to be less responsive to their infants, less stimulating verbally, and less accepting of their infants.[10] This same study also pointed out that the homes of the children with FTT tended to be more disorganized. Berkowitz and Senter[24] found a similar trend in reduced vocalizations of both infants and mothers in mother/nonorganic FTT infant dyads as compared to control pairs. Mothers of the nonorganic FTT infants were also less responsive to their infants' vocal cues.[24] When Mathisen et al.[25] compared the feeding situation in the home of FTT infants to a matched comparison group, they found that FTT infants had more delays in oral-motor performance and less ability to communicate needs during feeding session and were more temperamentally difficult, more likely to be fed in inappropriate positions for age, and surrounded with more distractions during mealtimes.

Fosson and Wilson[26] suggest that useful information can be obtained from an interview and feeding session with all of the family members present. One finding of their study of families with a child with nonorganic FTT was a decreased tendency of the mothers to respond to infants' cues. Additional factors affecting the feeding situation were sibling rivalry, displaced maternal anger, undermining of the mother, and a generally chaotic family life. A psychologist or therapist could be of much assistance in this type of evaluation and could help develop interventions to improve the manner in which the family functions during the feeding situation.[26]

Although the interaction between child and caregiver may be very different in the clinic than at home, it is important to try to obtain some clues about the nature of this relationship during the evaluation. It should be fairly easy to note whether the relationship appears relaxed and comfortable or tense. An infant who is overly friendly with unfamiliar staff and who turns to these strangers for comfort if distressed, could indicate emotional rejection and social deprivation in the home situation. Other signs to note include a parent's lack of visual attention to the infant, critical comments made by the parent concerning the infant, or whether the parent seems to ignore the infant.[6] The validity of the observations made of the parent-infant relationship could be tested by further observing the pair during a feeding situation.

Biochemical tests

Biochemical tests of significance in diagnosing FTT include complete blood count, serum electrolytes and acid-base status, urinalysis, lead levels, serum glucose, serum protein, BUN, and liver function tests. Stools should be checked for pH level, stool-reducing substance, fat, parasites and eosinophils.[15] Determining skeletal age can also be helpful.[19]

Dietary Management

Current views of FTT that emphasize consideration of both organic and nonorganic causes of this syndrome suggest a multidisciplinary approach that includes medical, nursing, nutritional, and social services,[3,6,20] as well as possible referrals to physical therapy, psychiatry, child development, gastroenterology, or other medical specialties.[3] Each member of the interdisciplinary team investigates the appropriate parameters so that a unified treatment plan can be devised.

Often, hospitalization is recommended initially to confirm the diagnosis, monitor weight, provide optimum nutritional intake, and observe caregiver-child interactions.[20] After the initial evaluation, the team develops treatment plans and continues to follow FTT children in the clinic setting. A member of the team will also help the family gain access to resources, such as WIC (Supplemental Food Program for Women, Infants, and Children), public welfare, public health nurses, homemaker services, support groups for the parents, child care, and transportation services. When babies repeatedly show good progress while in the hospital but do not gain weight when they are back in the home situation, foster placement may be recommended.[20]

Nutritional management of the child with FTT includes: (1) continued assessment of nutritional status and rate of growth; (2) provision of adequate calories, protein, and other nutrients for catch-up growth; (3) nutritional instruction to the family about exact amounts, types, and preparation of food; and (4) long-term monitoring and follow-up.[3]

When calories and protein are provided in amounts that are equal to normal age-specific requirements (Table 21-2),[27] the growth of that child will continue along the low percentile rank to which the child has fallen. Therefore, calories and protein in excess of normal needs must be provided for the weight and height of the child to catch up to a more normal level. Catch-up growth begins with a period

Table 21-2. Recommended Dietary Allowances (RDAs), 1989

Age	kcal/kg*	g Protein*
0–6 mo	108	13
6–12 mo	98	14
1–3 yr	102	16
4–6 yr	90	24

*Energy and protein allowances are based on median intakes of children of these ages followed in longitudinal growth studies.

of initial growth acceleration followed by a slowing of growth until the normal percentile for the child is reached. Nutritionists at the FTT clinic at the University Affiliated Cincinnati Center for Developmental Disorders use a formula to estimate calorie and protein needs for catch-up growth according to age (Table 21-3). Other methods to determine catch-up needs may also be used. After the amount of calories and protein is determined, the nutritionist must explain to the parents exactly what foods, in what amounts, will supply these needs. To provide the additional calories needed, it is often necessary to fortify foods by using a more concentrated formula or adding carbohydrate, fat, and protein sources. The individual needs of each FTT child must be further considered in relation to the medical condition, gastrointestinal tolerance, and renal solute load. Any nutritional treatment plan must be integrated into the overall care of the FTT patient and be developed in consultation with the primary physician.[3] Feeding problems and misconceptions of the parents about the proper amounts and/or types of foods that infants and toddlers need can be corrected by nutritional instruction.

Observing the caregiver-infant relationship or the feeding situation may suggest necessary behavioral interventions. The observer should note whether there is an atmosphere of tension or distraction, the tempo of the feeding (fast paced or too slow), the demonstrated readiness of the child for self-feeding, the position of the bottle or breast, and the technical ability and flexibility of the caregiver. More spe-

Table 21-3. Estimating Catch-Up Growth Requirements

$$\text{Catch-Up Growth Requirement (kcal/kg/day)} = \frac{\text{Calories Required for Weight Age (kcal/kg/day)} \times \text{Ideal Weight for Age (kg)}}{\text{Actual Weight (kg)}}$$

1. Plot the child's height and weight on the NCHS growth charts.
2. Determine at what age the present weight would be at the 50th percentile (weight age).
3. Determine recommended calories for weight age.
4. Determine the ideal weight (50th percentile) for the child's present age.
5. Multiply the value obtained in (3) by the value obtained in (4).
6. Divide the value obtained in (5) by actual weight.

Estimated protein requirements during catch-up growth can be calculated similarly:

$$\text{Protein Requirement (g/kg)} = \frac{\text{Protein Required for Weight Age (g/kg)} \times \text{Ideal Weight for Age (kg)}}{\text{Actual Weight (kg)}}$$

*Guidelines are used to estimate catch-up growth requirements; precise individual needs will vary and be mediated by medical status and diagnosis.

From Rathbun & Peterson,[30] with permission.

cifically, the observation should provide answers to these questions:

- How often does the parent glance at the baby?
- How does the parent hold the baby—loosely, awkwardly, closely, or comfortably?
- How does the parent verbally and nonverbally comfort or guard the baby or child when he or she is crying?
- How does the parent respond verbally and nonverbally to compliments about the baby? Does the parent look at the baby and smile?
- How does the parent act toward the child during feeding or mealtime?
- What does the parent do when asked to get the baby to smile?
- How does the parent discipline or punish the child?
- What does the parent do when a second child is present and seeks closeness?
- How does the child respond to the parent? Eye contact? Frightened or relaxed facial expression? Withdrawn from parent? Very quiet and shy? Clings to parent? Plays and cuddles with parent? Curious about environment? Apathetic?
- What is the child's reaction to younger or older siblings?
- Is the child's general behavior age-appropriate?
- What is the child's general appearance?
- What is the child's reaction to other adults?

Interventions to address problems discovered by the observation include: decreasing noise and tension at mealtimes, offering finger foods to toddlers who want more control when eating, and using a behavioral modification program to provide rewards or decrease rumination.[3]

When refusal of food occurs, several studies have found that a positive approach is preferable to the more traditional use of aversive techniques.[28,29] Larson's group[28] studied only three infants with FTT and maladaptive feeding behavior, but found that the feeding program using food and social reinforcers, a time-out period, and music to mask the introduction of food produced success with all three infants. The infants accepted food more readily and there was a reduction of vomiting and gagging at meals. Hilton[29] also suggests the use of preferred foods or liquids as reinforcers. Other successful techniques are making the eating process fun by entertaining the child or introducing toys and setting a predetermined amount of food or formula that must be consumed at a particular meal and sticking to that amount.

Follow-up

Uncontrolled, long-term follow-up studies of children with nonorganic FTT with hospitalization as the mode of treatment have shown a poor prognosis.[11] Hufton and Dates[4] followed 21 children for an average of 6 years after diagnosis of nonorganic FTT and found that the children remained at risk for problems with physical growth, educational development (two-thirds were 1 or 2 years behind in reading age), and personality (ten were classified as having abnormal personalities). Singer's review[5] of FTT infants at 3 years old who had received long-term hospitalization, although showing maintenance of the weight gains achieved in the hospital, also showed persistent intellectual delays, as measured by IQ, and continuation of significant health problems.

A team approach, including a pediatrician-coordinator, visiting or clinical nurse, nutritionist, social worker or mental health professional, and parents, is recommended for long-term treatment of FTT.[30] Few studies, however, document the long-term effects of an interdisciplinary team approach including intensive ongoing therapeutic interventions. One study by Kristiansson and Fallstrom,[2] did measure the long-term effects of intensive therapeutic intervention for infants with nonorganic FTT using growth in weight and height as indicators. Infants with nonorganic FTT were assigned a psychosocial score depending on the number of adverse family factors, such as single parent, drug or alcohol abuse, and dependence on welfare. At 4 years of age those children who had been assigned a score of three or less showed partial catch-up growth that was greater than the growth for children with four or more factors. For six children having four or more adverse social factors, intensive therapeutic intervention was provided, such as foster care placement, assistants at the day care center, and/or counselors at home. Seven others with high scores did not receive intensive treatment. Higher weights and heights were attained by the group receiving intensive intervention than by the seven with the high scores who did not receive special therapeutic intervention. The authors conclude that intensive therapeutic intervention, which aims to eliminate or counteract adverse familial social factors, does seem to enhance long-term growth in children with nonorganic FTT.

As an alternative to lengthy hospitalization for treatment of FTT, Karniski and his group[31] have reported an intervention including hospitalization when necessary, but in addition, placement in medical placement homes (MPH). The MPH program consisted of 12 individual homes with volunteer parents who received special training regarding the care of children with FTT and who were supervised periodically by a physician and nurse. The purpose of the program was to initiate change in the parent-infant interaction by modeling appropriate feeding and parenting techniques and by providing direct teaching to the parents of the FTT children. Although long-term results of this intervention were not included in this study, the cost effectiveness of the program was analyzed. Compared to the costs of medical care of FTT children treated in a more traditional manner, the MPH program was found to be less expensive. Costs per 100 grams of weight gained by FTT children was $308 for the MPH group compared to $1636 for the traditional treatment method group. The difference was found to be highly significant.

References

1. Berkowitz, C.D., Sklaren, B.C. Environmental failure to thrive: the need for intervention. *Am. Fam. Physician.* 1984; 29:101.
2. Kristiansson, B., Fallstrom, S.P. Growth at the age of 4 years subsequent to early failure to thrive. *Child Abuse Negl.* 1987; 11:35.
3. Peterson, K.E., Washington, J., Rathbun, J.M. Team management of failure to thrive. *J. Am. Diet. Assoc.* 1984; 84:810.
4. Hufton, I.W., Dates, K. Nonorganic failure to thrive: a long-term follow-up. *Pediatrics.* 1977; 59:73.
5. Singer, L. Long-term hospitalization of failure-to-thrive infants: developmental outcome at three years. *Child Abuse Negl.* 1986; 10:479.
6. Skuse, D.H. Non-organic failure to thrive: a reappraisal. *Arch. Dis. Child.* 1985; 60:173.
7. Vietze, P.M., Falsey, S., O'Connor, S., Sandler, H., Sherrod, K., Altemeier, W.A., eds. *High-Risk Infants and Children: Adult and Peer Interactions.* New York: Academic Press; 1980.
8. Casey, P.H. Failure-to-thrive: transitional perspective. *J. Dev. Behav. Pediatr.* 1987; 8:37.

9. Altemeier III, W.A., O'Connor, S.M., Sherrod, K.B., Vietze, P.M. Prospective study of antecedents for nonorganic failure-to-thrive. *J. Pediatr.* 1985; 106:360.

10. Casey, P.H., Bradely, R., Wortham, B. Social and nonsocial home environments of infants with nonorganic failure-to-thrive. *Pediatrics.* 1984; 73:348.

11. Casey, P.H., Wortham, B., Nelson, J.Y. Management of children with failure-to-thrive in a rural ambulatory setting. *Clin. Pediatr.* 1984; 23:325.

12. Bithony, W.G., Newberger, E.H. Child and family attributes of failure-to-thrive. *J. Dev. Behav. Pediatr.* 1987; 8:32.

13. Hergenroeder, A.C., Taylor, P.M., Rogers, K.D., Taylor, F.H. Neonatal characteristics of maltreated infants and children. *Am. J. Dis. Child.* 1985; 139:295.

14. Fomon, S.J., ed. *Infant Nutrition.* Philadelphia: W.B. Saunders; 1974.

15. Rudolph A.J. Failure to thrive in the perinatal period. *Acta Paediatr. Scand.* 1985; 319(suppl):55.

16. Pugliese, M.T., Weyman-Daum, M., Moses, N., Lifshitz, F. Parental health beliefs as a cause of nonorganic failure to thrive. *Pediatrics.* 1987; 80:175.

17. Tarnow-Mordi, W.O. Failure to thrive owing to inappropriate diet free of gluten and cow's milk. *Br. Med. J.* 1984; 289:1113.

18. Denton, R. An occupational therapy protocol for assessing infants and toddlers who fail to thrive. *Am. J. Occup. Ther.* 1986; 40:352.

19. Steele, S. Nonorganic failure to thrive: a pediatric social illness. *Iss. Comp. Pediatr. Nursing.* 1986; 9:47.

20. Showers, J., Mandelkorn, R., Coury, D.L., McCleery, J. Nonorganic failure to thrive: identification and intervention. *J. Pediatr. Nurs.* 1986; 1:240.

21. Frisancho, A.R. New norms of upper limb fat and muscle areas for assessment of nutritional status. *Am. J. Clin. Nutr.* 1981; 34:2540.

22. Edwards, A., Halse, P., Parkin, J., Waterson, A. Recognizing failure to thrive in early childhood. *Arch. Dis. Child.* 1990; 65:1263.

23. Powell, G.F., Low, J.F., Speers, M.A. Behavior as a diagnostic aid in failure-to-thrive. *J. Dev. Behav. Pediatr.* 1987; 8:18.

24. Berkowitz, C.D., Senter, S.A. Characteristics of mother-infant interactions in nonorganic failure to thrive. *J. Fam. Pract.* 1987; 25:377.

25. Mathisen, B., Skuse, D., Wolke, D., Reilly, S. Oral-motor dysfunction and failure to thrive among inner-city infants. *Develop. Med. Child. Neurol.* 1989; 31:293.

26. Fosson, A., Wilson, J. Family interactions surrounding feedings of infants with nonorganic failure to thrive. *Clin. Pediatr.* 1987; 26:518.

27. Food and Nutrition Board. *Recommended Dietary Allowance.* 10th ed. Washington, DC: National Academy of Sciences; 1989.

28. Larson, K.L., Ayllon, T., Barrett, D. A behavioral feeding program for failure-to-thrive infants. *Behav. Res. Ther.* 1987; 25:38.

29. Hilton, A. Approaches for feeding the young child with anorexia. *J. Pediatr. Nurs.* 1987; 2:45.

30. Rathbun, J.M., Peterson, K.E. Nutrition in failure to thrive. In: Grand, R.J., Sutphen, J.L., Dietz, W.H., eds. *Pediatric Nutrition.* Boston: Butterworths; 1987.

31. Karniski, W., Van Buren, L., Cupoli, J.M. A treatment program for failure to thrive: a cost/effectiveness analysis. *Child Abuse Negl.* 1986; 10:471.

Chapter 22
Rumination

Shirley Walberg Ekvall, Valli Ekvall, and Susan Dickerson Mayes

The American Psychiatric Association's diagnostic criteria[1] for rumination in infancy, as specified in the third revised edition of the Diagnostic and Statistical Manual of Mental Disorders (DSM-III-R), are twofold:

1. Repeated regurgitation, without nausea or associated gastrointestinal illness, for at least 1 month following a period of normal functioning
2. Weight loss or failure to make expected weight gain

Some aspects of the DSM-III-R criteria have been questioned based on a 1992 review of publications on rumination disorder.[2] Although 84% of ruminators described in the literature have problems with weight, 16% are not underweight or losing weight. The criterion, "following a period of normal functioning," is also questionable because most ruminators, particularly those with developmental delays, were clearly not normal before the onset of rumination. Lastly, the rationale for the diagnostic requirement of rumination being present "for at least 1 month" is unclear and may interfere with prompt diagnosis and treatment of this potentially life-threatening disorder. A definition of rumination consistent with the existing literature is *the voluntary and pleasurable repeated regurgitation of stomach contents without organic cause.*

Rumination disorder is noted in infants, but has been described more frequently in mentally retarded children and adults. Of the 123 cases of rumination reported in the literature, 38% are infant ruminators, and 62% are mentally retarded individuals of any age.[2] Rumination, or merycism, was first identified in adults during the 17th century by Fabricios ab Aquapendente. It was not until the 20th century that rumination was recognized in infants. Just as medical writers described this condition as having received little attention several centuries ago, this statement holds true today.

Rumination—the regurgitation or backward flowing of stomach contents—must be distinguished from vomiting—the forcible expulsion of stomach contents. Involuntary vomiting is a common symptom in young children and may be associated with such infections as salmonella, tonsillopharyngitis, and septicemia.[3] Psychogenic vomiting may be a feature or symptom of a variety of psychological problems, including anorexia and bulimia nervosa and anxiety disorder. However, it differs from rumination in that it is not a pleasurable or self-stimulating act.[2]

Rumination in infants differs from ordinary regurgitation or other organic problems that are involuntary and do not require effort on the part of the infant to induce regurgitation. Deliberate regurgitation is often achieved either by thrusting the fingers in the mouth, by a series of vigorous thrusting movements of the tongue backward and forward,[3]

or by the contraction of abdominal muscles.[4] However, the act of rumination often appears effortless. Rumination usually begins within 30 minutes after completion of a meal and continues for up to an hour or more, with rumination frequency decreasing thereafter. The decline with time may be related to the process of gastric emptying (and therefore the gradual decrease in amount of food to ruminate) and the increasingly unpleasant or acidic taste of the stomach contents.

Age at onset for rumination in infants is usually between 3 weeks and 12 months[5] (mean, 5.7 months[2]); for rumination in mentally retarded individuals, it is 0.25–21 years (mean, 5.7 years).[2] For both types of rumination, the disorder is about 3.5 times more common in males than in females.[2] Infants also frequently exhibit other self-stimulating behaviors, such as head rolling, head banging, body rocking, and excessive finger and thumb sucking.[6] Infants with rumination are often described as quiet, sad, and singularly wide eyed,[3] and some are irritable and hungry between episodes.[1] These infants seem to be lost in inner contemplation and are very detached from the environment, but are quick to respond to external stimulation. However, infant ruminators do not comprise a homogeneous group in terms of social, emotional, and behavioral functioning, and much variation is described in the literature.[2]

Etiology

Etiological theories of rumination that have had some currency at various times include heredity, dilation of the lower end of the esophagus or the stomach, overaction of the sphincter muscles in the upper portions of the alimentary canal, cardiospasm, pylorospasm, gastric hyperacidity, achlorhydria, movements of the tongue, insufficient mastication, pathological conditioned reflex, aerophagy, finger sucking, neuropathic constitution, motility neurosis, gastric neurosis, lack of occupation, and boredom. These theories only received limited acceptance mainly because they did not generate effective treatment strategies or described involuntary or organic problems, not true rumination, which is voluntary and nonorganic.[2,3]

Today, rumination is conceptualized according to one of two theories: a psychodynamic theory or a learning principle theory.[7] Although both of these theories—a psychodynamic or psychogenic theory in infants and a learning or self-stimulation theory in individuals or children who are mentally retarded—implicate different rewarding consequences, both are in accord with the causative factor of rumination; namely, the seeking of stimulation.[7,8]

The psychodynamic explanation has two central assumptions.[9] The first links ruminating behavior to infant characteristics, such as anxiety, depression, or neurotic tendencies. The second emphasizes maternal characteristics and mother-child interaction. Psychodynamic theory holds that, as a result of the mother's personality problems or psychosocial stress that influence her ability to interact with the baby, she cannot form an appropriate mother-child bond and interaction pattern. Thus, the infant seeks internal gratification because of a lack of external stimulation.[9] An infant who is unable to evoke appropriate responses from his or her mother is thought to resort to rumination as a tension-releasing or stimulation-producing activity.

The main emphasis of the behavioral approach, based on the learning or self-stimulation theory, is on the consequences of the behavior. Rumination is thought to be maintained as a result of positive reinforcement. In contrast to psychodynamic theories, which focus on the origin of the behavior, the behavioral theories look more at its maintenance. Chronic rumination is thought to be a self-stimulatory behavior independent of social reinforcement in individuals who are mentally retarded.[2] Rumination in such individuals who are mentally retarded may occur even though the caregiver or parents are warm and nurturing to the individual.[2]

By the time the diagnosis is made in infants, the child may be severely malnourished and have undergone extensive medical evaluations to rule out organic causes. Rumination occurs most frequently when the infant is alone, and thus the diagnosis may be frequently overlooked.

Although rumination does not appear to be linked to any organic abnormality, it is often confused with a variety of other disorders. Since rumination is fairly rare, many erroneous diagnoses may be made before the physician, by a process of elimination, labels the problem as rumination. For example, some diagnoses commonly considered before the symptom complex is recognized as rumination include adrenal insufficiency, pyloric stenosis, food allergy, duodenal ulcer, esophageal chalasia, and severe feeding problems of unknown origin.[3] Rumination was initially considered to be a symptom of gastroesophageal reflux caused by a physical disorder, such as chalasia or hiatal hernia. It was believed that activities associated with ruminating behavior—for example, tongue thrusting—are initiated as the result of an attempt to empty the esophagus of refluxed gastric contents or as a response to abnormal esophageal dilation. However, when a person with rumination is admitted to an inpatient facility with another diagnosis—for example, failure to thrive—close observation by clinicians, in conjunction with a detailed social history, usually enables the diagnosis of rumination.[6]

Complications

The chronic vomiting associated with rumination can lead to a rapid breakdown in bodily functions with serious repercussions; for example, dehydration and malnutrition, resulting in lowered resistance to disease.[10,11] If rumination is allowed to continue for a long period of time, it may result in weight loss or lack of weight gain, failure to thrive, electrolyte imbalance, dehydration, malnutrition, anemia, de-

pressed immunocompetence, aspiration, aspiration pneumonia, gastric disorders, and even death.[2,8] The mortality rate attributed to chronic rumination ranges from 12% to 20%,[12] although this rate has been declining. Progression of this condition may also detract from the child's physical appearance, lead to avoidance of the ruminator, impede developmental progress, and cause tooth decay. Gingivitis, etching of tooth enamel, and numerous cavities have been reported among persons who ruminate.[13] These dental manifestations are the result of exposure to acids, which subsequently results in demineralization, hemorrhagic gingiva, decreased salivary flow, erosion of the lingual surfaces of the maxillary anterior teeth, and temperature sensitivity.[13]

Biochemical and Behavioral Abnormalities

The behavior approach to the etiology and maintenance of rumination states that rumination is a conditioned behavior and thus can be eliminated by altering the antecedents or consequences of the behavior. Behavioral techniques have often been used to treat rumination, and the results have been quick, effective, and enduring when a rigorous behavioral program has been used. However, these techniques usually require one-to-one attention during the period of implementation, and they may be constrained by legal and regulatory restrictions. Behavioral treatments that have been used successfully to eliminate rumination include aversive conditioning (administering a taste-aversive substance or electric shock immediately after rumination), overcorrection, and the presentation or withdrawal or reinforcement contingent on rumination.[2,14,15] Studies conducted by Rast et al.[12,16] investigated the relationship between quantity of food ingested (food satiation) and frequency of ruminating behavior in residents who were institutionalized and retarded. The collected data revealed that rumination decreased significantly in frequency when ruminators were allowed to eat to satiation (three to eight times normal meal volume) and increased again when smaller "standard" portions were eaten. Thus, a satiation diet must be maintained indefinitely to control rumination, unlike behavior modification strategies that can be faded often without recurrence of rumination. Studies performed with persons with Prader-willi syndrome show that the incidence of rumination becomes more frequent with an increase in caloric restriction.[13]

Although not as effective as high-calorie satiation programs, satiation achieved through the consumption of low-calorie foods also has been found to decrease rumination. Thus, it has been suggested that oropharyngeal and esophageal stimulation due to chewing and swallowing might contribute to the etiology and maintenance of ruminating behavior.[17] A recent study that examined the role of chewing in rumination found that moderate decreases in ruminating occurred after the consumption of normal meals that were preceded by supplementary gum chewing.[17]

Frequency of rumination in a 12-year-old boy with profound mental retardation was investigated over a 4-week period. Less frequent rumination was significantly associated with individual attention (versus independent play or group activity), special education programming (versus non-school hours), time spent with caregivers who liked the child (versus those who liked him less), earlier time of day (versus later in the day), and increasing time following meals.[18]

The relationship between the assumed etiology and the method of treatment is complex. Those who see rumination as a learned conditioning problem are likely to recommend only behavioral treatment, particularly if the person is mentally retarded. Those who believe rumination to be a disturbance in the mother-child relationship may opt to arrange for a stimulating environment, nurturing mother substitute, and therapy for the mother, particularly for infant ruminators.

Factors to be Considered in Nutritional Evaluation

Nutritional assessment

Because of the frequent losses of nutrients through vomitus expulsions, the individual who ruminates is often malnourished. Thus, it is important to perform a nutritional assessment. Particular attention should be given to calorie and protein intake.[19] Anthropometric data, such as height, weight, waist circumference, and triceps skinfold (including muscle mass) measurements, should be taken during the initial evaluation, as well as periodically throughout the duration of the treatment program, to provide a baseline against which to monitor future developmental gains. Biochemical tests should include routine blood and urine analysis and serum nutrient analysis to identify any suspected nutrient deficiencies. Mothers of infants who ruminate are typically described as immature, dependent, and depressed[5,20] and may not provide adequate stimulation, which the infant requires for proper development. Thus, parent-child interaction should also be assessed during the evaluation.

Treatment

Because of confusion about etiology, several methods of treatment have been identified. Placing the child in a prone position at a 30- to 45-degree angle with head up on an "anti-reflux" board may be somewhat effective following meals. However this approach is more appropriate for treatment of an involuntary gastroesophageal reflux than for rumination. Similarly, medications that improve lower esophageal sphincter tone and accelerate gastric emptying (metoclopramide and bethanechol) may reduce rumination. However, if these medications are discontinued, rumination is likely to resume. Further, these medications do not prohibit rumination, but instead make it more difficult for the ruminator to regurgitate purposefully. Therefore, rumination can (and does) still occur while the individual is on these medications, although its frequency may be reduced.

A surgical treatment—a Nissen fundoplication used for the treatment of an involuntary gastroesophageal reflux—also has been used in an attempt to control rumination. However, this operative procedure has a significant rate of postoperative morbidity and mortality.[16] Additionally, one of the authors has treated a patient who continued to ruminate post-Nissen fundoplication. Again, the procedure makes it difficult but not impossible to ruminate. Considering these limitations and the existence of safer and more effective procedures (e.g., behavioral techniques), medication and surgery are not advised.

Psychodynamic or psychogenic treatment methods may involve one of two approaches. The first is aimed at changing the parent-child interactions. Substitute or surrogate mothers, who provide a stimulating and nurturing environment, have been used with success. At the same time the mother may be treated with psychotherapy and trained in parenting skills.

A review of behavioral literature reveals several effective interventions based on the principles of reinforcement and punishment. These include delivery of an aversive stimulus contingent on rumination (most commonly a taste-aversive substance, such as lemon juice or Tabasco sauce, or electric shock), overcorrection (requiring the ruminator to practice oral hygiene for an extended period after each episode of rumination, which is experienced as aversive), time-out from positive reinforcement, and differential reinforcement of other or incompatible behaviors. Other treatment approaches have involved contingent or noncontingent increased social attention and stimulation, satiation, peanut butter following consumption of food (which works in the same way as satiation by increasing caloric intake),[21] changing the consistency of food and decreasing the rate of feeding.[22] All of these techniques have been successful in some but not all cases. Therefore, what is effective with one ruminator may not work with another.

In choosing interventions, one should consider ethical issues, client rights, and social validation data. The factors that promote or hinder generalization of treatment effects and maintenance of effects after treatment are poorly understood and merit systematic research. Treatment needs to be individualized according to the ruminator's symptoms, rumination frequency and complications (which may justify aggressive treatment), and family or caregiver dynamics.

Dietary Management

A very promising new area of investigation is the nutritional and mechanical management of rumination. Previously, nutritional management consisted of decreasing the amount of food presented at each meal, giving clear liquids, and withholding fluids during the mealtime. However, these procedures proved to be ineffective in improving nutritional status, and instead produced weight loss and dehydration to the point of hospitalization. A combined effort of an interdisciplinary team that includes both psychologists and dietitians, has recently been reported to provide the highest degree of success.[14] Providing large quantities of food has resulted in a decrease in ruminating, an increase in weight, and an improvement in nutritional status. Although consumption to the point of satiation reduced rumination, it can cause weight gain above the estimated ideal body weight. Thus, weight should be monitored accordingly. Also, once satiation is discontinued, rumination often recurs.

Children who ruminate are typically found to ravenously consume their food. This condition is managed by providing the proper eating environment in which to decrease the rate of consumption and maintain a high-caloric, high-protein intake. Management techniques to be considered during treatment include[19]

- Provide relaxed and quiet mealtimes, to promote slow eating and adequate mastication of food.

- Avoid excessive fluid intakes during and soon after consumption of meals.
- Avoid consumption of raw or coarse foods.
- Decrease stimulation of gastric mucosa by providing bland foods only.
- Avoid high concentrated fat, which may cause diarrhea and dehydration.
- Avoid overloading the stomach or prolonged emptiness.
- Provide thicker liquids, which are more difficult to regurgitate.

A high-protein and high-calorie diet is usually needed; sometimes it may be as high as one-third above the recommended daily allowance.[19]

Follow-up

After successful treatment has been completed, anthropometric measurements, such as weight, height, waist circumference, and triceps skinfold (with muscle mass), should continue to be monitored and plotted on a grid. Food intake and loss must be recorded daily, with particular attention directed toward calorie and protein intake. If ruminating behaviors resume, both the frequency and amount of loss should be determined and attended to promptly.

References

1. American Psychiatric Association. *Diagnostic and Statistical Manual of Mental Disorders*, 3rd ed. rev. Washington, DC: APA; 1987.
2. Mayes, S.D. Eating disorders of infancy and early childhood. In: Hooper, S.R., Hynd, G.W., Mattisons, R.E., eds. *Child Psychopathology: Diagnostic Criteria and Clinical Assessment.* Hillsdale, NJ: Erlbaum; 1992.
3. Singh, N. Rumination. *Int. Rev. Res. Ment. Retard.* 1981; 10:139.
4. Chatoor, I., Dickson, L. Rumination: a maladaptive attempt at self regulation in infants and children. *Clin. Proc. CHNMC.* 1984; 40:107.
5. Chatoor, I., Dickson, L., Einhorn, A. Rumination-etiology and treatment. *Pediatr. Ann.* 1984; 13:924.
6. Sheagren, T.G., Mangurten, H.H., Brea, F., Lutostanski, S. Rumination—a new complication of neonatal intensive care. *Pediatrics.* 1980; 66:551.
7. Tierney, D., Jackson, H. Psychosocial treatment of rumination disorder: a review of the literature. *Austr. NZ. J. Dev. Disabil.* 1984; 10(2):81.
8. Mayes, S.D., Humphrey, F.J., Hanford, H.A., Mitchell, J.F. Rumination disorder: differential diagnosis. *J. Am. Acad. Child Adolesc. Psychiatr.* 1988; 27:300.
9. Lavigne, J.V., Burns, W.J., Cotter, P.D. Rumination in infancy: recent behavioral approaches. *Int. J. Eating Disord.* 1981; 1:70.
10. Mulick, J.A., Schroeder, S.R., Rojahn, J. Chronic ruminative vomiting: a comparison of our treatment procedures. *J. Autism Dev. Disord.* 1980; 10:203.
11. Davis, P.K., Curo, A.J. Chronic vomiting and rumination in intellectually normal and retarded individuals. *Behav. Res. Severe Dev. Disord.* 1980; 1:31.
12. Rast, J., Johnston, J.M., Drum, C., Conrin, J. The relation of food quantity to rumination behavior. *J. Appl. Behav. Anal.* 1981; 14:121.
13. Alexander, R.C., Greenswag, L.R., Nowak, A.J. Rumination and vomiting in Prader-Willi syndrome. *Am. J. Med. Genet.* 1987; 28:889.
14. Winton, A.S., Singh, N. Rumination in pediatric populations: a behavioral analysis. *J. Am. Acad. Child Psychiatr.* 1983; 3:269.
15. Singh, N.N., Manning, P.J., Angell, M.J. Effects of an oral hygiene punishment procedure on chronic rumination and collateral behaviors in monozygous twins. *J. Appl. Behav. Ann.* 1982; 15:309.
16. Rast, J., Ellinger-Allen, J.A., Johnston, J.M. Dietary management of rumination: four case studies. *Am. J. Clin. Nutr.* 1985; 42:95.
17. Rast, J., Johnston, J.M., Lubin, D., Ellinger-Allen, J. Effects of premeal chewing on ruminative behavior. *Am. J. Ment. Retard.* 1988; 93:67.
18. Humphrey, F., Mayes, S.D., Bixier, E.O. Variables associated with frequency of rumination in a boy with profound mental retardation. *J. Autism Dev. Disord.* 1989; 19:435.
19. Heinrichs, E., Rokusek, C., eds. *Nutrition and Feeding for the Developmentally Disabled.* Pierre, SD: Department of Education and Cultural Affairs; 1985.
20. Fleisher, D. Infant rumination syndrome. *Am. J. Dis. Child.* 1979; 133:266.
21. Greene, K.S., Johnston, J.M., Rossi, M., Rawal, A., Winston, M., Barron, S. Effects of eating peanut butter on ruminating. *Am. J. Ment. Retard.* 1991; 95:631.
22. Johnson, J., Greene, K. Relation between ruminating and quantity of food consumed. *Ment. Retard.* 1992; 30:7.

Chapter 23
Anorexia Nervosa and Bulimia

Valli Ekvall, Shirley Walberg Ekvall, and Michael Farrell

Both anorexia nervosa (AN) and bulimia nervosa (BN) are conditions characterized by abnormal behavior related to weight control. These eating disorders are illnesses that are caused by an interaction of biological, psychological, and social influences with an intense preoccupation with food.[1] There is diagnostic overlap between these two disorders. The physical effects of anorexia nervosa and bulimia are shown in Table 23–1.

The term "anorexia nervosa" (AN) was coined in 1874 by Sir William Gull to describe a nervous morbid disease characterized by a loss of appetite and severe wasting.[2] The most notable feature of AN is marked weight loss and maintenance of low weight.[3]

The third revised edition of the *Diagnostic and Statistical Manual* (DSM-III-R) of the American Psychiatric Association establishes these diagnostic criteria for AN:

A. Refusal to maintain body weight over a minimal normal weight for age and height, e.g., weight loss leading to maintenance of body weight 15% below that expected; or failure to make expected weight gain during period of growth, leading to body weight 15% below that expected.
B. Intense fear of gaining weight or becoming fat, even though underweight.
C. Disturbance in the way in which one's body weight, size, or shape is experienced, e.g., the person claims to "feel fat" even when emaciated, believes that one area of the body is "too fat" even when obviously underweight.
D. In females, absence of at least three consecutive menstrual cycles when otherwise expected to occur (primary or secondary amenorrhea). A woman is considered to have amenorrhea if her periods occur only following hormone, e.g., estrogen administration.

The term "bulimia" may be used to refer to a pattern of overeating even in a person without a psychiatric diagnosis or with anorexia nervosa. DSM-III-R,[5] however, reserves the term "bulimia" for an eating disorder that meets following criteria[5]:

A. Recurrent episodes of binge eating (rapid consumption of a large amount of food in a discrete period of time).
B. A feeling of lack of control over eating behavior during the eating binges.
C. The person regularly engages in either self-induced vomiting, use of laxatives or diuretics, strict dieting or fasting, or vigorous exercise in order to prevent weight gain.
D. A minimum average of two binge eating episodes a week for a least 3 months.
E. Persistent overconcern with body shape and weight.

The use of these criteria presents some problems. They blur the differences between a bulimic subgroup of AN and bulimia nervosa (BN). Currently, the practice is to separate these subgroups by body weight: a person is categorized as anorexia nervosa (bulimic subgroup) if the person is emaciated; a person may be classified as bulimia nervosa if she is of normal weight.[6] Children with both bulimia and anorexia tend to be older, less socially isolated, have a higher incidence of familial obesity, and show more evidence of premorbid social instability, than those children with restrictive anorexia. Some people with anorexia nervosa may meet bulimic characteristics, whereas some normal-weight people with bulimia may previously have met the criteria for a diagnosis of anorexia nervosa.

In earlier literature, anorexia nervosa was often seen as a form of rebellion against sexuality. Through maintenance of a low body weight, a young girl was able to delay sexual maturation. This view is still held today, although the higher rate of married women with AN[7] tends to disprove it. AN has been classified by some authors into primary and secondary or atypical anorexia. Patients with primary AN fear becoming obese, perhaps because of a disturbed body image, and they make a variety of attempts to lose weight. Secondary or atypical AN often results from psychiatric disorders—conversion reaction, depression from unipolar or bipolar affective mood disorders, or schizophrenia—or from other medical diseases involving a true loss of appetite. The person with AN may be brought to the health professional when body weight is 15% below normal. By that time the person may have bradycardia, edema, hypotension, neonatal-like or lanugo hair, and amenorrhea, but may well deny symptoms.[5] The person with AN may prepare elaborate meals, but limit food intake to a few low-calorie foods.

Certain factors suggest a favorable prognosis for BN: early age of onset, hysterical personality structure, short duration of symptoms, and diminution of disturbances of body perception following weight increase.[6] These factors suggest an unfavorable prognosis: vomiting, abuse of purgatives, bulimia, compulsive personality traits, numerous physical complaints, and psychological test results that are suggestive of psychosis.[6]

Two studies found that between 40% to 50% of persons with primary AN exhibit bulimic behaviors.[8,9] These people form a subgroup distinct from others with primary AN who control their weight exclusively by restriction of food intake. Those with bulimia and AN have an older age of onset; poorer impulse control; a higher incidence of alcohol and drug abuse and kleptomania; less severe weight loss; more symptoms of anxiety, guilt, and depression; and a poorer prognosis. Obesity also is more prevalent in the person with bulimia.[8,9]

Six theories have been proposed to explain the etiology of AN: sociocultural, family pathology, individual psychodynamic, developmental psychobiological, primary hypo-

Table 23–1. Biochemical and Physical Manifestations of Anorexia Nervosa and Bulimia

Manifestation	Anorexia Nervosa	Bulimia

Endocrine/metabolic	Amenorrhea
	Osteoporosis
	Decreased norepinephrine secretion
	Low somatomedin C
	Functional hypothyroidism—
	    high RT_3, normal T_4, TSH
	Elevated growth hormone
	Elevated cortisol
	Decreased/erratic vasopressin
	    secretion
	Prepubertal gonadotropin levels—
	    LH, FSH
		Menstrual irregularities

Cardiovascular	Bradycardia Hypotension Arrhythmias	
Renal	Renal calculi Edema	Hypokalemia— diuretic-induced Ipecac poisoning

Gastrointestinal	Early satiety
	Constipation
		Acute gastric dilation,
		    rupture
		Dental enamel erosion
		Esophagitis
		Mallory-Weiss tears
		    esophageal rupture
		Parotid enlargement

Biochemical	Hypokalemia
	Metabolic alkalosis
	Hypophosphatemia
	Hyperlipidemia
	Elevated SOT, SGPT
	Elevated bilirubin (Gilbert's
	    disease)
	Azotemia
	Hypercarotenemia
		Hypokalemia—
		    laxative-induced

Hematological	Bone marrow hypoplasia
	    Leukopenia
	    Thrombocytopenia	

Immunological	Hypocomplementemia Anergy	
Pulmonary		Aspiration pneumonia

From Michael Farrell, M.D., Children's Hospital Medical Center, Cincinnati, OH.

thalamic dysfunction, and an affective disorder.[10] Although some feel eating disorders may have a single cause, they are more likely to be the result of a multifactorial chain of events. The interacting causes are felt to have roots in three spheres: biological, psychological, and social.[4] Certain early experiences and family influences may create intrapsychic conflicts that create a psychological predisposition toward an eating disorder. Social influences and expectations of women to be thin play an important role in the development of eating disorders.[11] A stressful lifestyle and the striving for perfection, particularly in a family of achievers, can initiate some of the problems in this disorder.[5] The biological factors that initiate anorexia nervosa may be mediated by pubertal endocrine changes. Psychological conflicts lead to

personality and behavioral changes that promote and support dieting.

The effects of these variables are different for each individual. Some people appear to have a strong innate tendency to develop the disorder, despite a supportive family environment, whereas others react particularly to conflicted family experiences, and still others react primarily to the pressures of society.[1] Data indicate that about 60% of families of children with AN were rigid, overprotective, and enmeshed; 20% displayed extreme chaos and disorganization; and 20% appeared normal.

There is a high prevalence of dieting and abnormal eating behavior in adolescents and young adults. In some reports, up to 70% of young women feel fat, and 33% are dieting at any given time. Maloney et al.[12] reported that dieting behavior even exists in school-aged children. Of children in grades three through six, 45% wanted to be thinner and 37% had tried to lose weight. Seven percent scored in the AN range on the questionnaire.[12]

The constant media attention to the "slim look," as well as concerns about the "unhealthy" American diet, has resulted in "fear syndromes": an exaggerated fear of obesity or cholesterol. This fear results in severe restriction of nutrient intake,[13,14] which may produce poor weight gain, delayed puberty, and decreased linear growth. If nutrient intake is decreased sufficiently, amenorrhea and other metabolic disturbances may occur. The fear syndromes can be distinguished from anorexia nervosa by the lack of body image distortion and the prompt response to nutritional counseling.

Girls often begin to diet near the time of puberty, often shortly after menarche—a time of rapid physical and psychological change. There is less of an increase in AN as girls get closer to 14, so those who gain 20–30 pounds as a result of earlier maturation may tend to be more vulnerable to AN or bulimia.[15] The process often begins with relatively innocent dieting. For example, the young girl is acutely aware of the changes in her own body configuration and becomes concerned about the increasing circumference of her hips and thighs. The diet is difficult at first but with persistence, it becomes easier to follow, and she becomes accustomed to smaller and smaller portions of food at less frequent intervals. She persists in dieting because of her determination and eventual pleasure is achieving control over her body, unlike most of her peers. The person may receive compliments from family and friends on her willpower and slim figure. Exercise becomes a bigger part of her everyday activities. As she beings to lose some weight, she may want to lose more and more. She may become more secretive, compulsive, and particular about her diet habits. Physical and mental signs of AN begin to develop, but often are ignored or denied. She withdraws increasingly from social interaction, becomes quiet and seclusive, and immerses herself in achievement-oriented activities, as family and friends become worried. Eventually the individual becomes hostile toward her family. School performance may decline, despite excessive studying, as she becomes easily distractible and preoccupied and, ultimately, depressed and apathetic. Unsuppressible hunger (bulimia) may ensue as a reaction to chronic semistarvation, and 50% of people with AN go on to become bulimic. This urge may be effectively suppressed for months or even years, but may lead to rapid weight gain and obesity before stabilization at normal weight occurs. The bulimic person who continues to desire to be thin will resort to vomiting or purging through laxative and diuretic abuse. This practice leads to chronic anorexia and bulimia with serious consequences. Bulimarexia, a more specific category of bulimia involving binging followed only by purging, is a disorder that may persist considerably longer than AN.[16]

Incidence

The incidence of AN seems to have increased over the past 20 years.[6,17] It occurs most often among young (under 25 years) affluent white women of at least normal intelligence.

It is not as common in men (10% to 13%).[12,18] A retrospective study in Monroe County, New York, found the incidence increased from a rate of 0.35 per 100,000 from 1900–1969 to 0.64 per 100,000 from 1970–1976.[17] This higher incidence may, however, be due to the increased awareness of the condition. In a survey published in 1989, 750 female students at the University of California in Los Angeles completed questionnaire distributed to health care clinics, sororities, athletic teams, dance majors, and psychology classes regarding eating disorder symptoms. Prevalence of some symptoms was 7.5% to 46%, but active eating disorders had a prevalence of 2% and 5% during lifetime using DSM-III diagnostic criteria. Dance majors had the highest rate of symptoms and athletes the lowest. In the subgroup 25% had used diuretics and 14% laxatives for weight control.[19] Primary care clinic attendees, dance majors, and psychology majors scored highest on the "maturity fears" scale. Several studies have examined the prevalence of anorexia in high school and college-age students in the United States.[20] A college survey using DSM-III criteria for bulimia found a prevalence rate of 4% among women and 0.4% among men.[21] Students in disciplines that require an increased focus on body image (such as dancing or drama) versus exercise (such as physical education) showed a greater risk for developing AN when given the Eating Attitudes Test.[22] A second study found that adolescent ballet dancers reported characteristics of AN (underweight, distorted body image, amenorrhea, and binge eating) significantly more often than the controls,[23] in particular bulimic symptoms, such as fasting, binge eating, and other individual methods to control weight. Another study found anorexic like behaviors significantly higher in college students taking an elective nutrition course than in dietetic majors.[24] This finding suggests that some features of BN may be widespread in college populations, without there being a full illness syndrome present, with a commonly cited female-to-male ratio in both AN and BN of 10 to 1.[25]

AN and BN appear to be chronic conditions, although there may be quite a lot of variability in the severity of symptoms and illness over time. In anorexia the course of the disease may be episodic, unremitting, or most commonly a single episode. With BN, the course is usually chronic or intermittent over many years.[5] The mortality rate for AN is a notable 5%–20%, one of the highest rates among psychiatric disorders.[2,22]

Risk factors for the development of eating disorders are unclear, but may include having a family member with AN or BN and a possible family history of affective disorder or substance abuse. First-degree biological relatives of people with AN or BN may have had a major depression. Weight loss can occur in depression, but no disturbance in body image or intense fear of obesity is noted as in AN.[5] In bulimia, parents of the person affected are often obese, or the child may be obese in adolescence.

Biochemical and Clinical Abnormalities

The signs and symptoms and laboratory findings in AN and BN are understood most easily in the context of the stage of the illness and the diet pattern that has been followed. After the onset of the illness and for a considerable time depletion of adipose tissue and no abnormalities on laboratory tests. Yet, because AN and BN are associated with potentially serious medical complications.[2,26,27] The American College of Physicians recently urged that physicians need to become more familiar with eating disorders, especially since many of these people appear to be healthy on initial examination and frequently deny any illness or minimize the severity of their symptoms.[2,27] A significant number of people with bulimia nervosa may have normal body weight or weight above the normal range; hence, only suspicion will lead to the diagnosis of the disorder. People with AN often wear baggy clothes to hide their thinness.

Persons with AN and BN may present with determatological signs as a result of (1) starvation or malnutrition (e.g., brittle hair and nails, lanugolike body hair, asteatodic skin, and carotenodermia[28,29]); (2) self-induced vomiting with dental enamel erosion and gingivitis[28,29] and hand calluses[30-32]; and (3) other concomitant psychiatric illness, e.g., hand dermatitis from compulsive hand washing.[5] Obsessive-compulsive behaviors may be present as well. People presenting with dermatological complaints where there is minimal or no physical basis for the complaint frequently have a disturbed body image.[33] Suspicion of an underlying eating disorder may be justified in these people, as the disturbed body image may be associated with concerns about body weight and may predispose them to development of an eating disorder.

Laboratory studies are of greatest help in documenting the degree of physiological adaptation to undernourishment and the complications of AN and BN and in identifying other illnesses resembling eating disorders. There is no laboratory profile that is diagnostic, although hypoalbuminemia and hypercarotenemia are often present.[28] The presence of hypophosphatemia indicates a need for hospitalization.[34] When physical signs and laboratory findings not usually associated with AN, such as increased heart rate, erythrocyte sedimentation rate, or leukocyte count, are found, they should alert the physician to a possible medical complication or the presence of another disorder.[2]

The laboratory profiles vary considerably in different stages of the disorder and give only a picture of the variables at the time the tests are performed. Therefore, consideration of the stage of the disorder is important in evaluating the laboratory findings. Abnormalities may not be noticed until the illness is present for a long time. People with bulimia have abnormalities in the hypothalamic-pituitary-thyroidal axis as seen by the response of T_3 to thyrotropin-relasing hormone.[35] This response differs from hypothroidism in that a 25% body weight loss, increased growth hormones, normal gonadotropin, PBI, and T_3 tests are noted (Table 23–1). MRI findings provide further evidence of pituitary abnormalities in eating disorder patients; however, the deficiencies may be due to endocrine nutritional deregulation.[36] Also, the higher C-peptide excretion per kg body weight in AN compared with normal-weight children, indicates that insulin secretion is increased in relation to body weight.[37] Serum electrolyte values tend to be in the normal range, except in cases in which vomiting or laxative abuse is a feature. The reported values may be high because of dehydration, which may be serious and cause death. Because of changes in dehydration, the hematological picture is variable. Vomiting may result in decreased extracellular

and blood values, metabolic alkalosis, and a shift of blood potassium into the cells. Laxative abuse produces hypovolemia, hypokalemia, metabolic acidosis, and up to 60m Eq/L loss of K+ in the stool.[34]

Although many people with AN present with protein-energy malnutrition, deficiency of other nutrients are rare.[38] Serum protein or albumin values tend to remain normal until advanced stages of starvation are reached. Many of the features of anorexia are common to zinc deficiency and starvation. The zinc, copper, and iron-binding protein deficiency reflect starvation.[39] Assessing body zinc levels is difficult, and the option of zinc supplementation is controversial. Decreased levels of pyridoxine may be noted. Histidine given in quantities of 8 to 12 grams to animals has produced anorexia with a stripping of zinc from binding sites and increased urinary excretion at a level of 234 mg/24 hr.[40] The total body potassium to total body water is not decreased or the total exchangeable sodium to total exchangeable potassium elevated in people with AN, as is shown in clinical relevant malnutrition.[40] Thus, these body composition measures should not be evaluated as malnutrition in the nutritional management of people with AN.[40]

Growth hormone presynaptic and alpha-2 adrenegic receptor activity is elevated and synaptic norepinephrine and 3-methaxy-4-hydroxyphinylglycol activity decreased in malnourished people with AN.[41] With nutrition rehabilitation before weight gain occurs, the synaptic norepinephrine output is increased, and the postsynaptic alpha-2 receptor activity is reduced but sill remains higher than normal. Perhaps pathways in the medial hypothalmics are disturbed, which influences feeding behavior.[41] A decreased level of cortisol is noted in the brain in AN as increased levels of cortisol fuel the body and shrink the frontotemporal lobe, which may in turn cause rejection or gorging of food and produce a preoccupation with it.

Little documentation of the long-term complications of AN and BN has been done, although various cardiovascular arrhythmias leading to heart failure and renal complications caused by dehydration can occur.[2] Demineralization of bone (osteoporosis) can be a long-range consequence, especially if the individual is not physically active. However, in one study the subjects who exercised did not differ from the controls in bone density.[42] Mazess et al.[43] used dual photon absorptiometry to measure 11 patients aged 18- to 46-year old weighing 15 kg less than their normal peers, who had AN for 1–8 years. In comparison to normal females, these patients had fat mass (3.35 kg) and content of soft tissue (7.8%) four and three times lower, respectively; total skeletal mineral content (1921 g) of femoral and spinal about 25% less; total body bone mineral density 10%, 13%, and 25% lower, respectively, and bone mineral content as a fraction of lean tissue mass 1% lower (4.9%).[43] Bachrach et al.[41] found that adolescents (12–20 years of age) with AN had significantly lower lumbar spine and whole body bone mass, as well as a lower body mass index than normal. Kidney stones may be present. Gastrointestinal complications, such as constipation and delayed gastric emptying may occur. There may be difficulty in urination, causing an elevation in serum amylase levels[44] The skeletal system also may be involved, with myopathies related to ipecac abuse or hypokalemia in bulimia.[45] Water and electrolyte imbalances are major complications. Restoration of muscle electrolytes, are major complications. Restoration of muscle electrolytes, particularly potassium and sodium, produces a greater positive effect on muscle function in AN than repletion of body nitrogen.[46] Prolonged undernutrition usually causes a decrease in serum cholesterol, although patients with AN may have hyperlipidemia.[47] People with AN can have elevated serum carotene and vitamin A levels that may be due to the excessive intake of carotenoids or to an acquired defect in the utilization or metabolism of these compounds.[27] Overt vitamin deficiencies are rare.[36]

Factors to be Considered in Nutritional Evaluation

A detailed history including the onset of the disorder, early childhood nutrition, and current history, is essential. The AN person may be dieting on a low caloric or other restrictive diet, have a distorted self-image, exercise obsessively, occasionally abuse alcohol or other drugs, use body weight to determine self-worth, talk and think about food constantly, and be afraid of not being able to stop eating. Possible warning signals for AN or BN in adolescents are shown in Table 23–2. BN patients often show strong feelings of guilt and anger when eating high amounts of calories or fat.[48]

Behavior

Although it was generally thought that people with AN have similar diet patterns characterized by specific carbohydrate avoidance,[49] a study of diet patterns in a group of people with AN found much diversity.[50] All people restricted their caloric intake, but 38% maintained a satisfactory quality in the selection of their diets.[50] Of the 62% whose diets were unsatisfactory in quality, most had irregular meal patterns, and high proportions of this group indulged in binge eating, fasting, or vomiting.[50] Recognition of the great variability in diet preferences among people with AN has implications for planning individualized treatment. A laboratory to study feeding behaviors in humans by allowing BN patients to freely binge for 24 hours from an unlimited amount of food has been designed.[51]

When tested against laboratory analysis, the use of food composition lists and food exchange lists proved acceptable in evaluating food offered to people hospitalized with eating disorders. The caloric intake was a 2.4% difference; carbohydrate and fat intakes were overestimated by 4.5% and 5.4%, respectively; and protein intake was underestimated 1.1%.[52]

Laboratory

Very few tests are definitive, but hypoalbuminemia and hypercarotenemia may be present. However, serum albumin, prealbumin, and retinol-binding protein levels may be normal[53] or reduced if severe depression is present due to either primary or secondary malnutrition.[54] Complement proteins may be decreased.[55] Body potassium may be elevated and growth hormone and urinary zinc excretion increased. A complete blood cell count (CBC), electrolytes, blood urea nitrogen (BUN)/creatinine or transferrin tests, and osmolality of both serum and urine levels may be performed (Fig. 23–1).[34]

Anthropometric measures

Height, weight, muscle mass, triceps fatfold, and physical activity should be determined and records kept regularly. Weight loss appears to be a major marker (rather than other anthropometrics) especially if depression is present.[54] Prolonged undernutrition in early adolescence may affect the adolescent growth spurt and depress growth in stature.

Physical signs

It is important to evaluate the skin, hair, nails, lips and tongue, and skeletal appearance.

Dietary Management

Both anorexia and bulimia require a multifaceted treatment approach encompassing medical management and behavioral, individual, cognitive, and family therapy. A multidisciplinary team needs to work together to provide the best treatment for the person. The dietitian is a key member of this team since nutrition intervention is a main concern in these disorders (Tables 23–2 and 23–3). In eating disorders, the immediate aim should be to restore the person's nutritional state to normal. Dietitians can identify disordered eating patterns through these assessment instruments; Eating Disorder Inventory (EDI)[57] and Eating Attitude Test (EAT).[22,57] Skilled clinicians use DSM-III-R diagnostic criteria to properly categorize candidates for the multifaceted treatment approach.

Nutrition

The dietitian's responsibility is to determine immediate and long-term goals in nutrition rehabilitation during hospital and follow-up care. The dietitian may serve as co-facilitator or general practitioner in working on such areas as body image, fitness, relaxation, assertiveness, problem solving, and anger management with the psychotherapist. The outpatient dietitian prescribes, evaluates, and monitors the dietary regimen. The hospital dietitian works with those who have severe medical, psychological, and nutritional risks.

Dietitians working with eating disorders must have an understanding of healthy patterns of eating, the consequences of eating disorders, proper screening tools, drug-nutrient interaction, the needs of the vulnerable population, counseling tools, standards of care and quality assurance standards, research in nutrition rehabilitation, and compliance education using statistical tools. The dietitian must have good counseling and listening skills,[56] as mere weight loss can cause irritability, depression, preoccupation with food, and sleep disturbance. A good relationship with the therapist is essential before nutrition intervention can take place.[57]

It is best to encourage weight gain through normal self-feeding versus artificial products. Liquid supplements, however, have been useful as an intermediate step if the patient is unwilling to eat ordinary food.[56] In cases of severe AN (with weight loss of 40% to 60%), total parenteral nutrition (TPN), with close monitoring of electrolytes, has been found to be a successful method of treatment until the patient is able to regain normal oral uptake in 3–8 weeks[58] (Table

Table 23–2. Warning Signals for Anorexia Nervosa or Bulimia

Category of Warning Signals	Anorexia Nervosa	Bulimia Nervosa
Eating and related behaviors	Caloric intake < 100 kcal/day Calorie counting Denial of hunger cues Extreme physical activity Fasting or restrictive dieting Feels controlled by food Food avoidances or hoarding Food seen as good or bad Frequent meal skipping Frequent thoughts about food	Binge eating > twice/week Eating used as coping strategy Fasting or restrictive dieting Feels lack of control over eating Frequent meal skipping Frequent sweets, starches, cravings Frequent thoughts about food Guilt after eating/secret eating Purging behavior Regular alcohol use Wide variation in caloric intake
Body image and body satisfaction	Body-image disturbance Fear of weight gain Previously overweight Thinness as valued goal Weight goal < 85% expected weight	Current or previous obesity Fear of weight gain Overconcern with weight/shape Thinness as valued goal Unrealistic weight goal
Health status	Amenorrhea (≥ 3 months w/no menses) Bloating/nausea Cold intolerance Constipation Weight ≤85% expected weight	Bloating/nausea/abdominal pain Constipation Frequent menses (< 21 days or > 45 days)
Personal functioning	Delayed psychosexual development Depressed affect Individuation difficulties Negative self identity Perfectionistic Poor coping with life event Recent withdrawal from friends	Depressed affect Negative self-identity Perfectionistic Poor coping with life event Recent withdrawal from friends Substance use/early sexual activity
Environmental influences	Enmeshed or overinvolved family Family history of obesity, eating disorder, or weight focus Few close friends High achievement expectations Participation in body-focused activity	Chaotic or uninvolved family Family history of obesity, eating disorder, weight or fitness focus High achievement expectations Participation in body-focused activity

From Adams, L. B., Shafer, M. B. Early manifestations of eating disorders in adolescents: defining those at risk. *J. Nutr. Educ.* 1988, 20:307. Used with permission.

23–3). TPN may be accepted more readily than nasogastric tube feedings and also is able to bring about rapid correction in electrolyte balance and protein and mineral levels, although enteral nutrition/nasogastric tube feedings are often the first line of treatment. TPN is expensive and does require close monitoring because of the possible risks of sepsis and air embolus from deliberate tampering with the TPN line, especially if the patient is depressed.[59,60] It should *not* be considered as routine treatment for AN, but rather as a last resort for those who will not respond to reasonable corrective measures, such as enteral nutrition.[34] TPN must be combined with other psychosocial treatment.

When using TPN, the short-term weight gain is not an accurate indicator of successful nutritional repletion. Only long-term weight changes can be relied on as true indicators of nutritional adequacy during nutritional repletion.[61] Estimated basal caloric requirements should be adjusted on the basis of the measured basal metabolic rate.[62] Abnormal cardiac function often occurs in asymptomatic patients with AN undergoing refeeding therapy.[63] Improved cardiac functions may lag weight gain.[64]

Treatment has several phases: obtaining a detailed diet history; determining the calorie content of the initial diet by assessing requirements for height, weight, age, and sex growth, etc. (but only increasing 300 kcal/day over the current caloric intake in the beginning); developing a diet based on calorie and protein intakes, the patient's food dislikes versus aversion, weight changes, eating and exercise patterns, purging behaviors, and behavior nutrient patterns[57]; and designing an appropriate dietary plan including initial food weighing and measuring and a diet booklet exchange list. Because the patient is concerned with weight gain, encouraging her to eat large amounts is counterproductive. Rather the diet plan should emphasize behavior strategies

Table 23-3. Nutritional Management of Eating Disorders*

I. Nutritional assessment
  A. Anthropometry
    1. Height/weight; ideal weight range
    2. Skinfold measurements; percentage body fat
  B. Laboratory tests
    1. Hematocrit, hemoglobin
    2. Transferrin, albumin
  C. Physical signs of possible nutritional deficiencies
    1. Hair
    2. Skin
    3. Lips, tongue, gums
    4. Nails
  D. Dietary history
    1. Restrictive eating pattern
    2. Binging/fasting cycle
    3. Binging/purging
II. Nutritional support
  A. Establishing nutrient needs
    1. Calories
    2. Protein
    3. Vitamins and minerals
  B. Choosing feeding modality
    1. Parenteral
    2. Enteral
    3. Oral
  C. Guidelines for nutritional therapy
    1. Gradual increase in caloric intake
    2. Controlled carbohydrate load
    3. Small, frequent stools
  D. Goals for nutritional support
    1. Restoration or preservation of nutritional status
    2. Weight maintenance/controlled gain or loss
    3. Independently maintain nutritional intake
  E. Treatment plan
    1. Inpatient—behavioral program
    2. Outpatient
      a. Weekly or biweekly weight checks
      b. Intake and vomiting records
    3. Outcome goals
      a. Cessation of vomiting/laxatives
      b. Weight maintenance; controlled loss or gain
      c. Ability to maintain adequate and balanced intake
      d. Incorporation of exercise as tolerated

Protocol of the Arizona Health Sciences Center, University Hospital
*Nutrition Service.
From Comerci, et al.,[34] with permission.

that require self-care and self-monitoring.[62] The person may be instructed to keep a diet record, as well as to record the number of laxatives, diuretics, and binge vomiting episodes.[60] Such a plan should achieve weight maintenance and incorporate variety, moderation, and regularity of eating.[65]

Giving high potassium foods to correct electrolyte imbalance and high calcium foods for bone density may be a first approach.[49] Gradually adding foods that were recently omitted from the diet should be considered. Constipation, which may result from slowed gut mobility caused by energy conservation and a small intake of foods, should subside with increased food intake. The person may have engaged in laxative abuse to relieve constipation. An effective way to decrease laxative abuse may be to contract with the person to decrease the use of laxatives by a specific amount while increasing fiber and fluid intake and concurrently pro-

viding education about the limited value of laxatives in weight loss.[60]

The whole family should be involved in the nutrition intervention rather than focusing on the child's eating problem. The focus should be on the food preferences and nutritional needs of the whole family, not on the patient's eating habits. The family should be encouraged to eat wholesome foods and snacks, rather than junk food.

Mealtimes should be pleasurable and filled with conversation about happenings of the day, news of the world, and upcoming family outings. The more enjoyable the family conversation, the more the person with AN will associate food with pleasantness. The person with AN should be involved in meal planning. The mother should be encouraged to sit with her child once a week with recipe cards, cookbooks, and supermarket ads to devise menus for meals and snacks for the following week.

Outpatient therapy

Outpatient therapy may be tried if the person has lost less than 25% of body weight. The goal of dietary treatment is to re-establish a normal weight pattern. An individualized approach is needed to identify the specific areas that need modification. The common problems of bloating and early satiety may require extensive counseling and medication. The patient must also be convinced that weight gain will be neither too excessive nor too rapid. Therapy should also include a psychological component, focusing on the inner conflicts of the person, family dynamics, and supportive counseling of the parents. The typical family of a patient with AN is characterized by role confusion, virgility, conflict avoidance, and enmeshment.[34] Interactions with the patient and family should encourage trust and be nonjudgmental.[65]

Successful drug-dependent treatment programs utilizing a twelve step recovery method have been used by Overeaters Anonymous (OA). In OA, it focuses on group therapy, peer support, honesty (a spiritual awakening), and abstinence from specific trigger foods and other compulsive eating behaviors which reduce binging, starving and graze type eating.[66] Since those with combined AN and bulimia are more prone to chemical dependency, the effect of alcohol and drugs on nutritional status must be evaluated and treated.[67,68]

Nutrition education is also needed to help the person understand the relationship of food to growth and weight so she can make appropriate food choices.

Hospital treatment

It is generally believed that psychological disturbances underlie the severe dieting and food restriction that form the basis of AN. Self-starvation in turn affects the physiological process, as well as psychological functions, thereby creating a self-perpetuating cycle that maintains the disorder.[69] Pancreatic polypeptide have been found to increase in AN and decrease in obesity and thus may play a role in appetite control mechanisms.[70] Ending the secrecy of the eating disorder may be a first step in treatment. Because of the interaction between the psychological and physiological areas, an interdisciplinary approach is necessary in the treatment of both AN and bulimia while in the hospital. Treatment requires a well coordinated effort by the interdisciplinary team. The required members of the interdisciplinary team include a physician specializing in behavioral health, nutritionist/dietitian, registered nurse, clinical social worker, and consulting psychologist or psychiatrist.[34]

Weight loss of 30% to 40% of beginning body weight or decreased growth over a 3-month period or hypophosphatemia or significant abnormalities of electrolytes indicates the need for hospitalization.[34,55] Severe depression or attempted suicide, severe binging and purging, psychosis, family crisis, and lack or response to outpatient therapy are other reasons for hospitalization.[3] Initially, the dietitian or nutritionist should obtain a detailed diet, weight, and behavior history. The protocol of care should specify the parameters of nutrition rehabilitation, itemizing caloric requirements, activity level, weight goals, and supervision of meals.[57] A recent study suggest that weight gain can be increased and the cost of hospitalization decreased by restricting exercise during refeeding the AN clients.[71]

The hospital plan should include the family to help it understand the eating disorder and what is involved in the treatment of the person. Family involvement also will greatly ease the transition from the hospital to the home (Fig. 23-1). The use of a nasalgastric tube feeding or peripheral intravenous feeding should be limited to those who need both calories and medical treatment or those with severe electrolyte imbalance, hypophosphatemia, and fluid retention.[57] A gain of 3 lb/wk for an 8- to 12-week period on a regular diet is ideal. A maintenance diet must be determined a few weeks before discharge. Amenorrhea often is the last symptom seen prior to recovery. In one study it was shown to increase arm anthropometries and prealbumin and total

iron binding capacity but to cause a problem with a moderate rise in serum aspartate and alanine aminotransferase.[72]

Medications

Although numerous medications have been used, they do not have an established place in the treatment of eating disorders. Under certain circumstances some medications appear to be of some help; however, they should not be administered as the sole treatment for eating disorder patients. Fluoxetine is part of a common adjunctive treatment regimen in AN or bulimia when obsessive-compulsive traits are present. Weight or food nutrient changes may occur with some antidepressant, antianxiety, and antipsychotic agents (see Chapter 27). Further research is necessary in this area of treatment.

Behavior modification

Behavioral therapy forms the basis for most treatment regimens. In behavior modification the symptoms, rather than the possible underlying disturbances, are treated by reinforcement of patient behaviors that increase weight. The patients are given reasonable specific goals for which to aim and are rewarded with positive reinforcement. Behavior modification treatment programs demonstrate short-term benefits, but their long-term outcome is unknown. The person with AN must learn coping and interpersonal skills through the help of family, friends, and self-help groups and avoid relapses by choosing one or two confidants. Healthy exercise three times per week for 20–30 minutes must replace the obsessive exercise regimen. When females with

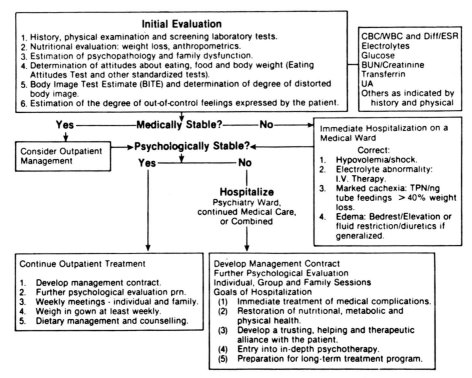

Fig. 23–1. Initial triage and management of the eating disorder patient. From Comerci et al.,[34] with permission.

bulimia described themselves as more capable of focused attention, they showed greater awareness of and responsiveness to cues signaling satiation while eating.[73] The person with bulimia must learn new eating habits to replace the alternating pattern of overfeeding and underfeeding and also may need medication to accomplish this change.[74] The nutritionist must be aware of the magnitude of change required during treatment and be knowledgeable of the relevant behavioral tools,[75] such as Multidimensional Inventory, Depression Inventory, Eating Attitudes Test, and Twelve Step Approach for Eating Disorders (Appendix 9).

Follow-up

No particular treatment has proved superior in long-term studies. Often the family of a patient with AN may think the patient is cured once she gains weight and does not realize her ongoing need for support. The treatment plan should be re-evaluated periodically (Table 23-3). In outpatient therapy, encouraging moderation of intake, variety of foods, regulation in mealtimes, and reintroducing feared foods will give the patient confidence in weight control and food selection. The dietitian or nutritionist can provide nutrition and behavior interventions to correct the cognitive distortions concerning food.[57] Providing continual nutrition education regarding nutrient needs for growth and weight control so the patient can make the proper food choices will encourage recovery.[57,76] Since the development of eating disorder behavior may begin with unsafe diets and unproven diet products, the patient should be made aware of the danger of fad diets and diet products.[77] Likewise, extreme dieting behavior in female elementary, junior high and high school students as well as in the general public should be examined and treated as early as possible.[78–80] The person with AN must learn to recognize the stressful events or people that trigger AN and have an emergency plan for such an incidence. If a weight loss of more than 5 pounds occurs, the physician should be notified. Quality assurance standards for nutrition practice of AN are being developed by the Pediatric Practice Group of the American Dietetic Association.

References

1. Herzog, D.B., Copeland, P.M. Eating disorders. *N. Engl. J. Med.* 1985; 313:295.
2. Lucas, A.R. Toward the understanding of anorexia nervosa as a disease entity. *Mayo Clin. Proc.* 1981; 56:254.
3. Abraham, S.F., Beumont, P.J.V. How patients describe bulimia or binge eating. *Psychol. Med.* 1982;12:625.
4. Anderson, A.E. Anorexia nervosa and bulimia: a spectrum of eating disorders. *J. Adoles. Health Care.* 1983; 4:15.
5. *American Psychiatric Association. Diagnostic and Statistical Manual of Mental Disorders.* 3rd ed. rev. Washington DC: APA; 1987.
6. Allen, J.R., Whichorexia: a disorder of inaccurate name, uncertain heterogeneity, questionable etiology variable course, and uncertain outcome. *J. Okla. State Med. Assoc.* 1987; 80:719.
7. Russell, G.F.M. The changing nature of anorexia nervosa: an introduction to the Conference. *J. Psychiatr. Res.* 1985; 19:101.
8. Woodside, D.B., Garfinkel, P.E. An overview of the eating disorders anorexia nervosa and bulimia nervosa. *Nutr. Today* 1989; 24:27.
9. Casper, R.C., Eckert, E.D., Halmi, K.A., Goldberg, S.C., Davis, J.M. Bulimia: its incidence and clinical importance in patients with anorexia nervosa. *Arch. Gen. Psychiatr.* 1980; 37:1030.
10. The aetiology of anorexia nervosa. *Psychol. Med.* 1983; 13:231. Editorial
11. Garner, D.M., Garfinkel, P.E., Schwartz, D., Thompson, M. Cultural expectations of thinness in women. *Psychol. Rep.* 1980; 47:483.
12. Maloney, M.J., McGuire, J., Daniels, S.R., Specker, B. Dieting behavior and eating attitudes in children. *Pediatrics.* 1989; 84:842.
13. Pugliese, M.T., Lifshita, F., Grad, G., Fort, P., Marks-Katz, M. Fear of obesity: A cause of short stature and delayed puberty. *N. Engl. J. Med.* 1983; 309:513–518.
14. Lifshitz, F., Moses, N. Growth failure: a complication of dietary treatment of hypercholesterolemia. *Am. J. Dis. Child.* 1989; 143:537.
15. Crisp, A.H. Premorbid factors in adult disorders of weight, with particular reference to primary anorexia nervosa (weight phobia). A literature review. *J. Psychom. Res.* 1970; 14:1.
16. Harris, R.T. Bulimarexia and related serious eating disorders with medical complications. *Ann. Intern. Med.* 1983; 99:800.
17. Jones, D., Fox, M., Babigan, H., Hutton, H. Epidemiology of anorexia nervosa in Monroe County. *Psychosom. Med.* 1980; 42:551.
18. Gwirtsman, H.E., Roy-Byrne, P., Lerner, L., Yager, J. Bulimia in men: report of three cases with neuroendocrine findings. *J. Clin. Psychiatr.* 1984; 45:78.
19. Kurtzman, F.D., Yager, J., Lundsverb, J., Weismeir, E., Bodurba, D.C. Eating disorders among selected female student populations at UCLA. *J. Am. Diet. Assoc.* 1989; 89:45.
20. Herzog, D. Focus on eating disorders. In: Herzog, D., ed. *Advanced in Psychiatry.* San Diego: Park Row; 1987.
21. Zuckerman, D.M., Colby, A., Ware, N.C., Lazerson, J.S. The prevalence of bulimia among college students. *Am. J. Public Health.* 1986; 76:1135.
22. Joseph, A., Wood, I.K., Goldberg, S.C. Determining populations at risk for developing anorexia nervosa based on selection of college major. *Psychiatr. Res.* 1982; 7:53.
23. Braisted, J.R., Mellin, L., Gong, E.J., Irwin, C.E. The adolescent ballet dancer: nutritional practices and characteristics associated with anorexia nervosa. *J. Adolesc. Health Care.* 1985; 6:365.
24. Johnston, C.S., Christopher, F.S. Anorexic-like behavior in dietetic majors and other student populations. *J. Nutr. Ed.* 1991; 23:148.
25. Yates, W.R., Sieleni, B. Anorexia and bulimia. *Prim. Care* 1987; 14:737.
26. Golden, N., Sacker, I.M. An overview of the etiology, diagnosis, and management of anorexia nervosa. *Clin. Pediatr.* 1984; 23:209.
27. Eating Disorders. Anorexia nervosa and bulimia. Position paper. Health and Public Policy Committee, American College of Physicians. *Ann. Intern. Med.* 1986; 105:790.
28. Schwabe, A.D., Lippe, B.M., Chang, R.J., Pops, M.A., Yager, J. Anorexia nervosa. *Ann. Intern. Med.* 1981; 94:371.
29. Lacey, J. Anorexia nervosa and a bearded female saint. *Br. Med. J.* 1982; 285:1816.
30. Williams, J.F., Friedman, I.M., Steiner, H. Hand lesions characteristic of bulimia. *Am. J. Dis. Child.* 1986; 140:28.
31. Joseph, A.B., Herr, B. Finger calluses in bulimia. *Am. J. Psychiatr.* 1985; 5:655.
32. Schwartz, B., Clendenning, W. A cutaneous sign of bulimia. *J. Am. Acad. Dermatol.* 1985; 12:725.
33. Cotterill, J.A. Dermatological non-disease: a common and potentially fatal disturbance of cutaneous body image. *Br. J. Dermatol.* 1981; 104:611.
34. Comerci, G.D., Kilbourne, K., Carroll, A.E. *Eating Disorders in Young Anorexia Nervosa and Bulimia: Part II.* Chicago: Year Book; 1985.
35. Kiyohara, K., Tamai, H., Kobayashi, N., Nakagawa, T. Hypothalmic-pituitary-thyroidal axis alterations in bulimic patients. *Am. J. Clin. Nutr.* 1988; 47:805.
36. Doraiswamy, P., Murali, K., Krishnan, R., Boyko, O.B., Mustafa, M.H., Figiel, G.S., Palese, V.J., Escalona, P.R., Sunjay, A.S., McDonald, W.M., Rockwell, W.J.K., Ellingwood, Jr., E.H.: Pituitary abnormalities in eating disorders: further evi-

dence from MRI studies. *Prog. Neuro-Psychopharmacol. Biol. Psychiat.* 1991; 15:351.

37. Wallensteen, M., Ginsburg, B.E., Dahlquist, G.: Urinary C-peptide excretion in obese and anorectic children. *Acta Paediatr. Scand.* 1991; 80:521.
38. Cainley, C., Cason, J., Carlsson, L., Thompson, R.P.H., Slavin, B.M., Norton, R.W. Short reports: zinc state in anorexia nervosa. *Br. Med. J.* 1986; 293:992.
39. Casper, R.C., Kischner, B., Sandstead, H.H., Jacob, R.A., Davis, J.M. An evaluation of trace metals, vitamins, and taste function in anorexia nervosa. *Am. J. Clin. Nutr.* 1980; 33:1801.
40. Dempsey, D.T., Crosby, L.O., Lusk, E., Oberlander, J.L., Pertschuk, M.J., Mullen, J.L. Total body water and total potassium in anorexia nervosa. *Am. J. Clin. Nutr.* 1984; 40:260.
41. Kaye, W.H., Gwirtsman. H.E., Lake, C.R., Siever, L.J., Jimerson, D.C., Ebert, M.H., Murphy, D.L. Disturbances of norepinephrine metabolism and alpha-2 adrenegic receptor activity in anorexia nervosa: relationship to nutritional state. *Psychopharmacol. Bull.* 1985; 21:419.
42. Rigotti, N.A., Nussbaum, S.R., Herzog, D.B., Neer, R.M. Osteoporosis in women with anorexia nervosa. *N. Engl. J. Med.* 1984; 311:1601.
43. Mazess, R.B., Barden, H.S., Ohlrich, E. Skeletal and body-composition effects of anorexia nervosa. *Am. J. Clin. Nutr.* 1990; 52:438.
44. Bachrach, L.K., Guido, D., Katzman, D., Litt, I.F., Marcus, R. Decreased bone density in adolescent girls with anorexia nervosa. *Pediatrics*, 1990; 86:440.
45. Mitchell, J.E., Seim, H.C., Colon, E., Pomeroy, C. Medical complications and medical management of bulimia. *Ann. Intern. Med.* 1987; 107:71.
46. Russell, D.M., Prendergast, P.J., Darby, P.L., Garfinkel, P.E., Whitwell, J., Jeejeebhoy, K.N. A comparison between muscle function and body composition in anorexia nervosa: The effect of refeeding. *Am. J. Clin. Nutr.* 1983; 38:229.
47. Mordasini, R., Klose, G., Greter, H. Secondary type II hyperlipidemia in patients with anorexia nervosa. *Metabolism.* 1978; 27:71.
48. Sunday, S., Einhorn, A., Holmi, K. Relationship of perceived macronutrient and caloric content to affective cognitions about food in eating-disordered, restrained, and unrestrained subjects. *Am. J. Clin. Nutr.* 1992; 55:362.
49. Garfinkel, P., Garner, D. *Anorexia Nervosa: A Multidimensional Perception.* New York: Brunner and Mazel; 1982.
50. Huse, D.M., Lucas, A.R. Dietary patterns in anorexia nervosa. *Am. J. Clin. Nutr.* 1984; 40:251.
51. Kaye, W., Weltzin, T., McKee, M., McCoraka, C., Hansen, D., Hsu, L. Laboratory assessment of feeding behavior in bulimia nervosa and healthy women: methods for developing a human-feeding laboratory. *Am. J. Clin. Nutr.* 1992; 55:372.
52. Peterson, R., Kaye, W.H., Gwirtsman, H.E. Comparison of calculated estimates and laboratory analysis of food offered to hospitalized eating disorder patients. *J. Am. Diet. Assoc.* 1986; 86:490.
53. Palla, B., Litt, I.F. Medical complications of eating disorders in adolescents. *Pediatrics.* 1988; 81:613.
54. Maes, M., Vandewoude, M., Scharpe, S., Clereq, L., Stevens, W., Lepoutre, L., Schotte, C. Anthropometric and biochemical assessment of the nutritional state in depression: evidence for lower visceral protein plasma levels in depression. *J. Affective Disord.* 1991; 23:25.
55. Wyatt, R.J., Farrell, M.K., Berry, P.L., Forristal, J., Maloney, M.J., West, C.D. Reduced alternative complement pathway control protein levels in anorexia nervosa: response to parenteral nutrition. *Am. J. Clin. Nutr.* 1982; 35:973.

56. Krey, S.H., Palmer, K., Porcelli, K.A. Eating disorders: the clinical dietitian's role. *J. Am. Diet. Assoc.* 1989; 89:41.
57. Position Paper of the American Dietetic Association. Nutrition intervention in the treatment of anorexia nervosa and bulimia nervosa. *J. Am. Diet. Assoc.* 1988; 88:68.
58. Croner, S., Larsson, J. Schildt, B., Symreng, T. Severe anorexia nervosa treated with total parental nutrition: clinical course and influence on clinical chemical analyses. *Acta Paediatr. Scand.* 1985; 74:230.
59. Maloney, M.J., Farrell, M.K. Treatment of severe weight loss in anorexia nervosa with hyperalimentation and psychotherapy. *Am. J. Psychiatr.* 1980; 137:310.
60. Gold, P.N., Goodwin, F.K., Chrousos, G.P. Clinical and biochemical manifestations of depression. Relation to the neurobiology of stress. *N. Engl. J. Med.* 1988; 319:348.
61. Dempsey, D.T., Crosby, L.O., Pertschuk, M.J., Feurer, I.D., Buzby, B.P., Mullen, J.L. Weight gain and nutritional efficacy in anorexia nervosa. *Am. J. Clin. Nutr.* 1984; 39:236.
62. Huse, D.M., Lucas, A.R. Dietary treatment of anorexia nervosa. *J. Am. Diet. Assoc.* 1983; 83:687.
63. Kahn, D., Halls, J., Bianco, J.A., Perlman, S.B. Radionuclide ventriculography in severely underweight anorexia nervosa patients before and during refeeding therapy. *J. Adolesc. Health.* 1991; 12:301.
64. Powers, P., Schocken, D., Feld, J., Holloway, J., Boyd, F. Cardiac function during weight restoration in anorexia nervosa. *Eating Disord.* 1991; 10:521.
65. Story, M. Nutrition management and the dietary treatment of bulimia. *J. Am. Diet. Assoc.* 1986; 86:517.
66. Devlin, C.L. Twelve step intervention in compulsive eating. *J. Am. Diet. Assoc.* 1991; 91:A81.
67. Mohs, M., Watson, R., Leonard-Green, T. Nutritional effects of marijuana, heroin, cocaine, and nicotine, *J. Am. Diet. Assoc.* 1990; 90:1261.
68. American Dietetic Association Position Paper: Nutrition intervention in treatment and recovery from chemical dependency. *J. Am. Diet. Assoc.* 1990; 90:1274.
69. Wakeling, A. Neurobiological aspects of feeding disorders. *J. Psychiatr. Res.* 1985; 19:191.
70. Uhe, A., Szmuckler, G., Collier, G., Hansky, J., O'Dea, K., Young, G. Potential regulators of feeding behavior in anorexia nervosa. *Am. J. Clin. Nutr.* 1992; 55:28.
71. Kaye, W.H., Gwirtsman, H.E., Obarzanek, W., George, D.T. Relative importance of calorie intake needed to gain weight and level of physical activity in anorexia nervosa. *Am. J. Clin. Nutr.* 1988; 47:989.
72. Bufano, G., Cervellin, G., Coscelli, C. Enteral nutrition in anorexia nervosa. *J. Pen.* 1990; 14:404.
73. Heilbrun, Jr., A.B., Worobow, A.L. Attention and disordered eating behavior: I. disattention to satiety cues as a risk factor in the development of bulimia. *J. Clin. Psychology.* 1991; 47:3.
74. Greene, G.W., Achterberg, C., Crumbaugh, J., Soper, J. Dietary intake and die practices of bulimic and non-bulimic female college students. *J. Am. Diet. Assoc.* 1990; 90:576.
75. Gray, G.E., Gray, L.K. Nutritional aspects of psychiatric disorders. *J. Am. Diet. Assoc.* 1989; 89:1492.
76. Clark, N. How to approach eating disorders among athletes. *Top. Clin. Nutr.* 1990; 5:41.
77. Kirkley, B.G. Bulimia: clinical characteristics, development and etiology. *J. Am. Diet. Assoc.* 1986; 86:468.
78. Stein, D. The prevalence of bulimia: a review of the empirical research. *J. Nutr. Ed.* 1991; 23:205.
79. Brownell, K. Dieting and the search for the perfect body: where physiology and culture collide. *Behav. Therapy* 1991; 22:1.
80. McDuffie, J., Kirkley, B. Eating disorders and management. *Semin. Ped. Gastro. Nutr.* 1992; 3:8.

Chapter 24
Feeding Problems of the Child With Special Health Care Needs

Harriet Cloud

The nutritional health of an infant and child is determined by food intake achieved through the act of feeding and/or eating. The amount of food intake is dependent, in turn, upon the infant's ability to suckle, suck, progress to the cup and solid food, and eventually self-feed the recommended mix of protein, fats, carbohydrates, vitamins, minerals, and water.

Through the consumption of adequate nutrients, infants and children grow in length and gain in weight at an appropriate rate and have adequate energy for basic metabolic needs, growth, and activity levels. Children with special health care needs often have feeding problems that result in altered growth either in height or weight, and they lack the energy needed to participate in activities associated with intervention (such as physical therapy, speech therapy, and education).[1]

Feeding problems are frequently found in children with cerebral palsy, cleft palate, Down's syndrome, seizures, hypotonia, prematurity, and other chronic medical disorders. To improve assessment of and intervention with these problems the therapist must understand the normal development of feeding.[1]

Normal Development of Feeding

Feeding is a multidimensional process that influences an infant's development.[2] It is part of the infant's interaction with the environment that promotes learning and development. Under 1 year of age, feeding occupies half of the time that the infant is awake.[2] The development of the feeding process involves oral motor, gross motor, fine motor, and behavioral skills.

The general terms used to describe the oral-motor process include suckling, sucking, swallowing, chewing and gagging, tongue elevation and lateralization, and biting.[3] Certain anatomical structures are associated with these processes. The oral cavity consists of the upper jaw or maxilla, the lower jaw or mandible, upper and lower lips, cheeks, tongue, teeth, floor of the mouth, hard and soft palates, uvula, and anterior and posterior faucial arches. Oral-motor structures are necessary for sucking and suckling, biting, and chewing (Fig 24-1). The structures involved in swallowing include the pharyngeal structures and the larynx. Pharyngeal structures include the superior, medial, and inferior pharyngeal constrictors, which function as a valve at the top of the esophagus. The juncture of the pharynx and the esophagus is known as the P-E juncture of the cricopharyngeal sphincter.[2] The larynx functions to keep food from entering the airway. In Figures 24-1 and 24-2 the various parts of the larynx are labeled.

The esophagus, the final component of the oral-motor system, is a hollow tube, approximately 23–25 cm long, and closed by a sphincter at each end. It is made up of a combination of smooth and striated muscles that together create the peristaltic action that directs food into the stomach.[2]

The normal infant is born ready to suck.[1] The first oral-motor reflex is the rooting reaction that is used to locate food (Table 24-1). If the infant's lips are touched from above, below, or from the side, the head will turn and the tongue extend toward the touch. Once the lips touch the nipple, a suck-swallow pattern is used to ingest the fluid. The suck-swallow reflex appears at or soon after birth. In suckling both the jaw and the tongue move in a forward and backward movement, propelling fluid from the external source to the back of the mouth. The oral cavity at this stage is nearly completely filled with the tongue, mandating that the tongue, lips, and cheeks work together. Fat pads in the cheeks aid in compressing the nipple, allowing the infant to consume 6–8 ounces of fluid within 20-30 minutes. The lip seal on the nipple at 1–2 months is not tight due to the decrease in total body flexion, allowing fluid to be lost at the sides of the mouth.[4]

At 4 months a true sucking pattern begins to emerge. Nose breathing is essential to normal nutritive sucking. The sucking pattern also involves separation of the jaw from the tongue. The oral patterns at this stage allow complete lip seal around the nipple and a great deal of suction to be generated.[1]

The phasic bite reflex is a rhythmical bite-and-release pattern seen as a series of jaw openings and closing, is present at birth, and continues until 3–5 months. It is a component of the early chewing pattern known as munching that appears when the child is 6–9 months of age. By 9 months, infants can hold a cookie or cracker between the gums or teeth. The jaw is stabilized in a closed position, and when the feeder breaks the cookie the child can chew and swallow the portion in the mouth. Chewing also requires tongue lateralization or the ability of the tongue to move food laterally to place it between the molars.

At 1 year of age children can achieve a controlled sustained bite through a soft cookie or cracker. A sustained bite is dependent upon jaw stability and the presence of upper and lower teeth, particularly the incisors. For children with special health care needs, lack of dentition at the usual milestones can delay chewing development.

By 18 months, chewing ability has progressed to the point that the child can bite through harder foods, such as an apple, with a controlled bite. Drooling may still be present

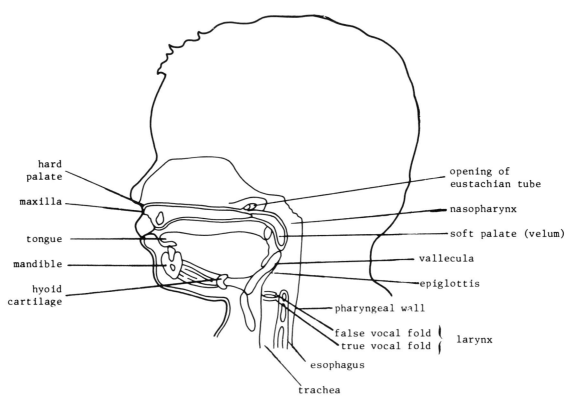

Fig. 24-1. The mouth and pharynx of the newborn (sagittal section). From Suzanne E. Morris and Marsha Dunn Klein, Pre-Feeding Skills, Therapy Skill Builders, 3830 E. Bellvue, P.O. Box 42050, Tucson, AZ. Used with permission.

when the child eats foods that are hard to bite and chew. By 24 months of age, the child becomes more experienced in biting and chewing foods of textures and hardness similar to those eaten by adults. Mature chewing has several phases: grading the jaw opening to the appropriate size for foods of different thicknesses, using fast closing strokes in rotary movement of the jaw, power closing, in which food is sheared and crushed between the teeth and an opening stroke.

To summarize, chewing is dependent upon the functioning of the jaw, tongue, lips, cheeks, and teeth. The chewing function progresses as these interdependent parts of the oral structure develop. This process prepares food for the swallowing function.

Swallowing has three phases: oral, pharyngeal, and esophageal. During the oral phase the food or liquid is organized into a bolus and moved from the front to the back of the mouth. The infant swallows liquids during the first month of life utilizing the suckle-swallow pattern. The tongue protrudes slightly from the lips with an extension-retraction movement. By 6 to 8 months liquids are swallowed from a cup with no observable elevated tongue tip position. By 12 months the infant swallows liquid from the cup with a tongue tip that is intermittently elevated. The lips may be open. By 2 years of age the child can swallow liquids from the cup with easy lip closure, and there is no liquid loss during drinking.

Solids are swallowed usually in a soft or pureed form around 4 months of age using a suckle-suck response. Initially, tongue protrusion occurs, along with periodic choking, gagging, or vomiting. By 6 to 7 months, the tongue

shows an extension-retraction pattern or simple protrusion between the teeth, and food is not pushed out by the tongue. The bolus of food moves to the posterior pharyngeal wall, past the epiglottis into the esophagus. The bolus then continues down the esophagus into the stomach.

By 12 months of age the infant swallows with easy lip closure; handles ground, mashed, or chopped table foods with noticeable lumps; and uses an intermittent tongue tip elevation (a pattern that continues until the child is around 2 years of age).

The growth and development of all oral skills is believed to continue until about the age of 3 years.[1] At this point the normal child should have all the basic components of oral skills that will be needed as an adult (Table 24-1).

Gross motor development

At birth infants are motorically dependent, receiving all stability from physiological flexion and external support[3]—being held for feeding in a position with the head and upper body elevated to less than a 45-degree angle. By 3 months of age most infants have achieved some head control, allowing them to lift and turn the head while lying on the stomach. At this age, infants usually are held in a more upright position for feeding. By 4 months the infant is visually more aware of the hands and inspects them intently. Around 5 months the infant reaches and grasps objects and brings them to the mouth.

By 6 months, babies are motorically ready to become more active participants in the feeding process.[3] They begin

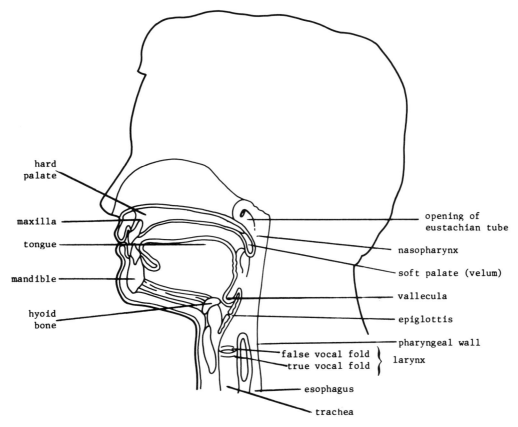

Fig. 24–2. The mouth and pharynx of the adult (sagittal section). From Suzanne E. Morris and Marsha Dunn Klein, Pre-Feeding Skills, Therapy Skill Builders, 3830 E. Bellvue, P.O. Box 42050, Tucson, AZ. Used with permission.

to sit without support, grasp for objects, and discover the world through their mouth exploring taste, shapes, weight, and texture.[3] At this point they may be fed in a high chair or infant feeding seat. As a stable feeding position develops at 6–8 months, infants are able to hold a small cup.

Motor development from 9–12 months varies, but the trend is toward increasing mobility and exploration of the environment. By 9 months sitting balance is usually improved, and the child can sit in a high chair without the need for propping devices. During the period from 9–12 months, the child can move about by pulling to stand, creeping, moving along holding onto furniture, and eventually walking independently. With good sitting ability and the increasing functionality of the hands and fingers, the infant reaches for the spoon, cup, or any food presented; puts fingers into the food; and takes it to the mouth or plays with it. As motor development progresses in the toddler and preschool years, independence in feeding continues. By 2 years of age in normal children the foundation has been set for a lifetime of skilled eating patterns.

Feeding position is an important component for all children. It is essential that the child has adequate support for the head, trunk, and legs. In the ideal position for feeding, the child has hip flexion of 90 degrees or more, thighs in neutral alignment or slight abduction, ankle dorsiflexion matching the degree of hip flexion, trunk in midline, elbows

flexed and resting in a tray, and head in midline with the chin slightly ventroflexed (Figs 24-3 and 24-4).

Behavioral aspects of feeding

Feeding is an important element of parental-child relations beginning in infancy and continuing through adolescence.[4] In a normal feeding situation the child should be in control of his or her food and fluid intake and should communicate to the mother and/or caregiver by furnishing cues related to satiety.[4] As infants mature they respond to their feeder's reaction to the cues they provide. This response may be positive or negative, causing either a decrease or increase of a certain feeding behavior, depending on the feeder's reaction to the infant.[4]

Positive behaviors that accompany feeding as the child matures include acceptance of a wide variety of foods and textures, remaining seated, keeping hands off other people, self-feeding at the appropriate level for age, eating at a moderate pace, eating and drinking quietly, using utensils appropriately, and chewing and swallowing with the mouth closed.[5] Negative behaviors include crying, refusal to accept an item of food, gagging and vomiting in response to food offered, and the inability or unwillingness to sit still during mealtime.[6] Studies of normal parent-infant interactions cited mealtime as a major avenue of parent-infant bonding, playing, and learning social games.[2,4]

Table 24–1. Feeding Development in Normal Infants

Age	Oral-Motor Skills	Self-Feeding
0–4 weeks	Rooting reflex Suckling pattern Suck-swallow reflex Jaw and tongue move up and down	
8 weeks	Tongue moves forward and back Suckling still primary action	
12 weeks	Corners of lips become active in sucking Tongue is extended out of mouth in feeding anticipation	
16 weeks	Sucking stage begins Tongue thrust still present	Sees bottle and becomes excited
20 weeks	Munching stage begins Smacks lips together Strained foods introduced	Pat or puts hands on bottle
24 weeks	Lips begin to close around spoon Progression of solid food continues	
28 weeks	Lips begin to move while chewing Vertical chewing stage begins Jaw and tongue move up and down	Plays with spoon May help spoon find mouth
32–36 weeks	Lip closure achieved Cup drinking begins	Feeds self crackers, cookies, etc. Holds bottle
40–52 weeks	Tongue lateralization leads to rotary chewing Licks food from lower lip	Can hold own bottle well Can hold cup but may spill contents

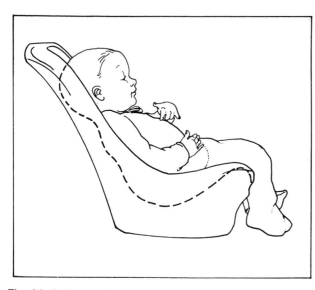

Fig. 24–3. Proper feeding position for the infant. From Cloud, H. *Team Approach to Pediatric Feeding Problems.* Chicago: American Dietetic Association, 1987. Used with permission.

Feeding Problems

Feeding problems are defined as the inability or refusal to eat certain foods because of neuromotor dysfunction, obstructive lesions, and/or psychosocial factors. Problems generally are classified as oral-motor, positioning, and behavioral. The nutritional consequences of feeding problems may include slow growth, inadequate weight gain, dental caries, anemia, vitamin and mineral deficiencies, developmental delay, and psychosocial problems (see Chapters 3 and 34).

Oral-motor problems

Generally oral-motor problems have been described by Lane[1] as an exaggeration of normal neuromotor mechanisms, leading to a disruption of rhythm and organization of oral-motor patterns and interference in the feeding process (Table 24-2).

Morris[3] has described the jaw as the most important component in the inner feeding process. Lack of stability to the jaw prevents the lips and tongue from operating from a stable, secure base. Food transfers in chewing cannot occur when abnormal or delayed control of the jaw is present.

Some neurologically impaired infants and children suffer from poor postural control and total body extension that contribute to jaw thrust, which makes it difficult for the infant to suck and for the young child to close the mouth for eating. In such children two types of bite reflexes may

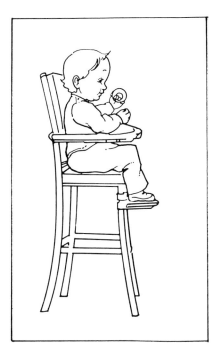

Fig. 24–4. Good feeding position for a child aged 6 months to 24 months, showing hip flexion, trunk in midline, and head in midline. Good foot support with a stool should continue throughout childhood. From Cloud, H. *Team Approach to Pediatric Feeding Problems*. Chicago: American Dietetic Association; 1987. Used with permission.

Table 24–2. Common Feeding Problems

Problem	Description
Tonic bite reflex	Strong jaw closure when teeth and gums are stimulated
Tongue thrust	Forceful and often repetitive protusion of an often bunched or thick tongue in response to oral stimulation
Jaw thrust	Forceful opening of the jaw to the maximal extent during eating, drinking, attempts to speak, or general excitement
Tongue retraction	Pulling back the tongue within the oral cavity at the presentation of food, spoon, or cup
Lip retraction	Pulling back the lips in a very tight smile-like pattern at the approach of the spoon or cup toward the face
Sensory defensiveness	A strong adverse reaction to sensory input (touch, sound, light)

Modified from Lane & Cloud.[1]

occur and interfere with eating. In the phasic bite reflex stimulation of the gums elicits a rhythmical opening and closing of the jaw. Oral stimulation elicits the tonic bite reflex, which results in tight closure of the jaw that the child cannot control. This action is often baffling to a parent who may interpret this abnormal feeding pattern as resistance to a certain food. Such a pattern interferes with all aspects of feeding.

Tongue thrust can make the placement of food in the mouth difficult and interfere with the child's ability to suck, chew, and swallow.[1] Tongue retraction can be identified easily when food can be placed in the front of the mouth in the hollow left by the pulled-back tongue.[1] Food is then pushed out of the mouth when the mouth closes and the tongue moves forward. Both tongue thrust and retraction interfere with the tongue's ability to organize food into a bolus and propel it to the back of the mouth for swallowing.

Lip retraction occurs when the lips are drawn back so they form a tight horizontal line over the mouth. Sucking from the bottle or breast, removing food from a spoon or liquid from a cup, transferring food, and retaining food in the mouth are all difficult. Lip pursing is often an attempt to compensate for retracted lips.

Whenever oral-motor problems occur, food intake is limited, and the possibility of severe nutritional problems exists. Slow growth and inadequate weight gain are common among children with oral-motor feeding problems and are often attributed to fatigue on the part of both the child and feeder.[1,7] In addition, oral-motor dysfunction often causes a disturbance in the normal progression of feeding development and food textures.

Problems with sensory processes

Sensory processes can be perturbed in the neurologically impaired infant and child with spina bifida, cerebral palsy, and seizure disorders. Morris and Klein[3] describe the deviations in normal sensory capacity into two broad categories: hypersensitivity and hyposensitivity.

The response in hypersensitivity is one of overreaction or hyperreaction.[3] The hyperreactive child has strong reactions to a variety of stimuli, resulting in increases in postural tone and abnormal reflex patterns. The author observed a typical reaction to the reintroduction of food in a 9-month-old infant who was fed by gastrostomy for 5 months. When strained fruit was offered and introduced onto the lips, the infant shuddered noticeably, a typical response. In contrast, children with hypersensitivity may also gag, vomit, or display delayed developmental skills.

Hyporeactions frequently are encountered in infants and children who are hypotonic or who have poor swallowing cues. A reduction in taste acuity, smell, and touch-pressure sensitivity in the mouth may occur. These sensory impairments contribute to severe motor feeding disorders and indifference toward eating.[3]

According to Lane, sensory defensiveness can occur alone or in combination with other feeding problems.[1] The most common type of defensiveness occurs in response to light touch around or in the mouth. An additional problem for the child with hyper- or hyporeaction is being subject to sensory overload.[3] When placed in an environment filled with many distractions (or even a normal environment), the neurologically damaged child may react with hyperactivity and display no attention to feeding. Therefore, control of the feeding environment to decrease sensory input is a key factor in nutrition intervention.

Problems with the feeding process

The feeding process involves suckling, sucking, swallowing, biting, and chewing. Generally, the disturbance in the feeding process stems from problems in oral-motor development and the positioning of the child.[3] Problems in the suckling process involve a suckle that may be arrhythmical, weak, poorly sustained, inefficient, or rapid, resulting in inadequate intake of formula or beast milk. Infants with this problem require a position for feeding that decreases extension, puts the trunk and pelvis in good alignment, and provides jaw stability.

A second problem in the feeding process involves an inability to make the shift from suckle to suck, which usually occurs around 6 to 9 months of age.[3] The child who is unable to progress to a suck may show poor control of the lips and cheeks; the lips are unable to create a seal to provide sucking. As a result, the frantic parent may use a small syringe for feeding or spend hours with each feeding. This condition may result in failure to thrive.

The usual result of poor control of the lips, tongue, cheeks, and jaw is an inability to remove food from a spoon by the upper lip and difficulty with the tongue propelling the food back to the swallowing position. Other problems include choking, abnormal swallowing patterns caused by absent or delayed swallowing reflexes, gagging on increased textures, and the inability to chew in a developmentally appropriate manner.

Other feeding problems stem from the child's inability or unwillingness to self-feed when he or she is developmentally able. For children with developmental disabilities, a delay in the process of self-feeding often occurs similarly to a lag in the overall developmental level or may be caused by motoric problems, such as found in cerebral palsy. In addition, some of the developmental lag may be attributed to a lack of expectation on the part of parents or caregivers, their aversion to the messiness of self-feeding, and their concern that inadequate food will be consumed if the child self-feeds.

In a child who is not developmentally disabled, finger feeding usually begins during the period from 9–12 months. At this time the child may be sitting alone or with minimal support, transferring objects from hand to hand, and using a hand-to-mouth pattern. In addition, the child has refinement of grasp, with increasing control of a mobile wrist, development of a pincer grasp, and graded hand pressure corresponding to the properties of the food. Independent cup drinking also begins at this age. The child attempts to use the spoon through grabbing and experimenting; however, independent spoon feeding usually develops between 24–30 months and is dependent on many factors: control of midrange movements in the humerus and elbow, ability to move the spoon through space, control of the midrange forearm rotation and wrist movements, and controlled overhand prehension of the utensil.

Children with neuromotor problems and developmental disabilities may be cognitively ready to self-feed, but are not ready to do so from a motor control standpoint. Positioning of the child to assist with trunk stability and head control, along with self-help devices, may enable independent feeding to occur (Figs 24-5 to 24-7). It is important to keep in mind that the developmentally disabled child requires time and many opportunities to develop these skills.

Assessment of feeding problems

The assessment and management of feeding problems lend themselves well to an interdisciplinary approach involving occupational therapists, physical therapists, speech pathologists, nutritionists, and, often, the special educator, nurse, and dentist.

A number of assessment forms have been developed for use in feeding evaluations; one interdisciplinary form is included in Table 24-3. This form, the Developmental Feeding Tool, was developed by the Child Development Center at the University of Tennessee in Memphis and is unique in its team application.[8]

One of the most effective techniques for assessing the child with developmental disabilities is to have the mother or caregiver feed the child in an environment familiar to the child while being observed through a one-way mirror. Videotaping the initial encounter is an effective way to establish baseline skills and problems and assist in evaluation of the progress made during intervention. The videotape is an effective teaching tool to use with parents in letting them see the feeding process they use.

Additional impressions of feeding strengths and needs can be obtained through discussing the questions and concerns of the parents and observing the child's interaction with the family or other caregivers. A careful interview should be conducted with the parent before observing the feeding session. The interview should cover such topics as positioning, types of food eaten (texture, consistency), number of times fed, amount of food consumed, amount of liquid consumed, vitamin/mineral supplement, appetite, food allergies/intolerance, temperature of food, where and who serves meals, length of time per meal, feeding utensils, and how food is prepared. In addition, at the initial assessment, anthropometric measures, hemoglobin and hematocrit should be obtained.

Assessment of oral-motor problems

Assessment of the oral-motor process is usually completed by an occupational therapist, physical therapist, or speech pathologist and is influenced by which discipline is available to the agency, school or developmental center (Tables 23-3 and 23-4). The assessment strategies utilized by the therapist are varied. Some assessments require specific tests such as videofluoroscopy using the barium swallow to evaluate swallowing problems.[9] The transit time, oral-motor skills, and amount of aspiration are monitored by the videofluoroscopy process. Barium (traditional and supine position) and foods of three different textures (modified in feeding position) are used in the testing.

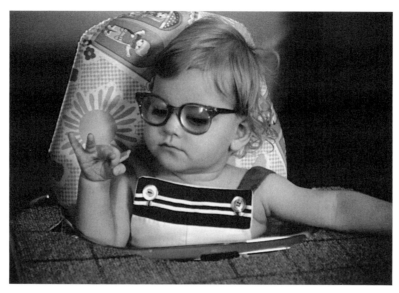

Fig. 24-5. Sixteen-month-old child with cerebral palsy just beginning to self-feed. Note that positioning provides head and trunk control and stability. Used with permission.

Although it is difficult to evaluate neurologically impaired children with the modified barium swallow, using good positioning techniques and keeping the procedure as close to normal feeding as possible for the child can facilitate its use.[9] The test provides valuable information for those therapists who plan to work on swallowing intervention in a safe manner. Where aspiration is not an issue and the individual has a very slow swallow, using thickened beverages enhances the ease of swallowing.

Assessing the position of the child is an important initial step in working with all oral-motor problems, but especially with swallowing. The child should be positioned to avoid extension of the head and particularly the neck. The trunk and pelvis should be in good alignment, the shoulder girdle and head forward, and the chin slightly tucked in.[1,10]

Individual oral structures

According to Morris,[3] the jaw is the most important component of the oral function team. It must be stable for the lips and tongue to operate from a stable base. Assessment of the jaw should include whether rotary chewing is present, jaw gradation is achieved, strong extension occurs with jaw thrusting, and a phasic bite reflex is present. The reflex is

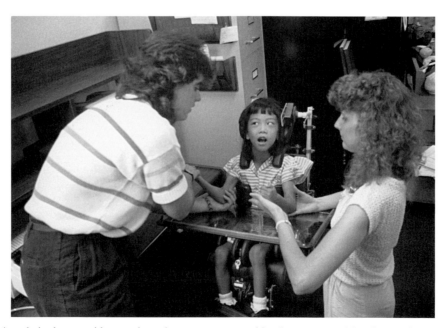

Fig. 24-6. A positioning chair that provides good trunk support, proper hip placement, and head control, all of which are necessary for working with oral-motor problems. Used with permission.

Table 24–3. Developmental Feeding Tool (DFT)

Parent/Guardian _____   Date _____
Address _____   Staff member _____
City _____ State _____ Zip _____   Child's name _____
County _____ Telephone _____ _____   Birth date _____ Age _____ Sex _____ Race _____
Referrer_____   Head circumference (cm) ____ (%ile NCHS) ____ Hand dominance ____
                                                   Height (cm) ____ (%ile NCHS) ____ Weight (kg) ____ (%ile NCHS) ____
                                                   Weight for height (%ile NCHS) ____ Hematocrit ____ Urine screen ____

PHYSICAL

Yes	No	Size
___	___	1. Weight (Avg. %ile NCHS)
___	___	2. Underweight
___	___	3. Overweight
___	___	4. Stature (Avg. %ile NCHS)
___	___	5. Short (below 5th %ile for ht. NCHS)
___	___	6. Tall (above 95th %ile for ht. NCHS)
___	___	7. Abnormal body proportions*
___	___	8. Head circumference (Avg. %ile NCHS)
___	___	9. Microcephalic
___	___	10. Macrocephalic

Laboratory

| ___ | ___ | 11. Hematocrit (Normal) |
| ___ | ___ | 12. Urine Screen (Normal)* |

Health Status

___	___	13. Bowel problems*
___	___	14. Diabetes
___	___	15. Vomiting
___	___	16. Dental caries
___	___	17. Anemia
___	___	18. Food allergies/intolerance*
___	___	19. Medications*
___	___	20. Vitamin/mineral supplements*
___	___	21. Ingests non-food items
___	___	22. Therapeutic diet*
___	___	23. General Appearance (Normal)*
___	___	24. Head (Normal)*
___	___	25. Eyes (Normal)*
___	___	26. Ears (Normal)*
___	___	27. Nose (Normal)*
___	___	28. Teeth/gums (Normal)*
___	___	29. Palate (Normal)*
___	___	30. Skin (Normal)*
___	___	31. Muscles (Normal)*
___	___	32. Arms/hands (Normal)*
___	___	33. Legs/feet (Normal)*

NEUROMOTOR/MUSCULAR

Yes	No	Tonicity
___	___	34. Body tone (Normal)*

Head and Trunk Control

___	___	35. Head control (Normal)*
___	___	36. Lifts head in prone
___	___	37. Head lags when pulled to sitting
___	___	38. Head drops forward
___	___	39. Head drops backward
___	___	40. Trunk control (Normal)*

Upper Extremity Control

___	___	41. Range of motion (Normal)*
___	___	42. Approach to object (Normal)*
___	___	43. Grasp of object (Normal)*
___	___	44. Release of object (Normal)*
___	___	45. Brings hand to mouth
___	___	46. Dominance established

Reflexes

___	___	47. Grossly normal
___	___	48. Asymmetrical tonic neck reflex*
___	___	49. Symmetrical tonic neck reflex*
___	___	50. Moro reflex*
___	___	51. Grasp reflex*

Body Alignment

___	___	52. Scoliosis
___	___	53. Kyphosis
___	___	54. Lordosis
___	___	55. Hip subluxation or dislocation, suspected

Position in Feeding

___	___	56. Mother's lap
___	___	57. Infant seat
___	___	58. High chair
___	___	59. Table and chair
___	___	60. Wheelchair
___	___	61. Other adaptive chair*

ORAL/MOTOR

Yes	No	Facial Expression
___	___	62. Symmetrical structure/function*
___	___	63. Muscle tone lips/cheeks (Normal)
___	___	64. Hypertonic muscle tone of lips
___	___	65. Hypotonic muscle tone of lips

Oral Reflexes

___	___	66. Gag (Normal)*
___	___	67. Bite (Normal)*
___	___	68. Rooting (Normal)*
___	___	69. Suck/swallow (Normal)*

Respiration

___	___	70. Mouth
___	___	71. Nose
___	___	72. Thoracic
___	___	73. Abdominal
___	___	74. Regular rhythm*

Oral Sensitivity

___	___	75. Inside mouth (Normal)*
___	___	76. Outside mouth (Normal)*
___	___	77. Hypersensitivity*
___	___	78. Hyposensitivity*
___	___	79. Intolerance to brushing teeth

FEEDING PATTERNS

Bottle-feeding

___	___	80. Suckling tongue movements
___	___	81. Sucking tongue movements
___	___	82. Firm lip seal*
___	___	83. Coordinated suck-swallow-breathing
___	___	84. Difficulty swallowing*

Cup-Drinking

| ___ | ___ | 85. Adequate lip closure* |
| ___ | ___ | 86. Loses less than 1/2 total amount* |

Yes	No	
___	___	87. Wide up-and-down jaw movements
___	___	88. Stabilizes jaw by biting edge of cup
___	___	89. Stabilizes jaw through muscle control
___	___	90. Drinks through a straw

Feeding patterns—Spoon-feeding

Yes	No	
___	___	91. Suckles as food approaches
___	___	92. Cleans food off lower lip
___	___	93. Cleans food off spoon with upper lip
___	___	94. Munching pattern

Lateralizes tongue:

| ___ | ___ | 95. When food placed between molars |

Yes	No	
___	___	96. When food placed center of tongue
___	___	97. To move food from side to side
___	___	98. Vertical jaw movements
___	___	99. Rotary jaw movements

Feeding patterns—Chewing

| ___ | ___ | 100. Lip closure during chewing* |

Table 24–3.. (*Continued*)

Isolated, Voluntary Tongue Movements
_____ _____ 101. Protrudes/retracts tongue
_____ _____ 102. Elevates tongue outside mouth
_____ _____ 103. Elevates tongue inside mouth
_____ _____ 104. Depresses tongue outside mouth
_____ _____ 105. Depresses tongue inside mouth
_____ _____ 106. Lateralizes tongue outside mouth
_____ _____ 107. Lateralizes tongue inside mouth
Special Oral Problems
_____ _____ 108. Drools*
_____ _____ 109. Thrusts tongue when utensil placed in mouth*
_____ _____ 110. Thrusts tongue during chewing/swallowing*
_____ _____ 111. Other oral-motor problem*

NUTRITION HISTORY
Past Status
_____ _____ 112. Feeding problems birth—1 year*
_____ _____ 113. Breast fed
_____ _____ 114. Bottle fed
_____ _____ 115. Weaned
Current Status
_____ _____ 116. Eats blended food
_____ _____ 117. Eats limited texture
_____ _____ 118. Eats chopped table foods
_____ _____ 119. Eats table foods
_____ _____ 120. Feeds unassisted
_____ _____ 121. Feeds with partial guidance
_____ _____ 122. Feeds with complete guidance
_____ _____ 123. Drinks from a cup unassisted
_____ _____ 124. Drinks from a cup assisted
_____ _____ 125. Finger-feeds
_____ _____ 126. Uses a spoon
_____ _____ 127. Uses a fork
_____ _____ 128. Uses a knife

_____ _____ 129. Average rate of eating
_____ _____ 130. Fast rate of eating
_____ _____ 131. Slow rate of eating
Diet Review
_____ _____ 132. Appetite normal
_____ _____ 133. Eats 3 meals/day
_____ _____ 134. Snacks daily
Dietary Intake, Current
_____ _____ 135. Milk/dairy products, 3-4/day
_____ _____ 136. Vegetables, 2-3/day
_____ _____ 137. Fruit, 2-3/day
_____ _____ 138. Meat/meat substitute, 2-3/day
_____ _____ 139. Bread/cereal, 3-4 day
_____ _____ 140. Sweets/snacks, 1-2 day
_____ _____ 141. Liquids, 2 cups/day

SOCIAL/BEHAVORIAL
Child-Caregiver Relationship
_____ _____ 142. Child responds to caregiver
_____ _____ 143. Caregiver affectionate to child
Social Skills
_____ _____ 144. Eye contact
_____ _____ 145. Smiles
_____ _____ 146. Gestures, i.e. waves byebye
_____ _____ 147. Clings to caregiver
_____ _____ 148. Interacts with examiner
_____ _____ 149. Responds to simple directions
_____ _____ 150. Seeks approval
_____ _____ 151. Toilet trained
_____ _____ 152. Knows own sex
Behavior Problems
_____ _____ 153. Self abusive
_____ _____ 154. Hyperactive
_____ _____ 155. Aggressive
_____ _____ 156. Withdrawn
_____ _____ 157. Other*
Play
_____ _____ 158. Plays infant games, i.e. pat-a-cake
_____ _____ 159. Solitary play
_____ _____ 160. Parallel play
_____ _____ 161. Cooperative play
_____ _____ 162. Additional comments*

Number COMMENTS

From Smith, M. A. H., Connolly, B., McFadden, S., Nicrosi, C. R., Muckolls, J., Russell, F. F., Wilson, W. M. *Feeding Management for a Child with a Handicap: A Guide for Professionals.* Memphis University of Tennessee Center for the Health Sciences Child Development Center, 1982. Used with permission.
*List or specify on comments section.

extinguished in the normal infant as chewing occurs; however, it may persist in the neurologically impaired child. The tonic bite reflex occurs as a hypertonic reaction and results in the child biting down on a spoon or cup and not releasing it. This pattern is common in children with strong flexor patterns in the neck, shoulder girdle, and arms (Table 24–2).

The tongue should be assessed for tongue thrust, retraction and cupping and for lack of tongue lateralization. These limiting tongue patterns can be assessed by observing the child when food is introduced. The tongue thrust is mani-

fested by the tongue pushing food or formula out when placed on the anterior third of the tongue. Tongue lateralization can be assessed by placing food in the corners of the mouth and asking the child to lick it off. Similarly, placing food on the upper lip and asking the child to lick it off can be used to evaluate tongue elevation.

Because the lips and cheeks work together, they should be assessed together. The cheek with poor muscle tone (hypotonia) does not contribute to chewing and may result in "squirreling," in which food is kept between the cheek and jaw. Poor lip tone reduces the ability to keep food in the

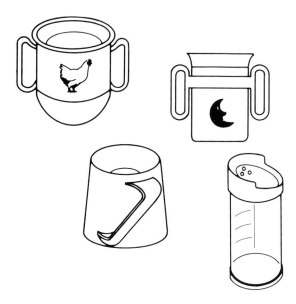

Fig. 24–7. Cups of varying shapes and weighted bottoms to assist in cup drinking during the transition from the bottle.

mouth. When there is increased tone, lip retraction results, and the lips are drawn back so that they form a tight horizontal line over the mouth. As a result, the child is unable to remove food from the spoon, use the cup well, or keep food in the mouth. One reaction to lip retraction is a process called lip pursing. The assessment process should include offering the child food from a spoon and cup and observing the lips' ability to close over the spoon and the lip of the cup.[3]

Consideration of the hard and soft palate is another important part of the oral-motor assessment. The obvious nature of a cleft in the hard palate interferes with the ability of the child to build up sufficient pressure in the mouth to obtain an efficient feeding pattern. Food or liquid may be lost through the cleft to the nose and make feeding frustrating and unpleasant for both the infant and feeder. Special nipples and bottles and proper positioning in an upright position are important (see Chapter 25).

Intervention for each oral-motor problem differs, dependent upon the nature of the problem and the developmental level of the child. The use of the interdisciplinary team and the involvement of the parent as a member of the team facilitate intervention. Some of the strategies that can be used for diagnosis and intervention of oral motor problems are shown in Table 24-4. Consultation with the occupational therapist, physical therapist, speech pathologist, and nutritionist for individualized help may be needed.

Positioning problems

Positioning is an important consideration for the child with oral-motor and self-feeding problems, as well as for the normal child. It provides stability to the child and increases the comfort level necessary for feeding intervention. Many children referred from physicians and agencies to feeding teams must be properly positioned before effective oral-motor intervention can occur. The assessment of major

feeding problems is conducted by a physical therapist and/or occupational therapist, whereas nutritionist or speech pathologist may assess minor feeding problems.

There are medical, orthopedic, respiratory, digestive and neurological components to all positions.[1,3,10] One should observe head control, trunk control, foot stability, placement of the hips and pelvis, shoulder girdle, knee flexion, and sitting base. Appropriate positioning varies, depending upon the problem identified and could include reclining on the stomach, side lying, sitting, or standing.[10] There are many types of therapeutic positioning devices available today that provide adequate trunk supports, place the hips and pelvis in a stable position, prevent shoulder retraction, and promote head control (Fig 24-5). Proper positioning also improves visual control by the child, which will improve food intake since the child may better see the food being offered, thereby enhancing his or her ability to self-feed.

Behavioral and environmental problems

An important consideration in working with children with feeding problems is the child's behavior related to eating and being fed, with particular consideration of the total environment.[1]

Often, parents misinterpret the child's oral-motor problem as "bad" behavior or lack of appetite. For that reason it is important to establish the child's readiness for certain foods by the assessment tools discussed. In addition to the appropriate position, environmental factors that must be evaluated include where the child is fed and the amount of noise and distractions present. Many children with neurological problems and short attention spans are fed in front of the television or next to a radio playing loud music. These distractions may interfere with the child's ability to concentrate on the feeding process.

Consideration should be given to the appearance of the food. Children respond to bright colors, small servings, and foods that are separated and not mixed. For visually impaired children the feeding area must be well lit, and the parents or caregiver must name the food being fed. Young children respond best to mild temperatures and bland flavors, but sharper, spicier flavors can be introduced as the child grows older. Certain medications distort taste and dull appetite.[2] The sense of smell also affects food and flavor acceptance.

An important behavioral consideration to assess during a feeding evaluation is the degree of structure in the child's environment, such as the regularity of bedtime, nap time, meal schedules, and snack time and the use of food as a reward.[11,12]. The child's use of the feeding situation to manipulate the family and environment should be evaluated. Children notice very quickly the anxious concern of the parent or caregiver about their food intake. A parental reaction to food avoidance may be to follow the child throughout the day and to offer food at frequent intervals. The intervention for such a behavior is to develop a schedule in which food is provided at well-timed intervals.

Feeding is successful when the parent attends to the child's rhythms and signals of hunger and satiety, works to calm him or her, and develops mechanics of feeding that are effective with the child's particular emotional make-up, skill,

Table 24–4. UACCDD Cincinnati, Strategies for Identification and Intervention of Oral-Motor Problems

Reflex	Diagnosis	Stimulation—Mechanics
Gag	1. Walk tongue blade back tongue until tongue bumps.	1. When spoon feeding, apply pressure on tongue with spoon. 2. Place spoon lateral to tongue. 3. Remove quickly.
Suck	1. Place pacifier or finger in mouth. Lips should elbow around it with strong suction applied.	1. Offer pacifier dipped in cold fruit juice. 2. Experiment with various nipple types. 3. Use fingers to stimulate, by pushing mouth open. 4. Encourage use of straw; use cold liquids.
Swallow	1. Offer drink of water. Swallow 2 oz without stopping.	1. Using fingers, vibrate from chin to enternal notch. 2. Keep head stable and in a downward position. 3. Position cup at side of mouth. Use other hand under chin to apply upward pressure so mouth closes on rim.
Tongue thrust	1. Use pretzel stick or small tongue blade dipped in fruit. Can also use pretzel stick if bite reflex is not over developed. 2. Place in mouth and observe. 3. Tongue section will push out solid food placed on anterior third of tongue.	1. Vibrate (carefully) under tongue on either side of freulum with pretzel stick. 2. Use fingers to vibrate under chin; keep teeth closed. 3. Place foods in corners of mouth between teeth. 4. a) When spoon feeding, use spoon with shallow bowl, with small amounts of food. b) When spoon is placed in mouth, give a slight downward pressure on tongue with spoon. 5. Use jaw control activities at non-eating times.
Tongue lateralization	*1. Place peanut butter at corners of mouth and ask patient to lick mouth.	1. Press against lateral sides of tongue with tongue blade or use popsicle stick, several times before feeding. Do this 1/2 to 1 hour before feeding time. 2. Play games—make faces, lick peanut butter, or lick ice cream cone. 3. Exercise tongue: place gauze on tongue and use fingers to move tongue (gently).
Tongue elevation	*1. Place peanut butter at center of upper lip and ask patient to lick mouth.	1. Using a small soft brush or tongue blade or pacifier, touch roof of mouth. 2. Play games, making faces; lick ice cream cone.
Bite	1. Overreactive: strong clamping on the feeding spoon. 2. Underreactive: drooling.	1. Stimulate the child's gums to stimulate bite reflex (use index finger or ear swab). 2. Offer cracker, bread, or vegetables in pieces that do not fit into the mouth unless bitten off.
Loose (slack) jaw	1. Place small piece of cracker between molars. 2. Observe chewing action for rotary movement.	1. Using fingers, vibrate over zygotic arch, near frontal ear lobe. 2. Use hands to guide jaw up and *inward* while patient chews. 3. Have patient imitate adult while feeling adult's jaw. 4. Use jaw control technique when child is at passive play.
Stable jaw— poor action	1. Place small piece of cracker between molars. 2. Observe chewing action for rotary movements.	1. Using fingers, vibrate masseters. 2. Introduce firm foods gradually; start with well cooked, progress to partially cooked, to *soft* raw foods. 3. Have patient imitate adult while feeling adult's jaw.
Chewing	1. Observe chewing for rotary motion, not loose vertical motion.	1. Massage gums with index finger before feeding. 2. Have patient imitate adult while feeling adult's jaw. 3. Play games before mirror: yawn, blow kisses. 4. Foods: progress slowly from well cooked to raw.
Finger feeding	1. Serve child thin slices of fresh peeled fruits and vegetables. 2. Serve child cubes of cheese. 3. Serve crackers/various shapes.	1. Play with stacking toys. 2. Play pegboards, push-pull toys, and pointing games (nose, eyes, ears, etc.) 3. Pour water or sand from cup to cup.

Cup drinking	1. Offer child drink of water and observe:
	  a. Cup should rest on lower lip, not teeth.
	  b. Upper lip should close over cup rim.
		1. Begin with weighted cup with handles and progress to plastic cup without handles.
		2. Stand behind child and use hand to bring lower jaw closed.

Table 24–4. (*Continued*)

Reflex	Diagnosis	Stimulation—Mechanics
Spoon feeding	1. Offer child applesauce in bowl and observe: a. Does spoon turn over or reach the mouth in upright position.	1. Offer child foods that stay on the spoon: — cooked cereal — mashed potatoes — puddings/custards — squash, cooked & mashed — sweet potatoes 2. Work from behind child when assisting him/her in grasping and using spoon. 3. Do not let spoon touch teeth.
Drooling	1. Accompanies poor swallowing reflex and/or jaw control.	1. Use jaw control actions at feeding and non-feeding times. 2. Stimulate swallowing reflex (see #3).

*May not use this technique in some children with cerebral palsy.

and limitations.[2] Until intervention has been implemented, it may not be always appropriate to feed the child with multiple feeding problems with the rest of the family. For good behavioral control, a quiet environment, with consistent handling, is mandatory. If the child is in a school-based feeding intervention program, the home and school must work together so that consistency between home and school is achieved.

Factors to be Considered in Nutritional Assessment and Intervention

Before any intervention program can be implemented, it is essential that a nutritional assessment be completed by a registered dietitian or nutritionist, if one is available to the team. The nutritional assessment is the same for any type of oral (not tube) feeding problem, and its aim is to determine nutrient needs related to energy, protein, fat and carbohydrates, vitamins, and minerals. In addition, the nutritional status of the child as defined by height, weight, skinfold thicknesses, and biochemical signs should be assessed initially and used as a baseline in monitoring intervention. Dietary intake, including both current and past intake; fluid intake; food texture; meal snacking, and sleep patterns; medications; elimination; and physical activity should be assessed, as well as the specific issues described in the earlier section, "Assessment of Feeding Problems" (see nutritional assessment forms in Appendices 4 and 5).

Assessment of growth may indicate that the child with a feeding problem is receiving inadequate nutrients and yet is limited in the volume of food that can be consumed. For this reason it is important to increase calories and other nutrients by modifying the food itself. Foods that can be added to pureed foods to increase calories and protein content are listed in Table 24–5.

Determination of the energy needs of the child with a serious feeding problem is essential when providing nutritional counseling to the parent who may be reluctant to follow intervention suggestions addressed to oral-motor problems. This reluctance may stem from concern for any change that results in a decrease in food intake and subsequent weight loss.

Table 24–5. Food That Can Be Added to Pureed Foods to Increase Calories and Protein

	Calories	Protein (g)
Infant cereal	9/T	0.25/T
Nonfat dry milk	25/T	1.3/T
Cheese	120/oz	5.0/oz
Margarine	101/T	–
Evaporated milk	40/oz	1.1/oz
Vegetable oils	110/T	–
Strained infant meals	100-150/jar	14.0/jar
Polycose, powdered	30/T	–

The recommended dietary allowances of the National Academy of Science[13] are not always applicable for the developmentally disabled population due to differences in growth rate and activity levels. The basal metabolic rates of infants and children ages 1 week to 16 years are shown in Table 24–6.[14] In general, this table can be used to determine basal metabolic needs with 50% to 75% added for activity or growth, but children usually need to be evaluated on an individual basis.

Another important nutritional consideration is medication and its impact on appetite, elimination, and nutrient utilization. Many children with handicaps take medications that depress appetite and cause nausea, dryness of the oral mucosa, gastrointestinal irritation, and constipation.[17] Anticonvulsant medications may interfere with the absorption of vitamins and minerals.[15]

Sleep patterns are a final consideration for the child with feeding problems. Many children with neurological disturbances have periods of wakefulness during the night, which fatigues both the child and the parent. This problem in turn makes the child difficult to work with during intervention times and makes participation difficult for the parent because of fatigue.

Tube feeding

Enteral support may be required by developmentally disabled children with a variety of conditions, especially if dysphagic and less than 75% of the nutrients and 90% of the fluid requirements are being maintained. Some of these clin-

Table 24–6. Basal Metabolic Rates: Infants and Children

Age 1 wk to 10 mo		Age 11 to 36 mo			Age 3 to 16 yr		
Weight (kg)	(kcal/hr) M/F	Weight (kg)	(kcal/hr) M	F	Weight (kg)	(kcal/hr) M	F
3.5	8.4	9.0	22.0	21.2	15	35.8	33.3
4.0	9.5	9.5	22.8	22.0	20	39.7	37.4
4.5	10.5	10.0	23.6	22.8	25	43.6	41.5
5.0	11.6	10.5	24.4	23.6	30	47.5	45.5
5.5	12.7	11.0	25.2	24.4	35	51.3	49.6
6.0	13.8	11.5	26.0	25.2	40	55.2	53.7
6.5	14.9	12.0	26.8	26.0	45	59.1	57.8
7.0	16.0	12.5	27.6	26.9	50	63.0	61.9
7.5	17.1	13.0	28.4	27.7	55	66.9	66.0
8.0	18.2	13.5	29.2	28.5	60	70.8	70.0
8.5	19.3	14.0	30.0	29.3	65	74.7	74.0
9.0	20.4	14.5	30.8	30.1	70	78.6	78.1
9.5	21.4	15.0	31.6	30.9	75	82.5	82.2
10.0	22.5	15.5	32.4	31.7			
10.5	23.6	16.0	33.3	32.6			
11.0	24.7	16.5	34.0	33.4			

From Altman, P. L., Dittmer, D. S. eds. Metabolism. *Fed Soc Exp Biol*. 1968:344. Used with permission.

ical conditions include failure to thrive, malabsorption, hypermetabolism, growth failure, prematurity, and a wide range of disorders of absorption, digestion, excretion, utilization, and storage of nutrients.[3] Formula selection depends on caloric density, nutrient composition and source, digestibility, accessibility, viscosity, osmolality, taste, and cost.[8] All of these indicators are influenced by the age and clinical need of the child and adolescent (see Chapter 34).

For the infant, breast milk or a variety of cow's milk, soy protein formulas, and "special" formulas are available; after 1 year of age, the formula Pedisure is available. For the older child and adult, available formulas include Ensure, Enrich, and Sustacal, which provide 30 cal/oz and show some variability in vitamins, minerals, and trace elements (Appendix 6).

Evaluation of formula selection should be ongoing to determine its appropriateness to the changing needs of the child or adolescent. Monitoring of physical status (especially growth parameters), hydration status, and biochemical indicators, including electrolytes, minerals, visceral proteins, indicators of organ function, and hematological factors,[16] should be done.

Orogastric, nasogastric, and gastrostomy are the most commonly used types of enteral tube feeding.[2] The tube should be viewed as a temporary measure for supporting life. This is an important concept for the family who may view the tube negatively, representing the family's fear about the severity of the child's disorder.[3]

To facilitate the transition to oral feeding, oral-motor and positioning treatment should be initiated when the tube feeding is begun. Such treatment is important to counteract the problems that occur when tube feeding is initiated for the infant: lack of stimulation, lack of opportunity to associate positive sensations in the mouth with reduction of hunger, and lack of social interaction with the mother during feeding. As a result of the disappearance of food from the child's sensory experience, coupled with negative and abrasive stimulation from the procedures of tube feeding, the face and mouth may become hypersensitive to touch, and taste and feeding may come to be viewed as extremely unpleasant.[3]

Children with feeding problems—poor tone and movement patterns, such as hyperextension, respiratory difficulties, disorganized sucking patterns, swallowing disorders, gastroesphageal reflux, and abnormal response to oral stimulation—who are being tube fed, still need to receive treatment for those problems. The use of the tube—whether oro-, nasal, or gastrostomy—works around those problems to sustain and improve nutritional status. However, for the return to oral intake to occur, the existing feeding problem will still need to be corrected (see Chapter 34). The components of an oral-motor treatment program for the tube-fed child are similar to those for the non-tube-fed child; however, the program may need to be instituted at a slower pace. All of the oral-motor treatment should be carried out before the transition is made from tube to mouth. Although some programs approach this aggressively, many programs concentrate on a gradual transition to reintroduce oral feeding as a pleasant experience.[17]

Occupational and physical therapy intervention normalizes muscle tone in the trunk, thereby developing postural stability that releases holding tension in the neck, shoulder, arms, and legs.[3] The therapist positions the child to assist in maintaining control of the pharyngeal airway. For some children, feeding may be carried out best when the child is lying on the side or in a prone position.

As oral-motor treatment proceeds, the therapist usually recommends to the parent that the infant be held for feeding (as for a non-tube-fed patient). This procedure includes holding the arms near the body, talking with the child, and stroking the cheeks and lips during the feeding through the tube.

Two major nutrients need to be monitored during the weaning process: calories and fluids. The registered dietitian or nutritionist calculates energy and protein needs and sets up an exchange list for food and tube feeding formula (Table

Table 24–7. Exchange System for Transition from Tube Feeding to Oral Feeding

1. Change the tube feeding schedule to after meals or nighttime.
2. Increase the volume of formula per feeding and decrease the number of tube feedings.
3. Exchange 1 oz of 30 cal/cc formula for

   • 2 oz strained fruit
   • 2 oz baby cereal
   • 1 oz beef

4. Continue with substitution until tube feedings are discontinued.

From Wolf & Green.[18]

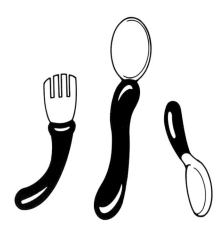

Fig. 24–8. Spoons of different lengths and shapes designed to enhance self-feeding.

24–7). As the amount of food by mouth increases, the formula fed per tube decreases,[18] especially if 100% of the fluid and 80% of the nutrient requirements are being maintained.

The successful transition from tube to oral feeding of the child with developmental disabilities requires consistency and commitment from the parent, caregivers in a developmental center or school, and health care providers. Parents need to expect that major changes in feeding will take a great deal of time to accomplish. In addition, the parent and/or practitioner must be reassured as progress is made.

Self-feeding

Self-feeding is defined as the ability and willingness of the individual to use a cup, fingers, or spoon in an act of independence. The normal child at 6 months begins to self-feed with a bottle. Many experiences help prepare the youngster for this independent function[19] (see UACCDD Nutrition Assessment in Appendix 3). Among the first steps in independent feeding is the ability to pick up and eat pieces of cereal or crackers. By 8 or 9 months, as a child is developing chewing patterns, self-feeding of crackers or small pieces of cheese provides excellent stimulation for biting, chewing, and hand and wrist control (Fig 24–6). Between 9 to 12 months, cup drinking develops, and the infant tries to grasp a spoon while being fed. Control of midrange movements in the humerus and elbow is important, as are the abilities to move the spoon in space, hold the posture of the abducted arm in space, and correct and verify these movements. Control of the forearm and wrist movements and of the overhand grasping of the spoon helps direct the spoon to the mouth. Children with neuromotor problems and developmental disabilities may be cognitively able to self-feed, but are unable to do so because of gross motor and fine motor inadequacies that interfere with control.[19]

Many types of spouted cups are available that are helpful when initiating the weaning process; generally, they prevent spillage (Fig 24–7). In addition a cup with a weighted base prevents tipping and may help stabilize movements for the child with poor coordination. The nosy or cut-out cup may be helpful for the child who tends to throw the head back during the drinking process.

Spoon feeding should begin in an orderly fashion when the child is developmentally ready. Generally, it follows finger feeding. Nylon-coated and plastic-coated spoons are available for protecting teeth and lips, come in all shapes and sizes depending upon the age and size of the child, and are angled for children (Fig 24–8). Spoons for the child who

has difficulty grasping may need built-up handles and velcro slings to go over the hand. The electric feeder may be needed for the child or adult whose arm and wrist are so involved that hand-to-mouth action cannot be attained successfully.

The bowl or plate used to assist self-feeding should have high sides so the food can be scooped. It may need to be anchored to the tray of the high chair with a non slip product, such as "dycem," clay, or suction cups. These devices can be ordered from AAMED Inc., Forest Park, IL; J. A. Preston Corporation, New York, NY; Special Education Materials, Inc., Yonkers, NY; Fairway King, Inc., Oklahoma City, OK; Cleo Living Aids, Cleveland, OH; Fred Sammons, Inc., Brookfield, IL, and Achievement Products, Inc., Mineola, NY.

Follow-Up

After the initial assessment the child may need to be seen weekly and later on a monthly basis for treatment and monitoring of feeding, anthropometry, and hemoglobin values. Oral feeding skills, gastrostomy feeding, positioning, nutrients, constipation, and behavior should be evaluated continually.[20]

The interdisciplinary approach is ideal in working with feeding problems, which require the skills of various disciplines, including physical therapy, occupational therapy, dentistry, nutrition, and speech pathology. The success of feeding intervention is determined by the degree of coordination of services between home and program (school or developmental center) and including the parent as an active member of the feeding team. An interdisciplinary team of nutritionist, nurse, and special educator (with parental input) can be of great benefit in facilitating the transition for the child fed by gastrostomy to school.

REFERENCES

1. Lane, S.J., Cloud, H.H. Feeding problems and intervention: an interdisciplinary approach. *Top. Clin. Nutr.*, 1988; 3:23.
2. Humphrey, R. Feeding problems and the mother-infant relationship. In: *Problems with Eating: Intervention for Children and Adults with Developmental Disabilities*. Rockville, MD: American Occupational Therapy Association; 1987.
3. Morris, S.E., Klein, M.D.: *Pre-Feeding Skills*. Tucson, AZ: Therapy Skill Builders; 1987.

4. Satter, E. Developing guidelines for feeding infants and young children. In: Urenos, E., ed. *Food Nutr. News. Natl. Livestock Meat Board*. 1984; 56:4.

5. Nagayda, J.M. Asocial feeding behaviors associated with severe mental impairment. In: *Problems with Eating, Intervention for Children and Adults with Developmental Disabilities*, Rockville, MD: American Occupational Therapy Association; 1987.

6. Cloud, H.H. *The Team Approach to Feeding* (study guide and audio cassette). Chicago: American Dietetic Association; 1987.

7. Krick, J., Van Dwyer, M.A.S. The relationship between oral-motor involvement and growth: a pilot study in a pediatric population with cerebral palsy. *J. Am. Diet. Assoc.* 1984; 5:555.

8. Smith, M.A.H., Connolly, B., McFadden, S., Nicrosi, C.R., Nuckolls, J., Russell, F.F., and Wilson, W.M.: Developmental feeding tool. In: Smith, M.A.H., ed. *Feeding Management for a Child with a Handicap*. Memphis: The Child Development Center, University of Tennessee, Center for Health Sciences; 1982.

9. Warren, L., Fax, R. Use of videoflourscopy in the evaluation and treatment of children with swallowing disorders. In: *Problems with Eating, Intervention for Children and Adults with Developmental Disorders*. Rockville, MD: American Occupational Therapy Association; 1987.

10. Bray, M., Beckman, D., Banks, L.S. Mealtime intervention for persons with compromised oral-motor functions. In: *Problems with Eating, Intervention for Children and Adults with Developmental Disorders*. Rockville, MD: American Occupational Therapy Association; 1987.

11. O'Neill, S.M. Management of mealtime behaviors. In: Pipes, P.L., ed. *Nutrition in Infancy and Childhood*. St. Louis: Mosby; 1985.

12. Rokusek, C., Heinrichs, E., eds. *Abnormal Mealtime Behavior in Nutrition and Feeding for the Developmentally Disabled*. Vermillion, SD: South Dakota University Affiliated Facility, Center for the Developmentally Disabled, University of South Dakota, School of Medicine; 1985.

13. National Research Council Food and Nutrition Board. 10th ed. Washington, DC: National Academy of Sciences Press; 1989.

14. Walker, W.A., Hendricks, K.M., eds. Estimation of energy needs. In: *Manual of Pediatric Nutrition*. 2nd ed. Philadelphia: B.C. Decker; 1990.

15. Roe, D. *Drug and Nutrient Interaction*. Chicago: American Dietetic Association; 1985.

16. McCrae, J.A.D., Hall, N.H. Current practices for home enteral nutrition. *J. Am. Diet. Assoc.* 1989, 89:2.

17. Rowe, J.S., Geggie, J. Intervention for a non-oral feeder. In: *Problems with Eating, Intervention for Children and Adults with Developmental Disorders*. Rockville, MD: American Occupational Therapy Association; 1987.

18. Wolf, D., Green, P. *A Practical Guide to Tube Feedings*. Baltimore: John F. Kennedy Institute for Handicapped Children Nutrition Division; 1983.

19. Boehme, R. Significant aspects of self-feeding. In: *Problems with Eating, Intervention for Children and Adults with Developmental Disorders*. Rockville, MD: American Occupational Therapy Association; 1987.

20. Isaacs, J., Davis, B., Montagne, M. Transitioning the child fed by gastrostomy into school. *J. Am. Diet. Assoc.* 1990; 90:982.

Chapter 25
Cleft Lip/Palate and Craniofacial Anomalies

Sheila Farnan

A cleft is an opening in the lip, hard palate, or soft palate. These openings are normally present in early fetal development, but close before birth.

The cleft space occurs when the bone, tissue, and/or muscles fail to fuse. Cleft lip is a unilateral (one side) or bilateral (two sides) separation of the upper lip occurring during the fifth week of fetal development. The severity may range from a slight notching of the lip (incomplete) to an opening that extends into the nasal cavity (complete). Clefts of the palate may occur in the bony hard palate or soft palate or in both, usually appearing in the midline, at approximately the seventh or eighth week of development. Clefts of the palate may also be unilateral or bilateral and can extend from a cleft of the soft palate only, to the hard palate, and on to the alveolus (upper gum ridge). There can also be a combination of cleft lip and cleft palate (Fig 25-1). The orofacial anatomy is distorted in shape and position by the cleft.

A related condition is the submucous cleft, which involves the muscles of the soft palate and part of the hard palate. An absence of bone in the posterior hard palate, a cleft in the midline of the soft palate, bifid or notched uvula, an intact but thin mucosal surface, and hypernasal voice quality are the usual findings in submucous cleft. Feeding is not a major problem, but milk may come through the nose, which is an indication to look for a submucous cleft. Since diagnosis is frequently overlooked until the preschool years when hypernasal speech is apparent, referral of children with nasal milk loss can accelerate early diagnosis.

There are well over 150 recognized disorders in which cleft lip, cleft palate, or both may represent one feature.[1] Pierre Robin oral formation sequence, usually characterized by clefting, micrognathia, and glossoptosis, is the congenital malformation seen most often is association with cleft palate. There is evidence to suggest that clefts with associated malformations are different epidemiological entities from those without associated malformations and possible syndromes.[1]

Clinical Abnormalities

Etiology. The specific causes of a cleft in a particular child are usually not known, but genetic and environmental factors are often associated with clefts. There is growing evidence that clefts are the result of susceptible genes being influenced by the environment. Thus, heredity or a combination of heredity and environmental conditions contributes to cleft conditions. A family history of clefts is reported by 15% to 25% of cases.[2]

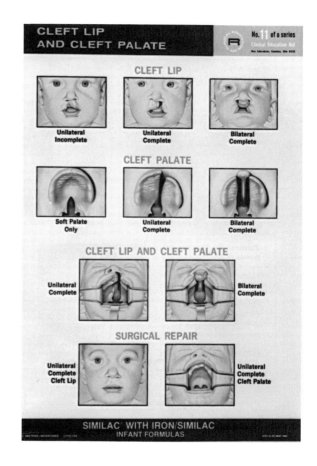

Fig. 25-1. Types of cleft lip and cleft palate. From Ross Laboratories. *Clinical Education Aid No. 11.* Columbus, OH: Ross Laboratories; 1962. Used with permission.

An increased incidence of congenital anomalies occurs in children born to women who have used cocaine.[3] Midline defects (i.e., craniofacial anomalies) are just beginning to be reported. Since drug and alcohol abuse are on the increase, this population warrants careful observation. The care of the children and the financial resources required are often overwhelming for those mothers, which can put the infants at further risk for nutritional problems.

Incidence. Clefts of the lip and palate are the most common orofacial defect and the fourth most frequent structural birth defect[4] Approximately 5000 children are born with cleft lip or palate in the United States each year. Differences exist in the incidence of cleft lip, cleft palate, and cleft lip and palate among races and sexes. It is frequently reported that some type of clefts occur in approximately 1 in every 700 live births in the white population, more often among Orientals and certain groups of American Indians, and less frequently among blacks.[5] The literature suggests that the risk of developing clefts in stillbirths and abortions is three times as frequent as in live births.[6]

Because studies are based on different sources of information, types of cleft, stillbirths or live births, great discrepancies appear in their findings. However, there does seem to be an increased occurrence of cleft lip, cleft lip with cleft palate, and isolated cleft palate with other malformations at late maternal ages. Only cleft lip with cleft palate and isolated cleft palate showed a relation to maternal age when reported as a sole defect.[7]

More males than females have cleft lip with or without cleft palate; a left-sided cleft is more frequent that a right-sided cleft. The recurrence risk for parents of having a second child with cleft lip with or without cleft palate is about 1 in 20 if there is no other family history of cleft. The recurrence risk is increased to about 1 in 10 after there have been two affected children

Clefts of the hard and soft palate or of the soft palate only are less frequent than is cleft lip with or without cleft palate, and occur in about 1 out of every 2200 live births. More females than males are affected. The risk that parents with one child born with cleft palate will have another such child is about 1 in 50.[4]

Interdisciplinary intervention. There is a wide range of oral involvement in a child with a cleft lip, palate, or both. Closure of clefts is accomplished through a sequence of staged surgical procedures. Although surgical repair and reconstruction timetables vary significantly throughout the country, the goal is to facilitate eating and speaking while improving appearance with a minimum of scarring and promoting normal facial growth.

The first treatment—surgical repair of the lip usually is done within the first month or when the child reaches a certain weight. Palate repair is done optimally within the first year before there has been much speech development. As the child matures, many surgical revisions, dental procedures, speech therapy, otological care, and possibly psychological therapy may be required. Intervention, treatment, and family support are complicated, so it is highly recommended that the children be cared for by a multidisciplinary team approach. Over 200 such treatment teams practice in the United States.[8]

Team composition varies throughout the country, but specialists representing each aspect of the child's total care include an audiologist, cosmetologist, dental hygienist, geneticist, nurse, oral surgeon, orthodontist, otolaryngologist, pediatric dentist, pediatrician, photographer, plastic surgeon, prosthodontist, psychologist, registered dietitian, social worker, and speech-language pathologist. All the members may not need to see the child at each clinic visit, but their expertise is important at some phase of the treatment plan and stage of the child's development. Since technology and research are rapidly changing, team members may differ on a management plan. When this occurs, parents will need support and guidance in selecting the most appropriate plan for their child.

Factors to be Considered in Nutritional Evaluation

The challenge immediately after birth is to reassure the parents that the child can be fed an adequate diet with no compromise in growth or health. Nutrient needs of children with cleft lip/palate are the same as those of other children, and they will experience the same appetite fluctuations, taste preferences, and food quirks. Depending on the location (lip, hard palate, soft palate, or combination) and the extent of the opening (bilateral or unilateral), feeding may or may not be a problem.

The first problem to present itself may be insufficient suction. However, a baby with a cleft lip and palate will start to suck when a nipple is placed in the mouth, just as any newborn baby does. This action occurs because the sucking and swallowing reflexes are present, even though the muscles are not able to operate as efficiently because of the cleft. The feeding difficulty is caused by a mechanical problem, in that the child is unable to suck adequately because a tight seal cannot be achieved. Without a seal, the infant must work very hard, using tongue and cheek muscles to compensate for the lack of normal suction. Poor sucking can lengthen feeding time, causing fatigue and the subsequent insufficient intake of formula or breast milk to satisfy the baby's appetite and nutrient needs.

Swallowing problems may occur in infants with the Pierre Robin malformation sequence, pharyngeal or esophageal abnormalities, or central nervous system (CNS) problems. Infants with cleft lip/palate as their sole health problem swallow normally, but because they may swallow excess air, need to be burped more frequently to decrease nasal regurgitation and possible aspiration.

In addition to promoting growth and development, good nutrition is essential in enabling the infant to

- build up resistance to infection
- acquire the necessary weight needed for surgery
- build up strength to meet the stress of surgery
- promote healing after surgery
- develop and maintain healthy oral structures

For these reasons, it is recommended that a nutrition assessment, including anthropometric measurements and dietary and hematological analysis, be part of the periodic team evaluation. The hemoglobin and hematocrit values should be greater than 11 g/dL and 33%, respectively.

Growth

Slow weight gain has been reported during the first few months of life.[9] When it occurs, this lag may be due to early feeding difficulties, frequent upper respiratory infections, middle ear disease, repeated surgical procedures, psychosocial dynamics, or some combination of these factors. In a study of 252 children, Bowers et al.[10] found that those with unilateral clefts and isolated clefts of the lip and palate were significantly shorter than their unaffected peers. Boys were also thinner. The study results indicate that congenital metabolic variation contributes to the orofacial clefting and influences postnatal development in certain types of cleft. There are reports in the literature of a higher incidence of growth hormone deficiency in children with cleft lip/palate.[11,12] However, this finding does not have total agreement.[13]

Even though research cannot currently resolve the debate, it is highly recommended that growth be measured and plotted routinely on a growth chart as a method of screening for growth disorder. It is also helpful to advise the parents of the importance of maintaining a growth chart. Only when anthropometric measurements appear on a chart can a clear picture be seen of an individual child's growth. A slowing down or leveling off of growth is an immediate sign for referral to a physician, and further referral to an endocrinologist may be indicated. Growth data are also important for the timing of surgery and prognosis for healing. Weight for length/height should be maintained between the 5th and 95th percentiles.

Dentition

Many children have malocclusion, crowding, and bite problems that can make eating difficult and thereby compromise adequate nutrition. Knowledge of the child's oral structure is imperative when planning adequate and realistic nutrient intake.

Dietary Management

Infancy

Feeding is an immediate and traumatic concern at the time of the child's birth. The methods of feeding vary, depending upon the type and extent of the cleft, as well as the philosophy of the hospital team members. An infant with a cleft lip may have difficulty closing tightly around the nipple. Cleft palate presents problems with suction, nasal regurgitation, and excessive air intake. Because early discharge of newborns may hinder the family from learning the types of equipment and/or techniques necessary to feed the baby, hospital discharge should be delayed until the child can feed successfully in approximately 30 minutes and the parent is confident about the feeding. If the child has difficulty sucking or swallowing, it may cause great anxiety and frustration for the adults during the feeding and subsequent problems for the child.

There are many approaches to feeding babies with cleft lip/palate, and parents need to be assured there is no right or wrong method. The goal is to find a method that allows the child to consume the liquid in a reasonable amount of time with few, if any physical problems, while developing the orofacial musculature needed for speech and chewing. In time, most infants learn methods of compensating for the physical defect. Some children squeeze or chew the nipple; others learn to direct the nipple to the side of their mouth. Some children need the assistance of the adult rhythmically squeezing the bottle so that the flow of liquid coincides with the child's swallow. After feeding, the oral area should be cleansed by giving a small amount of water. In addition, the teeth and gums should be wiped lightly with a clean damp gauze pad.

The most successful position for feeding is in a semi-sitting position (60 to 90-degree angle) to allow gravity to assist with swallowing. An infant should never be put to bed with a bottle since this habit can result in choking, ear infections, and tooth decay. In addition to the position of the child's body, the position of the nipple is important. Some children

are more successful at sucking when the liquid is directed toward the cheek, rather than the back of the throat. The nipple should not be placed into the cleft.

There may be a good deal of trial and error before achieving the optimal feeding situation, and even then, it may change as the child grows. A feeding method that works at birth may not be appropriate as the child matures and develops greater strength. The method should not be so effortless that there is no challenge to orofacial muscles. Each child is different and the parent should be guided toward allowing enough time to feed, developing a relaxed atmosphere, and being willing to adapt and change with their infant.

Although children with clefts are often weaned early from the bottle, the importance of weaning by 1 year of age should be stressed. Baby bottle tooth decay (BBTD) is a feeding-related oral health problem associated with prolonged bottle feeding, resulting in early and rampant caries. Prevention is the most effective strategy. Caregivers should be advised never to put the child to bed with a bottle. The use of a bottle containing decay-producing liquids as a pacifier should also be discouraged to avoid caries.

Most babies can be breastfed or bottle fed, but occasionally babies who have an exceptionally wide cleft or accompanying conditions or syndromes may need to be fed by tube feeding or gavage. Some babies may need to have a prosthetic feeding appliance inserted. An obturator (dental plate usually made of dental acrylic) can be constructed to fit an individual baby's mouth. It artificially restores the hard palate until surgery can be performed and often improves the feeding situation. An obturator may also prevent the tongue from entering the cleft, support dental arch integrity, guide the growth of alveolar ridges and alleviate maternal stress.[9] All surgeons do not agree about the value of this appliance, but parents have reported that it lessened choking, nasal regurgitation, and the amount of time needed to complete each feeding.[14] A very small study showed improved weight gain after insertion of an obturator.[9] This appliance must be reconstructed every 2 to 3 months as the child's oral area grows and changes.

Breastfeeding

Breastfeeding children with cleft lip or palate has traditionally been discouraged because of an anticipated failure to obtain good suction and the fear there could be deleterious effects after surgery. However, many women have nursed their children successfully, and a study by Weatherly-White et al.[15] reported no surgical complications. A baby with a cleft lip only may be able to obtain adequate suction because the mother's soft breast tissue may mold to the open area between the mouth and nose better than a firmer bottle nipple. A baby born with a bilateral cleft may have more difficulty breastfeeding, and it may not be successful.

Because of the benefits of breastfeeding (nutritional, immunological, and bonding), mothers should be made aware of all the feeding options so that they can make an informed decision. In addition to breastfeeding or formula, the choices for the mother are to express her milk with a breast pump and give it in a bottle or to use a Lact-Aid® device, which consists of a sterile plastic bag and a small capillary tube. The bag contains expressed breast milk or formula, and the tube is placed near the mother's nipple for the baby to suck. Mothers wishing to breastfeed may need additional education in the hospital, referral to a support group, or provision of printed material.[16]

Improved weight gain and shortened hospital stay among infants with cleft lip who were breastfed following lip repair as compared with infants who drank from a cup have been reported.[15] Another study indicated that children who were breastfed had improved resistance to middle ear infections.[17]

Bottle feeding

Babies use different techniques to suck from bottles than from breasts. Bottle fed infants use their gums and, to a lesser extent, their tongue and palate to stabilize the nipple and create negative pressure to draw the milk from the bottle. Breastfed babies use negative intraoral pressure to stabilize the nipple and the tongue to mechanically strip the milk from the nipple. Some nasal regurgitation is to be expected with many children.

It bottle feeding is chosen, the standard infant formula with iron is recommended, and the method should be as "normal" as possible. This is to foster the attitude that the child is not different and to enable all family members or child care providers to help with the feeding. However, it may be necessary to purchase special commercial products or modify regular equipment.

Some recommendations for bottle feeding

Several commercial products have been designed for children with cleft lip and/or palate (Fig. 25-2). The cleft lip/palate nurser produced by the Mead Johnson company is a very soft plastic 6-oz bottle with a cross-cut nipple. The bottle can be easily squeezed to aid the baby's weak suck. It is Stock #2001-01 and available from any major drug wholesaler. The cleft palate nipple produced by Ross Lab-

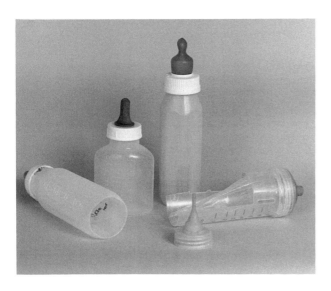

Fig. 25–2. Recommendations for bottle feeding: various types of nipples/bottles.

oratories is available at no cost from the company or hospital nurseries. This nipple operates on the gravity flow principle in which the formula is squeezed onto the back of the tongue. The child can then swallow without sucking. For this reason, this method is not advocated by all practitioners.[18] Standard commercial products that may be effective are soft regular nipples with a cross-cut or enlarged hole and the cross-cut preemie nipple. However, the nipple walls of the preemie nipple are softer and compress more easily, but may also collapse. Existing infant feeding equipment can be modified in the following ways:

- Playtex® bottle with opening on side enlarged to allow for squeezing of bag containing formula
- regular nipple with additional holes added
- nipple softened by boiling
- plastic bottle that has had the base removed and a plastic liner inserted; bag compresses as the child sucks and thus avoids excess air intake
- plastic bottle that has been softened by boiling or previous use; is usually too large for a newborn, but works well when the baby is older
- inverted Playtex® nipple, which creates a longer nipple

Toddler period

The addition of solid foods and cow's milk should progress the same as for any child. Spoon feeding and cup drinking should be started at the same age as other children. Solids should always be fed by spoon and never from a bottle or commercial syringe type infant feeder unless it is prescribed for a unique situation. Spoon and finger feeding are activities that contribute to a healthy diet, as well as strengthen the orofacial muscles. Surgeons may want the child weaned from the bottle before palate surgery.

Hard and sticky food or small particles that may get lodged in the palate opening should be avoided. Occasionally, acidic or spicy foods may cause irritation. Since all toddlers are so prone to food asphyxiation, foods that are small, round, slippery, or tough should be avoided or only given in a supervised setting.[19]

Because sound teeth and healthy gums are important for chewing, appearance, and speech, a child should be encouraged to eat wisely and to avoid constant snacking and sticky, retentive foods. The child should receive adequate ingested fluoride through the drinking water supply or a dietary fluoride supplement.

Even after the palate is surgically repaired, an opening or fistula into the hard palate may be present. Depending on the size and location, suction may be affected, and food regurgitation into the nasal cavity may still occur.

Childhood and adolescence

Depending on the degree of involvement, severe malocclusion can occur. There may be a cross-bite, missing and supernumerary teeth, and dental crowding and rotations. Some children's diets may be compromised by their inability to masticate a wide variety of foods. The child should be asked how well he or she can chew and which foods cause problems. The foods may need to be modified (cut smaller, moistened) or a substitute served until the adverse dental situation is corrected.

Poor appetite and the potential for decreased nutrients and calories may occur in some children. The prevalence of mouth breathing among individuals with cleft lip and palate is significantly higher than in the normal population.[20] This higher prevalence has been attributed to nasal abnormalities, such as septal deformities, atresia of the nostrils, mucosa hypertrophy, and a pharyngeal flap that is too wide; all of these abnormalities diminish airway size. The result may be a very dry mouth and difficulty in coordinating chewing, swallowing, and breathing.[117] They may need to be counseled to chew, pause, breathe, resume chewing etc. and parents should be aware of the fact that these children do chew with their mouths open. Often these children complain of excessive effort in eating or reduced taste due to their poor sense of smell. Another study reported olfactory deficits in boys with cleft palate,[21] which could result in decreased appetite and interest in food. Fetal surgery is an emerging modality that may alter treatment of craniofacial abnormalities.[22]

Hospitalization

When the child is hospitalized, the purpose of nutrition intervention is to maintain adequate nutritional status during the recovery period without a compromise in health or growth. Adequate calories and nutrients are essential during the recovery process to promote healing and normal growth and development. The diet will depend on the age of the child and the postsurgical regime of the surgery. Surgery during early infancy may necessitate feeding by aspepto syringe. With older children, the postsurgical diet advances from liquids to solids, and the routine or oral surgical dietary progression can usually be followed. If an older child must remain on semi-solids for an extended period, a nutritional supplement, increased caloric density, or small frequent feedings may be indicated. Nutrition and feeding education for the family is imperative if the child is going home on any dietary modifications or with new feeding equipment.

Follow-Up and Summary

The most important guideline for feeding children with cleft lip/palate is to individualize the feeding and nutrition information. All children will not develop at the same rate or require the same intervention strategies. Growth, diet, and biochemical values should be evaluated, as well as feeding problems. Team care is highly recommended, with the children and parents being vital contributing members of the team at all stages of treatment. Health care team members have important roles in the total care of children with craniofacial anomalies:

- learn the contributions of all team members and advocate for team assessment and treatment planning
- be informed about all facets of treatment
- be supportive of all the family during the lengthy and difficult phases of treatment

become knowledgeable about referral systems and resources[23–25]

References

1. Jones, M.C. Etiology of facial clefts: prospective evaluation of 428 patients. *Cleft Palate J.* 1988; 25:16
2. Starr, P., Pearman, W.A., Peacock, J.L. *Cleft Lip and/or Palate.* Springfield, Il: Charles C. Thomas; 1983.
3. Little, B.B., Snell, L.M., Klein, V.R., Gilstrap, L..C. Cocaine abuse during pregnancy: maternal and fetal complications. *Obstet. Gynecol.* 1989; 73:157.
4. American Cleft Palate Educational Foundation (ACPEF); *The Infant with Cleft Lip, Palate, or Both.* Pittsburgh: ACPEF; 1982.
5. March of Dimes Birth Defects Foundation. *Cleft Lip and Palate Information Sheet.* White Plains, NY: March of Dimes; 1988.
6. Hook, E.B. "Incidence" and "prevalence" as measures of the frequency of congenital malformations and genetic outcomes: application to oral clefts. *Cleft Palate J.* 1988; 25:101.
7. Vanderas, A.P. Incidence of cleft lip, cleft palate, and cleft lip and palate among races: a review. *Cleft Palate J.* 1987; 24:221.
8. American Cleft Palate Craniofacial Association Membership—Team Directory, Pittsburgh; Craniofacial Association; 1992.
9. Balluff, M.A., Udin, R.D. Using a feeding appliance to aid the infant with a cleft palate. *Ear Nose Throat J.* 1986; 65:316.
10. Bowers, E.J., Mayro, R.F., Whitaker, L.A., Pasquariello, P.S., LaRossa, D. Randal, P. General body growth in children with clefts of the lip, palate, and craniofacial structure. *Scand. J. Plast. Reconstr. Surg. Hand Surg.* 1987; 21:12.
11. Rudman, D., Davis T., Priest, J.H, Patterson, J.H., Kutner, M.H., Heymsfield, S.B., Bethel, R.A. Prevalence of growth hormone deficiency in children with cleft lip or palate. *J Pediatr* 1978; 93:378.
12. Duncan, P.A., Shapiro, L.R. Soley, R.L. Turet, S.E. Linear growth patterns in patients with cleft lip or palate or both. *Am. J. Dis. Child.* 1983; 137:159.
13. Jensen, B.L., Dahl, E., Kreiborg, S. Longitudinal study of body height, radius length and skeletal maturity in Danish boys with cleft lip. *Scand. J. Dent. Res.* 1983; 91:473.
14. Jones, J.E., Henderson, L., Avery, D.R. Use of feeding obturator for infants with severe cleft lip and palate. *Special Care Dent.* 1982; 2:120.
15. Weatherly-White, R.C.A., Kuehn, D.P., Miarrett, M.A., Gilman, J.I. Weatherly-White, C.C. Early repair and breast feeding for infants with cleft lip. *Plast. Reconstr. Surg.* 1987; 79:879.
16. Danner, S.C., Cerutti, E.R. *Nursing Your Baby with a Cleft Palate or Cleft Lip.* Rochester, NY: Childbirth Graphics; 1984.
17. Breast feeding prevents otitis media. *Nutr. Rev.* 1983; 41:241.
18. Paradise, J.L., McWilliams, B.J., Elster, B. Feeding of infants with cleft palate. *Pediatrics.* 1984; 74:316.
19. Harris, C.S., Baker, S.P., Smith, G.A., Harris, R.M. Childhood asphyxiation by food. *JAMA.* 1984; 251:2231.
20. Hairfield, W.M., Warren, D.W. Dimension of the cleft nasal airway in adults: a comparison with subjects without clefts. *Cleft Palate J.* 1989; 26:9.
21. Richman, R.A., Sheehe, P.R., McCanty, T., Vespasiano, M., Post, E.M., Guzi, S., Wright, H. Olfactory deficits in boys with cleft palate. *Pediatrics.* 1988; 82:840.
22. Strauss, R., Davis, J. Prenatal detection and fetal surgery of clefts and craniofacial anomalies of humans: social and ethical issues. *Cleft Palate J* 1990; 27:176.
23. Easter Seal Society. *Bright Promise*, Chicago, IL; Easter Seal Society; 1987.
24. Minnesota Department of Health. *Feeding Young Children with Cleft Lip and Palate.* Minnesota Dietetic Association; 1992.
25. American Cleft Palate Association. Telephone number: (800) 24-CLEFT.

Chapter 26
Pica and Lead Toxicity

Agnes Huber and Shirley Walberg Ekvall

Pica and lead intoxication may be associated conditions, but either can occur independently of each other. Although the etiology of pica is not well understood, an increased lead burden in children and adults is an environmental problem that is preventable by appropriate public health measures.

Pica has been defined in various ways. One author describes it as a repetitive search for and ingestion of nonfood substances.[1] Another applies the term "pica" to a pathological craving, both for items normally considered food (for example, a pregnant women consuming ten heads of lettuce daily) and for substances normally not regarded as food (clay or coal).[2] Some children and adults practice pica nondiscriminantly, some ingest several nonfood items, and others may seek out a very specific single substance. Various types of pica have been characterized: *geophagia*, the consumption of clay and dirt; *pagophagia*, the consumption of ice and refrigeration frost; and *coprophagia*, the ingestion of fecal material. A large variety of other pica substances have been reported, such as string, putty, ashes, plaster, crayons, laundry starch, cigarette butts, oak leaves, paper, cloth, and insects. In other countries pica is known under such terms as "hunger of pregnant women," clay-eating stomach illness, or indiscriminant craving.

Incidence

The prevalence of pica is difficult to establish because of inconsistent definition, reluctance to admit the practice, and the limited objective data reported. The craving for particular food items during pregnancy is widely recognized. In addition to the craving of such food items as fruit and other sweet-sour, sour, or sharp-tasting foods, pregnant women sometimes also crave or eat nonfood substances. Some pregnant women from the South eat clay and starch.[3] This type of pica also has been reported in other populations of black, white, and Mexican pregnant women. Some authors report a decline of pica from the 1960s to the 1980s, but the reasons are not clear. Although pica in men is said to be underreported, that incidence also seems to be decreasing.

Pica is most prevalent among children. It is said to occur in 50% of all children between the ages of 1–3 years.[1] Among psychotic, mentally retarded children, the incidence may exceed 50%. In a group of 991 adults with mental retardation, the incidence of pica was found to be 26%, greater than that of any other eating dysfunction, such as anorexia, rumination, or hyperphagia.[4]

Biochemical and Clinical Abnormalities

Etiology

Many hypotheses have been suggested to explain the cause of pica. One such hypothesis suggests that pica is a craving generated by nutrient deficiency. On the basis of animal studies, Snowdon[5] proposed that children deficient in calcium may discover that pica relieves some of the deficiency symptoms. Other specific nutrient deficiencies, such as of vitamin D, phosphorus, and vitamin C, have been thought to prompt the consumption of nonfood substances. However, pica did not decline in children given vitamin and mineral supplements.

Most attempts to link pica with nutritional states have concentrated on iron. Pagophagia in pregnant women consuming large amounts of ice (averaging 700 g/day) has been associated with iron deficiency. The low hemoglobin and low serum iron levels in these women responded to iron therapy, following which the pagophagia disappeared; whether the ice reduces iron deficiency remains unknown.[2] Other theories explaining pica are psychological, specifically the persistence of the infantile hand-to-mouth behavior patterns, a need to chew something solid, or a craving sensation related to texture, color, odor, or taste. Pica also may be cultural or familial. For example, clay eating was encouraged among male youths of Greece, eating the earth has frequently been associated with religious beliefs, and in African cultures consumption of earth during pregnancy is believed to suppress nausea. Pica may be practiced in an effort at self-medication. For example, pharmacological effects have been sought from extraordinarily large amounts of ground coffee, cigarette butts, oak leaves, and other substances.[4] This obsessive pica has been associated with a constant searching for and dreaming about the craved substance. Although geophagia is the most commonly reported and reviewed form of pica, the potential number of substances consumed is limitless.

Factors to be Considered in Evaluation

Nutritional and other

The health risks in pica are many. They range from the ingestion of toxic substances, such as lead, to interference with normal digestion and absorption, to the ingestion of life-threatening substances, such as glass. Surgery for foreign bodies, gastrointestinal obstruction, and vomiting after eating foreign substances have been reported frequently. Of special concerns in children and adults are pinworm and other parasitic infections and the risk of lead toxicity, especially in children and pregnant women.

Nutritional assessment of children and adults with pica has shown inadequacies in their diets. The iron-deficiency anemia associated with geophagia and pagophagia has already been mentioned. People with pica are reported to consume less meat and milk, fewer vitamin C-rich food sources, and a less varied diet. Geophagia specifically has been associated with low calorie, thiamin, niacin, and iron intakes. Nutritional status in general can be jeopardized by pica because the nonfood substance may replace the normal food intake that provides needed vitamins and minerals. When pica is complicated by lead toxicity, the nutritional status of children is compromised further by the detrimental effects of lead on hemoglobin and vitamin D metabolism; if lead toxicity is severe, urinary losses of nutrients will occur due to kidney damage.

The theory that some individuals may practice pica as self-medication has led to the belief that pica is a treatment for certain mineral deficiencies. The suggestion was made that iron and other essential trace elements may be obtained from clay and earths. However, this has not been borne out. Clays and earths consumed are cation exchangers that bind minerals, making them unavailable for intestinal absorption. The studies by Danford et al. in adults practicing geophagia have shown that, although calcium, iron, and zinc were adequate according to the RDA, low hemoglobin, serum iron, and serum zinc levels were found, indicating the decreased efficiency of absorption.

Dietary Management

The treatment of pica involves many health care disciplines. The dietitian and physician are involved because pica is frequently associated with a nutrient deficiency, specifically mineral absorption, and the risk for gastrointestinal obstruction, parasitic infections, and in some cases lead toxicity. Pica represents a behavioral challenge to the psychiatrist and psychologist. An anthropologist may be interested in the study of pica related to cultural patterns ingrained in the food habits of a region and possibly related to an ancestral food shortage. A public health nurse may be involved in the screening and identification of increased lead burden in children and pregnant women with pica. The dietitian must assess the diet, anthropometrics, and blood values, especially those relating to iron and zinc status. Improvement of diet, sufficient fluid, and a supplement with minerals and vitamins may lessen the pica behavior. However, not all types of pica are affected by diet, especially if they relate to a possible addictive behavior, such as the consumption of cigarette butts.

Lead exposure

Modern industrialization has markedly increased exposure to lead, and even children without pica are at increased risk for lead toxicity. The major sources of lead in the environment are lead-containing motor fuels, and flaking lead paint in old houses, but lead is even found in the diet and drinking water. All these sources increase the lead burden in children and adults.[7]

Epidemiological data from the HANES II, which were collected from 1976-1980,[8] indicate that 4% of children 6 months to 5 years old have blood lead levels greater than 30 µg/dL. High-risk children within this age group are black children, of whom 12% had increased blood lead levels; innercity children; and children of low-income families. However, increased lead levels in children may also occur in rural high-income families and other subpopulations. Screening programs to identify children with elevated blood lead levels should continue to focus on younger children, particularly among Puerto Ricans living in the New York City area and Mexican-Americans living in poverty in the southwestern United States, as well as the black population.[9] With the decrease in the use of leaded gasoline in the early 1980s, the average blood lead levels in children have been falling. In the United States, the number of children with blood levels greater than 40 µg/dL has been estimated as 53,000 and is comprised mostly of black children.

Diet, especially food from lead-soldered cans, and water running through lead pipes or from lead containing-water fountains can contribute significant amounts of lead, of which half is absorbed, according to Ziegler et al.[10] For children aged 6 months to 5 years, the FDA has estimated a mean lead intake from diet of 59-82 µg/day.[11] Variable amounts of lead are also obtained through drinking water. Although food, water, and gasoline lead in the air contribute significantly to an increased lead burden in the body, the main source of lead poisoning is lead paint.[12] Lead containing paints are now outlawed, but flaking paints and dust in old dwellings may be swallowed by children. Solubilized by stomach acidity, the lead is then absorbed.

Pathophysiological effects of lead

Lead interferes with many metabolic processes and normal physiological functions (Tables 26-1 and 26-2). The anemia of lead toxicity is due to the reversible inhibition of heme synthesis by lead. Kidney damage can occur in severe cases, resulting in excessive urinary nutrient losses. Lead depresses the immune response so that children with lead toxicity cannot fight infections efficiently.[13] Although these effects are reversible, the neurological consequences of lead toxicity are not.

Table 26–1. Effects of Lead on Health

Hematopoiesis
   Anemia due to decreased heme synthesis
   Elevated amino levulinic acid (ALA) and protoporphyrin in
     urine and erythrocytes
Kidney
   Aminoaciduria
   Glucosuria
   Reduced synthesis of calcitriol (1 25-dihydroxycholecalciferol)
Nervous System
   Peripheral nervous system damage (in adults)
   Central nervous system damage (in children)
   Low-level exposure
     Impaired psychological, behavioral and intellectual function
Immune System
   Host resistance to bacteria and viral infections decreased
   Possible other effects

Table 26–2. Effect of Nutritional Status on Lead Toxicity

Nutritional Factor	Effect
Fasting	Increases GI lead absorption
High-fat diets	Increases body lead burden
Lecithin	Increases GI lead absorption
Calcium	Liberal dietary intake protects
Iron deficiency	Increases susceptibility to lead toxicity
Zinc	Liberal dietary intake protects

The neurobehavioral effects of early lead exposure have been reviewed extensively.[14] Cross-sectional studies documenting such effects have been criticized because of their small effects and confounding variables. However, despite these problems, these studies clearly show that subclinical lead exposure (in the absence of symptoms of lead encephalopathy) carries the risk of permanent neuropsychological deficits. A study of an asymptomatic group of Head Start children, aged 3 to 7 years, showed a linear negative relationship between the children's IQ and their blood lead levels (47.4 μg/dL for the highest and 6.3 μg/dL for the lowest blood lead level) suggesting that lead at all levels has a detrimental effect on IQ.[14]

Nutritional factors

Nutrition is a consideration in the prevention and treatment of lead toxicity.[15] Table 26-2 summarizes the major lead-nutrient interactions. Overall, a child or adult in excellent nutritional status is partially protected from lead toxicity. Children who are anemic absorb a greater proportion of a lead dose than children who are not. When iron absorption is enhanced because of anemia, more lead may be absorbed as well. Similarly an increased intestinal lead absorption occurs when dietary calcium is low. Since deficiencies in body calcium, zinc, iron, and protein stores are all associated with an increased uptake of lead, optimizing nutrition enhances the resistance to lead[16] The high prevalence of lead toxicity in inner-city, poverty conditions is no doubt related to the presence of dilapidated, lead-containing structures. A second factor, which is a less recognized contribution, to the lead problem, may be the high prevalence of lactose intolerance in black children, which often results in a decreased calcium intake through dairy products. Furthermore, even with blood lead levels as low as 10-15 μg/dL, a significant reduction in serum 1, 25-dihydroxyvitamin D has been observed, further worsening calcium status.[17]

Because of their high metabolic rate, young children absorb more lead form the air they breathe. Because of their need for growth, the gastrointestinal absorption of mineral elements is also more efficient in children than in adults, as is the gastrointestinal absorption of lead. Furthermore, the exploratory mouthing behavior or pica may result in the ingestion of lead chips or dust. Thus the high growth rate with concomitant food intake and hand dust obtained from mouthing behavior may be the primary source of lead during the first year of life and may explain problems with lead toxicity in this age group. The need for measurements of growth in all surveys of the effect of lead and other environmental toxins on children is essential.[18] For all these reasons, preschool children are at the highest risk for lead intoxication. For similar reasons, pregnant women also are at risk for increased lead absorption, whereas lead exposure in the adult is of lesser concern except during occupational exposure.[19] Lead ingested by pregnant women crosses the placenta and has detrimental effects on fetal development.[20] Therefore, both children and pregnant women, should be exposed to the least lead dose possible, and be in optimal nutrient status for protection.

Screening, Treatment, Prevention, and Follow-up

Greater knowledge of the detrimental effects of subclinical lead levels in children has resulted in the lowering of the cut-off level for lead burden over the years. An elevated blood lead level is defined by the Centers for Disease Control as a whole blood lead concentration of 25 μg/dL or greater. Lead toxicity is present in a child if blood lead levels are equal or greater than 25 μg/dL, in conjunction with an erythrocyte protoporphyrin level of equal or greater than 35 μg/dl. Former cut-off points were 30 μg/dL and 50 μg/dL erythrocyte protoporphyrin.[11] However, erythrocyte protoporphyrin measurement is not sensitive enough to be recommended uniformly as a screening test for lead poisoning.[21]

All children should be screened for lead at regular intervals, but especially those with anemia, growth failure, and developmental or behavioral problems. Controlling the environment, strengthening the family's support systems, enhancing nutrition, and offering remedial education are essential to a successful therapeutic outcome.[16] This also applies for children with low to moderate lead exposure who have adequate nutritional status, significant alterations in vitamin D metabolism, calcium and phosphorus homeostasis and bone mineral content are not present.[22]

Children who are found to have lead toxicity need to be detoxified. Although vigorous chelation therapy can reduce morbidity and mortality, no therapy can replace the neurons destroyed by lead exposure.[23] Chelating agents bind lead, and the resultant chelate is excreted in urine. However, these drugs also bind essential mineral elements, such as zinc, markedly increasing their urinary excretion. Therefore, after chelation therapy, children need to be refed with adequate diets with special attention given to mineral content. An effort must also be made to remove the lead from the child's environment. As shown in Figure 26-1, chelation treatment alone had no lasting effect in one study. Only after removing the child from the high-lead environment did blood lead values stay in the lower ranges.[24]

Because of the irreversible, deleterious effects of lead toxicity in children, the Academy of Pediatrics Committee on Environmental Hazards and the Committee on Accident and Poison Prevention recommend that childhood lead poisoning be prevented by these treatment measures:[25]

- using the erythrocyte protoporphyrin (EP) test to screen children for lead toxicity and iron deficiency and to have hospital and clinical labs make EP available
- screening all preschool children for lead absorption; in cases where this is unrealistic, the Academy suggests screening children in a priority ranked order

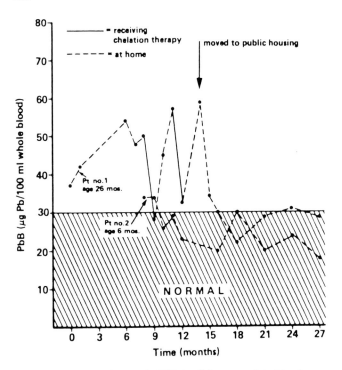

Fig. 26–1. Serial changes in PbB in siblings as related to changes in housing. Patient no. 1, the older sibling, received chelation therapy twice in the hospital, as indicated by the solid segments of the line showing trends in that patient's PbB. After each treatment course, this child returned to the same old house. Patient no. 2, the younger sibling, was first tested at the age of 6 months when the older sibling was hospitalized and was sent immediately to stay with an aunt in public "lead-free" housing. At the time that patient no. 1's PbB spiked for a third time; the family, including both siblings, moved to public housing. Patient no. 1's PbB promptly declined without additional chelation therapy. The shaded portion of the figure indicates the "normal" PbB range. From Chisholm,[24] with permission.

- closely monitoring any child who has an elevated venous blood level by means of repeat venous testing
- identifying and correcting those children with iron, calcium, and other nutritional deficiencies
- educating parents about the dangers of lead exposure

Government agencies should assume these responsibilities in lead poisoning prevention efforts:[25]

- mandating that all cases of lead poisoning be reported to the state health department
- systematically screening all living dwellings for lead hazards
- having state and local health departments require that lead base paint (exterior and interior) be removed from all living dwellings
- developing safer, more effective methods of lead abatement
- urging the U.S. government to recognize the prevalence and irreversibility of childhood lead poisoning and restore funding for screening, hazard identification, and abatement
- urging the EPA to persist in removing all lead from gas
- having blood lead and EP tests only done in laboratories that meet quality assurance criteria through proficiency testing programs

References

1. Singhi, P., Singhi, S Nutritional status and psycho-social stress in children with pica. *Indian Pediatr.* 1983; 20:345
2. Danford, D.E., Huber, A.M. Pica and nutrition. *Annu. Rev. Nutr.* 1982; 12:303.
3. Edwards, C.H., McDonald S., Mitchell, J.R., Jones, L., Mason, L., Kemp, A.M., Laing, D., Trigg, L. Clay and cornstarch-eating women. *J. Am Diet. Assoc.* 1959; 35:810.
4. Danford, D.E., Huber, A.M. Eating dysfunction in an institutionalized mentally retarded population. *Appetite*, 1981; 2:281.
5. Snowdon, C.T., Sanderson, B.A. Lead pica in rats. *Science.* 1974; 183:92.
6. Danford, D.E., Smith, J.C., Huber, A.M. Pica and mineral status. *Am. J. Clin. Nutr.* 1982; 35:958.
7. Chisholm, J.J., Jr. Pediatric exposures to lead, arsenic, cadmium, and methyl mercury. In: Chandra, R.K., *Trace Elements in Nutrition of Children.* New York; Vevey/Raven; 1985.
8. Mahaffey, K.R., Annest, J.L., Roberts, J., Murphy, R.S. National estimates of blood lead levels: United States, 1976-80: association with selected demographic and socioeconomic factors. *N. Engl. J. Med.* 1982; 307:573
9. Carter-Pokras, O., Pirkle, J., Chavez, G., Gunter, E. Blood lead levels of 4-11 year old Mexican American, Puerto Rican, and Cuban children. *Pub. Health Rep.* 1990; 105:388.
10. Ziegler, E.E., Edward, B.B., Jensen, R.I., Mahaffey, K.R., Fomon, S.J. Absorption and retention of lead by infants. *Pediatr. Res.* 1978; 12:29.
11. Beloian, A., McDowell M. Estimate of lead intake by children up to 5 years of age. 1973-1978 and 1980. Washington, DC: U.S. Food and Drug Administration Bureau of Foods, Division of Nutrition Final International Report; 1981.
12. Landrigan, R.J., Graef, J.W. Pediatric lead poisoning in 1987: the silent epidemic continues. *Pediatrics* 1987; 79:582.
13. Beisel, W.R. Single nutrients and immunity. *Am. J. Clin. Nutr.* 1982; 35(S):454.
14. Dietrich, K.M., Kraft, K.M., Shukla, R., Bornschein, R.L., Succop, P.A. The neurobehavioral effects of early lead exposure. In Schroeder, S.R., Ed. *AAMD Monographs, Toxic Substances and Mental Retardation*, Washington, DC: American Association on Mental Deficiency; 1987.
15. Mahaffey, K.R. Nutritional factors in lead poisoning. *Nutr. Rev.* 1981; 39:353.
16. The persistent threat of lead: medical and sociological issues. *Curr. Probl. Pediatr.* December, 1988; 703.
17. Mahaffey, K.R., Rosen, J.F., Chesney, R.W., Peeler, J.T., Smith, C.M., DeLuca, H.F. Association between age, blood lead concentration, and serum 1, 25-dihydroxycholechalciferol levels in children. *Am. J. Clin. Nutr.* 1982; 35:1327.
18. Angle, C.R., Kuntzelman, D.R. Increased erythrocyte protoporphyrins and blood lead—a pilot study of childhood growth patterns. *J. Tox. Environ. Health.* 1989; 26:149.
19. Goldman, R.H., Baker, E.L., Hannan, M., Kamerow, D.B. Lead poisoning in automobile radiator mechanics. *N. Engl. J. Med.* 1987; 317:214.
20. Bellinger, D., Leviton, A., Waternaux, C., Needleman, H., Rabinowitz, M. Longitudinal analyses of prenatal and postnatal lead exposure and early cognition. *N. Engl. J. Med.* 1987; 316:1037.
21. DeBraun, M.R., Sox, H.C. Setting the optimal erythrocyte protoporphyrin screening decision threshold for lead poisoning: a decision analytic approach. *Pediatrics* 1991; 88:121.
22. Koo, W.K., Succop, P.A., Bornschein, R.L., Krug-Wispe, S.K., Stenchen, J.J., Tsang, R.C., Berger, O.G. Serum vitamin D metabolites and bone mineralization in young children with chronic low to moderate lead exposure. *Pediatrics* 1991, 87:680.
23. Piomelli, S., Rosen, J.F., Chisolm, J.J., Jr. Graef, J.W. Management of childhood lead poisoning. *J. Pediatr.* 1984; 105:523.
24. Chisholm, J.J. Management of increased lead absorption and lead poisoning in children. In: Chisholm, J.J., Jr., O'Hara, D.M. *Lead Absorption in Children—Management, Clinical and Environmental Aspects.* Baltimore: Urban and Schwarzenberg; 1982.
25. Academy of Pediatrics Committee on Accident and Poison Prevention. *Pediatrics*; 1979; 79:3.

Chapter 27
Drug-induced Malnutrition

Ninfa Saturnino Springer and Marshal Shlafer

One of the major modes of intervention for handicapping conditions and chronic diseases is drug therapy. However, drug therapy is not without complications, and many drugs affect nutritional status. Those drugs used in handicapping conditions and that result in undesirable food-drug and nutrient-drug interactions are discussed in this chapter. The use of vitamins in pharmacological doses—popularly known as megavitamin or orthomolecular therapy—causes adverse physiological effects and is also discussed. This practice needs to be differentiated from the supplemental use of vitamins/minerals as presented in the last section of this chapter. Supplements used in this context compensate for adverse drug effects. The amounts used are based on individual needs and are supported by the data presented in this chapter.

In addition to drug-induced adverse nutritional effects, there is growing concern over the use of drugs among institutionalized[1] and community-based[2] residents with mental retardation. Drugs frequently prescribed by private physicians to 1369 group homes residents were surveyed and reported.[2] Although 63.6% of the residents were taking some kind of medication, 39.7% were on these psychoactive drugs as listed in decreasing frequency: anticonvulsants (22.5%), neuroleptics (13.6%), sedative/hypnotics (4.5%), antiparkinson drugs (3.4%), antidepressants (3.2%), and antimanic drugs (0.9%)

Drugs used for chronic diseases are too numerous to discuss in this chapter. The nutritional effects of drugs used in chronic diseases and in handicapping conditions, and substances that are commonly abused, are summarized in Table 27-1. In most cases only drugs generally prepared as prototypes of the class are listed in the table. When there are important differences among other members of a class, individual drugs are noted separately. Drug-drug interactions are not emphasized; the reader is encouraged to refer to a pharmacology textbook for additional information.[3]

Biochemical Abnormalities: Nutrition and Pharmacokinetics

The relationship between nutrition and pharmacokinetics, the fate of drugs and nutrients in the body, is important clinically. Pharmacokinetics encompasses the four major processes that affect the entry of exogenous substances into the systemic circulation, their ability to reach sites of action or use, and their elimination from the body: absorption, distribution, metabolism, and excretion. The integrity of each process, such as a person's ability to absorb and utilize nutrients and to respond in a predictable way to drugs that might be administered, is an important determinant of a person's overall wellness or illness. Conversely, nutritional deficiencies, illness, and the therapeutic agents used to treat or prevent them may have important effects on basic pharmacokinetics. Because of this important interrelationship, each component of pharmacokinetics is discussed briefly. The reader should consult a comprehensive pharmacology text[3,4] for more details about pharmacokinetics in general and for information about specific drugs and nutrients. Clark et al.[4] provide a useful table that summarizes the pharmacokinetic properties of drugs affected by these processes.

Absorption

The oral route is the most common administration route for drugs and nutrients. As is true for most drugs, many nutrients—most minerals and water-soluble vitamins—are absorbed into the circulation by passive diffusion through cell membranes. However, other nutrients are absorbed by other processes. For example, iron is absorbed mainly by active transport, and glucose is absorbed by an ATP-independent carrier-mediated phenomenon that has often been called facilitated diffusion.

Three key characteristics of drug/nutrient molecules affect absorption: lipid solubility, ionization, and size. Absorption is also affected by gut motility and by the local environment in various parts of the gastrointestinal tract. For example, the fat-soluble vitamins (A, D, E, K) depend greatly on the presence of adequate amounts of bile and bile salts for sufficient absorption. Vitamin B_{12}, a large water-soluble molecule, depends on the presence of intrinsic factor and normally low gastric acidity for absorption. Gut motility, whether altered by nutritionally related or other diseases or by drugs, influences the absorption of orally administered nutrients or drugs, potentially changing their bioavailability. For example, increases of gut motility associated with acute or chronic diarrhea or vomiting decrease the amount of time available for absorption. In persons with such a condition, nutrients may need to be administered by alternative routes to prevent or treat deficiencies. Conversely, if gut motility is decreased unduly, whether by a medical condition or by drug therapy, still other modifications of diet therapy may be required to reduce the risk of excessive drug absorption.

Alterations in pH from what is normal for parts of the gastrointestinal tract (mainly the stomach and duodenum) affect drug and nutrient absorption. Age is but one of the important factors that could affect absorption of orally administered drugs through gastric pH-related effects. For example, normal gastric pH is not reached until about age 2 or 3 years, and pH rises again in the older adult. At higher pH values, a greater proportion of acidic drugs are in the

Table 27-1. Adverse Nutritional Effects of Selected Drugs

Drug Category or Class	Generic Name (BRAND NAME)	Adverse Reactions	Comments
		DRUGS USED FOR ARTHRITIS OR OTHER INFLAMMATORY STATES	
Analgesics (non-narcotic; includes most nonsteroidal anti-inflammatory agents)	Aspirin	1. gastrointestinal distress (variable incidence, severity) 2. gastric mucosal damage may increase blood loss via gut, cause iron deficiency 3. potential increase of urinary vitamin C excretion 4. urinary acidification by high doses of vitamin C may reduce renal salicylate excretion, increase risk of toxicity	1. may alter taste sensitivity 2. administration with food or antacids may reduce GI distress, may also reduce absorption and therapeutic effects 3. buffered aspirin products may increase serum sodium levels
Anti-inflammatory drugs, nonsteroidal	Most generic and brand names	See 1 and 2 for aspirin above	
	Colchicine	1. decreases vitamin B_{12} absorption 2. gastric mucosal damage may increase fecal blood loss, cause iron deficiency	1. severe gastrointestinal intolerance may depress appetite
Corticosteroids (all administered orally or parenterally)	Many generic brand names	1. hypernatremia 2. hypokalemia 3. hyperglycemia 4. hypocalcemia 5. hypophosphatemia 6. hypertriglyceridemia, hypercholesterolemia 7. decreases protein synthesis, increases protein catabolism 8. potential deficiencies of Vitamins C, D, B_6 (pyridoxine), and folate	1. caused by increased renal sodium absorption, accompanied by water retention; may be sufficient to cause/worsen edema, congestive heart failure, hypertension 2. both a renal effect and due to reduced potassium absorption from gut (with oral administration); may be significant 3. contributes to muscle wasting with long-term therapy 4. may contribute to bone fragility with long-term high-dose use 5. if phosphorus supplements are indicated, use sodium-free salts to avoid exacerbating hypernatremia
Uricosuric drugs	Probenecid (BENEMID) Sulfinpyrazone (ANTURANE)	1. potential increase of renal excretion of calcium, magnesium, sodium, especially chloride salts	
		DRUGS USED FOR NEOPLASTIC DISEASES	
Alkylating agents	Cyclophosphamide (CYTOXAN)	1. metallic taste, nausea and vomiting	1. sucking hard candy may reduce sensation; drug is contraindicated in malnutrition 2. high fluid output needed to prevent sterile hemorrhagic cystitis
Antimetabolites	Methotrexate (FOLEX)	1. inhibits dehydrofolate reductase 2. nausea, anorexia, stomatitis	1. administer reduced folate 2. monitor fluid intake and output
Antitumor antibiotics	Doxorubicin (ADRIAMYCIN)	1. nausea, vomiting, and mucositis	1. interferes with nucleic acid synthesis
Hormonal and anti-hormonal agents	Diethystilbestrol (STILPHOSTROL)	1. nausea and occasional vomiting	1. monitor sodium intake, blood pressure, and cardiac status
Plant alkaloids	Vincristine (ONCOVIN)	1. constipation	1. use stool softeners, mild laxatives; increase dietary fiber and fluid
		DRUGS USED FOR CARDIOVASCULAR CONDITIONS	
Anticoagulants, oral	Warfarin (COUMADIN) Dicumarol, Phenprocouman	1. actions antagonized by vitamin K	1. vitamin K-rich foods that could interact if eaten in very large amounts include most green leafy vegetables, cauliflower, soy beans, tomatoes, liver 2. anemia, iron deficiency during anti-coagulant therapy should be assessed for underlying blood loss, as via gastrointestinal tract

Table 27–1. (*Continued*)

Drug Category or Class	Generic Name (BRAND NAME)	Adverse Reactions	Comments
Cholesterol-lowering agents	Cholestyramine (QUESTRAN) Colestipol (COLESTID)	1. decreases absorption of fat-soluble vitamins (A, D, E, K)	
	Clofibrate (ATROMID-S)	1. potential decrease of absorption of vitamins A and B_{12}, iron	1. may alter taste, cause aftertaste that could alter appetite

ANTIHYPERTENSIVE DRUGS

Drug Category or Class	Generic Name (BRAND NAME)	Adverse Reactions	Comments
Vasodilators	Hydralazine (APRESOLINE)	1. potential deficiency of vitamin B_6	1. may be symptomatic with long-term therapy, whether used for hypertension or heart failure
	Diazoxide (HYPERSTAT)	1. hyperglycemia	1. consequences may be important, especially for diabetic patients despite usual short-term use of this drug
	Nitroprusside (NIPRIDE)	1. potential deficiency of serum vitamin B_{12} levels	1. not likely to be significant with usual acute use
Catecholamine depletors	Reserpine (SERPASIL), others	1. potential gastric hyperacidity, dyspepsia; diarrhea due to predominant actions of parasympathetic nervous system on gut	

DIURETICS

Drug Category or Class	Generic Name (BRAND NAME)	Adverse Reactions	Comments
Thiazides	Hydrochloro-thiazide (many name brands and generic drugs)	1. hyponatremia 2. hypokalemia 3. hypercholesterolemia, hypertriceridemia 4. hyperglycemia, impaired glucose tolerance 5. hypercalcemia	1. these drugs are potassium-wasting; use potassium-rich foods or prescriptive oral potassium supplements 2. duretic-induced hypokalemia is major cause of digitalis toxicity in patients treated with cardiac glycosides concomitantly 3. administration to diabetic patients may require compensatory alterations of diet and/or antidiabetic drug therapy 4. reduced renal calcium; monitor accordingly, especially in patients taking digitalis
High-ceiling ("loop") diuretics	Furosemide (LASIX), others	1. hyponatremia 2. hypokalemia 3. hyperglycemia 4. hypocalemia 5. hypomagnesemia 6. dehydration, hypochloremic, hypokalemic (metabolic) acidosis, hyponatremia	1. more likely to occur and be severe than with any other diuretic classes; may be symptomatic (e.g., accompanied by hypotension due to concomitant renal water loss) 2. see thiazides #2 above 3. see thiazides #2 above 4. increased renal calcium excretion due to high-ceiling diuretics 5. may become symptomatic, monitor accordingly 6. due to excessive diuresis from acute or chronic overdose or lack of adequate fluid intake
Carbonic anhydrase inhibitors	Acetazolamide (DIAMOX)	1. hypokalemia 2. hyperglycemia 3. systemic (metabolic) acidosis	1. see thiazides above; may occur after diuretic effect subsides, treatment is continued (as for therapy of glaucoma, seizures) 2. see thiazides above 3. urine is alkalinized, thereby causing base deficit in blood; assess accordingly during chronic therapy, regardless of reason for use
Potassium-sparing diuretics	Triamterene (DYRENIUM)	1. hyponatremia	1. risk greatest when used adjunctively with other diuretics, as is often done

Table 27-1. (*Continued*)

Drug Category or Class	Generic Name (BRAND NAME)	Adverse Reactions	Comments
	Amiloride (MIDAMOR) Spironolactone (ALDACTONE)	2. hyperkalemia 3. hyperglycemia	2. risk greatest when oral potassium supplements are given concomitantly, which should be avoided ordinarily

DRUGS WITH PREDOMINANT CNS EFFECTS OR USES

Drug Category or Class	Generic Name (BRAND NAME)	Adverse Reactions	Comments
Alcohol	Ethyl alcohol	1. gastric irritation; high dose can cause ulcers, inhibits drug metabolism; low dose stimulates hepatic metabolizing enzymes 2. organ damage and malnutrition when ingesting large amounts at the expense of well-balanced diet 3. malabsorption of vitamins A, C, B_1, B_{12} and folic acid; increased excretion of folic acid, Ca, Mg, and Zn	1. rapidly absorbed; milk products slow absorption 2. enters fetal circulation and maternal milk 3. give diet of high nutritional quality 4. low dose stimulates hepatic metabolizing enzymes
Nicotine		1. decreases appetite, increases physical activity, can lead to weight loss, generalized nutritional deficiencies 2. decreases intake of sweets, increases intake of fatty foods 3. elevates LDL, VLDL, favors atherogenesis 4. stimulates hepatic metabolism, lowers blood levels of other drugs (e.g., theophylline, propranolol)	1. alters taste sensation 2. clear link with carcinogenesis 3. cardiovascular, metabolic effects increase risk, severity of cardiovascular diseases
Marijuana		1. increases appetite, food intake, weight gain 2. major effects as for tobacco smoking (nicotine)	1. heightens apparent taste sensations
Central nervous system stimulants or anorexigenics (peptide antagonists are under investigation)	Methylphenidate (RITALIN) Cocaine	1. nervousness, insomnia, headache, dizziness 2. anemia, scalp hair loss 3. loss of appetite, abdominal pain, nausea, weight loss	1. use cautiously with MAO inhibitors 2. inhibit metabolism of anticonvulsants, tricyclic antidepressants 1. no studies on pregnant women
	Dextroamphetamine (DEXEDRINE)	1. dermotoses, insomnia, irritability, hyperactivity, personality changes, psychosis, headache, dizziness 2. dryness of mouth, unpleasant taste, diarrhea, constipation	1. anorectic and adrenergic agent 2. not recommended for minimum brain dysfunction under 3 years 3. increased risk of birth defects 4. excreted in breast milk
Anticonvulsants	Phenytoin (DILANTIN)	1. nausea, vomiting, constipation 2. megaloblastic anemia 3. gingival hyperplasia 4. hyperglycemia 5. insomnia, dizziness, headache, fatigue	1. administer drug with or immediately after meal 2. poor water solubility
	Valproic acid (DEPAKENE)	1. transient nausea, vomiting, and indigestion at initiation of therapy 2. diarrhea, abdominal cramps, and constipation 3. hair loss	1. teratogenic during pregnancy 2. capsules should be swallowed, not chewed
	Carbamazepine (TEGRETOL)	1. drowsiness, dizziness, unsteadiness, nausea, and diplopia 2. blood dyscrasias	1. excreted in breast milk 2. teratogenic during pregnancy
Barbiturates	Phenobarbital	1. nausea, vomiting, constipation 2. stimulates breakdown of vitamin D 3. vitamin D and calcium deficiency may lead to osteomalacia or rickets 4. increases incidence of fractures 5. alters hepatic synthesis of vitamin K, hemorrhage of newborn when taken during third trimester	1. not very lipid soluble; enters CNS and tissues slowly 2. unmetabolized drug excreted through kidney and milk 3. long half-life, can inhibit seizures without marked sedation 4. give drug with meals 5. give high fiber and fluid diet

Table 27–1. (*Continued*)

Drug Category or Class	Generic Name (BRAND NAME)	Adverse Reactions	Comments
		6. fetal malformation when high doses are taken during early pregnancy	6. give vitamin K supplements to pregnant women 7. excreted in maternal milk
Benzodiazepines	Diazepam (VALIUM)	1. commonly reported: drowsiness, fatigue, and ataxia 2. infrequent: constipation, nausea, changes in salivation, skin rash, tremor, insomnia	1. avoid during pregnancy—may be teratogenic 2. 1–2 days half-life
Antidepressants, tricyclics, and related agents	Imipramine (TOFRANIL) Fluoxetine (PROZAC)	1. insomnia, dry mouth, constipation, paralytic ileus, skin rash, petechiae, nausea, vomiting, anorexia, epigastric distress, diarrhea or constipation, peculiar taste, stomatitis, abdominal cramps, fatigue, headache, alopecia 2. weight gain or loss 3. in enuretic children: nervousness, sleep disorders, tiredness, and mild GI disturbance usually disappear during continued drug therapy or when dosage is decreased	1. triclyic antidepressant used also for reducing enuresis in children; not recommended under 6 years 2. safe use in pregnancy not established 3. excreted in breast milk 4. Fluoxetine is serotoninergic and may be used for weight loss
Antidepressants, MAO inhibitors	Phenelzine (NARDIL)	1. dizziness, constipation, dry mouth, postural hypotension, drowsiness, weakness and fatigue, edema, GI disturbances, tremors and twitching	1. may result in hypertensive crisis—should not be given with foods containing high concentration of tryptamine or tyramine 2. safe use during pregnancy has not been established 3. not recommended for less than 16 years
Antimanic drug	Lithium (CIABALITH, others)	1. early effects related to blood drug levels include nausea, dry mouth, diarrhea, and thirst 2. effects unrelated to blood levels include weight gain, metallic taste, altered taste of some foods, edema of hands and ankle 3. constipation	1. absorbed quickly and well 2. metabolism closely associated with sodium (Na balance plays role in development of side effects and toxicity) 3. give with meals to reduce nausea 4. monitor electrolyte loss 5. monitor exercise for fluid loss 6. give high fiber and fluid diet
Antiparkinson drugs	Levodopa (DOPAR, LARODOPA)	1. nausea, vomiting, dry mouth, dysphagia	1. give drug with meals; however, high-protein diet will compromise effectiveness
	Carbidopa plus levodopa (SINEMET)	1. anorexia 2. headaches, dizziness, insomnia, fatigue	1. monitor weight; allow adequate time to eat
Narcotics	Morphine sulfate Heroin	1. hypotension 2. constipation, aggravation of hemorrhoids 3. nausea, vomiting 4. hyperglycemia	1. relieved by quietly lying in bed 2. encourage high-fiber and fluid diet; laxatives and stool softener may be indicated
Neuroleptics (antipsychotic drugs)	Chlorpromazine (THORAZINE)	1. drowsiness 2. persistent tardive dyskinesia—symptoms are irreversible after long-term therapy 3. weight loss 4. hyper- or hypoglycemia 5. occasional dry mouth, nasal congestion 6. constipation 7. skin pigmentation 8. inhibits insulin release and impair glucose tolerance 9. increases in appetite and weight	1. 30 hour half-life accounts for slow onset of antipsychotic action
	Thiordazine (MELLARIL)	1. drowsiness 2. dryness of mouth, blurred vision, con-	1. reproductive studies in animals failed to show teratogenic effect

Table 27–1. (*Continued*)

Drug Category or Class	Generic Name (BRAND NAME)	Adverse Reactions	Comments
		stipation, nausea, vomiting, nasal stuffiness, and pallor 3. dermatitis	
	Haloperidol (HALDOL)	1. tardive dyskinesia 2. lethargy 3. decreases thirst sensation	1. possible fetal damage during pregnancy

DRUGS USED FOR ENDOCRINE-METABOLIC DISORDERS

Drug Category or Class	Generic Name (BRAND NAME)	Adverse Reactions	Comments
Antidiabetic drugs	Insulin (all)	1. hypoglycemia resulting from hyperinsulinism; hunger, weakness 2. decreases serum potassium	1. give calorie modified diet planned according to person's nutritional needs
	Tolbutamide (ORINASE)	1. risk of hypoglycemia 2. nausea, vomiting, diarrhea, heartburn or abdominal pain 3. occasional GI bleeding	1. increased by excessive exercise, skipping of meals, poor nutrition; carry source of simple sugar for emergencies 2. age and excessive alcohol intake will increase risk of hypoglycemia; give drug with meals
Thyroid, antithyroid drugs	Levothyroxine (LEVOTHROID, SYNTHROID);	1. increases bowel activity if doses are excessive or increased too rapidly	1. monitor bowel habits
	Propylthiouracil, ("ptu"; METHIMAZOLE)	1. fever and nausea	1. give drugs with meals
	Iodine, iodides (LUGOL'S SOLUTION)	1. staining of teeth 2. diarrhea, pain in throat, mouth, and gums; vomiting	1. sip medication through straw; also helps mask poor taste 2. may indicate iodism; assess immediately, avoid iodine containing foods and drugs 3. bloody diarrhea or vomitus may indicate acute iodine poisoning
Drugs for hypercalcemia	Calcitonin-salmon	1. nausea with or without vomiting	1. contraindicated in osteoporosis 2. encourage fluid to decrease possibility of renal calculi 3. avoid multivitamin, mineral supplements and antacids
Androgens and anabolic steroids	Testosterone (ANDRO 100), others	1. hypercalcemia, renal calcium stone 2. constipation, vomiting	1. monitor serum calcium level
	Conjugated estrogens (PREMARIN)	1. anorexia or increased appetite, weight gain 2. nausea, bloating, vomiting 3. diarrhea, abdominal cramping 4. edema	1. monitor weight
	Medroprogesterone acetate (PROVERA)	1. changes in appetite, nausea, edema, weight gain	
	Oral contraceptives—estrogen-progestin combinations	1. low serum vitamin C; possible low vitamin B_1, B_{12}, B_6, B_2, folate, Mg, Zn 2. high hematocrit, hemoglobin, serum iron, Ca, vitamins A and E 3. increases absorption of vitamins A and Ca 4. may cause hyperglycemia	1. modify diet as appropriate and assess need for and amount of nutrient supplementation
Adrenocorticosteroids	Hydrocortisone (CORTEF)	See Corticosteroids page 230.	

Table 27–1. (*Continued*)

Drug Category or Class	Generic Name (BRAND NAME)	Adverse Reactions	Comments
		DRUGS USED FOR GI DISORDERS	
Antacids	All	1. may interfere with absorption of any orally administered vitamins 2. increases gastric pH may reduce iron absorption 3. may elevate serum sodium levels unless low-sodium or sodium-free products are used	1. discourage frequent or excessive use unless use can be monitored or supervised 2. sodium-free products preferred for chronic, intensive therapy, especially when hypernatremia is an added risk 3. magnesium-aluminum products generally preferred for long-term use (e.g., for ulcers) to minimize altered gut motility
	Aluminum salts (e.g., aluminum hydroxide gel)	1. potential hypercalcemia, hypophosphatemia with chronic high-dose use 2. constipation possible unless used in combination with magnesium salt	1. used in combination with magnesium salt to reduce risk of constipation
	Calcium carbonate	1. risk of hypercalcemia with frequent or high-dose use 2. constipation probable unless used in combination with magnesium salt; fecal impaction possible	1. used in combination with magnesium salt to reduce risk of constipation
	Magnesium hydroxide, oxide (e.g., milk of magnesia)	1. risk of hypermagnesemia, frank magnesium intoxication, especially in persons with renal dysfunction 2. diarrhea (dose-related) probable unless used in combination with constipating antacid (aluminum or calcium salt), with potential generalized fluid and electrolyte loss	1. discourage use of products containing only magnesium salt for frequent or high-dose use, especially by persons with poor renal function and the elderly 2. assess for excessive fluid and electrolyte loss, and neurological evidence of hypermagnesemia
	Sodium bicarbonate— baking soda	1. risk of hypernatremia and associated hypertension, circulating fluid overload, edema	1. discourage routine use as antacid unless under physician's supervision
Anticholinergics (parasympatholytics)	Atropine, many others	1. inhibits gastric acid secretion, increases gastric pH, may impair absorption of iron and vitamin B_{12}	1. decreased salivary secretions may cause dry mouth, dysphagia, decreased appetite, impaired ability to swallow 2. anticholinergic side effect common to many drug groups, including antihistamines (H_1-blockers), antidepressants, antipsychotics, etc.
Antihistamines (H_1-blockers)	Diphenhydramine (BENADRYL)	1. see anticholinergics, above	1. see anticholinergics, above
Antihistamines (H_2-blockers)	Cimetidine (TAGAMET)	1. inhibits gastric acid secretion, increased gastric pH, may interfere with absorption of iron and vitamin B_{12}	1. inhibits hepatic metabolism of many other drugs
Emetics	Syrup of ipecac	1. metabolic alkalosis, hypokalemia, other electrolyte imbalances; dehydration, hypotension from fluid loss 2. impairs nutrient and drug absorption, generalized malnutrition 3. damage to oral mucosa and teeth from frequent contact with acidic emesis	1. a major concern with emetic abuse, as by persons with anorexia nervosa-bulimia
Laxatives, cathartics	All	1. excessive and potentially significant fluid, electrolyte loss (especially of potassium), with laxative/cathartic abuse 2. impairs absorption of orally administered drugs and vitamins 3. loss of spontaneous bowel rhythm, especially if abused as part of laxative-antidiarrheal drug cycle	1. discourage frequent or high-dose use without physician's approval 2. if interacting drugs or nutrients must be administered (orally) separate administration by at least 2 hours if possible

Table 27–1. (*Continued*)

Drug Category or Class	Generic Name (BRAND NAME)	Adverse Reactions	Comments
	Bisacodyl, enteric-coated tablets (DULCOLAX)	1. gastric mucosal irritation if taken with antacids, alkaline foods	1. avoid interaction
	Bulk-forming agents (e.g., calcium polycarbophyl, psyllium), stool softeners (e.g., docusate)	1. potential constipation or gut obstruction; dysphagia during administration	1. administer with ample amounts of water or juice as recommended on label
	Magnesium salts (citrate, hydroxide, sulfate)	1. see antacids, above	
	Mineral oil	1. impairs absorption of fat-soluble vitamins (A, D, E, K)	1. discourage frequent or chronic use

DRUGS USED FOR INFECTIOUS DISEASES

Drug Category or Class	Generic Name (BRAND NAME)	Adverse Reactions	Comments
Antibiotics	Penicillin G (PENTIDS)	1. nausea, epigastric distress 2. vomiting, diarrhea 3. glossitis or black hairy tongue may occur	1. not absorbed well after oral administration; decreased acidity increases absorption
	Antifungals Isoniazid (INH, NYDRAZID)	1. peripheral neuropathy resulting from inhibition of pyridoxine's effect on nervous tissue 2. hypoglycemia 3. nausea and vomiting occur from gastric irritation 4. interferes with absorption of iron, folic acid, B_{12}; diminishes absorption of vitamin E; causes depletion of niacin 5. increases excretion of B_6 and folic acid 6. increases absorption of iron	1. give pyridoxine supplements 2. give drug with meals 3. multivitamins and iron supplements are recommended
	Chelating agents (Penicillamine)	1. malabsorption of Cu, Zn, Fe	1. monitor intake and supplement as needed

From Shlafer & Marieb,[3] Moore,[60] Roe,[61] Mohs, et al.,[62] Bray,[63] Wise,[64] Wellman.[65]

---

ionized and poorly diffusible form. Their absorption is reduced and their effects potentially diminished. Conversely, gastric absorption of weak bases is increased, with the potential for excessive effects or toxicity.

When malnutrition is generalized and severe, alterations of gut microvillar structure can affect the absorption of a variety of drugs and nutrients. Although the changes described above apply generally to many drugs, some specific consequences may occur; for example, vitamin B_{12} deficiency arising from diminished vitamin absorption secondary to achlorhydria.

Distribution

Many of the processes that affect the entry of molecules into the bloodstream also affect their ability to leave the blood for ultimate distribution to and utilization by parenchymal cells of tissue and organs. Important considerations include plasma protein binding, total body water content, and relative fat content.

Not all nutrient or drug molecules circulating in the bloodstream are free to interact with the cells of the body. Plasma proteins, particularly albumin, have the ability to bind a variety of nutrient and drug molecules. For a given total amount of nutrient or drug in the blood, a certain percentage or fraction will bind the plasma proteins, and the remainder will be free. Molecules that are bound to plasma proteins or other storage sites are pharmacologically inactive and remain that way until they become free. Only those molecules that are unbound can produce effects as they are metabolized or be excreted. The percentage of nutrient molecules that will be bound to plasma protein depends largely on the nutrient's chemical structure. That structure affects not only the extent (amount) of binding but also the strength of the interaction between the molecule and its binding site. Depending on the chemical nature of the molecule, the fraction of total molecules that is bound (or unbound) can range from nearly zero to nearly 100%.

The ability of drugs and nutrients to bind plasma protein may cause potential problems. In some diseases the liver is unable to manufacture normal amounts of plasma protein. In others, renal damage may cause excessive loss of plasma proteins in the urine. Both of these situations cause hypoalbuminemia, which is also relatively common in the elderly and in pregnant women. Other conditions, including advanced age, also appear to reduce the number of binding sites on plasma proteins. If the drug in question is highly (or almost completely) bound, such alterations of plasma protein levels or binding capacity will require dosage adjustments and careful measurement (when possible) of both total and free serum drug levels in laboratory tests to guide those adjustments. Drugs that are highly protein bound include many of the sedatives, hypnotics, and anxiolytic drugs (including most of the benzodiazepines and barbiturates); most of the anticonvulsants except for ethosuximide and primidone; most antidepressants, antipsychotics, and lithium; theophylline; the oral anticoagulants, and most of the beta-adrenergic blockers and calcium channel blockers.

Malnutrition, debility, and even aging in otherwise healthy individuals tend to increase relative total body water content and to decrease relative fat content. Since drugs and nutrients differ in their water and lipid solubility, these changes also may require therapeutic adjustments.

Metabolism

Metabolism is one of the two major processes (the other is excretion) that are largely responsible for reducing the amount of active drug or nutrient in the body. The liver is the major site of metabolism, and the hepatocyte's microsomal enzyme systems are the major cellular sites of biotransformation. Overall, metabolism serves two basic functions: (1) it transforms a drug or nutrient to one or more metabolites that are less active pharmacologically or biologically and therefore potentially less toxic to the body, and (2) it converts drugs or nutrients to metabolites that are more water soluble (or less lipid soluble) so that they can be eliminated more readily.

Some substances are totally metabolized to other compounds before they are excreted. Others undergo no metabolism and are excreted unchanged in the same chemical form in which they were administered. However, most absorbed substances are handled by both processes simultaneously, with some of the molecules being metabolized and the rest excreted without prior metabolism. Several important factors can alter the ability of the liver's enzymes to metabolize drugs and therefore can dramatically influence a patient's response to pharmacotherapy.

Age. Most hepatic drug metabolizing enzymes are poorly developed in the fetus and newborn, and "normal" enzyme activities are not reached until puberty when they peak and remain high until 60 years of age or so. After that, enzyme activity usually declines again. Age-related decreases of renal function may accompany declines of hepatic function.

Nutrition and Diet. The effectiveness of the liver's drug metabolizing enzymes depends upon the presence of relatively normal dietary levels of carbohydrates, lipids, amino acids, and vitamins. Marked and prolonged deficiencies of many nutrients can seriously impair liver function, including those functions that are necessary to eliminate therapeutic agents.

Disease. Any disease that damages the hepatocytes or reduces hepatic blood flow has the potential to seriously reduce drug or nutrient metabolism. Hepatitis and cirrhosis are examples of primary liver dysfunction; congestive heart failure is one extrahepatic cause of inadequate liver function.

Hormones. Hormones can have marked effects on hepatic drug metabolism. Deficiencies of insulin, thyroid hormone, or adrenal corticosteroids can significantly decrease hepatic drug metabolism. Fluctuations in progesterone and estrogen levels during the menstrual cycle and during pregnancy also seem to influence hepatic metabolic activity.

Drugs. Hepatic function clearly affects the disposition of many drugs and nutrients. Importantly, however, drugs may also affect hepatic metabolism, resulting in increased or decreased rates of metabolism of drugs and nutrients. Some drugs tend to inhibit metabolism, so that they or other extensively metabolized drugs accumulate unless proper dosage reductions are made. Other drugs stimulate the liver's drug metabolizing capacity mainly by inducing the synthesis of increased amounts of drug-metabolizing enzymes in the hepatocytes. The result is a greater capacity for the liver to metabolize many nutrients and drugs, which may contribute to apparent refractoriness or tolerance to interacting drugs or nutrients that also depend on hepatic metabolism unless proper dosage increases are made.

Drug-induced enzyme inhibition or induction appears to be a reversible process that disappears over days or weeks after discontinuing administration of the causative agent. The speed with which the interaction wanes depends on which hepatoactive agent has been administered. Proper monitoring of the therapeutic response, blood levels of the drug, and dosage adjustments are mandatory during such changes in combined drug administration.

Excretion

Most drugs and their metabolites are excreted by the kidneys and eliminated from the body in the urine. Depending on the agent under consideration, renal excretion involves glomerular filtration, tubular secretion, or both. Tubular reabsorption is the renal process that returns initially eliminated drug to the bloodstream, thereby counteracting the other two processes to varying degrees.

Renal excretion appears to be more resistant to malnutrition and other nutritional deficits than absorption, distribution, and metabolism. Conditions that decrease cardiac output to levels sufficient to reduce renal blood flow decrease glomerular filtration rates and hinder renal drug elimination in general. More common are alterations in drug elimination caused by changes of tubular reabsorption. One physical process that governs the tubular reabsorption of most molecules is passive diffusion. Just as pH affects absorption from the gut, urine pH influences tubular reabsorption. Both medical disorders and drugs used to treat them can affect urine pH and therefore have dramatic effects on the biological fate of drugs. For example, alkalinizing the urine through administration of sodium bicarbonate increases phenobarbital elimination by favoring the formation of ionized and poorly diffusible molecules that cannot undergo tubular reabsorption. The effects of urine pH on amphetamine, a weak base, are the opposite. Alkalinizing the urine reduces amphetamine excretion, and acidifying it increases excretion.

Although the phenobarbital-sodium bicarbonate interaction is relatively easy to avoid if the person is compliant and educated about the potential result, the amphetamine-urinary acidification interaction is somewhat more problematic. If the dosages are not timed properly with respect to meals, anorexia and a nutritional deficit may occur—the desired result when amphetamines are given for anorexigenic effects in grossly obese persons. Regardless of the drug's indication, altered nutrient utilization can lead to ketosis, which acidifies the urine, increases the drug's elimination, and decreases the drug's effects (tolerance). These effects, in turn, could lead to inappropriate administration of higher doses and an associated risk of causing drug-induced psychosis.

Adverse Nutritional Effects Of Psychoactive Drugs

Anticonvulsants

Anticonvulsants have been a subject of research for many years, primarily because of their many adverse effects on metabolism. They cause abnormalities in mineral and bone metabolism, resulting in rickets or osteomalacia, folate deficiency with or without macrocytosis, congenital malformations among infants born to mothers on anticonvulsants, and connective tissue disorders (gum hypertrophy and hyperplasia). Possible abnormalities in fat and protein metabolism and deficiencies in blood vitamins E and K, pyridoxine, vitamin B_{12}, biotin, and thyroid hormones have also been reported.

The influence of anticonvulsant drugs on bone metabolism is evidenced by decreased serum phosphate, calcitonin, calcium, and 25-$(OH)D_2$ levels; normal or increased alkaline phosphatase and 1,25-dihydroxy-vitamin D levels; and decreased bone density. Whether anticonvulsant-induced rickets or osteomalacia occurs, however, is dependent on the number of drugs taken,[5] the relative plasma concentration (dependent on drug dose),[6] and the duration of treatment.[7] The pathophysiological mechanism of rickets and osteomalacia is attributed to induction of the hepatic microsomal enzyme system,[8] resulting in vitamin D deficiency[9] or increased skeletal turnover of minerals.[10]

Gingival hyperplasia during phenytoin therapy is an adverse drug-induced effect that may involve more than systemic alterations of drug metabolism. In its most severe form, phenytoin-induced gingival hyperplasia can alter the dietary intake of many nutrients. Phenytoin, as do phenobarbital and many other drugs, stimulates the hepatic microsomal enzyme system. As a result, it speeds the metabolism of many drugs and nutrients. Gurian et al.[11] reported gingival hyperplasia in 20% to 63% of patients taking phenytoin. An interesting study by Drew et al.[12] showed that topical administration of folate inhibited further hyperplasia, whereas systemic folate administration did not. This finding suggests a local (gingival) and potentially treatable cause of phenytoin-induced gingival hyperplasia. Nevertheless, until further data are collected, the results do not min-

imize the importance of prophylactic oral hygiene and dental care for persons taking this common and effective anticonvulsant drug.

Studies on folate deficiency following anticonvulsant use are continuing, and several hypotheses underlying its causation have been proposed. Hendel and co-workers[13] suggested that intestinal folic acid absorption is inhibited during anticonvulsant therapy. It is also hypothesized that folic acid acts as a co-factor in the metabolism of phenytoin.[14] The causes of folate deficiency are summarized by Basu[15] and include decreased folate absorption, decreased metabolic activation of folate and decreased induction of drug metabolizing enzymes. Although all three mechanisms result in folate deficiency and impaired hematopoiesis, induction of drug enzymes (NADPH co-factor) may increase not only the requirement for the enzymes but also the rate of drug metabolism, resulting in an increase in drug dosage given.

An isolated study correlating anticonvulsant use, folate status, and memory dysfunction has been reported.[16] Results show significant positive correlations between memory performance and folate levels but not between memory performance and serum anticonvulsant levels.

Pregnant women are most vulnerable to alterations in folic acid metabolism since deficiency of this vitamin has been reported to cause congenital malformations and stillbirths.[17] Another nutritional risk for pregnant women on phenytoin is the possibility of hemorrhagic disease of the newborn, attributed to decreased levels of vitamin K-dependent clotting factors.

Hepatoxicity, because of hyperammonemia, is a common side effect of valproic acid (VPA) therapy. Treatment with a medium-length, straight-chain fatty acid diet is reported to abolish the VPA-induced hyperammonemia. Hypocarnitinemia, related to an alternation in fatty acid metabolism among persons receiving valproic acid, has also been reported. Coulter[18] has proposed that carnitine deficiency may be a possible mechanism for valproate hepatotoxicity. This deficiency, inversely correlated to VPA dose,[19] has been attributed to an alteration in fatty acid metabolism[20] and/or insufficient endogenous carnitine synthesis.[21] Avoidance of high-protein diets has been recommended by Laub.[22] Other abnormalities in fat metabolism resulting from anticonvulsant therapy include increases in serum triglycerides and/or cholesterol observed in persons on long-term multidrug therapy.[23] During monotherapy with carbamazepine or valproate, significant decreases in thyroid hormones were noted although no overt symptoms of hypothyroidism were observed.[24] Blood folic acid remained unchanged. Lower T_4 and higher retinol-binding capacity were found among children with delayed cognitive development who received diphenylhydantoin, phenobarbital, or anticonvulsant combinations, but vitamin A was higher among those receiving diphenylhydantoin. Vitamin A and retinol-binding protein were lower in children with infections, and vitamin A was lower among those with serum zinc less than 70 mcg/dL.[25]

Neuroleptics

Few studies have been reported linking neuroleptics (antipsychotic drugs) to abnormalities in nutrient metabolism.

Two vitamins, B_{12} and folic acid, were investigated,[26,27] and both were found to be unaffected by the drugs. That pyridoxine hydrochloride could alleviate toxicities resulting from phenothiazines was reported by Brooks et al.[28] More recently, Rebec[29] reported that ascorbic acid could play an important role in modulating the behavioral effects of haloperidol and related neuroleptics, which includes virtually all phenothiazines.

Other complications of neuroleptics that could affect nutritional status are the development of tardive dyskinesia and the accompanying dry mouth syndrome (xerostomia), caused by thickening of the saliva. The resulting reduction in saliva could lead to dental caries. Weight changes often are observed in patients during long-term neuroleptic use. Tardive dyskinesia could affect oral, jaw, tongue, and pharyngeal musculature, thereby impairing chewing and swallowing, decreasing food intake, and causing weight loss. Chlorpromazine also is known to promote weight gain attributed to an increase of appetite and water retention. A contributing factor to weight gain is glucose intolerance brought about by the inhibition of insulin release by the drug. Thus, diabetic persons may also be at greater risk.

CNS stimulants

Although methylphenidate is classified as a stimulant, it has a "sedating" effect on children with attention deficit hyperactivity disorder (ADHD). The use of drug therapy for ADHD has been a controversial issue among parents, educators, and other professionals. Children with learning problems appear to need drug therapy upon entering school, an environment in which their attention is demanded. Although there seems to be no evidence that methylphenidate interferes with the metabolism of any specific nutrient, its effects have not been investigated fully. There is, however, a significant suppression of growth in height and weight, possibly preceded by a reduction in appetite.[30,31] A rebound weight gain is often observed during the summer months when medication is discontinued. The same effects and their underlying mechanisms almost certainly apply to amphetamines used in lieu of methylphenidate.

Antidepressants

Antidepressants can also affect appetite and weight, as seen in mild to moderately depressed outpatients. After 6 weeks of clinical trials in one study, changes due to the treatment regimes were minimal, although significant associations with weight, appetite, and of carbohydrate preference at presentation and at the end of 6 weeks were observed.[32] The findings of the study suggest that, before long-term carbohydrate craving and increases in appetite and weight occur with antidepressant therapy, there is a simple reversal of the appetite and weight changes that occur with depression. The same investigators[33] in a subsequent study assessed seven antidepressant regimes. Subjects on combined imipramine and isocarboxazide and whose appetite was decreased at presentation showed marked increases in appetite and weight. The findings demonstrate that this combined therapy may be of particular use where weight increase is desirable.

The subclass of antidepressants known as monoamine oxidase (MAO) inhibitors is responsible for a unique and potentially lethal interaction with some foods and drugs. By inhibiting MAO in the central nervous system, these drugs alleviate depression symptoms by increasing the apparent activity of biogenic amines, such as norepinephrine and serotonin, which serve as important neurotransmitters. These drugs cause a similar biochemical effect in peripheral sympathetic nerves, although the overall response appears as if sympathetic neurotransmitter release is inhibited in response to normal nerve stimulation. Tyramine, a mixed-acting (catecholamine-releasing) sympathomimetic drug, triggers the release of accumulated neurotransmitters, causing such symptoms as headache, hypertension, tachycardia, and possibly death if hypertension or cardiac stimulation is too great. The severity of the reaction is related to the total dietary intake of tyramine. As little as 6 mg of tyramine can cause a measurable blood pressure increase, and 25 g can produce severe hypertension. Both prescription and nonprescription drugs containing tyramine-like catecholamine-releasing sympathomimetics (e.g., ephedrine, phenylpropanolamine, amphetamines, methylphenidate) interact similarly. Thus, tyramine-restricted diets must be prescribed for persons taking MAO inhibitors, whether for depression or hypertension. In addition, emphatic directions to adhere to the restrictions and written list of foods (see last section) and drugs to avoid should be given to such persons.

Lithium

Lithium, the major antimanic drug, is a naturally occurring element useful in the treatment of mania. Results of studies relating folic acid deficiency to lithium therapy for affective disorder are not consistent. In 1986, a report of a double-blind trial by Coppen et al.[34] demonstrated that patients whose plasma folate increased to 13 ng/mL or higher had a 40% reduction in their mania symptoms. They suggested a daily folate supplement of 300–400 mcg during long-term lithium prophylaxis. Most recently, however, Stern and co-workers[35] did not find any significant correlation between folate levels and lithium therapy in 17 outpatients.

In contrast to the uncertainty over the folate-lithium interaction, there is little or no controversy over the need for strict dietary control of sodium intake and periodic monitoring of serum sodium levels during lithium therapy. The two are chemically similar. In positive sodium balance (excessive sodium intake or reduced sodium loss) lithium blood levels are reduced; on the other hand, negative sodium balance prolongs lithium's half-life, possibly causing toxic blood levels. Excessive salting of food during preparation or at the table is liable to elevate serum sodium levels, thereby reducing blood lithium levels and the drug's antimanic effects. Drugs that elevate serum sodium levels (e.g., systemic corticosteroids and many antihypertensive drugs) may do the same. In contrast, dietary sodium restriction or administration of sodium-wasting drugs (notably, all diuretics) can raise serum lithium levels and increase the risk of potentially serious lithium toxicity. A summary of the adverse effects of psychoactive drugs is given in Table 27–1.

Vitamins Used in Pharmacological Doses (Megavitamins)

The importance of niacin in the diet was recognized during the early part of the century when it was found to cure pellagra, characterized by dementia, as well as other symptoms. The similarities of the mental symptoms of pellagra to those of schizophrenia led to the use of niacin in megadoses for the treatment of schizophrenia.

Presently, the term "megavitamin" or "orthomolecular" therapy encompasses the use of such other vitamins as thiamin, pyridoxine, B_{12}, biotin, E, ascorbic acid, and folic acid, singly or in combination, for treatment of nonspecific mental retardation, psychosis, autism, hyperactivity, dyslexia, Down's syndrome, and other learning disorders. Although occasional remarkable benefits of megavitamin therapy have been reported,[36] objective data have not documented these benefits sufficiently[37] to allow endorsement of this type of therapy by the American Psychiatric Association. For example, a vitamin B_6 supplementation study of mentally retarded children failed to show improvement in Stanford-Binet scores.[38] Another study,[39] with a 24-week multiple cross-over component, using megadoses of niacin, ascorbic acid, pyridoxine, and pantothenate, showed no beneficial effect on hyperactivity; instead, gastrointestinal complaints and hepatoxicity resulted.

The use of vitamins in pharmacological doses raises questions of safety and side effects. The toxic effects of excessive amounts of fat-soluble vitamins (A, D, E, and K) have long been established, whereas water-soluble vitamins are generally considered harmless. However, the latter generalization is not always correct, especially when amounts of up to 1000 times the normal requirements have been employed therapeutically. Megadoses of nicotinic acid, which has been used therapeutically to lower blood cholesterol, may result in skin erythema, pruritus, liver damage, and high blood sugar and uric acid levels. Another water-soluble vitamin, pyridoxine, has recently been shown to cause sensory neuropathy after daily consumption of 2–6 g.[40] Severe complications attributed to pharmacological doses of vitamins A, B, C, D, E, and K are described by Evans and Lacey[41] and Springer.[42] Birth defects associated with vitamin A occurred with maternal intake of 25,000 IU/day.[43]

Megavitamin therapy is accepted by the Committee on Nutrition of the American Academy of Pediatrics only for a group of "vitamin-responsive" or "vitamin-dependent" disorders and inborn errors of metabolism in which the requirements for a *specific* vitamin are increased. Remission and exacerbation of symptoms are demonstrated by administration and withdrawal, respectively, of the vitamin. Children with these disorders, although rare, require lifelong treatment consisting of pharmacological doses of the vitamin.[44]

Factors to be Considered in Nutrition Evaluation

Persons on drug therapy are at risk for nutrient deficiencies and require nutrition screening and/or evaluation. Evaluation methods may include dietary study, anthropometric measurements, physical examination, biochemical analysis, and observation of feeding and eating skills/behavior.[42]

Dietary study focuses on the intake of nutrients at risk of deficiency because of drug therapy. For example, if a person is on anticonvulsants, the emphasis of the dietary study would be on intake of foods rich in calcium, vitamins D and K, and folic acid. Furthermore, nonfood sources of vitamin D,

such as exposure to sunlight, and amount of activity, which increases utilization of vitamin D, should be considered.

Anthropometric measurements commonly used are height, weight and triceps skinfold for children. These measurements are useful in assessing growth and development. Monitoring of height and weight is recommended for children on methylphenidate, whereas monitoring of weight is recommended for persons on lithium or neuroleptics.

In conducting a physical examination, a person is screened for signs and symptoms of nutrient deficiencies, such as megaloblastic anemia accompanying folic acid deficiency or skeletal abnormalities observed in rickets.

Laboratory analysis of blood or urine for nutrient or enzyme levels could detect subclinical nutrient deficiencies. Low serum levels of inorganic phosphorus and elevated alkaline phosphatase may be indicative of rickets or osteomalacia.

Assessment of feeding and eating skills or behavior requires an understanding of normal infant development so that one could identify abnormal patterns at mealtimes. The sequential development of feeding patterns from birth to 52 months is given in Springer.[42]

Dietary Supplementation and Management

Drug therapy is an accepted mode of intervention. However, an understanding of the physiological mechanisms that cause adverse effects is important in providing nutritional care. In most cases, dietary modification or nutrient supplementation, as well as regulation of dosage and timing of drug administration, compensates for these adverse effects.[45]

Improving the nutrient quality of the diet is preferred to supplementation. However, in persons on anticonvulsant therapy, supplementation with vitamin D and folic acid has been recommended. Reversal of an abnormal serum profile with vitamin D_2 treatment has been demonstrated,[45] whereas an unchanged value of bone mass with vitamin D_3-treated patients on phenobarbital/phenytoin therapy has been reported.[46] On the other hand, slow and gradual improvement in bone mass was reported by Hahn et al.[47] and Hunt et al.,[48] who used calcitriol (1,25-dihydroxyvitamin D_3) at daily doses of 10,000 IU and 0.25 to 0.75 mcg/dL, respectively. Long-term, low-dose (400 IU vitamin D_3 daily) supplementation is recommended for the epileptic pregnant woman on anticonvulsant therapy.[49] Prophylactic vitamin K therapy has also been recommended for pregnant women taking phenytoin or barbiturates.[3] Studies in sunny regions of the world report that adequate ultraviolet light exposure, diet, and activity prevented the development of anticonvulsant-induced osteomalacia.[50,51] Since toxic effects of megadoses of vitamin D have been reported, a combination of these approaches is recommended. Surveillance of hypocalcemia during long-term anticonvulsant therapy is also recommended because hypocalcemic tetany may result in increased drug dosage.[52]

Although giving folic acid supplements to some epileptic persons has resulted in improvement of their mental state,[53] routine supplementation is not recommended. Supplementation with 1 mg oral folic acid to seven adult male folate-deficient patients on phenytoin resulted in significant decreases in serum concentration of the anticonvulsant. The reduction in serum phenytoin levels could contribute to an associated loss of control of the seizure disorder, leading to an increased drug dosage.[54] Studies among pregnant epileptic women showed that supplementation decreased the incidence of folate deficiency and negative outcomes of pregnancy[55] (see Chapter 5). Folate supplementation has also been suggested during lithium therapy. Supplementation based on individual needs and surveillance of serum folate and drug levels are recommended.

Fasting blood glucose levels of chlorpromazine-treated persons have to be monitored; appropriate exercise and dietary modifications assist in limiting weight gain.

Dietary modification can enhance or decrease the absorption of phenytoin. Using healthy volunteers, Johansson et al.[56] found that carbohydrate foods enhance and protein-rich foods reduce phenytoin absorption; fatty foods had no measurable influence. Persons on MAO-inhibiting antidepressants are advised to avoid foods high in tyramine—(an indirect-acting catecholamine-releasing sympathomimetic).[57] The following foods are natural and potentially important sources of tyramine.

- aged and strong-flavored cheeses
- avocado, banana
- beer, ale, wines
- chicken and beef livers
- chocolate
- cultured dairy products—yogurt, buttermilk, sour cream
- chocolate
- dried fruits—figs, raisins, prunes
- pickled herring and salted dried fish
- pole or broad beans—lima, Italian broad beans, lentils, snow peas
- salami, sausage
- soy sauce, monosodium glutamate
- vanilla

Some anorexic effects of methylphenidate can be offset by modifying the dose,[58,59] and by administering the drug with meals. Weekly monitoring of weight and energy intake is recommended so that drug therapy may be adjusted as needed. For additional suggestions in managing the adverse effects of specific drugs, see Table 27–1.

References

1. Poindexter, A.R. Psychotropic drug patterns in a large ICF/MR facility: A ten year experience. *Am. J. Ment. Retard.* 1989; 93:624.
2. Gowdey, C.W., Zarfas, D.E., Phipps, S. Audit of psychoactive drug prescriptions in group homes. *Ment. Retard.* 1987; 25:331.
3. Shlafer, M., Marieb, E. *The Nurse, Pharmacology, and Drug Therapy.* Redwood City, CA: Addison-Wesley; 1989.
4. Clark, W.G., Brater, D.C., Johnson, A.R. *Goth's Medical Pharmacology.* 12th ed. St. Louis: C.V. Mosby; 1988.
5. Tjellesen, L., Gotfredsen, A., Christiansen, C. Effect of vitamin D_2 and D_3 on bone-mineral content in carbamazepine-treated epileptic patients. *Acta Neurol. Scand.* 1983; 68:424.
6. Gascon-Barre, M., Villeneuve, J.P., Lebrun, L.H. Effect of increasing doses of phenytoin on the plasma. *J. Am. Coll. Nutr.* 1984; 3:45.
7. Wolschendrof, K., Vanselow, K., Moller, W.D., Schulz, H. A quantitative determination of anticonvulsant-induced bone demineralization by an improved x-ray densitometry technique. *Neuroradiology.* 1983; 25:315.
8. Christiansen, C., Rdbro, P., Tjellesen, L. Pathophysiology behind anticonvulsant osteomalacia. *Acta Neurol. Scand.* 1983; 94(suppl):21.
9. Hoikka, V., Alhava, E.M., Karjalainen, P., Keranen, T., Savolainen, K.E., Riekkinen, P., Korhonen, R. Carbamazepine and bone mineral metabolism. *Acta Neurol. Scand.* 1984; 70:77.
10. Weinstein, R.S., Bryce, G.F., Sappinton, L.J., King, D.W., Gallagher, B.B. Decreased serum ionized calcium and normal vitamin D metabolite levels with anticonvulsant drug treatment. *J. Clin. Endocrinol. Metab.* 1984; 58:1003.
11. Gurian, S., Ryan, P., Daniels, E. Gingival hyperplasia due to dilantin therapy. *J. Acad. Dent. Handicapped.* 1975; 1:11.
12. Drew, H.J., Vogel, R.I., Molofsky, W., Baker, H, Frank, O. Effect of folate on phenytoin hyperplasia. *J. Clin. Periodontol.* 1987; 14:350.
13. Hendel, J., Dam, M., Gram, L., Winkel, P., Jorgensen, I. The effects of carbamazepine and valproate on folate metabolism in man. *Acta Neurol. Scand.* 1984; 69:226.
14. Berg, M.J., Fincham, R.W., Ebert, B.E., Schottellius, D.D. Decrease of serum folates in healthy male volunteers taking phenytoin. *Epilepsia.* 1988; 29:67.
15. Basu, T.K., ed. *Drug-Nutrient Interactions.* New York: Croom Helm; 1988.
16. Butlin, A.T., Danta, G., Cook, M.L. Anticonvulsants, folic acid and memory dysfunction in epileptics. *Clin. Exp. Neurol.* 1984; 20:57.
17. Biale, Y., Lewenthal, H. Effect of folic acid supplementation on congenital malformations due to anticonvulsant drugs. *Eur. J. Obstet. Gynecol. Reprod. Biol.* 1984; 18:211.
18. Coulter, D.L. Carnitine deficiency: a possible mechanism for valproate hepatotoxicity. *Lancet.* 1984; 1:689. Letter.
19. Morita, J., Yuge, K., Yoshino, M. Hypocarnitinemia in the handicapped individuals who receive polypharmacy of antiepileptic drugs. *Neuropediatrics.* 1986; 17:203.
20. Laub, M.C., Paetzke-Brunner, I., Jaeger, G. Serum carnitine during valproic acid therapy. *Epilepsia.* 1986; 27:559.
21. Melegh, B., Kerner, J., Kispal, G., Acsadi, G., Dani, M. Effect of chronic vaproic acid treatment on plasma and urine carnitine levels in children: decreased urinary excretion. *Acta. Paediatr. Hung.* 1987; 28:137.
22. Laub, M.C. Nutritional influence on serum ammonia in young patients receiving sodium valproate. *Epilepsia.* 1986; 27:55.
23. Dastur, D.K., Dave, U.P. Effect of prolonged anticonvulsant medication in epileptic patients: serum lipids, vitamins B_6, B_{12}, and folic acid, proteins and fine structure of liver. *Epilepsia.* 1987; 28:147.
24. Bentson, K.D., Gram, L., Veje, A. Serum thyroid hormones and blood folic acid during monotherapy with carbamazepine or valproate. *Acta Neurol. Scand.* 1983; 67:235.
25. Kozlowski, B.W., Taylor, M.L., Baer, M.T., Blyler, E.M., Trahms, C. Anticonvulsant medication use and circulating levels of total thyroxine, retinol binding protein, and vitamin A in children with delayed cognitive development. *Am. J. Clin. Nutr.* 1987; 46:360.
26. Henderson, I.G., Dawson, A.A. Serum vitamin B_{12} levels in psychiatric patients on long-term psychotropic drug therapy. *Br. J. Psychiatr.* 1970; 116:439.
27. Gunderson, H.J. Serum folate in psychiatric patients under long-term treatment with tricyclic neuroleptic drugs. *Acta Psychiatr. Scand.* 1969; 45:133.
28. Brooks, S.C., D'Angelo, L., Chalmeta, A., Ahern, G., Judson, J.H. An unusual schizophrenic illness responsive to pyridoxine HCl (B_6) subsequent to phenothiazine and butyrophenone toxicities. *Biol. Psychiatr.* 1983; 18:1321.
29. Rebec, G.V., Centore, J.M., White, L.K., Alloway, K.D. Ascorbic acid and the behavioral response to haloperidol: implications for the action of anitpsychotic drugs. *Science.* 1985; 227:438.
30. Hoshino, Y., Kumashiro, H., Kaneko, M., Takahashi, Y. Effects of methylphenidate on early infantile autism and its relation to serum serotonin levels. *Folia. Psychiatr. Neurol. Jpn.* 1977; 31:605.
31. Safer, D., Allen, R., Barr, E. Depression of growth in hyperactive children on stimulant drugs. *N. Engl. J. Med.* 1972; 287:217.
32. Harris, B., Young, J., Hughes, B. Changes occurring in appetite and weight during short-term antidepressant treatment. *Br. J. Psychiatr.* 1984; 145:645.

33. Harris, B., Young, J., Hughes, B. Comparative effects of seven antidepressant regimes on appetite, weight and carbohydrate preference. *Br. J. Psychiatr.* 1986; 148:590.

34. Coppen, A., Chaudhry, S., Swade, C. Folic acid enhances lithium prophylaxis. *J. Affect. Disord.* 1986; 10:9.

35. Stern, S.L., Brandt, J.T., Hurley, R.S., Stagno, S.J., Stern, M.G., Smeltzer, D.J. Serum and red cell folate concentrations in outpatients receiving lithium carbonate. *Int. Clin. Psychopharmacol.* 1988; 3:49.

36. Griendman, D. Megascorbic therapy. *Aust. Nurs. J.* 1978; 8:5.

37. Kleijnen, J., Knipschild, E. Niacin and vitamin B_6 in mental functioning: a review of controlled trials in humans. *Biol. Psychiatry.* 1991; 29:931.

38. Coburn, S.P., Schaltenbrand, W.E., Mahuren, J.D., Clausman, R.J., Townsend, D. Effect of megavitamin treatment on mental performance and plasma vitamin B_6 concentration in mentally retarded young adults. *Am. J. Clin. Nutr.* 1983; 38:352.

39. Megavitamin and the hyperactive child. *Nutr. Rev.* 1985; 43:105.

40. Schaumburg, H., Kaplan, J., Windebank, A., Vick, N., Rasmus, S., Pleasure, D., Brown, J.J. Sensory neuropathy from pyridoxine abuse: a new megavitamin syndrome. *N. Engl. J. Med.* 1983; 309:445.

41. Evans, C.D.H., Lacey, J.H. Toxicity of vitamins: complications of a health movement. *Br. Med. J.* 1986; 292:509.

42. Springer, N.S. *Nutrition Casebook on Developmental Disabilities.* Syracuse, NY: Syracuse University Press; 1982.

43. Hatcock, J., Hattan, D., Jenkins, M., McDonald, J., Sundaresan, P., Wilkening, V. Evaluation of vitamin A toxicity. *Am. J. Clin. Nutr.* 1990; 52:183.

44. Rosenberg, L.E. Contrast between vitamin-responsive inherited metabolic disease and vitamin use in schizophrenia. In: Serban, J., ed. *Nutrition and Mental Function.* New York: Plenum; 1975.

45. Tjellesen, L., Christiansen, C., Rdbro, P., Hummer, L. Different metabolism of vitamin D_2 and vitamin D_3 in epileptic patients on carbamazepine. *Acta Neurol. Scand.* 1985; 71:385.

46. Tjellesen, L., Gotfredsen, A., Christiansen, C. Different actions of vitamin D_2 and D_3 on bone metabolism in patients treated with phenobarbitone/phenytoin. *Calcif. Tissue. Int.* 1985; 37:218.

47. Hahn, T.J., Shires, R., Halstead, L.R. Serum dihydroxyvitamin D metabolite concentrations in patients on chronic anticonvulsant drug therapy: response to pharmacologic doses of vitamin D_2. *Metab. Bone Dis. Relat. Res.* 1983; 5:1.

48. Hunt, P.A., Wu-Chen, M.L., Handal, N.J., Chang, C.T., Gomez, M., Howell, T.R., Hartenberg, M.A., Chan, J.C. Bone disease induced by anticonvulsant therapy and treatment with calcitriol (1,25-dihydroxyvitamin D_3) *Am. J. Dis. Child.* 1986; 140:715.

49. Marketstad, T., Ulstein, M., Strandjord, R.E., Aksnes, L., Aarskog, D. Anticonvulsant drug therapy in human pregnancy: effects on serum concentrations of vitamin D metabolites in maternal and cord blood. *Am. J. Obstet. Gynecol.* 1984; 150:254.

50. Williams, C., Netzloff, M., Folkerts, L., Vargas, A., Garnica, A., Frias, J. Vitamin D metabolism and anticonvulsant therapy: effect of sunshine on incidence of osteomalacia. *South. Med. J.* 1984; 77:834.

51. Bogliun, G., Beghi, E., Crespi, V., Delodovici, L., d'Amico, P. Anticonvulsant drugs and bone metabolism. *Acta Neurol. Scand.* 1986; 74:284.

52. Viukari, N.M.A., Tamamisto, P., Kauko, K. Low serum calcium levels in forty mentally subnormal epileptics. *J. Ment. Defic. Res.* 1972; 16:192.

53. Neubauer, C. Mental deterioration in epilepsy due to folate deficiency. *Br. Med. J.* 1970; 2:473.

54. Berg, M.J., Rivey, M.P., Vern, B.A., Fisher, L.J., Schottelius, D.D. Phenytoin and folic acid: individualized drug-drug interaction. *Ther. Drug. Monit* 1983; 5:395.

55. Dansky, L.V., Andermann, E., Rosenblatt, D., Sherwin, A.L., Andermann, F. Anticonvulsants, folate levels and pregnancy outcome: a prospective study. *Ann. Neurol.* 1987; 21:176.

56. Johansson, O., Wahlin, B.E., Lindberg, T., Melander, A. Opposite effects of carbohydrate and protein on phenytoin absorption in man. *Drug Nutr. Interact.* 1983; 2:139.

57. Christakis, G., Miridjanian, A. Diets, drugs, and their interrelationships. *J. Am. Diet. Assoc.* 1968; 52:21.

58. Eisenberg, L. Symposium: behavior modification by drugs. III. The clinical use of stimulant drugs in children. *Pediatrics.* 1972; 49:709.

59. Tec, L. An additional observation on methylphenidate in hyperactive children. *Am. J. Psychiatr.* 1971; 127:1424.

60. Moore, M.C. *Pocket Guide to Nutrition and Diet Therapy.* St. Louis: C. V. Mosby; 1988.

61. Roe, D.A. *Nutrient and Drug Interactions.* New York: Van Nostrand Reinhold/AVI; 1988.

62. Mohs, M.E., Watson, R.R., Leonard-Green, T. Nutritional effects of marijuana, heroin, cocaine, and nicotine. *J. Am. Diet. Assoc.* 1990; 90:1261.

63. Bray, J. Drug treatment of obesity. *Am. J. Clin. Nutr.* 1992; 55:538S.

64. Wise, S. Clinical studies with fluoxetine in obesity. 1992; 55:181S.

65. Wellman, P. Overview of adrenergic anorectic agents. *Am. J. Clin. Nutr.* 1992; 55:193S.

Chapter 28
Allergy and Immunological Disorders in Children

Thomas Fischer

The Immune System and Nutrition

The relationship between nutrition and the immune system is interlocking as manifested by diseases or conditions in which food or lack thereof produces altered immune function; for example, food allergies or secondary immunodeficiency in malnutrition syndromes. (Fig. 28-1).

The function of the immune system is to distinguish self from nonself and to eliminate the latter. Such a system is necessary for survival in all living creatures. A functioning immune system is required to prevent attack by internal forces (e.g., tumor cells, autoimmune phenomena) and from external forces (micro-organisms or toxic substances). Deficiency or dysfunction in the immune system leads to a variety of clinical diseases of varying severity, ranging from such disorders as food allergy and allergic rhinitis to immunodeficiency or malignancy. The immune system is made up of specific and nonspecific components that have distinct but overlapping and often interdependent functions (Fig. 28-2). The antibody (humoral) and cell-mediated immune systems provide specificity and a memory of previously encountered antigens; that is, substances (e.g., protein or polysaccharide) that can stimulate an immune response. Phagocytic cells capable of engulfing and eliminating foreign material serve as nonspecific cellular factors, and complement proteins are nonspecific humoral factors.

Cell-mediated immunity is mediated by two types of cells, T lymphocytes and monocytes-marcrophages. These cells carry out their immune functions either by direct cell-to-cell contact or by production of soluble factors, such as interleukins or interferon. These cells provide a primary defense against viruses, fungi, intracellular organisms, tumor antigens, and allograft rejection. Severe dysfunction of this system by such infectious agents as human immunodeficiency virus can produce disastrous consequences, such as AIDS (acquired immune deficiency syndrome).

Humoral-mediated immunity is mediated by immunoglobulins in the serum. These immunoglobulins, a major defense against bacterial infections, are derived from B lymphocytes. These immunoglobulin proteins are divided into five major classes: IgG, IgA, IgM, IgD, and IgE. Each of these immunoglobulin classes has characteristic features (Table 28-1).

Although the function of the immune system is to protect the host from foreign antigens, abnormal immune responses can result in tissue injury and disease. Gell et al.[1] have classified the mechanisms of immune tissue injury into four distinct types of reactions; this classification enables an improved understanding of the immunopathogenesis of disease.

Type 1: Anaphylactic or immediate hypersensitivity. Antigen binding to preformed IgE antibodies attached to the

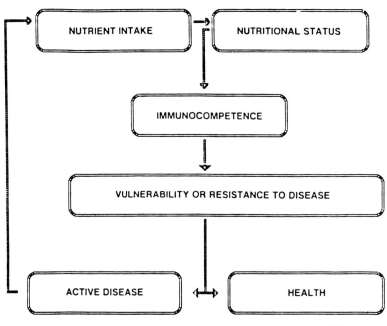

Fig. 28-1. The relationships among nutrition, immunocompetence, and health. From Sherman, A.R. Alterations in immunity related to nutritional status. *Nutr. Today.* 1986; 21:10. Used with permission.

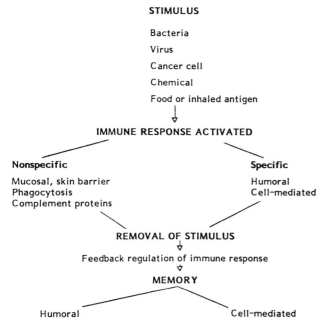

STIMULUS

Bacteria

Virus

Cancer cell

Chemical

Food or inhaled antigen

IMMUNE RESPONSE ACTIVATED

Nonspecific   **Specific**

Mucosal, skin barrier   Humoral
Phagocytosis   Cell-mediated
Complement proteins

REMOVAL OF STIMULUS

Feedback regulation of immune response

MEMORY

Humoral   Cell-mediated

Fig. 28–2. Overview of the nonspecific and specific components of the immune response. From Sherman, A.R. Alterations in immunity related to nutritional status. *Nutr. Today.* 1986; 21:10. Used with permission.

surface of the mast cell or the basophil causes release of mediators—histamine, leukotrienes, and the eosinophilic chemotactic factor of anaphylaxis (ECF-A)—which produce the clinical manifestations. Examples of type I diseases include anaphylactic shock, allergic rhinitis, allergic asthma, and acute penicillin allergy.

Type II: Cytotoxic reactions. Cytotoxic reactions involve the binding of either IgG of IgM antibody to cell-bound antigen. Antigen-antibody binding results in activation of the complement cascade and the destruction of the cell (cytolysis) to which the antigen is bound. Examples of tissue injury by this mechanism include immune hemolytic anemia and Rh hemolytic disease in the newborn.

Type III: Immune complex-mediated reactions. Immune complexes are formed when antigens bind to antibodies. They are usually cleared from the circulation by the phagocytic system. However, deposition of these complexes in tissues or in vascular endothelium can produce immune complex-mediated tissue injury. Two important factors

leading to injury by this mechanism include an increased quantity of circulating complexes and the presence of vasoactive amines, which increase vascular permeability and favor the tissue deposition of immune complexes. Immune complex deposition results in complement activation, anaphylatoxin (C3a, C5a) generation, chemotaxis of polymorphonuclear leukocytes, phagocytosis, and tissue injury. Clinical examples are serum sickness, certain types of nephritis, and certain features of bacterial endocarditis.

Type IV: Delayed hypersensitivity. Delayed hypersensitivity is mediated primarily by T lymphocytes. the classic examples are the tuberculin skin test reactions and contact dermatitis

Although IgE immunoglobulin is normally present in a very small concentration, it is the major antibody that produces anaphylactic type I or immediate hypersensitivity diseases. In allergic diseases, elevated levels of IgE, especially to specific antigens, are observed. Although Prausnitz and Kustner in 1921 first demonstrated the presence of this factor in serum (using fish allergy as the model), it was not until 1966 that Ishizaka and co-workers[2] demonstrated the identity of this serum factor (reagenic antibody) and termed it IgE. Subsequently, the role of IgE in immediate hypersensitivity disorders, such as food allergy, has been studied extensively.[3]

The final expression of immediate hypersensitivity (allergy) results from the culmination of the following sequence of reactions: (1) exposure to antigen (allergen); (2) development of an IgE antibody response to the antigen; (3) binding of the IgE to mast cells; (4) re-exposure to the antigen; (5) antigen interaction with antigen-specific IgE bound to the surface membrane of mast cells; (6) release of potent chemical mediators from sensitized mast cells in areas, such as the bronchi or the gastrointestinal tract; and (7) action of these mediators (e.g., histamine, leukotrienes, platelet-activating factor) on various organs and the production of symptoms[4] (Fig. 28-3)

The mast cell plays a critical role in this allergic response. Any mast cell can have bound to its surface IgE antibodies with multiple antigenic specificities that can react to a large variety of antigens. Mast cell stimulation is initiated by the cross-linking of two or more mast-cell -bound IgE molecules by an antigen. This stimulation transmits a signal to the cell interior that culminates in the release of preformed mediators (e.g., histamine, eosinophilic chemotactic factors of anaphylaxis) or synthesis of mediators, e.g., leukotrienes,

Table 28–1. Characteristic Features of the Five Classes of Immunoglobulins

Immunoglobulin	Adult serum concentration (mg/dL)	Serum half/life (days)	Placenta transfer	Biological function
IgG	1200	23	+	Neutralization, opsonization, bacteriolysis, agglutination, hemolysis
IgM	150	5	–	Neutralization, hemolysis, agglutination, bacteriolysis, opsonization, first detectable antibody, receptor on B lymphocyte
IgA	300	6	–	Neutralization, present in body secretions
IgD	3	3	–	Recepter on B lymphocyte
IgE	0.03	2	–	Mast-cell binding and increased vascular permeability on antigen exposure

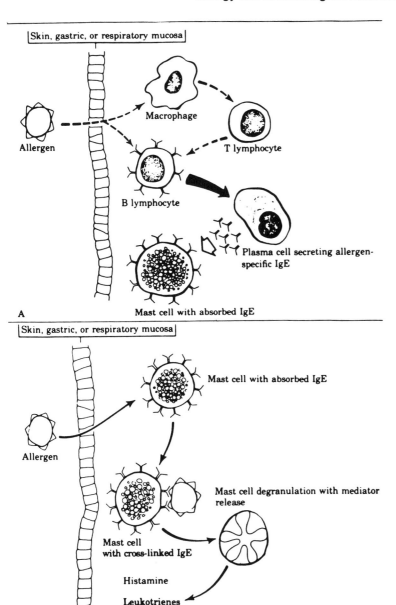

Fig. 28–3. *A*, Allergen sensitization. Allergen is absorbed. A macrophage takes up the allergen, processes it, and presents it to the T lymphocyte. A B lymphocyte exposed to the allergen is influenced by the T lymphocyte to mature into an allergen-specific IgE immunoglobulin-secreting plasma cell. Allergen-specific IgE antibodies are absorbed onto the surface of a mast cell (sensitization). *B*, Allergen stimulation of mediator release. Allergen is absorbed and cross-links with specific IgE antibody on the sensitized mast cell. The mast cell degranulates and mediators are released. From Lawlor, G.J., Fischer, T.J., eds. *Manual of Allergy and Immunology*, 2nd ed. Boston: Little Brown and Company; 1988. Used with permission.

prostaglandins, or platelet-activating factor. When released into tissues, these mediators can produce vasodilation, increased vasopermeability, smooth muscle contraction, increased mucus secretion, stimulation of pain receptors, and attraction of other inflammatory cells, such as neutrophils and eosinophils, which can augment the inflammatory process. Depending upon the organ system(s) involved, a variety of symptoms can be produced: hives or angioedema (swelling) in the skin, wheezing and cough in the lungs, sneezing and nasal congestion in the nasal passages, and vomiting, diarrhea, and abdominal pain in the gastrointestinal tract. Scientists have developed pharmacological agents to counteract or modulate these effects. These drugs include antihistamines, corticosteroids, adrenergic agents (adrenalin), methylxanthines (theophylline),and mast-cell stabilizing agents (cromolyn sodium).

In addition to drug therapy, additional strategies must also be considered to control allergic symptoms. Avoidance of food or inhaled materials (enviromental controls) known to stimulate symptoms should be a primary goal in the management of allergic disorders. Likewise, immunological modification by allergy immunotherapy (allergy shots or hyposensitization) attempts to reduce the sensitivity to an inhaled antigen(s) in such diseases as allergic rhinitis and asthma. For the complete control of symptoms, a combined approach is often required.

Food Allergy
Incidence

Food allergy is perceived by the public as a major health problem.[5] The actual prevalence of food allergy is difficult to determine, but true IgE-mediated allergy has previously been estimated to occur in between 0.3% to 7.5% of children.[6] With increasing age, it is believed that the incidence of food allergy decreases, although it is clearly evident that IgE-mediated allergies can develop in adults who previously tolerated foods without difficulty. To determine a more accurate incidence of food allergy, it is mandatory to distinguish IgE-mediated reactions from nonimmune adverse reactions, such as pharmacological or metabolic reactions, food toxicity, or food idiosyncrasy. These reactions are better termed *food intolerance* (see Table 28-2 for a categorization of nonimmunologically mediated adverse food reactions and commonly associated foods).[7]

The clinical manifestations of food allergy include (1) classic allergic symptoms, such as severe systemic anaphylaxis, asthma, allergic rhinitis, atopic dermatitis, urticaria, and angioedema, or (2) gastrointestinal symptoms, such as nausea and vomiting, diarrhea, and abdominal pain. The role of food allergy in such conditions as enuresis, migraine headaches, or attention deficit hyperactivity disorder is less clear. Of considerable concern is the role of allergy in the production of severe systemic anaphylaxis (shock-like syndromes) in response to eating certain foods. The first anaphylactic episode may be unexpected or may be only forewarned by minor symptoms, such as mild abdominal discomfort or hives on a previous exposure to the food.

Table 28-2. Food Intolerance: Nonimmunologically Mediated Adverse Food Reactions and Commonly Associated Foods

Pharmacological Adverse Food Reactions
Caffeine
Coffee, tea, cola, soft drink, cocoa
Theobromine
Chocolate, tea
Histamine*
Toxicity or poisoning (contaminated tuna or mackerel)
Histamine-releasing foods (strawberry, shellfish, egg white, Swiss cheese)
Tyramine
Cheese
Serotonin, tyramine, dopamine, phenylethylamine (in chocolate), norepinephrine
Food colors
Particularly tartrazine (yellow dye no. 5) in commercial foods

Metabolic Food Reactions
Disaccharidase deficiency
Bowel wall lactase—"lactose intolerance": sucrase, isomaltase (cow's milk, milk, milk products, fruits)
Gluten sensitivity
Celiac syndrome (wheat, rye)
Sugar and protein diet content
Normal diet
Phenylketonuria
Glucose-6-phosphate dehydrogenase deficiency
Ceruloplasmin deficiency
Wilson's disease
Hypoglycemia
Particularly, diabetes mellitus

Food Idiosyncratic Reactions
Reactions to food colors (dyes)*
Tartrazine (yellow dye no. 5)
In commercial foods
Reactions to food preservatives*
Sulfites and SO_2 (particularly in restaurant foods, such as fresh salads, fruits and seafood; commercial foods, such as dried fruits, potato chips, vinegar, cider, baked products, shrimp, beer, wine, and some fruit drinks)
Sodium benzoate, butylated hydroxyanisole (BHA), and butylated hydroxytoluene (BHT) (in commercial foods)
Reactions to flavor enhancers*
Monosodium-L-glutamate (MSG)—Chinese restaurant syndrome or shock; restaurant and home-cooked foods
Reactions to exercise
Following a meal or ingestion of a specific food, particularly shrimp and celery†

*Anaphylactoid reactions (mediator release, anaphylaxis-like reactions).
†May be anaphylactoid or anaphlactic.
From Anderson,[7] with permission.

Treatment of food-induced anaphylaxis must be immediate, and a plan must be developed to educate the patient and parents about sources of the implicated food to be avoided in the future.

Biochemical Abnormalities

Food represents the largest antigenic challenge confronting the human immune system. Virtually any food can cause allergic symptoms. In addition, several dyes, flavorings, and preservatives can elicit allergic-like reactions. Commonly implicated foods include cow's milk, eggs, wheat, tree nuts, peanuts, whitefish, and crustacea. As a general rule, cooked foods are less allergenic than raw foods. Also, families of foods can share common properties. Cross-reactivity is more common among some food families than others, e.g., crustaceans. Classifications of foods from both plant and animal sources according to shared allergenic properties are described in Sheldon's *Manual on Clinical Allergy*, (Appendix 6).

Several factors determine the molecular size of dietary breakdown products, including the sequential actions of stomach acids and pepsins, pancreatic secretions, and intestinal peptidases. The mucosal endothelial cells also actively absorb amino acids, small peptides, and intact proteins, and cellular lysozymes further degrade these proteins and peptides. These antigenic materials transverse through Peyer's patches or the mucosal endothelial cells, eliciting an immune response predominantly of the IgA class. These immunoglobulins form complexes with their respective food antigens, limiting further absorption of these materials. Allergic individuals, however, respond to these food proteins by producing antigen-specific IgE, which can predispose them to develop immediate allergic reactions. Additional factors that increase sensitization include such conditions as achlorhydria, mucosal injury following gastroenteritis, selective IgA deficiency, and immaturity with relative IgA deficiency.[8]

When ingested food antigens subsequently encounter IgE-coated mast cells, degranulation of mast cells occurs with release of preformed mediators and/or generation of secondary mediators. These mediators in turn produce a local change in vasopermeability, stimulation of mucus production, increased muscle contractions, stimulation of pain fibers, and recruitment of inflammatory cells.[9] In addition, this local intestinal reaction facilitates the passage of macromolecules through the GI tract barrier, allowing them to be distributed to other target organs and initiating degranulation of mast cells at these sites and subsequent symptom production.

Although IgE-mediated reactions explain many reactions to foods, additional evidence has shown that antigen-antibody complex mediated mechanisms can also be involved.[8] For example, IgG and IgM antibodies to food antigens have been seen in serum and gastrointestinal tract secretions. Likewise, complement protein deposition has been demonstrated, a process that when activated can result in mast cell degranulation through generation of C3a and C5a anaphylatoxins. Finally, cell-mediated delayed hypersensitivity reactions to ingested material occur, as noted in studies with ingested poison ivy antigen or the inedible portion of the Ginko tree fruit.

Factors to be Considered in Nutrition Evaluation and Diagnosis

A rational approach to the diagnosis of food allergy and food intolerance demands careful consideration in the patient of other etiologies for observed symptoms. For example, in infants and children, vomiting and diarrhea are common complaints that are often attributed to food allergy. Vomiting is a symptom, not a diagnosis, and has many causes outside the gastrointestinal tract. It is important to determine whether the vomiting is associated with other gastrointestinal symptoms, such as distention or diarrhea.[10] A differential diagnosis of vomiting is outlined in Table 28-3. Likewise, diarrhea is a common complaint that is often ascribed to food hypersensitivity and is often inappropriately treated by multiple dietary manipulations without regard to the cause of the diarrhea or the specific dietary component causing symptoms. Unfortunately, these manipulations can produce a diet that is insufficient to meet caloric requirements. Such a diet can perpetuate the diarrhea, causing decreased pancreatic enzyme synthesis and intestinal mucosal function. Weight loss and increasing diarrhea result in increasing malnutrition, thus setting up a vicious cycle. For young children, especially infants under 4 months of age, hypocaloric diets for periods longer than 48 hours should be avoided. If the diarrhea becomes chronic and persistent or if it is impossible to achieve adequate caloric intake, a more detailed evaluation should follow, keeping in mind the numerous possibilities shown in Table 28-3.

A rational diagnostic approach is needed for the patient with suspected food hypersensitivity. This approach includes an accurate history, a detailed physical examination, and application of approved laboratory methods. In particular, the nature and severity of the symptoms (respiratory or cutaneous symptoms versus gastrointestinal symptoms), the age of onset, suspected precipitating foods, and the temporal relationship between the ingestion of the suspected food and the symptom must be detailed. The frequency and duration of the attacks and any changes in their nature or frequency should be noted. Any previous evaluations must be reviewed to allow for a more efficient diagnosis with less discomfort and cost. Likewise, past and present treatments should be detailed carefully. Because allergic diseases have a strong propensity for familial incidence, a careful history to detect allergic disorders in other family members is necessary.

With gastrointestinal symptoms the possibility of intercurrent gastrointestinal infection should be considered, and possible exposure sources should be explored carefully, e.g., water sources, travel in underdeveloped areas. The role of food additives, such as tartrazine or sulfites, or antigenically cross-reacting foods in the patient's diet must be explored carefully. Foods can be contaminated by minute quantities of substances that can produce an allergic reaction in susceptible patients. For example, cow's milk has been and occasionally still is contaminated with antibiotics, such as penicillin.

Table 28–3. Causes ot Vomiting and Diarrhea

Vomiting

Gastrointestinal
  Gastroesophageal reflux (chalasia)
  Obstruction
    Pyloric stenosis, antral web
    Malrotation, superior mesenteric artery syndrome
  Peptic ulcer disease
  Hepatitis
  Pancreatitis
  Infections: acute gastroenteritis (usually occurs with diarrhea)
  Motility disturbances
    Idiopathic pseudo-obstruction
    Ileus from trauma, Addison's disease
    Hypokalemia, hypothyroidism
    Acute gastric dilation (trauma, body cast)
Psychogenic
  Psychogenic vomiting
  Anorexia nervosa, rumination
Extraintestinal
  Metabolic
    Reye's syndrome
    Metabolic acidosis, uremia, lead poisoning
    Disorders of fat oxidation
  Toxic
    Ingestion, drug toxicity (e.g., theophylline)
  Infectious
    Meningitis, encephalopathy
  Increased intracranial pressure
    Trauma, tumor, hydrocephalus

Diarrhea

Infections
  Viral (rotavirus), *Salmonella, Shigella, Amoeba, Yersinia, Campylobacter, Giardia, Cryptosporidia*
Chronic inflammation
  Crohn's disease, ulcerative colitis, tuberculosis, histoplasmosis
Abnormality of anatomy or motility
  Surgical short gut, malrotation, intestinal obstruction, Hirschsprung's disease, chronic constipation
    (overflow diarrhea), idiopathic intestinal pseudo-obstruction
Inadequate pancreatic function
  Cystic fibrosis, Schwachman-Diamond syndrome, malnutrition, lipase deficiency
Alteration of the enterohepatic bile salt circulation
  Metabolic immaturity of the liver (prematurity), cholestatic liver disease, ileal resection, Crohn's
    disease, bacterial overgrowth of the small bowel ("blind loop")
Abnormality of the intestinal mucosa
  Celiac disease, immune deficiencies, postgastroenteritis changes, drug toxicity, cow's milk or soy
    protein intolerance
  Primary and secondary disaccharidase deficiencies, monosaccharide intolerance
Miscellaneous
  Irritable bowel syndrome, chronic nonspecific diarrhea
  Endocrine
    Hypoparathyroidism, hyperthyroidism, neuroblastoma

From Lawlor, G.J., Fischer T.J., eds. *Manual of Allergy and Immunology.* 2nd ed. Boston: Little Brown and Company; 1988. Used with permission.

If gastrointestinal symptoms are present, careful recording of the patient's nutritional history is needed. Serial measurements of weight and height should be obtained and compared with standard growth curves. If the patient fails to follow normal growth curves despite an adequate diet, malabsorption must be considered. (With adequate diet and normal growth, malabsorption is unlikely.) In adolescence, calculation of growth velocity and assessment of the stages of sexual development are useful methods to establish normal adolescent growth and development (see Appendix 9).

Next, a complete physical examination is performed with specific attention directed to areas where allergic diseases are often manifested, such as the skin, conjunctiva, nose, and lungs. The entire skin should be examined to document important physical changes, such as atopic dermatitis (eczema). Reddened and swollen conjunctivae suggest allergy. The nose should be examined for an *allergic crease*—a transverse line across the nose occurring as a result of chronic upward nose rubbing (the allergic salute). The interior of the nose should be checked for nasal secretions, polyps, or foreign bodies. Because the mucosa of the oral pharynx is continuous with the nasal mucosa, allergic individuals can demonstrate findings in this area. A narrow, high-arched palate and elongated maxilla with overbite can result from chronic mouth breathing in allergic children. Changes of chronic lung disease or acute findings, such as acute wheezing, can be seen.

In the presence of gastrointestinal symptoms, muscle mass and the amount of subcutaneous tissue should be noted. The patient with malabsorption, especially the young child, often demonstrates protuberant abdomen, thin extremities, and wasting of the buttocks. Sparse hair growth and the appearance of lanugo on the back indicate continued caloric deprivation. Peripheral edema suggests hypoproteinemia; hepatomegaly occurs with fatty infiltration of the liver during malnutrition (see Chapter 4).

Laboratory diagnosis of food hypersensitivity

After a careful history and physical examination, laboratory tests can help document a clinical diagnosis of food allergy. These tests include methods designed to detect IgE antibodies to food, as well as tests used to exclude other causes for these symptoms. For example, a patient with diarrhea requires a stool culture to exclude common pathogens, such as *Salmonella* and *Shigella*, as well as rare pathogens, such as *Yersenia* and *Campylobacter*. A complete blood count looking for anemia and a stool analysis to detect occult blood should be obtained. In a child with poor weight gain and abnormal stools, a sweat chloride determination to exclude cystic fibrosis is warranted. In patients suspected of lactose intolerance, measurement of reducing substances in the stool or a lactose tolerance test is indicated. Finally, in complex cases, invasive procedures, such as esophagoscopy or intestinal biopsies, may be required.[10]

To help determine the presence of IgE-mediated food allergy, skin testing with commercially available food extracts is done by the prick method. If the patient has IgE antibody to a food material, a local hive reaction typical of immediate hypersensitivity is produced at the site of the skin test. Although patients can have positive skin test results in the absence of clinical food allergy (false-positive results), true IgE-mediated allergic reactions to foods are infrequent in the face of negative skin tests (false-negative results)[11,12] Epicutaneous skin tests for milk, egg, soy, fish, and nuts correlate well with clinical symptomatology. Intradermal testing is avoided because of the greater danger of systemic reactions and of nonspecific irritant reactions.

The RAST test (radioallergosorbent test) is an in vitro blood test designed to demonstrate the presence of serum IgE antibody to a specific antigen. This test or its variants (e.g., MAST, FAST, etc.) can be useful in the evaluation of patients with widespread skin disorders, such as eczema or dermographism, which preclude accurate skin testing. Also, in the evaluation of severe anaphylaxis the physician may not wish to expose the patient to the suspected food antigen with an in vivo test method for fear of inducing a severe allergic reaction. These in vitro tests are usually more expensive than skin tests, and also there is a delay of several days in obtaining results. In addition, a positive RAST result alone is no more diagnostic of food allergy than a positive skin test result.[13] Additional serum tests include hemagglutinating or precipitating antibodies, measurement of circulating IgG and IgE food immune complexes,[14] and measurement of IgG[15] for antibodies to food antigens. Although these techniques are of interest in food allergy research,[16] routine application of these assays for clinical practice is generally not warranted.[14,15]

Food challenges

Double- or single-blinded placebo-controlled oral food challenges are, at present, the only definitive procedures to diagnose food intolerance. However, if there is a clear history of major allergic symptoms (e.g., anaphylaxis; wheezing; swelling or the lips, tongue, or face; hoarseness; hypotension), this test should not be used. Because any food challenge has the possibility of side effects, the patient must be aware of these potential dangers, and the procedure should be done only under the supervision of a qualified physician in an appropriate setting.

Food challenges may also be performed in an open unblinded, an open single-blinded, or double-blinded manner. A positive challenge by itself does not prove that an immunological mechanism is responsible because adverse reactions can result from other conditions, e.g., disaccharide deficiency. In an open, unblinded food challenge, both the patient and the physician know which food is being given. In a single-blind food challenge, the patient (and parent) are unaware of which food is being given. Finally, in a double-blind food challenge both the patient (and parent) and a neutral observer, such as a physician, do not know what substance is being administered and a placebo is included. Because results are scored by the patient and the blinded medical observer, the double-blind, placebo-controlled challenge has the advantage of objectivity. Double-blind food challenges provide the most precise information for routine clinical care, although they are more time consuming and cumbersome, and are an absolute necessity for clinical research studies. The following double-blind food challenge method proposed by May[17] (or similar methods[18]) has been useful:

1. Two weeks before the challenge, eliminate suspected food from all diet using the temporary elimination diet given in Table 28–4.
2. Obtain dry foods (e.g., milk, egg, wheat flour, or peanuts). If necessary, wet foods can be freeze-dried and powdered.
3. Place the suspected food in opaque, colorless No. 1 pharmacy capsules (the capsules should be filled by someone other than the patient or observer). The initial dose, ranging from 20-2000 mg, depends on the suspected degree of hypersensitivity. Administer the capsule just before a meal consisting of the restricted diet.
4. In infants and young children unable to swallow capsules, have the suspected food hidden in the diet by someone other than the parent or observed.
5. Symptoms usually occur within 2 hours in immediate food hypersensitivity. If no reactions occur within 24 hours, increase the dose twice daily until a dose of 8000 mg of dried

Table 28–4. Elimination Diet

Foods allowed at mealtime	
Rice	Honey (2 oz/day)
Puffed Rice	Cane Sugar
Rice flakes	Salt
Rice Krispies	Oleomargarine without
Fruit or juice:	milk
Pineapple	Crisco, Spry
Apricots	A carbonated, dye-free
Cranberries	beverage
Peaches	Snacks
Pears	1 box rice cereal
Lamb	midmorning and
Chicken	midafternoon
Asparagus	Foods to avoid
Beets	Any food and drink
Carrots	suspected of causing
Lettuce	reactions or not on this
Sweet potato	list
Tapioca	Pepper and spices
White vinegar	Coffee
Olive oil	Tea
	Chewing gum

From Lawlor, G.J., Fischer, T.J., eds. *Manual of Allergy and Immunology*, 2nd ed. Boston: Little Brown and Company; 1988. Used with permission.

food is reached. This amount of dried food represents approximately 100 g (3.5 oz) of food in the wet state.

6. Assess questionable symptoms by the administration of glucose-filled capsules in the same manner, being sure to obscure the order of presentation.

7. A single unequivocal positive reaction is definitive. Failure to react to 8000 mg of a given food usually implies that this food can be included in the diet without any problem.

Elimination diet

Food diaries and elimination diets have been used for many years on an outpatient basis. This approach is based upon monitoring food intake, removing the suspected food from the diet of the individual patient, and observing if the food-induced illness resolves and then recurs upon reintroduction of the suspected food. In obvious cases of food-induced allergies, such as anaphylaxis, such diets are not necessary. In fact, in these situations the patient should be advised to carefully avoid the food suspected of causing this severe reaction. An elimination diet and subsequent reintroduction of suspected foods under controlled conditions should be applied in situations where symptoms are not life-threatening, e.g., chronic hives.

In this methodology, patients remain on their usual diet for approximately 10 to 14 days before the special diet is begun. During that time, the patient keeps a food diary listing the type and amount of foods ingested and the occurrence and character of any adverse reactions. In addition to searching for suspected foods, this food diary establishes baseline symptoms against which the success of the elimination diets can be measured. In some patients, if one or a few foods are prime suspects as the cause of symptoms, the initial elimination diet can consist of simply removing these foods. Also, the patient should be cautioned not to inadvertently eat suspected foods that are hidden in other foods; for example, eggs are commonly found in ice cream, salad dressings, or mayonnaise.

The initiation of a severely restricted elimination diet (Table 28–4) can be attempted if simple dietary removal is not successful in eliminating symptoms or if multiple food sensitivities are suspected. Severe elimination diets, especially in young children, however, can be used for only 1 to 2 weeks because these diets can lead to severe malnutrition. In complex cases, a professional dietitian must be consulted, and accurate monitoring of caloric intake, nutritional adequacy, weight, and other biochemical parameters must be performed. Products used in these elimination diets in young infants (younger than 3 months) should include milk substitutes, such as Nutramigen® or Pregestimil®; for children 3 to 6 months, the above milk substitute plus rice cereal; and for children 6 months to 2 years, these milk substitutes, with vitamin supplements, rice cereal, applesauce, pears, lamb, squash, and carrots. Older children and adults can follow the elimination diet in Table 28–4.

If food is indeed the cause of the patients symptoms, the symptoms should resolve on this restricted diet and recur if the foods are reintroduced. Foods eliminated, but not clearly implicated, should be returned to the diet every 3 to 4 days. Those returned to the diet without reinitiation of symptoms can remain in the diet. Unfortunately, this procedure is still unblinded and is subject to biased interpretation by the patient, physician, and nutritionist. Psychological factors can play a role. Single- or double-blinded placebo-controlled oral food challenges under direct medical supervision may still be necessary to diagnose food sensitivity in these situations.

Dietary Management

If food hypersensitivity has been documented, elimination of the incriminating food as well as possible cross-reacting food substances, is the primary method of treatment. At all times, a nutritionally adequate diet must be given. The practice of avoiding all foods within a botanical family when one of the members is suspected of provoking allergic symptoms appears to be undergoing study, and more specific diets based upon new research may make management of food allergy on an elimination basis more feasible.[19,20] (see Appendix 6).

In patients with marked food sensitivity, even trace residues of allergic foods can produce symptoms.[20] Foods may contain these offending traces because of inadequate cleaning of processing equipment or from direct or indirect contact between two foods, e.g., using the same utensil for several different entrees. Other hidden sources include exposure when opening packages, inhalation of vapors from cooking of offending foods (e.g., fish), kissing the lips of a person who is eating the offending food, or transfer of food allergens from mother to infant via breast milk. Microparticulated protein usage in place of fat (e.g., Simplesse or Beta IL) may produce allergic reactions in those individuals allergic to cow's milk and/or eggs.[21]

When using elimination diets, one must remember that food allergy is a dynamic process. Patients with food hypersensitivity, especially children, can lose their symptomatic reactivity. Especially in infants with milk allergy, the offending food can be cautiously reintroduced after an appropriate interval (usually after 2 years). The reintroduction should always be done cautiously in an appropriate medical setting and with adequate preparation for treatment of anaphylaxis. Patients with proven anaphylaxis, especially older children and adults, should generally not be rechallenged. It is also critical to have patients read labels on food products. Sample elimination diets for various foods can also be offered to the patient as noted in Tables 28-5 and 28-6 (see Table 49–1 in Chapter 49).

A major goal in medicine, especially in pediatrics, is prevention of the development of disease. The same approach applies with food allergy. It is known that food antigens can cross the placenta and that they are secreted in breast milk. Although there are several contradictory reports in the literature regarding the exact role of breastfeeding and prevention of food allergy, sufficient evidence exists that breastfeeding for at least 6 months may protect infants from developing food sensitivities at 1 year.[19] Avoidance of highly allergic foods (e.g., milk, egg, peanuts) by the breastfeeding mother may be of further benefit. However, dietary manipulation of the mother during the third trimester does not appear to modify allergic disease in infancy.[22] In addition, special caution must be taken not to compromise the mother's diet and health by unnecessary and possibly harmful restrictions.

Similarly, there is a sound rationale for avoiding exposure of the immature or inflamed intestinal mucosa or highly antigenic foods, e.g., after an episode of gastroenteritis or intestinal bowel syndrome.[23] If the ideal infant food, breast milk, cannot be given, one should consider artificial feeding using casein hydrolysate formulas in the following types of patients: (1) an infant with early manifestations of allergy, (2) an infant with a strong family history or a high incidence of allergic disease, and (3) an infant recovering from a severe bout of acute gastroenteritis. These casein hydrolysate formulas (e.g., Nutramigen), ingested in vitro by enzymatic hydrolysis, have been used for over 40 years in infants with defects of protein digestion or adverse reactions to intact cow protein. Treatment failures are rare although appropriately confirmed cases of reactions to Nutramigen have been published.[24] Recently introduced whey hydrolysates have been shown to produce anaphylactic reactions in cow milk sensitive infants challenged with formula.[25] These studies with both casein hydrolysate formulas and whey hydrolysates indicate that all infant formulas promoted as "hypoallergenic" must be tested in milk allergic patients prior to introduction by the manufacturer to assess their allergic potential. Likewise, practitioners must be keenly aware that "hypo-allergenic" does not mean "non-allergenic" and that exquisitely sensitive patients must be carefully monitored even with the introduction of casein hydrolysate formulas.[26]

Pharmacological management of food allergy

The only specific treatment of food allergy is avoidance. However, pharmacological therapy for food allergy can be attempted in patients with multiple food sensitivities that do not respond to elimination measures; in patients with accidental, unavoidable exposure to offending foods, especially when meals are eaten away from home; and in those in whom significant symptoms continue because the offending food is not recognized. If no medical contraindication exists for its use, the provision of epinephrine for self-admin-

istration or administration by a parent is mandatory for patients with severe, life-threatening food reactions. Individuals should also wear a bracelet or similar article identifying their sensitivities and reactions.

Antihistamines such as diphenhydramine (Benadryl®) can be helpful in adverse reactions to foods that involve histamine release, for example, urticaria, angioedema, conjunctivitis, or rhinitis. Use of these H-1 antihistamines for gastrointestinal symptoms is controversial. Although premedication with these drugs can be attempted to decrease allergic symptoms, H-1 antihistamines cannot be relied upon to prevent life-threatening, anaphylactic food reactions. Corticosteroids, because of their side effects with extended use, are used only for temporary treatment of a severe hypersensitivity response to food and for the treatment of eosinophilic gastroenteritis caused by food sensitivity. Sodium cromolyn has been used as an investigational drug for food allergy but further studies are required for the definitive criteria for the proper indication and the most effective dose.

Immunotherapy (allergy shots) and oral hyposensitization are of unproved effectiveness in the treatment of food allergy. An exception is the recommended trial of subcutaneous immunotherapy for respiratory sensitivity to inhaled food allergens (e.g., baker's asthma).

Controversial techniques

Several controversial and unproved procedures are often touted, often in the media, for the diagnosis and treatment of food allergy. Leukocytotoxic testing has been proposed for the in vitro diagnosis of food allergies. Likewise, intracutaneous and subcutaneous provocative testing, neutralization testing, and sublingual provocation testing with food extracts have been advocated for diagnosing allergies to foods. These procedures have also been advocated for the treatment of food allergies. The American Academy of Allergy and Immunology and the National Center for Health Technology have reported that these are unproved, unreliable, and without scientific basis.

Immunodeficiency

Alterations in immunologic function with increased susceptibility to infection can occur as a result of many local or systemic diseases. Secondary forms of immunodeficiency are considerably more common than primary immunodeficiencies. These patients with secondary immunodeficiency have an intact immune system but during or following the primary disease or process their host defenses become transiently or permanently impaired. The relationship among nutrition, immunocompetence, and health is very complex but the schematic representation in Figure 3 gives an overview of these processes. An appreciation of these abnormalities is important not only because of theoretic interests but of practical value in the management of the primary disorder.

These secondary immunodeficiencies are found in the newborn and patients on immunosuppressive therapy, patients with infectious disease (e.g., human immunodeficiency virus),[27] malignancies (e.g., leukemia), following surgery or trauma, and in a variety of hereditary and metabolic diseases (e.g., diabetes mellitus). See Appendix 6.

Table 28–5. Milk-, Egg-, and Wheat-Free Diets*

Milk-Poor Diet

Avoid:

Milk, buttermilk, cream as such and in prepared foods: ice cream, sodas, milk sherbet, Bavarian cream mousses, custards, gravies, cream sauces, soups, chowders

Prepared flour mixes for home cooking

Malted milk, hot chocolate, or cocoa prepared with milk

Cheese

Evaporated, powdered, condensed milk (bakery products, as pies, breads and cakes containing small amounts of cooked milk can often be tolerated)

Study the label on packaged foods for evidence of milk or milk products

Egg-Poor Diet

Avoid:

Eggs: Fresh, frozen, powdered, cooked in any form

Egg-containing foods, such as

Soups, broths made with egg

Prepared flour mixes for home cooking

Waffles, doughnuts, pretzels

Pancakes, griddle cakes, pastries, French toast

Macaroons, meringues, frostings

Cakes, cookies, unless known to be egg-free

Breads with glazed crust

Foods breaded with egg mixture

Sausages, croquettes, meat cakes containing egg as binder

Poultry, especially chicken, if fricasseed or in broth

Salad dressings, unless known to be egg free; Hollandaise, mayonnaise, and egg sauces

Ice cream and sherbets, unless known to be egg-free

Custards, cream candies, fondants, Bavarian cream

Marshmallows

Baking powder containing egg white

Prepared drinks containing egg or egg powder for insomnia or underweight

Study the labels on packaged foods for evidence of egg in any form

Avoid vaccine made in egg, as for influenza, yellow fever

Wheat-Poor Diet

Avoid:

White, whole wheat, cracked wheat flour in breads, waffles, griddle cakes, doughnuts, muffins, pastries, pies, cakes, crackers, spaghetti, macaroni, dumplings, pretzels, zwieback, noodles

Corn bread, unless known to be wheat-free

Soy bread, unless known to be wheat-free

Rye bread, unless known to be wheat-free

Gluten bread

Breakfast cereals, dry or cooked, containing wheat, whole wheat, cream soups, farina, or bran

Custards, gravies, sauces containing wheat

Breaded foods prepared with wheat

Coffee substitutes containing wheat; beer; ale

Prepared meats, as sausages, frankfurters, meat loaf, croquettes made with wheat

Prepared mixes for biscuits, muffins, pastries, pie crusts, cookies

Study the label on prepared foods for evidence of wheat or wheat products

COW'S MILK-FREE DIET†

All cow's milk and cow's milk products are eliminated from the diet. All labels on foods must be read for products containing milk or milk products

Instant nonfat dry milk powder	Margarine
Milk solids	Casein
Butter	Casein hydrolysate
Whey	Ice cream
Curd	Cheese
	Lactose

EGG-FREE DIET

All egg and egg products are eliminated from the diet. All labels on foods must be read for products containing eggs, egg powder, dried egg, or albumin. Read every label since it is impossible to list all sources of egg, and the composition of any food product may be changed without notice.

WHEAT-FREE DIET

All wheat and products made from wheat are eliminated from the diet. This includes any wheat flour (cake, whole wheat, etc.), graham flour, wheat germ, bran, farina, bread crumbs, cracker meal, or flour used as a thickening agent. All labels on foods must be read for products containing wheat or wheat products

*From Goodhart, R.S., Shils, M.E., *Modern Nutrition in Health and Disease*. 5th ed. Philadelphia: Lea & Febiger; 1973. Used with permission.
†From Lawlor, G.J., Fischer, T.J., eds. *Manual of Allergy and Immunology*. 2nd ed. Boston: Little Brown and Company; 1988. Used with permission.

Malnutrition falls into the category of metabolic disease. Protein/calorie malnutrition has been seen in two clinical extremes: marasmus (insufficiency of all food) and kwashiorkor (deficiency of protein in a diet usually high in calories). These conditions are a serious problem, especially in developing countries. (See chapter on Nutritional Assessment.) Marasmus generally occurs early in infancy; kwashiorkor is more common during the second year of life.

Overlap exists between the two syndromes and malnutrition of less severity is quite common. At autopsy, kwashiorkor patients show thymic and lymphoid atrophy.[28] Often there is an associated zinc deficiency which by itself can produce T-cell abnormalities.[29] Malnutrition can markedly increase susceptibility to infection, resulting in increased morbidity and mortality for many infectious diseases, including measles, herpes infections, tuberculosis, fungi, and parasites.

Table 28–6. Soy-Free Diet

All soybeans and soybean products are eliminated from the diet. **All labels on foods must be read** for products containing soy or ingredients that may contain soy. Soy is used freely as a filler and often is not marked on packages. Possible sources of soy in foods include vegetable protein, lecithin, flour, and vegetable oil. **Read every label** since it is impossible to list all sources of soy. The composition of any food product may be changed without notice. For nebulous ingredients, such as "vegetable protein," check with the food manufacturer for possible soy.

Types & Amounts of Food	Include	Omit
Soup—as desired	Soups prepared without soy or soy products	Soups containing soy or soy products
Meats & Meat substitutes 2–3 servings 5 oz total)	Beef, chicken, ham, kidney, lamb, liver, pork, turkey, veal, fish Eggs, cheese, cottage cheese	Cold cuts or sausage containing a soy additive Hamburger with soy protein "Vege burgers" made with textured vegetable protein Products fried in soy oil Fish canned in soy oil
Potato & Potato substitutes 1 or more servings (¼ cup each)	White & sweet potatoes, macaroni, noodles, rice, spaghetti	Spaghetti made with soy flour Products cooked with soy oil or soy margarine
Vegetables 2 or more servings (¼ cup each)	Any canned, cooked, frozen or raw vegetables (Include 1 serving dark-green or deep-yellow vegetable daily for a source of Vitamin A)	Soybeans, soybean sprouts Vegetables prepared with soy sauce
Breads 3 or more servings	Breads and rolls prepared without soybean flours	Soy bread "Cornmeal bread" Breads containing soy oil
Cereals 1 or more servings (½ cup each)	Cooked or ready-to-eat cereals without soy	Cereals containing soy flour, soy oil, vegetable protein
Fats 3 or more servings (1 tsp each)	Butter, cream, bacon, margarine, shortening or oils that do not contain soy	Soybean oil, margarine or shortening, salad dressing containing soybean oil as an ingredient
Fruits & Fruit Juices 2 or more servings 4 oz juice or ¼ cup fruit each)	All (Include 1 serving citrus fruit or juice daily for a source of Vitamin C)	None
Desserts In moderation	Gelatin, custard, cornstarch puddings Homemade ice cream, sherbet, cake, cookies, pastries, pie	Commercial ice cream Most commercial bakery products (Soybean flour is often added to bakery products to keep them moist)
Milk 3 or more servings (8 oz each)	Milk, 2% milk, skim milk, evaporated milk, non-fat dry milk powder	Soy milks, such as Isomil, Neo-Mull-Soy, ProSobee, Nursoy Commercial milk shakes
Beverages	Water as desired, tea, carbonated beverages, fruit drinks, coffee	Excessive use of sugared and caffeinated drinks
Miscellaneous	Salt (iodized), sugar, honey, jelly, syrup, chocolate, cocoa Catsup, mustard, olives, pepper, herbs, spices	Lecithin (derived from soybeans, often used in candy) Soy sauce, Worcestershire sauce, steak sauce Toasted soybeans Caramel candies Excessive use of salt or sugar

From Lawlor, G.J., Fischer, T.J., eds. *Manual of Allergy and Immunology*. 2nd ed. Boston, Little Brown and Company; 1988. Used with permission.

The spectrum of deficiencies involves various host defenses, including nonspecific immune factors, immunoglobulin levels, and specific antibody production, as well as abnormalities in cellular immunity.[30]

Both the quality and the quantity of protein ingested determine the extent of the immunological impairment in protein-calorie malnutrition. Although phagocytic activity and complement protein levels are diminished, cell-mediated immunity is more consistently impaired in protein nutritional deficiency. In malnutrition, lymphoid atrophy and impaired maturation result in decreased number of rosetting T lymphocytes in peripheral blood. About 15% of children with moderate to severe protein-energy malnutrition show lymphopenia. In addition to the reduction in the number of precursor T cells, there may be impaired differentiation that results in decreased thymic hormone activity.[31] A practical, inexpensive assessment of T-cell function is the use of delayed hypersensitivity skin tests with a variety of recall antigens injected intradermally into the skin and observed for development of a reaction at 24 and 48 hours. Commonly employed antigens include Candida, trichophyton, mumps, tetanus, and PPD. Streptokinase and streptodornase have been used in the past. A lack of response to these skin test antigens (anergy) may be due to a variety of defects, including failure of recognition of the antigen for processing, a decrease in the number and function of the responsible T lymphocytes, or a decrease in lymphokines or other soluble factors that bring about mobilization of the polymorphonucleocytes and macrophages into the test area. These tests, using an immunological response, can serve as a sensitive indicator of nutritional status (see Chapter 4). Other techniques to assess nutritional status include complement levels, the number of T cells and subsets, terminal transferase activity, and salivary secretory IgA. The advantages and disadvantages of these methodologies have been discussed elsewhere.[32-34]

Although much of the early work on nutritional regulation of immunity was done in young children in developing countries (often with malnutrition), these studies have been extended to other groups at risk for malnutrition, e.g., surgical patients. Likewise, recent work[35] indicates that nutrition may be a critical determination of immunocompetence in elderly patients at risk for illness. In Chandra's studies[35] he note the intriguing effect of severe emotional trauma on immunological function. In particular, the loss of a spouse has been shown to have an important and significant effect on the immunocompetence of the elderly. The lymphocyte stimulation index, natural killer cell activity, and delayed hypersensitivity were diminished from the pretreatment values in a group of 20 elderly subjects who were undergoing longitudinal studies of nutrition and immunity in old age and who subsequently lost a spouse.

In addition to cell-mediated immunity, other immune mechanisms can be important in controlling intestinal infections that can be disastrous for malnourished individuals. These mechanisms include antigen processing by macrophages and lamina propria lymphocytes, formation of IgA antibodies, and interaction between lymphocytes and cells of the immune system and the epithelium. In children with protein-calorie malnutrition, low levels of secretory IgA have been found in tears, nasopharyngeal secretions, and saliva. The mechanism for this decrease in secretory IgA activity

has not been determined, although it likely results from the impaired formation of the secretory dimer of this protein.[36] Nonspecific humoral factors, such as complement proteins, can also be affected by protein-calorie malnutrition. The increased incidence of serious Gram-negative infections including sepsis, the decreased inflammatory responses, or the decreased opsonic activity in sera of patients with protein-calorie malnutrition parallel the symptoms of patients with congenital or nutritionally associated deficiency of complement. Studies in experimental animals have shown that manipulation of protein, lipid, and vitamin E content in the diet of Balb/C mice for up to 24 weeks can cause variable changes in complement levels.[37]

Deficiencies of vitamins and trace minerals can influence immunocompetence. Deficiencies of vitamins A and B_6, folate, thiamine, and riboflavin occur frequently in children with protein-calorie malnutrition.[38] All these vitamins are required for normal immunological responses in laboratory animals. Isolated vitamin deficiencies may also induce clinically significant depression of immunological function. For example, isolated deficiencies of vitamin A or folate depress responses to tests of cell-mediated immunity in humans. Deficiency of vitamin A also may lead to decreases in the epithelial barrier functions, which can result in an increased susceptibility to infection. Individuals at increased risk for a single nutrient deficiency include patients with chronic disease, particularly those undergoing parenteral nutrition or hemodialysis, the elderly, pregnant women, growth-retarded or premature children, the obese, patients with chronic or recurrent infections, and food faddists.

In humans, the best evidence for an effect on immunological responses has been provided for folate, iron, and zinc.[39] Zinc deficiency has been shown to produce lymphoid atrophy and reduced capacity to respond to many T-cell-dependent antigens. Moderate to severe zinc deficiency is clinically observed in the syndrome of acrodermatitis enteropathica, which includes the clinical features of symmetrical mucocutaneous lesions, growth failure, hair changes, and frequent infections with viruses, fungi, and bacteria. Immunological studies of these patients have shown impaired delayed hypersensitivity skin tests and decreased lymphocyte proliferation. In addition, polymorphonuclear chemotaxis or directed cell movement is slowed. There also is a significant reduction in the proportion of T4 helper cells and decreased thymic hormone activity. Likewise, helper T-cell activity for B-cell function is decreased, as is suppressor T-cell function. These clinical and immunological changes in acrodermatitis enteropathica can be corrected by the administration of zinc supplements.[29]

Another common trace element deficiency is that of iron. Iron deficiency may predispose subjects to infections, although the association of iron and infection, must still be examined carefully. Several in vitro experiments have demonstrated the ability of added iron to reduce the microbiostatic function of serum. Extrapolation of the results of these in vitro experiments has aroused concerns about the benefits of iron treatment. As Chandra[30] points out, however, the notion that iron therapy predisposes the host to infection by increasing the virulence of pathogenesis is misleading. He contends that oral iron treatment or iron fortification of food neither saturates the circulating transferrin in vivo nor increases the presence of free ionic iron needed for microbial growth. Parenteral administration of iron, however, depending upon the dose used and the levels of iron-binding proteins of the individual, may exceed or equal the total iron-binding capacity and may increase the virulence of the pathogens. For children suffering from protein-calorie malnutrition with reduced levels of iron-binding protein, iron administration is delayed during initial feeding, thus giving the opportunity for repair of transferrin synthesis.[29]

In addition to zinc and iron, other trace elements may play a role in immune function. Although copper deficiency is rare in clinical practice, infants with congenital copper deficiency (Menkes' syndrome) often die in early life from infection, such as pneumonia. Selenium deficiency, particularly coexisting with vitamin E deficiency, can reduce antibody responses to red cells and the activity of thymic hormone.[40] This interaction between selenium and the immune system may play a role in the pathogenesis of cardiomyopathy of humans and animals seen in the Keshan region of China where the soil and water content of selenium is extremely low.[41]

Because severe malnutrition can occur in many clinical disorders, including gastrointestinal, hepatic, renal, and cardiopulmonary disease and malignancy, it can have an extensive impact on the day-to-day care of countless patients. In addition to an awareness of its import, diagnostic measures to monitor immune parameters and therapeutic regimens (including drugs and appropriate nutrition) designed to counteract the effect of malnutrition are required to ensure the complete care of these patients.

References

1. Gell, P.G.H., Coombs, R.R.A., Lachman, P.J. *Clinical Aspects of Immunology*. 3rd ed. London: Blackwell; 1977.
2. Ishizaka, T., Ishizaka, K. Biology of immunoglobulin E. *Prog. Allergy*. 1975; 19:60.
3. Buckley, R.H. IgE antibody in health and disease. In: Bierman, C.W., Pearlman, D.M., eds. *Allergic Diseases from Infancy to Adulthood*. Philadelphia: W.B. Saunders; 1988.
4. Kesarwala, H.H., Fischer T.J. Introduction to the Immune System. In: Lawlor, G.J., Fischer, T.J., eds. *Manual of Allergy and Immunology*. 2nd ed. Boston: Little, Brown, and Company; 1988.
5. Sloan, A.E., Powers, M.E. A perspective on popular perceptions of adverse reactions to foods. *J. Allergy Clin. Immunol.* 1986; 78:127.
6. Metcalfe, D.D. Food hypersensitivity. *J. Allergy Clin. Immunol.* 1984; 73:749.
7. Anderson, J.A. Adverse reactions to foods. In: Bierman, C.W., Pearlman, D.M., eds. *Allergic Diseases from Infancy to Adulthood*. Philadelphia: W.B. Saunders; 1988.
8. Sampson, H.A. Buckley, R.H., Metcalfe, D.D. Food allergy. *JAMA*. 1987; 258:2886.
9. Lemanske, R.F., Atkins, F.M., Metcalfe, D.D. Gastrointestinal mast cells in health and disease. *J. Pediatr.* 1983; 103:177.
10. Farrell, M.K. Food allergy. In: Lawlor, G.J., Fischer, T.J. eds. *Manual of Allergy and Immunology*. 2nd ed. Boston, Little, Brown, and Company; 1988.
11. Atkins, F.M., Steinberg, S.S., Metcalfe, D.D. Evaluation of immediate reactions to foods in adults: I. Correlation of demorgraphic, laboratory, and prick skin test data with response to controlled oral food challenge. *J. Allergy Clin. Immunol.* 1985; 75:348.
12. Sampson, H.A., McCaskill C.M. Food hypersensitivity and atopic dermatitis. Evaluation of 113 patients. *J. Pediatr.* 1985; 107:669.
13. Yuninger, J.W. Proper application of available laboratory tests for adverse reactions to foods and food additivies. *J. Allergy Clin. Immunol.*1986; 78:220.
14. Sheffer, A.L., Lieberman, R.L., Aaronson, D.W., Anderson, J.A., Kaplan, A.P., Pierson, W.E., Ellis, E.F., Lichtenstein, L.M., Lockey, R.F., Salvaggio, J.E., Zweiman, B. Measurement of circulating IgG and IgE food immune complex. *J. Allergy Clin. Immunol*, 1988; 81:759.
15. Practice Standards Committee, American Academy of Allergy and Immunology. Measurement of specific and non-specific IgG4 levels as diagnostic and prognostic tests for clinical allergy. American Academy of Allergy and Immunology. News and Notes, *American Academy of Allergy and Immunology*, Spring, 1989.
16. Kemeny, D.M., Price, J.F., Richardson, V., Richards, D., Lessof, M.H. The IgE and IgG subclass antibody response to food in babies during the first year of life and their relationship to feeding regimen and the development of food allergy. *J. Allergy Clin. Immunol.* 1991; 87,5:920.
17. May, C.D., Black, S.A. Adverse reactions to foods due to hypersensitivity. In: Middleton, E., Reed, C.E., Ellis, E.F., eds. *Allergy. Principles and Practice*. St. Louis, C.V. Mosby, 1978.
18. Leinhaus, J.L., McCaskill, G.G., Sampson, H.A. Food allergy challenges: Guidelines and implications. *J. Am. Diet. Assoc.* 1987; 87:604.
19. Sampson, H.A. Food sensitivity in children. In: Lichtenstein, L.M., Fauci, A.S., eds. *Current Therapy in Allergy, Immunology, and Rheumatology-3*. Toronto: Decker; 1988.
20. Taylor, S.L., Bush, R.K, Busse, W.W. Avoidance diets—How selective should we be? *N. Eng. Reg. Allergy Proc.* 1986; 7:527.
21. Sampson, S., Cooke, S. Food allergy and potential allergenicity of microparticulated egg and cow's milk proteins. *J. Am. Coll. Nutr* 1990; 9:410.
22. Zeiger, R.S., Heller, S., Mellon, M.H., Forsythe, A.B., O'Connor, R.D., Hamburger, R.N., Schatz, M. Effect of combined maternal and infant food allergen avoidance on development of atopy in early infancy: a randomized study. *J Allergy Clin. Immunol.* 1989; 84:72.
23. Barau, E., Dupont, C. Modifications of intestinal permeability during food provocation procedures in pediatric irritable bowel syndrome. *J. Pediatr. Gastrointest. Nutr.* 1990; 11:72.
24. Lifshitz, C.H., Hawkins, H.K., Guerra, C., Byrd, N. Anaphylactic shock due to cow's milk protein hypersensitivity in a breast-fed infant. *J. Pediatr. Gastroenterol. Nutr.* 1988; 7:141.
25. Businco, L., Cantani, A., Longhi, M.A., Giampietro, P.G. Anaphylactic reactions to a cow's milk whey protein hydrolysate (Alfa-Re, Nestle) in infants with cow's milk allergy. *Ann. Allergy* 1989; 62:33.
26. Sampson, H.A., Bernhisel-Broadbent, J., Yang, E., Scanlon, S.M. Safety of casein hydrolysate formula in children with cow milk allergy. *J. Pediatr.* 1991; 118:520.
27. Falloon, J., Eddy, J., Wiener, L., Pizzo, P.A. Human immunodeficiency virus infection in children. *J. Pediatr.* 1986; 114:1.
28. Smythe, P.M., Schonland, M., Brereton-Stiles, C.G., Coovadia, H.M., Grace, H.J., Loening, W.E.K., Mafoyane, A., Parent, M.A., Vos, G.H. Thymolymphatic deficiency and depression of cell-mediated immunity in protein-calorie malnutrition. *Lancet.* 1971; 2:939.
29. Chandra, R.K. Trace element regulation of immunity and infection. *J. Am. Coll. Nutr.* 1985; 4:5.
30. Shearer, W.T., Anderson, D.C. In: Stiehm, E.R., ed. *Immunologic Disorders in Infants and Children*. 3rd ed. Philadelphia: W.B. Saunders; 1989.
31. Chandra, R.K. Of nutritional status and disease outcome. Immunocompetence assessment. *Sem. Immunopathol. Oncol.* 1987; 172:2.
32. Chandra, R.K. Immunodeficiency as a functional index of nutritional status. *Br. Med. Bull.* 1981; 37:89.
33. Chandra, R.K., Scrimshaw, N.A. Immunocompetence in nutritional assessment. *Am. J. Clin. Nutr.* 1980; 33:2694.
34. Puri, S., Chandra, R.K. Nutritional regulation of host resistance and predictive value of immunologic tests in assessment of outcome. *Pediatr. Clin. North Am.* 1985; 32:499.

35. Chandra, R.K. Nutritional regulation of immunity and risk of infection in old age. *Immunology*. 1989; 67:141.

36. Sherman, A.R. Alterations in immunity related to nutritional status. *Nutr. Today*. 1986; 21:7.

37. Watson, R.R., McMurray, D.N. CRC-critical. *Rev. Food Science Nutr*. 1979; 12:113.

38. Rogers, A.E., Newberne, P.M. Nutrition and immunological responses. *Cancer Detection Prevent. Suppl*. 1987; 1:1.

39. Beisel, W.R., Edeman, R., Nauss, K., Suskin, R.M. Single nutrient effects on immune functions. *JAMA*. 1981; 245:53.

40. Chandra, R.K., Dayton, D.H. Trace element regulation of immunity and infection. *Nutr. Res*. 1982; 2:721.

41. Xhen, X.S., Yang, G.O., Chen, I.S., Chen, X.L., Wen, Z.M. Studies on the relations of selenium and Keshan disease. *Biol. Trace Element Res*. 1980; 2:91.

Chapter 29
Pediatric Acquired Immune Deficiency Syndrome

Mildred Bentler

When acquired immune deficiency syndrome (AIDS) was first observed in 1981,[1] it was thought to be a disease limited to homosexual men. In the following year, the first cases of pediatric AIDS were noted and reported in the United States.[2,3] Since the first observations, the reported number of cases of AIDS in children has increased rapidly. As of February, 1991, 2841 children under 13 years of age (1.5% of total reported cases) have been reported to the Centers for Disease Control (CDC). The majority of these cases (56%) have been reported in three states—New York, New Jersey, and Florida—with the highest concentration of cases coming from large urban areas of these states.[4]

AIDS is caused by the human immunodeficiency virus (HIV) and is transmitted by the exchange of blood or blood products or sexual contact. In children, HIV is acquired perinatally from high-risk HIV-infected mothers (78%) or through receipt of blood or blood products (19%).[4] High-risk mothers are identified as either intravenous (IV) drug users, sexual partners of HIV-positive men, or recipients of HIV-contaminated blood products. Transfusion-related transmission accounts for a much smaller percentage of cases since the development of the enzyme-linked immunosorbent assay (ELISA) test for screening HIV-infected blood donors. HIV also has been isolated from cell-free breast milk,[5,6] and there have been three reports of transmission of HIV via breast milk to infants of women receiving postpartum blood transfusions.[7,8] To date, there has been no evidence to support the transmission of HIV through casual contact or ordinary household activity.[9,10] Risk factors for pediatric AIDS include *maternal or paternal IV drug abuse, paternal bisexuality, maternal or paternal promiscuity, exposure to HIV-contaminated blood or blood products, exposure to HIV-contaminated breast milk, sexual abuse, and IV drug abuse.*

Biochemical Abnormalities

Diagnosis of AIDS is based on laboratory and clinical criteria. A child who fits the case definition of AIDS set by the CDC (Tables 29–1 and 29–2) is considered HIV infected.

Serology for HIV antibody (ELISA, Western Blot) is effective in diagnosing AIDS in children over 15 months of age; however, these tests are not definitive for children under 15 months since they may still carry HIV antibody acquired from their mother transplacentally without actually being infected. In infants, therefore, the presence of clinical disease is also necessary to confirm HIV infection.[11]

AIDS has a relatively long incubation period. The median age of CDC-defined diagnosis is 10 months for perinatal

Table 29–1. Definition of HIV Infection in Children

Infants and children under 15 months of age with perinatal infection

1) Virus in blood or tissues
   or
2) HIV antibody
   and
   evidence of both cellular and humoral immune deficiency
   and
   one or more categories in Class P-2 (see Table 29–2)
   or
3) Symptoms meeting CDC case definition for AIDS

Older children with perinatal infection and children with HIV infection acquired through other modes of transmission

1) Virus in blood or tissues
   or
2) HIV antibody
   or
3) Symptoms meeting CDC case definition for AIDS

acquisition, 42 months for transfusion-acquired HIV infection, and 9 years for children with hemophilia who acquired HIV via factor VII concentrate. From this data, the incubation period has been estimated as a median of 8 months for perinatal acquisition and 19 months for transfusion-acquired HIV infection.[12,13]

Prognosis has been poor. Fifty-eight percent of CDC reported cases have died. Rarely do symptomatic HIV-positive children live longer than 38 months after diagnosis.[12–14]

As a member of the retrovirus family, HIV enters the cell and causes cell dysfunction or death. Since HIV affects mainly those cells of the immune system, immunodeficiency results. There is a characteristic but not universal depletion of the number of T-helper/inducer lymphocytes which results in a reversal of the T4/T8 ratio. Abnormalities of the B-lymphocyte system are also common. Hypergamma-globulinemia, especially of IgM and IgG, is reported frequently.[15,16]

Clinical Abnormalities

Major clinical findings in children with HIV infection are *failure to thrive, oral candidiasis, parotitis, chronic or recurrent diarrhea, malabsorption, lymphoid interstitial pneumonitis (LIP), bacterial and viral infections, opportunistic infections, hepatomegaly, splenomegaly, encephalopathy and*

257

Table 29-2. CDC Classification of HIV Infection in Children under 13 Years

Class P-0. Indeterminate infection

Class P-1. Asymptomatic infection

    Subclass A. Normal immune function
    Subclass B. Abnormal immune function
    Subclass C. Immune function not tested

Class P-2. Symptomatic infection

    Subclass A. Nonspecific findings
    Subclass B. Progressive neurologic disease
    Subclass C. Lymphoid interstitial pneumonitis
    Subclass D. Secondary infectious diseases
        Category D-1. Specified secondary infectious diseases listed in the CDC surveillance definition for AIDS
        Category D-2. Recurrent serious bacterial infections
        Category D-3. Other specified secondary infectious diseases
    Subclass E. Secondary cancers
        Category E-1. Specified secondary cancers listed in the CDC surveillance definition for AIDS
        Category E-2. Other cancers possibly secondary to HIV infection or associated with HIV infection

CLASSIFICATION SYSTEM

Children fulfilling the definition of HIV infection discussed above may be classified into one of two mutually exclusive classes based on the presence or absence of clinical signs and symptoms. Class Pediatric-1 (P-1) is further subcategorized on the basis of the presence or absence of immunologic abnormalities, whereas Class P-2 is subdivided by specific disease patterns. Once a child has signs and symptoms and is therefore classified in P-2, he or she should not be reassigned to class P-1 if signs and symptoms resolve.

Perinatally exposed infants and children whose infection status is indeterminate are classified into class P-0.

Class P-0. Indeterminate infection. Includes perinatally exposed infants and children up to 15 months of age who cannot be classified as definitely infected according to the above definition but who have antibody to HIV, indicating exposure to a mother who is infected.

Class P-1. Asymptomatic infection. Includes patients who meet one of the above definitions for HIV infection but who have had no previous signs or symptoms that would have led to classification in Class P-2.

These children may be subclassified on the basis of immunologic testing. This testing should include quantitative immunoglobulins, complete blood count with differential, and T-lymphocyte subset quantitation. Results of functional testing of lymphocytes (mitogens, such as pokeweed) may also be abnormal in HIV-infected children, but it is less specific in comparison with immunoglobulin levels and lymphocyte subset analysis, and it may be impractical.

Subclass A—Normal immune function. Includes children with no immune abnormalities associated with HIV infection.

Subclass B—Abnormal immune function. Includes children with one or more of the commonly observed immune abnormalities associated with HIV infection, such as hypergammaglobulinemia, T-helper (T4) lymphopenia, decreased T-helper/T-suppressor (T4/T8) ratio, and absolute lymphopenia. Other causes of these abnormalities must be excluded.

Subclass C—Not tested. Includes children for whom no or incomplete (see above) immunologic testing has been done.

Class P-2. Symptomatic infection. Includes patients meeting the above definitions for HIV infection and having signs and symptoms of infection. Other causes of these signs and symptoms should be excluded. Subclasses are defined based on the type of signs and symptoms that are present. Patients may be classified in more than one subclass.

Subclass A—Nonspecific findings. Includes children with two or more unexplained nonspecific findings persisting for more than 2 months, including fever, failure-to-thrive or weight loss of more than 10% of baseline, hepatomegaly, splenomegaly, generalized lymphadenopathy lymph nodes measuring at least 0.5 cm present in two or more sites, with bilateral lymph nodes counting as one sitel, parotitis, and diarrhea (three or more loose stools per day) that is either persistent or recurrent (defined as two or more episodes of diarrhea accompanied by dehydration within a 2-month period).

Subclass B—Progressive neurologic disease. Includes children with one or more of the following progressive findings: 1) loss of developmental milestones or intellectual ability, 2) impaired brain growth (acquired microcephaly and/or brain atrophy demonstrated on computerized tomographic scan or magnetic resonance imaging scan), or 3) progressive symmetrical motor deficits manifested by two or more of these findings: paresis, abnormal tone, pathologic reflexes, ataxia, or gait disturbance.

Subclass C—Lymphoid interstitial pneumonitis. Includes children with a histologically confirmed pneumonitis characterized by diffuse interstitial and peribronchiolar infiltration of lymphocytes and plasma cells and without identifiable pathogens, or, in the absence of a histologic diagnosis, a chronic pneumonitis—characterized by bilateral reticulonodular interstitial infiltrates with or without hilar lymphadenopathy—present on chest X-ray for a period of at least 2 months and unresponsive to appropriate antimicrobial therapy. Other causes of interstitial infiltrates should be excluded, such as tuberculosis. *Pneumocystis carinii* pneumonia, cytomegalovirus infection, or other viral or parasitic infections.

Subclass D—Secondary infectious diseases. Includes children with a diagnosis of an infectious disease that occurs as a result of immune deficiency caused by infection with HIV.

Category D-1. Includes patients with secondary infectious disease due to one of the specified infectious diseases listed in the CDC surveillance definition for AIDS: *Pneumocystis carinii* pneumonia; chronic cryptosporidiosis; disseminated toxoplasmosis with onset after 1 month of age; extra-intestinal strongyloidiasis; chronic isosporiasis; candidiasis (esophageal, bronchial, or pulmonary); extrapulmonary cryptococcosis; disseminated histoplasmosis; noncutaneous, extrapulmonary, or disseminated mycobacterial infection (any species other than leprae); cytomegalovirus infection with onset after 1 month of age; chronic mucocutaneous or disseminated herpes simplex virus infection with onset after 1 month of age; extrapulmonary or disseminaled coccidioidomycosis; nocardiosis; and progressive multifocal leukoencephalopathy.

Category D-2. Includes patients with unexplained, recurrent, serious bacterial infections (two or more within a 2-year period) including sepsis, meningitis, pneumonia, abscess of an internal organ, and bone/joint infections.

Category D-3. Includes patients with other infectious diseases, including oral candidiasis persisting for 2 months or more, two or more episodes of herpes stomatitis within a year, or multidermatomal or disseminated herpes zoster infection.

Subclass E—Secondary cancers. Includes children with any cancer described below in categories E-1 and E-2.

Category E-1. Includes patients with the diagnosis of one or more kinds of cancer known to be associated with HIV infection as listed in the surveillance definition of AIDS and indicative of a defect in cell-mediated immunity: Kaposi's sarcoma, B-cell non-Hodgkin's lymphoma, or primary lymphoma of the brain.

Category E-2. Includes patients with the diagnosis of other malignancies possibly associated with HIV infection.

Subclass F—Other diseases. Includes children with other conditions possibly due to HIV infection not listed in the above subclasses, such as hepatitis, cardiopathy, nephropathy, hermatologic disorders (anemia, thrombocytopenia), and dermatologic diseases.

developmental delay, loss of development milestones, cardiomyopathy, and nephropathy. These findings are similar to those found in adult AIDS patients with some exceptions. Features that are most common in pediatric AIDS include pulmonary lymphoid hyperplasia (PLH), parotid enlargement, developmental delays, serious bacterial sepsis, and chronic lymphocytic interstitial pneumonia (LIP). Less common findings in HIV-positive children are Kaposi's sarcoma, B-cell lymphoma, and lymphopenia.[17]

Bacterial infections are common and include bacteremia, meningitis, pneumonia, septic arthritis, osteomyelitis, and urinary tract infections. These infections are caused by common organisms, such as *Streptococcus pneumoniae, Hemophilus influenzae type B, Staphylococcal aureas* and *epidermis, Salmonella, Escherichia coli, Enterobacter,* and *Pseudomonas.*[17,18] Because of the impaired immune system, children with AIDS are vulnerable to opportunistic infections. Pneumocystis carinii pneumonia (PCP) is the most frequently seen opportunistic infection and is associated with a poor prognosis and high morbidity and mortality rate.[16,18] Oral thrush or candidiasis is frequently found in children with HIV infection. It should be noted that oral thrush is also common among healthy infants under 1 year of age and those who are receiving antibiotic treatment. It is also prevalent in infants born to drug-abusing mothers. In AIDS children, however, the infection can extend into the esophagus and cause fever, poor appetite, weight loss, and vomiting.[17,18]

Failure to thrive, malabsorption, and intermittent or chronic diarrhea are common, devastating problems associated with pediatric AIDS. Early studies report that up to 90% of children with AIDS failed to thrive.[2,19] A profile of 55 children with HIV infection revealed 50% of patients had a height at or below the 10th percentile and 66% had a weight below the 10th percentile.[20] Gastrointestinal disease in AIDS children may be due to idiopathic villus atrophy, bacterial overgrowth, or opportunistic infection.[2,21] Diarrhea may persist despite total parenteral nutrition (TPN) or fasting[22] and is not always present with malabsorption. Cases have been reported in which, despite the presence of severe diarrhea and weight loss, malabsorption was not documented by laboratory evidence.[23] Other studies have documented weight loss in the absence of diarrhea.[24] Malabsorption and infection may lead to a self-perpetuating form of malnutrition, with resulting nutrient deficiencies exacerbating gut dysfunction and nutrient losses through diarrhea.[25]

Central nervous system dysfunction has been documented in up to 90% of children with AIDS.[26] This dysfunction is manifested as deficits in language and fine and gross motor skills. Bilateral pyrimidal tract signs (gait changes, bilateral weakness of the extremities, ataxia) are also documented. The encephalopathy of pediatric AIDS is progressive and is characterized by loss of developmentcal milestones in younger children, loss of higher cortical function in older children, deterioration of play, progressive apathy, and progressive bilateral pyrimidal tract signs. Several factors have been implicated in the cause of AIDS encephalopathy, the foremost being infection of the central nervous system (CNS) either by HIV itself or other organisms, such as cytomegalovirus (CMV) and *Candida albicans.* Calcification of the basal ganglia and cortical atrophy have been documented in numerous patients.[26–28] Other factors that may contribute to developmental delays include maternal drug use, poor prenatal care, frequent and lengthy hospitalizations, reverse isolation procedures, and poor home environments. Multiple medications, chronic hypoxia secondary to lung disease, and malnutrition also have been implicated.[29]

Hepatic abnormalities have been reported in children with AIDS and can be related to coincident hepatotrophic virus exposure, complications of the immunosuppressed state—either infectious, malignant, or iatrogenic—or nonspecific changes associated with a chronic debilitating illness.[30] Hepatitis is frequently found and may be secondary to CMV infection. Hepatic injury also may result from potentially hepatotoxic drugs, such as ketoconazole and pentamidine, which are commonly used in the treatment of AIDS-related infections. Malnutrition, common in AIDS patients, may exacerbate the toxic effect of some drugs by affecting the plasma binding and hepatic metabolism of these drugs.[31] Liver damage has also been associated with the long-term use of total parenteral nutrition (TPN)[32] Nephropathy, associated with AIDS, including glomerular sclerosis and nephrotic syndrome, has been linked to immune complex deposits in glomeruli[33] and the use of nephrotoxic drugs.

The existence of an HIV-associated facial dysmorphism has remained a controversial issue. In 1986, Marion et al.[34] reported common dysmorphic features in AIDS children that included growth failure, microcephaly, hypertelorism, prominent box-like forehead, flat nasal bridge, upward obliquity of the eyes, long palpebral fissures with blue sclera, a short nose with flattening of the columnella, a well-formed triangular philtrum, and markedly patulous lips. In a later study, Marion and co-workers[35] were able to show a high correlation of the severity of dysmorphism with the age of onset of immune deficiency. The younger the onset of symptoms, the more severe the dysmorphism. These findings have not been universal. Some researchers argue that many of the listed facial features are common in black and Hispanic children, and the evaluation of features is subjective.[36] However, the possibility of an HIV-associated facial dysmorphism should not be ruled out, and further investigation is needed.

Factors to be Considered in Nutritional Evaluation

In considering the child with AIDS, it is important to be aware of the detrimental effect that malnutrition can have on the immune system. Protein-calorie malnutrition has been shown to impair delayed cutaneous hypersensitivity and to decrease the number of T cell lymphocytes. Deficits of iron; magnesium; vitamins A, C, D, and E, pyridoxine; and folate are also known to impair immunity.[37,38] Zinc, in particular, has been shown to affect immune response, and several studies have reported reduced serum zinc levels in AIDS patients.[39,40]

Other consequences of malnutrition include decreased K_{40}, indicating decreased lean body mass (LBM) or muscle wasting (54% of normal LBM and 66% of ideal body weight at death).[41] Decreased LBM may produce decreased cardiac function secondary to heart muscle atrophy. Respiratory muscle can also be affected and may result in an inability of the lungs to clear infectious secretions, thereby increasing the child's susceptibility to pneumonia.[25] Malnutrition also may contribute to cortical degeneration[28] and has been shown to impair digestion through decreased production of pancreatic enzymes and flattened intestinal villi.[22]

In children with AIDS, many factors can contribute to malnutrition. The numerous infections seen in pediatric AIDS can affect the immune system by altering vitamin and mineral metabolism and electrolyte and water balance by the overutilization, diversion, or sequestration of various nutrients. There is an increase in gluconeogenesis, causing an overutilization of protein. Nitrogen, potassium, magnesium, phosphorus, and zinc are lost. Sodium and iron are sequestered, leading to fluid overload and anemia.[42]

Fever in AIDS children can be intermittent or persistent and low grade. Calorie expenditure can increase 7% for each degree Fahrenheit above normal, and dehydration is possible. Fever also can increase protein utilization. Respiratory difficulties caused by pneumonia can increase energy expenditure dramatically and can limit intake.

Gastrointestinal manifestations of AIDS are among the most common and the most devastating to nutritional status. Oral and esophageal candidiasis and herpes gingivostomatitis cause painful lesions, making eating and swallowing difficult. Infants are unable to suck, and older children refuse food and fluids. In more severe cases, some children even avoid swallowing their own saliva. The diarrhea that affects a majority of the children with AIDS can cause a decrease in oral intake and an increase in nutrient losses. There is a danger of dehydration, and as previously discussed, this diarrhea can lead to malabsorption and gut failure.

Encephalopathy of AIDS and developmental delays frequently affect feeding abilities. In a study of 55 children with AIDS, 45% exhibited dysphagia. Of the 45%, 44% were classified as mild to moderate, and 56% were classified as severe.[43]

Psychosocial issues also affect the maintenance of nutritional status. The majority of AIDS children come from homes where one or both parents and possibly other siblings may be HIV infected and are either in various stages of the disease themselves or are deceased. Home environments may not be optimal, and care may be inconsistent. Many are placed in foster care and are living in poverty, which also may play a role in the quality of care given outside the hospital setting. It also has been this author's observation that several children with AIDS exhibit a complete disinterest in food or eating independent of any organic explanation.

Nutritional assessment should include a detailed diet history. In addition to the usual questions dealing with food preferences, use of supplements, and food intolerances, information regarding methods of feeding, developmental milestones, usual appetite and bowel habits, and home environment should be obtained.

Anthropometric measurements—head circumference, weight and height for age, and weight for height—are necessary to monitor nutritional adequacy and the effect of nutritional intervention (see Chapter 4). Serum albumin or transferrin is useful in evaluating visceral protein status; however, total iron-binding capacity (TIBC) can only be used in the absence of anemia (see Chapter 4). In addition, a complete blood count, serum potassium, blood urea nitrogen (BUN), creatinine, and liver function tests should be monitored where indicated. Weight should be reassessed weekly for older children and daily for infants. Appetite and intake can be erratic and need to be evaluated frequently. Drugs, either therapeutic or maintenance, should be reviewed for any possible nutrient interactions.

Dietary Management

The goal of dietary intervention in the child with AIDS is to manage each problem as it occurs with an ultimate goal of preventing nutritional deficits and maximizing the child's nutritional status.

To determine calorie requirements, a formula similar to that used in failure to thrive is used (Table 29–3). First, the weight for actual height and the weight for age at the 50th percentile are determined. The recommended daily allowance (RDA)[44] for the patient's age is then applied to these weights, giving a range of optimal caloric intake. By dividing these figures by the patient's actual weight, a range for Kcal/kg can be determined. For example, a 9-month-old female with a weight of 5 kg and a length of 63 cm would require a range of 702 kcal to 928 kcal or 140 to 185 kcal per kilogram of actual body weight. More calories are needed for catch-up-growth (see Chapter 21, Table 21–3). The resting energy expenditure is increased in AIDS but decreased caloric intake appears to be the more significant cause of short-term weight loss. Rapid weight loss and anorexia in AIDS requires the investigation for a secondary infection.[45]

Protein requirements can be estimated by substituting the RDA for protein into the same formula. The same 9-month-old infant would require 13–17 g/day of protein. Another method to determine protein needs is to increase the RDA for protein by 50% to 100% to provide for increased needs and nitrogen losses as long as renal function is satisfactory.[18] For more accurate estimates of protein needs, nitrogen balance studies may be helpful (see Chapters 4 and 21).

Vitamin supplementation of one to two times the RDA may be necessary to replace deficits and balance losses caused by increases in metabolism or excretion.[25] Supplemental zinc may also be beneficial in view of reduced serum levels and their relationship to immune status. In patients with a low TIBC, supplemental iron is contraindicated to avoid proliferation of iron-dependent organisms.[46] Folate deficiency and thiamine deficiency may contribute to neurological degeneration produced by medications; thus, folate- and thiamine-[47] rich foods should be encouraged.[48] Cardiac function improved on selenium supplementation.[49]

Oral feeding should be individualized for the patient and his or her specific problems. For infants with a limited intake, calorically dense formula (24–27 kcal/oz) is commonly used. These formulas are commercially available or can be prepared by adding carbohydrate and/or fat or by reducing the amount of water added to powdered or concentrated formulas. However, the renal solute load must be evaluated. Frequent feedings also may be beneficial, but each feeding should not exceed 30 minutes. HIV positive women in the U.S. should not breast feed; women however may differ in breast feeding in underdeveloped countries where sanitation is a major problem.[50]

For the child with oral lesions, good oral hygiene and topical medication can decrease discomfort.[43] Such foods as

Table 29–3. Guide for Determining Optimal Calorie Range

$$\frac{\text{Minimum: Weight (kg) at 50th percentile for actual height} \times \text{RDA for calories per kilogram based on age}}{\text{Actual Weight}} = \text{kcal/kg}$$

$$\frac{\text{Maximum: Weight (kg) for age at 50th percentile} \times \text{RDA for calories per kilogram based on age}}{\text{Actual Weight}} = \text{kcal/kg}$$

From Bentler & Stanish,[25] with permission.

pudding, ice cream, and nonacidic juices are well accepted because of their soothing quality. Ice pops, particularly if taken before a meal, provide a numbing effect and a source of calories and fluid. Favorite foods should also be considered.

Frequent, high-calorie, nutrient-dense snacks can increase caloric intake and prevent overwhelming the child at mealtimes. Peanut butter, cheese, pudding, yogurt, and cereal seem to be preferred snacks. Commercial supplements should be evaluated for patient acceptance and tolerance. For dysphagic children, evaluation by a dysphagia team or therapist is valuable. Changes in position, food consistency, feeding nipples, and utensils and desensitization therapy for feeding aversions resulted in an improvement in 76% of AIDS children evaluated in a study by Pressman.[43]

Consistency in care and stimulation also can improve the child's intake. For example, one clinician noted that hospitalized children would eat well and progress developmentally when cared for by a familiar nurse on a regular schedule; however, when less stimulation was received from one shift, they would become less responsive and would decrease their food intake.[51]

Management of diarrhea and malabsorption due to AIDS is difficult, and these conditions may never resolve completely. Elemental products may be beneficial in maximizing the absorption of nutrients and minimizing abdominal distention. A lactose restriction may help in some cases; however, long-term dietary restrictions should be avoided to prevent limitations on an already poor appetite.[52] Fluid intake needs to be encouraged to prevent dehydration, and adequate potassium should be provided in the presence of chronic diarrhea. One should avoid gas formers—bran, prunes, and caffeine-rich beverages that stimulate the bowels. Food sanitation is essential to reduce infection. Cooked foods and those with a low bacteria count are preferred.[48]

Oral or tube feedings

When a child with AIDS is unable to maintain adequate oral intake, enteral feedings, either via nasogastric, gastrostomy, or jejunostomy tube, should be considered. Tube feedings can be used to provide supplemental or total nutrition and can be combined with oral or parenteral nutrition to maximize intake. Feedings by slow continuous drip may improve tolerance and decrease diarrhea. Nighttime tube feedings have been helpful in the management of some cases by allowing the child freedom to eat as desired during the day without affecting caloric intake. Oral feedings or oral stimulation (as with a pacifier) should be continued at least therapeutically to maintain feeding abilities and improve

absorption. Adjustment of calorie requirements under stress should be 25% for diarrhea, 12% per degree rise in centigrade temperature, 20% minor operation, 60% for sepsis.[53]

If oral or tube feedings are inadequate, unsuccessful, or contraindicated, parenteral nutrition can be instituted to maintain or improve nutritional status. Although there is an increased risk of catheter-associated infection in an immune-compromised patient, complications from central line TPN have been reported to be only 10%.[16] Oral or tube feedings should be continued for the patient receiving TPN to maintain feeding abilities and to promote repair of the gastrointestinal mucosa. Therapeutic feedings can prevent or ameliorate cholestasis,[32,54] and there is some evidence that enteral stimulation during TPN can maintain or improve mucosal immunity.[55]

Follow-up

Evaluation of nutrition support should include anthropometric measurements, appetite, daily food intake, and blood chemistries, e.g. complete blood count, serum albumin, and electrolytes. Drugs should be reviewed regularly for nutrient interactions.

Optimal nutrition can improve the quality of life for the AIDS patient. An AIDS education program for low-income Afro-American and Latino women (administered through the Women, Infants, and Children's Nutrition Program) was beneficial in changing knowledge and attitudes.[56] Nutrition support for the child with AIDS should be aggressive and prevention of nutritional deficiencies a major priority.

References

1. Gottleib, M.S. Pneumocystitis carinii pneumonia and mucosal candidiasis in previously healthy homosexual men. *N. Engl. J. Med.* 1981; 305:1426.
2. Oleske, J., Minnefor, A., Cooper, R. Jr., Thomas, K., Dela Cruz, A., Ahdieh, H., Guerrero, I., Joshi, V., Desposito, I. Immune deficiency syndrome in children. *JAMA.* 1983; 249:2345.
3. Rubenstein, A. Acquired immunodeficiency syndrome in infants. *Am. J. Dis. Child.* 1983; 137:825.
4. *HIV/AID Surveillance.* Atlanta, GA: Centers for Disease Control; 1991. US Dept. of Health and Human Services.
5. Wasserberger, J., Ordog, G.J. AIDS and breast milk. *JAMA.* 1986; 255:464. Letter.
6. Thiry, L., Sprecher-Goldberger, S. Isolation of AIDS virus from cell-free breast milk of three healthy virus carriers. *Lancet.* 1985; 2:891.
7. Zeigler, J.B., Cooper, D.A. Postnatal transmission of A.I.D.S. associated retrovirus from mother to infant. *Lancet.* 1985; 1:896.
8. Lepage, P. Perinatal transmission in Rwanda. Presented at International Conference on AIDS in Children, Adolescents and Heterosexual Adults; February 19, 1987, Atlanta, GA.

9. Friedland, G.H., Saltzman, B.R. Lack of transmission of HTLV-III/LAV infection to household contacts of patients with AIDS or ARC with oral candidiasis. *N. Engl. J. Med.* 1986; 314:344.

10. Kaplan, J.E., Oleske, J.M. Evidence against transmission of human T lymphotropic virus/lymphadenopathy associated virus (HTLV III/LAV) in families of children with acquired immune deficiency syndrome. *J. Pediatr. Infect. Dis.* 1985; 4:468.

11. Connor, E.M. *Human Immunodeficiency Virus (HIV) Infection in Infants and Children.* London: Wiley; 1986.

12. Rogers, M.F. Pediatric HIV infection: epidemiology, etiopathogenesis and transmission. *Pediatr. Ann.* 1988: 17:324.

13. Oleske, J., Connor, E., Boland, M. A perspective on pediatric AIDS. *Pediatr. Ann.* 1988; 17:319.

14. Scott, G.B., Hutto, C., Makuch, R.W., et al. Survival in children with perinatally acquired human immunodeficiency virus type I infection. *N. Engl. J. Med.* 1989; 321:791.

15. Ryan, B., Connor, E., Minnefore, A., Desposito, F., Oleske, J. Human immunodeficiency virus (HIV) infection in children. *Hematol. Oncol. Clin. North Am.* 1987; 1:381.

16. Oleske, J., Connor, E., Grobenau, M., Minnefore, A. Treatment of HIV infected infants and children. *Pediatr. Aids.* 1988; 17:332.

17. Rubenstein, A. Pediatric AIDS. *Curr. Probl. Pediatr.* 1986; 16:361.

18. Scott, G. Clinical manifestations of HIV infection in children. *Pediatr. Ann.* 1988; 17:365.

19. Shannon, K.M., Amman, A.J. Acquired immune deficiency syndrome in childhood. *J. Pediatr.* 1985; 106:332.

20. Boland, M., Klug, R. AIDS: the implications of home care. *Maternal Child Nurs.* 1986; 11:404.

21. McLoughlin, L., Nord, K., Joshi, V., Oleske, J., Connor, E. Severe gastrointestinal involvement in children with acquired immunodeficiency syndrome. *J. Pediatr. Gastroenterol. Nutr.* 1987; 6:517.

22. Weinstein, W.M. The gastrointestinal tract as a target organ. In: Gottlieb, M.S., Groopman, J.E., Weinstein, W.M., eds. The acquired immunodeficiency syndrome. *Ann. Intern. Med.* 1983; 99:208.

23. Benkov, K., Stawski, C., Sirlin, S., Klapholz, M., Siegal, F., Le Leiko, N. Atypical presentation of childhood acquired immune deficiency syndrome mimicking Crohn's disease: nutritional considerations and management. *Am. J. Gastroenterol.* 1985; 80:260.

24. Kotler, D., Gaetz, H., Lange, M., Klein, E., Holt, P. Enteropathy associated with the acquired immunodeficiency syndrome. *Ann. Intern. Med.* 1984; 101:421.

25. Bentler, M., Stanish, M. Nutrition support of the pediatric patient with AIDS. *J. Am. Diet. Assoc.* 1987; 87:488.

26. Belman, A., Diamond, G., Dickson, D. Pediatric acquired immunodeficiency syndrome. Neurologic syndromes. *Am. J. Dis. Child.* 1988; 142:29.

27. Epstein, L., Sharer, L., Joshi, V., Fojas, M., Koenigsberger, M., Oleske, J. Progressive encephalopathy in children with acquired immune deficiency syndrome. *Ann. Neurol.* 1985; 17:488.

28. Belman, A., Ultmann, M., Horoupian, D., Novick, B., Sprio, A., Rubinstein, A., Kurtzberg, D., Wesson, B. Neurological complications in infants and children with acquired immune deficiency syndrome. *Ann. Neurol.* 1985; 18:560.

29. Ultmann, M., Belman, A., Ruff, B., Novick, M., Wesson, B., Cohen, H., Rubinstein, A. Developmental abnormalities in infants and children with acquired immune deficiency syndrome (AIDS) and AIDS related complex. *Dev. Med. Child. Neurol.* 1985; 27:563.

30. Lebovics, E., Dworkin, B., Heier, S., Rosenthal, W. The hepatobiliary manifestations of human immunodeficiency virus infection. *Am. J. Gastroenterol.* 1988; 83:1.

31. Hathcock, J. Metabolic interactions of nutrients and drugs. *Fed. Proc.* 1985; 44:123.

32. Merrit, R. Cholestasis associated with total parenteral nutrition. *J. Pediatr. Gastroenterol. Nutr.* 1986; 5:9.

33. Pardo, V., Aldana, M., Colton, R. Glomerular lesions in the acquired immunodeficiency syndrome. *Ann. Intern. Med.* 1985; 103:704.

34. Marion, R., Wiznia, A., Hutcheon, G., Rubinstein, A. Human T-cell lymphotropic virus type III (HTLV-III) embryopathy. *Am. J. Dis. Child.* 1986; 140:638.

35. Marion, R., Wiznia, A., Hutcheon, G., Rubinstein, A. Fetal AIDS syndrome score. Correlation between severity of dysmorphism and age at diagnosis of immunodeficiency. *Am. J. Dis. Child.* 1987; 141:429.

36. Nicholas, S. Controversy: is there an HIV associated facial dysmorphism? *Pediatr. Ann.* 1988; 17:353.

37. Chandra, R. Cell-mediated immunity in nutritional imbalance. *Fed. Proc.*, 1980; 30:88.

38. Chandra, R. Effect of macro and micronutrient deficiencies and excesses on immune response. *Food Technol.* 1985; 39:91.

39. Diarrhea and malabsorption associated with the acquired immunodeficiency syndrome (AIDS). *Nutr. Rev.* 1985; 43:235.

40. Fabris, N., Mocchegiani, E., Galli, M., Irato, L., Lazzarin, A., Moroni, M. AIDS, zinc deficiency and thymic hormone failure. *JAMA.* 1988; 259:839. Letter.

41. Kotler, D.P., Tierney, A.R., Wang, J., Pierson, R.N. Magnitude of body-cell mass depletion and the timing of death from wasting in AIDS. *Am. J. Clin. Nutr.* 1989; 50:444.

42. Grant, A., Dehoog, S., eds. *Nutritional Assessment and Support.* Seattle: Grant and DeHoog; 1985.

43. Pressman, H., Morrison, S. Dysphagia in the pediatric AIDS population. *Dysphagia.* 1988; 2:166.

44. Food and Nutrition Board. *Recommended Daily Allowances.* 9th rev. ed. Washington, DC: National Academy of Science; 1980.

45. Grunfeld, C., Pang, M., Shimizu, L., Shigenaga, J., Jensen, P., Feingold, K. Resting energy expenditure caloric intake and short term weight change in human immunodeficiency virus infection and the acquired immunodeficiency syndrome. *Am. J. Clin. Nutr.* 1992; 55:455.

46. Beisel, W.R. Infectious diseases. In: Schneider, H., Anderson, C., Coursin, D., eds. *Nutritional Support of Medical Practice.* New York: Harper and Row; 1983.

47. Leung, J. An approach to feeding HIV-infected infants and toddlers. *Top. Clin. Nutr.* 1989; 4:27.

48. Butterworth, R., Gaudreau, C., Vincelette, J., Bourgault, A., Lamother, F., Nutini, A. Thiamine deficiency in AIDS. Lancet 1991; 338:1086.

49. Kavanaugh-McHugh, A.L., Ruff, A., Perlman, E., Hutton, N., Modlin, J., Rowe, S. Selenium Deficiency and Cardiomyopathy in Acquired Immunodeficiency Syndrome. *J. Parenteral Enteral Nutr.* 1991; 15:347.

50. Mendez, H. Ambulatory care of HIV-seropositive infants and children. *J. Pediatr.* 1991; 119:S14.

51. Krener, P. Impact of the diagnosis of AIDS on hospital care of an infant. *Clin. Pediatr.* 1987; 26:30.

52. Miller, T.L., Orav, J.E., Martin, S.R., Cooper, E.R., McIntosh, K., Winter, H.S. Malnutrition and carbohydrate malabsorption in children with vertically transmitted human immunodeficiency virus 1 infection. *Gastroenterology* 1991; 100: 1296.

53. Nicholas, S.W., Leung, J., Fennoy, I. Guidelines for nutritional support of HIV-infected children. *J. Pediatr.* 1991; 119:S59.

54. Silverman, A., Roy, C. *Pediatric Clinical Gastroenterology.* St. Louis: C.V. Mosby; 1983.

55. Alverdy, J., Chi, H.S., Sheldon, G. The effect of parenteral nutrition on gastrointestinal immunity. The importance of enteral stimulation. *Ann. Surg.* 1985; 202:681.

56. Flasherud, J., Nyamathi, A. Effects of an AIDS education program on the knowledge, attitudes and practices of low income black and Latina women. *J. Comm. Health.* 1990; 15:343.

Chapter 30
Juvenile Rheumatoid Arthritis

Daniel Lovell and Carol Henderson

Juvenile rheumatoid arthritis (JRA) is the most common pediatric rheumatic disease and the most common cause of chronic arthritis in childhood. It is estimated that between 60,000 to 250,000 children in the United States have JRA.[1,2] Currently reported prevalence rates establish JRA as one of the more common chronic diseases of childhood[3] (Table 30–1).

The diagnosis of JRA is established entirely on clinical grounds. It is based on the observation of persistent arthritis of one or more joints of at least 6 weeks duration in a patient 16 years or less in age and the exclusion of all other causes of chronic arthritis in childhood.[4] Onset before 6 months of age is unusual, but the peak age of onset is young—between 1–3 years. However, a substantial number of cases begin later in childhood.[2]

Common constitutional symptoms include joint stiffness in the morning and after periods of inactivity. A very common presentation in the younger child is increased irritability and assumption of a guarded posture or refusal to walk. Fever, anorexia, weight loss, failure to grow, and fatigue may occur in all subtypes of JRA.[5] Three distinct subtypes have been described: systemic, polyarticular, and oligoarticular (Table 30–2). Systemic JRA patients manifest daily or twice-daily spiking fevers greater than 103° F and the appearance of a characteristic fleeting erythematous rash, in addition to the arthritis. These patients commonly develop pericarditis, pleuritis, hepatosplenomegaly, and generalized lymphadenopathy, but are at low risk for the development of chronic iritis (inflammation of the anterior chamber of the eye). Polyarticular JRA (arthritis in five joints or more) occurs in slightly less than half of the cases of JRA (Fig. 30–1) and carries an increased risk for chronic iritis. The largest proportion have pauci- or oligoarticular

Table 30–1. Prevalences of Selected Childhood Chronic Diseases

Disease	Rates per 1000 children
Asthma (moderate to severe)	10.00
Congenital heart disease	7.00
Diabetes mellitus	1.80
Cleft lip/palate	1.50
Juvenile rheumatoid arthritis	1.00
Sickle-cell anemia	0.25
Cystic fibrosis	0.20
Hemophilia	0.15
Acute lymphocytic leukemia	0.11
Chronic renal failure	0.08
Muscular dystrophy	0.06

From Gortmaker & Sappenfield,[3] with permission.

Table 30–2. Clinical Subtypes of Juvenile Rheumatoid Arthritis and Corticosteroid Use*

Parameter	Systemic	Polyarticular	Oligoarticular
Percent of all JRA cases	10%–20%	50%	30%–40%
Number of joints involved	Varies	≥5	≤4
Chronic iritis	<5%	5%–10%	20%
Rheumatoid factor positive	Rare	10%	Rare
Antinuclear antibody positive	<10%	40%	60%
Outcome 10 years after disease onset			
No functional limitations	25%	50%	40%
Mild to moderate limitations	60%	25%	60%
Wheelchair or crutches	15%	25%	0%
Corticosteroid Usage			
Number of patients	84	150	227
Number treated with steroids	45	23	20
Percentage†	54%	15%	9%

*Data from Children's Hospital Medical Center, Cincinnati, OH.
†Overall percentage, 22%

JRA (four joints or fewer involved), which carries the greatest risk for the development of iritis.

JRA serves as the prototype for inflammatory chronic arthropathy in childhood. Patients with JRA represented approximately half of the caseload in a national sample of pediatric rheumatic disease clinics[6] and have served as the stimulus for the development of a health care team approach to address the broad spectrum of medical and psychosocial problems arising from the condition. Despite growing evidence that a significant proportion of JRA patients have nutritional problems, data from two national surveys of university-based pediatric rheumatology centers performed in 1985 and 1986 demonstrated that less than 8% of the patients with JRA were seen by dietitians[6,7] (Fig. 30–2).

Biochemical and Anthropometric Abnormalities

The occurrence of malnutrition in JRA patients should not be unexpected. The chronic inflammatory process in arthritis dramatically alters the type of tissue that accounts for

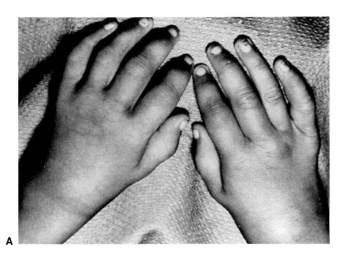

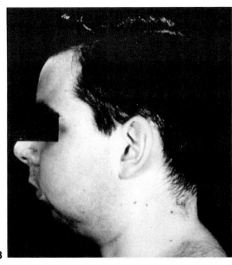

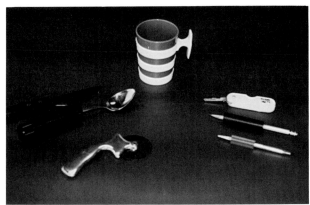

Fig. 30–1. A, Polyarticular JRA involving the hands and wrists. B, Hypoplasia of the mandible. C, Adaptive eating utensils.

losses in body weight.[8] In starvation without an underlying inflammatory process—so-called simple starvation—adipose tissue accounts for approximately 90% of the observed weight loss. However, in the presence of inflammation, known as "complicated starvation," over 50% of the weight loss comes from lean body mass, such as skeletal muscle. This predisposition for loss of lean body mass can make even a small percentage of total body weight loss significant. It requires that nutritional assessment be performed in a comprehensive fashion to assist in determining body composition, including the relative proportions of fat, somatic protein, and visceral protein stores.

Such a comprehensive assessment was performed in a randomized sample of JRA patients.[9] A randomized selection of all JRA patients seen in a university-based pediatric rheumatology center were studied to avoid any bias introduced by using consecutive clinical patients, which would select for more severely ill patients. In the 19 patients studied (Table 30–3), 15 were girls, the average age was 12.6 years, average disease duration was 6.7 years, and the JRA course type was systemic in three, pauciarticular in six, and polyarticular in 10. Six had active JRA, five were in partial remission, and eight were in total remission. In these 19 JRA patients, four were less than the 5th percentile for height, four were less than the 5th percentile for weight,

seven weighed less than 80% of the recommended weight for observed height (adjusted height-for-weight index, an indicator of strong nutritional risk), three were less than the 5th percentile for arm circumference, ten were less than the 5th percentile in both arm muscle circumference and arm muscle area, and seven had serum levels of the short half-life visceral proteins (retinol-binding protein and prealbumin) that were significantly below age-matched norms. However, only 1 of 19 was less than the 5th percentile for subcutaneous fat stores. This work confirms Johansson's[10] study by demonstrating a propensity for the development of significant depletion of somatic and visceral protein stores in JRA patients even in the face of no or only mild depletion of subcutaneous fat stores. It also found a high prevalence of protein-energy malnutrition in this randomly selected population. In Johansson's study comparing 26 Swedish girls with juvenile chronic arthritis (JCA) aged 11 to 16 years to 28 age- and sex-matched normal controls,[10] the JCA patients were found to be similar in height and weight to the controls, but had significantly lower values for midarm and arm muscle circumference, significantly higher values for triceps skinfold thickness, and lower serum albumin and prealbumin levels. These changes were more pronounced in patients with active articular disease and were observed only in those with systemic or polyarticular disease. The authors judged 5 of 26 JCA patients (19%) and none of the controls to be malnourished. This malnutrition occurred even though the two groups were similar in their dietary intake.

Blood

Children with active arthritis often have a normocytic hypochromic anemia that may be moderate to severe, with a hemoglobin in the range of 4–11 g/dL. The anemia is primarily due to chronic disease, but iron deficiency may play a role in some cases.[11] Serum ferritin has been advocated as a useful means for the estimation of total body iron stores.

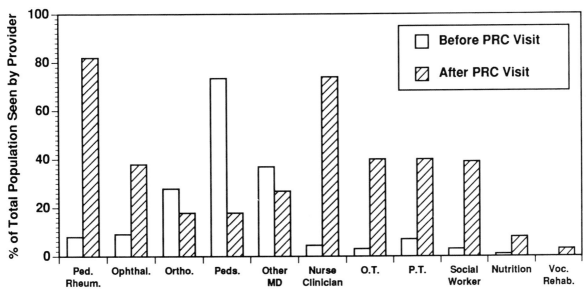

Fig. 30–2. Health care providers seen before and after visits to pediatric rheumatology clinics (PRC). Data from Lovell,[6] and Lovell et al.[7]

Elevation of serum ferritin has been found in children with active JRA.[12] Iron utilization by reticuloendothelial cells is impaired in a chronic active inflammatory state.[12] In one study, 13 of 15 children with JRA who were anemic responded to supplemental oral iron therapy for a 6-month period by a rise in hemoglobin of 1 g/dL or more.[13] However, studies have demonstrated an association between the amount of iron deposited in synovial tissue and the degree of erosive joint damage, thus raising questions concerning the desirability of supplemental iron therapy. In a pilot study, treatment with deferoxamine, an iron-chelating agent with anti-inflammatory properties, resulted in improvement in disease activity in five patients with rheumatoid arthritis. Improvement lasted up to 8 weeks after the cessation of treatment.[14]

Transferrin is a hepatically synthesized transport glycoprotein, the major physiological function of which is to bind and transport iron. Depressed serum transferrin concentrations can occur secondary to protein-energy malnutrition. However, the usefulness of serum transferrin in detecting protein-energy malnutrition is limited due to wide variations in serum concentration and confounding variables, such as the presence of iron-deficiency anemia, which causes an elevation in serum transferrin concentrations.[15]

Leukocytosis is not uncommon in children with active articular inflammation, and patients with systemic JRA may commonly demonstrate white blood cell counts of 30,000 to 50,000/mm³. Other commonly seen indicators of active inflammation are increased platelet count, elevated sedimentation rate, elevated C-reactive protein, elevated levels of immunoglobulins (IgG, IgA, IgM), and serum complement components. Rheumatoid factor tests are positive in only 15% to 20% of children with JRA and are most frequently found in girls with an onset of polyarticular disease during adolescence. Antinuclear antibodies (ANAs) are found in 40% to 65% of patients depending upon the method used.[11,16] The frequency of ANA positivity is increased in girls with a younger age of onset and decreased in boys and in children

with systemic subtype JRA.[11] Children with both pauciarticular JRA and iritis are most likely to have a positive ANA (65%–85%).[17]

Hormonal

Despite several studies documenting normal baseline serum growth hormone levels and normal growth hormone secretion responses to pharmacological stimulation,[18-21] 15 of 21 JRA patients with growth failure treated with growth hormone demonstrated normalized linear growth.[18,20] Six of 22 children with JRA demonstrated serum somatomedin levels more than two standard deviations below age-matched normal controls. All six of these had heights below the 5th percentile.[21] Somatomedin peptides are growth factors thought to mediate the effects of growth hormone on several tissues, including cartilage, muscle, and adipose tissue. The endocrine response in humans to marasmus and kwashiorkor malnutrition is characterized by impaired generation of somatomedin, despite high growth hormone levels.[22]

Factors to be Considered in Nutritional Evaluation and Diagnosis

The diagnosis of JRA is entirely clinical. There is no diagnostic laboratory test, and normal or negative results on any laboratory test should never be used to eliminate JRA as a diagnostic possibility.

In a recent study, 36% of JRA patients (n=28) were found to have protein-energy malnutrition based on results obtained using a standardized pediatric comprehensive nutritional profile.[23] Of those patients referred to a pediatric dietitian by the managing rheumatologist, 70% were found to have protein-energy malnutrition, whereas almost 20% of the JRA outpatients screened at random and not thought to be at nutritional risk by the managing rheumatologist were protein-energy malnourished[24] (Table 30–3).

Table 30–3. Nutritional Parameters in JRA Patients

Anthropometric Measurements and Selected Biochemical
Parameters in 19 Randomly Selected JRA Patients*

Parameter	< 5th Percentile
Height	4/19
Weight	4/19
Arm circumference	3/19
Arm muscle circumference (most predictive of risk for PEM)[37]	10/19
Arm muscle area	10/19
Triceps skinfold thickness	1/19
Prealbumin	7/19
Retinol-binding protein	7/19
Adjusted weight-for-height index (actual weight/ideal weight for current height < 0.80)	7/19

Comprehensive Nutritional Assessment in 28 JRA Patients

Nutritional referral status	Nutritional status Protein-energy malnourished (PEM)
Referred: n = 10	7 (70%)
Screened: n = 18	3 (17%)

Daily Caloric Need Estimates in JRA Patients
(no significant difference in kcals/day)

Method	Mean	Median	SD
Indirect calorimetry	2096	2227	654
Height age for actual height	2058	2007	336
Weight age for actual weight	2093	2076	452
Weight age for ideal body weight	2344	2416	553
Actual intake	1958	1942	404

Growth Velocities in Seven JRA Patients Before and After
Nocturnal Nasogastric Tube Feedings

Parameter	Six months before	Six months after
Height velocity (mean)	0.15 cm/month	1.62 cm/month
Weight velocity (mean)	−0.22 kg/month	0.8 kg/month

*Data from Lovell et al.[9]

In a recent study, total calorie intake was found to be below the recommended dietary allowance (RDA) only in systemic JRA patients, who also had a significantly lower vitamin E intake than other JRA patients.[25] However, another study demonstrated that the mean caloric intake for JRA patients of all three subtypes ranged from 50% to 80% of that of healthy children of comparable age and sex, as reflected in the RDA. These patients also had suboptimal dietary intakes of calcium and iron.[26] Vitamin C, which is stored in leukocytes and platelets, was found to be low in rheumatoid arthritis patients receiving high doses of aspirin (a commonly prescribed drug for arthritis) who did not receive vitamin C supplementation.[27] Not only does the metabolic demand for vitamin C increase secondary to an active inflammatory process[28] but it has also been suggested that aspirin competes for ascorbic acid receptors in the leukocyte membrane and thus inhibits uptake of the vitamin.[29]

JRA patients were not found to be hypermetabolic. No statistical differences were detected between metabolic caloric needs measured via indirect calorimetry and a variety of standard methods to estimate caloric needs.[9,30] Often, JRA patients have depleted somatic and visceral protein stores and increased subcutaneous fat stores despite proportional weight for height. This situation is only worsened by the use of corticosteroids. Corticosteroids not only stimulate the degradation of muscle to provide amino acids that serve as the substrate for gluconeogenesis but also promote increased fat deposition and bone demineralization.[31] Increased deposition of subcutaneous fat concurrent with depletion of somatic protein stores and often serum protein concentrations is observed most frequently in patients with active systemic and polyarticular JRA subtypes, but has also been seen in patients with oligoarticular and inactive JRA. This increased frequency may occur due to the greater use of corticosteroids in systemic and polyarticular JRA subtypes (Table 31–2).

Alterations in body composition resulting in obesity—defined as triceps and subscapular skinfold thickness greater than the 85th percentile for age- and sex-matched norms or when current weight is > 120% of ideal body weight for current height—also require aggressive nutritional intervention measures.[32] Patients receiving corticosteroids are instructed to follow a low-calorie and sodium-restricted diet adequate in all nutrients, especially protein, calcium and iron.

It is often difficult to prescribe forms of exercise as a means by which obese JRA patients can increase energy expenditure or non obese JRA patients can improve muscle tone and facilitate increased lean body mass. Children with JRA are often denied participation in weight-bearing activities (i.e., contact sports, jumping) to avoid excessive mechanical stress to the joints. Children with less severe arthritis can participate in more forms of exercise. Alternative non-weight-bearing exercises can improve both joint range of motion and function. Biking and swimming are two recommended physical activities that can improve a child's muscle strength and cardiovascular fitness.[33] The amount and form of exercise should be individualized to each child with JRA and depend on the type, number, and severity of joints involved.

Recent immunological research suggests that increased cytokine levels, specifically of interleukin-1 and tumor necrosis factor (TNF), can contribute to the metabolic aberrations, altered body composition, and anorexia seen in JRA patients.[34] Depletion of protein stores in animals during TNF administration has been shown to be similar to the muscle wasting that occurs in the presence of an active inflammatory condition.[35]

Given the high risk for the development of nutritional problems in this population, all newly diagnosed JRA patients should be evaluated by a dietitian to determine the adequacy of dietary intake and to obtain standard anthropometric and biochemical measures. This comprehensive nutritional assessment should be repeated at regular intervals in all patients, but most definitely at times of worsening articular inflammation when unintentional weight loss is experienced or in patients demonstrating poor linear growth.

Dietary Treatment

The major objectives in dietary management of JRA patients are consistent ingestion of a diet meeting age- and sex-matched RDAs, the promotion of normal growth and prevention of obesity, and the avoidance of unconventional dietary regimens as a treatment method.

Many children with JRA have persistent or intermittent anorexia, which may result from a variety of causes. Chronic inflammation causes fatigue and poor appetite (perhaps related to increased cytokine production, see above); many arthritis medications can cause nausea, abdominal pain, and cramping; arthritis in the temporomandibular joint can limit mouth opening and cause pain with chewing; patients sometimes develop hypoplasia of the mandible resulting in difficulties in chewing and swallowing (Figure 30-1) and arthritis in the upper extremities can make meal preparation and the use of eating utensils difficult (Figure 30-1). Maximization of nutrient intake may be best achieved through the combined efforts of a dietitian and occupational therapist who can provide parents and older children with basic nutritional guidelines, suggestions for nutritional supplementation, and recommendations for energy-conserving meal preparation methods and use of adaptive eating utensils (Figure 30-1). Patients with temporomandibular joint involvement should be referred to an experienced physical therapist or orthodontist.

In the pediatric rheumatology center at the Children's Hospital Medical Center in Cincinnati, seven children with JRA received aggressive nutritional intervention. All seven children developed profound protein-energy malnutrition secondary to anorexia, with poor linear growth, despite intensive and long-standing efforts by a pediatric dietitian to maximize volitional intake. These patients were nutritionally repleted through the use of outpatient nocturnal nasogastric tube feedings and adjunct volitional intake. This treatment program was well tolerated by the patients and easily administered by the parents and resulted in normalization of somatic and visceral protein stores in all patients. On average, for the seven patients, during the 6 months before the initiation of the nocturnal nasogastric drip feedings, the growth velocity was 0.15 cm/month and the weight gain velocity was −0.22 kg/month. For these same seven patients, during the 6 months after the initiation of nocturnal drip feedings, the average growth velocity was 1.62 cm/month and weight gain velocity was 0.8 kg/month (Table 30-3). These preliminary results suggest that, for the subset of JRA patients with moderate to severe protein-energy malnutrition, aggressive nutritional repletion can improve depleted protein stores and growth rates. Patients generally require nocturnal drip feedings for prolonged periods of time—months to years—and usually until the arthritis becomes less actively inflamed.

According to a recent survey, approximately 40% of JRA patients and families had used unconventional therapies, with unproven dietary manipulations being the most frequently used.[36] Almost all parents of children with JRA are frequently approached by well-intentioned individuals with dietary "cures" for arthritis. Demonstration of an active and supportive interest in the child's nutrition and growth by the rheumatology team and forewarning to the parents concerning the frequency and inaccuracy of unsolicited treatment testimonies are usually adequate to prevent inappropriate dietary manipulations.

Follow-up

JRA is a disease characterized by frequent fluctuations in the severity of the inflammatory process. Patients commonly experience periods of spontaneous remission and then relapse. Dietitians need to be aware of the patient's disease status and the increased risk for nutritional depletion with worsening disease activity. To identify potential nutritional deficits, nutritional screening should be conducted at each visit on all children seen in the pediatric rheumatology clinic. It should include the child's weight percentile, height percentile (inaccuracies in height measurement may be due to the child's inability to stand erect; obtaining height in a segmented manner may be useful), and brief dietary history to determine the adequacy of the child's typical intake, eating patterns, and use of nutritional supplements or vitamin preparations. In addition, routine, periodic, comprehensive nutritional assessment—an evaluation comprised of four integral parts: anthropometry, biochemical analyses, clinical examination, and dietary history—should be performed to identify further nutritional inadequacies. The importance of a well-balanced diet and the avoidance of unconventional dietary practices should be emphasized, as well as dietary counseling and support given to parents and patients for their continued efforts.

References

1. Gewanter, H.L. The prevalence of juvenile arthritis. *Arthritis Rheum.* 1983; 26:599.
2. Towner, S.R., Michet, C.J. Jr., O'Fallon, W.M. The epidemiology of juvenile arthritis in Rochester, Minnesota. 1960–1979. *Arthritis Rheum.* 1983; 26:1208.
3. Gortmaker, S.L., Sappenfield, W. Chronic childhood disorders: prevalence and impact. *Pediatr. Clin. North Am.* 1984; 31:3.
4. Brewer, E.J., Bass, J., Baum, J., Cassidy, J., Fink, C., Jacobs, J., Hanson, V., Levinson, J., Schaller, J., Stillman, J. Current proposed revision of JRA criteria. *Arthritis Rheum.* 1977; 20(suppl):195.
5. Cassidy, J.T. Juvenile rheumatoid arthritis. In: Kelley, W.N., Harris, E.D., Ruddy, S., Sledge, C.B., eds. *Textbook of Rheumatology.* 2nd ed., Philadelphia: W.B. Saunders; 1985.
6. Lovell, D.J. Health care services, school performance and needs in pediatric rheumatology. *Arthritis Rheum.* 1987; 30(suppl):S35.
7. Lovell, D.J., Levinson, J.E, Lindsley, C., Members of the SPRANS Centers. Pediatric rheumatology as a special project of regional and national significance. *J. Rheumatol.* 1986; 13:978.
8. Mascioli, E.A., Blackburn, G.L. Nutrition and rheumatic diseases. In: Kelly, W.N., Harris, E.D., Ruddy, S., Sledge, C.B., eds. *Textbook of Rheumatology.* 2nd ed. Philadelphia: W.B. Saunders; 1985.
9. Lovell, D.J., Gregg, D., Heubi, J.E., Levinson, J.E. Nutritional status in juvenile rheumatoid arthritis (JRA)—an interim report. *Arthritis Rheum.* 1986; 29(suppl):S67.
10. Johansson, V., Portinsson, S., Akesson, A., Svantesson, H., Ockerman, P.A., Akesson, B. Nutritional status in girls with juvenile chronic arthritis. *Hum. Nutr. Clin. Nutr.* 1986; 40:57.
11. Cassidy, J.T. *Textbook of Pediatric Rheumatology.* New York: Wiley; 1982.
12. Craft, A.W., Eastham, E.J., Bell, J.I. Serum ferritin in juvenile chronic polyarthritis. *Ann. Rheum. Dis.* 1977; 36:271.
13. Koerper, M.A., Stempel, D.A., Dallman, P.R. Anemia in patients with juvenile rheumatoid arthritis. *J. Pediatr.*, 1978; 92:930.
14. Marcus, R.E. Treatment of rheumatoid arthritis with deferoxamine: pilot study. *Arthritis Rheum.* 1987; 30:S95.
15. Guidelines for interpreting nutritional assessment data. In: Jansen, T.G., Enghert, D.M., Dudrick, S.J., eds. *Nutritional Assessment: A Manual for Practitioners.* Norwalk, CT: Appleton-Century-Crofts; 1983.

16. Rosenberg, A.M., Prokopchuk, P.A. Antibodies to HEP-2 nuclei in juvenile rheumatoid arthritis analyzed by immunoblotting. *Arthritis Rheum.*, 1989; 32(suppl):S151.

17. Cassidy, J.T., Sullivan, D.B., Petty, R.E. Clinical patterns of chronic iridocyclitis in children with juvenile rheumatoid arthritis. *Arthritis Rheum.*, 1977; 20:224.

18. Ward, D.J., Hartog, M., Ansell, B.M. Corticosteroid-induced dwarfism in Still's disease treated with human growth hormone—clinical and metabolic effect including hydroxyproline excretion in two cases. *Ann. Rheum. Dis.* 1966; 26:416.

19. Sturge, R.A., Beardwell, C., Hartog, M., Wright, D., Ansell, B.M. Cortisol and growth hormone secretion in relation to linear growth: patient's with Still's disease on different therapeutic regimens. *Br. Med. J.* 1970; 3:547.

20. Butenandt, O. Rheumatoid arthritis and growth retardation in children: treatment with human growth hormone. *Eur. J. Pediatr.* 1979; 130:15.

21. Allen, R., Jimenez, M., Cowell, C. Physiologic growth hormone secretion and somatomedin levels in juvenile rheumatoid arthritis. *Arthritis Rheum.* 1988; 31(suppl):S118.

22. Kirschner, B.S., Sutton, M. Somatomedin-C levels in growth-impaired children and adolescents with chronic inflammatory bowel disease. *Gastroenterology.* 1986; 91:830.

23. Hess, L.V. The development and use of a serial nutritional assessment form. *Nutr. Supp. Serv.* 1986; 6:60.

24. Henderson, C.J., Lovell, D.J. Assessment of protein-energy malnutrition in children and adolescents with juvenile rheumatoid arthritis. *Arthritis Care Res.* 1989; 2:108.

25. Bacon, M.C., White, P.H., Raiten, D.J., Craft, N., Margolis, S., Levander, O., Taylor, M., Lipnick, R., Sami, S. Nutritional status and growth in juvenile rheumatoid arthritis. *Arthritis Care Res.* 1990; 2:97.

26. Miller, M.L., Chacko, J.A., Young, E.A. Dietary deficiencies in children with juvenile rheumatoid arthritis. *Arthritis Care Res.* 1989; 2:22.

27. Sahud, M.A., Cohen, R.J. Effect of aspirin ingestion on ascorbic acid levels in rheumatoid arthritis. *Lancet.* 1971; 1:937.

28. Loh, H.S., Wilson, C.W.M. The interactions of aspirin and ascorbic acid in normal men. *J. Clin. Pharmacol.* 1975; 15:36.

29. Loh, H.S. The effects of aspirin on the metabolic availability of ascorbic acid in human beings. *J. Clin. Pharmacol.* 1973; 13:480.

30. Beal, V.A. Nutritional intake. In: McCammon, R.W., ed. *Human Growth and Development.* Springfield, IL: Charles C. Thomas; 1970.

31. Seale, J., Compton, M. Side effects of corticosteroid agents. *Med. J. Aust.* 1986; 144:139.

32. Dietz W.H., Jr. Childhood obesity. *Acad. Ann. NY. Sci.* 1987; 499:47.

33. Giannini M.J. Exercise and arthritis in children. *Arthritis Rheum.* 1988; 31(suppl):S154.

34. Martini, A., Ravelli, A., Notarangelo, L.P. Enchanced interleukin-1 and depressed interleukin-2 production in juvenile arthritis. *J. Rheumatol.* 1986; 13:598.

35. Tracey, K.J., Wei, H., Manogue, K.R. Cachectin/tumor necrosis factor induces cachexia, anemia and inflammation. *J. Exp. Med.* 1988; 167:1211.

36. Hoyeraal, H.M., Brewer, E.J. Jr., Giannini, E.H., Goolsbee, C.B., Lovell, D.J., Person, D.A., Stillman, C. Unconventional therapies in pediatric rheumatology. *Scand. J. Rheum.* 1984; 53(suppl):S113.

37. Henderson, C., Lovell, D., Gregg, D. Nutritional screening tool for use in children and adolescents with juvenile rheumatoid arthritis. *J. Rheumatol.* In press, 1992.

Chapter 31
Children With Neoplastic Diseases (Cancer)

Karyl Rickard

Within the last decade, significant advances have been made both in treating children with neoplastic diseases and in providing proper nutrition support. Enlightened, quality nutrition care is now possible for children with cancer. An improved understanding of the significance and prevalence of protein-energy malnutrition (PEM) in such children has led to more attention to the staging and assessment of nutritional status and the efficacy and limitations of various options for nutrition support. Ethical considerations related to maximizing survival potential, assuring normal growth and development (physical, cognitive, and emotional), and assuring quality of life (e.g., energy and desire to play) require a positive and definitive stance toward nutrition care.

This chapter provides a brief review of childhood neoplasms and respective oncological treatment, as well as a more extensive discussion of factors to be considered in nutritional diagnosis or evaluation and nutritional management of children with cancer. Its intent is to provide a practical perspective gained from careful monitoring of patients on nutrition study protocols (more than 125 newly diagnosed patients). The approach to the nutritional care of children at James Whitcomb Riley Hospital for Children, Indianapolis, IN, has evolved over 13 years of cumulative experience through the collaborative efforts of a pediatric surgeon, pediatric dietitian, nurse clinician specialist, social worker, pharmacist, pedodontist, and the family of the child with cancer. Our approach to nutritional care of children with cancer has been described extensively in two previous publications[1,2] that form the basis for this chapter.

Pathological Abnormalities

Overview of oncological treatment of childhood neoplastic diseases

Childhood cancer, although an infrequent occurrence in absolute numbers, is the second most common cause of death in children older than 6 weeks of age. The overall incidence of neoplastic disease in children under the age of 15 is 12 per 100,000 population among white children and nine per 100,000 among black children.[3] The type and prognosis of malignancies in children differ from those seen in adults. Table 31–1 lists the most frequently occurring childhood tumor types. Approximately 50% of the cases of childhood cancer are leukemias and lymphomas. The remaining cases are other solid tumors.

The recent development of effective multimodal therapy protocols necessitates referral of children with cancer to specialized diagnostic and treatment centers. Since the frequency of each tumor type is relatively low at each pediatric

Table 31–1. Frequency of Tumor Types, by Site, for White and Black Children under 15 Years of Age in the United States

Site	White	Black
	←% of total→	
Leukemia	30.9	24.3
Acute lymphocytic leukemia (90%)*		
Acute nonlymphocytic leukemia (10%)*		
Central nervous system	18.3	21.6
Lymphomas	13.8	11.3
Hodgkin's lymphoma		
Non-Hodgkin's lymphoma		
Sympathetic nervous system	6.8	5.4
Neuroblastoma		
Soft tissue	6.2	8.6
Rhabdomyosarcoma		
Kidney	5.7	8.1
Wilms' tumor		
Bone	4.7	3.6
Osteosarcoma		
Ewing's sarcoma		
Eye	2.5	4.1
Retinoblastoma		
Germ cell	2.4	4.1
Liver	1.3	
Others	7.4	8.9
All sites	100.0	100.0

*Percent of childhood leukemias.
Adapted from Altman & Schwartz.[3]

cancer center, large cooperative groups have been established to evaluate treatment adequately. Currently, the Children's Cancer Study Group (CCSG) and Pediatric Oncology Group (POG) are the two major multi-institution groups involved in the study of pediatric cancer. The National Wilms' Tumor Study (NWTS) and Intergroup Rhabdomyosarcoma Study (IRS) are two of the largest intergroup studies for solid tumor malignancies.

Multi-institution protocols have rapidly improved treatment outcome of many malignancies over the past 15 to 20 years. Membership in CCSG, NWTS, and IRS has facilitated our evaluation of the efficacy of various nutrition regimens because treatment in each category of tumor is relatively uniform.

Proper treatment requires establishment of the tumor type (tissue diagnosis) and extent of dissemination (stage). Type of cancer and stage of disease determine the oncological treatment and nutrition support program. Treatment often includes operative procedures, irradiation, and chemotherapy.

In many instances of childhood cancer, initial treatment is curative because of an extraordinary response to multimodal treatment. Prognosis depends upon tumor histology, stage of disease, age of patient, certain laboratory indexes, and nutrition stage (nutritional status) at diagnosis.[4,7] Table 31–2 provides an example of the clinicopathological staging criteria and prognosis of two common pediatric solid tumors that are associated with PEM—Wilms' tumor and neuroblastoma.

Significance of protein-energy malnutrition

Nutritional status at the time of diagnosis of neoplastic disease has been clearly associated with treatment outcome in adults,[4,5] as well as in children.[6,7] This association may reflect an advanced disease state or may suggest that nutritional status at the beginning of treatment actually influences outcome. PEM is associated with impaired immune competence,[8-10] increased susceptibility to infections,[8-10] major organ dysfunctions,[11-13] and increased morbidity and mortality.[14,15] The organ systems most readily affected by PEM are the hematopoietic,[11,16-18] gastrointestinal,[13] and immunological systems.[8-10] Those organ systems are also the most sensitive to oncological treatment. One of the results of effective prevention or reversal of PEM is the maintenance or improvement of the function of those organ systems.

PEM in children with cancer has documented effects upon major organ functions, including immune competence, ability to resist infections, and bone marrow suppression. In an initial study[19] of children with newly diagnosed advanced solid tumors and relapsed leukemia-lymphoma, anergy was documented in 17 of 18 patients considered malnourished. Anergy was defined as the inability to respond to any one of four recall skin test antigens. Anergy was reversed with 28 days of central parenteral nutrition (CPN) support in approximately two-thirds of the patients (7 of 11 retested), despite continuing oncological treatment.

In a group of patients who received CPN, van Eys et al.[20] documented significantly higher rates of infectious complications in malnourished compared with nourished children with metastatic disease involving bone. Additionally, Hughes et al.[21,22] documented an association of *Pneumocystis carinii* with PEM (under weight for height, hypoalbuminemia) in children with cancer. Finally, current data suggest that bone marrow suppression may be attenuated by parenteral nutrition support in patients with stages III and IV neuroblastoma,[7,23] acute nonlymphocytic leukemia (ANLL),[24] and metastatic disease involving bone.[20] PEM may be also associated with lethargy, irritability, and lack of interest in playing, which affect the child's day-to-day quality of life.

Biochemical Abnormalities

Several biochemical abnormalities may be associated with either the diagnosis or treatment of cancer. These include low serum proteins (albumin, transferrin, prealbumin, and retinol-binding protein) that are associated with malnutrition, phosphate abnormalities associated with tumor lysis syndrome, and hypokalemia associated with amphotericin B. The incidence of PEM and factors that place a patient at a higher risk for the development of PEM are further discussed in the next section. Depending on the problem, biochemistry tests may be obtained to assess these parameters: electrolytes, zinc, magnesium, calcium, phosphorus, hemoglobin/hematocrit, and liver and kidney function.

Table 31–2. Examples of Clinicopathological Staging Criteria for Wilms' Tumor and Neuroblastoma and Associated Prognosis

	Wilms' tumor			Neuroblastoma	
Group	Criteria	2-Year survival	Stage	Criteria	2-Year survival
I.	Tumor limited to kidney and completely excised	95%	I.	Tumor confined to organ or structure of origin	84%
II.	Tumor extends beyond kidney but is completely excised	90%	II.	Tumor extends beyond organ of origin but not across midline. Regional lymph nodes may be involved on homolateral side.	65%
III.	Residual tumor confined to abdomen	84%	III.	Tumor extends beyond midline. Regional lymph nodes may be involved bilaterally.	33%
IV.	Tumor metastases beyond the abdomen to lung, liver, bone, and/or brain	54%	IV.	Tumor metastases involving skeletal, soft tissues, distant lymph nodes, liver, or skin	5%
			IV-S.	Patients who would otherwise be stage I or II but have remote disease confined only to one or more of the following sites: liver, skin, or bone marrow (without radiographic evidence of bone metastases on complete skeletal survey) in children less than 1 year of age	84%

*With or without disease. D'Angio et al.,[64] and Evans et al.[65]

Factors to be Considered in Nutritional Diagnosis or Evaluation

Childhood neoplasms at high risk for PEM

PEM is a common occurrence in certain high-risk populations of children with neoplastic diseases.[25] The incidence of PEM at diagnosis depends upon tumor type, stage of disease, and criteria for PEM.[26] It varies from 6% in children with newly diagnosed leukemia[27] to as high as 50% in children with newly diagnosed stage IV neuroblastoma.[7] Furthermore, PEM may occur during specific types of treatment.[19,23,28,29] The factors that place a patient at a higher risk for the development of PEM were determined from sequentially monitoring nutritional status indexes (Table 31–3) of children with newly diagnosed neoplastic diseases during initial phases of treatment.[19,23,28,29] Table 31–4 lists tumor types associated with high and low nutritional risk. Data from the M.D. Anderson Hospital and Tumor Institute, Houston, TX,[30] suggest that patients with newly diagnosed Ewings's sarcoma often are nutritionally depleted at diagnosis and that patients with soft tissue sarcomas and osteosarcomas are at high risk for nutritional depletion during the first 6 months of oncological treatment.

Some of the factors that contribute to high and low nutritional risk are understood. In general, patients with advanced disease during initial intense treatment[19,23,28] and those who relapse or do not respond to treatment[23,28] are most likely to develop PEM. Additionally, certain types of treatment promote the development of PEM; for example, major operative procedures of the abdomen[19,27]; irradiation to the head, neck, esophagus, abdomen, and pelvis[19,28]; or intense, frequent courses of chemotherapy (3 week intervals or less) in the absence of corticosteroids.[19,23,31] Finally, complications, such as pain, fever, and frequent or severe infections, decrease appetite and may increase energy requirements.

In the past, treatment of acute lymphocytic leukemia has not involved drugs with significant gastrointestinal toxicity. In addition, protocols often contained prolonged courses of corticosteroids, which stimulate the appetite when given longer than 1 week. In contrast, the treatment of acute nonlymphocytic leukemias uses drugs that have significant gastrointestinal toxicity, e.g., a 7-day infusion of cytosine arabinoside. Newer treatment protocols for acute lymphocytic leukemia with a poor prognosis now use drugs with significant gastrointestinal toxicity. Solid tumor protocols frequently use multiple drugs and abdominal irradiation, which have associated gastrointestinal toxicity, such as mouth sores, diarrhea, adynamic ileus, nausea, and vomiting.

A supportive health care team is essential for the patient's and the family's understanding and acceptance of the treatment program, including nutrition support. Knowledge of the specific oncological treatment protocol and the potential for success with various options for nutrition support is essential to provide effective long-term nutrition care.

Nutrition staging and assessment

Nutrition staging and assessment provide the cornerstones for recognizing the value of nutrition support in preventing depletion and sustaining growth and other nutrition functions and for determining an appropriate nutritional management strategy.

Identification of PEM (nutrition staging) at diagnosis. Criteria for staging patients as malnourished at diagnosis include greater than or equal to 5% weight loss, weight for height less than 5th percentile[32] when height is equal to or greater than 5th percentile for age,[32] or serum albumin less than 3.2 g/dL. When a patient does not meet any of those criteria, he or she is staged as *nourished*. In growing children, these criteria may be conservative estimates of true depletion. This is especially true in children with large abdominal masses since the tumor itself may weigh as much as 3% of the child's weight. Since changes in weight and weight for height are limited in specificity, serum albumin is used as a biochemical indicator of protein nutrition. The serum albumin concentration that the author uses as an indicator of PEM (3.2 mg/dL) is the lowest percentile of healthy children.[33] These criteria for PEM identify patients who are somewhat less malnourished than those identified by criteria used by other researchers (80% of the median weight/height percent).[6] A weight/height percent of less than 90 was suggested also as a criterion for an inadequate weight for height.[30] The weight/height percent is derived from this formula: Weight/height percent = patient's weight × 100 ÷ patient's height × S where S = median weight divided by median height of similar age and sex standards from a healthy population.

The significance of nutrition staging at diagnosis was emphasized in a study[7] of 18 of our children with newly diagnosed stage IV neuroblastoma. Although the number of malnourished and nourished patients was equal at diagnosis, significantly more malnourished patients relapsed or died by 180 days after treatment began ($P < 0.05$). The difference in survival between the two groups of patients approached significance ($P = 0.08$) at 1 year into treatment. The median survival of the malnourished group was 5 months compared with 12 months for the nourished group. It remains to be determined whether the patients considered to be malnourished at diagnosis had a more aggressive or advanced form of neuroblastoma or whether nutritional status influenced the outcome.

Ongoing nutrition assessment. The criteria for nutrition staging of patients at diagnosis may not be sensitive enough to detect ongoing depletion. Earlier indicators of nutritional depletion and repletion allows one to intervene in a timely fashion relative to the patient's treatment protocol and nutritional risk, thereby reducing the cost, complexity, and length of hospitalization associated with nutritional repletion.

Weights, heights, and weight-for-height measurements plotted sequentially on growth grids[32] are well-accepted tools for documenting the adequacy of children's growth. In children with cancer, care must be taken to avoid incorrect weight assessments that may occur secondary to edema, dehydration, or large fluid infusions given with certain drugs. Weight loss expressed as a percentage of body weight lost provides a more accurate estimate of the true significance of the weight lost in children. It should not be more than 5% body weight.

Skinfold measurements—triceps and subscapular—compared to nationally accepted norms[34] for healthy children

Table 31-3. Ongoing Nutrition Assessment Measurements That Identify Real or Impending Nutritional Depletion in Children with Cancer

Measurements	Risk criteria and interpretation	Comments
Nutrient intakes		
Energy (kcal/kg) % of healthy children	<80% of median intake: Low intake	Energy intakes calculated from records kept by trained parents or personnel and reviewed by a dietitian for completeness, explicitness, and use of acceptable measures
		Adjust for emesis: emesis within half-hour–do not include in calculations; emesis 1 to 2 hours after eating—calculate as half intake; emesis 3 to 4 hours later—calculate as all intake
		Energy intakes >80% of medium intake may be low when diarrhea occurs
Anthropometric		
Height		
Height for age	<5th percentile: growth stunting that may be due to chronic PEM.*	
Weight		
% change	>5% loss: acute PEM (with adequate hydration state)	Percentage weight loss derived from highest previous weight. Weight is inaccurate when child has edema, large tumor masses and organs extensively infiltrated with tumor, effusions or organ congestion, solid mass or excess fluid administration (twice maintenance) for chemotherapy.
Weight for age	<5th percentile: acute or chronic PEM.	Weight losses of >2% a day suggest dehydration
Weight for height	<5th percentile: acute PEM when height for age is <10th percentile[28]	
Skinfold thickness measurements		Steroid therapy may increase fat deposition. Measurements are inaccurate when child has edema or untrained, inexperienced or different personnel measure the same patient
Triceps	<10th percentile: depleted body fat stores.	
Subscapular	>0.3 mm decrease: subclinical PEM.†	
Arm muscle area	<10th percentile: severe acute PEM or chronic PEM	Measurements (skinfold thickness and arm muscle circumference from which arm muscle area is derived) are inaccurate when child has edema or untrained personnel measure the patient
Biochemical		
Albumin	<3.2 g/dL: acute or chronic PEM	Biological half-life of 14 days. May be decreased in presence of overhydration, severe liver dysfunction, or zinc deficiency
% change	>10% decrease#: subclinical PEM	
Transferrin	<200 mg/dL: subclinical PEM.	Biological half-life of 8 days. May be decreased in the presence of liver dysfunction; may be elevated in the presence of infection or iron deficiency.
% change	>20% decrease#: subclinical PEM	
Prealbumin	<20 mg/dL: subclinical PEM	Biological half-life of 2 days. May be decreased in the presence of severe liver dysfunction, vitamin A deficiency, or zinc deficiency; can be useful in assessing adequacy of nutrition support regimens.
% change	>20% decrease#: subclinical PEM	
Retinol-binding protein	<4 mg/dL: subclinical PEM	Biological half-life of 12 hours. May be elevated in the presence of renal failure; can be useful in assessing adequacy of nutrition support regimens.
% change	>20% decrease#: subclinical PEM	

*PEM = protein-energy malnutrition.
†More than twice coefficient of variation (method error) determined from 265 data sets of measurements obtained by two trained examiners.
‡Lowest percentile of healthy children.
#More than twice coefficient of variation.
Adapted from Rickard et al.[1]

Table 31–4. Types of Neoplastic Diseases Associated with High and Low Nutritional Risk

High Nutritional Risk
Advanced diseases during initial intense treatment
Stages III and IV Wilms' tumor and unfavorable histology
Wilms' tumor
Stages III and IV neuroblastoma
Pelvic rhabdomyosarcoma or Ewing's sarcoma
Some non-Hodgkin's lymphoma*
Acute nonlymphocytic leukemia
Some poor prognosis acute lymphocytic leukemias
Multiple relapse leukemia
Medulloblastoma

Low Nutritional Risk
Good prognosis acute lymphocytic leukemia
Nonmetastatic solid tumors
Advanced diseases in remission during maintenance treatment

*Tumor, the extent of which significantly impairs gastrointestinal function.

provide an estimate of fat reserves in children. Furthermore, changes in skinfold measurements, especially truncal measurements, are a valuable indicator of subtle, subclinical changes in nutritional status. The author found that subscapular skinfold decreases greater than 0.3 mm in children who initially had skinfold measurements in the normal range correlated with low energy intakes—more than two standard deviations below the mean of Beal's data for healthy children[35]. Changes greater than 0.3 mm were more than twice the coefficient of variation determined from 265 data sets of measurements obtained by two trained examiners.

In several children who had no evidence of edema, low energy intakes (more than two standard deviations below the mean of healthy children)[35] and decreases in subscapular skinfold measurements were the first indicators of nutritional depletion that occurred despite weight gain. This phenomenon is similar to that described in the classic study of Fomon et al.[36] of infants fed skim milk, which provided only 67% of their energy requirements. The infants as a group had significant decreases in triceps and subscapular skinfold measurements (approximately 25%), even though they gained weight at a slower rate than normal. Fomon et al.[36] hypothesized that the babies were mobilizing calorically dense fat stores to resynthesize fat-free tissues at a lower caloric cost.

For ongoing nutrition assessment, albumin is a useful indicator of protein nutrition[37-39] in some patients. We have found that decreases in albumin greater than twice method error (10% coefficient of variation) correspond to very low protein or energy intakes and may be observed before significant weight loss occurs. However, an adaptive phenomenon[40,41] that preserves concentrations at marginally low ranges of normal (2.9 to 3.2 g/dL) may occur during severe caloric restrictions. Transferrin, prealbumin, and retinol-binding proteins—serum proteins that have shorter half-lives and different synthetic rates than albumin[39]—may be useful indicators of subclinical PEM. (Table 31–3) Preliminary data from a recent study[42] support the use of prealbumin and retinol-binding protein as early indicators of successful repletion of PEM with parenteral nutrition.

Table 31–5 shows nutrition quality assurance criteria for children with cancer who are receiving conventional or phase III oncological treatment, for leukemias, lymphomas or solid tumors.[43] Children who are receiving bone marrow transplantation and end-stage disease management are not included in the target population for these criteria sets. The criteria were developed and field tested by the Quality Assurance Committee of the Dietitians in Pediatric Practice Group of the American Dietitic Association.[43] They provide useful guidelines for evaluating both the process of providing nutritional care and the nutritional outcome of children with cancer.

Dietary Management

A position paper[44] from the American Academy of Pediatrics provides an authoritative review of various options, including enteral and parenteral nutrition, for nutrition management of children with malignancies. The benefits and limitations of both methods of nutrition support were reviewed by Rickard et al.[45] and by the Task Force on the Special Needs of Children with Malignancies from the American Academy of Pediatrics.[44] In addition, ASPEN has recently developed guidelines for the nutritional support of children with cancer.[46]

Enteral nutrition

Several modes of nutrition support are available for the pediatric patient. Enteral nutrition, defined as the provision of nutrients to the gastrointestinal tract with volitional oral feedings, is the preferred method of feeding children with cancer who are at low nutritional risk. Our comprehensive enteral nutrition program consists of an individualized feeding program that uses the child's favorite nutritious foods during treatment-free periods to prevent aversive conditioning associated with nausea and vomiting[47] and liquid nutritional supplements taken voluntarily. Delicious, high-nutrient density recipes popular with children and educational cooking projects[48,49] encourage eating in a positive and fun way. Vitamin supplements are given only when patients are unable to consume adequate nutrients through foods; iron supplements are given only for documented iron-deficiency anemia. The impact of aversive conditioning in children receiving chemotherapy may be reduced by using a strongly flavored candy, such as rootbeer Life Savers®, as a scapegoat when given between the consumption of a meal and administration of chemotherapy. The strong flavored candy is considered the cause of nausea and vomiting and thus the child does not avoid more nutritious favorite foods.[50]

Enteral nutrition has numerous practical and psychological advantages over parenteral nutrition, including a lower risk of infection or other catheter-related complications, and enabling more normal play activities and a life style that provides a positive way for the parent and child to be involved in the child's care. In addition, enteral feeding is more economical.

High nutritional risk patients. In our experience, enteral feeding programs have not been effective in either preventing or reversing PEM in most high-risk children during initial, intense treatment. In a study of 21 children with advanced cancer who received a comprehensive enteral nu-

Table 31–5. Nutrition Quality Assurance Criteria for Children with Cancer who are being Treated with Conventional or Phase III Oncologic Treatment for Leukemias, Lymphomas, or Solid Tumors Excluding Patients who are Undergoing Bone Marrow Transplantation and End-Stage Disease Management

Criteria*	Critical time	Exceptions
(P) 1. Nutrition screening completed according to established protocol.	Duration of treatment	
(P) 2. Nutrition assessment completed according to established protocol.	Duration of treatment	
(P) 3. Patient maintains weight/height between the 5th and 95th percentiles according to National Center for Health Statistics (NCHS) growth charts or detailed tables.	Duration of treatment	Initial obesity; chronic sepsis; fluid shifts during critical care period; prolonged high-dose steroid treatment
(O) 4. Patient does not lose > 5% body weight.	Duration of treatment	Initial obesity; chronic sepsis
(O) 5. Patient maintains serum albumin level according to established protocol.	Duration of treatment	Chronic sepsis; extensive hepatic tumor involvement; other extensive hepatic disease (eg, fungal abscesses); critically ill patients with fluid shifts or other nonnutrition-related explanation for depressed serum albumin level
(P) 6. Estimates of patient's fat reserves and/or lean body mass documented according to established protocol.	Duration of treatment	Well-nourished patients at low risk for malnutrition
(P) 7. Nutrition care plan developed, based on assessment data according to established protocol.	Within 24 h of completion of nutrition assessment	Well-nourished patients at low risk for malnutrition
(P) 8. Nutrition care plan implemented as written or revised.	Duration of therapy	
(O) 9. Patient/caregiver can state rationale for nutrition care plan.	When nutrition care plan implemented or revised	Well-nourished patients at low risk for malnutrition
(P) 10. Patient referred to home nutrition support and/or food/nutrition resources, based on identified patient needs.	Within 1 wk of need identification	Well-nourished patients at low risk for malnutrition

*P, process; O, outcome.
Adapted from Burgess.[43]

trition program,[19] energy intake averaged only 48% ± 24% of the Recommended Dietary Allowance (RDA), and weight loss averaged 16% in less than a month of treatment.[51] Nutritional depletion was most dramatic in nine of the children with advanced Wilms' tumor, whose average weight loss was 22% in 26 ± 17 days of treatment.

Likewise, a recent study of 32 children with stages III or IV neuroblastoma[23] documented significant loss of fat reserves and weight during the initial 4 weeks of treatment when enteral nutrition alone was provided. Energy intakes of the children with neuroblastoma were low (less than two standard deviations below the mean of healthy children[35]) for 10 to 21 days between chemotherapy courses given at the beginning of weeks 1 and 4. Children with neuroblastoma who became malnourished were unable to make nutritional gains thereafter, despite numerous delays in treatment.[23]

Low nutritional risk patients. Enteral nutrition is generally effective in low nutritional risk groups unless complicating factors, such as relapse, sepsis, or major abdominal procedures, occur. Those findings were documented[28,29] in children with Wilms' tumor in remission who were successfully past the first 40- to 60-day high nutritional risk portion of their oncological treatment and were into maintenance treatment. During maintenance treatment (3 to 15 months after diagnosis), a comprehensive enteral nutrition program maintained appropriate weights for heights[32] and skinfold thickness measurements,[34] despite continuing 5-day cycles of chemotherapeutic treatment.

Nutrient intakes, weights, and skinfold thicknesses were significantly lower during the 5-day periods of chemotherapy.[1,52] Energy intakes were less than those for the 10th percentile of healthy children,[35] and intakes of other nutrients were less than 66% of the RDAs for most of the children. The nutrient intakes improved within 1 to 2 weeks after chemotherapy.[1,52] Apparently, the length of time between treatment was adequate to allow recovery from those short periods of nutritional depletion. During the 5 days before chemotherapy, energy intakes were greater than the 50th percentile for the majority of the patients and greater than the 90th percentile for a third of the children.[1,52] Intakes of other nutrients were also adequate before chemotherapy.[1,52] Calcium and iron intakes were low 20% to 25% of the time before chemotherapy, but were not consistently low for any single patient.[1,52] The data emphasize the changing nature of nutrient intakes of young children relative to oncological treatment and suggest a continuing need for nutrition counseling and positive reinforcement throughout treatment, which may last several years.

Data from Carter et al.[53] of 277 pediatric cancer patients suggest that energy and iron intakes were lower than the RDAs (75% to 80% and 70% to 78%, respectively) at diagnosis and at 6 months into treatment, although the intakes were not different from those of healthy children reported in the NHANES survey. In the Carter et al. study,[53] the effect of specific oncological treatment regimens upon enteral (ad libitum) nutrient intake was not evaluated.

It generally has been assumed that PEM could be reversed with nutritional counseling and oral foods in children with stage I disease who received treatment considered to be associated with a low nutritional risk. Recent data,[29] however, suggest that an enteral nutrition program is not effective initially in reversing PEM, even in children with less advanced solid tumors. Children with stage I Wilms' tumor who were considered malnourished at diagnosis had further nutritional depletion during the first month of treatment that included operative removal of the tumor and chemotherapy.[29] Subsequently, an enteral nutrition program was successful in reversing the PEM, i.e., nutritional status improved throughout the next 5 months of treatment. Thus, children with stage I Wilms' tumor may benefit from parenteral nutrition support during the first 7 to 10 days of treatment and thereafter may be successfully managed with enteral nutrition.

Oral supplements. Oral supplements were tried in every patient as part of our comprehensive enteral nutrition program.[19,23,28] Milk base, soy base, and other liquid oral supplements were used to provide every possible ad libitum option for improving the effectiveness of enteral nutrition. We found that the children who had a reduced intake and therefore the highest need for supplements were the least likely to accept them. Furthermore, when patients were in the low nutritional risk portions of their treatment program, they were less interested in using supplements than in eating favorite nutritious foods. The choice of foods preferred during treatment-free periods often changes, possibly because of taste changes associated with treatment[51,54] or the changing nature of healthy young children's likes and dislikes. We have noticed that children request more salty or spicy foods, such as salted nuts, pretzels, chips, spaghetti sauce, ravioli, pizza, and tuna, during the most intense treatment.

The contribution made by supplements to the energy intake during the first 22 weeks of treatment of 10 children with newly diagnosed neuroblastoma has been documented.[1,31] The average percentage of energy intake provided by supplements before, during, and after chemotherapy for all 10 patients was only 10%, 18%, and 15%, respectively. Only five children consumed a supplement for more than 4 days; three of them were older infants or young toddlers who drank from a bottle and obtained as much as 30% of their energy intakes from supplements either during or immediately after chemotherapy. Thus, supplements to drink may be valuable in select subpopulations of children during certain periods of low intake.

Nasogastric tube feeding

Nasogastric tube feedings of infant formulas or meal replacement formulations are appropriate when the infant or child is unable to take adequate nutrition voluntarily, but has a functional gastrointestinal tract. In general, the use of nasogastric tube feedings is more prevalent in children with nononcological disorders. Reasons for the lower usage in cancer patients include concerns regarding the trauma associated with passing catheters in patients who may be thrombocytopenic, concerns about infectious complications in neutropenic patients, and difficulties in acceptance of this procedure by parents and children who frequently have multiple other invasive procedures. If utilized, this route would be most appropriate for younger infants or children old enough to cooperate who have minimal gastrointestinal symptoms from the oncological treatment and have adequate platelet counts. Some older children may be taught to pass their own nasogastric tube for intermittent or continuous nighttime feedings at home.

Nutritionally complete formulas that contain protein, carbohydrate, and fat in a high molecular weight form have a relatively low osmolality and residue and are appropriate for patients with normal digestive function. Elemental formulas that contain amino acids or peptides as the protein source, oligosaccharides or monosaccharides as the carbohydrate source, and either a lower fat content or medium-chain triglycerides as a portion of the fat source are an appropriate choice for patients with abnormal digestive function. A gastrostomy or a jejunostomy may be appropriate for a few selected patients, such as those with head and neck neoplasms.

Parenteral nutrition

Nutritional and immunological benefits. Parenteral nutrition is both safe[29,55,56] and effective in children with advanced neoplastic diseases. The effectiveness of central parenteral nutrition (CPN) in reversing PEM and restoring immunity was documented in a group of 18 of our malnourished patients who had stage III or IV solid tumors or second relapse leukemia-lymphoma.[19] These patients received CPN for a mean of 24 days (average caloric intake of 90% of the RDA during weight gain). Initially, patients were randomized to either 10 days or 28 days CPN. The 10-day randomization was abandoned after three of the patients rapidly returned to their initial malnourished state because of continuing oncological treatment. Review of data[19] from patients who received shorter (9 to 14 days) or longer intervals (28 or more days) of parenteral nutrition indicated that shorter intervals did not restore an appropriate weight for height and fat reserves or normalize albumin concentrations (greater than or equal to 3.2 g/dL). An improvement in transferrin concentration at 9 to 14 days suggested that transferrin was more responsive than albumin. Another short-term benefit was a significant improvement in the child's general state of well-being. Twenty-eight days of CPN normalized weight-for-height percentiles, subscapular skinfold percentiles, and albumin and transferrin concentrations.

Curtailment of parenteral nutrition support before reversal of PEM and completion of intensive oncological support reduced the benefits of previous nutrition support. Therefore, parenteral nutrition support is continued for several days beyond the cessation of chemotherapy or irradiation treatment, which induces anorexia, nausea, and vomiting. Adequate reversal of PEM is defined as a weight that is 1 kg greater than the 50th percentile weight for the child's height,[32] subscapular skinfold measurements greater than the 10th percentile (less than or equal to 2 years[57]; greater than 2 years[34]), and serum albumin concentrations equal to or greater than 3.2 g/dL. The weight gain objective allows for fluid readjustment and adaptation to eating at the cessation of parenteral fluid administration. Nutritional benefits from effective parenteral nutrition support are maintained after completion of the intense treatment unless complicating factors, such as relapse, sepsis, or major abdominal procedures, occur in the patient's clinical course.[23,28]

The effectiveness of parenteral nutrition provided by either central venous catheters or via peripheral veins has been studied in malnourished children with advanced neuroblastoma or Wilms' tumor. An initial report[56] documented the fact that both routes effectively reversed PEM (significant and similar increases in anthropometric measurements and albumin) when adequate energy and protein were provided over a 21- to 28-day period. The effectiveness of peripheral parenteral nutrition (PPN) was dependent upon an oral intake of calories that provided an average of 25% additional energy to meet the RDA. Although both routes effectively reversed PEM, PPN was associated with significant psychological trauma related to the repeated venipunctures that were necessary to replace the intravenous catheters. The incidences of anemia, fever episodes (with and without documented sepsis), and mildly elevated serum glutamic oxalic transaminase (SGOT) concentrations were similar for both groups. In subsequent reports,[29,58] PPN was not as effective in reversing PEM in children with advanced Wilms' tumor because of the children's inability to tolerate oral foods during the period of abdominal irradiation and their potentially higher energy requirements that could not be provided with

PPN. This finding was substantiated by a significantly higher weight, arm muscle area, and serum retinol-binding protein in the CPN than in the PPN group of patients. These data suggest that CPN is preferable for long-term support (more than 7 days) and that PPN is preferable as a temporary substitute for CPN. When PPN is used as a temporary substitute for CPN, it is important to provide a nutrient mixture that includes glucose, amino acids, and the energy-dense fat component to meet the total energy needs within the fluid limitations and to meet even higher energy needs in the presence of fever.

Treatment Tolerance Benefits. Treatment tolerance benefits from parenteral nutrition compared with oral nutrition were documented in several recent prospective randomized studies of children with specific tumors. In our initial report[7] of 17 patients with stage IV neuroblastoma, those with a favorable nutrition course during the first 21 days of therapy had significantly fewer treatment delays and fewer drug dose reductions throughout the first 10 weeks of treatment. Treatment delays were secondary to absolute granulocyte counts less than or equal to 1000/ul or platelets less than or equal to 75,000/ul. Treatment consisted of 5-day cycles of dimethyl-triaminoimidazole-carboxamide (DTIC), vincristine, and cyclophosphamide given at 3-week intervals. The treatment tolerance benefits from effective reversal or prevention of PEM were further documented in 32 patients with stages III and IV neuroblastoma.[23]

Three other prospective randomized studies of children with cancer also documented benefits from CPN in comparison with oral nutrition in improving tolerance to chemotherapy (35 children with metastatic disease involving bone),[20] in improving adherence to chemotherapy schedules (25 children who received abdominal irradiation),[59] or in accelerating recovery of normal marrow function (10 children with acute nonlymphocytic leukemia).[24] In contrast to those findings, Shamberger et al.[60] failed to document benefit from CPN in comparison with oral nutrition in improving recovery from bone marrow suppression in a series of 27 patients who received extremely aggressive treatment for poor-prognosis sarcomas. Patients in that study[60] included older teenagers and young adults (median age, 17; range, 11 to 33 years). In a multi-institutional study[61] of 25 children who received abdominal irradiation, the CPN and oral nutrition groups of patients did not differ in their ability to adhere to the radiotherapy schedule or in irradiation toxicities. Thus, the value of CPN in improving treatment tolerance is directly related to the type and stage of tumor, specific treatment, and adequacy of nutrition support.

Complications and limitations.   Complications can be minimized or controlled safely with careful patient management and adherence to a parenteral nutrition protocol.[62] Mullen[63] reported data from a multi-institutional study of complications of adults with cancer randomized to either CPN (125 patients) or control groups (126 patients). The CPN group had an increased incidence of fever ($P < 0.003$), anemia ($P < 0.09$), and pulmonary dysfunction ($P < 0.12$). However, both groups had a similar incidence of documented infections (25%) at distant sites.

A randomized prospective cooperative study[55] of 64 children with neoplastic diseases confirmed also that complications (except for fever) that might be attributed to CPN were seen in both CPN and control groups. Approximately 25% of our patients with newly diagnosed, advanced solid tumors [56] had major medical problems or complications during initial intense treatment that limited their fluid and nutrient intake. Those complications, which were unrelated to CPN, limited our ability to provide adequate parenteral nutrition support.

The possibility that CPN in excess of host repletion stimulates tumor growth needs to be considered, although clinically that has not been observed when aggressive oncological treatment is given simultaneously. In fact, CPN may beneficially stimulate cell replication and increase the effectiveness of cell-cycle-specific drugs. However, nutrition support is not oncological treatment,[71] and the effectiveness of primary oncological treatment far outweighs other supportive factors as a determinant of ultimate survival.

Follow-up

The benefits of nutrition support are inherently important independent of their potential benefit related to improved survival. Proper nutrition support in children with cancer has value in improving growth and organ system function (e.g., immunological, hematopoetic, and gastrointestinal) and appears to have value in improving treatment tolerance. Nutrition support also facilitates the treatment of the "whole" child, including enhancing the day-to-day quality of life, e.g., energy to facilitate playing. Parents welcome help in "living" with cancer and in providing adequate nutrition support.

References

1. Rickard, K.A., Grosfeld, J.L., Coates, T.D., Weetman, R.M., Baehner, R.L. Advances in nutrition care of children with neoplastic disease: a review of treatment, research and application. J. Am. Diet. Assoc. 1986; 86:1666.
2. Detamore, C.D., Rickard, K.A., Jaeger, B.J. Planning and implementing a nutrition program for children with cancer. Topics Clin. Nutr. 1986; 1:71.
3. Altman, A.J., Schwartz, A.D. Malignant Diseases of Infancy, Childhood and Adolescence. 2nd ed., Philadelphia: W.B. Saunders; 1983.
4. DeWys, W.D., Begg, C., Lavin, P.T., Band, P.R., Bennett, J.M., Bertino, J.R., Cohen, M.H., Douglass, H.O., Engstrom, P.F., Exdinli, E.Z., Horton, J., Johnson, G.J., Moertel, G.G., Oken, M.M., Perlia, C., Rosenbaum, C., Silverstein, M.N., Skeel, R.T., Sponzo, R.W., Tormey, D.C. Prognostic effect of weight loss prior to chemotherapy in cancer patients. Am. J. Med. 1980; 60:491.
5. Freeman, M., Frankmann, C., Beck, J., Valdiviesco, M. Prognostic nutrition factors in lung cancer patients. JPEN. 1982; 6:122.
6. Donaldson, S.S., Wesley, M.N., DeWys, W.D., Suskind, R.M., Jaffee, N., van Eys, J. A study of the nutritional status of pediatric cancer patients. Am. J. Dis. Child. 1981; 135:1107.
7. Rickard, K.A., Detamore, C.M., Coates, T.D., Grosfeld, J.L., Weetman, R.M., White, N.M., Provisor, A.J., Boxer, L.A., Loghmani, E.S., Oei, T.O., Yu, P., Baehner, R.L. Effect of nutrition staging on treatment delays and outcome in stage IV neuroblastoma. Cancer. 1983; 52:587.
8. Scrimshaw, N.S. Interactions of malnutrition and infection: advances in understanding. In: Olson, R.E., ed. Protein-Calorie Malnutrition. New York: Academic Press; 1975.
9. Edelman, R. Cell-mediated immune response in protein calorie malnutrition: a review. In: Suskind, R.M., ed., Malnu-

trition and the Immune Response. New York: Raven Press; 1977.
10. Chandra, R.K. Interaction of nutrition, infection and immune response: immunocompetence in nutritional deficiency, methodological considerations and intervention strategies. Acta Paediatr. Scand. 1979; 68:137.
11. Keys, A., Brozek, J., Henschel, A., Mickelsen, O., Taylor, H.L. The Biology of Human Starvation. Vols. 1 and 2. Minneapolis: University of Minnesota Press; 1950.
12. Gardner, L.I., Amacher, P., eds. Endocrine Aspects of Malnutrition, Santa Ynez, CA: Kroc Foundation; 1973.
13. Viteri, F.E., Schneider R.E. Gastrointestinal alterations in protein-calorie malnutrition. Med. Clin. North Am. 1974; 58:1487.
14. Obi, J.O. Morbidity and mortality of children under five years old in a Nigerian hospital. JAMA. 1979; 71:245.
15. Chen, L.C., Chowdhury, A., Huffman, S.L. Anthropometric assessment of energy protein malnutrition and subsequent risk of mortality among preschool aged children. Am. J. Clin. Nutr. 1980; 33:1836.
16. Finch, G.A. Erthropoieses in protein-calorie malnutrition. In: Olson, R.E., ed., Protein-Calorie Malnutrition. New York: Academic Press; 1975.
17. Viart, B. Blood volume (51Cr) in severe protein-calorie malnutrition. Am. J. Clin. Nutr., 1976; 29:25.
18. Vilter, R.W. The anemia of protein-calorie malnutrition. In: Olson, R.E., ed. Protein-Calorie Malnutrition. New York: Academic Press; 1975.
19. Rickard, K.A., Grosfeld, J.L., Kirksey, A., Ballantine, T.V.N., Baehner, R.L. Reversal of protein-energy malnutrition in children with advanced neoplastic disease. Ann. Surg. 1979; 190:771.
20. Van Eys, J., Copeland, E.M., Cangir, A., Taylor, G., Teitell-Cohen, B., Carter, P., Ortiz, C. A clinical trial of hyperalimentation in children with metastatic malignancies. Med. Pediatr. Oncol. 1980; 8:63.
21. Hughes, W.T., Price, R.A., Sisko, F., Havron, W.S., Kafatof, A.G., Schonland, M., Smythe, P.M. Protein-calorie malnutrition: a host determinant for Pneumocystis carinii infection. Am. J. Dis. Child. 1974; 128:44.
22. Hughes, W.T., Sanyal, S.K., Price, R.A. Signs, symptoms and pathophysiology of Pneumocystis carinii. Pneumonitis. Natl. Cancer Inst. Monogr. 1976; 43:77.
23. Rickard, K.A., Loghmani, E.S., Grosfeld, J.L., Detamore, C.M., White, N.M., Foland, B.B., Coates, T.D., Yu, P., Weetman, R.M., Provisor, A.J., Oei, T.O., Baehner, R.L. Short-and long-term effectiveness of enteral and parenteral nutrition in reversing protein energy malnutrition in advanced neuroblastoma. A prospective randomized study. Cancer. 1985; 56:2881.
24. Hays, D.M., Merritt, R.J., Ashley, J., White, L., Siegel, S.E. Effect of total parenteral nutrition on marrow recovery during induction therapy for acute nonlymphocytic leukemia in childhood. Med. Pediatr. Oncol. 1983; 11:134.
25. Smith, D.E., Stevens, M.C.G., Booth, I.W. Malnutrition at diagnosis of malignancy in childhood: common but mostly missed. Eur. J. Pediatr. 1991; 150:318.
26. Rickard, K.A., Baehner, R.L., Coates, T.D., Weetman, R.M., Provisor, A.J., Grosfeld, J.L. Supportive nutritional intervention. Cancer Res. 1982; 42(suppl):766.
27. Ramirez, I., van Eys, J., Carr, D., Arter, P., Coody, D., Taylor, G. Malnutrition in children with malignancies. Proc. Am. Assoc. Cancer Res. 1980; 21:378.
28. Rickard, K.A., Kirksey, A., Baehner, R.L., Provisor, A.J., Weetman, R.M., Ballantine, T.V.N., Grosfeld, J.L. Effectiveness of enteral and parenteral nutritional in the nutritional management of children with Wilms' tumor. Am. J. Clin. Nutr., 1980; 33:2622.
29. Rickard, K.A., Godshall, B.J., Loghmani, E.S., Becker, M.C., Grosfeld, J.L., Weetman, R.M., Coates, T.D., Lingard, C.D., White, N.M., Foland, B.B. Integration of nutrition support into oncologic treatment protocols for high and low nutritional risk children with Wilms' tumor: a prospective randomized study. Cancer. 1989; 64:491.
30. Carter, P., Carr, D., van Eys, J., Coody, D. Nutritional parameters in children with cancer. J. Am. Diet. Assoc. 1983; 82:616.

31. Detamore, C.M. Nutrition regimens for children with advanced neuroblastoma. Bloomington, In: *M.S. Thesis*, Indiana University School of Medicine; 1981. Thesis.

32. Hamill, P.V., Drizd, T.A., Johnson, C.L.: NCHS growth curves for children birth to 18 years, United States. *Vital and Health Statistics. Series II. Data from the National Health Survey*. No. 165. Washington, DC: Government Printing Office; 1977. VS DHEW Publication 78-1650.

33. Trevorrow, V.E. Serum proteins. In: McCammon, R.W., ed., *Human Growth and Development*. Springfield, IL: Charles C. Thomas; 1970.

34. Owen, G.M. Measurement, recording, and assessment of skinfold thickness in childhood and adolescence: report of a small meeting. *Am. J. Clin. Nutr.* 1982; 35:629.

35. Beal, V.A. Nutritional intake. In: McCammon, R.W., ed., *Human Growth and Development*. Springfield, IL: Charles C. Thomas; 1970.

36. Fomon, S.J., Filer, L.J., Ziegler, E.E., Bergmann, K.E., Bergmann, R.L. Skim milk in infant feeding. *Acta Paediatr. Scand.* 1977; 66:17.

37. Hoffenberg, R., Black, E., Brock, J.F. Albumin and β-globulin tracer studies in protein depletion states. *J. Clin. Invest.* 1966; 45:143.

38. Stead, R.H., Brock, J.F. Experimental protein-calorie malnutrition: rapid induction of protein depletion signs in early-weaned rats. *J. Nutr.* 1972; 102:1357.

39. Olson, R.E. The effect of variations in protein and calorie intake on rate of recovery and selected physiological responses in Thai children with protein-calorie malnutrition. In: Olson, R.E., ed. *Protein-Calorie Malnutrition*. New York: Academic Press; 1975.

40. James, W.P., Hay, A.M. Albumin metabolism: effect of the nutritional state and the dietary protein intake. *J. Clin. Invest.* 1969; 47:1958.

41. Waterlow, J.C. Adaptation to low-protein intakes. In: Bianchi, R., Mariani, G., McFarlane, A.S., eds. *Plasma Protein Turnover*. London: Macmillan; 1976.

42. Rickard, K.A., Foland, B.B., Grosfeld, J.L., Loghmani, E.S., Yu, P., Detamore, C.M., Coates, T.D., Weetman, R.M., Provisor, A.J., Oei, T.O., Baehner, R.L.: Prealbumin and retinol-binding protein: early biochemical indicators of nutritional repletion in children with neuroblastoma or Wilms' tumor. *Fed. Proc.* 1984; 43:468.

43. Burgess, J. Oncology patients, age 0 to 18 years. In: Woolridge, N.H., ed. *Quality Assurance Criteria for Pediatric Nutrition Conditions: A Model*. Chicago: American Dietetic Association; 1988.

44. Mauer, A.M., Burgess, J.B., Donaldson, S.S., Rickard, K.A., Stallings, V.A., van Eys, J., Winick, M. Special nutritional needs of children with malignancies: a review. *JPEN*. 1990; 14:315.

45. Rickard, K.A., Coates, T.D., Grosfeld, J.L., Weetman, R.M., Baehner, R.L. The value of nutrition support in children with cancer. *Cancer*. 1986; 58:1904.

46. Klein, G., Farrell, M., Gottschlich, M., Rickard, K., Schandler, R. *Pediatric Clinical Guidelines, American Society Parenteral and Enteral Nutrition*. Rockville: Aspen, in press.

47. Berstein, I.L. Learned taste aversions in children receiving chemotherapy. *Science*. 1978; 200:1302.

48. Rickard, K., Farnum, S. Food for fun and thought: nutrition education in a children's hospital. *J. Am. Diet. Assoc.* 1974; 65:294.

49. Dixon, G., Rickard, K.A. Nutrition education for young patients. *Child. Today*. 1975; 4:7.

50. Broberg, D.J., Bernstein, I.L. Candy as a scapegoat in the prevention of food aversions in children receiving chemotherapy. *Cancer*. 1987; 60:2344.

51. Food and Nutrition Board. *Recommended Dietary Allowances*. 10th rev. ed. Washington DC: National Academy of Sciences; 1989.

52. White, N.M. Nutritional management of children with neuroblastoma and Wilms' tumors. Bloomington, IN: Indiana University School of Medicine; 1979. Thesis.

53. Carter, P., Carr, D., van Eys, J., Ramirez, I., Coody, D., Taylor, G. Energy and nutrient intake of children with cancer. *J. Am. Diet. Assoc.* 1983; 82:610.

54. DeWys, W.D. Changes in taste sensation and feeding behavior in cancer patients. A review. *J. Hum. Nutr.* 1978; 32:447.

55. Van Eys, J., Wesley, M.N., Cangir, A., Copeland, E.M. Donaldson, S.S., Ghavimi, F., Shils, M., Suskind, R., Jaffe, N., Filler, R. Safety of intravenous hyperalimentation in children with malignancies: a cooperative group trial. *JPEN*. 1982; 6:291.

56. Rickard, K.A., Foland, B.B., Detamore, C.M., Coates, T.D., Grosfeld, J.L., White, N.M., Weetman, R.M., Provisor, A.J., Loghmani, E.S., Oei, T.O., Yu, P., Baehner, R.L. Effectiveness of central parenteral nutrition vs. peripheral parenteral nutrition plus enteral nutrition in reversing PEM in children with advanced neuroblastoma and Wilms' tumor: a prospective randomized study. *Am. J. Clin. Nutr.* 1983; 38:445.

57. Karlberg, P., Taranger, J., Engstrom, E., Lichtenstein, H., Svenbergreden, I. The somatic development of children in a Swedish urban community. *Acta Paediatr. Scand.* 1976; 258(suppl):1.

58. Rickard, K.A., Becker, M.C., Loghmani, E.S., Godshall, B.J., Grosfeld, J.L., Weetman, R.M., Coates, T.D., Lingard, C.D., White, N.M., Foland, B.B. Effectiveness of two methods of parenteral nutrition support in improving muscle mass of children with neuroblastoma or Wilms' tumor: a randomized study. *Cancer*. 1989; 64:116.

59. Ghavimi, R., Shils, M.E., Scott, B.F., Brown, M., Tamaroff, M. Comparison of morbidity in children requiring abdominal radiation and chemotherapy with and without total parenteral nutrition. *J. Pediatr.* 1982; 101:530.

60. Shamberger, R.D., Pizzo, P.A., Goodgame, J.T., Lowry, S.F., Maher, M.M., Wesley, R.A., Brennan, M.F. The effect of total parenteral nutrition on chemotherapy-induced myelosuppression. *Am. J. Med.* 1983; 74:40.

61. Donaldson, S.S., Wesley, M.N., Ghavimi, F., Shils, M.E., Suskind, R.M., DeWys, W.D. A prospective randomized clinical trial of total parenteral nutrition in children with cancer. *Med. Pediatr. Oncol.* 1982; 10:129.

62. Kerner, J.A., ed. *Manual of Pediatric Parenteral Nutrition*. New York: Wiley; 1983.

63. Mullen, J. Complications of total parenteral nutrition in the cancer patient. *Cancer Treat. Rep.* 1981; 65(suppl 5):107.

64. D'Angio, G.J., Evans, A., Breslow, N., Beckwith, B., Bishop, H., Farewell, V., Goodwin, W., Leape, L., Palmer, N., Sinks, L., Sutow, W., Tefft, M., Wolff, J. The treatment of Wilms' tumor: results of the second national Wilms' tumor study. *Cancer*. 1981; 44:2302.

65. Evans, A.E., D'Angio, G.J., Randolph, J. A proposed staging for children with neuroblastoma. *Cancer*. 1971; 27:374.

66. Frisancho, A.R. New norms of upper limb fat and muscle areas for assessment for nutritional status. *Am. J. Clin. Nutr.* 1981; 34:2540.

67. Rickard, K.A., Matchett, N., Ballantine, T.V.N., Kirksey, A., Grosfeld, J.L., Baehner, R.L. Serum transferrin: an early indicator of nutritional status in children with advanced cancer. *Surg. Forum.* 1979; 30:78.

68. Ingenbleek, I., De Visscher, M., De Nayer, P.H. Measurements of prealbumin as index of protein-calorie malnutrition. *Lancet*. 1972; 1:106.

69. Ogunshina, S.O., Hussain, M.A. Plasma thyroxine binding prealbumin as an index of mild protein-energy malnutrition in Nigerian children. *Am. J. Clin. Nutr.* 1980; 33:794.

70. Ingenbleek, Y., Van Den Schrieck, H.G., De Nayer, P.H., De Visscher, M. The role of retinol-binding protein in protein-calorie malnutrition. *Metabolism*. 1975; 24:633.

71. Holcomb, G.W., Ziegler, M.M. Nutrition and cancer in children. *Surg. Annu.* 1990; 22:129.

Chapter 32
Children With Chronic Congenital Heart Disease and Renal Disease

Alison Hull

Congenital Heart Disease

The prevalence of congenital heart disease (CHD) in the general population is 8 per 1000 live births, or approximately 1%, not including the heart disease associated with premature infants.[1] Congenital heart disease accounts for 12% of all congenital anomalies.[2] It has a hereditary component; the incidence (not risk) increases to 3% with one first-degree relative (parent or sibling) affected, to 9% with two affected relatives, and to 50% with three affected first-degree relatives.[1] Of the 1% of all live births with congenital heart disease, half have ventricular septal defect (VSD), and half have a combination of other abnormalities.

Many genetic syndromes and inborn errors of metabolism are also associated with congenital cardiovascular malformations. For example, over 50% of individuals with Down's syndrome have congenital heart disease.[1] Tables 32-1 and 32-2 illustrate the relationship between disease syndromes and various cardiac abnormalities. Substances ingested during pregnancy may act as cardiovascular teratogens (Table 32-3). Most teratogenic agents require an interaction with a genetic predisposition toward malformation in order to have an effect upon the heart. The majority of cardiovascular malformation cases are still best explained by a combination of multifactorial inheritance patterns and environmental triggers.

Table 32–1. Congenital Heart Diseases in Selected Chromosomal Aberrations

Population	Incidence of CHD (%)
General population	1
Trisomy 21	50
Trisomy 18	99 +
Trisomy 13	90
Trisomy 22	67
Partial trisomy 22	40
4p-	Approximately 40
5p- (Cri-du-chat)	Approximately 20
Trisomy 8 (mosaic)	Approximately 50
Trixomy 9 (mosaic)	≥ 50
13q-	Approximately 25
+14q-	≥ 50
18q-	≤ 50
XO Turner	35
XXXXY	14

Adapted from Nora J., Nora A. The evolution of specific genetic and environmental counseling in congenital heart diseases. *Circulation.* 1978; 57:2. Used with permission.

Heart disease in children may be categorized as *cyanotic* (hypoxic), such as tetralogy of Fallot, pulmonary atresia, and transposition of the great arteries (TGA), or as *acyanotic*, e.g., patent ductus arteriosis, ventricular septal defect (VSD), aortic stenosis, and coarctation of the aorta. As a general rule, patients with cyanotic or hypoxic heart disease are more severely growth retarded than patients with acyanotic lesions. Successful cardiac surgical intervention typically brings a dramatic improvement in nutritional status. One disease from each category is considered as an example.

Ventricular septal defect (VSD) is the most common heart defect.[3] The closure of the ventricular septum is a critically timed event during development that may be affected by genetic or environmental factors. Closure normally occurs at 44 days gestation. Spontaneous closure of the ventricular septal defect frequently occurs later in life, suggesting a yet undefined back-up mechanism.[4] Children with this defect may or may not experience congestive failure in infancy.[3] Mean height and weight were found to be subnormal in many children with small defects,[4] with weight usually more regarded than height. Weights around the 3rd percentile and heights at the 20–25th percentile are characteristic.[4]

Transposition of the great arteries (TGA) is an example of a hypoxic disorder. Although birth weight is normal, significant failure to thrive is very common.[4] TGA tends to cause the most severe growth failure among the cyanotic lesions. However, the degree of cyanosis does not seem to correlate with the severity of growth failure.[4]

Biochemical abnormalities and etiology

The mechanisms underlying delayed growth and development in children with CHD are poorly understood. Genetic factors independent of the heart disease, hypoxia, hemodynamic abnormalities, and nutritional/metabolic factors are all implicated. The hypoxia associated with many forms of congenital heart disease causes growth failure, perhaps because of direct effects on cell multiplication and growth.[5]

Congestive heart failure (CHF) is strongly linked with failure to thrive and malnutrition.[4] Impaired caloric intake and hypermetabolism are both postulated as causes of the malnutrition, similar to adult cardiac cachexia.[4] This equivalent to cardiac cachexia is a more serious problem in children since they must struggle not only to maintain body weight but also to sustain linear growth.[4]

Table 32–2. Cardiovascular Abnormalities and Their Modes of Inheritance

Syndrome	Autosomal mode of inheritance
Adrenogenital syndrome (21 & 3)	Recessive
Alkaptonuria	Recessive
Apert	Dominant
Carpenter	Recessive
Chondrodysplasia punctata	Recessive
Conduction defects, familial	Dominant
Crouzon	Dominant
Cutis laxa	Recessive
Cystic fibrosis	Recessive
Ehlers-Danlos	Dominant
Ellis-van Creveld	Recessive
Fanconi pancytopenia	Recessive
Forney	Dominant
Friedreich's ataxia	Recessive
Holt-Oram	Dominant
Idiopathic hypertophic subaortic stenosis (IHSS)	Dominant
Ivemark	Recessive
Jervell and Lange-Nielsen	Recessive
Laurence-Moon (Bardet-Biedl)	Recessive
Leopard	Dominant
Marfan	Dominant
Meckel-Gruber	Recessive
Mitral click-murmur	Dominant
Mucolipidosis II & III	Recessive
Mucopolysaccharidosis (IH, IS, IV, VI)	Recessive
Muscular dystrophy I, II	Recessive
Myocardial disease (non-obstructive)	Dominant
Myotonic dystrophy (Steinert)	Dominant
Neurofibromatosis	Dominant
Noonan	Dominant
Osteogenesis imperfecta	Dominant
Periodic paralysis (hypo- and hyperkalemic)	Dominant
Primary pulmonary hypertension	Dominant
Pseudoxanthoma elasticum	Recessive
Refsum	Recessive
Romano-Ward	Dominant
Seckel	Recessive
Sickle-cell disease	Recessive
Smith-Lemli-Opitz	Recessive
Supravalvar aortic stenosis (with or without elfin facies)	Dominant
Thalassemia major	Recessive
Thrombocytopenia absent radius (TAR)	Recessive
Thyroid defects	Recessive
Treacher Collins	Dominant
Tuberous sclerosis	Dominant
Waardenburg	Dominant
Weill-Marchesani	Recessive
Zellweger	Recessive

Adapted from Nora, J., Nora, A. The evolution of specific genetic and environmental counseling in congenital heart disease. *Circulation*. 1978; 57:2. Used with permission.

Gastrointestinal abnormalities are seen in 29% of all cases of CHD,[6] implicating malabsorption. A mild degree of exudative enteropathy in the presence of a positive nitrogen balance has been found, as well as fat malabsorption.[3]

As a result of malabsorption, underlying metabolic derangements, malnutrition, and some vitamin and mineral abnormalities have been noted. Riboflavin and folic acid deficiencies are quite possible.[6] Calcium is apparently poorly absorbed.[2]

Factors to be considered in nutritional evaluation

Caloric Intake. A characteristic feeding pattern is found in infants with cyanotic large left-to-right shunts and congestive failure. They are ravenous at first, as if starved, and initially take the feeding very rapidly. They then become more tachypneic and exhausted as they feed and gradually slow down. Next, they become irritable and refuse further feedings or just fall asleep, having finished only one-quarter to one-third of the necessary amount. An hour or two later the entire pattern is repeated.[2] The inadequate intake is a by product of illness. The dyspnea and tachypnea of CHF, the fatigue from hypoxia, and the difficulty sucking when the baby needs ancillary muscles to breath make achieving an adequate intake very difficult.[4] In addition, over time, the caloric requirements for catch-up growth outstrip the infant's ability to consume them. Concomitant pulmonary infections increase energy requirements for respiration and thus necessitate additional calories. Intake may have a cyclical pattern. During "healthy times," the child selects and eats larger amounts. Unfortunately, the increase in intake volume during the healthy period may be so great that it worsens the CHF, causing another sequence of sick days and decreased intake. After surgery, in what has become known as "postoperative television syndrome," compensatory overfeeding has resulted in obesity.[6] This apparently is most common in the repair of relatively mild left-to-right shunts.

Energy requirements. As stated earlier, energy requirements may be higher because of the demands from an enlarged heart, increased cardiac output, increased oxygen consumption, and accelerated respiratory rate. Whether there is an overall increase in the basal metabolic rate (BMR) is debatable; however, the BMR seems to be similar to that in malnourished infants.[4] In one study, the BMR rose sharply during recovery from surgery and malnutrition; it was speculated that this increase was the "energy cost of growth."[6] Another study, which sought to determine the most effective nutritional regimen given for correction of growth failure, found that only 24-hour enteral infusions of a supplemental formula (to 1 kcal/mL) significantly improved nutritional status.[7]

Other dietary components. Water balance is of particular concern and should be monitored closely because losses through the lungs due to tachypnea, fever, or warm hospital rooms are higher than in the normal child. Conversely, fluids may need to be restricted to avoid fluid overload in acute congestive heart failure.

The sodium content of the diet should not exceed that of normal infants (7–8 mEq/day). Sodium should be restricted in the acute phase of CHF to 250–1000 mg/day. The actual estimated requirement is 2.1–2.6 mEq/day. Because the frequent use of diuretics can cause hypokalemia, the potassium content of the diet should be monitored.

Having parents or caregivers complete a food recall covering at least several days to one week is recommended to gauge cyclical intake patterns and vitamin and mineral nu-

Table 32–3. Cardiovascular Teratogens, Their Prevalence and Effect

Potential teratogen	Frequency of cardiovascular disease (%)	Most common malformations
Drugs		
Alcohol	25–30	VSD, PDA, ASD
Amphetamines	5–10	VSD, PDA, ASD, TGA
Anticonvulsants		
Hydantoin	2–3	Pulmonary stenosis, aortic stenosis, coarctation of aorta, PDA
Trimethadione	15–30	TGA, tetralogy, hypoplastic left heart
Lithium	10	Epstein, tricuspid atresia, ASD
Sex hormones	2–4	VSD, TGA, tetralogy
Thalidomide	5–10	Tetralogy, VSD, ASD, truncus
Infections		
Rubella	35	Peripheral pulmonary artery stenosis, PDA, VSD, ASD
Maternal conditions		
Diabetes	3–5 (30–50)	TGA, VSD, coarctation of aorta (for cardiomegaly and cardiomyopathy)
Lupus	?	Heart block
Phenylketonuria	25–50	Tetralogy, VSD, ASD

Adapted from Nora J., Nora A. The evolution of specific genetic and environmental counseling in congenital heart diseases. *Circulation*. 1978; 57:2. Used with permission.

trition adequately. One should consider the potential for deficiency states when assessing the diet.

Medications. The child with heart disease usually receives medication, which should be reflected in assessment and management. Three of the most commonly prescribed drugs are discussed in this section. *Digoxin*® may inhibit glucose absorption and may cause anorexia and nausea. When renal disease is also a concern, a vitamin-D-induced hypercalcemia may potentiate the effects of the drug. It should not be combined with high-fiber foods. Natural licorice (usually only the imported variety) should be avoided. Because many herbal teas have components that are cardiac stimulants or are derivatives of the foxglove plant (from which digitalis was first isolated), they should be used with caution. The diet should provide at least RDA levels of potassium and magnesium and be low in sodium. *Indomethacin*, now given intravenously, decreases the absorption of amino acids, but hyperglycemia and hyperkalemia may be seen, as well as edema and weight gain. *Propranolol (Inderal)*® is another drug that requires the avoidance of natural licorice. Fatigue, constipation, and gastrointestinal distress are common side effects. Over a period of time, a decreased carbohydrate tolerance is seen. High-density lipoprotein (HDL) decreases, triglyceride levels increase, and many other changes in serum values occur. A calorie-restricted, low-sodium diet is important to assist the action of Inderal. Diuretics, such as Lasix®, enable the patient to consume adequate calories and fluid, but also may cause hypokalemia, hyponatremia, and hypochloremia. Close monitoring is essential (see Chapter 27 for other diuretics).

Dietary management

Dietary management should be flexible, based on the individual patient's degree of illness and level of medication.

Calories. The capacity of many infants is only 450 mL/day of fluid, which is usually less than what is necessary for their increased energy needs. A formula concentrated to 24 kcal/day does not jeopardize fluid status.[6] Extra carbohydrate (Polycose, Karo syrup) or fat (vegetable oil) may be added to a formula to increase calories.[8] However, the addition of calories in this fashion to regular infant formula does not provide enough protein in the available volume. Therefore, preemie (24 kcal/oz) formulas should be used as a base. Butterfat-based formulas (evaporated milk) should not be given because butterfat is not well digested, and most is excreted, along with its calories, in the stool. If fat malabsorption is present, a formula containing medium-chain triglycerides (MCT) oil may be used. MCT oil does not contain linoleic acid, however, and should not be used as the sole fat source. Calorie levels are 120–135 kcal/kg/day for maintenance and may reach 150–175 kcal/kg/day for growth. By comparison, normal infants only require 105–115 kcal/kg/day.

Protein. Approximately 2.0–2.5 g/kg of protein should be provided. Calories must be sufficient to keep protein from being used as an energy source.

Other dietary components. Most pediatricians recommend that fluids be supplied in sufficient amounts to preserve urine osmolarity to less than 400 mOsm/L. For growth, 8 mEq/day of sodium is provided. Potassium should be monitored and kept within normal limits. A vitamin supplement containing iron and calcium should be given. If fat malabsorption occurs, water-soluble forms of vitamins A, D, E, and K are available.

Counseling. Family dynamics play an important role in counseling these patients and their families. Children who turn blue when they cry cause everyone around them to react quickly to their needs. Children with heart disease may well become the center of attention in their families and be quite manipulative. Parents may continue to treat their child as if he or she were a helpless infant long after the need has passed. In addition, they may see all weight gain as edema and therefore something to be avoided. Social workers can often offer excellent insights into the family situation that will allow the clinician to advise the family and patient more appropriately.

Follow-up

Follow-up in children with cardiovascular disease includes evaluating cardiovascular function and treating the symptoms. Measuring growth and evaluating nutrients, as listed in the section on dietary management, will need to be done on a regular basis and will be influenced by the severity of the disease.

Long-term cardiovascular health is as much a concern for children with CHD as it is for the general population. Atherosclerosis has been called a "pediatric problem"[9] since lifestyle patterns that will have a profound effect on the progression of the disease are determined during childhood. Appropriate amounts of exercise, fat, salt, fiber, copper, and zinc[10] and the control of contributing factors, such as diabetes and hypertension, are essential in the pediatric population if the goal of lessened adult mortality and morbidity is to be achieved.

Renal Disease

Chronic renal insufficiency is a progressive decline in the number of functioning nephrons that results ultimately in the loss of kidney function. The kidney is an excretory organ, filtering, reabsorbing, and excreting electrolytes, protein byproducts, glucose, amino acids, and toxic substances. The kidney also functions as an endocrine gland, producing hormones involved with growth (somatomedin), regulation of blood pressure (renin), red blood cell production (erythropoietin), and the absorption of calcium (1,25-dihydroxycholecalciferol). Chronic renal insufficiency (CRI) is generally considered to be the point at which the glomerular filtration rate (GFR) is less than 50% of normal. Chronic renal failure (CRF) is a continuous process, the various clinical stages of which merge into one another. The incidence of chronic renal failure in children less than 16 years of age is 1.5–3.0 children per million total population. The rate of deterioration is fastest in children with glomerulonephropathies, followed by hereditary nephropathies and renal dysplasia, and is slowest in children with urinary tract malformations.[11]

Growth failure is the major manifestation and primary nutritional management problem in the child with renal disease. It can be the result of any of the impaired excretory or endocrine functions of the kidney and may be exacerbated by malnutrition or the use of corticosteroids.[11] The overall incidence of growth failure in children with CRF is 35% to 65%.[5] Children with the congenital nephropathies may experience the most severe growth failure if onset occurs in infancy. Salt and bicarbonate wasting are major

contributors to the growth failure seen in infants with obstructive disease or renal dysplasia.[12] An infant's growth is particularly sensitive to uremic renal insufficiency, as manifested by achieved adult heights below the 5th percentile.[9] Growth failure, electrolyte imbalance, and metabolic problems occur more frequently and with greater severity as the GFR declines.[13]

It is rare that children with early severe renal failure achieve their growth potential. Growth lost during infancy is growth potential lost. Since children grow one-third of their total height in the first 2 years, disruption in this period may result in the short stature so commonly seen in older affected children. Children with open epiphyses and renal osteodystrophy show less linear growth than expected and are shorter as adults.[5] Most children receiving dialysis treatments grow at below average weights and have no catch-up growth.[9] By the time dialysis is begun, a significant deficit in height is usually observed, despite equivalent bone maturation, suggesting again a loss of growth potential due to uremia.

Children with congenital CRF can sometimes have normal growth velocity if properly managed, even in infancy and even if GRF is severely reduced.[14] Many children under 12 years of age are supplemented with 1,25 dihydroxy vitamin D_3 and its analog, based on a study showing accelerated growth in at least 73% of supplemented children.[15] However, the preliminary report of the Growth Failure in Children with Renal Diseases Study indicates that, despite osteodystrophy and height deficits, their unsupplemented subjects show an "inclination to catch-up growth."[16]

Transplantation has an uneven success record with regard to growth. Corticosteroids used in transplantation inhibit growth and may accelerate demineralization of bone,[17] but some success has been seen with alternate-day dosage.[9]

Biochemical abnormalities

Uremia produces a constellation of symptoms, showing the widespread effects of the toxins. Neurological signs, gastrointestinal distress, cardiovascular problems, hematological disorders, and immune system changes may be observed. Acute severe uremia results in an acceleration of the normal catabolic response seen in starvation.[18] Uremia may cause metabolic derangement of amino acid transport into the cells and the process of glucose utilization through peripheral insulin resistance.[19] Protein degradation and synthesis are therefore affected.[18] An imbalance in amino acid patterns progresses to a more distorted amino acid ratio. This disproportion affects amino acid transport and synthesis throughout the body. It is hypothesized that plasma amino acid patterns seen in CRF may be both a cause and an effect of uremia.[18]

Renal osteodystrophy is found with uremia and may affect growth profoundly. Phosphorus homeostasis is regulated by the kidney. As GFR drops, serum phosphate rises. Serum calcium is lowered through calcium phosphate complexes, but the decrease results in an increased parathyroid hormone concentration. Phosphate reabsorption is decreased in the presence of increased parathyroid hormone. Thus, phosphate and calcium levels are maintained at near-normal levels at the expense of a secondary hyperparathyroidism and its effects on bone.

Vitamin D deficiency is equally important as a factor in renal osteodystrophy and may precede the phosphorus retention. The kidney is the site for synthesis of 1,25-dihydroxyvitamin D, which has a critical influence on the intestinal absorption of vitamin D. Hyperphosphatemia reduces the rate of conversion of 25-hydroxyvitamin D_3 to 1,25-dihydroxyvitamin D_3 and may be an important factor in Vitamin D resistance.[13] Vitamin D resistance diminishes bone density by decreasing the absorption of calcium in the gut.[13]

Acidosis, through its symptom of anorexia and/or by its effect upon the skeleton, is also a growth inhibitor. Bone mineralization is less easily accomplished in an acidic extracellular environment.[11] Persistent metabolic acidosis is a factor in failure to thrive during infancy.[13] Bone calcium may also be liberated to act as a serum buffer for the acidosis, which, over time, weakens the bone. Kleinknecht et al.[14] believe acidosis to be the major cause of growth retardation in nondialyzed children with congenital disease, although its effects could not be separated clearly from those of chronic dehydration, sodium depletion, and malnutrition. In patients with CRI, overly strict dietary control of phosphorus may lead to hypophosphatemia, impairing bicarbonate production and contributing to metabolic acidosis.[20] Secondary abnormalities associated with renal tubular acidosis—out of proportion to or occurring in the absence of glomerular insufficiency—may also be involved. These conditions include hypovolemia, dehydration, sodium and potassium wasting, or abnormalities in calcium and phosphate metabolism.[21]

Dialysis has an effect upon the biochemical status of the patient. Amino acids are lost in the dialysate, particularly in the peritoneal forms of dialysis. The younger the child, the greater the insulin sensitivity and glucose tolerance. Conversely, more insulin resistance and glucose intolerance are observed in older children.[19] Sodium losses to the dialysate in continuous peritoneal dialysis (CPD) may result in hyponatremia, particularly in infants, and threaten growth. There is increasing evidence in adults that controlling the characteristic hyperlipidemia seen in ESRD will inhibit the development of glomerulosclerosis.[22] Both dietary and pharmacologic therapies are effective.[23] Although this has not been studied in children, it seems reasonable to modify the lipid content of therapeutic diet, provided other, primary objectives (such as weight gain) have been met.

Hypertriglyceridemia is seen in children, and it is speculated that its cause may be increased hepatic production and decreased removal of triglycerides.[24] Carnitine, a critical factor in the oxidation of fatty acids, is synthesized and clearly by the kidneys. Predialysis patients have elevated serum levels. However, dialysis removes carnitine, and a deficiency state is thought to play a role in the accelerated atherosclerotic disease seen with CRF.[13] Several studies have shown that low-dose supplementation of L-carnitine improves lipid metabolism in dialyzed children.[25]

When renal function decreases to one-third of normal, a normocytic, nomochromic anemia is seen, paralleling the severity of the renal failure.[26] It is a direct result of a decrease in the rate of red blood cell production and a shortened life-span of circulating red cells. Decreased erythropoietin activity and inhibited heme synthesis by uremic substances may be two causal factors.[26] In general, anemia

does not develop until creatinine clearance is less than 35 mL/min/1.73 m, although the correlation is not as strong as previously thought.[27] Folacin is bound to protein in uremia and is utilized poorly. In addition, significant quantities are lost during dialysis, as are all of the water-soluble vitamins.[24]

Young CPD patients lose more albumin and total protein per kilogram to the dialysate than older children.[26] Protein loss may be as high as 0.35 g/kg/day in patients less than 6 years old and from 0.11 to 0.19 g/kg/day in older children.[28] Hyperglycemia, hypercholesterolemia, and hypertriglyceridemia are all more marked in younger CAPD patients.[29]

Children with CRF due to obstruction or reflux nephropathy are very sensitive to fluctuations in water balance because of their inability to concentrate urine. Obstructive disorders also result in a decreased tolerance for dietary variations in sodium and potassium. Because fluid requirements are high, a relatively minor disruption in fluid intake may cause dehydration, hypernatremia, and acute renal failure.[26] Patients with interstitial nephritis, obstructive disorders, and diabetic nephropathy are also very sensitive to flucuations in potassium and are at risk for hyperkalemia.[26]

Even subtle levels of sodium chloride deficiency may interfere with growth. Some factors that may result in the increased excretion of sodium chloride are changes in cardiac output, renal perfusion pressure, extracellular fluid volume, or colloid osmotic pressure.[20] Chloride, independently of sodium, has been implicated as an agent in cases of failure to thrive or poor growth.[20]

Aluminum administration to infants and children in the form of phosphate binders or via dialysate may contribute to renal osteodystrophy and brain intoxication. Whether this outcome is the result of increased absorption or a function of the large quantities of aluminum involved is unclear.[26]

Factors to be considered in nutritional evaluation

Anorexia and altered taste acuity are common in patients with renal disease.[29] Compliance with strict dietary regimens is usually variable and often poor. Fine and Salusky[27] found that the majority of their patients on CAPD and CPD consumed less than 75% of the prescribed energy intake, even when glucose absorption from the dialysate was included.[30] Completion of a 3- to 4-day dietary recall is recommended. When less than 80% of the recommended daily allowance for specific nutrients or overall calories is consumed, further investigation is needed to determine whether the decreased intake is short term or a long-standing pattern (Table 32-4).

Dry weight and height for age are the main anthropometric measures used to assess nutritional status. Midarm circumference and triceps skinfold thickness may be taken to calculate muscle status for an ongoing assessment of muscle wasting, yet rarely provide more information about malnutrition than does weight for height or weight for age.[31] However, skinfold thickness below the 5th percentile and a decrease in the rate of growth are cause for concern.

Growth failure creates its own set of measurement difficulties. Because there are no specific growth grids for children with CRF, the standard National Center for Health Statistics growth charts may be used (Appendix 2). Increasingly, standard deviation scores are used to compare the growth rate of children over defined intervals of time. At-

Table 32–4. Daily Nutrient and Fluid Recommendations for the Child with End-Stage Renal Disease

	Energy	Protein	Sodium	Potassium	Calcium	Phosphorus	Vitamins	Trace minerals	Fluid
Predialysis (>15% GFR)									
Infants	Minimum of RDA for statural age	RDA for statural age	1–3 mEq/kg if necessary	1–3 mEq/kg if necessary	Supplement as necessary	Restrict high content foods, use low content formula if necessary	1 cc multivitamin drops if necessary + vitamin D metabolite if needed	Supplemental zinc, iron, or copper if necessary	Minimum of maintenance levels
Children/adolescents	Minimum of RDA for height age	Minimum of RDA for height age	1–3 mEq/100 kcal expended if necessary	Unrestricted until K elevated	Supplement as necessary	500–1000 mg/day when <50% GFR	Multivitamin preparation if necessary + vitamin D metabolite if needed	Supplemental zinc, iron, or copper if necessary	When edema develops, give insensible + urinary output
Predialysis (<15% GFR)									
Infants	Minimum of RDA for statural age	1.5–1.6 g/kg	1–3 mEq/kg if necessary	1–3 mEq/kg	Supplement as necessary	Restrict high content foods, use low content formula	Same as when GFR>15% normal	Same as when GFR >15% normal	When edema develops, give insensible + urinary output
Children/adolescents	Minimum of RDA for height age	Maximum of RDA for height age	1–3 mEq/100 kcal expended if necessary	Unrestricted until K elevated <10% GFR	Supplement as necessary	500–1000 mg/day	Same as when GFR >15% normal	Same as when GFR >15% normal	Same as when GFR >15% normal
Hemodialysis									
Infants	Minimum of RDA for statural age	RDA for statural age	1–3 mEq/kg if necessary	1–3 mEq/kg	Supplement as necessary	Restrict high content foods, use low content formula	1 cc multivitamin drops, 1 mg folic acid + vitamin D metabolite if needed	Same as during predialysis period	Insensible + ultrafiltration + urinary output (if any)
Children/adolescents	Minimum of RDA for height age	RDA for height age	1–3 mEq/100 kcal expended if necessary	25–50 mEq/day when necessary	Supplement as necessary	500–1000 mg/day	1 mg folic acid, 50–100 mg vitamin C, B-coplex + vitamin D metabolite as needed	Same as during predialysis period	Insensible + urinary output
Peritoneal dialysis (IPD)									
Infants	Minimum of RDA for statural age	2.5–3 g/kg	1–3 mEq/kg if necessary	1–3 mEq/kg	Supplement as necessary	Same as for hemodialysis	Same as for hemodialysis	Same as during predialysis period	Same as for hemodialysis
Children/adolescents	Minimum of RDA for height age	Usually midway between hemodialysis and CAPD recommendations	1–3 mEq/100 kcal expended if necessary	25–50 mEq/day when necessary	Supplement as necessary	Same as for hemodialysis	Same as for hemodialysis	Same as during predialysis period	Same as for hemodialysis
Peritoneal dialysis (CAPD)									
Infants	Minimum of RDA for statural age	3–4 g/kg	3 mEq/kg based upon edema, BP	3 mEq/kg and possibly not necessary	Supplement as necessary	May be liberalized based upon serum levels	Same as for hemodialysis	Same as during predialysis period	Same as for hemodialysis

Table 32-4. (*Continued*)

	Energy	Protein	Sodium	Potassium	Calcium	Phosphorus	Vitamins	Trace minerals	Fluid
Children/ adolescents	Minimum of RDA for height age	3.0 g/kg-ht age 2–5 yr 2.5 g/kg-ht age 5–10 yr 2.0 g/kg-ht age 10–12 yr 1.5 g/kg-ht age > 12 yr	Usually unlimited, 85–174 mEq/ day if necessary	Usually unlimited, 25–50 mEq/ day if necessary	Supplement as necessary	Generally 240 cc milk/day or equivalent in milk products	Same as for hemodialysis	Same as during predialysis period	Usually not necessary
Transplant Infants	RDA for statural age after ideal weight/ length is achieved	3 g/kg	1–3 mEq/kg	Unlimited	Ad libitum	May need very high intakes—supplement as necessary	Usually not necessary unless severe malnutrition prior to transplant-vitamin D if needed	Should not be necessary	Usually not necessary
Children/ adolescents	RDA for height age—no concentrated sweets for 6 weeks posttransplant	2–3 g/kg	130–174 mEq/ day and less if edema and BP are present	Unlimited	Ad libitum	May need very high intakes—supplement as necessary	Usually not necessary unless severe malnutrition prior to transplant-vitamin D if needed	Should not be necessary	Usually not necessary

From Nelson, P., Strover, J. Principles of nutritional assessment and management of the child with ESRD. In: Fine, R.N., Gruskin, A.B., eds. *End Stage Renal Disease in Children*. Philadelphia: W.B. Saunders; 1984, p. 212. Used with permission

tained height age is expressed as the height standard deviation score, which is the difference between the individual height and mean height for normal children of the same age and sex divided by the population standard deviation. Height velocity standard deviation scores, derived in a similar manner, are used to compare average rates of growth.[32] The standard deviation score (SDS) is calculated according to this formula:

$$ SDS = \frac{height\ (cm)\ -\ mean\ height\ for\ age^{33}}{SD\ of\ mean\ height} $$

Transferrin may be depressed in chronic renal failure, and an increase in the concentration of this transport protein commonly correlates with improvement in other measures of nutritional status.[26] However, in CAPD patients, transferrin may not be as accurate as prealbumin, plasma albumin, and thyroxin-binding globulin levels.[28] Losses of total protein and albumin to the CPD dialysate are higher per kilogram in younger than older children.[13] Although low-protein diets are widely considered to delay the progression of renal disease, very low-protein (0.3–0.4 g/kg/day) diets result in a negative nitrogen balance.[12] The use of ketoacids and essential amino acids as adjuncts to conventional dietary therapy is now being investigated in clinical trials. No benefit or harm from their use has yet been established. Jureidini et al.[34] used a low-protein and low-phosphorus diet supplemented with a mixture of keto and amino acids and histidine with ten CRF children for 3 years; they found an overall improvement in health and an apparent reduction of the rate of deterioration of renal function.

Iron deficiency may result from an inadequate intake of iron, blood loss in hemodialysis patients from the procedure, malabsorption of iron secondary to iron-chelating nonabsorbed aluminum gels, excessive blood loss from laboratory studies, and blood loss secondary to bleeding diathesis associated with uremia. However, children with mild chronic renal failure are usually not anemic and should receive the recommended daily allowance for iron. Iron stores are best monitored using serum ferritin.[26] Because children with CRF are also at risk for iron overload because of all the blood transfusions required, they should be provided with supplemental iron only when serum ferritin is indicative of depleted iron stores.[26] Patients with uremia have reduced plasma and cellular levels of pyridoxine.[23] Children with uremia may also have low plasma levels of zinc, especially if their appetites are poor or muscle wasting is occurring.[24]

Phosphorus intake may be partially controlled by a low-protein diet, but in time, orally administered phosphate binders will be required. Calcium carbonate, lactate, or gluconate are commonly given to children to avoid problems with aluminum toxicity.[26] If hypercalcemia occurs, the binders are discontinued temporarily until serum calcium returns to within normal limits.[26] Adequate calcium intake and absorption are important in the control of renal osteodystrophy.

Frequent monitoring of calcium and phosphorus is helpful in deciding when to begin therapy. Although the most effective and appropriate assessment and intervention techniques are as yet unclear, one can assume that mineral metabolism is abnormal when the GRF is at or below 20% of normal, even if serum calcium, phosphorus, and alkaline phosphatase levels are acceptable.[26] Typically, vitamin D analogs are given to enhance the intestinal transport of calcium. If hypercalcemia or hypermagnesemia occurs, the vitamin D compounds and oral calcium are discontinued. The potential for toxicity from vitamin D should be considered.[13] A predialysis BUN, creatinine, potassium, phosphorus, and albumin biochemistries should be obtained.

Patients on long-term hemodialysis or peritoneal dialysis are at risk for a carnitine deficiency because carnitine is lost to the dialysate and is chiefly found in animal products, which are restricted on a low-protein diet. It is therefore recommended that carnitine status be evaluated (tissue or serum) in patients showing signs of cardiomyopathy. In addition, the diet should be evaluated for lysine and methionine, the amino acid precursors for carnitine.[26]

Medications influence nutritional status. Three of the most commonly drugs used are discussed in this section. *Bactrim (Septra)*® increases the need for fluids and decreases the absorption of folacin and vitamin K over a long period of time. It contains 3.5 g sucrose /5 mL, which should be calculated into the diabetic exchanges for brittle individuals. It causes many gastrointestinal side effects, including diarrhea, stomatitis, and anorexia. *Hypdrocortisone (Prednisone)*® decreases the absorption of calcium and phosphorus, and prolonged use interferes with carbohydrate metabolism. Growth is suppressed in children, and wound healing may be impaired. Weight fluctuations secondary to the medication are difficult to control. The diet is particularly important, one rich in potassium, pyridoxine, vitamins C and D, folacin, calcium, and phosphorus, yet low in sodium is recommended. Gastrointestinal distress is common. *Furosemide (Lasix)*® is a strong diuretic. Loss of magnesium, potassium, and chloride should be expected and monitored and the diet constructed to provide good sources of magnesium and potassium. Again, gastrointestinal symptoms, such as diarrhea, vomiting, and nausea, are common. Zinc stores drop, yet it is noteworthy that serum values increase, as do blood urea nitrogen and glucose, perhaps due to slight dehydration.

Dietary management

The goals of dietary management are to preserve renal function, treat symptoms, prevent deficiency or excess states, and promote growth and development. Table 32-4 presents dietary specific requirements according to age and intervention. This section describes dietary management in detail.

Calories. Caloric requirements for the predialysis child are at least equivalent to those for the unaffected child—38–115 kcal/kg/day. Recovery from malnutrition may require a larger amount of calories. The most important period for growth is the first 3–12 months of life, and a special effort to meet caloric demands then should be made.[35] Infants provided with 9–12 kcal/cm/day will grow and yet not exceed their kidney function limits.[31] The common practice of concentrating infant formulas by mixing them with less water results in a higher renal solute load than is tolerable. (See Appendix 6 for commercial formulas to reduce renal solute load.) Vegetable oils and carbohydrate supplements may be added to standard formulas to raise calories. If the proportion of carbohydrate or fat is too high, vomiting or diarrhea will result. It is best to make changes slowly. Older children should be encouraged to use margarine and other fats on their foods for extra calories.

Children receiving hemodialysis and CPD have approximately the same caloric requirements as the predialysis child. Approximately 12% of daily calories are derived from glucose in the dialysate for the child on CPD.[13] A caloric intake of 10 kcal/cm/day contributes to positive nitrogen balance and does not increase hemodialysis requirements.[29] CPD patients should consume more complex carbohydrates than simple sugars for extra calories because of the increased incidence of hypertriglyceridemia.[31] Some centers recommend a caloric intake of 120–150% RDA for young infants and children with severe CRF.

Protein. Protein intake for all patients should be at least the minimum recommended daily allowance for normal children of the same age and should comprise 8% of total calories.[11] CPD patients may require slightly higher amounts since more is lost to the dialysate. Protein intake is related to and affects the urinary excretion of creatinine, potassium, phosphate, sulfate, calcium, and net acid in CRI.[36] Dialysate losses are also higher in metabolic stress.[13] Fifty to 75% of the total protein intake for pre dialysis patients, especially infants, should be high biological value (HBV) for optimal utilization. Sixty to 70% HBV is adequate for hemodialysis and CPD patients. HBV protein with a low saturated fat content, such as poultry or fish, is recommended for CPD patients because of their risk for the hyperlipidemias. Carnitine supplementation in CPD patients should be considered if serum and or tissue levels are abnormally low. Daily amounts of 100–200 ng/kg/day are recommended.[13] Carnitine status should be evaluated regularly in anyone on dialysis. The BUN should also be closely monitored.

Dietary components. To prevent hyperphosphatemia, one should first decrease the intake of phosphorus and monitor its serum levels. Infants should receive breast milk or formulas with a calcium:phosphorus ratio of 1.4:1 to 2:1. Second, calcium carbonate, lactate, and gluconate should be used as binders. Hypercalcemia is more common when vitamin D analogs are used.

The RDA for all minerals and vitamins is recommended for individuals receiving CPD therapy,[13] with the exception of folic acid (1 mg/day), B6 (5–10 mg/day) and vitamin C (75–100 mg/day). The RDA for iron should be given in mild CRF, with the levels being monitored by serum ferritin.[13] One should not give oral iron with phosphate binders.

Follow-up

Follow-up in children with renal disease includes evaluating renal function, treating symptoms, measuring growth, and evaluating the diet for all nutrients. The frequency of evaluation is determined by the severity of the disease. Should transplant occur, assessment and evaluation do not cease, but continue at regular intervals until the transplant is well established.

Acknowledgments

The author would like to thank Robert Fildes, M.D., Elliot Gersh, M.D., and John Cocherham, M.D. for their review and assistance with this paper.

References

1. Park, M. *Pediatric Cardiology for Practitioners*. Chicago: Year Book; 1988.

2. O'Leary, M. Nutritional care in diseases of infancy and childhood. In: Krause, M., Mahan, L., eds. *Food, Nutrition and Diet Therapy*. 7th ed. Philadelphia: Saunders; 1984.

3. Praagh, R., Takao, A., eds. *Etiology and Morphogenesis of Congenital Heart Disease*. Mount Kisco, NY: Futura Publishing; 1990.

4. Neill, J. Hemodynamic growth retardation. In: Accardo, P., ed. *Failure to Thrive in Infancy and Early Childhood*. Baltimore: University Park Press; 1982.

5. Kreiger, I. *Pediatric Disorders of Feeding, Nutrition and Metabolism*. New York: Wiley; 1982.

6. Nadas, A., Rosenthal, A., Crigler, J. Nutritional considerations in the prognosis and treatment of children with congenital heart disease. In: Suskind, R., ed. *Textbook of Pediatric Nutrition*, New York: Raven Press; 1981.

7. Schwarz, S.M., Gewitz, M.H., See, C.C., Berezin, S., Glassman, M.S., Medow, C.M., Fish, B.C., Newman, L.J. Enteral nutrition in infants with congenital heart disease and growth failure. *Pediatrics*. 1990; 86:368.

8. Jackson, M., Poskitt, E.M.E. The effects of high-energy feeding on energy balance and growth in infants with congenital heart disease and failure to thrive. *B. J. Nutr.* 1991; 65:131.

9. Haust, M.D. The genesis of atherosclerosis in the pediatric age group. *Pediatr. Pathol.* 1990; 10:253.

10. Laitinen, R., Vuori, E., Viikari, J. Serum zinc and copper: associations with triglyceride levels in children and adolescents. Cardiovascular risk in young Finns. *J. Am. Coll. Nutr.* 1989; 8:400.

11. Roskes, S. Growth failure in renal disease. In: Accardo, P., ed. *Failure to Thrive in Infancy and Early Childhood*. Baltimore: University Park Press; 1982.

12. Murakani, K., Kitagawa, T., Yabuta, K., Sakai, T., eds. *Recent Advances in Pediatric Nephrology: Proceedings of the Seventh International Congress of Pediatric Nephrology*. New York: Excerpta Medica; 1986.

13. Hellerstein, S., Holliday, M., Grupe, W., Fine, R., Fennell, R., Chesney, R. Chan J. Nutritional management of children with chronic renal failure. *Pediatr. Nephrol.* 1987; 1:195.

14. Kleinknecht, C., Broyer, M., Huot, D., Marti-Henneberg, C., Dartois, A-M. Growth and development of nondialyzed children with chronic renal failure. *Kidney Int.* 1983; 24(suppl 15):S-40.

15. Chan, J., Greifer, I., Boineau, F., Mendoza, S., McEnergy, P., Strife, F., Abitbol, C., Stapleton, B., Roy, S., Strauss, J., Rationale of the growth failure in children with renal diseases study. *J. Pediatr.* 1990; 116:S11.

16. Abitbol, C., Bradley, A., Massie, M., Balvarte, H., Fleischman, L., Geary, D., Kaiser, B., McEnery, P., Chan, J. Linear growth and anthropometric and nutritional measurements in children with mild to moderate renal insufficiency: a report of the growth failure in children with renal diseases study. *J. Pediatr.* 1990; 116:S46.

17. Chesney, R., Mehls, O., Anast, C., Brown, E., Hammerman, M., Portale, A., Fallon, M., Mahan, J., Alfrey, A. Renal osteodystrophy in children: the role of vitamin D, phosphorus, and parathyroid hormone. *Am. J. Kidney Dis.* 1986; 7:275.

18. Wassner, S., Bergstrom, J., Brusilow, S., Harper, A., Mitch, W. Protein metabolism in renal failure: abnormalities and possible mechanisms. *Am. J. Kidney Dis.* 1986; 7:285.

19. Mak, R., Haycock, G., Chantler, C. Glucose intolerance in children with chronic renal failure. *Kidney Int.* 1983; 24:S-22.

20. Rodriguez-Soriano, J., Arant, B.S., Brodehl, J., Norman, M.F. Fluid and electrolyte imbalances in children with chronic renal failure. *Am. J. Kidney Dis.*, 1986; 7:268.

21. Donckerwolcke, R., Yang, W.N., Chan, J. Growth failure in children with renal tubuler acidosis. *Sem. Nephrol.* 1989; 9:72.

22. Schreiner, G., Kalahr, S. Diet and kidney disease: The role of dietary fatty acids. *Proc. Soc. Exp. Biol. Med.* 1991; 197(1):1.

23. Schnutz, P.G., Kasilke, B.L., O'Donnell, M.P., Keane, W.F. Lipids and progressive renal injury. *Semin. Nephrol.* 1989; 9:354–369.

24. McVicar, M. Nutritional consequences of kidney disease. In: Lifshitz, F., ed. *Pediatric Nutrition, Infant Feedings-Deficiencies-Diseases*. New York: Marcel Dekker; 1982.

25. Gloggler, A., Bulla, M., Furst, P. Effect of low dose supplementation of L-carnitine on lipid metabolism in hemodialyzed children. *Kidney Int.* 1989; 36:S256.

26. American Academy of Pediatrics. *Nutritional Management of Children with Chronic Renal Failure*. Chicago: American Academy of Pediatrics; 1986.

27. Boineau, F., Lewy, J., Baharte, G., Pomrantz, A., Waldo, B. Prevalence of anemia and correlation with mild and chronic renal insufficiency. *J. Pediatr.* 1990; 116:S60.

28. Broyer, M., Niaudet, P., Champion, G., Jean, G., Chopin, N., Czernichow, P. Nutritional and metabolic studies in children on continuous ambulatory peritoneal dialysis. *Kidney Int.* 1983; 24:S-106.

29. Grupe, W., Harmon, W., Spinozzi, N. Protein and energy requirements in children receiving chronic hemodialysis. *Kidney Int.* 1983; 24:S-6.

30. Fine, R., Salusky, I. CAPD/CCPD in children: four year's experience. *Kidney Int.* 1986; 10:(S-7).

31. Stover, J., Nelson, P. Nutritional recommendations for infants, children, and adolescents with ESRD. In: Gillit, D., Stover, J., Spinoi, N. *A Clinical Guide to Nutrition Care in End-Stage Renal Disease*. Chicago: American Dietetic Association; 1987.

32. Barrett, T., Broyer, M., Chatler, C., Gilli, G., Guest, G., Marti-Henneberg, C., Preece, M., Rigden, S. Assessment of growth. *Am. J Kidney Dis.* 1986; 7:340.

33. Abitbol, C., Foreman, J.W., Strife, C.F., McEnery, P.T. Quantitation of growth deficits in children with renal diseases. *Sem. Nephrol.* 1989; 9:31.

34. Jureidini, K.F., Hogg, R.J., van Renen, M.J. Southwood, T.R., Henning, P.H. Cobiac, L., Daniels, L., Harris, S. Evaluation of long-term aggressive dietary management of chronic renal failure in children. *Pediatr. Nephrol.* 1990; 4:1.

35. Rizzoni, G., Broyer, M., Guest, G., Fine, R., Holliday, M. Growth retardation in children with chronic renal disease: scope of the problem. *Am. J. Kidney Dis.* 1986; 7:256.

36. Nakano, M., Alon, U., Jennings, S., Chan, J. Protein intake and renal function in children. *Am. J. Dis. Child.* 1989; 143:160.

Chapter 33
Nutrition in Sickle-Cell Anemia

Karen Kalinyak

Sickle-cell anemia is an inherited disorder in which the person inherits a sickle gene (Hb S) from each parent. Persons with sickle-cell trait (Hb AS) carry the sickle gene, but under normal circumstances are completely asymptomatic. The sickle gene is prevalent in people of black African ancestry, Italians, Sicilians, Egyptians, Turks, Arabs, and Asiatic Indians. About 1 out of every 12 black Americans carries the sickle-cell trait, and 1 out of approximately 625 black Americans actually has the disease.[1]

Biochemical, Pathological, and Clinical Abnormalities

The sickle hemoglobin is the result of a single amino acid substitution of valine for glutamic acid in the sixth position of the beta globin chain. In contrast to the usual adult hemoglobin (Hb A), the sickle hemoglobin tends to polymerize when it undergoes deoxygenation. This process affects the shape of the red blood cell, forming an elongated stiff, less deformable sickle-shaped cell that is rapidly destroyed and removed from the circulation.

The diagnosis of sickle-cell anemia, as well as other hemoglobinopathies, is usually made using a technique called hemoglobin electrophoresis. Using this method, the different hemoglobins migrate various distances on a gel and form separate bands, which can then be identified. Other available techniques include high-pressure liquid chromatography and isoelectric focusing. A rapid screening test that is used frequently is the solubility test. The decreased solubility of deoxy-Hb S forms the basis for this test, which only indicates whether or not sickle hemoglobin is present. Thus, it is only a fast screen, and one of the other above-listed techniques should be done to confirm the results. Prenatal diagnosis is available and can be performed very early in a pregnancy for those couples at genetic risk for sickle-cell disease.

The two primary manifestations of sickle-cell anemia are severe hemolytic anemia and widespread vaso-occlusion and infarction of various organs and tissues. The hemolytic anemia is a result of the markedly shortened life-span of the sickle cells, which survive in the circulation only 9–11 days as compared to 120 days for normal red cells. The clinical manifestations that reflect this ongoing hemolytic process include jaundice, pallor, weakness, and easy fatigability. The widespread vaso-occlusion is a result of the adherence of the stiff, less deformable sickled cells to the lining of blood vessels, which virtually plugs up the small vessels and thus obstructs blood flow to a particular tissue or organ. This adherence results in decreased oxygen supply to that particular area, which leads to tissue death or infarction. The decreased oxygen supply causes the pain so characteristic of sickle-cell anemia. The pain may be localized to one area or extremity or may become diffuse. Certain factors are known to trigger painful episodes and include infection, hypoxia, extremes in temperature, and acidosis. Frequently, however, there is no obvious precipitating factor.

Symmetrical, painful swelling of the hands and feet (hand-foot syndrome) may be the initial manifestation of a vaso-occlusive episode in the infant or toddler. As the child grows, the painful episodes may involve the abdomen or extremities or chest. Strokes caused by occlusion of the cerebral vessels occur in approximately 8% to 17% of children with sickle-cell anemia.[2,3] Acute chest syndrome, in which there is extensive pulmonary infarction, can be rapidly progressive if not treated aggressively.

Virtually every organ of the body can be affected in sickle-cell anemia. Intrahepatic sickling may damage the liver, causing subsequent liver impairment. Gallstones have been seen in patients as young as 3 years of age and are the result of the chronic hemolytic anemia. Renal function may become progressively impaired in the adult patients. Chronic leg ulcers occur in a small percentage of patients. Involvement of the eye with a sickle-cell retinopathy can be progressive and lead to blindness in the older patient. The spleen undergoes an autoinfarction process very early in life, leaving the patient functionally asplenic. This process accounts, at least in part, for the markedly increased susceptibility to infection, in particular infections caused by *Streptococcus pneumoniae*. The incidence of overwhelming pneumococcal sepsis is 400 times greater in children less than 5 years of age with sickle-cell anemia than in those children without this condition.

Other complications include splenic sequestration, which is a sudden decrease in the hemoglobin caused by sudden massive trapping of red blood cells in the spleen. This condition is usually seen in the young toddler-aged child. An aplastic episode, which can also cause a sudden drop in the blood count, occurs when the bone marrow temporarily stops making red blood cells. The parvovirus is one of the agents that has been implicated as a cause of the aplastic episodes in these patients.

Finally, growth is also affected. Approximately one-third of sickle-cell patients are below the 5th percentile for height and/or weight.[4] Deficits in height and weight are associated with a delayed onset of puberty.[4,5] The mean age of menarche in girls with sickle-cell anemia is 15.4 years compared to 12.6 years in normal controls.[6] Delayed sexual maturation has also been seen in boys with sickle-cell anemia. The etiology of this poor growth and delayed sexual maturation is not clearly understood. Growth hormone and thyroid hormone are not deficient in these children, and no abnormality of the pituitary-hypothalamic axis has been found. Therefore, there is no need for hormone replacements.

Factors to be Considered in Nutritional Evaluation and Dietary Management

The role of nutrition in the care of persons with sickle-cell anemia and other hemoglobinopathies is only now beginning to receive attention. Historically, adults with sickle-cell anemia were noted to be short, thin, and eunuchoid in appearance.[7] Early reports of children with sickle-cell anemia suggested the presence of decreased height, weight, and hypogonadism. Anthropometric measurements showed that these children were indeed shorter and weighed less than their siblings.[8] In addition, skeletal maturation was delayed in 25% of the study population.[9] Infants with sickle-cell anemia who were identified at birth are not different initially with regard to weight, length, or head circumference from full-term black newborns without hemoglobinopathies.[10] However, significant deficits can be demonstrated at 35–70 months of age, with these deficits increasing over time.[10]

Many studies have clearly shown that height and weight are significantly reduced in many patients with sickle-cell anemia, that this reduction is more pronounced in boys, and that weight is more affected than height.[4,6] Skinfold thickness measurements are within normal limits, suggesting that good nutritional status is maintained, despite low body weight (see growth grids in Appendix 2).[6]

Zinc

In experimental animals zinc deficiency has been recognized to result in growth retardation and testicular atrophy. The sequelae of zinc deficiency in humans include growth retardation, hyperammonemia, abnormal dark adaptation, hypogonadism, and cell-mediated immune dysfunction. Prasad et al. have shown that zinc deficiency occurs in adult sickle-cell patients, as determined by plasma, red blood cells, and neutrophils[11-13] (Table 33-1). Other biochemical evidence of zinc deficiency is the decreased activity of zinc-dependent enzymes.[14]

Hyperzincuria has been well documented to occur in sickle-cell anemia,[13,15] as well as in other hemolytic anemias. It is thought to be a result of the chronic hemolysis. It is not certain whether the hyperzincuria fully accounts for the low zinc levels in sickle-cell patients or if other factors, such as decreased intake or malabsorption also, play a role.

The role that zinc plays in the growth and pubertal development of sickle-cell children is not known. Studies at

Table 33–1. Mean Zinc Levels in Sickle-Cell Patients

	Plasma	RBC (μg/dL)	Neutrophils
Patients (n = 27)	96.3 + 11.6	32.5 + 6.3	82.0 + 12.5
Controls (n = 25)	115 + 11.7	38.4 + 4.9	108.4 + 10.9
P value	<0.001	<0.001	<0.001

From Prasad & Cossack,[12] used with permission.

the Children's Hospital of Philadelphia confirm the low zinc levels, but showed no correlation to growth parameters.[16] Those patients who were growth retarded were not necessarily those who had the lower zinc values. On the other hand, studies done by Prasad and Cossack[12] showed that zinc supplementation did stimulate growth and increased basal serum testosterone levels in a small group of growth-retarded boys with sickle-cell anemia.

In summary, the incidence of zinc deficiency in sickle-cell patients is unknown at this time. How much of a role zinc deficiency plays in the growth retardation and delayed puberty is again unknown. From the reported studies, zinc deficiency appears to be prevalent among boys with sickle-cell anemia, and supplementation appears to positively affect growth and gonadal function. Further implications of zinc deficiency, which need to be studied, include impaired wound healing, T-cell immune dysfunction, and possible anti-sickling effects. Until more information is available, zinc supplementation should only be prescribed to those patients with documented deficiency.

Other trace metals

Other trace elements investigated in sickle-cell anemia include copper and magnesium. Copper and zinc compete for similar binding sites in the body, and data confirm a mild increase in plasma copper in those patients who were zinc deficient.[13] Changes in plasma and erythrocyte magnesium levels were also observed in sickle-cell subjects,[13] although they are likely a result of a redistribution phenomenon. Levels of plasma selenium were significantly lower than those of controls, which is consistent with increased oxidative stress as previously reported in sickle-cell anemia.

Vitamin A

Vitamin A levels have been reported to be low in sickle-cell patients. In a study at Children's Hospital of Philadelphia, vitamin A levels less than 20 mg/dL, which is the level considered to indicate risk for vitamin A deficiency in children, were noted in 70% of growth-retarded sickle-cell patients, 44% of growth-normal sickle-cell patients, and 20% of control patients.[16] The mean level of retinol-binding protein (RBP) was significantly lower for the growth-retarded group of sickle-cell patients when compared to both the control group and the growth-normal sickle-cell group. Levels below 3 mg/dL—the normal range in children is 3.5–7.0 mg/dL—were found in 55% of the growth-normal patients, in 85% of the growth-retarded patients, and in only 30% of the controls.[16] Again, the full implications of these studies are as yet uncertain.

Vitamin E

Sickle erythrocytes are more susceptible to peroxidation than are normal red blood cells. This may be due to the membrane phospholipid reorganization during the sickling process[18] or to a deficiency in the normal antioxidant systems, such as vitamin E, glutathione peroxidase, catalase, and/or superoxide dismutase. The peroxidative damage can produce abnormal cellular properties, i.e., potassium leakage and decreased cell deformability. These factors may initiate the formation of irreversibly sickled cells, as well as increase hemolysis. Low serum levels of vitamin E have been identified in sickle-cell patients.[19,20] Furthermore, the susceptibility of sickle red blood cell to peroxidation was reduced in vitro by preincubation with vitamin E.[20] Confirmation of the value of vitamin E supplementation is pending. However, other studies in sickle-cell children reported normal vitamin E levels in both growth-retarded and growth-normal sickle-cell patients.[17,21]

Folate

As a result of severe hemolytic disease, folic acid stores may be compromised and daily requirements increased.[22] Actual folate deficiency occurring as a result of a deficient diet has rarely been documented in sickle-cell anemia, but may result from increased utilization to meet the demands of accelerated erythropoiesis. Minimum daily doses of 500–1000 μg/day have been required to achieve a good hematological response.[22,23] Routine supplementation with folate at a dose of 1 mg/day is recommended by some hematologists.

Iron

The final aspect of replacement therapy in sickle-cell anemia is iron therapy. It has been generally assumed that patients with sickle-cell anemia acquire an increased total body iron burden as a result of hemolysis and blood transfusions and that iron deficiency was rare. O'Brien[24] was one of the first to report that the majority of sickle-cell patients he studied under age 20 years did not have an excessive iron burden.[24] The incidence of iron-deficiency anemia in pediatric sickle-cell patients is 16% in nontransfused patients and 0% in transfused patients.[25] The most reliable tests in discriminating iron deficiency in sickle-cell patients are serum ferritin and mean corpuscular volume (MCV). Although there is some theoretical evidence that iron deficiency prevents sickling of the red blood cell and could in theory make the clinical manifestations less severe, this hypothesis lacks clinical verification. However, the nonhematological implications of iron deficiency in a developing infant or toddler are important enough to warrant the prevention and aggressive treatment of iron deficiency. Therefore, patients should be screened periodically using a CBC (complete blood count), which includes the hemoglobin determination and the MCV, and, when indicated, a serum ferritin. Nontransfused infants should be on iron-fortified formula, or if breastfed, they should be supplemented with vitamins with iron similar to the recommendations for normal infants. If iron deficiency is documented, a therapeutic trial of iron should be initiated.

Protein and caloric needs

Because growth also depends on the normal metabolism of nutritional components, nitrogen utilization has recently been studied as a factor in the somatic growth retardation of sickle-cell disease. There is some evidence that nitrogen economy is impaired in sickle-cell patients with poor growth.[26] When a group of sickle-cell teenagers was compared to a group of normal controls of comparable ages, the mean urinary nitrogen excretion was significantly higher in the sickle-cell patients at all three levels of intake tested. More-

over, the sickle-cell patients were in negative nitrogen balance at all levels.[26] Is there any evidence that inadequate intake of calories may also be associated with the poor growth? This question prompted a recent investigation of absorptive function and nutritional supplementation.[26] Five growth-retarded boys with sickle-cell disease were evaluated; in all of them the daily calorie and protein intakes were deemed adequate by careful dietary history. Visceral protein status, assessed by serum albumin, was normal in all patients. Somatic protein depletion was documented in three patients by midarm muscle circumference less than the 5th percentile. Intestinal function was normal in all patients. Two of the patients were supplemented only with zinc, iron, folate, and vitamin E. One patient received nightly oral Ensure® supplements, and the remaining two patients were supplemented by nocturnal nasogastric feedings. Those two patients receiving only iron, zinc, folate, and vitamin E supplements had no change in growth rate. Likewise, there was no change in the patient on oral formula supplements. In the two patients receiving nasogastric (NG) feedings, there was a dramatic increase in growth both in height and weight. Hospital admissions for infection and painful crises also decreased significantly. This suggests that inadequate caloric intake rather than specific nutritional deficiencies may be involved in the growth retardation of children with sickle-cell disease. This finding is consistent with the increased metabolic requirements of sickle-cell disease resulting from vaso-occlusive episodes, repeated infections, or hyperactivity of the hematopoietic system. Significantly, all three patients on caloric supplementation experienced a marked reduction in hospitalizations related to sickle-cell disease. In other studies, the dietary intake of calories and some micronutrients (vitamins E and C, beta-carotene) exceeded the recommended daily allowances (similar to healthy controls). Thus, the reduced serum plasma level was not due to the low dietary intake of these nutrients.[27,28]

Follow-up and Summary

In summary, growth retardation and pubertal delay occur in a significant number of sickle-cell patients. The etiology is unknown, but trace elements have been implicated and used with some success therapeutically. Recently, attention has turned to the increased metabolic requirements of these patients and the possible use of caloric supplementation for some. However, controlled therapeutic trials with large numbers of patients will be important in determining the need for supplementation. Hormonal replacement is unnecessary. Nutritional support may be one of the most promising therapeutic interventions available. Dietary, nutrient, biochemical, and anthropometric assessment should be evaluated at each routine clinic visit.

References

1. Whitten, C.F., Nishiura, E.N. Sickle cell anemia. In: Hobbs, N., Perrin, J.M., eds. *Issues in the Care of Children with Chronic Illness.* San Francisco: Jossey-Bass; 1985.
2. Portnoy, B., Herion, J. Neurologic manifestations in sickle-cell disease. *Ann. Intern. Med.* 1972; 76:643.
3. Powars, D., Wilson, B., Imbus, C., Pegelow, C., Allen, J. The natural history of stroke in sickle cell disease. *Am. J. Med.* 1978; 65:461.

4. Phebus, C., Gloninger, M., Maciak, B. Growth patterns by age and sex in children with sickle cell disease. *J. Pediatr.* 1984; 105:28.
5. Abbasi, A.A., Prasad, A.S., Ortega, J., Congo, E., Oberleas, D. Gonadal function abnormalities in sickle cell anemia: studies in adult male patients. *Ann. Intern. Med.* 1976; 85:601.
6. Luban, N., Leikin, S., August, G. Growth and development in sickle cell anemia. *Am. J. Pediatr. Hematol. Oncol.* 1982; 4:61.
7. Ashcroft, M.T., Serjeant, G.R. Body habitus of Jamaican adults with sickle cell anemia. *South. Med. J.* 1972; 65:579.
8. Jimenez, C.T., Scott, R.B., Henry, W.L., Sampson, C.C., Ferguson, A.D. Studies in sickle cell anemia. XXVI. Sickle cell disease on the onset of menarche, pregnancy, fertility, pubescent changes, and body growth in Negro subjects. *Am. J. Dis. Child.* 1966; 111:497.
9. Whitten, C.F. Growth status of children with sickle cell anemia. *Am. J. Dis. Child.* 1961; 102:355.
10. Kramer, M.S., Rooks, Y., Washington, L.A., Pearson, H.A. Pre- and postnatal growth and development in sickle cell anemia. *J. Pediatr.* 1980; 96:857.
11. Prasad, A.S., Abbasi, A., Rabbani, P., DuMouchelle, E. Effect of zinc supplementation on serum testosterone level in adult male sickle cell anemia subjects. *Am. J. Hematol.* 1981; 10:119.
12. Prasad, A.S., Cossack, Z. Zinc supplementation and growth in sickle cell disease. *Ann. Intern. Med.* 1984; 100:267.
13. Prasad, A.S., Ortega, J., Brewer, G., Oberleas, O. Trace elements in sickle cell disease. *JAMA.* 1976; 235:2396.
14. Ballester, O.F., Prasad, A.S. Energy, zinc deficiency, and decreased nucleoside phosphorylase activity in patients with sickle cell anemia. *Ann. Intern. Med.* 1983; 98:180.
15. Niell, H.B., Leach, B.E., Kraus, A.P. Zinc metabolism in sickle cell anemia. *JAMA.* 1979; 242:2686.
16. Finan, A.C., Elmer, M.A., Sasanow, S.R., McKinney, S., Russell, M.O., Gill, F.M. Nutritional factors and growth in children with sickle cell disease. *Am. J. Dis. Child.* 1988; 142:237.
17. Natta, C., Chen, L., Chow, C. Selenium and glutathione peroxidase levels in sickle cell anemia. *Acta Haematol.* 1990; 83:130.
18. Chiu, D., Lubin, B., Shohet, S. Erythrocyte membrane lipid reorganization during the sickling process. *Br. J. Haematol.* 1979; 41:223.
19. Natta, C., Machlin, L. Plasma levels of tocopherol in sickle cell anemia subjects. *Am. J. Clin. Nutr.* 1984; 40:235.
20. Chiu, D., Vichinsky, E., Yee, M., Kleman, K., Lubin, B. Peroxidation, vitamin E, and sickle cell anemia. *Ann. NY. Acad. Sci.* 1982; 393:323.
21. Broxson, E., Sokal, R., Githens, J. Normal vitamin E status in sickle hemoglobinopathies in Colorado. *Am. J. Clin. Nutr.* 1989; 50:497.
22. Pearson, H., Colab, W. Folic acid studies in sickle cell anemia. *J. Lab. Clin. Med.* 1964; 64:913.
23. Lindenbaum, J., Klipstein, F. Folic acid deficiency in sickle cell anemia. *N. Engl. J. Med.* 1961; 265:1033.
24. O'Brien, R. Iron burden in sickle cell anemia. *J. Pediatr.* 1978; 92:579.
25. Vichinsky, E., Kleman, K., Embury, S., Lubin, B. The diagnosis of iron deficiency anemia in sickle cell disease. *Blood.* 1981; 58:963.
26. O'Donkor, P., Addae, S., Yamamoto, S., Apatu, R. Effect of dietary nitrogen on urinary excretion of non-protein nitrogen in adolescent sickle cell patients. *Hum. Nutr. Clin. Nutr.* 1984; 38:23.
27. Tangrey, C., Phillips, S., Bell, R., Fernadis, P., Hopkins, R., Wu, S. Selected indices of micronutrient status in adult patients with sickle cell anemia. *Am. J. Clin. Hematol.* 1989; 32:161.
28. Chire, D., Vichinsky, E., Ho, S., Lice, T., Lubin, B. Vitamin C deficiency in patients with sickle cell anemia. *Am. J. Pediatr. Hematol. Oncol.* 1990; 12:262.

Chapter 34
Nutrition in Gastrointestinal Disorders of Infancy and Childhood

Michael Farrell

For a child to grow and develop normally, food must be ingested, digested, and absorbed. Obviously the gastrointestinal (GI) tract is crucial in this process. This chapter describes primary and secondary conditions that interfere with the normal digestive and absorptive functions of the GI tract. The past decade has seen the development of a variety of nutrition support modalities that allow the child with any type of GI dysfunction to grow and develop normally. An understanding of the physiology of digestion and the pathophysiology of GI diseases allows the selection of the appropriate method of nutrition support.

Gastroesophageal Reflux

Gastroesophageal reflux, the spontaneous passage of gastric contents from the stomach into the esophagus, is the most common cause of vomiting in infants.[1] However, the differential diagnosis of vomiting is vast; the practitioner must remember that it is a symptom, not a disease.

Biochemical and clinical abnormalities

Certain signs and symptoms warn of potentially serious conditions. Vomiting in the neonate must always be investigated. Bilious or projectile vomiting mandates the exclusion of anatomical disorders, such as pyloric stenosis or malrotation. Failure to thrive or fluid and electrolyte disturbances, such as metabolic alkalosis or acidosis, are worrisome and warrant further evaluation. However, the majority of infants have gastroesophageal reflux; that is, the effortless postprandial spitting or regurgitation of feedings with no associated symptoms. In one study, up to 50% of infants 2 months of age vomited more than two times per day. The regurgitation is the result of an immature lower esophageal sphincter.[2] Carré[3] studied the natural history of gastroesophageal reflux; 60% of infants improved spontaneously by 18 months of age, and only 10% developed severe complications. Numerous subsequent studies have demonstrated the benign nature of infantile gastroesophageal reflux.

Factors to be considered in nutritional evaluation

When the vomiting persists, food allergy may be considered, and a cow milk formula may be changed to a soy-based formula.[4] However, if the vomiting persists after several formula changes, other causes should be sought (see Chapter 28). During the time of formula manipulation, adequate nutrition must be maintained. Prolonged hypocaloric or clear liquid intake is never appropriate in an infant.

Management

A detailed feeding history must be obtained. The volume and frequency of feeding, as well as the formula concentration, must be examined. There is a tendency, particularly among young mothers, to overfeed infants, which results in postprandial vomiting.

The primary treatments for gastroesophageal reflux are time and position[5]; in 90% of infants, symptoms resolve within the first year. After feeding, the child should be placed in the prone position, not in an infant seat because the sitting position increases intra-abdominal pressure and thus reflux. The use of thickened feedings is controversial; recent studies have yielded conflicting results.[6,7] In one study there was less vomiting, but another found delayed gastric emptying and increased reflux. Medical therapy of gastroesophageal reflux is usually expectant and supportive. Adequate nutrition for growth and development must be provided.

The neurologically impaired child, however, presents a different set of problems. Approximately 15% of severely handicapped institutionalized children have chronic vomiting.[8] Sondheimer[8] demonstrated that 80% of these infants have significant gastroesophageal reflux. These children may have a myriad of symptoms: vomiting, pain, anemia, hypoalbuminemia, malnutrition, bizarre contortions (Sandifer syndrome) have been reported. These children are often at great nutritional risk. Any neurologically impaired child who has anemia should be investigated for iron deficiency. If iron deficiency is documented, it is likely that blood loss from esophagitis is the source. Factors that place the neurologically impaired child at greater risk for severe gastroesophageal reflux are scoliosis, severe impairment, a nonambulatory status, and intractable seizures.

Unfortunately, medical therapy for these children is not very effective. In one study, Sondheimer[9] demonstrated approximately 20% mortality from medical therapy and poor response in the remaining patients. Surgery frequently becomes the only method for controlling severe reflux.[10] However before the child undergoes an antireflux procedure, nutritional status must be assessed and improved. The author uses a combination of medical and nutritional therapy to prepare these children for surgery. The esophagitis is controlled with antacids or H_2 blockers, such as ranitidine. If gastric emptying is delayed or other motility disturbances are present, metoclopramide or cisapride (not available yet in the United States) may improve motility. Short-term nasojejunal feedings have been used to promote positive nitrogen balance and weight gain, as well as to correct the iron-deficiency anemia and hypoalbuminemia so often found in these patients before surgery.

Neurologically impaired children are often referred for gastrostomy because of feeding difficulty. Gastroesophageal reflux must be excluded, as placement of the gastrostomy will aggravate reflux.[10] If no reflux is detected and a gastrostomy is performed, 25% to 40% of these children will develop reflux later. Hence, the decision to place a gastrostomy in a neurologically impaired child is complex and should involve the nutritionist, physician, and surgeon.

Follow-up

With intensive medical care and nutritional support, symptoms will improve in approximately 85% of neurologically impaired children.

Liver Disease

The estimated incidence of neonatal cholestatic liver diseases—neonatal hepatitis, biliary atresia, biliary hypoplasia, and various metabolic disorders—is 1 in 8000–10,000 live births. Growth failure is a frequent complication.[11] Currently there are very few medical therapies for these disorders and liver transplantation has become the major treatment.[12] However, donor availability is a function of recipient weight; therefore, maintaining optimal nutritional status is crucial.

Biochemical and clinical abnormalities

Most liver diseases encountered in infants and children have a significant cholestatic component.[13] Serum total and direct bilirubin are elevated, as are the aminotransferases. Bile flow is obstructed from the hepatocyte into the biliary system and hence the intestine; there is a marked decrease in concentration of intraluminal bile acids, often below the critical micellar concentration necessary for micelle formation and fat absorption.[14] The result is fat and fat-soluble vitamin malabsorption. These patients, as do many infants with chronic disease, may also have anorexia, which results in protein-calorie malnutrition, as well as specific nutrient deficiencies.

Hepatic portoenterostomy (the Kasai procedure) attempts to restore bile flow in the infant with biliary atresia.[15] It is successful in approximately 20% of infants. However, even if bile drainage is established, cholestasis often persists, despite declining serum bilirubin concentrations.

The natural history of these disorders is progression to cirrhosis and end-stage liver disease. As the seriousness of the liver disease increases, ascites develops. The child becomes very fluid and sodium sensitive. The ongoing destruction of functioning liver cells makes processing of nutrients difficult. Therefore, nutrition intervention must be accomplished early in the course of the disease as soon as a deviation from normal growth patterns is detected.

Factors to be considered in nutritional evaluation

Long-chain fatty acids are poorly absorbed in the absence of bile acids. Medium-chain triglycerides (MCT) do not require micelle formation and are absorbed into the portal system directly. Therefore, any formula used in cholestatic liver disease should contain sufficient long-chain fats to prevent essential fatty acid deficiency and should use MCT as a caloric source. Portagen has been used frequently, but it has several limitations. Its linoleic acid content is suboptimal, and essential fatty deficiency has been reported in infants with cholestatic liver disease.[16] A formula containing approximately half MCT oil and half long-chain fats and 10% to 12% of its total calories as linoleic acid (Pregestimil®, Alimentum®) is preferable. No controlled studies support the superiority of high-branched chain amino acid diets. They may be useful in the treatment of acute decompensation and/or encephalopathy, but the lack of data and their expense preclude their routine use for children with chronic liver disease.[17]

Growth and nutrition must be monitored carefully; any deviation from established percentiles must be investigated promptly. Nutritional status is difficult to assess since weight may be affected by edema, ascites, and organomegaly. Anthropometric measurements may be unreliable due to fluid retention. Linear growth and growth velocity are the best indicators.

Management

Breastfeeding should be encouraged and allowed as long as the infant is gaining weight appropriately. If weight gain decreases, supplementation with a MCT-containing formula should be initiated. The caloric intake of any infant who is failing to gain appropriately should be assessed; if it is inadequate, supplementation should be begun. Although a gastrostomy tube may be placed, in the face of portal hypertension there frequently is peristomal variceal bleeding. Therefore, we prefer nasogastric feeding, in which small-bore Silastic or polyurethane tubes are inserted and the formula is delivered continuously throughout a specified time of the day to provide the needed calories. The use of small soft tubes decreases the chances of variceal bleeding. Oral feeding should continue during the tube feeding.

If weight gain does not occur on 20 cal/oz formula, caloric density may be increased by the addition of Polycose or MCT. The formula may be concentrated, but adequate free water must be provided. Most infants can tolerate protein concentrations to 3 g/kg/day. Therefore, if necessary, concentration of the formula to 30 cal/oz is possible.

Vitamin Supplementation

Vitamin A. Chronic malabsorption results in fat-soluble vitamin deficiency. If cholestyramine is being administered in an attempt to control pruritus, further vitamin malabsorption may occur. The usual supplement is 50,000 units per day of a water-miscible compound (Aquasol A).[18] Clinical vitamin A deficiency also occurs despite supplementation if zinc deficiency is present.[19] However, because vitamin A toxicity may occur, serum concentrations should be monitored. If cholestasis resolves, supplementation should be promptly discontinued.

Vitamin D. Vitamin D is essential for bone formation and calcium and phosphorus homeostasis. Deficiency of vitamin D results in osteopenia, rickets, and fractures. Exposure to sunshine should be encouraged as a major source of vitamin D[20] because orally administered vitamin D_2 is poorly absorbed in cholestasis. The vitamin D metabolites,

25-hydroxyvitamin D and 1,25 dihydroxy-vitamin D, are more polar compounds and are therefore absorbed better.[21] The serum concentration of 25-hydroxyvitamin D level is the best indicator of total vitamin D status. If there is no response to sunlight exposure or vitamin D supplementation, 25-hydroxyvitamin D should be administered at a dose of 5–7 μg/kg/day. Serum concentration should be monitored. A bone radiograph or an assessment of bone mineral density also provides an adequate indication of mineralization.

Vitamin E. Vitamin E requires bile for absorption.[22] A vitamin E deficiency syndrome of peripheral neuropathy, ataxia, and ophthalmoplegia has been described in patients with cholestasis.[23,24] The early neurological findings are reversible, but as the deficiency progresses they become irreversible. Vitamin E deficiency occurs before any clinical symptoms are detectable and may develop by 18 months. The initial clinical findings are loss of deep tendon reflexes and vibratory sense.

Vitamin E supplementation should be initiated when cholestasis is diagnosed (50-400 IU Aquasol E/day). The patient's ability to absorb vitamin E can be determined by an oral vitamin E tolerance test. Vitamin E levels should be determined at 3-month intervals, rather than waiting for clinical deficiency states to develop. Since vitamin E is transported in serum by the lipid fraction, the vitamin E:total lipid rates should be determined (<0.8 indicates deficiency).[23] If serum E:lipid ratios are <0.8, supplementation should be given by intramuscular vitamin E or oral tocopherol polyethylene glycol-1000 succinate (15–25 IU/kg/day).[25]

Vitamin K. Hemorrhage, secondary to vitamin K deficiency, may be the initial sign of cholestatic liver disease.[26,27] Children with cholestasis are particularly at risk for bleeding due to portal hypertension, gastroesophageal varices, and exteriorized conduits. Absorption of either dietary vitamin K or the vitamin K synthesized by intestinal bacteria requires bile-acid-containing micelles. Therefore, coagulation status should be monitored carefully by the prothrombin time and vitamin K supplementation provided. The initial dose therapy is 2.5–5 mg orally every 1–3 days. Vitamin K_1 has minimal side effects compared to other forms. If no absorption occurs or if intraluminal bile acids concentrations are very low, synthetic water-soluble vitamin K_3 (Synkavite®) may be necessary. Parenteral vitamin K may be necessary to reverse prolonged prothrombin times in the face of bleeding or in the child who does not improve on oral therapy.

Water-Soluble Vitamins. Deficiencies of water-soluble vitamins have been reported in adult liver disease[28]; there are currently no data available in children. It is reasonable to provide a daily dose of a standard multivitamin preparation.

Minerals

Iron. Malabsorption of iron, as well as ongoing bleeding, may result in iron deficiency. However, the judicious use of iron supplementation is warranted because iron overload may injure the liver. Early in iron deficiency, the serum ferritin decreases, followed by an increase in transferrin. The mean corpuscular volume (MCV) decreases as intracellular iron content decreases. Unfortunately, cirrhosis itself increases serum ferritin concentrations. Therefore MCV,

serum iron concentration, and saturation index should be examined; the saturation index should be kept greater than 16%.

Calcium. Calcium is malabsorbed in infants with cholestasis.[29] The exact mechanisms remain to be elucidated, but calcium malabsorption is believed to be due to binding of calcium in fatty acids, which results in insoluble soaps. Calcium supplementation should be provided only if bone disease or a low serum concentration persists after the correction of vitamin D deficiency.

Zinc. Zinc deficiency accompanies chronic malnutrition, cirrhosis, and any stress state. However, identification of zinc deficiency is difficult. The serum zinc concentration is at best an imprecise measure of total body zinc status. This concentration is directly correlated to the serum albumin concentration, which is frequently lowered in chronic liver disease. If there is persistent vitamin A deficiency, poor growth, or persistent anorexia, zinc supplementation at 1 mg/kg/day should be begun.[30]

Infants with chronic liver disease are difficult to manage. Because of fat malabsorption they should be begun on formulas containing MCT. Fat-soluble vitamin supplementation should be begun immediately and should be monitored both clinically and biochemically at 3-month intervals.

Follow-up

Growth parameters, including height, weight, and anthropometric measurements, should be followed serially. Aggressive intervention is warranted at the first indication of growth failure.

Inflammatory Bowel Disease

The incidence of inflammatory bowel disease is 3.5–7.9 per 100,000 and appears to be increasing. The peak age of onset is the second and third decade of life; approximately 20% of patients are under 21 years of age.[31]

Biochemical and clinical abnormalities

Malnutrition and growth failure frequently complicate inflammatory bowel disease. Delayed sexual maturation and decreased linear growth are present in 20% to 30% of affected children.[32]

Ulcerative colitis usually begins with the acute or semiacute onset of bloody diarrhea, which then persists. Often, fever, abdominal pain and cramps, and tenesmus occur. There may be extraintestinal manifestations, such as arthritis, recurrent mouth sores, and such dermatological disorders as pyoderma gangrenosum. Characteristically, mucosal involvement begins at the anal verge and spreads continuously to involve varying amounts of the colon. The diagnosis of ulcerative colitis is established by excluding infectious causes for the bloody diarrhea and demonstrating the typical endoscopic and histological features.[33]

Crohn's disease, in contrast, usually has an insidious onset and follows a chronic course of relapses and exacerbations. Any portion of the GI tract, from the mouth to anus, may be involved. Abdominal pain and/or diarrhea are not necessary for the diagnosis, and they are frequently absent initially. Presenting symptoms may include unexplained fever, anemia, growth failure, delayed sexual maturation, amenorrhea, and joint symptoms; perianal disease is frequently a problem, and its presence in a child or adolescent should prompt the search for inflammatory bowel disease.[34]

The cause of the growth failure is multifactorial[35] and includes enteric losses of blood and protein, malabsorption of carbohydrate and fat, (depending on the area and length of small bowel involvement), and increased needs due to the inflammatory process. However, the major cause of poor growth is inadequate caloric intake.[36] Several studies have shown that the usual intake is 60% to 70% of the recommended intake for age.

Factors to be considered in nutritional evaluation

The child or adolescent with suspected inflammatory bowel disease should have a detailed nutritional evaluation. Serial height and weight data are invaluable and should be plotted on standard growth charts with any deviation noted. Growth velocity (cm/year) should be determined and compared to standards since a decline in growth velocity is frequently the initial nutritional disorder. The degree of sexual development in adolescents should be estimated and expressed as Tanner ratings (see Appendix 9).

Anthropometric measurements may show depleted somatic protein stores and decreased subcutaneous fat. Useful biochemical determinations include the blood count (looking for evidence of iron deficiency) and serum albumin and prealbumin to estimate visceral protein status. Specific nutrient deficiencies that may develop include vitamin B_{12} deficiency if there is extensive ileal involvement; folic acid depletion occurs secondary to the rapid turnover of mucosal cells (sulfasalazine interferes with folate metabolism). Calcium and magnesium malabsorption may occur as a result of malabsorption and the formation of soaps with fatty acids within the intestinal lumen. Zinc deficiency frequently develops due to stress, protein losses and the use of corticosteroids, which increase the urinary excretion of zinc.

Dietary intake should be evaluated by a 7-day food recall, although it frequently is inadequate. Energy needs should be estimated; the recommended daily allowance (RDA) provides an approximate estimate. Although there may be increased energy requirements due to fever and inflammation, the hypermetabolic state is uncommon. Rather, anorexia and insufficient intake are more common. If there is no response to what appears to be adequate caloric intake, indirect calorimetry can be used to define actual energy needs.

Dietary and nutritional management

Management begins with the recognition that nutrition is crucial in patients with inflammatory bowel disease.[37] Because no specific foods have been implicated in these diseases, no food should be excluded unless there is evidence that it causes problems in a particular patient.

There is little specific nutritional therapy for ulcerative colitis.[38] Therapy is medical or surgical, and adequate nutrition should be provided. Patients are at risk for iron deficiency due to chronic bleeding, and sulfasalazine therapy increases folic acid requirements. Parenteral nutrition has not been shown to be effective in ulcerative colitis and should not be used as a primary therapy.

In contrast, Crohn's disease has a significant nutritional component. Every attempt should be made to maximize nutritional intake.[39] If counseling is not effective, supplementation should be considered. The most effective means is nocturnal (10–12 hours)[40] nasogastric feedings. The patient is taught to insert the nasogastric tube nightly; a non-lactose-containing formula is infused at a constant rate using a pump. The rate of the enteral feedings should be adjusted according to the patient's needs and average daily oral intake.

The choice of enteral product is controversial. In most cases, a specialized formula is not required. Some patients have lactose intolerance due to small bowel disease and benefit from a nonlactose formula.[41] Recent studies suggest that an elemental formula may induce remission; this action is based on the theory that absorption of intact proteins aggravate inflammation. However, these studies have not compared the effects of improved nutrition alone.[42,43] The author uses a standard formula for caloric supplementation and reserves the semi-elemental formulas for refractory situations. Total parenteral nutrition (TPN) should be reserved for patients with extensive intestinal resection, those who are obstructed, or those who are immediately postoperative. TPN should not be used as a primary therapy unless the GI tract is nonfunctional. Long-term nutritional needs can be met by nocturnal enteral feedings at home.[44] Severely affected patients who cannot tolerate enteral feedings can be treated with home parenteral nutrition.[45]

Follow-up

Regardless of which nutrition modality is used, there must be close follow-up; particular attention must be paid to linear growth and sexual maturation. If adequate nutrition is provided, the vast majority of patients with inflammatory bowel disease can grow and lead useful functioning lives.

Short Bowel Syndrome

Biochemical and clinical abnormalities

The short bowel syndrome is a malabsorptive disorder secondary to extensive small bowel resection. Modern surgical techniques and advances in nutrition support have allowed infants to survive previously lethal resections.[46] Loss of absorptive surface is the primary problem, but motility disturbances, bile acid deficiency, and bacterial overgrowth are additional complications. A precise anatomical definition is difficult since measurements are notoriously inaccurate. A useful functional definition is "the gut is short when it acts short."

The most common causes of short gut in infants are congenital anomalies and necrotizing enterocolitis. In older children, Crohn's disease is the major cause. Factors affecting outcome include the extent and site of resection, the presence or absence of the ileocecal valve, the absorptive capacity of the remaining bowel, and the potential for adaptation. Most neonatal intestinal growth occurs in the last trimester so premature infants have a greater capacity to lengthen their bowel.[47]

Currently, the overall survival of these infants is 85%; the minimum amount of viable bowel necessary is 17 cm with an ileocecal valve and 30 cm without a valve.[48] The major complications of current therapy are those of parenteral nutrition; namely, infection and cholestatic liver disease.

Factors to be considered in nutritional evaluation

Crucial factors to be determined are the site and extent of involvement and/or resection, since each portion of the bowel has distinct functions. The colon absorbs water and electrolytes and acts as a "scavenger," absorbing the fatty acid byproducts of carbohydrate digestion and fermentation. The ileum specifically absorbs vitamin B_{12} and bile acids; these functions cannot be assumed by the jejunum. The jejunum is the major source of carbohydrate and fat absorption, but the ileum can partially adapt to these functions.

Small bowel involvement results in carbohydrate malabsorption and osmotic diarrhea.[49] Steatorrhea is common; its causes include insufficient mucosal surface area, bacterial overgrowth, and bile acid deficiency due to the lack of ileal absorption. If the colon is absent, there may be excessive loss of cations.[50,51] Sodium (90–120 mEq/L) and zinc (8–12 mg/L) losses are the most common problems, but increased losses of magnesium, calcium and phosphorus may occur.

The infant's nutritional status should be assessed and growth and weight gain closely monitored. New techniques of body compartment measurements, such as bioelectric impedance, may be available in the future (see chapter 4.) The goal of therapy is normal gain and growth and adaptation of the remaining bowel. The major stimulus to mucosal adaptation is intraluminal nutrients.[52]

Nutritional management

Management is based on the phase of the infant's response and the clinical factors in each phase.

Initial phase. Immediately after resection, the major problem is the replacement of ongoing fluid and electrolyte losses, which may be extensive. Total parenteral nutrition should be begun within the first few postoperative days. Usually a central venous catheter is required to deliver the necessary volume. Caloric needs should be determined based on age, losses, and nutritional status. Serum electrolyte, urea nitrogen, glucose, and phosphorus concentrations should be monitored frequently. Hepatic status should be followed weekly to detect cholestasis. Elevation of serum bile acids may be the first indicator of cholestasis,[53] before there is an increase in serum direct bilirubin or aminotransferase concentrations.

Phase 2. After initial stabilization has occurred and GI motility returns, enteral feedings should be begun. It is important to begin enteral feeding as soon as possible in any amount since it is a major factor in preventing TPN-associated cholestasis. They are best delivered by continuous infusion via a nasogastric tube, gastrostomy, or jejunostomy, depending on clinical indications. Stool volume, pH, and reducing substances must be monitored. Stool pH less than 5 or reducing substances greater than 1% indicate carbohydrate malabsorption. This phase may last for months.

The choice of formula is controversial. A hydrolyzed protein, consisting of di- and tripeptides, allows easier absorption and avoids sensitization from the absorption of intact protein. Peptides are reabsorbed more efficiently than amino acids. Many patients have lactose intolerance so lactose should be avoided (see Chapter 46). Formulas containing glucose polymers and sucrose are preferred. The choice of fat is problematic: MCTs are absorbed more efficiently especially if there is bile acid deficiency. However, long-chain triglycerides appear to provide better mucosal hyperplasia in animal studies.[54] The best approach is to use a formula that contains both fat sources. The preferred formula is semi-elemental; it should be started at 3% to 5% of caloric needs. Enteral feedings are increased as tolerated; parenteral nutrition is reduced isocaloricly. After 1 or 2 months, if TPN is still required, home therapy should be considered.[55]

Phase 3. There are long-term problems associated with therapy of the short bowel syndrome. A recently recognized complication is feeding refusal after prolonged TPN.[56] The best treatment appears to be prevention of this problem by the early introduction of small oral feedings and by the encouragement of nonnutritive sucking.

When the patient is gaining weight on enteral feedings and all his or her nutrition needs are met, the central line can be removed. Solid feedings can then be begun. Introduction of bolus feedings should be gradual as the continuous feedings are decreased. During this phase, the major problems encountered are deficiencies of trace metals and vitamins. If there has been extensive ileal resection, vitamin B_{12} supplementation may be necessary. Fat-soluble vitamin malabsorption resulting in rickets, osteopenia, and other clinical symptoms may be present.[57] Intermittent parenteral supplementation may be necessary. Patients who have steatorrhea and an intact colon are at risk for renal oxalate stones and should avoid high oxalate containing foods. Medication-nutrient interaction should also be identified.

Follow-up

With attention to detail and the use of a multidisciplinary team, these children can survive their intestinal resection and lead normal lives.

Enteral and Parenteral Nutrition

Parenteral nutrition allows the provision of adequate nutrition to patients who cannot or will not eat. Although many patients have functioning GI tracts, anorexia, weakness, or neurological impairments prevent adequate oral intake. Recently, it has been recognized that the primary stimulus to gut health and repair is nutrition, specifically intraluminal nutrients. A variety of methods to obtain access to the gastrointestinal tract and many formulas have been developed. There has been an unfortunate tendency to view parenteral and enteral nutrition as exclusive rather than complementary therapies. What matters most is that the child receive adequate *total* nutrition and that some be administered enterally.

Parenteral nutrition should be initiated only when the child's caloric needs cannot be met through enteral or oral feedings. It may be administered via either peripheral or central veins (see Chapter 3). The peripheral route can be started quickly; however, peripheral veins tolerate hyperosmolar fluids poorly so *total* caloric support is difficult to achieve. The maximum dextrose concentration that can be administered via a peripheral vein is 10%; therefore, the use of lipid emulsions is mandatory to achieve reasonable caloric intake. For example, 10% dextrose parenteral fluid provides 0.34 kcal/cc, and 10% lipid emulsion provides 1.1 kcal/cc.

The central venous route should be used for those patients requiring prolonged support (Table 34-1). Many complications have been reported, such as infections, thrombosis, pneumothorax, and metabolic derangements. Therefore, catheters should be placed only by experienced physicians. Several studies have shown that institutions with nutrition support teams that carefully follow protocols have much lower complication rates.[58]

Nutritional support is begun as soon as the child is identified as being at risk. Methods of nutrition support include: oral supplementation, an increase in formula density, enteral feedings—nasogastric (continuous or bolus) or nasojejunal—and parenteral nutrition: total or partial, peripheral or central (see Appendix 6). Risk factors include present nutritional status, disease process, anticipated medical or surgical therapy, current caloric intake and past history. If possible, oral supplementation is recommended either with specific supplements or by increasing the caloric density of the formula. If the caloric density is increased, care must be taken to provide adequate free water to excrete the increased renal solute load.

When oral supplementation is unsuccessful and the GI tract is functional, a nasoenteric tube is placed. Small-bore (5,8 French) soft Silastic catheters are easily inserted and well tolerated and may be placed in the stomach or jejunum. Nasogastric feedings are simple to administer, and the tube can be placed by the child or caregivers. Placement in the stomach allows normal digestive processes and hormonal response. Nasogastric feedings can be administered as a bolus or continuously. They allow greater freedom and mobility for the child. An intact gag reflex is an absolute requirement for intragastric feedings to prevent aspiration. Transpyloric feedings are indicated in patients with gastroesophageal reflux, impaired gag reflex, vocal cord paralysis, gastric motor abnormalities, or intractable vomiting. A weighted tube may be allowed to pass out of the stomach into the small bowel and its position verified radiographically. Alternatively, the tube may be passed through the pylorus under fluoroscopic or endoscopic guidance. If a gastrostomy tube is in place and jejunal feedings are necessary, the tube can be passed through the gastrostomy tube into the jejunum under fluoroscopy. Jejunal feedings generally are administered continuously for a specified time period to meet caloric needs. Oral stimulation is needed during enteral and parenteral feedings (see Chapter 24).

Follow-up

If nutritional therapy is chosen appropriately and the child's nutritional needs are met, children with a wide variety of GI disorders can be discharged from the hospital, grow normally and lead normal lives. An interdisciplinary team of nutritionist, nurse, parent, and special educator can facilitate the transition of the child fed by gastrostomy to school. Growth, nutrients, oral feeding skills, gastrostomy feeding, behavior, constipation, and positioning should continue to be evaluated.[59]

Table 34-1. Electrolyte and Mineral Requirements in Total Parenteral Nutrition

	Infant (per kg/day)	Child-adult
Sodium	2–4 mEq	1–2 mEq/kg
Potassium	2–3 mEq	0.5–1.0 mEq/kg
Calcium	3–4 mEq	1–2 mEq/kg
Phosphate	1–2 mM	0.3–1 mM/kg
Magnesium	0.25–0.5 mEq	0.25–0.5 mEq/kg
Chloride	2–5 mEq	2–3 mEq/kg
Zinc*	400 µg (premature) 100 µg (term)	2.5–4 mg*†
Copper‡	20 µg	0.5–1.5†
Chromium	0.14–0.2 mcg	10–15 µg†
Manganese	2–10 µg (total)	0.05–0.2 mg
Molybdenum	0.25 µg/kg	
Selenium	2.0 µg/kg	

*Increase zinc if excessive GI losses (8–12 mg/L intestinal fluid).
†Maximum recommended adult concentrations.
‡Decrease copper (10 mcg/kg) if liver disease is present.

References

1. Sondheimer, J.M. Gastroesophageal reflux: update on pathogenesis and diagnosis. *Pediatr. Clin. North Am.* 1988; 35:103.
2. Boix-Ochoa, J., Canals, J. Maturation of the lower esophagus. *J. Pediatr. Surg.* 1976, 11:749.
3. Carre, I.J. The natural history of the partial thoracic stomach ("hiatus hernia") in children. *Arch. Dis. Child.* 1960; 35:481.
4. Proujansky, R., Winter, H.S., Walker, W.A. Gastrointestinal intestinal syndromes associated with food sensitivity. *Adv. Pediatr.* 1988; 35:219.
5. Orenstein, S.R., Whitington, P.F. Positioning for prevention of infant gastroesophageal reflux. *J. Pediatr.* 1983; 103:534.
6. Orenstein, S.R., Magill, S.R., Brooks, P. Thickening of infant feedings for therapy of gastroesophageal reflux. *J. Pediatr.* 1987; 110:181.
7. Bailey, D.J., Andres, J.M., Danek, G.D., Pinerio-Carrero, V.M. Lack of efficacy of thickened feedings as treatment for gastroesophageal reflux. *J. Pediatr.* 1987; 110:187.
8. Sondheimer, J.M. Gastroesophageal reflux among severely retarded children. *J. Pediatr.* 1979; 94:710.
9. Wilkinson, J.D. A comparison of medical and surgical treatment of gastroesophageal reflux in severely retarded children. *J. Pediatr.* 1981; 99:202.
10. Vane, D.W., Harmel, R.P., King, D.R., Boles, E.T. The effectiveness of Nissen fundoplication in neurologically impaired children with gastroesophageal reflux. *Surgery.* 1985; 98:662.
11. Kaufman, S.S., Murray, N.D., Wood, P., Shaw, B.W., Vanderhoof, J.A. Nutritional support for the infant with extrahepatic biliary atresia. *J. Pediatr.* 1987; 110:679.
12. Shaw, B.W., Wood, R.P., Kauffman, S.S., Williams, L., Antonson, D.L., Kelly, D.A., Vanderhoof, J.A. Liver transplantation therapy for children. *J. Pediatr. Gastroenterol. Nut.* 1988; 7:157.
13. Balistreri, W.F. Neonatal cholestasis. *J. Pediatr.* 1985; 106:171.
14. Weber, A., Roy, C.C. The malabsorption associated with chronic liver disease in children. *Pediatrics.* 1972; 50:73.
15. Kasai, M. Treatment of biliary atresia with special reference to hepatic porto-enterostomy and its modifications. *Prog. Pediatr. Surg.* 1974; 6:5.

16. Gourley, G.R., Farrell, P., O'Dell, G.B. Essential fatty acid deficiency after hepatic portoenterostomy for biliary artesia. *Am. J. Clin. Nutr.* 1982; 36:194.

17. Christie, M.L., Sack, D.M., Pomposelli, J., Horst, D. Enriched branched chain amino acid formula versus a casein-based supplement in the treatment of cirrhosis. *JPEN.* 1985; 9:671.

18. Amedee-Manesme, O., Mourey, M.S., Therasse, J., Couturier, M., Alverez, F., Hanck, A., Bernard, O. Short and long term vitamin A treatment in children with cholestasis. *Am. J. Clin. Nutr.* 1988; 47:690.

19. Smith, J.C. The vitamin A-zinc connection. *Ann. NY. Acad. Sci.* 1980; 355:62.

20. Kook, S.W., Jones, G., Reilly, B.J., Fraser, D. Pathogenesis of rickets in chronic hepatobiliary disease in children. *J. Pediatr.* 1979; 94:870.

21. Sokol, R.J., Iannaccone, S., Heubi, J.E., Bove, K.E., Balistreri, W.F. Mechanism causing vitamin E deficiency during chronic childhood cirrhosis. *Gastroenterology.* 1983; 85:1172.

22. Guggenheim, M.A., Ringel, S.P., Silverman, A., Grabert, B.E. Progressive neuromuscular disease in children with chronic cholestasis and vitamin E deficiency: diagnosis and treatment with alpha tocopherol. *J. Pediatr.* 1982; 100:51.

23. Sokol, R.J., Guggenheim, M.A., Iannaccone, S.T., Barkhaus, P.E., Miller, C., Silverman, A., Balistreri, W.F., Heubi, J.E. Improved neurologic function after long-term correction of vitamin E deficiency in children with chronic cholestasis. *N. Engl. J. Med.* 1985; 313:1580.

24. Sokol, R.J., Butler-Simoin, N.A., Bettis, D., Smith, D.J., Silverman, A. Tocopherol polyethylene glycol 1000 succinate therapy for Vitamin E deficiency during chronic childhood cholestasis neurologic outcome. *J. Pediatr.* 1987; 111:830.

25. Payne, N.R., Hasegawa, D.K. Vitamin K deficiency in a newborn: a case report in alpha-1-antitrypsin deficiency and a review of factors predisposing to hemorrhage. *Pediatrics.* 1984; 73:712.

26. Suttie, J.W. Recent advances in hepatic vitamin K metabolism and function. *Hepatology.* 1987; 7:367.

27. Rossourn, J., Labadarios, D., Davis, M., Williams, R. Water soluble vitamins in severe liver disease. *S. Afr. Med. J.* 1979; 54:183.

28. Bengoa, J.M., Setrin, M.D., Meredith, S., Kelly, S.E., Shak, N., Baker, A.L., Rosenberg, I.H. Intestinal calcium absorption and vitamin D status in chronic cholestatic liver disease. *Hepatology.* 1984; 4:261.

29. Barness, L.A., Mauer, A.M., Anderson, A.S. Zinc. *Pediatrics.* 1978; 62:408.

30. Kanof, M.E., Lake, A.M., Bayless, T.M. Decreased height velocity in children and adolescents before the diagnosis of Crohn's disease. *Gastroenterology.* 1988; 95:1523.

31. Whelan, G. Epidemiology of inflammatory bowel disease. *Med. Clin. North Am.* 1990; 74:1.

32. Michner, W.M., Wyllie, R. Management of children and adolescents with inflammatory bowel disease. *Med. Clin. North Am.* 1990; 74:103.

33. Markowitz, J., Daum, F., Aiges, H., Kahn, E., Silverberg, M., Fisher, S.E. Perianal disease in children and adolescents with Crohn's disease. *Gastroenterology.* 1984; 86:829.

34. Kirschner, B.S. Nutritional consequences of inflammatory bowel disease on growth. *J. Am. Coll. Nutr.* 1988; 7:301.

35. Kelts, D.G., Grand, R.J., Shen, G., Watkins, J.B., Werlin, S.L., Boehme, C. Nutritional basis of growth failure in children and adolescents with Crohn's disease. *Gastroenterology.* 1979; 76:720.

36. Nishi, Y., Lifshitz, F., Bayne, M.A., Daum, F., Silverberg, M., Aiges, H. Zinc status and its relation to growth retardation in children with chronic inflammatory bowel disease. *Am. J. Clin. Nutr.* 1980; 33:2613.

37. McIntyre, P.B., Powell-Tuck, J., Lennard-Jones, J. E., Lerebours, E., Hecketsweiler, P., Galmiche, J.P., Colin, R. Controlled trial of bowel rest in the treatment of severe acute colitis. *Gut.* 1986; 27:481.

38. Kleinman, R.E., Balistreri, W.F., Heyman, M.B., Kirschner, B.S., Lake, A.M., Motil, K.J., Seidman, E., Udall, J.N. Nutritional support of pediatric patients with inflammatory bowel disease. *J. Pediatr. Gastroenterol. Nutr.* 1989; 8:8.

39. Morin, C.L., Roulet, M., Roy, C.C., Weber, A. Continuous elemental enteral alimentation in children with Crohn's disease and growth failure. *Gastroenterology.* 1980; 79:1205.

40. Kirschner, B.S., DeFavaro, M.V., Jensen, W. Lactose malabsorption in adolescents with inflammatory bowel disease. *Gastroenterology.* 1981; 81:829.

41. Belli, D.C., Seidman, E., Bouthillier, Weber, A.M., Roy, C.C., Pletincx, M., Beaulieu, M., Morin, C.L. Chronic intermittent elemental diet improves growth failure in children with Crohn's disease. *Gastroenterology.* 1988; 94:603.

42. Sanderson, I.R., Udeen, S., Davies, P.S.W., Savage, M.O., Walker-Smith, J. Remission induced by an elemental diet in small bowel Crohn's disease. *Arch. Dis. Child.* 1987; 61:123.

43. Aiges, H., Markowitz, J., Rosa, J., Daum, F. Home nocturnal supplemental nasogastric feedings in growth-retarded adolescents with Crohn's disease. *Gastroenterology.* 1989; 97:905.

44. Strobel, C.T., Byrne, W.J., Ament, M.E. Home parenteral nutrition in children with Crohn's disease: an effective management alternative. *Gastroenterology.* 1979; 77:272.

45. Dorney, S.F.A., Ament, M.E., Berquist, W.E., Vargas, J.H., Hassall, E. Improved survival in very short small bowel of infancy with use of long term parenteral nutrition. *J. Pediatr.* 1985; 107:521.

46. Caniano, D.A., Starr, B.S., Ginn-Pease, M.E. Extensive short-bowel syndrome in neonates in the 1980's. *Surgery.* 1989; 105:119.

47. Touloukian, R.J., Walker Smith, G.J. Normal intestinal length in preterm infants. *J. Pediatr. Surg.* 1983; 18:720.

48. Wilmore, D.W. Factors correlating with a successful outcome following extensive intestinal resection in newborn infants. *J. Pediatr.* 1972; 80:88.

49. Ameen, V.Z., Powell, G.K., Jones, V.Z. Quantitation of fecal carbohydrate excretion in patients with short bowel syndrome. *Gastroenterology.* 1987; 92:493.

50. Ladefoged, K., Olgaard, K. Fluid and electrolyte absorption and renin-angiotensin-aldosterone axis in patients with severe short bowel syndrome. *Scand. J. Gastroenterol.* 1979; 14:729.

51. Naveh, Y., Lightman, A., Zinder, O. Effect of diarrhea on serum zinc concentrations in infants and children. *J. Pediatr.* 1982; 101:730.

52. Lentze, M.J. Intestinal adaptation in short-bowel syndrome. *Eur. J. Pediatr.* 1989; 148:294.

53. Balistreri, W.F., Suchy, F.J., Farrell, M.K., Heubi, J.E. Pathologic versus physiologic cholestasis: elevated serum concentration of a secondary bile acid occurs only in the presence of hepatobiliary disease. *J. Pediatr.* 1981; 98:399.

54. Vanderhoof, J.A., Grandjean, C.J., Kaufman, S.S., Burkley, K.T., Antonson, D.L. Effect of high percentage medium chain triglyceride diet on mucosal adaptation following massive bowel resection in rats. *JPEN* 1984; 8:685.

55. Nuty, S.F.A., Byrne, W.J., Ament, M.E. Case of congenital short small intestine: survival with use of long term parenteral feedings. *Pediatrics.* 1986; 77:386.

56. Tinscheid, T.R., Tarnowski, K.J., Rasnake, L.K., Brams, J.S. Behavioral treatment of food refusal in a child with short-gut syndrome. *J. Pediatr. Psychol.* 1987; 12:451.

57. Markestad, T., Akones, L., Finne, P.H., Aarskog, D. Decreased vitamin D absorption after limited jejunal resection in a premature infant. *J. Pediatr.* 1982; 101:1001.

58. Nehme, A.E. Nutritional support of the hospitalized patient: the team concept. *JAMA.* 1980; 243:1906.

59. Isaacs, J., Davis, B., Montagne, M. Transitioning the child fed by gastrostomy into school. *J. Am. Diet. Assoc.* 1990; 90:982.

Chapter 35
Constipation and Fiber

Shirley Walberg Ekvall

Constipation is a common complaint in infancy and childhood. It also is one of the oldest gastrointestinal problems in this age group. Pediatric gastroenterologists report that approximately 10% to 25% of private practice visits and 3% of outpatient pediatric clinic visits are made because of constipation problems.[1] Normal defecatory pattern may range from three bowel movements a day to one movement every other day.

Formula-fed infants usually have only one bowel movement daily, whereas breastfed infants have two or three. Constipation exists only when the stools are hard and dry and eliminated with difficulty. It is frequently seen in children with developmental disorders or mental retardation.[1]

Gabriel et al.[2] classify the causes of constipation into five categories.

1. *Conditions causing a change in stool character:* Undernutrition, cystic fibrosis, and insufficient dietary fiber and/or fluid may cause scanty, viscid, or hard stools.
2. *Local organic problems:* Anorectal malformations, anal fissure, and external rectal compression by an abscess or neoplasm are some of the conditions included in this category.
3. *Intrinsic motility disorders:* Metabolic and endocrine disorders, including hypercalcemia, hyperkalemia, hyperthyroidism, and hyperparathyroidism, and pharmacologicol agents, such as phenothiazines and opiates, may temporarily affect intestinal motility and cause constipation.
4. Extrinsic neurological or muscular disorders: Myelomeningocele, spinal injury, or tumor may interfere with extrinsic intestinal innervation. Abdominal wall or diaphragmatic muscular weakness or paresis prevents the voluntary increase in intra-abdominal pressure that is necessary for defecation.
5. *Functional constipation:* Habitual inhibition of the defecation reflexes is the most common cause of childhood constipation. In time, delayed elimination weakens normal peristalsis, and the stools become dry and hard and difficult to eliminate.

Anal irritation or parents' references to stools as "dirty" stools may also produce constipation.[3]

Biochemical, Anatomical, and Other Abnormalities

A stool weighs approximately 25 grams, depending on diet and fiber intake, with a transit time of 33 hours.[1] The emptying of the rectum occurs when there is increased abdominal pressure caused by peristasis in the rectal wall. This increased pressure is accomplished through synchronization of autonomic and voluntary muscles and sensory fibers.[1] As the infant matures, the rectum length increases and rectal valves develop. By 39 weeks of functional age, the internal anal sphincter reflex appears. Infants who have chronic constipation tend to have increased tonus in the distal colon

with delay in storage passages and dryness in the intraluminal contents. At 1–2 years of age, a change in diet, such as from breast milk to cow's milk, which has a higher phosphorus to calcium ratio, may produce constipation.[4] At 2.5 years of age, these muscles and fibers are mature, which is a good time for toilet training.[1]

Chronic constipation may have a major genetic component, as has been shown in studies of identical versus fraternal twins. Boys tend to be more constipated than girls, and the age of peak incidence is 2 to 4 years, with an onset about 1 year of age.[5] Functional idiopathic constipation without an associated abnormality is the most frequent type of constipation.[4] Some children do not understand how to defecate, some have had a painful experience with dry, hard stools, and others have a maturational abnormality.[5]

Factors to be Considered in Nutritional Evaluation

Determining the cause of constipation is important for its proper treatment. For example, poor muscle tone, such as in Down's syndrome, or increased muscle tone as is found in cerebral palsy can cause the problem. A thorough dietary, medical, and social history is needed. A combination dietary intake and bowel movement or stool evaluation can delineate the personal elimination pattern and dietary intake. Fluid and fiber intake and BM frequency and consistency should be assessed by a 7-day food, fluid, BM, and physical activity list, as is shown in Figure 35-1.

Dietary Management

Fiber, fluid, and physical activity or exercise are three major modes of treatment for constipation. For children under 2 years, milk content may also be a concern, with cow's milk producing greater constipation.[4]

Fiber

A wide variety of foods, including whole grains, fruits, vegetables, nuts, legumes, and various parts of these foods,[6] supply significant amounts of dietary fiber. The following foods are recommended[1]:

- whole grains and whole-grain products
- vegetables that retain a crunchy texture when properly cooked— broccoli, carrots, cabbage, corn, cauliflower, and others
- tuberous root vegetables—beets, carrots, white potatoes (and skins), sweet potatoes, and turnips
- tough-skinned fresh fruits, vegetables, and/or those containing seeds; dried fruits, such as prunes, plums, and apricots

DATE	KIND OF FOOD	AMOUNT	BOWEL MOVEMENT				
Breakfast Time: ____ Where: ____ With Whom: ____			**T I M E**		**G A S**		
			S I Z E	Large (Bulky)	Medium	Small	Very Small
			A M O U N T	Approx. 1/8 C	Approx. 1/4 C	Approx. 1/2 C	Approx. 3/4 C
Mid-morning Snack			**C O N S I S T E N C Y**	Hard Pebbles	Large Hard Stool	Soft	Runny
Lunch Time: ____ Where: ____ With Whom: ____							
			P A S S A G E	Very Difficult	Difficult	Relatively easy	Easy (No Effort)
Afternoon Snack			FOR OFFICE USE ONLY				
Supper Time: ____ Where: ____ With Whom: ____			**P H Y S. A C T.**	1 2 3	4 5	6 7	
Evening Snack							

Fig. 35-1. Dietary intake and bowel movement evaluation. From Turnbull, E., Ekvall, S. *Guide for Assessment of Dietary Intake and Bowel Movement.* Cincinnati: University Affiliated Cincinnati Center for Developmental Disorders; 1977.

- pod vegetables—peas and green beans, dried peas and beans, and lima beans
- nuts of all kinds; crunchy peanut butter
- miscellaneous—tortilla chips (if made with whole corn and water), popcorn, sunflower seeds, pumpkin seeds, and toasted soybeans

Despite popularly held misconceptions, lettuce, celery, and other salad greens are not as high in fiber as the aforementioned foods. Rice-based cereals are especially low in fiber. In both fresh vegetables and fruits, total dietary fiber appears to be relatively low because of the high water content, but it represents a substantial portion of the solid content. Potatoes and starchy vegetables supply significant amounts of fiber if consumed in fairly large quantities.

Physiological effects of fiber are not uniform and depend on its capacity to dissolve the contents in aqueous solutions.

Fiber in food comes in two forms: dietary (soluble or insoluble) and crude fiber. All components of plants resistant to human digestive enzymes are dietary fiber. The small fraction of the plant that remains after the exposure to alkali or acid is crude fiber. Dietary fiber is the more helpful form in constipation management[7] (Table 35-1). Intake of approximately 5–8 g/day of crude fiber[8] or 25–30 g/day of dietary fiber is recommended.[9] Food sources of dietary fiber are shown in Tables 35-1 and 35-2. The addition of sufficient bran to muffins increases stool volume and decreases the total amount of intestinal transit time. Fruits and vegetables have a similar effect of increasing the fecal output, but bran appears to be the most popular food product.[10]

Several objections have been raised to an increased fiber intake for children.[11] First, because children have a small

Table 35–1. Comparison of Soluble and Insoluble Dietary Fiber in Certain Foods

	Dietary fiber (g/100 g)		
	Total	Soluble	Insoluble
Breads and Cereals			
White bread	3.22	1.58	3.08
Whole wheat bread	9.26	2.03	8.15
All Bran cereal® Kellog Co.	31.60	5.24	28.43
Cornflakes® Kellog Co.	1.65	0.48	1.06
Puffed wheat	7.20	3.40	6.68
Rice Krispies® Kellog Co.	1.21	0.32	0.81
Fiber 1® General Mills	44.02	3.10	40.98
Rolled oats	10.51	5.43	9.47
Graham crackers	2.47	1.22	2.29
Vegetables			
Broccoli, frozen	30.40	13.63	28.94
Beets, canned	24.27	7.50	23.67
Carrots, raw	23.76	11.32	22.75
Lettuce, raw	21.02	4.70	19.00
Sweet corn, cooked	9.43	1.24	8.88
Potatoes, white, raw	9.48	4.91	8.58
Tomatoes, raw	13.13	2.13	11.44
Fruits			
Apple, raw	12.73	4.48	10.50
Banana, raw	7.35	2.14	4.13
Orange, raw, seedless, California navel	11.45	6.70	11.14
Peach, canned	18.80	7.60	17.06
Pear, canned	32.18	6.89	27.24
Pineapple canned	9.54	1.22	9.33
Plums, purple, canned	22.81	9.92	19.71
Legumes			
Green beans, canned	33.97	8.13	31.42
Kidney beans, canned	20.90	5.26	17.53
Pinto beans, canned	24.10	7.52	21.42
Pork and beans, canned	15.67	7.70	14.88
White beans, dried, cooked	18.16	5.29	17.21
Lentils, dried, cooked	12.71	1.32	10.61
Green peas, canned	21.30	3.00	20.40

Modified from Anderson & Bridges.[17]

stomach capacity and the caloric density of high-fiber foods is low, a high-fiber diet may not provide sufficient calories. To avoid this problem, particularly for those on highly restricted vegetarian diets, nuts and legumes, which are relatively high in both protein and fat, should be added to the diet.

The second objection is that dietary fiber may influence adversely the absorption of certain essential minerals, such as calcium, iron, copper, magnesium, phosphorus, and zinc. Many foods that are good sources of fiber—primarily whole-grain products—are also high in phytate. Phytate may form insoluble compounds with those minerals, thereby rendering them unavailable. If the intake of these minerals is low and the small amount consumed is chelated, a deficiency may occur. Using large amounts of fiber as a laxative may also inhibit vitamin and mineral levels in children.[10] However, high-fiber diets are often enriched in iron, magnesium, chromium, potassium, calcium, copper, zinc, and selenium.[12,13] Mineral deficiencies occur less frequently in Western diets.

The major constituents of dietary fiber are structural materials of plant cell walls: cellulose, hemicellulose, pectin, mucilages, lignin, and gums. These fibers generally can be classified either as highly fermentable with low indigestible residue or less fermentable with high indigestible residue[14] (Table 35-3). In general, the fiber constituents of fruits and vegetables are much more fermentable than are cereal brans, which display thicker cell walls and a high degree of lignification. Crude fiber is composed primarily of lignin and cellulose. Dietary fiber contains both soluble and insoluble fractions (Table 35-1). Present methods now permit more accurate and precise definition of the amounts and types of dietary fiber polymers in various foodstuffs and of those that might be used for experimental studies.

The extent of fiber degradation in the colon is dependent on the nature of the colonic bacterial flora, the transit time through the colon, and the physical and chemical composition of the fiber. Digestion of polysaccharides varies from 30% to more than 90%. Pectin, mucilages, gums and hemicellulose are almost completely lost during passage through the stool; cellulose is digested somewhat less completely. Lignin, by virtue of its polymeric cross-linked structure, is

Table 35-2. Sample Menu for the High Fiber Diet

	Sunday	Monday	Tuesday	Wednesday	Thursday	Friday	Saturday
Breakfast	Orange juice Pancakes with bran and blueberries in the batter Margarine Milk	Tomato juice Poached egg WW toast Milk	Orange sections Oatmeal sprinkled w/bran and raisins Milk	Prune juice Hard cooked egg WW toast Milk	Orange juice Bran Cereal Milk	Tomato juice Scrambled egg WW toast Milk	Orange juice WW French toast Strawberries Milk
Midmorning snack	Pineapple juice	Grape juice	Apple juice	Water	Pineapple juice	Orange juice	Cranberry juice
Lunch	Roast beef Baked potato with skin Squash Peas Orange sections and pineapple salad Oatmeal cookie Milk	Crunchy peanut butter on WW bread Carrot and celery strips Diced peaches canned or fresh Milk	Turkey sandwich on WW bread Fresh pear or canned pear Milk	Bean soup Hamburger WW roll Tomato (optional) Fruit cocktail Milk	Potato soup Crunchy peanut butter on WW bread Tomato wedges Carrot strips Milk	Vegetable soup Ry-Krisp® Pineapple rings Milk	Egg salad sandwich on WW bread Celery strips Fruit cocktail with bran Milk
Midafternoon snack	Apple juice	Orange juice Raisins	Lemonade Dried apricots	Cranberry juice Walnuts	Water Dates	Grape juice Sunflower seeds	Water Prunes
Dinner	Fish sandwich*/ sauce Corn on the cob or canned corn Cole slaw 1/2 apple with skin Milk	Tomato soup Meatloaf WW Grapes Milk	Chili with beans Carrot/raisin salad Baked apple or fresh apple Milk	Chicken noodle casserole Broccoli Bran muffin Lettuce salad/ dressing Strawberries Milk	Pork chop Brown rice Brussel sprouts Apple Brown Betty made with bran Milk	Chicken Spinach Waldorf salad Bran muffin Milk	Meatloaf w/ bran Hashed potatoes Peas and carrots Fresh plums or canned plums Milk
Evening snack	Water and the other 1/2 of the apple	Cranberry juice Popcorn	Pineapple juice Mixed nuts	Lemonade	Cranberry juice Peanuts	Pear juice	Grape juice
Dietary fiber	30	34	49	30	47	24	24
Crude fiber	10	11	13	13	16	11	9

*WW = whole wheat
Modified from Turnbull et al.,[6] 1990

resistant to bacterial degradation and is almost completely recovered in the stool.[14] The physical structure of plant fiber also determines access to bacterial enzymes. Polysaccharides from older, highly lignified plant tissues are less well digested since physical encrustation and chemical bonding to lignin occur.

Fiber effects the *water-holding capacity* and has important physiological effects in both the upper and lower intestine. Hydration of fiber occurs by adsorption to the surface of the macromolecules and by entrapment within the interstices of the fibrous or gel matrix. The fiber saturation capacity is determined by the chemistry and morphology of the macromolecules and by the pH and electrolyte concentration of the surrounding medium.[12]

Adsorption occurs at the surface of the fiber when substances are taken from the surrounding medium.[14] The forces that bind the adsorbed layer to the surface may be physical or chemical in nature. In addition to fiber's ability to adsorb water, a number of organic materials, such as bile acids, other steroids, various toxic compounds, and bacteria, may be reversibly bound to fiber as it passes along the gastrointestinal tract.

The existence of *cation-exchange properties* of dietary fiber is well established.[14] The effect is related to the number of free carboxyl groups on the sugar residues. Formation of cation complexes with acidic polysaccharides affects mineral balance, electrolyte absorption, and heavy metal toxicity.[12]

The *bulkier* or larger the stool, the greater the pressure against the intestinal wall. This pressure activates the peristaltic motion, resulting in a more rapid movement or reduced transit time of the stool. As the stool moves down the intestine, water is reabsorbed into the body. If the stool

Table 35–3. Types of Dietary Fiber

Fiber type	Food sources	General character
Cellulose—absorbs water	Vegetables Fruits, Legumes, Nuts, Seeds Bran Whole grains	Carbohydrate of plant cell walls (polymer of B-linked glucose)
Hemicellulose—absorbs water and increases peristalsis	Vegetables Whole grains	Carbohydrate of plant cell walls (polymer of galactose and other simple sugar units)
Lignin—absorbs water and increases peristalsis	Vegetables Fruits Whole grains	Noncarbohydrate compounds of plant cell walls (composed of phenyl propane units)
Pectin—absorbs water and binds cell walls	Fruits, especially apples and whites of citrus fruits	Carbohydrates with gel properties (polymers of galacturonic acid units)
Mucilages—absorbs water and lubricates	Oat Bran Psyllum seeds	Carbohydrates and proteins with gummy properties (composed of galacturonic acid, xylose and arabinose)
Gums—absorbs water, ferments, and increases bile acid excretion	Legumes Guar	Carbohydrates with gel and gummy properties (composed of monosaccharide units through glycosidic linkages)

Adapted from Reed, P.B. *Nutrition: An Applied Science.* St. Paul: West Publishers, 1980.

moves too slowly, then more water is absorbed and the stool becomes hard, impacted, and difficult to eliminate. When transit time is reduced, the stool moves more quickly and less water is reabsorbed.[6]

Stephen and Cummings[15] demonstrated that 48% of the increase in stool bulk and water content in subjects fed wheat fiber could be accounted for by the water-holding capacity of the hydrated fiber. Only 36% of the wheat fiber fed was bacterially degraded. By contrast, when an almost completely digestible (92%) fiber (cabbage) was fed, stool bulk and water content also increased, but much of this increase (35%) was due to enhanced bacterial output. Although large amounts of fermentable fibers enhance fecal bulk and water content, they are somewhat less effective than less fermentable types. Stasse-Wolthuis et al.[16] demonstrated in a carefully controlled study that the mean increase in stool weight was 4.1 grams per gram of added fiber for coarse wheat bran (fermentation resistant) as compared to 1.9 grams per gram of added fiber when fruit and vegetables (highly fermentable) were used as a fiber source. The total fiber, polysaccharides and lignin components and the sugar constituents of selected foods were measured by Anderson and Bridges[17] and Marlett[18] in two studies. Sol-

uble fiber content as percentage of total fiber averaged 32% for cereal products, 32% for vegetables, 25% for dried beans and 38% for fruits.[17] (See Table 35–1). Marlett[18] found the soluble fiber content to be 23% for refined grains, 3% for nuts and 13–20% for other food groups. Pectin was 15–30% in fruits, vegetables, legumes and nuts and 0% in grains; whereas hemicellulose was 50% in grains and 30% in other foods. Cellulose was 30% for most foods and 50% in legumes.

Fiber and diseases or disorders

Diverticular disease of the sigmoid colon is characterized by thickening of the circular muscle and contraction of the teniae coli, resulting in the formation of pouches (diverticula). This condition is often accompanied by pain on the lower left side, alternating diarrhea and constipation, and flatulence. A diet that provides little colonic residue results in a small hard stool that requires vigorous segmentation for propulsion along the colon, eventually culminating in circular muscle hypertrophy, high colonic pressure, and production of diverticula. In contrast, populations that ingest a diet high in fiber, have bulky stools and low colonic pressure, and the disease incidence is low. Thus, diverticulosis is now frequently treated with a high-fiber diet with good results.[19] A key factor in reducing symptoms in irritable bowel syndrome (IBS) is dietary manipulation.

Esophageal reflux symptoms can be reduced by eliminating foods that lower the esophageal sphincther pressures such as chocolate, alcohol, peppermint and coffee. Esophageal mucosal irritants such as tomatoes, citrus juices, sharp condiments, also may need to be limited. Treatment with rapid or delayed gastric emptying or gastric acid secretions might be useful in gastric-duodenum IBS (diabetes mellitus, anorexia nervosa and collagen diseases may be confused with IBS however). Gastric emptying and small bowel motility appear to be slowed by soluble dietary fiber (pectin, gum, psyllium, oat bran which ferment) and fatty foods. Insoluble fiber (lignin, cellulose, hemicellulose such as in cereals and whole grains) may be helpful due to increased distention and peristalsis. Metoclopramide, domperidone, cisapride also may be used to alleviate delayed gastric emptying. Small bowel problems may be exaggerated by the ingestion of lactose, sorbitol and fructose. Complex carbohydrates or soluble fiber may relieve symptoms that originate in the small bowel.[20]

Fiber as well as other nutrients may reduce the incidence of *colon cancer*. "The mechanisms to inhibit mutagenesis and carcinogenesis at the *extracellular level* in the grastrointestinal tract include: deactivation of mutagens; modification of metabolism during enterohepatic circulation; protection of the mucosal barrier: inhibition of transepithelial absorption; dilution and complexation of mutagens and carcinogens; acceleration of transit time; maintenance of optimal pH; inhibition of nitrasation; increased production of short bowel fatty acids; inhibition of metabolic activation by gut colonizing bacteria; decreased fecal pH. At the *cellular level* mechanisms of inhibitors of mutagenesis and carcinogenesis include: favoring sequestration in nontarget cells; inhibiting uptake by target cells and metabolic activation; stimulating detoxification; reacting with electrophiles; scavengering reactive oxygen species; protecting nucleophilic sites of DNA; inhibiting cell proliferation before DNA repair and favoring repair of DNA damage: inhibiting error-prone repair pathways; increasing fidelity of DNA replication and controlling gene expression."[21] Examples of these mechanisms follow in diseased state.

Dietary fiber may lower *cardiovascular disease (CVD) and blood lipid levels* by reducing the transit time through the gastrointestinal tract, resulting in the decreased absorption of dietary lipids. There is also a widespread conviction that the effect of dietary fiber on serum lipids may be largely mediated by enhanced fecal excretion of bile acids. In a long-term study in humans, legumes (high in guar gum) enhanced fecal bile output in accordance with bile acid adsorption observed in vitro. Wheat bran demonstrated moderate bile acid affinity in vitro, yet few human studies have indicated an effect on fecal bile acid excretion. Oat bran, however, did significantly increase fecal bile acid loss. In contrast to wheat bran, oat bran is more mucilaginous in nature because of a high content of B-glucans. Other mucilaginous fibers, such as pectin, guar gum, and psyllium seed colloid, have consistently been shown to increase bile acid excretion by 33% to 300%.[12,22] Overall, mucilaginous fibers appear to have the greatest effect on decreasing total serum cholesterol concentrations. Beet and psyllium fiber

(soluble dietary fiber) produced the greatest reduction in LDL cholesterol and serum glucose in healthy men eighteen to fifty-five years of age.[23] The use of 2.5 g of psyllium fiber twice daily with a diet for children from three to seven years and 3.5 g twice daily in children over seven years with 8 oz. of water was found safe and effective in reducing total and LDL cholesterol in Type II A hyercholesterolemia.[24] (Weights and heights of these children at desirable body weight were not significantly changed over a six month period.) Antioxidants found in vegetables and fruits may also be beneficial in CVD.[25]

Dietary fiber shortens the transit time and may lower the concentration of fecal carcinogens or change the bacterial flora by modifying bile acids, thereby reducing the incidence of *colorectal cancer*.[26] It is conceivable that fermentable fiber may alter the production of secondary sterols through its effects on colonic pH, since most bacterial enzymes acting on acidic and neutral sterols have pH optima of 6.5 or greater. Bacterial modification of fecal steroids is apparently reduced in individuals consuming high-fiber diets.[27] Some reports indicate specific benefits for pentose sugars in reducing colon cancer and thus the sugar components of the polysaccharides are being determined.[17,18] In wheat products pentose sugars were the major component of the soluble fractions whereas in all cereals pentose sugars were the major component of the insoluble fractions.[17] The wise choice of using high antioxidant foods in reducing colon cancer should also be considered (see Appendix 5). Several plant phenolic compounds have been shown to have anticancer properties in experimental cancer models.[28] Perhaps the lignin fraction of dietary fiber is responsible for the anticarcinogenic activity in fiber.[18] (Indoles, plant sterols, thiols, and protease inhibitors have been mentioned as well.)

Several studies have found that normal adults and persons with mild cases of *diabetes mellitus*—those taking oral hypoglycemic agents or less than 20 units of insulin per day—may benefit from a higher fiber diet because their glucose tolerance is improved.[29] Soluble dietary fibers appear to have the greatest glycemic effect.[17]

The hypothesis linking *obesity* with the ingestion of an excessive proportion of fiber-depleted carbohydrates is supported by the following arguments[30]: (1) fiber-depleted food is calorically more concentrated than fiber-intact food; (2) food fiber promotes chewing, thereby increasing the effort required to eat and retarding the rate of food ingestion; (3) diets rich in fiber tend to decrease absorptive efficiency; and (4) fiber-depleted food is less satiating than a calorically equivalent amount of high-fiber food.[30] These arguments appear to have validity, but ongoing research is required before firm conclusions can be drawn. Likewise, research related to the modification of the fiber by processing or cooking is being developed.[31]

Recently, the use of fiber in *enteral nutrition* has been studied on a international basis. In the United States, the effect of dietary soy polysaccharide (18–24 g/day) fiber and vitamin D on 11 profoundly retarded institutionalized youth who were fed by gastrostomy and received anticonvulsants for 1 year was assessed by determining plasma levels and balances of zinc, magnesium, calcium, and phosphorus. Nitrogen and phosphorus levels improved, but zinc and calcium were reduced (to require) or equal to 150% of the RDA.[32] In England, the use of a pectin-supplemented predigested diet in animals with short bowel syndrome maintained body weight and serum albumin, although mineral supplementation was reduced and required supplementation.[33] The diet, however, liberated acetate, proprionate, and butyrate during colonic fiber digestion and enhanced intestinal adaptation. A single-blind cross-over study in Denmark—using a nongeling water-insoluble fiber (30 g/day plant cellulose) for marked obesity added to a very low-calorie nutrition powder formula (388 calories for women and 466 calories for men) that was adequate in protein, vitamins, and minerals—produced an increased number of bowel movements and reduced hunger without impairment of absorption of calcium, magnesium, or iron. However, it did not increase weight loss or decrease the levels of plasma cholesterol, triglycerides, or glucose.[30,34] Fiber may be used as part of a standard tube-feeding regimen to provide gut mucosal integrity but not specifically to treat constipation/diarrhea. Soy polysaccharide (hemicellulose, cellulose and pectin) are frequently used as fiber sources. More research is needed regarding the administration of soluble versus insoluble fibers.[35]

Glycerin suppositories and stool softeners should be used in infants less than 1 year of age. Some children after age two who are developmentally delayed and have diminished stool reflexes may need ½ t/day of bran or Metamucil® (a natural vegetable source high in psyllium) with 6 oz. of water and with frequent medical assessment[6] to assess intestinal blockage and height and weight measurements. Increased fiber in snacks is a good way to relieve constipation. When solid foods are introduced into the diet of the older child, care should be taken to include whole-grain cereals, breads, fruits, and vegetables. If whole grains are used for breads or cereals, raw fruits and vegetables for that group, and nuts (if tolerated) or legumes are used one time each day as a meat source, adequate fiber should be obtained. A one week high fiber sample menu is shown in Table 35–3.

In addition, raw wheat bran, a concentrated source of dietary fiber, with the addition of plenty of water, should be used to promote further stool bulk. The bran should be gradually incorporated into the diet. When excessive amounts are given initially, they may irritate a sensitive alimentary tract and cause flatulence, loose stools, or intestinal blockage. A child aged 3–5 years with constipation may need only about ½ t/day daily, whereas a child aged 5–13 years with constipation may need one-half teaspoon two ot three times a day.[6] The bran can be included in the diet in several ways: sprinkling it on top of cereals, puddings, or mashed fruit; mixing it with peanut butter and jelly; or adding it to pancakes, hamburgers, casseroles, or other cooked foods during preparation.

Prunes and prune juice have been found to stimulate intestinal motility. The laxative substance found in prunes is dihydroxyphenyl isatin. Other foods may have this same ability, but data on pharmacological laxative properties of food are very limited.[36]

Diet plays an important role in the treatment of *chronic constipation*. In a study of 60 cases, control by diet alone was found to be more effective than other treatment plans.[36] The anticonstipation diet should include enough bulk (vegetables, fruits, and whole-grain products) so that the fiber residue left in the bowel after digestion will encourage the movement of the intestinal contents and stimulate periodic evacuation. Six to eight servings from the fruit and vegetable group and six to eleven servings from the whole grain bread and cereal group will add a significant amount of fiber to the stool. Certain foods implicated in the delay in stool passage, such as applesauce, bananas, rice cereal, and tea, should be restricted until the constipation resolves.

Fluid

Because water is absorbed by the colon, a fluid intake of six to eight glasses a day is necessary to form a soft, bulky stool. This amount includes beverages and the water present in foods, i.e., soups, cereal with milk, fruits, and raw vegetables. Ingesting adequate amounts of fluid is also important when using bran or an impaction can occur.

Physical activity and regimen

Physical activity can be effective in relieving constipation, particularly for the child with a handicap. In the sample regimen below, exercises are included to increase intestinal motility, and regular mealtimes and sleep patterns are established.[6]

7:30 a.m.	Rise
7:35 a.m.	Fluid
8:00 a.m.	Bathroom
8:30–9:00 a.m.	Breakfast with fluid
9:30 a.m.	Bathroom
10:30 a.m.	Fluid
12:00–12:30 p.m.	Lunch with fluid
1:00 p.m.	Bathroom
3:30 p.m.	Fluid
4:00 p.m.	Exercises
4:30 p.m.	Bathroom
5:00–6:00 p.m.	Supper with fluid
6:30 p.m.	Bathroom
7:30 p.m.	Fluid
8:30 p.m.	Bed

Other treatment

A variety of treatment programs, including medical, behavioral, pharmacological, dietary, and surgical approaches, have been used in the treatment of encopresis bowel incontinence. Treatment of most encopretic children should consist of counseling and education about the medical treatment, retraining, monitoring, and follow-up. Explaining the physiological abnormalities found in the child (if applicable) to the parents helps decrease guilt and blame. Retraining should include frequent toilet use after meals and regulating bowel habits with the use of high-fiber foods and laxatives, when indicated by a physician. With this interdisciplinary approach, a marked decrease of soiling episodes can be achieved in every child. In addition, disappearance of irritability, moodiness, and abdominal pain and often an improvement of behavioral symptoms also have been observed.[37] Biofeedback control over anal splinter function also may be used to treat fecal incontinence. "The decreased ability of the anal splinter to relax helps recovered patients be at less risk for recurrence of constipation."[38]

Although medical, behavioral, pharmacological, dietary, and surgical modalities have been used to treat constipation, preventing it by anticipating the problem and providing proper counseling is the best treatment method. Most physicians agree that the colon must be cleaned out initially with enemas, fiber, laxatives, or surgical treatment in extreme cases before any regimen is established to manage chronic constipation. Physicians often prescribe Metamucil® or psyllium. Long-term management is usually necessitated to include all forms of therapy.[39] Occasionally mineral oil is used but is not recommended. It is a mixture of liquid hydrocarbons obtained from petroleum, is undigestible, and is absorbed only to a limited extent. Thus, it softens fecal contents by lubrication and retardation of water resorption.[40] Mineral oil is not recommended because it appears to decrease the absorption of fat-soluble vitamins (vitamins A, D, E, and K), which are attracted to the mineral oil and are then excreted in the feces. Therefore, mineral oil should be used only with the supervision of a physician and not for long periods of time. Cisapride appears to improve gastrointestinal motility and bowel habits in children with chronic idiopathic constipation.[41]

An effective program called "Smart Choice" which significantly decreased dietary fat by increasing dietary fiber in the diets of school children in Connecticut is available from the State of Connecticut Department of Health.[42] American children need more food based information regarding low fat and high fiber foods.[43]

Follow-up

A dietary, physical activity, fluid, and bowel movement record is recommended weekly or for 1 month if constipation is severe. The 7-day food list is a good tool to use in evaluating the beneficial effects of the diet.[6] An increase in fibrous foods, fluid intake, and physical activity should correlate with an increase in bowel movement frequency and/or volume.

References

1. Hatch, T.F. Encopresis and constipation in children. *Pediatr. Clin. North Am.* 1988; 35:257.
2. Gabriel, D., Zahavi, I., Rosenbach, Y., Nitzan, M. Constipation as a presenting symptom in childhood—a diagnostic problem. *Am. J. Proctol. Gastroenterol. Col. Rect. Surg.* 1981; 32:16.
3. Levine, M.J. Colic, constipation and diarrhea—old symptoms, new approaches. *Pediatr. Ann.* 1987; 16:765.
4. Pettei, M.J. Chronic constipation. *Pediatr. Ann.* 1987; 16:796.
5. Wald, A., Chandra, R., Chiponis, D., Gabel, D. Anorectal function and continence mechanisms in childhood encopresis. *J. Pediatr. Gastroenterol. Nutr.* 1986; 5:346.
6. Turnbull, E., Llenado, M., Ekvall, S. *The Problem of Constipation in the Developmentally Disabled Child.* Cincinnati: University Affiliated Cincinnati Center for Developmental Disorders; 1977.
7. Chicago Dietetic Association and The South Suburban Dietetic Association. *Manual of Clinical Dietetics.* Chicago: American Dietetic Association; 1988.
8. Columbus Dietetic Administrative Council. *Manual of Clinical Dietetics,* Columbus: Dietetic Administrative Council; 1985.
9. Stephen, A.M., Cummings, J.H. Water-holding by dietary fiber in vitro and its relationship to fecal output in man. *Gut.* 1979; 20:722.
10. Floch, M.G. The pharmacology of dietary fiber for laxation. *Am. J. Gastroenterol.* 1987; 82:1259.
11. American Academy of Pediatrics Committee on Nutrition. Plant fiber intake in the pediatric diet. *Pediatrics.* 1981; 67:574.
12. Kay, R.M. Dietary fiber. *J. Lipid Res.* 1982; 23:221.
13. Hanson, C.F., Kopel, B.H., Hermann, J.R. Intake of trace minerals and fiber by healthy elderly people. *J. Am. Diet Assoc.* 1991; 91(9):A118.
14. Spiro, H.M. Medical aspects of dietary fiber. In: Spiller, G.A., Kay, R.M., eds. *Dietary Fiber.* New York: Plenum; 1980.
15. Stephen, A.M., Cummings, J.H. Mechanism of action of dietary fiber in the human colon. *Nature.* 1980; 284:283.
16. Stasse-Wolthuis, J.G., Albers, J.F., Vand Jevesen, J., DeJong, Hautvast, M.D., Hermus, R.J., Katan, M.B., Brydon, W.G., Eastwood, M.A. Influence of dietary fiber from vegetables and fruits, bran or citrus pectin on serum lipids, fecal lipids, and colon function. *Am. J. Clin. Nutr.* 1980; 33:1745.
17. Anderson, J.W., Bridges, S.R. Dietary fiber content of selected foods. *Am. J. Clin. Nutr.* 1988; 47:440.
18. Marlett, J. Content and composition of dietary fiber in 117 frequently consumed foods. *J. Am. Diet Assoc.* 1992; 92:175.
19. Brodribb, A.J.M. Treatment of symptomatic diverticular disease with a high fiber diet. *Lancet.* 1977; 1:665.
20. Friedman, G. Diet and the irritable bowel syndrome. *Gastroenterol. Clin. N. Am.* 1991; 20:313.
21. Hayatsu, H. *Mutagens in Food: Detection and Prevention.* Boca Raton, FL: CRC Press; 1990.
22. Kritchevsky, D. Dietary fiber and atherosclerosis. In: Vahouny, G., Kritchevsky, D., eds. *Dietary Fiber—Basic and Clinical Aspects,* New York: Plenum Press, 1986.
23. Spiller, G.A., Freeman, H.J. Recent advances in dietary fiber and colorectal disease. *Am. J. Clin. Nutr.* 1981; 34:1145.
24. Spark, A., Glassman, M.S., Newman, L.J. A psyllium-supplemented simplified diet for treatment of primary type II-A hypercholesterolemia in children. *J. Am. Diet Assoc.* 1990; 91:A112.
25. Kritchevsky, D. Antioxidant vitamins in the prevention of cardiovascular disease. *Nutr. Today* 1992; 27:30.
26. Sugerman, S.B., Bowen, P.E., Tiongson, B.B., Tan, N.T. Physiological effects of four types of dietary fiber in healthy subjects. *J. Am. Diet Assoc.* 1990; 91(9):A112.
27. Augerinos, G.C., Fuchs, H.M., Floch, M.H. Increased cholesterol and bile acid excretion during a high fiber diet. *Gastroenterology.* 1977; 72:1026.
28. Newmark, H. Plant phenolics as inhibitors of mutational and precarcinogenic events. *Can. J. Physiol. Pharmacol.* 1987; 65:461.
29. Trowell, H. Diabetes mellitus and dietary fiber of starchy foods. *Am. J. Clin. Nutr.* 1978; 31:553.
30. Van Itallie, T.B. Dietary fiber and obesity. *Am. J. Clin. Nutr.* 1978; 31:S45.
31. Eastwood, M., Morris, E. Physical properties of dietary fiber that influence physiological function: a model for polymers along the gastrointestinal tract. *Am. J. Clin. Nutr.* 1992; 55:346.
32. Van Calcar, S.C., Liebl, B.H., Fischer, M.H., Marlett, J.A. Long-term nutritional status of an enterally nourished institutionalized population. *Am. J. Clin. Nutr.* 1989; 50:381.
33. Progress report. fibre and enteral nutrition. *Gut.* 1989; 30:246.
34. Astrup, A., Vrist, E., Quaade, F. Dietary fibre added to very low calorie diet reduces hunger and alleviates constipation. *Int. J. Obesity.* 1990; 14:105.
35. Frankenfield, D.C., Beyer, P.L. Dietary fiber and bowel function in tube-fed patients. *Perspect. Pract.* 1991; 91:590.
36. Olness, K., Tobin, J. Chronic constipation in children—can it be managed by diet alone? *Postgrad. Med.* 1982; 72:149.
37. Loening-Baucke, V., Cruikshank, B., Savage, C. Defecation dynamics and behavior profiles in encopretic children. *Pediatrics.* 1987; 80:672.
38. Weber, J., Ducrotte, P.H., Touchais, J.Y., Roussignol, C., Denis, P. Biofeedback training for constipation in adults and children. *Dis. Col. Rect.* 1987; 30:844.

39. Katz, C., Drongowski, R.A., Coran, A.G. Long-term management of chronic constipation in children. *J. Pediatr. Surg.* 1987; 22:976.

40. Clark, J.H., Russell, G.J., Fitzgerald, J.F., Nagamori, K.E. Serum carotene, retinol, and tocopherol levels during mineral oil therapy for constipation. *Am. J. Dis. Child.* 1987; 141:1210.

41. Staiano, A., Salvatore, C., Andreotti, M.R., Raffaele, M., Manzi, G. Effect of cisapride on chronic idiopathic constipation in children. *Dig. Dis. Sci.* 1991; 36:733.

42. Cobb, K.F., Berger, N.E., Zamore, P.R., Gebo, S.C. Smart choice: effective program to decrease fat and increase fiber in school meals. *J. Am. Diet Assoc.* 1991; 91(9):A76.

43. Resnicow, K., Reinhardt, J. What do children know about fat, fiber, and cholesterol—a survey of 5116 primary and secondary school students. *J. Nutr. Ed.* 1991; 23:65.

Part III
Hereditary Metabolic Disorders

Helen Berry

The successful prevention of mental retardation, death, or serious disease by the early detection and treatment of inborn errors of metabolism stands as a milestone in medicine equal to the prevention of diseases caused by nutritional deficiencies and infections.

The concept of inborn errors of metabolism was introduced by Sir Archibald Garrod in 1908, based on studies of alkaptonuria, albinism, cystinuria, and pentosuria.[1] He reasoned that these defects were present at birth and persisted throughout life. They resulted from a failure in the series of chemical changes that constitute metabolism, and he viewed them as biochemical counterparts of structural malformations. He noted that the disorders often occurred in several members of the same family, frequently in collateral relatives of the same generation, and that parents of affected individuals were often related. Garrod's description is now recognized as that of autosomal-recessive inheritance.

Simply put, inborn errors of metabolism are defects in the internal mechanisms of the body through which food chemicals are converted to body chemicals or tissue. Each of several thousand different molecules in a cell is capable of reacting with other cellular molecules. Unaided, the reactions are slow but they can be accelerated by special molecules called enzymes. Enzymes are proteins with a unique catalytic function. Each is so specific that it catalyzes a single type of reaction. Synthesis of each enzyme is controlled by a single gene made up of deoxyribonucleic acid (DNA). Specific arrangements of the bases that make up DNA correspond to specific amino acids. The genetic code specifies the order in which amino acids are assembled to make a protein in the body. A change in the sequence of these bases within the gene can result in production of an altered protein or enzyme that cannot carry out its catalytic function. The result is an alteration of the ability of the cell to carry out a particular reaction; hence, a metabolic block.

In the body, these errors, or mutations, may occur in critical areas of the cell, such as energy production, and the cell dies. Or, the block may occur in a less sensitive area, and the cell survives with the defect. Mutations that occur in germ cells are passed on to the next generation. They may remain hidden for many generations, since a recessive gene can only exert an effect when it occurs in a double dose; that is, the mutated gene must be present in both parents.

Inborn errors of metabolism might have remained curiosities known only to geneticists, if not for the recognition in the 1950s that the alteration of dietary intake of components that the body was unable to metabolize might prevent or minimize the pathological consequences of meta-bolic blocks. In this section are discussed inborn errors of metabolism that respond to dietary therapy. For the most part, treatment is based on restriction of essential amino acids that cannot be degraded and the accumulation of which results in toxic effects on brain development and physical growth. In some instances co-factor replacement is beneficial.

Phenylketonuria (PKU) has long been the model on which treatments for other disorders are based. Experience over the past 35 years has revealed both successes and problems in the dietary therapy of inborn errors of metabolism. If dietary treatment of PKU is stopped, intellectual ability, so carefully attained, may be lost. Behavioral complications prevent affected individuals from holding jobs and functioning in adult society. Women with untreated PKU are at risk of bearing defective, mentally retarded children as a result of teratogenic effects of phenylalanine in the maternal circulation during gestation.

Other metabolic defects have not responded to dietary treatment as well as has PKU. Costs of treatment and management can be great. Nevertheless, nutritional intervention will continue as the mainstay of treatment for patients with inherited metabolic disorders for the present time. Dietary supplements have been improved, and a wider variety of products are now available. The Orphan Product Development Program of the U.S. Food and Drug Administration may encourage the development of innovative treatments for these rare diseases. Organ transplantation may help some patients with inborn errors of metabolism. Gene therapy will surely be a new modality of treatment. Until that time nutritionists have both great opportunities and great challenges in their task of treating patients from infancy through adulthood for a wide variety of inborn errors of metabolism.

Complete information on the products available for treatment of patients with metabolic disorders can be obtained from their manufacturers, e.g., Mead Johnson Nutritionals, Evansville, IN 47721; Ross Laboratories, Columbus, OH 43216; and Scientific Hospital Supplies, Gaithersburg, MD 20877. Nutrition quality assurance criteria for management of patients with inborn errors of metabolism have been developed by the American Dietetic Association.[2] Examples of protocols for nutrition support of patients with inborn errors of metabolism are also available.[3]

References

1. Garrod, A. E. Inborn errors of metabolism. Croonian lectures. *Lancet* 1908; 2:1, 73, 142, 214.
2. Spinozzi, N., ed. *Quality Assurance Criteria for Pediatric Nutrition Conditions: A Model.* Chicago: American Dietetic Association; 1990.
3. Acosta, P. *The Ross Metabolic Formula System Nutrition Support Protocols.* Columbus, OH: Ross Laboratories; 1989.

Chapter 36
Homocystinuria

Helen Berry, Alison Hull, and Nina Scribanu

Homocystinuria was described independently in 1962 by Gerritsen, Vaughn, and Waisman[1] in the United States and by Carson and Neill[2] in Northern Ireland. In the course of screening urine specimens from mentally retarded children, Carson and Neill found two sisters with dislocated lenses, a malar flush, skeletal changes, and excretion of large amounts of homocystine, an amino acid not usually found in human urine. This form of homocystinuria was shown to result from a deficiency of cystathionine-beta-synthase, the enzyme that normally converts methionine to cystathionine and subsequently to cysteine.[3] Blocks in the methyltetrahydrofolate-homocysteine methyltransferase reaction, either acquired or inherited, can result in homocystine accumulation.[4] Cystathionine-beta-synthase deficiency is inherited as an autosomal-recessive trait.[5] Although the incidence of abnormal homocystine excretion among mentally retarded subjects in Northern Ireland was relatively high, with 10 cases being detected among 2920 specimens,[6] the incidence of homocystinuria determined from neonatal screening programs is approximately 1 in 200,000 live births.[7]

Biochemical and Clinical Abnormalities

Cystathionine-beta-synthase deficiency is characterized biochemically by elevated plasma concentrations of methionine and homocystine. Plasma methionine concentrations may be as high as 2 mM (normal < .03 mM).[8,9] Homocystine, which is not normally detected in plasma, may be as high as 0.2 mM.[8,9] Plasma cystine is low, reflecting the enzymatic defect. Homocystine, not usually found in urine, may exceed 1 mM/L. In addition to homocystine, the mixed disulfide of homocysteine and cysteine is usually excreted, along with methionine and methionine sulfoxide.[10,11]

The clinical symptoms of homocystinuria that were initially reported were considered characteristic of the disorder: mental retardation, ectopia lentis with secondary glaucoma, cataracts and retinal degeneration, skeletal deformities, and thromboembolic and cardiovascular disease, often leading to early death. Subsequent experience has shown that these features are not constant; for example, about half the patients with ectopia lentis have normal intelligence.[12] In many instances the diagnosis is not suspected until after repeated thromboembolic episodes.[13] A listing of the clinical abnormalities is shown in Table 36-1.

The vascular pathology has been attributed to the accumulation of homocysteine or its derivatives[14] or to increased platelet adhesiveness.[15] Skeletal abnormalities have been attributed to a defect in cross-linkage between the polypeptide chains of collagen, as evidenced by a greater proportion of soluble collagen.[16] Disruption of disulfide bonds has also been implicated in the pathogenesis of the connective tissue disorders.[17]

Therapeutic measures based on the restriction of dietary methionine have been proposed to eliminate substances accumulating beyond the block that may have toxic effects (homocystine) and to supply substances that may become deficient (cystine). In addition, administration of pyridoxine (vitamin B_6) reverses biochemical abnormalities in over half the patients.[18,19] Residual cystathionine synthase activity has been found in all livers examined from B_6-responsive patients, but not from B_6-nonresponsive patients.[4]

Mudd et al.[7] reviewed data on 629 patients with homocystinuria. B_6-responsive patients had higher intellectual ability (IQ mean = 79) than those who did not respond to B_6 (IQ mean = 57). B_6-responsive patients also had a lower frequency of dislocation of optic lenses, thromboembolic events, and osteoporosis and lower mortality compared to B_6-nonresponsive patients. Earlier studies suggested that mortality among patients with cystathionine synthase deficiency was about 75% at age 30, primarily as a consequence of thromboembolic episodes.[12] The more recent survey by Mudd et al.[7] found that more than 75% of B_6-nonresponsive patients were alive at age 30.

A methionine-restricted diet begun in infancy prevented mental retardation, retarded the rate of lens dislocation and reduced the frequency of seizures in the study of Mudd and co-workers.[7] Experience with the early treatment of homocystinuria is still too limited to assess the effectiveness of dietary restriction in preventing thromboembolic events.[7] A recent report suggested that signs of vascular disease appear early.[20] Data from the survey suggest that screening programs that identify methionine elevations during the newborn period may not identify B_6-responsive patients. However, infants with a more severe enzyme defect can also be missed.[21]

Analysis of pregnancies in women with cystathionine synthase deficiency, most of whom were B_6-responsive, showed that most full-term pregnancies resulted in normal children, with none of the abnormalities similar to those seen in offspring of women with PKU. However, the rate of fetal loss was high.[7] Prenatal diagnosis has been accomplished by the measurement of cystathionine synthase activity in cultured amniocytes.[22]

Methylcobalamin is the co-factor for the reaction by which homocysteine is remethylated to methionine and catalyzed by 5-methyltetrahydrofolate:homocysteine methyltransferase. A defect in the intestinal absorption of vitamin B_{12} has been reported in patients with the combination of homocystinuria, methylmalonic aciduria, and megaloblastic ane-

Table 36–1. Clinical Abnormalities in
Cystathionine-Beta-Synthase Deficiency

Eye
  Frequent
    Ectopia lentia
    Myopia
  Less frequent
    Glaucoma
    Optic atrophy
    Retinal degeneration
    Retinal detachment
    Cataracts
    Corneal abnormalities

Skeletal system
  Frequent
    Osteoporosis
    Biconcave ("codfish") vertebrae
    Scoliosis
    Increased length of long bones
    Irregular, widened metaphyses
    Metaphysical spicules
    Abnormal size and shape of epiphyses
    Growth arrest lines
    Pes cavus
    High-arched palate
  Less freqent
    Arachnodactyly
    Enlarged carpal bones
    Abnormal bone age
    Pectus carnatum or excavatum
    Genu valgum
    Kyphosis
    Short fourth metacarpal

Central nervous system
  Frequent
    Mental retardation
    Psychiatric disturbances
  Less frequent
    Seizures
    Abnormal EEG
    Extrapyramidal signs

Vascular system
  Frequent
    Vascular occlusions
    Malar flush
    Livedo reticularis

Other involvements
  Fair, brittle hair
  Thin skin
  Fatty changes in liver
  Inguinal hernia
  Myopathy
  Endocrine abnormalities
  Reduced clotting factors

From Mudd et al.,[4] with permission

mia.[23] Defective synthesis of the active forms of the vitamin (methylcobalamin, adenosylcobalamin) also gives rise to homocystinuria and methylmalonic acidemia.[24,25] These patients usually have severe, often fatal illness beginning in infancy.[26] Survivors are usually retarded. The presence of methylmalonic acid with homocystine and low or normal serum methionine should arouse suspicion of one of these defects.

Biochemical abnormalities associated with malabsorption or dietary deficiency of vitamin B_{12} are readily corrected by its administration parenterally.[23] Administration of hydroxycobalamin may be beneficial in the deficiency of 5-methyltetrahydrofolate:homocysteine methyltransferase. It is not known whether cobalamin therapy will prevent clinical deterioration.

Factors to be Considered in Nutritional Evaluation and Dietary Management

Initial treatment should consist of the administration of pyridoxine–150 mg/day in the young infant and 300—500 mg/day in an older child—in several divided doses. Higher doses may be required to obtain a response in some patients. The success of treatment is monitored by a rise in plasma cystine and a decrease in plasma methionine, which should occur within 5—21 days. If no response is observed, low-methionine diets supplemented with cysteine should be instituted. Folic acid deficiency may occur, and in some patients it must be corrected before a pyridoxine response is observed.[21,27] In some instances it has been suggested that a supplement of vitamin B_{12} might be beneficial.[28]

Several commercial methionine-restricted formulas are available: Methionaid® (Scientific Hospital Supplies, Gaithersburg, MD), Analog XMet® (Ross Laboratories, Columbus, OH), and Hom-1® and Hom-2® (Mead Johnson Nutritionals, Evansville, IN). Essential requirements for methionine can be supplied by small amounts of milk and later by low-protein foods. Recommended daily intakes of methionine range from 35 mg/kg at 0—3 months to 25 mg/kg at 1 year; in older children intakes of 15—20 mg/kg/day are suggested.[29] Cystine is an essential amino acid for affected patients and must be present in the diet. Calcium cysteinate is a soluble form of cystine that may be used. Alternatively, the more soluble cysteine may be added to the formula immediately before use. On standing, cysteine is readily converted to cystine, which has limited solubility.

Betaine has been used to enhance remethylation of methionine in patients who are not responsive to vitamin B_6 or who have difficulty maintaining biochemical control on a low-methionine diet. In two studies, its administration at a dose of 6 g/day in two divided doses brought about a significant decrease in plasma total homocysteine and an increase in plasma cysteine levels.[30,31] In most patients plasma methionine concentrations rose two- to fourfold. The biochemical response was accompanied by clinical improvement and there were no apparent ill effects. Betaine was used to correct hypomethioninemia and homocystinemia in a patient who failed to respond to the administration of hydroxycobalamin or methyl cobalamin.[32]

Follow-up

Frequent measurement of plasma and urinary concentrations of methionine and homocystine is recommended until it is determined whether the biochemical abnormalities are altered by pyridoxine administration. Some patients who respond to pyridoxine may still need methionine restriction. As with other diseases in which an essential amino acid is restricted, careful attention must be paid to providing enough methionine and cystine for growth and to prevent tissue catabolism. Serum methionine should be kept between 20 and 100 umol/L. Adjustments in intake of the restricted amino acid are made on the basis of plasma concentrations. Measurements should be made at monthly intervals in the early years when frequent dietary adjustments are required. Measurements at quarterly intervals may be sufficient in older patients.

Cardiac, ophthalmologic, and radiological evaluations at yearly intervals are recommended for monitoring the effectiveness of treatment in preventing the clinical symptoms of homocystinuria.

References

1. Gerritsen, T., Vaughn, J.G., Waisman, H. A. The identification of homocystine in the urine. *Biochem. Biophys. Res. Commun.* 1962; 9:493.
2. Carson, N.A.J., Neill, D.W. Metabolic abnormalties detected in a survey of mentally backward individuals in Northern Ireland. *Arch. Dis. Child.* 1962; 37:505.
3. Mudd, S.H., Finkelstein, J.D., Irreverre, F., Laster, L. Homocystinuria:an enzymatic defect. *Science* 1964; 143:1443.
4. Mudd, S., Levy, H., Skorby, F. Disorders of transsulfuration. In: Scirver, C.R., Beaudet, A.L., Sly, W.S., Valle, D., eds. *The Metabolic Basis of Inherited Disease.* 6th ed. New York: McGraw-Hill; 1989.
5. Finkelstein, J.D., Mudd, S.H., Irreverre, F., Laster, L. Homocystinuria due to cystathionine synthase deficiency: the mode of inheritance. *Science* 1964; 146:785.
6. Gaull, G.E., Carson, N.A.J., Dent, C.E., Field, C.M.B. Homocystinuria: clinical and pathological description of 10 cases. Presented at the International Copenhagen Congress on the Scientific Study of Mental Retardation; August 7–14, 1964; Denmark.
7. Mudd, H.S., Skovby, F., Levy, H.L., Pettigrew, K.D., Wilcken, B., Pyeritz, R.E., Andria, G., Boers, G.H.J., Bromberg, I.L., Cerone, R., Fowler, B., Grobe, H., Schmidt, H., Schweitzer, L. The natural history of homocystinuria due to cystathionine-B-synthase deficiency. *Am. J. Hum. Genet.* 1985; 37:1.
8. Brenton, C.P., Gaull, G.E. Homocystinuria: metabolic studies on three patients. *J. Pediatr.* 1965; 67:58.
9. Perry, T.L., MacDougall, L., Warrington, P.D. Sulphur-containing amino acids in the plasma and urine of homocystinurics. *Clin. Chim. Acta.* 1967; 15:490.
10. Sardharwalla, I.B., Jackson, S.H., Hawke, H.D., Sass-Kortsak, A. Homocystinuria: a study with low-methionine diet in three patients. *Can. Med. Assoc. J.* 1968; 99:731.
11. Laster, L.G., Mudd, S.H., Finkelstein, J.D., Irreverre, F. Homocystinuria due to cystathionine-synthase deficiency: the metabolism of L-methionine. *J. Clin. Invest.* 1965; 44:1708.
12. McKusick, V.A., Hall, J.G., Char, F. The clinical and genetic characteristics of homocystinuria. In: Carson, N. A. J., Raine, D. N. eds. *Inherited Disorders of Sulfur Metabolism.* London: Churchill Livingstone, 1971; 179.
13. van den Berg, W., Verbraak, F.D., Bos, P.J. Homocystinuria presenting as central retinal artery occlusion and longstanding thromboembolic disease. *Br. J. Ophthalmol.* 1990; 74:696.
14. McCully, K.S. Vascular pathology of homocysteinemia: implications for the pathogenesis of arteriosclerosis. *Am. J. Pathol.* 1969; 56:111.
15. McDonald, L., Bray, C. Field, C., Love, F., Davies, B.: Homocystinuria, thrombosis, and the blood-platelets. *Lancet.* 1964; 1:745.
16. Kang, A.H., Trelstad, R.L.A collagen defect in homocystinuria. *J. Clin. Invest.* 1973; 52:2571.
17. Irreverre, F., Mudd, S.H., Heizer, W.D., Laster, L. Sulfite oxidase deficiency: studies of a patient with mental retardation, dislocated ocular lenses, and abnormal urinary excretion of 5-sulfo-L-cysteine, sulfite, and thiosulfate. *Biochem. Med.* 1967; 1:187.
18. Barber, G.W., Spaeth, G.L. Pyridoxine therapy in homocystinuria. *Lancet.* 1967; 1:337.
19. Barber, G.W., Spaeth, G.L. The successful treatment of homocystinuria with pyridoxine. *J. Pediatr.* 1969; 75:463.
20. Rubbad, P., Faccenda, F., Pauciullo, P., Carbone, L. Strisciuglio, P. Carrozzo, R., Sarrtorio, R., del-Giudice, E., Andria, G. Early signs of vascular disease in homocystinuria: a noninvasive study by ultrasound methods in eight families with cystationine-beta-synthase deficiency. *Metabolism.* 1990; 39:1191.
21. Wagstaff, J., Korson, M., Kraus, J.P., and Levy, H.L. Severe folate deficiency and pancytopenia in a nutritionally deprived infant with homocystinuria caused by cystathionine beta-synthase deficiency. *The Journal of Pediatrics,* 1991; 118(4)I:569.
22. Fowler, B., Borresen, A.L., Boman, N. Prenatal diagnosis of homocystinuria. *Lancet.* 1982; 2:875.
23. Hollowell, J.G., Coryell, M.E., Hall, W.K., Findley, J.K., Thevaos, T.G. Homocystinuria as affected by pyridoxine, folic acid and vitamin B_{12}. *Proc. Soc. Exp. Biol. Med.* 1968; 129:327.
24. Goodman, S.I., Moe, P.G., Hammond, K.B., Mudd, S.H., Uhlendorf, B.W. Homocystinuria with methylmalonic aciduria: two cases in a sibship. *Biochem. Med.* 1970; 4:500.
25. Levy, H.L., Mudd, S.H., Schulman, J.D., Dreyfus, P.M., Abeles, R.H. A derangement in B_{12} metabolism associated with homocystinuria, cystathioninemia, hypomethioninemia and methylmalonic aciduria. *Am. J. Med.* 1970; 48:390.
26. Brandstetter, Y., Weinhouse, E., Splaingard, M.L., Tang, T.T. Cor pulmonale as a complication of methylmalonic acidemia and homocystinuria. *Am. J. Med. Genet.* 1990; 36:167.
27. Morrow, G., Barness, L. Combined vitamin responsiveness in homocystinuria. *J. Pediatr.* 1972; 81:946.
28. Selhub, J., Miller, J. The pathogenesis of homocysteinemia: interruption of the coordinate regulation by S-adenosylmethionine of the remethylation and transsulfuration of homocysteine. *Am. J. Clin. Nutr.* 1992; 55:131.
29. Elsas, L.J., Acosta, P.B. Nutrition support of inherited metabolic disorders. In: Skhils M.E., Young, V.R., eds. *Modern Nutrition in Health and Disease.* 7th ed. Philadelphia: Lea and Febiger; 1988.
30. Smolin, L.A., Benevenga, N.J., Berlow, S. The use of betaine for the treatment of homocystinuria. *J. Pediatr.* 1981; 99:467.
31. Wilcken, D.E.L., Wilken, B., Dudman, N.P.B., Tyrrell, P.A. Homocystinuria—the effects of betaine in the treatment of patients not responsive to pyridoxine. *N. Engl. J. Med.* 1983; 309:448.
32. Ribes, A., Briones, P., Velaseca, M. A., Lluch, M., Rodes, M., Maya, A., Campistol, J., Pascual, P., Suormala, T., Baumgartner, R. Methylmalonic aciduria with homocystinuria; biochemical studies, treatment, and clinical course of a Cbl-C patient. *Eur J Pediatr* 1990; 149:412.

Chapter 37
Maple Syrup Urine Disease

Nina Scribanu, Alison Hull, and Helen Berry

Maple syrup urine disease (MSUD) exemplifies the concept of an inborn error of metabolism first proposed in 1908 by Sir Archibald Garrod.[1] His concept of metabolic blocks, together with the later hypotheses of gene-enzyme-chemical reaction, laid the foundation for the science of biochemical genetics. Garrod reasoned that inborn errors of metabolism resulted from an interruption in the series of chemical changes that constitute metabolism. Later it was recognized that blocking of a specific reaction was caused by the absence or deficiency of a specific enzyme.

Biochemical and Clinical Abnormalities

Maple syrup urine disease results from a defect in branched-chain amino acid (BCAA) metabolism. The initial transamination of leucine, isoleucine, and valine to alpha-keto acids occurs normally, but the second step, oxidative decarboxylation of the branched-chain ketoacids (BCKA), is defective[2] (Figure 37-1). The consequence of the defect is accumulation of amino acids and their corresponding ketoacids in blood, cerebrospinal fluid, and urine.

In 1954, Menkes et al.[3] described four siblings with a progressive neurological disorder in which their urine had an odor reminiscent of maple syrup. His patients demonstrated the clinical features of the classical form of the disease. The first symptom is usually lethargy, which appears during the first days of life. Loss of appetite, feeding difficulties, and a constant shrill cry are followed by apnea, loss of reflexes, and alternating periods of hyperactivity and flaccidity leading to convulsions, coma, and respiratory disturbances. Once neurologic symptoms are apparent, progression of the disease is rapid. Diagnosis as late as 10 to 12 days may be too late to prevent irreversible damage to the central nervous system.[4]

Emergency measures, including peritoneal dialysis and exchange transfusion, may be necessary during the early stages of the disease.[5] A parenteral nutrition solution free of BCAA can be especially useful in the treatment of acute acidotic episodes.[6] Ongoing treatment requires restriction of BCAA in the diet.[7,8] The untreated patient who survives the first weeks of life has EEG abnormalities, severe psychomotor retardation, generalized dystonic posturing, and other manifestations of structural brain dysfunction.[9,10]

The toxic effects of increased BCAA and BCKA are not well understood. Among the theories for pathogenesis are

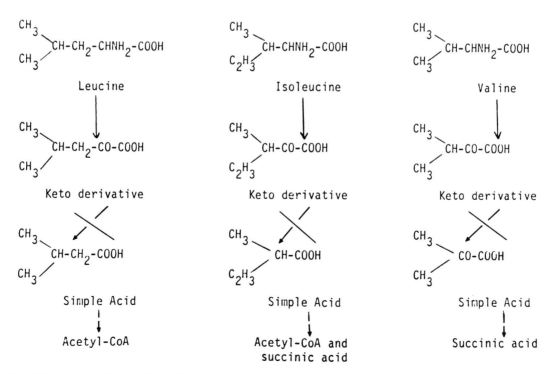

Fig. 37-1. Simplified version of metabolism of branched-chain amino acids demonstrating the site of block in maple syrup urine disease.

decreased energy sources for brain[11-13] decreased neuro-transmitters,[14,15] and interruption of myelin production and oligodendroglial migration.[16,17] The seventh of these changes depends on the degree and duration of exposure of the developing brain to BCAA and BCKA and the time in development at which the insult occurs.

Seven forms of MSUD can be differentiated by clinical and biochemical features (Table 37-1). The classification is based on clinical presentation and outcome. The classical form has a severe clinical course with onset in the neonatal period. It is inherited as an autosomal-recessive trait. The incidence varies from 1:760 in an inbred Mennonite population[18] to 1:290,000 in a New England population.[19] In general the branched-chain keto acid dehydrogenase (BCKD) complex has no detectable activity in the classical form, the greatest degree of activity in the intermittent form, and intermediate levels in the intermediate and thiamine-responsive variants.[20,21] Different mutations in the same gene may result in different degrees of impaired BCKD function; mutations in entirely different genes may result in the decreased metabolism of BCKA and BCAA.[22]

The intermittent and intermediate forms are characterized by variable onset and outcome.[23-25] In the intermediate variant, there is persistent elevation of BCAA and BCKA in body fluids.[26,27] Untreated subjects are mentally retarded. In the intermittent form enzyme activity is sufficient to maintain BCAA concentrations in the normal range, except in times of stress. The postnatal course may be uneventful; clinical signs appear between 2 months and 40 years of age and are triggered by infections, immunizations, surgery or trauma, or a sudden increase in dietary protein. Symptoms include ataxia, irritability, and progressive lethargy. The characteristic maple syrup odor may be noted during acute episodes when BCAA and BCKA concentrations increase in blood and urine. Under stress these children can be as sick as those with classical MSUD, and unless recognized and treated, the outcome can be fatal.[28]

The thiamine-responsive form of MSUD was first described in 1971.[29] Thiamine-responsive patients have residual enzyme activity, and clinical presentations are less severe than in patients with the classical form of the disease.[30] Duran[31] found that a minimum of 3 weeks was required before responses were seen to the thiamine therapy.

Recently, cDNA probes for the genes encoding the proteins of the branched-chain keto acid dehydrogenase complex have been isolated.[32,33] Mutations have been identified

Table 37-1. Clinical Classifications of Maple Syrup Urine Disease

Phenotypic Classification	Clinical Features		Prognosis	Biochemical Features		Specific Features
	Age of Onset	Symptoms		Plasma Leu (μM)	Leucine Decarboxylation by Intact Cells (% of control)	
Classic	Neonatal to early childhood	Poor feeding, apnea, ketoacidosis seizures, hypoglycemia	Death to mild central nervous system impairment	1000–5000	0–2	BCKD proteins present
Intermediate	Infant to adult	Ataxia, failure to thrive, usually no acidosis, progressive	Severe psychomotor delay to normal	400–2000	2–20	BCKD proteins present
Intermittent	Childhood to adult	Intermittent ataxia and ketoacidosis during infection or protein ingestion, normal intervals	Death to normal	50–4000	2–40	BCKD proteins present
Thiamine	Infant to adult	Generally milder than classic onset	Recurrent ataxic attacks to psychomotor delay	50–5000	2–40	Increased specific activity of BCKD after one month of 10–200 mg/kg per day thiamine orally
E1 deficiency	Neonatal	Severe classic symptoms	Death	4000	0–1	In Mennonite population, cell GM 1654
E2 deficiency	Neonatal	Apnea, coma, ketoacidosis	Death in infancy	4000	<1	Absent E2 by immunoblot, specific for BCKD deficiency
E3 deficiency	Neonatal	Hypotonia with progressive impairment of CNS	Death in early childhood	400–600	0–10	Absent E3 by immunoprecipitation: combined deficiency of PDH, KGDH, and BCKD

From: Danner & Elsas,[22] with permission.

Table 37–2. Composition and Commercial Sources of Chemically Defined Medical Foods for Branched-Chain Amino Acid Restricted Diets

Nutrient (g/100 g powder)	Branched-Chain Amino Acid Free Products				
	Analog X* Ile, Leu, Val	Maxamaid* MSUD	MSUD diet† powder	MSUD‡ 1	MSUD‡ 2
Energy, kcal	475.00	360.00	466.00	286.00	307.00
Protein equivalent, g	13.50	25.00	8.20	40.90	54.30
Alanine, g	0.79	1.40	0.44	2.40	3.10
Arginine, g	1.40	3.00	0.49	2.00	2.70
Aspartic acid, g	1.31	2.53	1.14	5.70	7.60
Carnitine, g	0.006	0.00	0.008	0.00	0.00
Cystine, g	0.52	0.97	0.25	1.40	1.80
Glutamic acid, g	1.95	3.27	2.10	12.00	16.00
Glutamine, g	0.16	0.30	0.00	0.00	0.00
Glycine, g	1.25	2.40	0.60	1.40	1.80
Histidine, g	0.80	1.74	0.25	1.40	1.80
Isoleucine, g	0.00	0.00	0.00	0.00	0.00
Leucine, g	0.00	0.00	0.00	0.00	0.00
Lysine, g	1.44	3.03	0.51	4.00	5.40
Methionine, g	0.32	0.65	0.25	1.40	1.80
Phenylalanine, g	0.94	1.75	0.55	2.40	3.20
Proline, g	1.50	2.80	0.89	5.40	7.10
Serine, g	0.92	1.70	0.60	3.00	4.00
Taurine, g	0.03	0.00	0.028	0.00	0.00
Threonine, g	1.04	1.94	0.55	2.70	3.60
Tryptophan, g	0.42	0.77	0.20	1.00	1.40
Tyrosine, g	0.94	1.74	0.65	2.90	3.90
Valine, g	0.00	0.00	0.00	0.00	0.00
Carbohydrate, g	57.00	62.00	63.30	30.50	22.50
Fat, g	23.20	0.00	20.00	0.00	0.00
Calcium, mg	300	810	491	2400	1312
Chloride, meq	8.00	12.90	10.50	47.10	28.20
Chromium µg	15.00	0.00	0.00	0.00	0.00
Copper, mg	0.40	2.00	0.40	6.70	2.00
Iodine, µg	47.00	134.00	33.00	234.00	120.00
Iron, mg	5.50	12.00	9.00	34.00	15.00
Magnesium, mg	34.00	200.00	52.00	521.00	156.00
Manganese, mg	0.39	1.60	0.70	2.40	0.70
Molybdenum, µg	25.00	0.06	0.00	107.00	32.00
Phosphorus, mg	226	810	268	1860	1014
Potassium, meq	10.20	21.50	8.60	59.80	34.10
Selenium, µg	15.00	0.00	0.00	0.00	0.00
Sodium, meq	5.30	25.20	9.70	46.40	27.80
Zinc, mg	3.90	13.00	3.00	26.00	7.80
Vitamin A, µg	533	300	357	841	468
D, µg	7.50	12.00	7.40	25.00	33.00
E, mg	4.90	5.90	7.00	34.00	18.00
K, µg	45.00	0.00	74.00	167.00	167.00
Ascorbic acid, mg	41.00	135.00	39.00	234.00	80.00
Biotin, mg	0.03	0.012	0.04	0.10	0.30
B₆, mg	0.34	1.00	0.30	2.20	1.50
B₁₂, µg	1.00	4.00	1.50	7.90	3.00
Choline, mg	65.00	110.00	63.00	434.00	261.00
Folate, µg	38.00	150.00	74.00	340.00	400.00
Inositol, mg	100.00	56.00	22.00	500.00	300.00
Niacin, mg	4.50	12.00	5.90	54.00	24.00
Panthothenic acid, mg	1.70	3.70	2.20	25.00	11.00
Riboflavin, mg	0.60	1.20	0.45	4.00	2.00
Thiamine, mg	0.40	1.08	0.37	2.70	1.40

*Scientific Hospital Supply Ltd., PO Box 117, Gaithersburg, MD 20877, (301)840–0408.
†Mead Johnson, Nutritional Division.
‡Milupa Company, 397 Boston Post Road, Darien, CT 06820, (203)655–6004.
From: Danner & Elsas,[22] with permission.

Table 37–3. Approximate Daily Requirements for Infants and Children with Classic MSUD*

Nutrient	Unit	<6 mo	6 to 12 mo	1 to 4 yr	4 to 7 yr	7 to 11 yr	11 to 15 yr	15 to 19 yr
					Age			
Fluid	ml/kg	120–150	100	95	90	75	50	50
Energy	kcal/kg	150–170	80–135	—	—	—	—	—
	kcal/day (range)	—	—	1300 (900–1800)	1700 (1300–2300)	2400 (1650–3300)	2200–2700 (1500–3700)	2100–2800 (1200–3900)
Protein	g/kg	1.5–2.5	2.2	—	—	—	—	—
	g/day	—	—	25	30	35	45–50	45–55
Carbohydrate (4 kcal/g)	% of kcal	— Approximately 35% of kcal —			Approximately 50% of kcal			
Fat (9 cal/g)	% of kcal	— Approximately 50% of kcal —			Approximately 35% of kcal			
Isoleucine†	mg/kg/day	30–90	30–80	20–80	20–80	20–30	20–30	20–30
Leucine†	mg/kg/day	40–100	35–60	30–60	30–65	30–60	30–50	15–40
Valine†	mg/kg/day	35–95	30–60	30–60	30–50	25–30	20–30	20–30

*All known other essential amino acids, essential fatty acids, minerals, and vitamins must be provided in adequate amounts.
†Adjustments in these ranges must be made by assessment of plasma aminograms, physical examination, growth, and development.
From Danner & Elsas,[22] with permission.

affecting both E_1 alpha and E_1 beta subunits of the BCKD complex.[34,35] Molecular heterogeneity seems to be a feature of the disease. Some affected individuals have been shown to be compound heterozygotes for two different mutations.[36] Further analyses at the gene level should provide more accurate assessment of the defects. Prenatal diagnosis is possible in the first trimester through chorionic villus biopsy, as well as through amniocentesis at 16 weeks gestation.

Factors to be Considered in Nutritional Evaluation

During gestation the mother metabolizes BCAA and BCKA. Affected infants are normal at birth, but during the first days of life they become listless, refuse to eat, and vomit. The characteristic urine odor may not be present until 4–5 days of age. Lethargy progresses to loss of reflexes, alternating hypertonicity and hypotonicity, convulsions, coma, and death unless intervention occurs. Emergency treatment with peritoneal dialysis or exchange transfusion can produce temporary improvement by quickly reducing BCAA and BCKA concentrations.[7,37] However, chronic management entails the dietary restriction of BCAA.[6]

Dietary Management

Dietary management of MSUD is complicated because the intake of three essential amino acids must be regulated carefully, so that sufficient amounts of each are provided to meet needs for net body protein accretion without allowing an excess to bring about a recurrence of symptoms. Deficiency of any one of the three BCAA can bring about tissue catabolism, with a consequent accumulation of the other two amino acids. An intake of 155–175 cal/kg is recommended to prevent the catabolism of endogenous protein and the release of additional amino acids.[38] Infections and febrile illness in the neonatal period result in rapid metabolic imbalances. Acidosis, hypoxia, and hypoglycemia may occur. Frequent monitoring of plasma BCAA and urinary BCAA and BCKA therefore is necessary.

Dietary therapy of affected infants with a diet that restricts BCAA intake must begin early in life. Infants are fed protein from a source lacking these amino acids along with the small amounts of natural foods to provide the required amounts of essential amino acid. The objective is to produce anabolism and prevent catabolism. A number of proprietary formulas are available that are nutritionally complete but are free of BCAA (Table 37-2), including MSUD Diet Powder[R], (Mead Johnson), MSUD 1[R] and MSUD 2[R] (Milupa), MSUD-Aid[R] (Scientific Hospital Supplies), Maxamaid MSUD[R] (Ross Laboratories). A protein-free diet powder (Product 80056, Mead Johnson) can be used with the amino acid mixtures to provide supplemental energy. Milk may be used to provide essential BCAA for infants, and table foods can be provided for the older child.

Follow-up

Although the recommended nutrient intake will vary depending on the age, growth rate, and degree of residual enzyme activity of each patient, approximate daily requirements are shown in Table 37-3. In general, patients on amino acid mixtures may need a slightly higher protein intake than normal individuals, since L-amino acids are not utilized as efficiently as whole protein. BCAA requirements for affected and normal infants are similar early in life, but the requirement drops rapidly with age. Monitoring of BCAA in blood and urine permits dietary adjustment to accommodate these decreasing requirements. For the variant forms that are symptomatic only in acute situations, protein restriction with attention to fluid, electrolytes, and glucose should be sufficient to maintain biochemical control.[38] A therapeutic trial of 5 to 20 mg/kg/day of thiamine is suggested in all patients with MSUD as an adjunct to dietary treatment. In patients with thiamine-responsive MSUD, plasma amino acid levels may be normalized by supplements, permitting liberalization of the diet.

Patients with MSUD present complications in diagnosis, treatment, and long-term management.[39] A childhood illness, which may be minor in a normal child, becomes a major crisis. Although dietary treatment has been lifesaving for affected children, many children only survive with severe handicaps, both physically and neurologically. Preventive approaches should focus on early diagnosis and treatment, genetic counseling, and prenatal diagnosis.

References

1. Garrod, A. Inborn errors of metabolism. Croonian lectures. *Lancet* 1908; 2:1, 73, 142, 214.
2. Dancis, J., Levitz, M., Westall, R.G. Maple syrup urine disease: branched-chain keto-aciduria. *Pediatrics*. 1960; 25:72.
3. Menkes, J.H., Hurst, P.L., Craig, J.M. A new syndrome: progressive familial infantile cerebral dysfunction associated with an unusual urinary substance. *Pediatrics*. 1965; 14:462.
4. Snyderman, S.E. Medical and nutritional aspects of maple syrup urine disease. In: Koch, R., Shaw, K.N.F., Durkin, R. eds. *Maple Syrup Urine Disease Symposium: Issues and Perspectives* Rockville, MD: Department of Health, Education, and Welfare; 1979. US DHEW publication (HSA) 79-5294:18–33.
5. Saudubray, J.M., Ogler, H., Charpentier, C. Neonatal management of organic acidurias. Clinical update. *J. Inher. Metab. Dis.* 1984; 7 (suppl 1):2.
6. Berry, G.T., Heidenreich, R., Kaplan, P., Levine, F., Mazur, A., Palmieri, M.J., Yudkoff, M., Segal, S. Branched-chain amino acid-free parenteral nutrition in the treatment of acute metabolic decompensation in patients with maple syrup urine disease. *N. Engl. J. Med.* 1991; 324:175.
7. Westall, R.G. Dietary treatment of a child with maple syrup urine disease (branched-chain ketoaciduria). *Arch. Dis. Child.* 1963; 38:485.
8. Snyderman, S.E., Norton, P.M. Roitman, E., Holt, L.E. Maple syrup urine disease with particular reference to dietotherapy. *Pediatrics.* 1964; 34:454.
9. Dent, C.E., Westall, R.G. Studies in maple syrup urine disease. *Arch. Dis. Child.* 1961; 36:259.
10. Holt, L.E., Jr., Snyderman, S.E., Dancis, J., Norton, P.M. The treatment of a case of maple syrup urine disease. *Fed. Proc.* 1969; 19:10.
11. Land, J.M., Mowbray, J., Clark, J.B. Control of pyruvate and beta-hydroxybutyrate utilization in rat brain mitochondria and its relevance to phenylketonuria and maple syrup urine disease. *J. Neurochem.* 1976; 26:823.
12. Bowden, J.A., McArthur, C.L. The inhibition of pyruvate decarboxylation in rat brain by alpha-ketoisocaproic acid. *Biochem. Med.* 1971; 5:101.
13. Patel, M.S. Inhibition by the branched-chain-2-oxo acids of the 2-oxoglutarate dehydrogenase complex in developing rat and human brain. *Biochem. J.* 1974; 144:91.
14. Tashian, R.E. Inhibition of brain glutamic decarboxylase by phenylalanine, leucine and valine derivatives. A suggestion concerning the neurological defect in phenylketonuria and branched-chain ketoaciduria. *Metabolism.* 1961; 10:393.
15. Yuwiler A., Geller E. Serotonin depletion by dietary leucine. *Nature* (Lond) 1965; 208:83.
16. Silberberg, D.H. Maple syrup urine disease metabolites studied in cerebellum cultures. *J. Neurochem* 1969; 16:1141.
17. Harper, P.A.W., Healy, P.J., Dennis, J.A.: Ultrastructural findings in maple syrup urine disease poll hereford calves. *Acta Neuropathol.* (Berlin) 1986; 71:316.
18. Naylor, E.W. Newborn screening for maple syrup urine disease (branched-chain ketoaciduria). In: Bickel, H., Guthrie, R., Hammersen, G., eds. *Neonatal Screening for Inborn Errors of Metabolism.* Berlin: Springer-Verlag; 1980.
19. Levy, H.L. Genetic screening. *Adv. Hum. Genet.* 1973; 4:389.
20. Dancis, J., Jansen, V., Hutzler, J., Levitz, M. The metabolism of leucine in tissue culture of skin fibroblasts of maple syrup urine disease. *Biochim. Biophys. Acta.* 1963; 77:523.
21. Dancis, J., Hutzler, J., Snyderman, S.E., Cox, R.P. Enzyme activity in classical and variant forms of maple syrup urine disease. *J. Pediatr.* 1972; 81:312.
22. Danner, D.J., Elsas, L.J. Disorders of branched-chain amino acid and keto-acid metabolism. In: Scriver, C.R., Beaudet, A.L., Sly, W.S., Valle, D., eds. *The Metabolic Basis of Inherited Disease.* 6th ed. New York: McGraw-Hill; 1989.
23. Kiil, R., Rokkones, T. Late manifesting variant of branched-chain ketoaciduria (maple syrup urine disease). *Acta Pediatr. Scand.* 1964; 53:356.
24. Morris, M.D., Fisher, D.A., Fiser, R. Late-onset branched-chain ketoaciduria (maple syrup urine disease). *Lancet.* 1966; 86:149.
25. Dancis, J., Hutzler, J., Rokkones, T. Intermittent branched-chain ketonuria. *N. Engl. J. Med.* 1967; 276:84.
26. Schulman, J.D., Lustberg, T.J., Kennedy, J.L., Museles, M., Seegmiller, J.E. A new variant of maple syrup urine disease (branched-chain ketoaciduria). *Am. J. Med.* 1970; 49:118.
27. Van Der Horst, J.L., Wadman, S.K. A variant form of branched-chain ketoaciduria. *Acta. Pediatr. Scand.* 1971; 60:594.
28. Kodoma, S., Seiki, A., Hanabusa, M., Morista, Y., Sakurai, T., Matsuo, T. Mild variant of maple syrup urine disease. *Eur. J. Pediatr.* 1976; 124:31.
29. Scriver, C.R., Clow, C.L., MacKenzie, S., Delvin, E. Thiamine-responsive maple-syrup-urine disease. *Lancet* 1971; 1:310.
30. Duran, M., Tielens, A.G.M., Wadman, S.K., Stigter, J.C. M., Kleijer, W.J. Effects of thiamine in a patient with a variant form of branched-chain ketoaciduria. *Acta Pediatr. Scand.* 1978; 67:367.
31. Duran, M., Wadman, S.K. Thiamine-responsive inborn errors of metabolism. *J. Inher. Metab. Dis.* 1985; 8:70.
32. Litwer, S., Danner, D.J. Identification of a cDNA clone in gtll for the transacylase component of branched-chain keto acid dehydrogenase. *Biochem. Biophys. Res. Commun.* 1985; 131:961.
33. Paxton, R., Harris, R.A. Isolation of rabbit liver branched-chain B-ketoacid dehydrogenase and regulation by phosphorylation. *J. Biol. Chem.* 1982; 257:1443.
34. Matsuda, I., Nebukuni, Y., Mitsubuchi, H., Indo, Y., Endo, F., Asaki, J., Harada, A. A T to A substitution in the E1 alpha subunit gene of the branched-chain alpha-ketoacid dehydrogenase complex in two cell lines derived from Mennonite maple syrup urine disease patients. *Biochem. Biophys. Res. Comm.* 1990; 172:646.
35. Nebukuni, Y., Mitsubuchi, H., Endo, F., Akaboshi, I., Asaka, J., Matsuda, I. Maple syrup urine disease. Complete primary structure of the E1 beta subunit of human branched chain alpha-ketoacid dehydrogenase complex deduced from the nucleotide sequence and a gene analysis of patients with this disease. *J. Clin. Invest.* 1990; 86:242.
36. Harris, R.A., Zhang, B., Goodwin, G.W., Kuntz, M.J. Shimomura, Y., Rougraff, P. Regulation of the branched-chain alpha ketoacid dehydrogenase and elucidation of a molecular basis for maple syrup urine disease. *Adv. Enzyme Regul.* 1990; 30:245.
37. Gaull, G.E. Pathogenesis of maple syrup urine disease: observations during dietary management and treatment of coma by peritoneal dialysis. *Biochem. Med.* 1969; 3:130.
38. Bickel, H., Schmidt, H. Dietary and coenzyme therapy. In: Crawford, M.d'A., Gibbs, D.A., Watts, R.W.E., eds. *Advances in the Treatment of Inborn Errors of Metabolism.* Chicester, England: Wiley; 1982.
39. Watts, R.W.E. The treatment of inborn errors of metabolism. In: Crawfurd, M.d'A., Gibbs, D.A., Watts, R.W.E., eds. *Advances in the Treatment of Inborn Errors of Metabolism.* Chicester, England: Wiley; 1982.

Chapter 38
Methylmalonic Acidemia

Helen Berry

Excretion of methylmalonic acid is recognized as a valuable indicator of acquired vitamin B_{12} deficiency or pernicious anemia.[1,2] However, acquired vitamin B_{12} deficiency is not the only cause of methylmalonic aciduria. Oberholzer et al.[3] and Rosenberg et al.[4] first described critically ill infants with profound metabolic ketoacidosis who excreted large amounts of methylmalonic acid.

Methylmalonic acidemia (MMA) is characterized by a clinical picture of metabolic acidosis, which may be accompanied by hyperammonemia, hypoglycemia, and the presence of methylmalonic acid in serum, urine, and cerebrospinal fluid. The ketoacidosis is caused by large amounts of acetoacetic and 3-hydroxybutyric acids. Hyperglycemia may also be present.[5] Patients usually have overwhelming illness early in life, typically with vomiting, acidosis, dehydration, and lethargy proceeding to coma and death unless there is intervention.[6] Patients with less severe onset typically grow poorly and develop neutropenia and pancytopenia.[7] Candidiasis, which can look almost like a thermal burn, is common.[8]

Biochemical Abnormalities

Methylmalonic acidemia is an array of different biochemical and clinical disturbances caused by defective conversion of methylmalonyl-CoA to succinyl-CoA. Table 38-1 outlines the enzymatic defects. Defects in the apoenzyme of methylmalonyl-CoA mutase, either absence (Mut[0]) or structural alteration of the protein (Mut[−]), and in adenosylcobalamin synthesis (cb1A, cb1B) result in severe clinical symptoms.[9] In this group of patients during acute phases of the condition, urinary methylmalonic acid excretion may range from 8 to 35 mg/mg creatinine and serum methylmalonic acid may range from 10 to 30 mg/dL. Serum cobalamin concentrations are normal. Some patients respond to cobalamin supplementation, but usually need dietary protein restriction as well. Another group of patients (cb1C, cb1D, cb1F) with impaired synthesis of adenosylcobalamin and methylcobalamin and resulting deficient activity of both methylmalonyl-CoA mutase and N^5methyltetrahydrofolate methyltransferase, have both methylmalonic aciduria and homocystinuria.[10,11] They excrete lesser amounts of methylmalonic acid and are more likely to respond to the administration of cyanocobalamin or hydroxocobalamin.[12]

The observed hypoglycemia and hyperammonemia are secondary to an accumulation of methylmalonic acid as the co-enzyme A (CoA) ester. In large amounts CoA esters inhibit key enzymes in gluconeogenesis—pyruvate carboxylase,[13] the transmitochondrial shuttle of malate,[14] and ureagenesis (N-acetylglutamate synthetase and, secondarily, carbamylphosphate synthetase).[15,16] Methylmalonic acid has been shown to inhibit the proliferation of stem cells in bone marrow cultures,[7] which may account for some of the hematological abnormalities.

The phenotypic and biochemical heterogeneity observed in patients with MMA has its basis in a number of mutations in the gene for methylmalonyl CoA mutase.[17] Fibroblasts from a patient with MMA were shown to contain compound heterozygous mutations for the gene.[18] Other patients, who were indistinguishable clinically, have mutations that result in an unstable protein.[19]

Table 38–1. Biochemical Defects Associated with Methylmalonic Acidemia

Mut[0]	Methymalonyl-CoA (MM-CoA) mutase apoenzyme deficiency	Blocks conversion of MM-CoA to succinyl-CoA; adenosylcobalamin (Adocbl) is co-factor
Mut[−]	MM-CoA mutase with altered structure and reduced affinity for AdoCbl	
cblA	Deficiency of a mitochondrial cobalamin reductase	Blocks synthesis of hydroxycobalamin (OHCbl) to AdoCbl
cblB	Deficiency of cobalamin adenosyltransferase	
cblC cblD cblF	Defective synthesis of AdoCbl and methylcobalamin (MeCbl)	Inhibits methyltransferase which results in methylmalonic acidemia with homocystinuria and hypomethioninemia

Table 38–2. Recommended Daily Intakes of Nutrients for Children with Methylmalonic Acidemia

Age	Isoleucine (mg/kg)	Methionine (mg/kg)	Valine (mg/kg)	Threonine (mg/kg)	Protein (mg/kg)	Energy (cal/kg)
0–12 mo	54–81	22–33	62–93	50–75	2.2–2.5	110–120
1–4 yr	30–65	10–25	30–75	35–75	1.8–2.0	100–110
4–7 yr	25–60	10–25	30–60	30–70	1.5–2.0	85–100
7–10 yr	20–40	8–15	20–50	25–55	1.0–1.5	75–100

Factors to be Considered in Nutritional Evaluation and Treatment

Emergency treatment measures may be needed for the acutely ill newborn infant. Peritoneal dialysis is the treatment of choice. Protein feeds should be stopped and sufficient carbohydrate provided to treat hypoglycemia and to spare the catabolism of body proteins. Large amounts of electrolytes may be needed to treat the acidosis. Patients should be tested for their response to vitamin B_{12}. In responsive patients, methylmalonic acid excretion should decrease after parenteral administration of 1 mg cyanocobalamin daily for 7 days. In B_{12}-sensitive patients MMA excretion falls within 24 hours. Oral B_{12} therapy is usually as effective as parenteral administration. Some degree of dietary restriction may be necessary even in B_{12}-responsive patients. Patients with defects in synthesis of both adenosylcobalamin and methylcobalamin (cb1C, cb1D, cb1F) may not respond to cyanocobalamin, but do respond to hydroxocobalamin.

Dietary Management

Dietary treatment aimed at lowering the endogenous production of methylmalonic acid should begin as soon as the acute symptoms are corrected and the infant can tolerate oral feedings. The objective of treatment is to reduce methylmalonic acid excretion to 0.05–2.0 mg/mg creatinine (normal = < .005) and to decrease serum methylmalonic acid to < 1 mg/dL (normal < .01 mg/dL). These objectives can be accomplished by reducing the dietary intake of four essential amino acids that are precursors of methylmalonic acid: threonine, isoleucine, valine, and methionine. Carnitine supplementation may be useful both in preventing accumulation within cells of toxic methylmalonyl-CoA and carnitine deficiency, which occurs secondary to its increased excretion as methylmalonylcarnitine.[20] Investigators attribute the continued excretion of large amounts of MMA, in spite of dietary restriction in amino acid precursors, to production of propionate by gut bacteria and to catabolism of odd-chain fatty acids.[21,22] Fasting should be avoided in patients with MMA to prevent the mobilization of fatty acids.[22]

Table 38-2 shows suggested nutrient intakes for treatment of methylmalonic acidemia, based on the author's experience and on others.[22,23] The diet consists of an amino acid mixture lacking threonine, isoleucine, valine, and methionine; a source of fat, carbohydrate, vitamins, and minerals; and small amounts of natural foods to provide the requirements for the amino acids that must be restricted in the diet. The recommended amounts of the restricted amino acids are approximately 50% of the infant requirement. Amino acid intakes may have to be adjusted for individual patients. The content of these amino acids in different foods varies, and crystalline L-amino acid supplements may be needed.

When dietary methionine is restricted, cystine becomes an essential amino acids. However, cystine may not dissolve well in the amino acid mixture and may be left behind. Cysteine, which is more soluble in water than cystine, can be used as a substitute. Energy requirements are often higher when amino acids serve as the nitrogen source. Fluid intake is important in organic acidemias. The nutrient composition of commercial amino acid modified products is shown in Table 38-3.

Follow-up and Outcome

Frequent monitoring of serum and plasma amino acids concentrations is used to adjust intake of the restricted amino acids to prevent either excess or deficiency. Both can lead to the increased excretion of methylmalonic acid. For protein synthesis to occur, all essential amino acids must be present in adequate amounts. If a single one of the four precursors of methylmalonic acid is deficient, the other three will not be utilized efficiently, and methylmalonic acid will be produced from the excess. Other essential or semi-essential amino acids may become limited if too little formula is ingested, which similarly may lead to the accumulation of methylmalonic acid.

The long-term outcome of 45 patients with methylmalonic acidemia was assessed in a 1983 survey.[5] Patients in the largest group, Mut[0], were either impaired or dead. Patients in the cblA group, who were responsive to cobalamin supplements, had the best outcome. Equal numbers of patients with cblB and Mut[-] defects were alive and well, alive and impaired, or dead. CblC, cblD, and cblF patients have not done well: many patients in these groups died in infancy, with hemolytic anemia or congestive heart failure as complications.[9]

Table 38-3. Nutritive Composition of Special Dietary Products for Methylmalonic Acidemia

Nutrients (per 100 g powder)	Analog® XMET, THRE, VAL, ISOLEU*	Maxamaid® XMET, THRE, VAL, ISOLEU*	OS1®	OS2®	Protein-Free† Diet Powder®
Calories	475	350	280	300	486
Protein (g)	13	25	42	56	0
Fat (g)	20.9	< 1	0	0	22
Carbohydrate (g)	59	62	29	20	72
L-Amino Acids (mg)					
Isoleucine	< 35	< 70	100	150	0
Leucine	2000	3900	5700	7600	0
Lysine	1360	2650	4000	5400	0
Methionine	Tr	Tr	Tr	Tr	0
Phenylalanine	880	1720	2400	3200	0
Threonine	Tr	Tr	Tr	Tr	0
Tryptophan	390	760	1000	1400	0
Valine	Tr	Tr	Tr	Tr	0
Cystine	490	950	1400	1800	0
Histidine	900	1750	1400	1800	0
Tyrosine	800	1720	2900	3900	0
Arginine	1330	2590	2000	2700	0
Aspartate	1180	2300	5700	7600	0
Glutamine	110	280	0	0	0
Glutamate	1470	2860	12000	16000	0
Glycine	590	1160	1400	1800	0
Proline	590	1160	5400	7100	0
Serine	830	1620	3000	4000	
Vitamins					
Vitamin A, IU	1760	1000	9300	5200	1800
Vitamin D, IU	340	480	1000	1310	360
Vitamin E, IU	4.9	605	34	18	18
Vitamin K, ug	21	0	167	167	90
Thiamine, mg	0.50	1.1	2.7	1.4	0.45
Riboflavin, mg	0.60	1.2	4.0	2.0	0.54
Vitamin B_6, mg	0.52	1.0	2.2	1.5	0.36
Vitamin B_{12}, mcg	1.25	4.0	7.9	3.0	1.8
Niacin, mg	4.25	12	54	24	7.2
Folic acid, mcg	38	150	340	400	90
Pantothenic acid, mg	2.65	3.7	25	11	2.7
Biotin, mcg	26	120	100	300	45
Ascorbic acid, mg	40	135	230	80	47
Choline, mg	50	110	430	260	76
Inositol, mg	100	56	500	300	27
Minerals					
Calcium, mg	325	810	2400	1310	540
Phosphorus, mg	230	810	1860	1010	300
Magnesium, mg	34	200	520	156	63
Iron, mg	7.0	12	34	15	10.8
Zinc, mg	5.0	13	26	7.8	4.5
Manganese, mg	0.60	1.3	2.4	0.7	0.18
Copper, mg	0.45	2.0	6.7	2.0	0.54
Iodine, mcg	47	134	234	120	40
Sodium, mg	120	580	1070	640	85
Potassium, mg	420	840	2300	1330	340
Chloride, mg	290	450	1650	990	135

*Analog® XMET,THRE,VAL,ISOLEU and Maxamaid® XMET,THRE,VAL,ISOLEU are products of Ross Laboratories, Columbus, OH 43216. Information may be obtained by calling 1–800–848–2607 or 1–614–438–6200.
†OS1® and OS2® are produced by Milupa A.G., and distributed in the United States by Mead Johnson Nutritionals, Evansville, IN 47721. Protein-Free Diet Powder is a product of Mead Johnson Nutritionals. Information may be obtained by calling 1–800–457–3550.

References

1. Cox E.V., White, A.M. Methylmalonic acid excretion: index of vitamin B¹² deficiency. *Lancet.* 1963; 2:853.
2. Barness, L.A., Young, D., Mellman, W.J., Kahn, S.B., Williams, W.J. Methylmalonate excretion in a patient with pernicious anemia. *N. Engl. J. Med.* 1963; 268:144.
3. Oberholzer, V.G., Levin, B., Burgess, E.A., Young, W.F. Methylmalonic aciduria: inborn error of metabolism leading to chronic metabolic acidosis. *Arch. Dis. Child.* 1967; 42:492.
4. Rosenberg, L.E., Lilljeqvist, A., Hsia, Y.E. Methylmalonic aciduria. An inborn error leading to metabolic acidosis, long-chain ketonuria and intermittent hyperglycinemia. *N. Engl. J. Med.* 1968; 278:1319.
5. Matsui, S.M., Mahoney, M.J., Rosenberg, L.E. The natural history of the inherited methylmalonic acidemias. *N. Engl. J. Med.* 1983; 308:857.
6. Morrow, G., Barness, L.A., Auerbach, V.H., DiGeorge, A.M., Ando, T., Nyhan, W.L. Observations of the coexistence of methylmalonic acidemia and glycinemia. *J. Pediatr.* 1969; 74:680.
7. Inoue, S., Krieger, I., Sarnaik, A., Ravindranath, Y., Fracassa, M., Ottenbriet, M. J. Inhibition of bone marrow stem cell growth *in vitro* by methylmalonic acid: a mechanism for pancytopenia in a patient with methylmalonic acidemia. *Pediatr. Res.* 1981; 15:95.
8. Nyhan, W.L. Understanding inherited metabolic disease. *Clin. Symp.* 1980; 32:2.
9. Rosenberg, L.E., Fenton W.A. Disorders of propionate and methylmalonate metabolism. In: Scriver, C.R., Beaudet, A.L., Sly, W.S., Valle, D. eds. *The Metabolic Basis of Inherited Disease.* 6th ed. New York: McGraw-Hill; 1989.
10. Mudd, S.H., Levy, H.L., Abeles, R.H. A derangement in B₁₂ metabolism leading to homocystinemia, cystathioninemia and methylmalonic aciduria. *Biochem. Biophys. Res. Comm.* 1969; 35:121.
11. Goodman, S.I., Moe, P.G., Hammond, K.B., Mudd, S.H., Uhlendorf, B.W. Homocystinuria with methylmalonic aciduria: two cases in a sibship. *Biochem. Med.* 1970; 4:500.
12. Carmel, R., Bedros, A.A., Mace, J.W., Goodman, S.I. Congenital methylmalonic aciduria-homocystinuria with megaloblastic anemia: observations on response to hydroxocobalamin and on the effect of homocysteine and methionine on the deoxyuridine suppression test. *Blood.* 1980; 55:570.
13. Utter, M.F., Keech, D.B., Scrutten, M.L. A possible role for acetyl-CoA in the control of gluconeogenesis. In: Webber, G., ed. *Advances in Enzyme Regulation.* Vol 2. New York: Pergamon; 1964.
14. Halperin, M.L., Schiller, C.M., Fritz, I.B. The inhibition by methylmalonic acid of malate transport by the dicarboxylate carrier in rat liver mitochondria. *J. Clin. Invest.* 1971; 50:2276.
15. Stewart, P.M., Walser, M. Failure of the normal ureagenic response to amino acids in organic acid loaded rats: a proposed mechanism for the hyperammonemia of propionic and methylmalonic acidemia. *J. Clin. Invest.* 1980; 66:484.
16. Shapiro, L.J., Bocian, M.E., Raijman, L., Cederbaum, S.D., Shaw, K.N.F. Methylmalonyl-CoA mutase deficiency associated with severe neonatal hyperammonemia: activity of urea cycle enzymes. *J. Pediatr.* 1978; 93:986.
17. Ledley, F.D., Crane, A.M., Lumetta, M. Heterogeneous alleles and expression of methylmalonyl CoA mutase in *mut* methylmalonic acidemia. *Am. J. Hum. Genet.* 1990; 46:539.
18. Jansen, R., Ledley, F.D. Heterozygous mutations at the *mut* locus in fibroblasts with *mut⁰* methylmalonic acidemia identified by polymerase-chain reaction cDNA cloning. *Am. J. Hum. Genet.* 1990; 47:808.
19. Ledley, F.D., Jansen, R., Nham, S.U., Fenton, W.A., Rosenberg, L.E. Mutation eliminating mitochondrial leader sequence of methylmalonyl CoA mutase causes *mut⁰* methylmalonic acidemia. *Proc. Natl. Acad. Sci. USA.* 1990; 87:3147.
20. Roe, C.R., Hoppel, C.L., Stacey, T.E., Chalmers, R.A., Tracey, B.M., Millington, D.S.: Metabolic response to carnitine in methylmalonic aciduria. *Arch. Dis. Child.* 1983; 58:916.
21. Thompson, G.N., Walter, J.H., Bresson, J.L., Ford, G.C., Lyonnet, S.L., Chalmers, R.A., Saudubray, J.M., Leonard, J.V., Halliday, D. Sources of propionate in inborn errors of propionate metabolism. *Metabolism* 1990; 39:1133.
22. Thompson, G.N., Chalmers, R.A. Increased urinary metabolite excretion during fasting in disorders of propionate metabolism. *Pediatr. Res.* 1990; 27:413.
23. Yanicelli, S. Nutrition support of methylmalonic acidemia. *Metab. Curr.* 1988; 1:10.
24. Ney, D., Bay, C. Saudubray, J-M., Kelts, D.G., Kulovich, S., Sweetman, L., Nyhan, W.L. An evaluation of protein requirements in methylmalonic acidemia. *J. Inher. Metab. Dis.* 1985; 8:132.

Chapter 39
Phenylketonuria

Melanie Hunt and Helen Berry

Phenylketonuria (PKU) may be the most thoroughly studied inherited metabolic disorder. It affects all nationalities, but is predominantly found in Western Europe and North America. Classical PKU has an overall incidence of about 1 in 11,000 newborns.[1]

Phenylketonuria (PKU) was first described by a Norwegian physician, Osbjorn Folling, in 1934, after a persistent and observant mother asked him to determine the cause of mental retardation in her two children. Folling recognized that the peculiar, clinging odor about the children might be a clue to the cause of their mental retardation. He first examined urine from the children for a possible chronic infection; when none was found, he tested for diacetic acid by adding ferric chloride solution to the urine.[2] The test resulted not in the anticipated red-brown color, but rather in a green color, a reaction now known to be characteristic of phenylpyruvic acid.

Phenylketonuria remained a somewhat obscure biochemical curiosity for nearly 20 years. In 1951 Woolf and Vulliamy[3] suggested that there might be a relation between excess phenylalanine and brain damage. If the amount of phenylalanine in the diet could be decreased, thereby preventing its accumulation, normalization of serum phenylalanine might improve the conditions of patients with phenylketonuria. About the same time Armstrong in Utah[4] began studies on the effects of phenylalanine-restricted diets. Bickel et al.[5] who were caring for a young patient found to have PKU, published the first report in 1953 describing marked clinical improvement after use of a phenylalanine-restricted diet.

Characteristic features of untreated individuals with PKU are mental retardation, diminished pigmentation, eczema, hypertonicity, seizures, a musty odor, and an abnormal electroencephalogram. Untreated patients may be irritable, subject to temper tantrums, and have erratic, aggressive behavior.[6] Many never learn to walk nor talk. The only symptoms to arouse suspicion in newborn infants are vomiting, feeding difficulties, and a high incidence of pyloric stenosis. In 1963 Guthrie and Susi[7] described a bacterial inhibition assay for phenylalanine in blood that led to widespread screening programs for PKU in newborn infants. Early detection and well-managed treatment allow an affected child to develop normally, both physically and mentally.[8] (Figs. 39-1 and 39-2).

Biochemical Abnormality

The biochemical defect in phenylketonuria is a deficiency of the liver enzyme, phenylalanine hydroxylase, which catalyzes the para-hydroxylation of phenylalanine to yield ty-

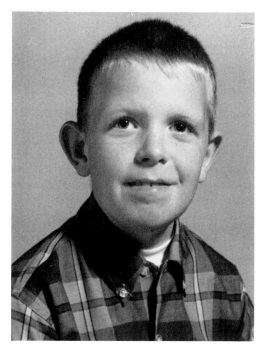

Fig. 39-1. Phenylketonuria was recognized at age 3 years when moderate retardation was noted. At age 8 he remains moderately retarded. Used with permission.

rosine.[9] The hydroxylase system is complex, consisting of a co-factor, tetrahydrobiopterin, and another enzyme, dihydropteridine reductase, which keeps the co-factor in its active (tetrahydro) form.[10] Metabolic blocks may occur in any component of the system.[11] Classical PKU occurs when phenylalanine hydroxylase activity is lacking entirely.[12] Serum phenylalanine concentrations on an unrestricted diet are usually above 20 mg/dL, and the characteristic metabolites of phenylalanine (phenylpyruvic acid, phenylacetic acid, phenyllactic acid, 2-hydroxyphenylacetic acid, and phenylethylamine) are excreted in the urine.[13] Phenylacetic acid is responsible for the odor associated with untreated or poorly controlled PKU. In variant forms of PKU, phenylalanine hydroxylase activity is present, although in greatly reduced amounts; serum phenylalanine levels are lower than in classical PKU, and excretion of metabolites is less consistent.[14] Recent studies on the phenylalanine hydroxylase gene suggest that a number of different mutations produce the clinical symptoms of classical PKU.[15]

Accumulation of phenylalanine results in a series of direct and indirect biochemical changes that occur during early stages of development of the central nervous system and

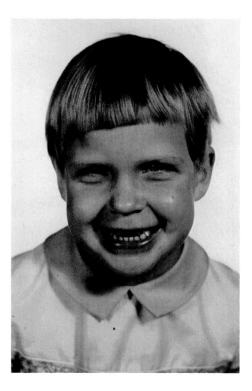

Fig. 39–2. PKU was detected in a sibling at birth. At age 6 years after treatment, she has normal intellectual development. Used with permission.

contribute to a pathogenic pattern that, without treatment, results in severe mental retardation by a still unknown mechanism. Among the hypothesized pathogenic mechanisms are monoamine depletion and impairment of brain protein synthesis through inhibition by phenylalanine or one of its by-products or through a relative deficiency of other essential amino acids. It is generally agreed that excess phenylalanine exerts a permanent deleterious effect on the brain during development and a reversible toxic effect subsequently.[15]

Factors to be Considered in Nutritional Evaluation

Specific nutrients

The dietary treatment of phenylketonuria consists of providing a nutritionally balanced diet containing enough phenylalanine to meet the needs of a growing child without exceeding the child's limited capacity to utilize phenylalanine. As an essential amino acid, phenylalanine must be included in the diet in sufficient amounts to allow for protein synthesis. The diet includes low-phenylalanine or phenylalanine-free protein substitutes, natural foods to provide the requirement for phenylalanine, and low-protein products. The objective of treatment is to reduce serum phenylalanine from concentrations above 15 mg/dL to a range between 3 and 8 mg/dL.

Holt and Snyderman[16] carried out the initial studies to define infant requirements for essential amino acids, including phenylalanine. The need for phenylalanine (per kilogram body weight) is greatest during infancy and diminishes significantly with age; by school age, a child needs less than

half as much as an infant and the adult requirement is about 10% of the infant requirement. Recommended daily intakes of nutrients for subjects with phenylketonuria are shown in Table 39-1. The recommendations for protein and phenylalanine are based on our own experiences, as well as those of others[16–18] and the recommended caloric intake is based on the RDA[19] (see Appendix 1).

The protein requirement is provided by a low-phenylalanine or phenylalanine-free protein substitute. These special dietary products are nutritionally designed to meet the needs for carbohydrate, fat, vitamins, and minerals. Supplements of natural foods provide essential phenylalanine, as well as additional calories, minerals, and vitamins. Sufficient calories must be offered to prevent utilization of protein for energy. Foods low in protein but high in fat or carbohydrate provide extra calories. When dietary phenylalanine is restricted in the diet, tyrosine becomes an essential amino acid. Although commercial low-phenylalanine preparations contain tyrosine, some individuals may require additional supplements of L-tyrosine.

Vitamin supplements are a prudent adjunct to the diet. Requirements for thiamine, riboflavin, niacin, and folacin increase significantly during times of rapid growth; vitamins A, C, and E are needed for structural and functional properties of new cells; and vitamin D is needed for skeletal growth. Because foods of animal origin are seldom used, intake of vitamin B_{12} may not meet the RDA requirement[20] and a vitamin B_{12} supplement should be given. Supplementary iron is recommended for the same reason.

Studies show that zinc and calcium concentrations in hair may be low in patients with PKU who are on predominantly synthetic diets.[21,22] Recommended dietary allowances have not been established for many trace elements, and no clinical consequences of deficiencies of these nutrients have been described in PKU patients. Commercial formulas for treatment of PKU vary considerably in their content of vitamins, minerals, and trace minerals. The degree to which vitamin and mineral requirements are met depends on which phenylalanine-restricted formula is selected.

In summary, requirements for essential amino acids, including phenylalanine and tyrosine, must be met for protein to be synthesized (see Appendix 8). Calories are essential and must be provided in sufficient amount to ensure that protein is not catabolized as a source of energy. Phenylalanine should be distributed evenly throughout the waking

Table 39–1. Recommended Daily Intake of Selected Nutrients for Individuals with Phenylketonuria

Age	Phenylalanine (mg/kg)	Protein (g/kg)	Energy (cal/kg)
0–3 mo	50–60	2.2–2.5	108
4–6 mo	40–50	2.0–2.5	108
7–12 mo	30–40	2.0–2.5	98
2 yr	25–30	1.8–2.0	102
3 yr	20–25	1.8–2.0	102
4–6 yr	15–25	1.5–2.0	90
7–10 yr	15–25	1.0–1.5	70
11–14 yr	10–25	1.0–1.5	47–55
15–18 yr	5–15	1.0–1.3	40–55
Adult	5–10	1.0–1.3	36–40

Table 39–2. Nutritive Compositions of Special Dietary Products for Phenylketonuria

Nutrient per 100 g Powder	Lofenelac (MJ)	Phenyl-Free (MJ)	PKU-1 Milupa	PKU-2 Milupa	PKU-3 Milupa	Analog XP (Ross)	Maxamaid XP (Ross SHS)	Maxamum XP (Ross SHS)	PKU-Aid (Milner)
Energy, Cal	460	410	280	300	290	475	350	340	240
Protein equiv (g)	15.1	20	50	67	68	13	25	39	60
Fat(g)	18	6.8	–	–	–	20.9	<1	<1	–
Carbohydrate (g)	60	66	19	7	3	59	62	45	–
Amino Acids (mg)									
Cystine	60	350	1400	1800	1800	380	710	1110	1500
Histidine	480	470	1400	1800	1800	590	1270	1710	1800
Isoleucine	870	1100	3400	4500	4500	900	1700	2660	2600
Leucine	1660	1730	5700	7600	7600	1550	2910	4560	6100
Lysine	1650	1890	4000	5400	5400	1060	2220	3490	6100
Methionine	540	630	1400	1800	1800	250	480	730	1500
Phenylalanine	75	–	–	–	–	Trace	Trace	Trace	Trace
Taurine	27	–	–	–	–	19	–	140	–
Threonine	780	940	2900	3600	3600	760	1420	2230	4800
Tryptophan	195	280	1000	1400	1400	300	570	890	900
Tyrosine	800	940	3400	4500	6000	1370	2560	4030	6000
Valine	1380	1260	4000	5400	5400	990	1850	2920	4600
Minerals									
Calcium (mg)	430	510	2400	1310	1310	325	810	670	2500
Phosphorus (mg)	320	510	1860	1010	1010	230	810	670	1500
Magnesium (mg)	50	152	520	156	540	34	200	285	300
Iron (mg)	8.6	12.2	34	15	21	7	12	23.5	25
Zinc (mg)	3.6	7.1	26	7.8	24	5	13	13.6	15
Manganese (mcg)	144	1020	2400	700	4800	600	1300	1700	3500
Copper (mcg)	430	610	6700	2000	3600	450	2000	1400	2500
Iodine (mcg)	32	46	230	120	143	47	134	107	150
Sodium (mg)	220	410	1070	640	640	120	580	560	1400
Potassium (mg)	470	1370	2300	1330	1330	420	840	700	2600
Chloride (mg)	320	930	1650	990	1000	290	450	560	2800
Chromium	–	–	–	–	–	15	–	50	–
Selenium (mcg)	10.4	6.1	–	–	–	15	–	50	–
Molybdenum (mcg)	–	–	107	32	476	35	60	110	–
Vitamins									
Vitamin A (IU)	1440	1220	9300	5200	4000	1760	1000	2350	–
Vitamin D (IU)	290	152	1000	1310	480	340	480	320	–
Vitamin E (IU)	14.4	10.2	34	18	12	4.9	6.5	7.8	–
Vitamin K (mcg)	72	102	167	167	167	21	–	70	–
Thiamine (mg)	.36	.61	2.7	1.4	1.8	.5	1.1	1.4	2
Riboflavin (mg)	.43	1.02	4.0	2.0	1.8	.6	1.2	1.4	2.5
Vitamin B_6 (mg)	.29	.91	2.2	1.5	3.2	.52	1.0	2.1	2
Vitamin B_{12} (mcg)	1.44	2.5	7.9	3.0	5.0	1.25	4	4	20
Niacin (mg)	5.8	8.1	54	24	18	4.5	12	13.6	25
Folic acid (mcg)	72	127	340	400	950	38	150	500	400
Pantothenic acid (mcg)	2200	3000	25000	11000	8300	2650	3700	5000	20000
Biotin (mcg)	36	30	100	300	179	26	120	140	600
Vitamin C (mg)	37	53	230	80	100	40	135	90	–
Choline (mg)	61	86	430	260	260	50	110	320	–
Inositol (mg)	22	30	500	300	300	100	56	86	–
Carnitine (mg)	8.6	–	–	–	–	9.5	–	19	–
Renal solute load (m Osm), approx	91	160	352	358	362	76	160	214	447

Calculation for estimating potential renal solute load: [Protein(g) × 41 + [Na(mEq) + K(mEq) + Cl(mEq)]

MJ = Mead Johnson Company, Evansville, IN.
Milupa = Milupa A. G. West Germany/Mead Johnson
Ross = Ross Laboratories, Columbus, OH.
SHS = Scientific Hospital Supplies, Liverpool, England/Ross Laboratories
Milner = Scientific Hospital Supplies, Inc., Gaithersburg, MD 20877.

Table 39–3. Method for Determining the Amount of Formula and Supplemental Phenylalanine Needed to Provide for Growth and Development

1. Based on the age of the child or adult, or the age and weight of the infant, determine the individual's protein and calorie needs as established by the recommended dietary allowance (RDA) (see Appendix 1).

2. Based on the age and weight of the infant, child or adult, determine the amount of phenylalanine (PHE) required.

3. Using the following calculation, determine the amount of prescribed formula needed to meet the recommended amount of protein:

$$\frac{grams\ protein\ needed\ daily}{gram\ protein/10\ grams\ prescribed\ dry\ powder} = grams\ prescribed\ powder\ daily$$

4. Determine the phenylalanine prescription of natural foods as follows:

mg total PHE − mg PHE in formula = mg PHE from natural foods.

5. Add phenylalanine-free foods, such as sugar or fat, to formula, if necessary to adjust calories.

Example 1   Age: 2 years
             Weight: 12.5 kg
             (1) RDA: 25 g protein
             (1) RDA: 1200 calories
             (2) PHE requirement: 25 mg/kg body weight

(3) *25 g protein = 166 grams* Lofenalac powder daily
    1.5 g pro/10 g Lofenalac powder

(4) 25 mg PHE × 12.5 kg = 312.5 mg PHE Total
    .75 mg PHE/g Lofenalac × 166 g = *124.5 mg* PHE/166 g Lofenalac powder
    188.0 mg PHE Natural Foods

(5) 4.6 calories/g Lofenalac × 166 g = 764 calories
    Additional calories will be provided from natural foods and may need to include free foods, e.g., fat or sugar.

Example 2   Age: 25 years, male
             Weight: 70 kg
             (1) RDA: 56 g protein
             (2) RDA: 3010 calories, estimated
             (3) FHE requirement: 8 mg/kg body weight

(3) *56 g protein = 144 g* Maxamum XP powder
    3.9 g pro/10 g Maxamum XP powder

(4) 8 mg PHE × 70 kg = 560 mg PHE Total
    0 mg PHE/g Maxamum XP × 144 g = *0 mg* PHE/144 g Maxamum XP
    560 mg PHE Natural Foods

(5) 3.4 calories/g Maxamum XP × 144 g = 490 calories
    Additional calories must be provided from natural foods; a significant amount of calories will need to come from free foods, e.g., lo-pro pasta, lo-pro bread, sugar and fat.

hours for best utilization of other amino acids. A multiple vitamin supplement with iron is recommended.

Components of the diet

The low-phenylalanine or phenylalanine-free formula is the most important part of the dietary treatment for PKU. If an inadequate amount of formula is consumed, serum phenylalanine concentrations may increase from tissue catabolism, growth will be inhibited, and mental development may be impaired.

The first commercial product for treatment of PKU, Lofenalac®, became available in the United States in 1958. Only in the 1970s were phenylalanine-free products with higher protein and lower calorie content introduced from Europe. These products together with Phenyl-Free®, offer a broader selection to meet individual protein and energy needs in children, adolescents, and adults. The nutritive composition of these products is shown in Table 39-2.

Lofenalac® is based on an enzymatic hydrolysate of casein that is processed to remove most of the phenylalanine. Fat, carbohydrate, vitamins, minerals, and L-tyrosine, L-tryptophan, L-methionine, and L-histidine are added to provide amounts similar to those in milk-based infant formula. Lofenalac® provides a disproportionate amount of calories when it is used to supply protein needs for older children and adults. Phenyl-Free® provides 33% more protein than an equal amount of Lofenalac®, allowing a decrease in calories without decreasing protein intake. Other products, such as PKUaid®, Maxamum®, and PKU-1®, contain all essential and nonessential amino acids except phenylalanine, but little carbohydrate and no fat. Vitamins and minerals are provided in varying amounts. If these products are used, extra attention must be given to energy requirements. Calories may be added to any of these formulas by using low-phen-

Table 39–4. A Sample Menu for an Older Infant

	Non PKU Diet	Phenylalanine (mg)	PKU Diet	Phenylalanine (mg)
Breakfast	2 T barley cereal, dry	28	2 T rice cereal, dry	16
	3 T banana/tapioca, jr.	12	3 T banana/tapioca, jr.	12
	2 T egg yolk, str.	108	2 T grits/egg yolk, str.	30
	4 oz milk	204	Prescribed formula	*
	Total	352	Total	58
Lunch	4 T creamed corn, jr.	40	4 T carrots, jr.	12
	2 T plums/tapioca, jr.	4	2 T plums/tapioca, jr.	4
	2 T chocolate custard, jr.	28	2 T dutch apple dessert, jr.	2
	4 oz milk	204	Prescribed formula	*
	Total	276	Total	18
Snack	2 animal crackers	16	2 animal crackers	16
	2 oz apple-grape juice	4	2 oz apple-grape juice	4
	Total	20	Total	20
Dinner	2 T turkey, jr.	188	1 T turkey, jr.	94
	2 T green beans, str.	18	2 T green beans, str.	18
	3 T peaches, jr.	12	3 T peaches, jr.	12
	4 oz milk	204	Prescribed formula	*
	Total	422	Total	124
Bedtime	4 oz milk	204	Prescribed formula	*
	Total for day	1274	Total for day	220

*Supplemental phenylalanine may need to be added to the prescribed formula. Usually the supplemental phenylalanine is in the form of homogenized milk. The amount varies according to need, but must be considered as part of the total phenylalanine requirement.
From Hunt, M.M., ed. *Phenylalanine, Protein and Calorie Content of Selected Foods.* Cincinnati: The Children's Hospital Research Foundation; 1977. Used with permission.

ylalanine or phenylalanine-free foods, such as cream or corn syrup.

All appropriate formulas used for treatment PKU are concentrated forms of protein, and all but Lofenalac® are composed of L-amino acids and simple sugars. The products consequently have high osmolalities at standard dilutions. The practice of making formulas more concentrated to increase consumption exacerbates this problem. To compensate, the individual is encouraged to drink additional water or other fluids. Increasing fluid intake helps eliminate phenylalanine and its metabolites and prevents symptoms of diarrhea, vomiting, and abdominal cramping, which are associated with hyperosmolar solutions.[23]

Natural foods—that is, any edible food other than the formula that might be included in the diet—not only provide essential amounts of phenylalanine but also additional calories, bulk, a variety of textures and flavors, and vitamins and minerals. The formula and other foods should be offered within the same time frame (about an hour) for optimal use of all essential amino acids. Fruits and vegetables are essential foods in the diet. Legumes, grains, and potatoes may be used, but in limited amounts because of their relatively high phenylalanine content. High-phenylalanine foods, meat, dairy products, and eggs should be omitted or limited severely. No food is strictly forbidden, but all foods are restricted to some degree.

Commercially available low-protein or protein-free products are an important adjunct to the low-phenylalanine diet. Aproten® pasta, Prono® (a gelatin), low-protein breads, and flour help make the diet palatable and interesting. Low-protein recipes have been compiled into cookbooks, and handbooks listing the phenylalanine content of foods are available. These resources are an invaluable aid in managing a low-phenylalanine diet.

Low-calorie diet foods warrant special attention because many contain Aspartame®. Aspartame®, under the brand name of NutraSweet®, is a dipeptide, L-aspartyl-L-phenylalanyl methyl ester, which metabolizes to aspartic acid and phenylalanine. Any product that contains this sweetener is contraindicated for individuals who have PKU.

Dietary Management

The diet may be implemented by one of two methods. The more common system is the equivalent method, which is similar to an exchange list. The other method, which requires an individual and/or caregiver to learn the phenylalanine content of foods, has the advantage of providing greater flexibility in selecting the diet. Each method requires the individual with PKU or the caregiver to select foods as desired to remain within a specific prescription for phenylalanine, which is determined by the nutritionist or physician.

A method for determining the necessary amount of phenylalanine and special formula is shown in Table 39-3. Once this amount is known, families can include foods with which they are familiar (Tables 39-4 and 39-5).

Table 39–5. A Sample Menu for an Adult

Non PKU Diet		Phenylalanine (mg)	PKU Diet	Phenylalanine (mg)
Breakfast	1 C Grape-nuts flakes	176	1/2 C cornflakes	48
	1/4 lg. cantaloupe	35	1/4 lg. cantaloupe	35
	1 sli. whole-wheat toast	117	1 sli. low-protein toast	15
	2 t margarine	3	2 t margarine	3
	2 C coffee	–	1 C Coffee	–
	4 oz 2% Milk	204	Prescribed formula	*
	Total	535	Total	101
Lunch	1 hamburger bun	134	1 sli. bread, regular	109
	4 oz hamburger	896	1 t margarine	2
	1 oz American cheese	351	1/2 sm. carrot, raw	10
	15 potato chips	75	1/2 C green beans	24
	1 peach, raw	30	1 peach, raw	30
	2 Oreo cookies	52	2 sugar wafter cookies	12
	12 oz Coke	–	Prescribed formula	*
	Total	1538	Total	187
Dinner	1 1/2 C spaghetti	384	2 rolls Lo-pro spaghetti	12
	1/2 C sauce/mushroom	160	1/4 C sauce/mushroom	80
	3 oz meatballs	672	1 med. tomato, sliced	46
	1 T Parmesan cheese	135	1/2 Parmesan cheese	68
	1 sli. garlic bread	100	1 sli. garlic bread	100
	1 C lettuce salad	18	1 C lettuce salad	18
	2 T salad dressing	10	2 T salad dressing	10
	8 oz 2% Milk	408	Prescribed formula	*
	Total	1887	Total	334
	Total for day	3960	Total for day	622

*Supplemental phenylalanine is seldom added to the prescribed formula for an adult or adolescent. However, if it is added, the supplemental phenylalanine, usually in the form of milk, must be considered a part of the total phenylalanine requirement.
From Hunt, M.M., ed. *Phenylalanine, Protein and Calorie Content of Selected Foods.* Cincinnati: The Children's Hospital Research Foundation; 1977. Used with permission.

The diet must be monitored continually and adjustments made when necessary. Elevated or depressed serum phenylalanine levels reflect an imbalance between the essential amino acids in the formula and phenylalanine from natural foods. An imbalance may result from an inadequate intake of formula, excessive intake of phenylalanine from natural foods, deficient intake of phenylalanine from natural foods, or illness.[24]

During the first year of life, the number of bottles of formula taken by the infant gradually decreases, as does the total volume of intake. The decrease in fluid intake is most prominent when an infant is weaned from bottle feeding to cup feedings. Unless the formula is made more concentrated, an insufficient amount of formula will be consumed, with a corresponding rise in serum phenylalanine. Regardless of age, low-fluid consumption requires a more concentrated formula plus supplemental fluids in the form of water, juice, or other beverages.

An excess of phenylalanine from natural foods is likely to cause serum phenylalanine levels to increase. During periods of rapid growth, a child or adolescent may be able to consume more phenylalanine from natural foods than during periods of lesser growth. Serum phenylalanine levels may also rise when phenylalanine from natural foods is so restricted that the body breaks down its own tissues to provide phenylalanine.

Illness and infections cause elevated serum phenylalanine levels because of protein catabolism. Colds, sore throat, ear infections, fever, vomiting, and diarrhea are common illnesses that may result in a temporary biochemical imbalance. Appetite and formula consumption are usually affected by illness. Broth, soup, juice, tea with sugar, gelatin, and carbonated beverages may be offered. These foods provide much needed fluid during fever and replace fluids lost because of vomiting or diarrhea. Although the phenylalanine content of some of these foods is high, the amounts consumed are usually small. After the illness, ordinary eating habits and formula should resume.

For an overnight hospital stay, as for minor surgical procedures, children and adults may have the diet usually prescribed for such procedures. If hospitalization is prolonged for more than several days, then the metabolic nutritionist should be consulted and the appropriate diet implemented.

Termination of the diet is not recommended; most individuals with classical PKU should remain on the phenylalanine-restricted diet throughout their life. Certainly, termination of treatment should not be considered for women with PKU during the childbearing years (see chapter 40).

Follow-up and Outcome

The nutritional assessment should include nutrient intake, anthropometric measurements, biochemical data, and clinical examination.[25] The individual diet prescription must be evaluated frequently to ensure that protein, phenylalanine, and calorie requirements are met. Nutritional progress is monitored by monthly serum phenylalanine determinations, and if possible, other amino acids, especially tyrosine, should be periodically evaluated. Most authorities agree that a serum phenylalanine concentration between 5–10 mg/dL is indicative of good dietary control, although many adolescents and young adults appear to tolerate serum phenylalanine levels between 10 and 15 mg/dL without adverse behavioral changes. Clinical well-being, adequate height and weight parameters, normal hemoglobin values, and normal bone growth indicate that nutritional requirements are met. Periodic psychological assessments monitor the outcome of treatment.

Although intellectual development within the normal range has been achieved in PKU patients in whom early diagnosis led to appropriate early treatment, investigators have found a small but significant deficit in intellectual ability of PKU children compared to unaffected family members.[26,27] The deficit was inversely related to serum phenylalanine concentrations, reinforcing the need for careful management of the diet.[26] The low-phenylalanine diet is fairly easy to maintain during periods of rapid growth in infancy and early childhood. However, dietary restriction of phenylalanine as a means of achieving and maintaining low serum phenylalanine concentrations becomes very difficult for the adolescent and adult because of significantly lower phenylalanine requirement and a declining growth rate. Termination of the low-phenylalanine diet in most patients with PKU, whether deliberately or from lack of compliance, has been accompanied by deterioration in intellectual and neuropsychological functioning.[29–33] Agorphobia, anxiety, and depression are other complictions.[34]

A promising development in dietary therapy is a regimen of valine, isoleucine, and leucine (VIL), which may help individuals maintain a lower phenylalanine concentration. In a double-blind cross-over trial of VIL as an adjunct to dietary treatment of phenylketonuria, better performance on a complex task of attention and mental process requirements was observed with VIL supplements than at baseline or when a control amino acid mixture was given.[28]

References

1. Veale, A.M.O. Screening for phenylketonuria. In: Bickel, H., Guthrie, R., Hammersen, G., eds. *Neonatal Screening for Inborn Errors of Metabolism*. Berlin: Springer-Verlag; 1980.
2. Centerwall, S.A., Centerwall, W.R. The discovery of phenylketonuria. In: Lyman, F.L., ed. *Phenylketonuria*. Springfield, IL: Charles C. Thomas; 1963.
3. Woolf, L.I., Vulliamy, D.G. Phenylketonuria with a study of the effect upon it of glutamic acid. *Arch. Dis. Child.* 1951; 26:487.
4. Armstrong, M.D., Tyler, F.H. Studies on phenylketonuria. I. Restricted phenylalanine intake in phenylketonuria. *J. Clin. Invest.* 1955; 34:565.
5. Bickel, H., Gerrard, J., Hickmans, E.M. The influence of phenylalanine intake on the chemistry and behavior of a phenylketonuric child. *Lancet.* 1953; 2:812.
6. Knox, W.E. Phenylketonuria. In: Stanbury, J.B., Fredrickson, D.S., Wyngaarden, J.B., eds. *The Metabolic Basis of Inherited Disease*. New York: McGraw-Hill; 1960.
7. Guthrie, R., Susi, A. A simple phenylalanine method for detecting phenylketonuria in large populations of newborn infants. *Pediatrics.* 1963; 32:338.
8. Williamson, M.L., Koch, R., Azen, C., Chang, C. Correlates of intelligence test results in treated phenylketonuric children. *Pediatrics.* 1981; 68:161.
9. Jervis, G.A. Phenylpyruvic oligophrenia: deficiency of phenylalanine oxiding system. *Proc. Soc. Exp. Biol. Med.* 1953; 82:514.
10. Kaufman, S. The phenylalanine hydroxylating system in PKU and its variants. *Biochem. Med.* 1976; 15:42.
11. Kaufman, S. Differential diagnosis of variant forms of hyperphenylalaninemia. *Pediatrics.* 1980; 65:840.
12. Berry, H., Hsieh, M., Bofinger, M., Schubert, W. Diagnosis of phenylalanine hydroxylase deficiency (phenylketonuria). *Am. J. Dis. Child.* 1982; 136:111.
13. Armstrong, M.D., Centerwall, W.R., Horner, F.A., Low, N.L., Weil, W.B. The development of biochemical abnormalities in phenylketonuric infants. In: Folch-Pi, J., ed. *Chemical Pathology of the Nervous System*. New York: Pergamon; 1961.
14. Hsieh, M.C., Berry, H.K., Bofinger, M.K., Phillips, P.J., Guilfoile, M.B., Hunt, M.M. Comparative diagnostic value of phenylalanine challenge and phenylalanine hydroxylase activity in phenylketonuria. *Clin. Genet.* 1983; 23:415–421.
15. Scriver, C.R., Kaufman, S., Woo, S.L.C. The hyperphenylalaninemias. In: Scriver, C.R., Beaudet, A.L., Sly, W.S., Valle, D., eds. *The Metabolic Basis of Inherited Disease*. 6th ed. New York: McGraw-Hill; 1989.
16. Holt, L.E., Jr., Snyderman, S.E. The amino acid requirement of children. In: Nyhan, W.L., ed. *Amino Acid Metabolism and Genetic Variation*. New York: Blakiston; 1967.
17. Berry, H.K. Hyperphenylalaninemias and tyrosinemias. *Clin. Perinatol.* 1976; 3:15.
18. Ruch, T., Kerr, D. Decreased essential amino acid requirements without catabolism in phenylketonuria and maple syrup urine disease. *Am. J. Clin. Nutr.* 1982; 35:217.
19. Food and Nutrition Board. *Recommended Dietary Allowances.* 10th ed. Washington, DC: National Academy Press; 1989.
20. Hunt, M.M., Berry, H.K., White, P.P. Phenylketonuria, adolescence and diet. *J. Am. Diet. Assoc.* 1985; 85:1328.
21. Acosta, P.B., Fernhoff, P.M., Warshaw, H.S., Elsas, L.J. Zinc status and growth of children undergoing treatment for phenylketonuria. *J. Inher. Metab. Dis.* 1982; 5:107.
22. Taylor, C.J., Moore, G., Davidson, D.C. The effect of treatment on zinc, copper and calcium status in children with phenylketonuria. *J. Inher. Metab. Dis.* 1984; 7:160.
23. Anderson, K., Acosta, P.B., Kennedy, B. Osmolality of enteral formulas for maternal phenylketonuria. *J. Inher. Metab. Dis.* 1986; 9:39.
24. Hunt, M.M., Sutherland, B.S., Berry, H.K. Nutritional management in phenylketonuria. *Am. J. Dis. Child.* 1971; 122:1.
25. Rohr, F.J. Inborn errors of metabolism. In: Wooldridge, N.H., ed. *Quality Assurance Criteria for Pediatric Nutrition Condition—A Model*. Chicago: American Dietetic Association; 1988.
26. Brunner, R.L., Jordan, M.K., Berry, H.K. Early treated phenylketonuria: neuropsychological consequences. *J. Pediatr.* 1983; 102:831.
27. Koch, R., Azen, C., Friedman, E.G., Williamson, M.L. Paired comparisons between early treated PKU children and their matched sibling controls on intelligence and school achievement test results at eight years of age. *J. Inher. Metab. Dis.* 1984; 7:86.
28. Berry, H., Brunner, R., Hunt, M., White, P. Valine, isoleucine, and leucine: a new treatment for phenyketonuria. *Am. J. Dis. Child.* 1990; 144:539.
29. Krause, W., Halminski, M., McDonald, L., Dembure, P., Salvo, R., Friedes, D., Elsas, L. Biochemical and neuropsychological effects of elevated plasma phenylalanine in patients with treated phenylketonuria. *J. Clin. Invest.* 1985; 75:40.
30. Seashore, M.R., Friedman, E., Novelly, R.A., Bapat, V. Loss of intellectual function in children with phenylketonuria after relaxation of dietary phenylalanine restriction. *Pediatrics.* 1985; 75:226.
31. Lou, H., Guttler, F., Lykkelund, C., Bruhn, P., Niederwieser, A. Decreased vigilance and neurotransmitter synthesis after discontinuation of dietary treatment for phenylketonuria (PKU) in adolescents. *Eur. J. Pediatr.* 1985; 144:17.

32. Pennington, B.F., van Doorninck, W.J., McCabe, L.L., McCabe, E.R. Neuropsychological deficits in early treated phenylketonuric children. *Am. J. Ment. Defic.* 1985; 89:467.

33. Holtzman, N.A., Kronmal, R.A., van Doorninck, W., Azen, C., Koch, R. Effect of age at loss of dietary control on intellectual performance and behavior of children with phenylketonuria. *N. Engl. J. Med.* 1986; 314:593.

34. Waisbren, S.E., Levy, H.L. Agoraphobia in Phenylketonuria. *J. Inher. Metab. Dis.* 1991; 14:755.

Chapter 40
Maternal Phenylketonuria

Helen Berry and Melanie Hunt

Legislation requiring the screening of infants for phenyl-ketonuria (PKU) was enacted by most states during the period from 1963 to 1966. The screening identified affected infants soon after birth, who were then treated with low-phenylalanine formulas; normal intellectual attainment was the outcome. However, the success of screening and treatment programs uncovered an unexpected problem: the harmful effects of phenylalanine are not limited to those who inherit the disease directly. During a conference held in 1956, Dent[1] described a phenylketonuric mother who had three retarded children by three separate fathers. He speculated that if excess phenylalanine or its products can damage the developing brain of an infant with PKU, the mother's high phenylalanine level, circulating through the developing fetus, may have a similar effect in utero. In 1963, Mabry and co-workers[2] called attention to the significance of maternal PKU and the toxic effect of phenylalanine on the fetus. They described three elderly phenylketonuric mothers, identified by screening patients in institutions for mentally retarded who together had six mentally retarded children in the same institution.

Description of the full spectrum of effects on the fetus of maternal PKU/hyperphenylalaninemia came from a retrospective survey of the literature by Lenke[3] and Levy in 1980. Their review of 524 pregnancies and 423 offspring of 155 women with PKU or hyperphenylalaninemia revealed that the frequencies of mental retardation, microcephaly, and congenital heart disease were greatly increased over those in the normal population and that the increases correlated with the mother's blood phenylalanine level, but were unrelated to the maternal tyrosine level. Other authors described pecular facies in infants of PKU mothers characterized by facial bone hypoplasia, especially maxillary hypoplasia; thin upper lip; underdeveloped nasal philtrums; short nasal bridges; upturned noses; epicanthal folds; and micrognathia.[4] The appearance was similar to that of infants of alcoholic mothers.[5]

The relation between the level of maternal phenylalanine concentrations and the degrees of damage to the fetus led to the hypothesis that the risk to the unborn child may be reduced by reducing its exposure to maternal phenylalanine. Allan[6] in 1968 described a phenylketonuric woman, who was identified because her three children were mentally retarded. She was treated with a phenylalanine-restricted diet during the last 5 months of a fourth pregnancy. The fourth child had normal birth weight, slightly reduced head circumference, and was reported to have normal intelligence. Rohr and co-workers[7] in New England studied 12 pregnant women with PKU, 5 of whom had live-born infants. The offspring of two women with poor diet compliance or late onset of treatment had microcephaly and/or poor growth and mental retardation. The infants of women who had good control of their phenylalanine levels (120-730 umol/L) were normal at birth and remained normal. A recent study in England, western Europe and Australia used head circumference at birth as an outcome indicator.[8] In this collaborative study, 64 live births to 48 mothers with PKU were analyzed. Seventeen infants of mothers who were on a diet before conception and were well controlled during gestation had normal birth weight and normal head circumference. In 29 infants whose mothers started a strict diet sometime during pregnancy, and in 18 infants whose mothers were untreated, birth weights and head circumferences were below normal, and there was an excess of malformations, particularly cardiac defects. The data showed a clear inverse relation between birth weight or head circumference and maternal phenylalanine concentration around the time of conception.

In sum, treatment by dietary restriction of phenylalanine during pregnancy, particularly if initiated before conception, seems to offer some protection to the fetus.

Biochemical Abnormalities

Pregnancy is of greatest concern in women with classical PKU, which is defined as an absence or inactivity of phenylalanine hyxroxylase, which normally catalyzes the conversion of phenylalanine to tyrosine.[9] The pathogenesis of the mental defect is probably the same whether infants are exposed to excess phenylalanine in utero or after birth. Excess phenylalanine interferes with the hydroxylation of tyrosine to dihydroxyphenylalanine and of tryptophan to 5-hydroxytryptophan, as well as with their subsequent decarboxylation, so that the production of catecholamines from tyrosine and serotonin from tryptophan is diminished.[10,11] Active transport systems that carry phenylalanine across membranes also carry other large neutral amino acids, such as valine, isoleucine, leucine, methionine, tyrosine, and tryptophan.[12] When the transport system is overloaded by excess phenylalanine, other amino acids are excluded from transport.[13] Impairment of amino acid transport is sufficient to produce significant disruption of growth and other processes.

Ideally, dietary treatment during pregnancy should be a continuation of treatment begun early in life. Unfortunately, in the past long-term dietary treatment of PKU was not considered essential, and with few exceptions, in the United States treatment was terminated at ages ranging from 3 to 10 years. Although the current recommendation is to continue dietary treatment indefinitely, many women were lost to follow-up. Reinstatement of a phenylalanine-restricted diet has been difficult at best. Michals et al.[14] found that, of 43 patients with PKU returned to diet therapy, 23 were unable to maintain dietary restrictions after a trial of 1 to 6 months. Hogan et al.[15] concluded that, in the absence of a powerful external motivating factor, compliance with the appropriate dietary regimen would be virtually impossible to maintain.

Factors to be Considered in Nutritional Evaluation and Management

A phenylalanine-restricted diet for women with PKU is similar to that prescribed for children or adolescents. Diet during pregnancy should be a continuation of the control of serum phenylalanine begun before conception. The goal of treatment is to lower blood phenylalanine to the range of 2 to 6 mg/dL while providing adequate prenatal nutrition.

The prescription for a phenylalanine-free diet during pregnancy is established following recommended guidelines for nutrients, which are shown in Table 40–1. The diet is based on a phenylalanine-free protein substitute, which provides about 1.3 g/day protein (see Tables 40–2 and 39–2, in Chapter 39). A phenylalanine requirement during pregnancy has not been established, but seems to be in a range from 5 to 10 mg/kg/day before and during the early stages of pregnancy and 10-15 mg/kg/day by the third trimester. It is important to recognize the increasing tolerance for phenylalanine as pregnancy progresses.[16] High-protein foods are limited; low protein fruits and vegetables provide the greatest amount of variety in the diet.

Because energy needs may not be met by the formula and the small amounts of natural foods permitted, patients may require special low-protein foods and other free foods (sugars and fats) as caloric supplements. Part of the fat should be in the form of safflower oil or corn oil to provide the essential fatty acid, linoleic acid. Vitamin-mineral supplements may not be needed, unless the prescribed phenylalanine-free formula clearly provides inadequate amounts.

Serum phenylalanine and tyrosine concentrations should be monitored at least weekly throughout the pregnancy. A full profile of serum amino acids should be obtained at least monthly. Tyrosine becomes an essential amino acid in phenylketonuria, and its concentration should be above 0.5 mg/dL.[17] If the prescribed formula does not contain adequate amounts of tyrosine, supplements are added.

Weight gain is the best assessment of dietary adequacy; at term, an optimal amount is between 24 and 28 pounds, although it may need to be greater for patients whose initial weight is below ideal for height. An inadequate intake of essential amino acids from the phenylalanine-free product or an inadequate intake of phenylalanine can be responsible for a low weight gain. An optimal serum phenylalanine level is maintained by adjusting the amount of natural foods that provide the increasing phenylalanine requirement as the fetus grows.

Ideally, the treatment team for women with PKU during pregnancy should include health care professionals in the metabolic treatment center and the high-risk obstetrical program. Educational inservice sessions may help obstetrical personel understand the need for the strict dietary regimen during pregnancy. Nausea and vomiting associated with pregnancy can become a problem as the formula may be rejected or lost through emesis with consequent tissue catabolism. Serum phenylalanine rises following the breakdown of body protein.

Follow-up

Monitoring during pregnancy includes routine prenatal examinations, laboratory tests, nutritional evaluations, and ultrasound for the determination of gestational age and intrauterine growth.

The National Institute of Child Health and Human Development initiated a 7-year collaborative effort in 1985—the Maternal PKU Collaborative Study—involving 50 states, the District of Columbia, and all the provinces of Canada.[18] This effort is a prospective, longitudinal, observational investigation designed to evaluate the efficacy of a phenylalanine-restricted diet in reducing the morbidity associated with maternal hyperphenylalaninemia. Offspring will be followed from birth to 6 years of age to assess their physical, neurological, cognitive, and psychosocial development.

Preliminary results from the US/Canada Collaborative Study suggested that the circumference at birth was small relative to length and weight.[19] Major malformations tended to decrease in frequency with lower phenylalanine levels during pregnancy. Phenylalanine levels below 360 μmol/L (6.4 mg/dL) were recommended.[20] Only treatment prior to conception resulted in normal fetal growth.[21] Cognitive development of offspring of women with preconceptual, strict treatment was normal.[22]

A good outcome cannot be assumed even if the diet of the woman with PKU is well controlled both before and after conception. In- utero control must be more rigid than previously supposed because the immature brain is more vulnerable than that of the infant postnatally. The toxicity is probably on going.

Table 40–1. Guidelines for the Intake of Nutrients by Pregnant Women with PKU

	Phenylalanine (mg/kg/day)	Tyrosine (mg/kg/day)	Protein (g/kg/day)	Energy (kcal/kg/day)
Preconception	5–10	110	1.0–1.3	40
Trimester				
First	5–10	110	1.3	35–55
Second	8–10	110	1.3	35–55
Third	10–15	110	1.3	35–55

Table 40–2. Nutritive Compositions of Special Dietary Products for Phenylketonuria

Nutrient per 100 Powder	Lofenelac (MJ)	Phenyl-Free (MJ)	PKU-1 Milupa	PKU-2 Milupa	PKU-3 Milupa	Analog XP (Ross)	Maxamaid XP (Ross SHS)	Maxamum XP (Ross SHS)	PKU-Aid (Milner)
Energy, cal	460	410	280	300	290	475	350	340	240
Protein equiv (g)	15.1	20	50	67	68	13	25	39	60
Fat (g)	18	6.8	–	–	–	20.9	< 1	< 1	–
Carbohydrate (g)	60	66	19	7	3	59	62	45	–
Amino acids (mg)									
Phenylalanine	75	–	–	–	–	Trace	Trace	Trace	Trace
Tyrosine	800	940	3400	4500	6000	1370	2560	4030	6000

MJ = Mead Johnson Company, Evansville, IN.
Milupa = Milupa A.G. West Germany/Mead Johnson.
Ross = Ross Laboratories, Columbus, OH.
SHS = Scientific Hospital Supplies, Liverpool, England/Ross Laboratories.
Milner = Scientific Hospital Supplies, Inc., Gaithersburg, MD 20877.

Management of the personal lives of women with PKU is a significant problem. Women diagnosed and treated in the 1960s and 1970s were taken off the diet, and many are lost to follow-up, placing them at risk during their childbearing years. These women must be found and warned of the risks if they become pregnant without treatment. Otherwise, in a single generation the frequency of PKU-related retardation could escalate beyond that of the years before screening was instituted. An important first step is to develop a registry in the Unitest States, similar to that in Canada, to track women with PKU so services and information can be made available to them.[23]

Maternal PKU presents a moral and ethical dilemma.[24] The fetal damage caused by untreated PKU can be compared to that resulting from drug and alcohol abuse for which coercive measures have been suggested. In women with PKU, when education and counseling fail, irreversible damage may already be caused by the time they become aware of their pregnancy.

References

1. Dent, C.E. Relation of biochemical abnormality to development of mental defect in phenylketonuria. In: Omesti, S.J., Jr., ed. *Etiological Factors in Mental Retardation.* Columbus, OH: Ross Laboratories; 1957.
2. Mabry, C.C., Denniston, J.C. Nelson, T.L., Son, C.D. Maternal phenylketonuria: a cause of mental retardation in children without the metabolic defect. *N. Engl. J. Med.* 1963; 269:1404.
3. Lenke, R.R. Levy, H.L. Maternal phenylketonuria and hyperphenylalaninemia. An international survey of the outcome of untreated and treated pregnancies. *N. Engl. J. Med.* 1980; 303:1202.
4. Lipson, A., Beuhler, B., Bartley, J., Walsh, D., Yri, J., O'Halloran, M., Webster, W. Maternal hyperphenylalaninemia, fetal effects. *J. Pediatr.* 1984; 104:216.
5. Lipson, A.H., Yu, J.S., O'Halloran, M.T., Williams, R. Alcohol and phenylketonuria. *Lancet.* 1981; 1:717.
6. Allan, J.D., Brown, J.K. Maternal phenylketonuria and foetal brain damage. An attempt at prevention by dietary control. In: Holt, K.S., Coffey, V.P., eds. *Some Recent Advances in Inborn Errors of Metabolism.* London: Livingstone; 1968.
7. Rohr, F.J., Doherty, L.B., Waisbren, S.E., Bailey, I.V., Ampola, M.G., Benacerraf, B. Levy, H.L. New England Maternal PKU Project: prospective study of untreated and treated pregnancies and their outcome. *J. Pediatr.* 1987; 110:391.
8. Drogari, E., Smith, I., Beasley, M., Lloyd, J.K. Timing of strict diet in relation to fetal damage in maternal phenylketonuria. *Lancet.* 1987; 2:927.
9. Berry, H, Hsieh, M., Bofinger, M., Schubert, W. Diagnosis of phenylalanine hydroxylase deficiency (phenylketonuria). *Am. J. Dis. Child.* 1982; 136:111.
10. Scriver, C.R., Kaufman, S., Woo, S.L.C. The hyperphenylalaninemias. In: Scriver, C.R., Beaudet, A.L., Sly, W.S., Valle, D., eds. *The Metabolic Basis of Inherited Disease.* 6th ed. New York: McGraw-Hill; 1989.
11. Vorhees, C.V., Butcher, R.E., Berry, H.K. Progress in experimental phenylketonuria: a critical review. *Neurosci. Biobehav. Rev.* 1981; 5:177.
12. Pardridge, W.M., Oldendorf, W.H. Transport of metabolic substrates through the blood-brain barrier. *J. Neurochem.* 1977; 28:5.
13. Oldendorf, W.J. Saturation of blood brain barrier transport of amino acids in phenylketonuria. *Arch. Neurol.* 1973; 28:45.
14. Michals, K., Dominik, M., Schuett, V. Brown, E., Matalon, R. Return to diet therapy in patients with phenylketonuria. *J. Pediatr.* 1985; 106:933.
15. Hogan, S.E., Gates, R.D., MacDonald, G.W., Clarke, J.T.R. Experience with adolescents with phenylketonuria returned to phenylalanine-restricted diet. *J. Am. Diet. Assoc.* 1986; 86:1203.
16. Hyanek, J., Viletova, H., Soukup, J., Kobikova, J., Kubik, M., Kunova, V. Changes in tolerance while monitoring the dietetic treatment of pregnant women suffering from hyperphenylalaninaemia. *J.Inher. Metab. Dis.* 1988; 11:427.
17. Acosta, P.B., Castiglioni, L., Michals-Matalon, K., Rohr, F., Wenz, E. *Protocol for Nutrition Support of Maternal PKU,* Bethesda, MD: National Institute of Child Health and Human Development; 1985.
18. Koch, R., Friedman, E.G., Wenz, E., Jew, K., Crowley, C., Donnell, G. Maternal phenylketonuria. *J. Inher. Metab. Dis.* 1986; 9 (suppl 2):15%.
19. Koch, R., Hanley, W., Levy, H., Matalon, R., Rouse, B., Cruz, D.F., Azen, C., Friedman, E.G. A preliminary report of the collaborative study of maternal phenylketonuria in the United States and Canada. *J. Inher. Metab. Dis.* 1990; 13:641.
20. Rouse, B., Lockhart, L., Matalon, R., Azen, C., Koch, R., Hanley, W., Levy, H., Dela Cruz, F., Friedman, E. Maternal phenylketonuria pregnancy outcome: a preliminary report of facial dysmorphology and major malformations. *J. Inher. Metab. Dis.* 1990; 13:289.
21. Smith, I., Glossop, J., Beasley, M. Fetal damage due to maternal phenylketonuria: effects of dietary treatment and maternal phenylalanine concentrations around the time of conception. *J. Inher. Metab. Dis.* 1990; 13:651.
22. Guttler, F., Lou, H., Andresen, J., Kok, K., Mikkelsen, I., Nielsen, K.B., Nielsen, J.B. Cognitive development in offspring of untreated and preconceptually treated maternal phenylketonuria. *J. Inher. Metab. Dis.* 1990; 13:665.
23. Waisbreau, S., Shiloh, S., St. James, P., Levy, H. Psychosocial factors in maternal phenylketonuria: prevention of unplanned pregnancies. *Am. J. Pub. Health.* 1991; 81:299.
24. Robertson, J.A. Schulman, J.D. *Pregnancy and Prenatal Harm to Offspring: The Case of Mothers with PKU.* Hastings, NY: Hastings Center Report; 1987.

Chapter 41
Tyrosinemia

Marietta Llenado, Helen Berry, and Shirley Walberg Ekvall

The term "tyrosinosis" was first used in 1932 to describe a single patient with constant urinary excretion of large quantities of tyrosine and tyrosine metabolites, p-hydroxyphenyllactic (p-HPLA) and p-hydroxyphenylpyruvic acids (p-HPPA).[1] The relation of biochemical abnormalities in this patient to more recently described aberrations remains unclear. Subsequently it became apparent that several conditions resulting from different defects produced the biochemical features of tyrosinemia and tyrosyluria.

Biochemical and Clinical Abnormalities

Tyrosinemia type I

Hereditary tyrosinemia, or tyrosinemia type I, was first recognized as a clinical entity by Baber in 1956.[2] It is an autosomal-recessive disorder that produces severe and usually fatal liver disease in infants and children. It is characterized by a marked elevation of tyrosine and methionine in plasma; increased urinary excretion of tyrosine and its metabolites, p-HPLA and p-HPPA; abnormal excretion of delta-aminolevulinic acid; and marked elevation of serum alphafetoprotein.[3-8] The presence of succinylacetone and succinylacetoacetate in urine is an essential finding to confirm the diagnosis.[9] The defect is a deficiency of the enzyme fumarylacetoacetase (fumarylacetoacetate hydrolase).[10] Measurement of enzyme activities in lymphocytes and fibroblasts can separate homozygotes from heterozygotes and these from normal individuals.[11]

The incidence of tyrosinemia type I varies worldwide. Screening studies revealed a range of incidence of 1 in 50,000 to 1 in 100,000 in most populations,[12] except for the Chicoutine-Lac St. Jean region in Quebec, Canada, which has a prevalence of 1 in 685.[4]

In the acute form of hereditary tyrosinemia, symptoms appear in infancy and include vomiting, jaundice, failure to thrive, and abdominal enlargement, together with a peculiar (methionine or cabbage-like) odor.[4] Hepatomegaly, splenomegaly, edema, and bleeding episodes occur due to progressive liver failure and renal tubular dysfunction. Death from liver failure occurs in 90% of patients by 1 year of age. In those who survive, later sequelae are hypophosphatemic rickets, hypertension from increased production of catecholamines,[13] and porphyria with abdominal cramps. Hepatoma is a frequent later complication.[14] Walking may be delayed because of vitamin-D-resistant rickets and hypokalemia.

Laboratory findings, in addition to those noted above, include plasma tyrosine levels up to 6–12 mg/dL, methionine up to 1–5 mg/dL, and increases of other amino acids.[12,15]

Renal tubular abnormalities are manifested by generalized aminoaciduria, proteinuria, glycosuria, phosphaturia, and increased potassium loss.[4] Elevated serum methionine is thought to result from the severe liver disease,[16] although Gaull et al.[17] demonstrated decreased activities of methionine-activating enzyme (ATP:L-methionine-S-adenosyltransferase). As a consequence of liver damage, there is usually hyperbilirubinemia, leukopenia, thrombocytopenia, hypoproteinemia, and reduced blood clotting factors. Platelet count, hepatic enzymes, and plasma renin are elevated, and prothrombin time is extended.[18] Red cell reduced glutathione and plasma cysteine levels are decreased.[19]

The secondary enzyme deficiencies seen in tyrosinemia type I of delta-aminolevulinic acid dehydratase and methionine adenosyl transferase result from inhibition by succinylacetone and fumarylacetoacetate, which accumulate because of a primary deficiency of fumarylacetoacetate hydrolase.[7] The renal tubular damage has been attributed to accumulation of the toxic compounds, fumarylacetoacetate and maleylacetoacetate, which are precursors of succinylacetoacetate and succinylacetone.[20]

Tyrosinemia type II

Tyrosinemia type II, or Richner-Hanhart syndrome, is also known as oculocutaneous tyrosinemia, which refers to the most frequent findings of corneal ulcers and skin lesions. Corneal erosions and plaques, palm and sole erosions, and hyperkeratosis occur during the first month of life and do not respond to conventional therapy.[4,21-24] Eye lesions include lacrimation, photophobia, microfollicular conjunctivitis, and dendritic keratosis. It has been postulated that the keratosis is due to tyrosine crystal formation within the cell from the high tyrosine levels.[25] Long-term effects include corneal scarring, nystagmus, and glaucoma. Skin lesions are more variable, occurring with or after the eye lesions. Initial blister-like lesions form on the hands and feet, become crusty, and are finally hyperkeratotic. These painful lesions can hinder mobility. Mental retardation occurs in about half the patients, some of whom have microcephaly and convulsions.[4]

The site of the defect in tyrosinemia type II is hepatic tyrosine aminotransferase[26] (Fig. 41–1). There are two separate tyrosine aminotransferases, one in the cytosol and one in the mitochondria. The cytosolic enzyme is defective in this disorder.[27]

Plasma tyrosine levels in tyrosinemia type II range from 14 to 62 mg/dL.[28] Younger patients have higher levels than adults. In one study, mean plasma tyrosine levels for patients up to 7 years old were 43.4 mg/dL ± 10.97, as com-

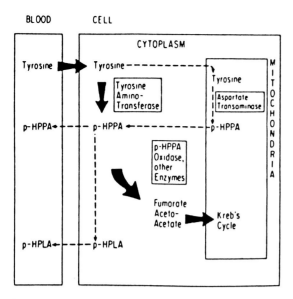

Fig. 41–1. The site of the defect in tyrosinemia type II.

pared to 23.0 ± 5.3 for those 8 to 55 years old.[4] Older patients had eye and skin lesions at blood tyrosine levels that produced no symptoms in younger patients. These data suggest that plasma tyrosine levels decrease with age, which may be related to the decreased protein intake relative to body size; alternative pathways may become more efficient.[4,29] Most patients with oculocutaneous tyrosinemia are lesion-free when the plasma tyrosine concentration is below 10 mg/dL.

Tyrosine is the only amino acid increased in the urine of patients with type II; other amino acids are normal. Urinary tyrosine and its metabolites—p-HPLA, p-HPPA, and N-acetyltyrosine—are increased. Tyramine is also found.[26,30] The presence of tyrosine metabolites in the absence of tyrosine aminotransferase is explained by the presence of mitochondrial amino transferase in such tissues as muscle where accumulated tyrosine is converted to p-HPPA and reduced to p-HPLA, but cannot be converted to homogentisic acid and further oxidized.[31,32]

Tyrosinemia type II is rare, with fewer than 20 cases reported. It is transmitted as an autosomal-recessive trait.

Transient neonatal tyrosinemia

Transient neonatal tyrosinemia is generally asymptomatic, although anorexia and lethargy, prolonged jaundice, and reduced motor activity have been reported.[33,34] Intellectual deficits have also been reported as a sequelae.[35] It is most common in the immature infant who is receiving a high protein diet and an inadequate amount of ascorbic acid.[4] It results from the inhibition of p-hydroxyphenylpyruvate oxidase by its substrate, tyrosine. The activity of the enzyme may be restored by ascorbic acid.[36]

Biochemical features of neonatal tyrosinemia are similar to those in the hereditary tyrosinemias: elevation of plasma and urinary tyrosine and excretion of the tyrosine metabolites, p-HPPA and p-HPLA. It can be distinguished from tyrosinemia type I by the absence of aminoaciduria and proteinuria and from tyrosinemia type II by a secondary

elevation of plasma phenylalanine. The biochemical abnormalities are rapidly corrected by the reduction of dietary protein intake and administration of 100 mg/day of ascorbic acid.

Prenatal diagnosis

Prenatal diagnosis of fetuses affected with tyrosinemia type I was reported by Gagne et al.[37] who demonstrated succinylacetone in amniotic fluid between 15 and 21 weeks gestation. Prenatal diagnosis was also accomplished by analyzing fumarylacetoacetase activity in cultured amniotic fluid cells between 16 and 20 weeks of pregnancy.[38] Normal erythrocytes and chorionic villus biopsy material contain fumarylacetoacetase activity so that prenatal diagnosis should be possible as early as the 8th week of gestation.[39] The assay can be performed directly, and results are available with 1 or 2 days.

Methods of heterozygote detection and prenatal diagnosis of tyrosinemia type II are not available.

Factors to be Considered in Nutritional Evaluation

In the acute form of tyrosinemia type I, dietary restriction of tyrosine, phenylalanine, and methionine has been effective in lowering plasma elevations of these amino acids, reducing the excretion of tyrosine metabolites, and correcting the renal tubular abnormalities.[40] However, despite the correction of biochemical abnormalities, treatment does not reverse the liver disease nor alter the progression to liver failure. Dietary treatment has also been beneficial in the chronic form, although hepatoma is a frequent complication. Benefit from any treatment other than liver transplantation is questionable.[41,42] Succinylacetone excretion continues even after liver transplantation.[43]

Treatment of tyrosinemia type II by restriction of tyrosine and phenylalanine effectively lowers tyrosine concentration in body fluids, and symptoms resolve promptly.[44]

Caloric requirements

Because of the severe vomiting and diarrhea during the first few months of life, provisions should be made for a higher caloric intake than the RDA, using dietary sources in which tyrosine and its precursor, phenylalanine, are avoided. Small frequent feedings are indicated to alleviate severe vomiting and diarrhea.

Low phenylalanine and tyrosine diet

The regimen calls for a restricted intake of phenylalanine and tyrosine. The dietary principles applied to phenylketonuria (PKU) are followed (see Chapter 39). Commercial products, protein hydrolysates from which most of the phenylalanine and tyrosine have been removed, or mixtures of crystalline amino acids omitting tyrosine and phenylalanine are used to provide the necessary amino acids in the diet. Maxamaid® XPHEN, TYR (Ross Laboratories)[45] and Mead Johnson Nutritionals' Low Phe/Tyr powder (Product 3200 AB®) are dietary supplements specific for tyrosinemia (Table 41–1).

Table 41–1. Nutritive Composition of Special Dietary Products for Tyrosinemia

Nutrients (per 100 g powder)	Analog XPHEN, TYR	Analog XPHEN, TYR, MET	Maxamaid XPHEN, TYR	Low Phe/Tyr Diet Powder	Tyr 2
Calories	475	475	350	460	300
Protein (g)	13	13	25	15	63
Fat (g)	20.9	20.9	<1	18	0
Carbohydrate (g)	59	59	62	60	12
L-Amino Acids (mg)					
Isoleucine	1000	1020	1960	870	4500
Leucine	1720	1750	3360	1660	7600
Lysine	1170	1190	2280	1650	5400
Methionine	270	Tr	540	540	1800
Phenylalanine	Tr	Tr	Tr	75	0
Threonine	840	860	1640	780	3600
Tryptophan	340	340	660	1950	1400
Valine	1100	1120	2140	1380	5400
Cystine	420	430	820	60	1800
Histidine	650	660	1260	4500	1880
Tyrosine	Tr	Tr	Tr	Tr	0
Arginine	1130	1150	2210	560	0
Aspartate	940	960	1840	1400	7600
Glutamine	110	110	240	0	0
Glutamate	1260	1280	2460	4000	16000
Glycine	1000	1020	1960	380	1800
Proline	1220	1240	2380	1420	7100
Serine	750	760	1460	940	4000
Vitamins					
Vitamin A (IU)	1760	1760	1000	1440	5200
Vitamin D (IU)	340	340	480	290	1310
Vitamin E (IU)	4.9	4.9	6.5	14.4	18
Vitamin K (ug)	21	21	0	72	167
Thiamine (mg)	0.50	0.50	1.10	0.36	1.40
Riboflavin (mg)	0.60	0.60	1.20	0.43	2.00
Vitamin B_6 (mg)	0.52	0.52	1.0	0.29	1.50
Vitamin B_{12} (mcg)	1.25	1.25	4.0	1.44	3.0
Niacin (mg)	4.5	4.5	12.0	5.80	24.0
Folic acid (mcg)	38	38	150	72	400
Pantothenic acid (mg)	2.65	2.65	3.7	2.20	11.0
Biotin (mcg)	26	260	120	36	300
Ascorbic acid (mg)	40	40	135	37	80
Choline (mg)	50	50	110	61	260
Minerals					
Calcium (mg)	325	325	2400	1310	540
Phosphorus (mg)	230	230	1860	1010	300
Magnesium (mg)	34	34	520	156	63
Iron (mg)	7.0	7.0	34	15	10.8
Zinc (mg)	5.0	5.0	26	7.8	4.5
Manganese (mg)	0.60	0.60	2.4	0.7	0.18
Copper (mg)	0.45	0.45	6.7	2.0	0.54
Iodine (mcg)	47	47	234	120	40
Sodium mg(meq)	120(5.2)	120(5.2)	1070	640	85
Potassium mg(meq)	420(10.7)	420(10.7)	2300	1330	340
Chloride mg(meq)	290(8.2)	290(8.2)	1650	990	135

Analog XPHEN, TYR, Analog XPHEN, TYR, MET, and Maxamaid XPHEN, TRY, MET are products of Ross Laboratories, Columbus, OH 43216. Information may be obtained by calling 1-800-848-2607 or 1-614-438-6200.
Low-Phe/Tyr Diet Powder is a product of Mead Johnson Nutritionals. Information may be obtained by calling 1-800-457-3550. Tyr 2 is produced by Milupa A.G., and distributed in the United States by Mead Johnson Nutritionals, Evansville, IN 47721.

Vitamin C and vitamin D

Vitamin C is important in the oxidation of p-hydroxyphenylpyruvic acid. Vitamin C alone is of no benefit in the treatment of the hereditary tyrosinemias.

Vitamin D must undergo two enzymatic hydroxylations, one in the liver and the other in the kidney, before it can function at the target cells.[46] Patients with tyrosinemia type I may have disturbed vitamin D metabolism with diminished hydroxylation because of progressive liver and renal damage. Although it is evident that the prophylactic administration of vitamin D does not prevent rickets or promote normal growth in these infants, additional oral supplementation has brought about good response.[47]

Phenylalanine and tyrosine requirements

The phenylalanine requirement for normal growth for infants is 90 mg/kg/day in the presence of tyrosine. This requirement increases in the absence of tyrosine.[48] The combined phenylalanine and tyrosine requirement for infants 3 to 4 months of age is estimated to be 125 mg/kg/day, and the adult minimum daily requirement is estimated to be 14 mg/kg/day.[49] About 70% of phenylalanine is converted to tyrosine.

Dietary Management and Follow-up

The objective of dietary therapy for the hereditary tyrosinemias is to provide adequate nutrition for normal growth and development while strictly controlling the intake of tyrosine and its precursor, phenylalanine. Patients with tyrosinemia type I may also require dietary methionine restriction.[50] To monitor the effectiveness of dietary restrictions, blood and urine levels of tyrosine and its metabolites should be measured weekly during the first 3 months, biweekly thereafter until 1 year of age, and monthly thereafter. Dietary intake, anthropomometric measures, and physical signs should be evaluated at the same time.

In tyrosinemia type I, plasma phenylalanine and tyrosine concentrations should be maintained at 40–80 umol/L and 50–150 umol/L, respectively. Serum alphafetoprotein should be monitored at least monthly, since increases in its concentration may signal the onset of hepatic carcinoma, requiring liver transplantation.

Most patients with tyrosinemia type II are free of symptoms as long as the plasma concentration of tyrosine is below 10–13 mg/dL. A combined intake of phenylalanine and tyrosine of less than 100 mg/kg/day may be necessary to achieve plasma tyrosine concentrations less than 10 mg/dL.[21]

References

1. Medes, G.A new error of tyrosine metabolism: tyrosinosis. The intermediary metabolism of tyrosine and phenylalanine. *Biochem. J.* 1932; 26:917.
2. Baber, M.D. A case of congenital cirrhosis of the liver with renal tubular defects akin to those in the Fanconi syndrome. *Arch. Dis. Child.* 1956; 31:335.
3. Scriver, C.R. The phenotype manifestations of hereditary tyrosinemia and tyrosyluria. *Can. Med. Assoc. J.* 1967; 97:1079.
4. Goldsmith, L.A., LaBerge, C. Tyrosinemia and related disorders. In: Scriver, C.R., Beaudet, A.L., Sly, W.S., Valle, D., eds. *The Metabolic Basis of Inherited Disease.* 6th ed., New York: McGraw-Hill; 1989.
5. Nordle, S., Antener, I., Kaeser, M., Gatti, R. Hepato-tubular syndrome with tyrosinuria-tyrosyluria. *Ann. Pediatr.* (Basel), 1966; 207:201.
6. Pettit, B.R., Kvittingen, E.A., Leonard, J.V. Early prenatal diagnosis of hereditary tyrosinemia. *Lancet.* 1985; 1:1038.
7. Berger, R. Biochemical aspects of type I hereditary tyrosinemia. In: Bickel, H., Wechtel, U., eds. *Diseases of Amino Acid Metabolism.* Stuttgart: Thieme; 1985.
8. Gentz, J., Johansson, S., Lindblad, B., Lindstedt, S., Zetterstrom, R. Excretion of delta aminolevulinic acid in hereditary tyrosinemia. *Clin. Chim. Acta.* 1969; 23:27.
9. Tazawa, Y., Kikuchi, M., Kurobane, I., Watanabe, A., Nakai, H., Narisawa, K., Tada, K. An acute form of tyrosinemia type I with multiple intrahepatic mass lesions. *J. Pediatr. Gastroenterol. Nutr.* 1990; 10:536.
10. Lindblad, B., Lindstedt, S., Steen, G. On enzymatic defects in hereditary tyrosinemia. *Proc. Natl. Acad. Sci. USA.* 1977; 74:4641.
11. Kvittingen, E.A., Halvorsen, S., Jellum, E. Deficient fumarylacetoacetate fumarylhydrolase activity in lymphocytes and fibroblasts from patients with hereditary tyrosinemia. *Pediatr. Res.* 1983; 14:541.
12. La Du, B.N., Gjessing, L.R. Tyrosinosis and tyrosinemia. In: Stanbury, J.B., Syngaarden, J.B., Fredrickson, D.S., Goldstein, J.L., Brown, M.S., eds. *The Metabolic Basis of Inherited Diseases.* 4th ed. New York: McGraw-Hill; 1978.
13. Sassa, S., Kappas, A. Hereditary tyrosinemia and the heme biosynthetic pathway. *J. Clin. Invest.* 1983; 71:625.
14. Weinberg, A.G., Mize, C.E., Worthen, H.G. The occurrence of hepatoma in the chronic form of hereditary tyrosinemia. *J. Pediatr.* 1976; 88:434.
15. Scriver, C.R., Rosenberg, L.E. Tyrosine. In: Scriver, C.R., Rosenberg, L.E., eds. *Amino Acid Metabolism and Its Disorders.* Philadelphia: W.B. Saunders; 1973: 338.
16. Kogut, M.D., Shaw, K.N., Donnell, G.N. Tyrosinosis. *Am. J. Dis. Child.* 1967; 113:47.
17. Gaull, E.D., Rassin, D.K., Solomon, G.E., Harris, R.C., Sturman, J.A. Biochemical observations on so-called hereditary tyrosinemia. *Pediatr. Res.* 1970; 4:337.
18. Evans, D.I.K., Sardharwalla, I.B. Coagulation defect of congenital tyrosinemia. *Arch. Dis. Child.* 1984; 59:1088.
19. Soirdahl, S., Lie, S.O., Jellium, E., Stokke, O. Increased need for L-cysteine in hereditary tyrosinemia. *Pediatr. Res.* 1979; 13:74.
20. Fallstrom, S.P., Lindblad, B., Steen, G. On the renal tubular damage in hereditary tyrosinemia and on the formation of succinylacetoacetate and succinylacetone. *Acta Pediatr. Scand.* 1981; 70:315.
21. Ney, D., Bay, C., Schenider, J.A., Kelts, D., Nyhan, W.L. Dietary management of oculocutaneous tyrosinemia in an 11-year old child. *Am. J. Dis. Child.* 1983; 137:995.
22. Hunziker, N. Richner-Hanhart syndrome and tyrosinemia type II. *Dermatologica.* 1980; 160:180.
23. Goldsmith, L.A. Tyrosinemia II: Lessons in molecular pathophysiology. *Pediatr. Dermatol.* 1983; 1:25.
24. Balato, N., Francesco, C., Lembo, G., Santoianni, P. Tyrosinemia type II in two cases previously reported as Richner-Hanhart syndrome. *Dermatologica.* 1986; 173:66.
25. Benevanga, N.J., Steele, R.D. Adverse affects of amino acids. *Annu. Rev. Nutr.* 1984; 4:157.
26. Kennaway, N.G., Buist, N.R.M. Metabolic studies in a patient with hepatic cytosol tyrosine aminotransferase deficiency. *Pediatr. Res.* 1971; 5:287.
27. Fellman, J.H., Vanbellinghen, P.J., Jones, R.T., Koler, R.D. Soluble and mitochondrial forms of tyrosine aminotransferase. Relationship to human tyrosinemia. *Biochemistry.* 1969; 8:615.
28. Fois, A., Borgogni, M., Cioni, M., Molinelli, M., Frezzotti, R., Vardelli, A.M., Lasorella, G., Barberi, L., Durand, P., DiRocco, M., Romano, C., Parini, R., Corbetta, C., Giovannini, M., Riva, E., Balato, N., Sartorio, R., Mollica, F., Zammarchi, E., Battini, M.L. Presentation of the data of the Italian Registry for oculocutaneous tyrosinemia. *J. Inher. Metab. Dis.* 1986; 9:262.
29. Hunziker, N. Richner-Hanhart syndrome and tyrosinemia type II. *Dermatologica.* 1980; 160:180.

30. Hill, A., Zaleski, W.A. Tyrosinosis: biochemical studies of an unusual case. *Clin. Biochem.* 1971; 4:263.
31. Kennaway, N.G., Buist, N.R.M., Fellman, J.H. The origin of p-hydroxyphenylpyruvate in a patient with hepatic cytosol tyrosine aminotransferase deficiency. *Clin. Chim. Acta.* 1972; 41:157.
32. Weber, W.W., Zannoni, V.G. Reduction of phenylpyruvic acids to phenyllactic acids in mammalian tissues. *J. Biol. Chem.* 1969; 241:615.
33. Light, I.J., Sutherland, J.M., Berry, H.K. Clinical significance of tyrosinemia of prematurity. *Am. J. Dis. Child.* 1973; 125:243.
34. Partington, M.W., Campbell, D., Kuyer, J. Motor activity in early life. *Biol. Neonate.* 1971; 18:121.
35. Manunes, P., Prince, P.E., Thornton, N.H., Hunt, P.A., Hitchock, E.S. Intellectual deficits after transient tyrosinemia. *Pediatrics.* 1976; 57:675.
36. Zannoni, V.G. The tyrosine oxidations system of liver. The ability of various quinones to reactivate inhibited p-hydroxyphenylpyruvic acid oxidase. *J. Biol. Chem.* 1962; 237:1172.
37. Gagne, R., Lescault, A., Grenier, A., Laberge, C., Melancon, S.B., Dallaire, L. Prenatal diagnosis of hereditary tyrosinemia: measurement of succinylacetone in amniotic fluid. *Prenatal. Diagn.* 1982; 2:285.
38. Kvittingen, E.A., Steinman, B., Gitzelmann, R., Leonard, J.V., Andria, G., Borrosen, A.I., Mossman, J., Micara, G., Lindblad, B. Prenatal diagnosis of hereditary tyrosinemia by determination of fumarylactoacetase in cultured amniotic fluid cells. *Pediatr. Res.* 1985; 19:334.
39. Holme, E., Lindblad, B., Lindstedt, S. Possibilities for treatment and for early prenatal diagnosis of hereditary tyrosinemia. *Lancet.* 1985; 1:527.
40. Michals, K., Matalon, R., Wong, P.W.K. Dietary treatment of tyrosinemia type I. *J. Am. Diet. Assoc.* 1978; 73:507.
41. Fische, R.O., McCabe, E.R.B., Doeden, D., Koep, L.J., Kohlhoff, J.G., Silvrman, A., Starzyl, T.E. Homotransplantation of the liver in a patient with hepatoma and hereditary tyrosinemia. *J. Pediatr.* 1978; 93:592.
42. Kvittingen, E.A. Tyrosinaemia type I—an update. *J. Inher. Metab. Dis.* 1991; 14:554.
43. Ramnaraine, M.L., Ulstrom, R.A., Najarian, J.S., Archer, N. Persistent succinylacetone excretion after liver transplantation in a patient with hereditary tyrosinemia type I. *J. Inher. Metab. Dis.* 1985; 8:21.
44. Buist, N.R.M., Kennaway, N.G., Fellman, J.H. Tyrosinemia type II: hepatic cytosol tyrosine amino-transferase deficiency (The "Richner-Hanhart Syndrome"). In: Bickel, H., Wechtel, U., eds. *Diseases of Amino Acid Metabolism.* Stuttgart: Thieme; 1985.
45. Acosta, P. *Ross Metabolic Formula System Nutrition Support Protocols.* Columbus, OH: Ross Laboratories; 1989.
46. Scriver, C.R. Vitamin-responsive inborn errors of metabolism. *Metabolism.* 1973; 10:1319.
47. Frazer, D. Pathogenesis of hereditary vitamin D dependent rickets. *N. Engl. J. Med.* 1973; 289:817.
48. Cohn, R.M., Yardkoff, M., Yost, B., Segal, S. Phenylalanine-tyrosine deficiency syndrome as a complication of the management of hereditary tyrosinemia. *Am. J. Clin. Nutr.* 1977; 30:209.
49. Food and Nutrition Board. *Recommended Dietary Allowances.* 10th ed., Washington, DC, National Academy of Sciences; 1989.
50. Levy, H.L. Nutritional therapy for selected inborn errors of metabolism. *J. Am. Coll. Nutr.* 1989; 8(S):54.

Chapter 42
The Urea Cycle Disorders

Kathleen Huntington

The function of the urea cycle is twofold: (1) it rids the body of toxic ammonia, an end product of protein catabolism, and (2) it provides the enzymatic mechanism for the synthesis of arginine.[1] This metabolic pathway operates primarily in the liver and is compartmentalized between the cellular cytosolic and mitochondrial compartments.

The main purpose of dietary protein is to supply essential amino acids for protein biosynthesis and nitrogen to form nitrogenous cellular constituents. However, only a small amount of the daily amino acids used in protein metabolism is supplied through the diet. The majority of amino acids used in protein synthesis come from the breakdown of endogenous protein. Human beings cannot store nitrogen in excess of the body's requirements. Therefore, the balance of unneeded essential and nonessential amino acids is converted to energy intermediates in a manner that involves the loss of the alpha-amino group to the formation of ammonia. Ammonia is thought to be toxic, especially to the brain, through the promotion of glutamate synthesis from alpha-ketoglutarate, which thereby depletes the TCA cycle of an essential intermediate and impedes aerobic metabolism. The process of ureagenesis converts toxic ammonia to the water-soluble nontoxic urea molecule.

Biochemical Abnormalities

The urea cycle is a multi-enzyme pathway of some complexity as illustrated in Figure 42–1. The first enzyme of the pathway, *carbamyl phosphate synthetase*, forms the activated intermediate carbamyl phosphate from ammonia, a molecule of CO_2, and the gamma-phosphate group of ATP. This enzyme is located in the mitochondria and is allosterically activated by N-acetylglutamate, a metabolite that is generated from acetyl CoA and glutamate by *N-acetylglutamate synthetase*. Carbamyl phosphate is then condensed with ornithine, an intermediate of the urea cycle to form citrulline, a reaction catalyzed by the mitochondrial enzyme, *ornithine transcarbamylase*. Citrulline then diffuses into the cytosol where it combines with aspartate to form argininosuccinate, a reaction catalyzed by *argininosuccinate synthetase*. Argininosuccinate is cleaved into arginine and fumarate, a TCA cycle intermediate, by *argininosuccinate lyase*. *Arginase* then liberates a molecule of urea from arginine, a process that regenerates ornithine. The ornithine formed in the cytosol is then transported back into the mitochondria, where it can serve as a substrate for another round of the urea cycle. The urea exits from the hepatic cells and is transported to the kidneys via the blood and is excreted in the urine.

Genetic malfunction of any one of the six enzymes interferes with ureagenesis by this cyclic system (Fig. 42–1). The cumulative frequency of urea cycle defects as a whole has not been identified, owing to a number of undiagnosed deaths, but the incidence may approach 1 in 50,000.[2]

Factors to be Considered in Nutritional Evaluation

Clinical symptoms for each of the enzyme defects are similar: lethargy, vomiting, seizures, hyperventilation, reduced sensitivity to pain, ataxia, convulsions, and coma.[3,4] Without an appropriate diagnosis and treatment, permanent brain damage or death can result. Presentation may be in the neonatal period or anytime thereafter. Otherwise normal female carriers of the mutant ornithine transcarbamylase allele are also known to be at serious risk for abnormalities of nitrogen metabolism.[5] Malfunction of each enzyme is characterized by hyperammonemia. Depending on the specific malfunction, plasma amino acid analysis will aid in identifying the specific disorder. Differential diagnosis and monitoring of therapy for each enzyme defect are dependent upon laboratory findings and phenotypic markers (Table 42–1). Measurement of urinary orotidine excretion after allopurinol administration is recommended for establishing the carrier status of women at risk for ornithine transcarbamylase deficiency.[6]

Dietary and Biochemical Management

Reducing and maintaining the concentration of serum ammonia at normal or near-normal levels and the provision of sufficient nitrogen for optimal growth are the overriding principles for the treatment of these disorders. After stabilization of the acute medical crisis, treatment has three main objectives[3,7]: (1) reduction of the ammonia precursor, e.g., dietary protein; (2) provision of the deficient cyclic intermediates, e.g., arginine or citrulline; and (3) utilization of alternative pathways for the excretion of waste nitrogen through amino acid acylation.

Reduction of dietary protein

Limiting protein intake as a chronic therapeutic measure reduces the production of waste nitrogen and serves to maintain the concentration of ammonia at a physiological level. The supply of protein must meet the growth needs of the infant and child, but should not exceed minimum nitrogen requirements.[8]

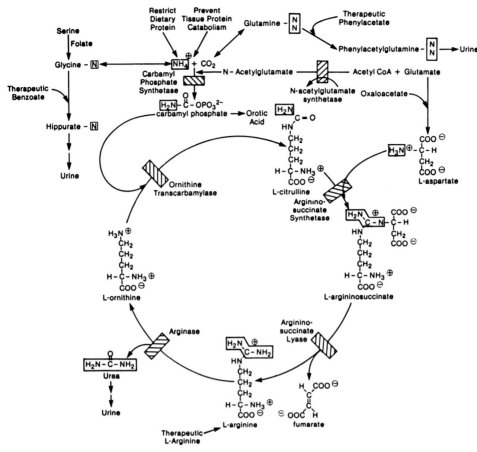

Fig. 42-1. The urea cycle. From Elias & Acosta[7] with permission.

Table 42-1. Urea Cycle Enzyme Defects*

Lab Parameters and Phenotypic Markers	CPS	OTC	AS	AL	Arginase
Relative hyperammonemia	+ +	+ + + +	+ +	+ +	+
Glutamine	+	+	+	+	+
Alanine	+	+	+	+	
Citrulline	Low	Low	+ +	+	+
Arginine	Low	Low	Low	Low	+
Orotic acid		+	+		−
Trichorrhexis nodosa†				+	

CPS = carbamyl phosphate synthetase; OTC = ornithine transcarbamylase; AS = argininosuccinate synthetase; AL = argininosuccinate lyase

*Note: N-Acetylglutamate synthetase deficiency has been cited in the literature only once; laboratory parameters are not completely elucidated.[1]

†Hair abnormality consisting of diffuse brittle hair related to arginine deficiency.

However, the minimum protein requirements of infants and children are not precisely known due to the difficulty of measuring growth needs and determining maintenance nitrogen specifications. A joint FAO/WHO report provides theoretically safe levels of protein intake relative to milk or eggs.[9] Based on these guidelines, safe protein intake levels have been suggested.[7,8,10] Recommendations for protein intake without an allowance for individual variability are found in Table 42-2.[7,8] Caloric intake should be more generous than standard recommendations for normal children to prevent a catabolic response and to supply sufficient carbohydrate for the synthesis of nonessential amino acids from alpha-ketoacids.[7] Given an adequate caloric intake from carbohydrate and fat, dietary amino acids can be spared to provide the nitrogen for protein synthesis. If caloric needs are not met, protein is catabolized to meet energy requirements, which in turn generates an ammonia load that exacerbates the risk of metabolic decompensation.

Supplementation with essential amino acids decreases the requirement for a dietary protein source of high biological value. In combination, the dietary protein and essential amino acid supplement should provide the minimum dietary pro-

Table 42-2. Protein and Energy Recommendations

Age	Protein (g/kg)	Energy (kcal/kg)
< 3 months	1.2–1.8	130–145
3 < 6 months	1.0–1.4	125–145
6 < 9 months	1.0–1.3	120–125
9 < 12 months	0.9–1.2	115–135
1 < 4 years	0.7–1.0	110–120
4 < 7 years	0.6–0.8	100–110
7 < 11 years	0.5–0.7	80–90
11 < 18 years	0.4–0.6	55–65
> 18 years	0.3–0.5	35–50

From Elsas & Acosta[7] and Bell et al.[8]

tein for growth.[10] (See Table 42–3 for the suppliers of essential amino acids.) Reducing whole dietary protein alone, rather than combining a mixture of essential amino acids and whole protein, may be sufficient. The use of supplements to increase essential amino acid intake further may not always be beneficial. Regardless of suggested intake, the prescribed protein should be based on monitored serum ammonia levels, plasma amino acids, orotic acid levels in the urine, and growth parameters. The discrepant enzyme activities among patients with urea cycle defects, in addition to the use of adjunct therapy, precludes rigid adherence to dietary protein guidelines for any given urea cycle defect.

Because of the severe protein restriction needed to reduce serum ammonia, commercially prepared formula at normal dilution or even breast milk, which has a lower protein content, cannot be used exclusively. Specialty products, referred to as medical foods, must be used in place of or in conjunction with the commercial formulas. Tables 42–4 and 42–5 give the nutrient composition of several medical foods. Product 80056 (Mead Johnson Co., Evansville, IN) supplies carbohydrate, fat, vitamins, and minerals. When combined with commercial formula that is adjusted to supply the minimum protein requirements, all other nutritional needs can be met. Because Product 80056 is low in sodium (180 mg/quart), the adequacy of dietary sodium intake should be assessed in infancy when formula comprises the total diet. Essential amino acid mixtures, UCD-1 and UCD-2 (Mead Johnson Co., Evansville, IN), are intended for the infant and child, respectively, and contain sugar, minerals, vitamins, and L-amino acids. UCD-2 does not contain L-cystine and L-tyrosine. Neither contains chromium, selenium, or fat. Another essential amino acid mixture, Amin-Aid (Kendall-McGaw, Irvine, CA) contains fat and carbohydrate with minimal electrolytes in addition to the amino acids, but has no vitamins or minerals. Osmolarity is high when it is prepared at full strength. An example of a low-protein dietary

Table 42–3. Dietary Resources

Suppliers of L-Amino Acids	Suppliers of L-Carnitine
Ajinomoto, U.S.A., Inc. (Eastern Distributor) Glenpoint Century West 500 Franks West Burr Blvd Teaneck, NJ 07666-6894 (201)488-1212	Sigma Tau, Inc. 723 North Beers Homedale, NJ 07733 (201)264-1200
Ajinomoto, U.S.A., Inc. (Western Distributor) Glenpoint Century West 19675 Mariner Avenue Torrance, CA 90503 (213)370-2500	Kendal-McCaw 2525 McGaw Avenue Irvine, CA 92714 (800)241-7703
Tanabe, U.S.A., Inc. P.O. Box 85132 San Diego, CA 92138 (619)571-8410	Tanabe, U.S.A., Inc P.O. Box 85132 San Diego, CA 92138 (619)571-8410

Low-Protein Specialty Outlets		
Ener-G-Foods, Inc. ?901 Fox Ave., South P.O. Box 24723 Seattle, WA 98124 (800)331-5222	Med Diet, Inc. 1409 Fairfield Rd., South Minnetonka, MN 55343 (800)633-3438 (612)546-3285	Kingsmill Foods Co., Ltd. 1399 Kennedy Rd., Unit 17 Scarborough, Ontario Canada, M1P 2L6 (416)755-1124
Dietary Specialties P.O. Box 227 Rochester, NY 14601 (800)544-0099 (716)263-2787	Scientific Hospital Supplies, Inc. P.O. Box 117 Gaithersburg, MD 20877 (301)840-0408	

Dietary Resources

Dietary References	Dietary Analysis
Lo Pro Diet Guide[11] Low Protein Food List[12] Know-Low-Pro, An Overview of Low Protein Products[13] Low Protein Cookery[14]	Nutrition & Diet Services 927 SE Rim Rock Lane Portland, OR 97267
Dietary Psychology	Amino Acid Analyzer III Nutrient Management System 1916 Wahalaw Ct. Tallahassee, FL 32301
Special Diets and Kids[42]	

Table 42–4. Nutrient Composition of Medical Foods

Product 80056	Per 100 g Powder	UCD #1	Per 100 g Powder	UCD #2	Per 100 g Powder
Protein (g)	0	Protein (g)	56	Protein (g)	67
		Amino acids (g)	68	Amino acids (g)	81
Carbohydrate (g)	72	Carbohydrate (g)	8	Carbohydrate (g)	6
Fat (g)	22	Fat (g)	0	Fat (g)	0
Water (g)	3	Water (g)	2	Water (g)	2
Linoleic acid (mg)	11,500	Vit. & min. (g)	20.2	Vit. & min. (g)	9.7
Calories	490	Calories	260	Calories	290
Vitamin A (IU)	1,800		11,200		5,200
Vitamin D (IU)	360		1,200		1,310
Vitamin E (IU)	18		41		18
Vitamin K (g)	90		200		167
Thiamine (vitamin B_1) (g)	450		3,200		1,400
Riboflavin (vitamin B_2) (g)	540		4,800		2,000
Vitamin B_6 (g)	360		2,600		1,500
Vitamin B_{12} (g)	1.8		8		3
Niacin (g)	7,200		65,000		24,000
Folic acid (folacin) (g)	90		400		400
Pantothenic acid	2,700		30,000		11,000
Biotin (g)	45		120		300
Vitamin C (ascorbic acid) (mg)	47		280		80
Choline (mg)	76		510		260
Inositol (mg)	27		590		300
Calcium (mg)	540		2,800		1,130
Phosphorus (mg)	300		2,200		1,010
Magnesium (mg)	63		0		0
Iron (mg)	10.8		40		15
Zinc (mg)	4.5		31		7.8
Manganese (g)	180		2,800		700
Copper (g)	540		8,000		2,000
Iodine (g)	40		270		120
Sodium (mg)	85		1,260		640
Potassium (mg)	340		2,800		1,330
Chloride (mg)	135		1,940		990
		L-Histidine	3.1g		3.6g
		L-Isoleucine	7.6g		8.9g
		L-Leucine	2.8g		15.0g
		L-Lysine	9.0g		10.7g
		L-Methionine	3.1g		7.1g
		L-Phenylalanine	5.3g		14.1g
		L-Threonine	6.0g		7.1g
		L-Tryptophan	2.2g		2.8g
		L-Valine	9.0g		10.7g
		L-Cystine	3.1g		
		L-Tyrosine	6.5g		

menu is shown in Table 42–6 for both a 9-month-old infant and a young child 24 months of age. The advantage of using formula through the toddler stage is that it provides a dependable source of high biological protein and calories. Children at this age are notorious for fluctuating appetites and cannot be expected to eat prescribed solids for protein intake; hence, the formula is a reliable source of nutrition for part of the child's diet at this age. When cow's milk is substituted for formula, fewer calories are available per equal amounts of protein at normal dilution. Cup drinking should be encouraged at the appropriate developmental stage of feeding, rather than relying on the bottle. Normal feeding practices should be encouraged, despite the continued reliance on infant formula as a nutritional source. Introduction of low-protein specialty products at an early age provides the opportunity for flavor acceptance and more flexibility in meeting the calorie demands of an older and more active child. Several companies offer low-protein products (Table

Table 42-5. Nutrient Composition of Amin-Aid (146 g/package)

	Grams Per Package	Calorie Contribution
Protein (as amino acids)	6.6	4.0%
Carbohydrate	124.3	74.8%
Fat	15.7	21.2%

L-Leucine 1.10
L-Methionine 1.10
L-Phenylalanine 1.10
L-Valine 0.80
L-Lysine 0.79
L-Isoleucine 0.70
L-Threonine 0.50
L-Tryptophan 0.25
L-Histidine 0.25
Total calories: 665 (640 nonprotein calories)
Osmolarity: 510 mOsm/L

42-3). Resources developed for management of various amino acidopathies can be useful for low-protein menu planning and intake analysis (Table 42-3).[11-14]

Provision of cyclic intermediates

With the exception of arginase deficiency, arginine becomes an indispensable amino acid for individuals with urea cycle defects.[1] If arginine is removed from the diet, affected individuals show nitrogen accumulation in the form of ammonia and/or glutamine, as well as orotic aciduria, which is associated with OTC and AL deficiencies specifically.[15] For those with functional urea cycle systems, controlled arginine-deficient diets do not induce hyperammonemia.[16] However, a deficiency of arginine as an essential amino acid can result in: (1) protein catabolism and an increased nitrogen load; (2) further diminution of residual activity of ornithine transcarbamylase (OTC), resulting in ornithine becoming rate limiting; and (3) reduced carbamyl phosphate synthetase (CPS), activity due to a lessened stimulatory effect of arginine on N-acetylglutamate synthetase.[3]

Administration of free-base arginine (175-700 mg/kg) is recommended for all urea cycle defects, except in the case of arginase deficiency.[1,10] Arginine is generally not considered part of the total protein intake.[1] For CPS and OTC deficiencies, citrulline may be substituted at 175 mg/kg for arginine.[3]

Amino acid acylation

Despite the restriction of protein and the supplementation of essential amino acids or nitrogen-free analogs, before 1979, most children who survived the acute crisis later succumbed to episodic hyperammonemia.[17,18] Adjunct therapies have since improved the survival rate. The failure of dietary therapy alone can be attributed to the incapacity for ureagenesis from waste nitrogen that results from an intake of nitrogen that exceeds growth needs and that of nitrogen retention from protein turnover.[1,19]

Table 42-6. Sample Menus

	9-Month-Old Infant*				24-Month-Old Child†			
	Measure	Wt (g)	Pro (g)	Energy (kcal)	Measure	Wt (g)	Pro (g)	Energy (kcal)
Formula								
Similac with iron, powder	9.5 T	83	10	425	8.5 T	75	88.5	385
Prod. 80056, powder	5 T	50	0	245	5 T	50	0	245
Fluid, to make	30 oz				24 oz			
Food								
Pear nectar	4 oz	125	.1	75	4 oz	125	.1	75
Rice cereal	4 T	14	1.2	60	–	–	–	–
Rice Chex	–	–	–	–	1/2 c	12 gr	.7	49
Bread, low protein	–	–	–	–	2 sl	–	.8	218
Annellini, low protein	1/4 c	55	.1	49	1/2 c	110	.2	98
Green beans	2 T	15	.3	5	3 T	24	.5	8
Broccoli	–	–	–	–	2 T	23	.7	7
Carrots	2 T	19	.2	8	–	–	–	–
Applesauce	1/4 c	61	.1	49	1/2 c	122	.2	98
Animal crackers	2	5	.3	17	–	–	–	–
Choc. chip cookies, low protein	–	–	–	–	2	–	.4	112
Butter	2 tsp	10	trc	72	2 tsp	10	trc	72
¹Total formula	30 oz	–	10	670	24 oz	–	8.5	630
Food	–	–	2.3	335	–	–	3.6	737
TOTAL	–	–	12.3	1,005	–	–	12.1	1,367

*Weight = 8.4 kg (25th percentile). Maximum protein/kg: 1.5 g. Minimum kcal/kg: 120.
†Weight = 12 kg (30th percentile). Maximum protein kg: 1.0 g. Minimum kcal/kg: 110.
Nutrient data from Nutrition and Diet Services, Portland, Oregon: *Low Protein Cookery*; Ross Nutrition Support Protocols.[49]

Glycine, alanine, glutamine, and glutamate comprise 80% of the total alpha amino acid pool.[20] There are compounds that can help rid the body of some of this nitrogen. Sodium benzoate combines with glycine to form hippurate, which is then excreted by the kidneys at five times the glomerular filtration rate.[3] Conjugation of sodium phenylacetate with glutamine forms phenylacetylglutamine, which is also excreted through the kidneys. Acylation of glutamine has three advantages over that of glycine[21]: (1) it disposes of twice the molar quantity of nitrogen; (2) plasma glutamine levels are increased in all urea cycle defects and are therefore readily available; and (3) glutamine is in equilibrium with glutamate, which is the normal nitrogen donor for urea synthesis.

In combination, these two methods of amino acid acylation account for more than 50% of the total urinary waste nitrogen.[22] However, the strong odor of sodium phenylacetate precludes enthusiastic compliance with its use. Ucephan, (Kendall McGaw, Irvine, CA) combines both benzoate and phenylacetate in equal proportions. Acceptance is still an issue, but the number of medications required is reduced. For some patients, sodium benzoate alone can excrete sufficient nitrogen.

There are reports of toxicity with doses of either benzoate or phenylacetate over 5 mmol/kg.[23] Symptoms related to toxicity include irritability, anorexia, lethargy, and coma and similar to those of a hyperammonemic crisis.[22,23] High levels of serotonin in the cerebrospinal fluid have been attributed to benzoate intoxication.[24] This effect may be caused by interference with albumin-binding sites for tryptophan, which is manifested in decreased appetite and anorexia.[24,25] Sodium benzoate may also potentiate ammonia toxicity and inhibit residual ureagenesis.[26] Protocols for maintenance therapy should include drug monitoring and avoidance of doses higher than the recommended 250 mg/kg/day.[1,27]

Inefficient hippurate synthesis hinges on glycine availability, which limits the utility of benzoate therapy for treatment of urea cycle disorders.[28] Folate (0.5 mg/day) and pyridoxine (5 mg/day) supplementation have been recommended for the purpose of averting glycine depletion[10]; both vitamins are required for serine conversion to glycine.

Carnitine

In addition to dietary protein restriction, cyclic intermediate supplementation, and amino acid acylation, it has been recommended that carnitine supplementation be included as a therapeutic measure in the treatment of urea cycle defects.[29] Carnitine, synthesized from methionine and lysine, is involved in the transport of activated fatty acids across the mitochondrial inner membrane both to and from the cytosol. Secondary carnitine deficiency may be expressed as an increased ratio of acylcarnitine to free carnitine in both serum and urine,[30] which has been identified in patients with OTC deficiencies.[33] During catabolism, as protein and fatty acids are broken down, toxic organic acyl-CoA derivatives become augmented; carnitine serves as a buffer by acylating these acyl-CoA metabolites.[30] Sodium benzoate therapy may affect the production of diacarbozylic acid derivatives, resulting in secondary depression of free carnitine levels in urine and plasma.[32] The administration of L-carnitine has reduced the number of hyperammonemic attacks in OTC patients.[31] There have been no identified toxic effects of therapeutic carnitine, but further research in this area is warranted.[3,33]

Neonatal hyperammonemia

Hemo- and peritoneal dialysis or continuous arteriovenous hemofiltration can be used for the rapid reduction of severely elevated ammonia levels and other problematic metabolites in patients with neurotoxic symptoms.[1,7,34,35] Hospital staff expertise usually dictates the choice of treatment. Except for the addition of L-arginine (350–700 mg/kg/day),[1,7] protein-free calories are supplied in the form of a nasogastric glucose infusion (10–12 mg/kg/min)[36] or orogastric perfusion of Mead Johnson Product 80056 (150 kcal/kg).[7] Sodium benzoate (250 mg/kg)[1,7] or Ucephan[36] is administered. After 72–96 hours of this regimen, the intravenous administration of essential amino acids (250 mg/kg/day)[36] should be initiated and gradually increased as tolerance allows; if orogastric delivery is being used, 1.0–1.5 g protein/kg/day is administered.[7]

Nutritional and behavior management

Personality and environment affect feeding behavior and thus nutritional management. Often, children with urea cycle disorders fail to thrive and demonstrate aberrant behavior around eating and food selection.[37] Both neurochemical and behavioral components have been suggested as causal factors.[37,38] Too much emphasis on obsessional dietary control to avoid hyperammonemia crises can overshadow the importance of focusing on developmental feeding skills. Artificial feeding methods, such as nasogastric tube feeding and in some instances gastrostomies, are sometimes used to ensure appropriate dietary therapy and nutritional adequacy. However, these strategies do not promote effective feeding behavior.[39] Behavioral responses that include vomiting, gagging, crying, and fighting may reflect lack of the development of normal oral feeding skills.[40] Successful feeding patterns often involve extensive and continuing intervention of an interdisciplinary team with nutritional, medical, occupational therapy, speech pathology, physical therapy, and psychological expertise.[41] Reviewing the issues surrounding the psychosocial dilemmas of contending with a prescribed diet can be helpful to the parent, as well as to the health care professional (Table 42–3).[42]

Monitoring and Follow-up

Since 1967, the American Academy of Pediatrics has published four reports on the dietary treatment of genetic disorders and has suggested a protocol for determining the safety of dietary products that are developed for the treatment of specific metabolic defects.[43–46] This protocol can be useful in establishing patient management guidelines. Its recommendations include the following:

- *Evaluation of dietary adequacy.* Periodic food diaries completed by the parent or child can serve two purposes: to establish the nutritional adequacy for energy, nutrients, vitamins, minerals, and amino acids and to provide an educational tool for the energy and protein content of specific foods.

- *Assessment of growth parameters.* Protein-restricted diets do not diminish the genetic potential for growth, as long as protein and energy intake are adequate. Downward deviations in height and weight reflect the same inadequacies seen in children without urea cycle disorders.
- *Plasma ammonia analyses.* Normal values should be 20–60 μg/dL. An adaptive tolerance for higher ammonia concentrations necessitates regular monitoring. Portable ammonia analyzers are available for home use.[1,47]
- *Plasma amino acid analyses.* Plasma amino acid levels can suggest a hyperammonemic condition.[4] Abnormally high levels of glutamine and alanine reflect increased transamination as an attempt at metabolic compensation via an interorgan relationship between the muscle tissue and liver. These two amino acids serve as the mechanism for the transport of excess nitrogen to the liver. An increase of ammonia may be precipitated by: catabolic responses generated by the need for energy through gluconeogenesis, fever, or the oxidation of amino acids in the liver or kidney. Chronic protein-deficient diets produce a depression of essential amino acids and stimulate an increase of nonessential amino acids in the plasma.[48]
- *Urine metabolite analyses.* The finding of orotic acid in the urine indicates that the cycle is overloaded and suggests that the prescribed treatment plan for OTC deficiency, patient adherence to the recommendations, or an intervening illness require attention.
- *Neurological evaluation and developmental assessment.* Children with urea cycle defects are at risk for developmental delay at least partly due to the hyperammonemic damage to the central nervous system.[1] Regular developmental evaluations are suggested. Special needs should be addressed within local school programs. Cognitive, speech, and hearing assessments serve to determine school and community programs appropriate for specific patients.

Acknowledgments

The author would like to extend special thanks to Neil Buist, M.B., Ch.B, D.C.H.; Buddy Ullman, Ph.D.; and Annie Prince, Ph.D., R.D. for their critical review of this manuscript.

References

1. Brusilow, S.W., Horwich, A.L. Urea cycle enzymes. In: Scriver, C.R., Beaudet, A.L., Sly, W.S., Valle, D., Stanbury, J.B., Wyngarrden, J.B., Fredrickson, D.S., eds. *The Metabolic Basis of Inherited Disease.* 6th ed. New York: McGraw-Hill; 1989.
2. Talbot, H.W., Sumlin, A.B., Naylor, E.W., Guthrie, R.A neonatal screening test for argininosuccinic acid lyase deficiency and other urea cycle disorders. *Pediatrics.* 1982; 70:526.
3. Batshaw, M.L., Monahan, P.S. Treatment of urea cycle disorders. *Enzyme.* 1987; 38:242.
4. Bachman, C. Diagnosis of urea cycle disorders. *Enzyme.* 1987; 38:233.
5. Arn, P.H., Hauser, E.R., Thomas, G.H., Herman, G., Hess, D., Brusilow, S.W. Hyperammonemia in women with a mutation at the ornithine carbamoyltransferase locus. *N. Engl. J. Med.* 1990; 322:1652.
6. Hauser, E.R., Finkelstein, J.E., Valle, D., Brusilow, S.W. Allopurinol-induced orotidinuria. *N. Engl. J. Med.* 1990; 322:1641.
7. Elsas, L.J., Acosta, P.B. Nutrition support of inherited metabolic disorders. In: Shils, M.E., Young, V.R., eds. *Modern Nutrition in Health and Disease.* 7th ed. Philadelphia: Lea & Febiger; 1988.
8. Bell, L., Chan, L., Sherwood, G., McInnes, R. Use and design of low protein diets for children with inborn metabolic disorders. *Can. Diet. Assoc.* 1982; 43:342.
9. FAO/WHO/UNU: *Energy and Protein Requirements.* Geneva: World Health Organization; 1985. Technical Series Report 724.
10. Valle, D.L. Dietary management of inborn errors of metabolism. In: Walser, M., Imbembo, A.L., Margolis, S., Elfert, G.A., eds. *Nutritional Management, The Johns Hopkins Handbook.* Philadelphia: W.B. Saunders; 1984.
11. Roberts, S., Meyer, B.A., eds. *Lo-Pro Diet Guide.* Indianapolis: Metabolism Clinic, James Whitcomb Riley Hospital for Children; 1987.
12. Schuett, V.E. *Low Protein Food List.* Madison, WI: Metabolic Clinic, Waisman Center on Mental Retardation and Human Development, University of Wisconsin; 1981.
13. Prince, A., Huntington, K.L., Cho-Youn, O.K. *Know-Low-Pro. An Overview of Low Protein Products.* Portland, OR: Child Development and Rehabilitation Center, Oregon Health Sciences University; 1988.
14. Schuett, V.E. *Low Protein Cookery.* Madison, WI: University of Wisconsin Press; 1988.
15. Brusilow, S.W. Arginine, an indispensable amino acid for patients with inborn errors of urea synthesis. *J. Clin. Invest.* 1984; 74:2144.
16. Carey, G.P., Kime, Z., Rogers, Q.R., Morris, J.G., Hargrove, D., Buffington, C.A., Brusilow, S.W. An arginine deficient diet in humans does not evoke hyperammonemia or orotic aciduria. *J. Nutr.* 1987; 117:1734.
17. Brusilow, S.W., Valle, D.L., Batshaw, M.L. New pathways of nitrogen excretion in inborn errors of urea synthesis. *Lancet* 1979; 2:452.
18. Brusilow, S.W., Tinker, J., Batshaw, M.L. Amino acid acylation: a mechanism of nitrogen excretion in inborn errors of urea synthesis. *Science.* 1980; 207:659.
19. Brusilow, S.W. Inborn errors of urea synthesis. In: Lloyd, J.K., Scriver, C.R., eds. *Genetic and Metabolic Diseases in Pediatrics.* Stoneham: Butterworth & Co.; 1985.
20. Munro, H.N. Free amino acid pools. In: *Mammalian Protein Metabolism.* Vol. 4. New York: Academic Press; 1970.
21. Batshaw, M.L., Thomas, G.H., Brusilow, S.W. New approaches to the diagnosis and treatment of inborn errors of urea synthesis. *Pediatrics.* 1981; 68:290.
22. Brusilow, S.W., Danney, M., Waber, L.J., Batshaw, M.L., Burton, B., Levitsky, L., Rothe, K., McKeethren, C., Ward, J. Treatment of episodic hyperammonemia in children with inborn errors of urea synthesis. *N. Engl. J. Med.* 1984; 310:1630.
23. Batshaw, M.L., Brusilow, S.W., Waber, L.J., Blow, W., Brubakk, A.M., Burton, B.K., Cann, H.M., Kerr, D., Mamunes, P., Matalon, R., Myerberg, D., Schafer, I.A. Treatment of inborn of urea synthesis: activation of alternative pathways of waste nitrogen synthesis and excretion. *N. Engl. J. Med.* 1982; 306:1387.
24. Hyman, S.L., Coyle, J.T., Qureshi, I.A., Batshaw, M.L. Sodium benzoate increases free tryptophan in blood and serotonin flux in cortex of OTC deficient spf mice. *Pediatr. Res.* 1987; 21:34A.
25. Blundell, J.E. Serotonin and appetite. *Neuropharmacology.* 1984; 23:1573.
26. O'Connor, J.E., Costell, M., Grisolia, S. The potentiation of ammonia toxicity by sodium benzoate is prevented by L-carnitine. *Biochem. Biophys. Res. Comm.* 1987; 145:817.
27. Batshaw, M.L., Hyman, S.L., Coyle, J.T., Robinson, M.B., Qureshi, I.A., Mellits, E.D., Quaskey, S. Effect of sodium benzoate and sodium phenylacetate on brain serotonin turnover in the OTCD sparse-fur mouse. *Pediatr. Res.* 1988; 23:368.
28. Barshop, B.A., Breuer, J., Holm, J., Nyhan, L. Excretion of hippuric acid during sodium benzoate therapy in patients with hyperglycinaemia or hyperammonaemia. *J. Inher. Metab. Dis.* 1989; 12:72.
29. Ohtani, Y., Ohyanagi, K., Yamamoto, S., Matsuda, I. Secondary carnitine deficiency in hyperammonemia attacks of OTC deficiency. *J. Pediatr.* 1988; 112:409.
30. Stumpf, D., Parker, W.D., Angelini, C. Carnitine deficiency, organic acidemias and Reyes' syndrome. *Neurology.* 1985; 35:1041.
31. Matsuda, I., Ohtani, Y., Ohyanagi, K., Yamamoto, S. Hyperammonemia related to carnitine metabolism with particular emphasis on ornithine transcarbamylase deficiency. *Enzyme.* 1987; 38:251.

32. Michalak, A., Qureshi, I.A. Plasma and urinary levels of carnitine in different experimental models of hyperammonemia
and the effect of sodium benzoate treatment. *Biochem. Med.
Metab. Biol.* 1990; 43:163.

33. O'Connor, J.E., Costell, M., Grisolia, S. Protective effect of
L-carnitine on hyperammonemia, *FEBS.* 1984; 166:331.

34. Rutledge, S.L., Havens, P.L., Haymond, M.W., McLean, R.H.,
Kan, J.S., Brusilow, S.W. Neonatal hemodialysis: effective
therapy for the encephalopathy of inborn errors of metabolism.
J. Pediatr. 1990; 116:125.

35. Ring, E., Zobel, G., Stockler, S. Clearance of toxic metabolites during therapy for inborn errors of metabolism. *J. Pediatr.*
1990; 117:349.

36. Williams, J.C. Diagnosis and acute care of infants and children
with urea cycle disorders. Presented at Current Issues in Nutrition Support of Inherited Metabolic Disorders, June 1–3,
1989; Los Angeles, CA.

37. Hyman, S.L., Porter, C.A., Page, T.J., Iwata, B.A. Kissel,
R., Batshaw, M.L. Behavior management of feeding disturbances in urea cycle and organic disorders. *J. Pediatr.* 1987;
111:558.

38. Hyman, S.L., Coyle, J.T., Park, J.C., Porter, C., Thomas,
G.H., Jankel, W., Batshaw, M.L. Anorexia and altered ser-
otonin metabolism in a patient with orininosuccinic aciduria.
J. Pediatr. 1986; 108:705.

39. Riordan, M.M., Iwata, B.A., Finney, J.W., Wohl, M.K.,
Stanley, A.E. Behavioral assessment and treatment of chronic
food refusal in handicapped children. *J. Appl. Behav. Anal.*
1984; 17:327.

40. Illingsworth, R.S., Lister, J. The critical or sensitive period
with special reference to certain feeding problems in infants
and children. *J. Pediatr.* 1964; 65:839.

41. Blackman, J.A., Nelson, C.L.A. Re-instituting oral feedings
in children fed by gastrostomy tube. *Clin. Pediatr.* 1985; 24:434.

42. Taylor, J.F., Latta, R.S. *Special Diets and Kids.* New York:
Dodd Mead & Co.; 1987.

43. American Academy of Pediatrics Committee on Nutrition.
*Guidelines for the Clinical Evaluation of New Products Used
in the Dietary Management of Infants, Children and Pregnant
Women with Metabolic Disorders. Final Report.* Evanston, IL:
AAP; 1987.

44. American Academy of Pediatrics Committee on Nutrition.
*Monitoring Oral Amino Acids for the Diagnosis and Dietary
Management of Inborn Errors of Amino Acid Metabolism. Fi-
nal Report.* Evanston, IL: AAP; 1979.

45. American Academy of Pediatrics Committee on Nutrition.
Special diets for infants with inborn errors of amino acid metabolism. *Pediatrics.* 1976; 57:783.

46. American Academy of Pediatrics Committee on Nutrition. Nutritional management in hereditary metabolic disease. *Pediatrics.* 1967; 40:289.

47. Ratnaike, R.N., Buttery, J.E., Hoffman, S. Blood ammonia
measurement using a simple reflectometer. *J. Clin. Chem. Bioch.*
1984; 22:105.

48. Abumrad, N., Miller, B. The physiologic and nutritional significance of plasma-free amino acid levels. *JPEN.* 1983; 7:163.

49. Acosta, P.B. Ross metabolic formula system. *Nutrition Support Protocols.* Columbus, OH: Ross Laboratories; 1989.

Chapter 43
Hereditary Fructose Intolerance

Shirley Hack

Hereditary fructose intolerance (HFI) was first described in 1956 by Chambers and Pratt[1] and in 1957 by Froesch et al.[2] Other cases have been reported in the literature since 1978.[3-12] This inborn error of fructose metabolism is inherited as an autosomal-recessive trait with an incidence estimated at approximately 1 in 20,000 in Switzerland.[13] HFI is a distinct disorder from two other inherited abnormalities of fructose metabolism: essential fructosuria and fructose–1,6-diphosphatase deficiency.

Although HFI is not common, it can be treated. Diagnosis is based on medical history, the response to a fructose-free diet, fructose tolerance test, and liver or intestinal mucosal biopsy. Growth and development of the treated infant or child are normal. If untreated, complications and death can occur.

Signs and symptoms at the time of diagnosis depend on the age of the individual, the duration of exposure to fructose, and the amount of fructose ingested. More severe symptoms occur in younger patients who ingest a larger fructose load. Signs and symptoms in HFI are, however, nonspecific and may be either acute or chronic. Nausea, vomiting, abdominal pain, and hypoglycemia are seen after acute ingestion of fructose. Poor feeding with recurrent vomiting, failure to thrive, hepatomegaly, jaundice, and bleeding disorders occur in infants and young children with HFI who continue to receive fructose. Severe liver and renal tubular damage is seen in those patients who go undiagnosed. Increased levels of serum transaminases, hepatomegaly, abdominal distention, ascites, low serum albumin levels, and deficiency of clotting factors result from the liver damage. Renal tubular damage is manifested by proteinuria, aminoaciduria, and acidosis. Patients are free of symptoms when fructose- and sucrose-containing foods/formula are eliminated from the diet. Chronic fructose intoxication can occur in children without symptoms. These patients have hepatomegaly, variable liver dysfunction, abdominal distention, and growth retardation. Tables 43–1 and 43–2 list the clinical and laboratory findings in HFI.

Biochemical Abnormalities and Manifestations

The primary biochemical defect in HFI is deficiency or absence of the enzyme fructose-1-phosphate aldolase B. This aldolase is present in the liver, small intestine, and renal cortex—the main sites of fructose metabolism. The other aldolase enzymes, A and C, are not affected. Aldolase B acts on fructose-1-phosphate and fructose–1,6–diphosphate. Figure 43–1 depicts the pathway for fructose metabolism. Fructose is normally metabolized to glucose and lactic

Table 43–1. Symptoms and Clinical Findings in Hereditary Fructose Intolerance

Acute	Chronic
Nausea	Recurrent vomiting, poor feeding
Vomiting	Failure to thrive
Abdominal pain	Jaundice
Lethargy	Abdominal distention
Sweating	Hepatomegaly
Trembling	Pallor, anemia
Seizures	Hemorrhage
	Edema, ascites
	Aversion to sweet foods
	Lack dental caries
	Growth retardation

acid. The activity of the aldolase enzyme in HFI is absent or reduced (0–15% normal) for fructose-1-phosphate and reduced to a lesser degree for fructose-1,6-diphosphate (10% to 50% normal).[13-17] Aldolase A in muscle and C in brain are available to act on the substrate fructose-1,6-diphosphate. A direct pathway of fructose conversion to glucose that bypasses the aldolase enzyme has been reported.[18]

As a result of the enzyme deficiency in the liver, intestine, and kidney, fructose-1-phosphate cannot be metabolized further and accumulates. This accumulation causes a cellular depletion of phosphorus. This depletion leads in turn to a breakdown of purine nucleotides to uric acid and an increase of serum and urinary uric acid.[19,20] The decrease in ATP probably causes the release of magnesium, with resultant increased serum levels. Energy metabolism and protein synthesis are altered because of the inorganic depletion of phos-

Table 43–2. Laboratory Findings in Untreated Hereditary Fructose Intolerance

	Decreased Levels	Increased Levels
Serum	Glucose	Magnesium
	Phosphorus	Uric acid
	Potassium	Lactic acid (acidosis)
	Protein	Fructose
	Hemoglobin	Transaminases
		Bilirubin
		Prothrombin Time
Urine		Fructose, glucose
		Proteins, amino acids
		Uric acid
		Phosphorus
		Potassium
		Bicarbonate (acidosis)

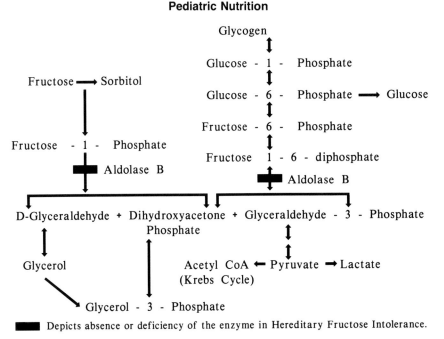

Fig. 43–1. Pathways for fructose metabolism.

phorus and ATP. A decrease in serum potassium is caused by a shift of potassium from the extracellular space. Metabolic acidosis is largely caused by the build-up of lactic acid.[21] Hypoglycemia—present in about 30% of infants and children but often of short duration—results from an inhibition of gluconeogenesis and a breakdown of glycogen.[13] Fructose-1-phosphate and phosphate depletion inhibit glycogen breakdown at the phosphorylase level. Secondary inhibition of fructose–1,6–diphosphate aldolase decreases glucose formation. The depletion of ATP, which is necessary for gluconeogenesis, may also contribute to the hypoglycemia.

Factors to be Considered in Nutritional Evaluation

Diagnosis can be suspected by a careful and detailed nutritional history. Symptoms indicating feeding difficulties begin with the introduction of fructose into the diet—usually by sucrose-containing formula, fruits, fruit juices, and vegetables. With the popularity of breastfeeding, the onset of the disease is often delayed until weaning. Symptoms can also begin if honey or corn syrup is added to a lactose-based cow-milk formula. This practice is not recommended due to the danger of botulism. With time, the infant will begin to refuse fructose-containing foods. By 2 years of age, children have an aversion to sweets and fruits. This distaste for these foods may delay the age of diagnosis to adulthood. Older children are free of dental caries as the causative agents—sweets, fructose, and sucrose—have been removed from the diet. Newbrun et al.[22] reported a dental caries-free incidence of 59% for 17 patients with HFI compared to 0% for 14 control subjects.

Diagnosis can be easily missed in pediatric practice as careful and detailed feeding histories are often not done. Diagnosis of HFI should be strongly suspected if there is

vomiting within 20 to 60 minutes after the intake of fructose-containing foods.[12]

As mortality is high in infancy, prompt diagnosis is important. If the diagnosis is suspected fructose should be removed immediately from the diet. The clinical response to the diet restriction needs to be evaluated as beneficial effects should be evident within days. Recovery of liver and renal dysfunction takes longer. Hepatomegaly may persist for months after initiating the diet. Hemophagocytosis was recently reported in HFI.[23]

An intravenous (IV) fructose tolerance test (FTT) confirms the diagnosis. The challenge should be done after the child has been on a fructose-free diet for several weeks. A dose of 200–300 mg fructose/kg body weight is used for the test.[3,13] Blood phosphorus and glucose levels are measured at 0 minutes and at intervals up to 120 minutes. The administration of fructose produces a decrease in serum phosphorus and glucose levels and a rise in blood lactate, uric acid, fructose, and magnesium levels. The increases in blood lactic and uric acids following the IV FTT in HFI patients are greater than those seen in normal children. There is an increase in the urinary excretion of lactic and uric acids, fructose, and magnesium. Others report fructose-induced hyperuricemia has not been demonstrated in children who receive an IV dose of fructose lower than 500 mg/kg body weight.[24] Urine chromatography can be used to demonstrate aminoaciduria and fructosuria. As the clinical symptoms are also evoked by the FTT, fructose or sorbitol solutions given intravenously to an undiagnosed infant or child, other than for challenge purposes, can be very dangerous and even lethal.[25]

Oral fructose tolerance tests are not recommended as they cause nausea and vomiting, which are not necessarily seen after IV infusion. Furthermore, variable absorption rates of fructose from the gastrointestinal tract affect the reliability of test results.

For definitive diagnosis, measurement of aldolase B activity from the liver or a small intestinal biopsy should be performed. A radioisotope method for enzyme assay is available.[16] Small intestinal mucosal biopsy is being recommended as an alternative to the standard liver biopsy because it is free of some of the complications seen with a liver biopsy. If a liver biopsy is done, fibrosis and fatty changes are also seen. The ratio of fructose-1,6-diphosphate aldolase to fructose-1-phosphate in tissue from liver or intestine is normally 1.0 to 1.5. In patients with HFI this ratio can range from 3 to 11 or greater.[13] Children with liver disease from other causes may have reduced aldolase activity. Mutations in the aldolase B gene have been identified. Diagnosis by direct testing for the presence of these mutations has been suggested as a less invasive test procedure.[26]

Dietary Management

Fructose (also known as levulose, fruit sugar) and sucrose are major sugars in the American diet. The normal intake of fructose for the adult is about 65 g/day. Dietary fructose is derived from free fructose, sucrose, and sorbitol. Fructose is naturally present in honey (20% to 40%), fruits, fruit juices (20% to 40%), vegetables (<1.0% to 2%), and other plant foods.[24] It is often added to foods and medications as a sweetening agent. High fructose corn syrups are being used today in increasing amounts by the food industry as sweetening agents. Crystalline fructose is recommended as an alternative sweetener to sucrose as it is sweeter than table sugar and hence cuts calories. Upon hydrolysis, sucrose, a disaccharide, yields 50% glucose and 50% fructose. Sucrose is found in the diet in the form of sugar, syrups (including those used in medicines), candies, desserts, carbonated beverages, and as a natural ingredient in fruit (<1.0% to 12%), fruit juices, and many vegetables and plants (<1.0% to 6%).[24] The sucrose/fructose content of fruits and vegetables varies depending on the growing conditions. Storage after harvest also affects sugar content. Sucrose is also often added during the manufacture of convenience foods. Invert sugar is derived from the acid hydrolysis of sucrose. Sorbitol, which is converted to fructose in the liver, provides another source of this sugar. Sorbitol is present in fruits, vegetables, and as a sweetener in dietetic foods.

Treatment for HFI consists of a diet containing almost no fructose, sucrose, invert sugar, and sorbitol.[27] Raffinose and stachyose are complex carbohydrates that contain fructose.[27,28] They are found in legumes and in small quantities in grains, nuts, seeds, and vegetables.[28–31] Foods containing them should be eliminated from the diet as it is unknown to what extent, if any, these sugars are hydrolyzed in the digestive tract. The ingredient list on food labels should be checked carefully to avoid foods containing sucrose, fructose, sorbitol, invert sugar, fruits, juices, and other forbidden foods. Tables 43–3 and 43–4 provide a listing of foods to include and exclude on this diet. There are few comprehensive tables listing the sucrose and fructose content of foods.[28–32] The most recent one (1987) is available from the U.S. Government Printing Office.[29] There is only one current discussion of dietary treatment of HFI in the literature.[27]

The diet allows foods from all food groups, although the fruit and vegetable group is severely restricted. When first introduced into the diet of the infant with HFI, solids should consist of strained meats, poultry, and egg yolk. No fruits or juices are allowed; vegetables in the diet are mainly the green leafy kind. Potatoes should be freshly harvested since storage of potatoes converts the starch to sucrose. Meats, poultry, fish, eggs, milk, and cheese provide adequate protein in the diet. Only a few kinds of breads and cereals are allowed. Products containing wheat germ are to be avoided due to the presence of sucrose in this part of the grain. Most baked products contain added sucrose. Cereal grains and flours contain small amounts of sugars. Breakfast cereals without added sugar contain only small amounts of natural free sugar, typical of the flours from which they are derived. As desserts are excluded, allowed sweeteners can be used in the preparation of special desserts for the older child and adolescent. The alternative carbohydrate sources in the diet are glucose, lactose from milk and milk products, and allowed starches. Glucose polymers (Polycose®, Moducal®, and Sumacal®) are available commercially for use in special recipes. The artificial sweeteners Equal®, Sugar Trim®, Sweet One®, Sweet'n Low®—can also be used.

Because the diet is deficient in vitamin C as all good sources of this vitamin are excluded, supplementation with a non-fructose-, non-sucrose-containing product is required. Newbrun et al.[22] reported, however, that their adult subjects with HFI were able to obtain sufficient amounts of vitamin C in their diets. When food records of the subjects were analyzed by computer, 86% of the recommended daily allowance for vitamin C was provided.

If there is acute liver dysfunction a restricted protein intake may be necessary in conjunction with the fructose-free diet. Once liver function returns to normal, protein intake appropriate for age should be given.

There is a lack of agreement about what constitutes optimal diet therapy and particularly about the following issues: foods allowed in the diet, the quantity of fructose intake that is considered safe, and liberalization of the diet in the older child and adolescent. Although small amounts of fructose are allowed, no specific maximum level of intake has been determined. Mock et al.[10] report that no more than 20–40 mg/kg/day should be given in order to prevent growth retardation. According to their research, a fructose intake of 130–160 mg/kg/day can retard growth and alter uric acid metabolism without causing symptoms of nausea, vomiting, or liver/renal dysfunction. Bell and Sherwood[27] recommend an intake of less than 1.5 g/day of fructose. Newbrun et al.,[22] in their dental study, analyzed the diets of HFI patients and control subjects. They found that carbohydrate intake was essentially the same in the two groups. The diets of patients with HFI contained an average of 2.5 g/day of sucrose. No data were given for fructose intake. The strictness of the diet in HFI can be understood by realizing that 1 teaspoon of sugar contains 2.5 grams of fructose. Liberalization of the diet during adolescence can be done by adding a larger variety of vegetables. The effects of any further additions to the diet need to be assessed by clinical symptoms, liver size, and growth patterns.

Sucrose, fructose, and sorbitol are frequently used as binders, diluents, and fillers or as sweetening agents for pediatric oral medications.[33] Physicians and other health

Table 43–3. Sucrose- and Fructose-Free Diet*

Food	Include	Avoid
Milk, milk products	Whole, low-fat, non-fat, acidophilus, buttermilk, evaporated, dry milk; plain yogurt; cream, cream cheese, sour cream, plain cottage cheese, unprocessed cheese	Milk drinks containing sugar, chocolate; vanilla, or fruit yogurt; nondairy liquid creamers; condensed milk; cottage cheese with fruit, some cheese spreads, and processed cheese
Meat, fish, poultry	Plain meat, veal, lamb, pork, organ meats, chicken, turkey, fish, seafood	Sugar-cured meats; some lunch meats and frankfurters; breaded meats and fish using bread made with sugar
Eggs	All	None
Vegetables	Beansprouts, celery, endive, escarole, kale, lettuce, spinach, Swiss chard, greens, shallots, fresh yam (check to make sure it is *not* sweet potato) In small amounts: cucumber, green pepper, radish, summer squash, onion used in recipes only	All others
Potato, substitutes	Fresh harvested white potato, macaroni, noodles, spaghetti, rice, other plain pasta; certain potato chips	Sweet potato, commercial rice, noodle and pasta mixes
Fruits, juices	Avocado, lime juice In small amounts, lemon juice, rhubarb	All others
Breads, cereals	Puffed rice, puffed wheat, shredded wheat, cream of rice; matzo, degermed cornmeal; certain breads, crackers, tortillas, saltines, English muffins, pretzels; rice bran, wheat bran In small amounts: cream of wheat, oats, oatmeal	All cereals, breads and crackers made with sugar or containing wheat germ; tortillas made with sugar
Fats	Butter, margarine, vegetable oil, shortening; salad dressings made without sugar	Commercial salad dressings and mayonnaise
Desserts	Dietetic desserts made without sorbitol or fructose; D-Zerta® low-calorie gelatin dessert	All other desserts, candy
Miscellaneous	Spices and herbs; gravy; homemade soup made with allowed foods; diet soda and sugar-free Kool-Aid® containing allowed sugar substitutes, (aspartame, NutraSweet®, Equal®; saccharin, Sugar Trim®, Sweet One®, Sweet 'n Low®); plain gelatin, distilled white vinegar; cocoa, baking chocolate In small amounts; popcorn	Dried peas and beans; coconut, nuts; seeds; peanut butter; honey, syrups, jam, jelly, sugars, molasses; vanilla flavor; soy flour; ketchup and other commercial sauces; sweet pickles; corn tortilla chips; chewing gum

*Note: As food manufacturers do change the ingredients in their products, an "allowed" product at the present time could become a "not allowed" food item. All labels on food cans and packages must be checked to make sure that *foods to avoid* have not been added.
Portion sizes of "allowed foods" need to be monitored to prevent excessive intake of fructose.

care professionals should therefore check the amount present in any medications that are prescribed. Parents need to be aware of the possible presence of fructose in over-the-counter medications. The contents of these and other products must be checked by a pharmacist.

Folic acid may increase the activity of the glycolytic enzymes, including fructose-1-phosphate aldolase. This vitamin in pharmacological doses has been suggested as a method of treatment in HFI.[34]

Follow-up

Follow-up of the infant or child with HFI is an important part of medical therapy as diet therapy is lifelong. During routine clinic visits, a registered dietitian should assess compliance with the diet. No simple test is available to measure the adequacy of the fructose restriction. Other supplementation, in addition to vitamin C, may be necessary in the diet. By use of computer nutrient analysis, the dietitian can determine any nutrient deficiencies based on analyses of

Table 43—4. Sucrose- and Fructose-Free Diet for Infants*

Food	Include	Avoid
Infant formulas, milk, milk products	Breast milk, Similac®, Enfamil®, SMA®, Pregestimil®, Nutramigen®, Good Start®, Carnation Follow-Up®, Isomil SF®, ProSobee®; whole milk, evaporated milk, plain yogurt	Nursoy®, Soyalac®, Isomil®, Portagen®, Alimentum®; formulas using condensed milk, honey, or Karo® corn syrup
Other fluids	Glucose water	All others
Fruits, juices	None	All
Cereals, breads	In small quantities; dry infant cereals without fruit, cream of rice; saltines, certain breads, crackers	All others
Vegetables	Pureed spinach	All others
Meat, egg yolks	Beef, chicken, turkey, veal, lamb, pork, plain egg yolks	All others; meat, chicken, or turkey sticks
Dinners	None	All
Desserts, other sweets	None except special prepared custards, puddings using glucose as the sweetener	All commercial desserts; honey, syrups, jam, jelly, sugar, molasses; vanilla flavor

*Vitamin C supplement must be provided unless a commercial infant formula is used. Other supplementation may also be necessary. Check food labels for inclusion of any "foods to avoid."

home diet records. Repeat nutrition counseling may be necessary to ensure the appropriate intake of foods and medications. The importance of the diet should be re-emphasized and continued support given to parents and children. Others (schoolteachers, babysitters, or relatives) who care for the infant or child with HFI need to be aware of the diagnosis and the importance of the diet restrictions. Children need to be taught about forbidden foods early in life. As chronic fructose ingestion in children can lead to growth retardation, monitoring of the velocity of growth in length and weight should be done at each clinic visit.

Long-term prognosis is very good for treated infants and children. The intelligence of children is normal. Often, liver and kidney damage can be reversed if the diagnosis is made early and there is strict adherence to the diet.

References

1. Chambers, P.A., Pratt, R.T.C. Idiosyncracy to fructose. *Lancet.* 1956; 2:340.
2. Froesch, E.R., Prader, A., Labhart, A., Stuber, H.W., et al. Die hereditare Fructosein-toleranz, eine bisher nicht bekannte kongenitale Staffwechselstorung. *Schweiz. Med. Wochenschr.* 1957; 87:1168.
3. Odievre, M., Gentil, C., Gautier, M., et al. Hereditary fructose intolerance in childhood. *Am. J. Dis. Child.* 1978; 132:605.
4. Baerlocher, K., Gitzelmann, R., Steinmann, B., et al. Hereditary fructose intolerance in early childhood: a major diagnostic challenge. *Helv. Paediatr. Acta.* 1978; 33:465.
5. Rampa, M., Froesch, E.R. Eleven cases of hereditary fructose intolerance in one Swiss family with a pair of monozygotic and dizygotic twins. *Helv. Paediatr. Acta.* 1981; 36:317.
6. Steinmann, B., Gitzelmann, R. The diagnosis of hereditary fructose intolerance. *Helv. Paediatr. Acta.* 1981; 36:297.
7. Ruecker, A.V., Endres, W., Shin, Y.S., et al. A case of fatal hereditary fructose intolerance. *Helv. Paediatr. Acta.* 1981; 36:599.
8. Cox, T.M., Camilleri, M., O-Donnell, M.W., et al. Pseudo-dominant transmission of fructose intolerance in an adult and three offspring. *N. Engl. J. Med.* 1982; 307:537.
9. Maggiore, G., Borgna-Pignatti, C. Disseminated intravascular coagulation associated with hereditary fructose intolerance. *Am. J. Dis. Child.* 1982; 136:169.
10. Mock, D.M., Perman, J.A., Thaler, M.M., et al. Chronic fructose intoxication after infancy in children with hereditary fructose intolerance. *N. Engl. J. Med.* 1983; 309:764.
11. Menahem, S., Adams, A. Severe acidosis in a neonate with pulmonary valve stenosis: a possible stress inducer of a fatal syndrome of fructose-1,6-biphosphatase and aldolase deficiency. *Acta Paediatr. Scand.* 1989; 78:800.
12. Edstrom, C. Hereditary fructose intolerance in the vomiting infant. *Pediatrics.* 1990; 85:600.
13. Gitzelmann, R., Steinmann, B., Von Den Berghe, G. Essential fructosuria, hereditary fructose intolerance, and fructose-1,6-diphosphatase deficiency. In: Stanbury, J.B., et al., eds. *The Metabolic Basis of Inherited Disease.* 5th ed. New York: McGraw-Hill; 1983.
14. Streb, H., Posselt, H.G., Walter, K., et al. Aldolase activities of the small intestinal mucosa in malabsorption states and hereditary fructose intolerance. *Eur. J. Pediatr.* 1981; 137:5.
15. Cox, T.M., O'Donnell, M.W., Camilleri, M., et al. Isolation and characterization of a mutant liver aldolase in adult hereditary fructose intolerance. *J. Clin. Invest.* 1983; 72:201.
16. Shin, Y.S., Moro, V., Doliwa, H., et al. A radioisotopic method for fructose-1-phosphate adolase assay that facilitates diagnosis of hereditary fructose intolerance. *Clin. Chem.* 1983; 29:1955.
17. Lerner, L., Cooper, M., Gronot, E., et al. Fructose-1-phosphate and fructose-1,6-biphosphate aldolases in the small intestinal mucosa. *Israel J. Med. Sci.* 1987; 23:185.
18. Lapidot, A. Inherited disorders of carbohydrate metabolism in children studied by ^{13}C-labelled precursors, NMR and GC-MS. *J. Inher. Metab. Dis.* 1990; 13:466.

19. Morris, R.C., Jr., Nigon, K., Reed, E.B. Evidence of the severity of depletion of inorganic phosphate determines the severity of the disturbance of adenine nucleotide metabolism in the liver and renal cortex of the fructose-loaded rat. *J. Clin. Invest.* 1978; 61:209.

20. Morris, R.C., Jr., Brewer, E.D., Brater, C. Evidence of a severe phosphate-depletion dependent disturbance of cellular metabolism in patients with hereditary fructose intolerance (HFI). *Clin. Res.* 1980; 28:556A. Abstract.

21. Richardson, R.M., Little, J.A., Patten, R.L., et al. Pathogenesis of acidosis in hereditary fructose intolerance. *Metabolism.* 1979; 28:1137.

22. Newbrun, E., Hoover, C., Mettraux, G., et al. Comparison of dietary habits and dental health of subjects with hereditary fructose intolerance and control subjects. *J. Am. Dent. Assoc.* 1980; 101:619.

23. Mandel, H., Gozal, D., Aizin, A., Tavori, S., Jaffe, M. Haemophagocytosis in hereditary fructose intolerance: a diagnostic dilemma. *J. Inher. Metab. Dis.* 1990; 13:267.

24. Reiser, S., Hallfrisch, J. *Metabolic Effects of Dietary Fructose.* Boca Raton, FL: CRC Press; 1987.

25. Schulte, M.J., Lenz, W. Fatal sorbitol infusion in patient with fructose-sorbitol intolerance. *Lancet.* 1977; 2:188.

26. Dazzo, C., Tolan, D.R. Molecular evidence for compound heterozygosity in hereditary fructose intolerance. *Am. J. Hum. Genet.* 1990; 46:1194.

27. Bell, L., Sherwood, W.G. Current practices and improved recommendations for treating hereditary fructose intolerance. *J. Am. Diet. Assoc.* 1987; 87:721.

28. Lee, C.Y., Shallenberger, R.S., Vittum, M.T. Free sugars in fruits and vegetables. *NY. Food Life Sci. Bull.* 1970; 1:1.

29. Matthews, R.H., Pehrsson, P.R., Farhat-Sabet, M. *Sugar Content of Selected Foods: Individual and Total Sugars.* Washington, DC: US Government Printing Office; 1987. USDA Home Economics Research Report Number 48.

30. Hardinge, M.G., Swarner, J.B., Crooks, H. Carbohydrates in foods. *J. Am. Diet. Assoc.* 1965; 46:197.

31. Southgate, D.T., Paul, A.A., Dean, A.C. et al. Free sugars in foods. *J. Hum. Nutr.* 1978; 32:335.

32. Li, B.W., Schuhmann, P.J. Gas liquid chromatographic analysis of sugars in ready-to-eat breakfast cereals. *J. Food Sci.* 1980; 45:138.

33. Hill, E.M., Flaitz, C.M., Frost, G.R. Sweetener content of common pediatric oral liquid medications. *Am. J. Hosp. Pharm.* 1988; 45:135.

34. Greene, H.L., Stifel, F.B., Herman, R.H. Hereditary fructose intolerance-treatment with pharmacologic doses of folic acid. *Clin. Res.* 1972; 20;275. Abstract.

Chapter 44
Insulin-Dependent Diabetes in Youth

Barbara Mathis Prater

Diabetes mellitus is an international health problem affecting societies at all stages of development. At least 30 million people have this disease, and the number of cases reported are increasing rapidly with the aging of populations, changes in lifestyles, and improvement in diagnostic techniques.[1] It is estimated that over 6 million Americans or 2.5% of the population have diabetes, with an additional 5 million as yet undiagnosed. These figures represent both non-insulin-dependent diabetes mellitus (NIDDM) and insulin-dependent diabetes (IDDM).[2]

Prevalence and Incidence

Limited data concerning the prevalence of IDDM in the United States are available, and research on prevalence has focused on the younger age groups (under 20 years of age). In the school-aged population, about 1 child in 600 has IDDM. This figure represents about 120,000 children under 18 years of age with IDDM in the United States. Thus, IDDM is the third most common chronic illness in children and adolescents.[3] Drash[4] reported that IDDM incidence figures (number of new cases appearing in a 1-year period per 100,000 population) varied from 3.1 in Japan, to 30 in Finland. His figures from Allegheny County, Pennsylvania represent a midpoint incidence rate of 14.6 new cases in children under 19 years of age.[4]

Clinical and Biochemical Abnormalities

Classification and clinical characteristics

IDDM is also known as type I diabetes. Formally called juvenile onset or ketosis-prone diabetes, IDDM has its onset predominantly in childhood. The peak incidence occurs between ages of 6 and 11 years and declines after puberty.[5] It presents with rapid clinical symptoms of polyuria, polydipsia, polyphagia (the three Ps of diabetes), and weight loss.

A predominant number (well over 95%) of children and adolescents developing diabetes mellitus in the Western world have the insulin-dependent form of diabetes resulting from beta cell damage and destruction in the islets of Langerhans. This primary insulin deficiency produces an imbalance resulting in major disturbances of carbohydrate, protein, and lipid metabolism that lead to the predictable and classical symptoms (three Ps of diabetes). Fatigue, visual disturbances, and progression to central nervous system depression, somnolence, and edema may occur if diagnosis is not made and proper therapy instituted.[4] The length of time from onset of symptoms to acute stages is commonly 3 to 4 days, but may be either shorter or up to 2 weeks.

The etiology of IDDM suggests that both genetic and environmental factors are involved in determining the susceptibility to the disease. Destruction of the beta cells resulting in an insulin deficiency is the cause of endogenous insulin deficiency. An exogenous source of insulin must be administered to replace this deficiency.

Components of treatment

Insulin treatment is directed toward correction of the acute and the chronic metabolic disturbance. Goals of that treatment are to bring blood glucose levels into as close a range of normal as possible without producing hypoglycemia. The insulin deficiency leading to hyperglycemia also affects lipid metabolism as it promotes lipid synthesis, thereby preventing excess mobilization from adipose tissue stores. With inadequate insulin secretion, lipid metabolism is increased, and elevation of triglyceride and total cholesterol levels is observed.[4]

Insulin is a synergist with pituitary growth hormone and promotes physical growth by stimulating cell growth and replication. The primary action promotes amino acid movement from extracellular to intracellular space, increased protein synthesis, and decreased protein degradation. It has been reported that linear growth is impaired as a result; however, Drash[4] questions this finding as ambiguous. Several reports indicate that, at the time of diagnosis, children are observed to be tall for their age, and a relationship between excessive growth hormone and insulin deficiency has been speculated. The period of absolute insulin deficiency may have been too short to affect growth adversely. However, impaired growth over a period of months and years is a clinical sign of poor metabolic control.[4]

Replacement of insulin is conventionally accomplished with one or two injections per day, usually with a mixture of short-acting insulin and intermediate-acting insulin at each injection.[6] Toddlers may also require two injections to limit nocturnal hyperglycemia and erratic swings in plasma glucose.[7] Some children may be maintained on a single injection.

Factors to be Considered in Nutritional Evaluation

The major emphasis of the nutritional intake in IDDM in the young is to achieve as near normal glycemia as possible by matching the action of insulin with carbohydrate distribution. In the nondiabetic state, when the child eats, insulin levels rise to match the need. The reverse occurs in IDDM. Therefore, insulin replacement is initiated, and food intake is calculated to attempt this physiological match. An additional dimension—physical activity—further complicates the synergism of insulin to food intake. Careful attention to timing and consistency in food intake can attempt to compensate for these derangements. Carbohydrate distribution and kilocalorie and protein intake need to be individualized for each child. Meal plans and nutritional intake should also be reviewed frequently—at least every 6 months—by the registered dietitian together with the health care team.[8]

Quality assurance nutritional criteria have been written to provide guidelines to the practitioner regarding standards of care and education of the population with IDDM from birth to 18 years of age.[9] The stated goals of nutritional care are to

- Provide optimal nutrition through an individualized meal plan that is modified as needed. The patient and/or caregiver states the rationale and demonstrates understanding of the treatment plan (diet in relation to activity and insulin).
- Promote normal growth and development. Patient maintains weight/height between the 5th and 95th percentiles according to the National Center for Health Statistics (NCHS) growth charts or detailed tables. The patient should not deviate more than one channel from the established pattern of weight/height growth.
- Maintain the best possible glucose control with prevention of glycemic excursions.
- Maintain the best possible lipid profile, which includes cholesterol and triglycerides.

Nutritional controversies

In Nuttall's[10] extensive 1983 review on diet and the individual with diabetes, he reports that the metabolic consequences of various dietary regimens, the composition of a diet that will result in optimum blood/glucose levels, and whether dietary changes significantly delay or prevent long-term complications of diabetes are not yet known. The American Diabetes Association 1984 policy statement on the glycemic effect of carbohydrates supported Nuttall's thesis.[11] Questions relating to the optimal carbohydrate intake, the differences between simple and complex carbohydrates, and the amounts that are acceptable still remain unanswered. Fortunately with the use of monitoring devices, the individual response to food intake can be determined, and glycemic excursions in the child can be better controlled.

The importance of individualized and flexible diets in facilitating dietary adherence has long been acknowledged.[12,13] Crapo stresses the importance of meal planning being a joint venture with the individual and with the family. Nuttall et al.[13] urge individualization of meal plans (diets), with the primary goal being encouragement of a reasonable consistency in the times that meals are eaten and the quantities of food ingested at each meal. If the diet is otherwise nutritionally sound, there can be considerable flexibility in the proportion of food energy that is supplied as carbohydrate acceptable. Severe restriction of carbohydrates no longer is considered either necessary or desirable.

In the past decade, patient management has entered a sphere beyond that of simple survival from ketoacidosis. With the increased longevity of patients and the consequent concern for long-term complications, new emphasis is being placed on limiting fat intake and protein to the recommended daily allowances. Careful attention to sodium intake and increased use of complex carbohydrates have been recommended.[8] Short-term consumption of legumes and low-glycemic index foods by Caucasian diabetics has resulted in improved glycemic control and glucose tolerance.[14] The soluble viscous fibers that are absorbed slowly in the small intestine delay gastric emptying and decrease upper gastrointestinal motility, whereas insoluble fiber, such as found in corn, appears to have little effect on glycemic response.[15]

Because definitive data about the optimum combinations, inclusion, or avoidance of the various macro- and micronutrients are not yet available, Crapo and Vinik[16] urge dietitians not to turn new ideas into dogma but rather to remain open-minded, to stay abreast of new knowledge, to develop the necessary skills to participate in total diabetes care, to try new approaches with their patients, and to experiment with the individual "based upon his or her responses to determine what works best."

Dietary and Nutritional Management

The American Dietetic Association's 1986 position statement on the management of IDDM in youth includes these four goals:

1. Restore normal blood glucose and optimal lipid levels. Maintain blood glucose as near to physiological level as possible to (1) prevent hyperglycemia and/or hypoglycemia and (2) prevent or delay the development of long-term cardiovascular, renal, retinal, and neurological complications associated with diabetes mellitus.
2. Maintain normal growth rate in children and adolescents, as well as attaining and maintaining reasonable body weight in adolescents. Any abnormal or unexplained deviation in growth rate or weight gain and/or loss as plotted on standard grids warrants an assessment of diabetes control, eating behavior, and caloric intake, as well as consideration of alternative problems.
3. Be consistent in the timing of meals and snacks to prevent inordinate swings in blood glucose levels for those using exogenous insulin.
4. Determine a meal plan appropriate for the individual's lifestyle and based upon a diet history of current food intake. Blood glucose monitoring results can then be used to integrate insulin therapy with the usual, as well as unanticipated, eating and exercise pattern.

The practitioner, in developing a specific nutritional care plan, should follow these broad recommendations.

- Calories prescribed to achieve and maintain a desirable body weight
- Carbohydrate should be liberalized, ideally up to 55% to 60% of total calories, and individualized, with the amount dependent on the impact on blood glucose and lipid levels
- Foods containing unrefined carbohydrate with fiber should be substituted for refined carbohydrate
- Modest amounts of refined sugars may be acceptable contingent upon metabolic control (and individual response)
- Protein intakes not to exceed the recommended daily allowance (RDA) for infants, children, and adolescents
- Total fat and cholesterol intake should be restricted. Total fat <30% of total calories; cholesterol <300 mg/day.

Table 44–1. Exchanges for Diabetic Meal Planning

	CHO (g)	PRO (g)	Fat (g)	Calories
Starch-bread*				
Cereals, grains, pasta; lentils, dried beans and peas; starchy vegetables, bread, crackers, snacks without fat	15	3	trace	80
Meat†				
Lean—1 oz	—	7	3	55
Medium Fat—1 oz	—	7	5	75
High Fat—1 oz	—	7	8	100
Vegetables				
1/2 c serving cooked or 1 c raw	5	2	—	25
***Fruit**				
Fresh, frozen, and unsweetened canned fruit; fruit juice and dried fruits	15	—	—	60
Milk				
Skim <1% fat, 1 c serving	12	8	trace	90
Low-fat—2% fat, 1 c serving	12	8	5	120
Whole—3.5% fat, 1 c serving	12	8	8	150
†Fat				
Saturated and unsaturated, including nuts and seeds	—	—	5	45
Free				
Any food or drink that contains less than 20 calories, such as vegetables	—	—	—	20

*Fiber identified if 3 grams or more per serving.
†Sodium identified if 400 mg or more per serving.
From *Exchange Lists for Meal Planning*.[18]

• Alternative sweeteners acceptable in the management of diabetes, but to be used in moderation
• Salt intake limited
• Vitamins and minerals to meet the RDA for age

By using sound principles of nutritional assessment, including appropriate anthropometric measures (at least height and weight), individualization of the meal plan can be achieved. Nutritional intake and food habits before diagnosis can provide the basis for the meal plan and approximate food intake. Successful integration of the change in lifestyle into the patient's routine will produce more adherence. In the life of a child, that integration is essential. Because the challenge of coping with the daily regimen may be overwhelming to the family, as well as the child, an ongoing educational counseling process is essential.

The basis for the successful management of diabetes is education.[4] The individual (if he or she is able to comprehend), the family, and significant others in the environment must have a thorough understanding of the underlying cause of diabetes and its management. An understanding of the role of nutrition, insulin, and physical activity in bringing about the best possible metabolic control is the overall initial goal of this educational process. Specific detailed information and knowledge will flow from this understanding.

1986 exchange lists

The meal plan should divide carbohydrates over the waking hours to match the peaking time of the insulin and the peaks

of physical activity. Although there exist other food grouping systems and methods for teaching nutrition in diabetes to the child and family,[17] the exchange system has been universally accepted in the United States.[18]

In 1950 a joint committee of the American Diabetes/Dietetic Association and the U.S. Public Health Service published the first exchange system for use in teaching diabetic patients about the energy-containing nutrients of foods. The system was in use until 1976 when a revised edition was published. This publication was an outgrowth of the work of the U.S. Commission on Diabetes, which was created to address the scope of the problem of diabetes in the United States. The Commission's report was made to the U.S. Congress in 1976. A decade later, the exchange system was again revised to reflect the latest concepts of nutrition and diabetes,[18,19] thereby enabling more effective nutrition education. The 1986 revision stresses the modification of fat intake, as well as decreasing sodium intake and increasing fiber consumption (Table 44–1). It is assumed to be appropriate for children. The British Dietetic Association also has prepared recommendations related to sucrose and fructose in the diet.[21] The *Exchange Lists for Meal Planning* recommends a variety of approaches to teach the individual effectively.[17] The approach used should be dependent upon the learning needs, abilities, nutritional needs, age, lifestyle, and personal needs of the patient. Individualized education is particularly necessary with the diabetic child.

Research is now being conducted into the prevention of IDDM by dietary means.[22]

Follow-up and Summary

IDDM in the infant, child, and adolescent affects dramatically the everyday life of the family and child. This chronic condition, which will be present for a lifetime, demands daily attention to insulin injection in correct dosage, food intake in appropriate amounts at prescribed times consistent with the insulin peaking time, and fairly predictable activity periods.

Illness and poor metabolic control upset the routine, with additional adaptations and arrangements necessary to prevent diabetic ketoacidosis. If frequent hospitalizations are necessary due to ketoacidosis and illness, the emotional imbalance of the child and family is exacerbated. The maintenance of a metabolic balance is paralleled by the need for psychological balance in relation to the chronic illness and its demands. Loss of metabolic control simply due to the capricious nature of the disease may be experienced. Hypoglycemia is an acute nuisance that can be prevented. IDDM requires special treatment of diabetic gastroparesis and related disorders[23] (see Chapter 34).

The treatment of IDDM children involves a complex interaction of metabolic, physical, psychological, social, environmental, and familial variables. Cerreto and Travis[24] explored these relationships and concluded that well-controlled experimental investigations of various educational and/or psychotherapeutic intervention strategies, utilizing randomized control or single-subject design, will yield cause-and-effect information regarding the efficacy of intervention. In the meantime, assisting the child and family to live fully and adjust and cope as necessary to the impositions of a chronic condition is the goal of care. Anticipating changes in the daily routine will help prevent glycemic excursions.[25] Providing adequate nutrition and maintaining best possible glycemic control without impairing the physical growth and emotional development are shared goals of both the family and health care team members.

References

1. World Health Organization. Expert Committee on Diabetes Mellitus. Geneva: WHO; 1980. Second Report, Technical Series.
2. Harris, M.D. Prevalence of non-insulin-dependent diabetes and impaired glucose tolerance. In: Harris, M., Hamman, R., eds. *Diabetes in America.* Washington, DC: US Government Printing Office; 1985. NIH publication 85-1468.
3. LaPorte, R.E., Tajima, N. Prevalence of insulin-dependent diabetes and impaired glucose tolerance. In: Harris, M., Hamman, R., eds. *Diabetes in America.* Washington, DC: US Government Printing Office; 1985. NIH publication 85-1468.
4. Drash, A.L. Diabetes mellitus in the child and adolescent. *Curr. Probl. Pediatr.* 1986; 16:479.
5. National Diabetes Data Group. Classification and diagnosis of diabetes and other categories of glucose intolerance. *Diab.* 1979; 28:139.
6. Thorp, F.K. Infants and children. In: Powers, M., ed. *Handbook of Diabetes Nutritional Management.* Rockville, MD: Aspen; 1987: 305.
7. Golden, M.P., Russel, B.P., Ingersoll, G.M., Gray, D.L., Hummer, K.M. Management of diabetes mellitus in children younger than 5 years of age. *Am. J. Dis. Child.* 1985; 139:448.
8. American Diabetes Association Position Statement. Nutrition recommendations and principles for individuals with diabetes mellitus, 1986. *Diab. Care.* 1987; 10:126.
9. American Dietetic Association. *Quality Assurance Criteria for Pediatric Nutrition Conditions, Children with Insulin Dependent Diabetes Mellitus.* Chicago: ADA; 1989.
10. Nuttall, F.Q. Diet and the diabetic patient. *Diab. Care.* 1983; 6:197.
11. Policy statement. Glycemic effects of carbohydrates. *Diab. Care.* 1984; 7:607.
12. Crapo, P.A. *Diet and Nutrition in Diabetes: A Statement-of-the-Art Review.* Washington, DC: US Government Printing Office, 1983. US Dept of Health and Human Services, Public Health Service.
13. Nuttall, F.Q., Maryniuk, M.D., Kaufman, M. Individualized diets for diabetic patients. *Ann. Intern. Med.* 1983; 99:204.
14. Jenkins, D., Wolever, T., Buckley, G., Lam, K., Giudici, S., Kalmusky, J., Jenkins, A.L., Patten, R.L., Bird, J., Wong, G.S., Josse, R.G. Low-glycemic-index starchy foods in the diabetic diet. *Am. J. Clin. Nutr.* 1988; 48:248.
15. Brand, J.C., Snow, B.J., Nabhan, G.P., Truswell, A.S. Plasma glucose and insulin responses to traditional Pima Indian meals. *Am. J. Clin. Nutr.* 1990; 51:416.
16. Crapo, P., Vinik, A.I. Nutrition controversies in diabetes management. *J. Am. Diet. Assoc.* 1987; 87:25.
17. Diabetes Care and Education Practice Group. *Meal Planning Approaches in the Nutrition Management of the Person with Diabetes.* Chicago: American Dietetic Association; 1987.
18. American Diabetes Association and American Dietetic Association. *Exchange Lists for Meal Planning.* Arlington, VA: American Diabetes Association; 1986.
19. Franz, M.J., Barr, P., Holler, H., Powers, M.A., Wheeler, M.L., Wylie-Rosett, J. Exchange lists: revised 1986. *J. Am. Diet. Assoc.* 1987; 87:28.
20. Chiarelli, F., Verrotti, A., Tumini, S., Morgese, G. Effects of normal carbohydrate, low fat diet on lipid metabolism in insulin-dependent diabetes mellitus in childhood. *Diab. Nutr. Metab.* 1989; 2:285.
21. Nutrition Subcommittee of the British Diabetic Associations Professional Committee. Sucrose and fructose in the diabetic diet. *Diab. Med.* 1990; 7:764.
22. Riccardi, G., Rivellese, A. Can diabetes mellitus be prevented by diet? *Diab. Nutr. Metab.* 1989; 2:259. Editorial.
23. Nompleggi, D., Bell, S.J., Blackburn, G., Bistrian, B. Overview of gastrointestinal disorders due to diabetes mellitus: emphasis on nutritional support. *JPEN.* 1989; 13:84.
24. Cerreto, M.C., Travis, L.B. Implications of psychological and family factors in the treatment of diabetes. *Pediatr. Clin. North Am.* 1984; 31:689.
25. Connell, J., Thomas-Dobersen, D. Nutritional management of children and adolescents with insulin-dependent diabetes mellitus: a review by the Diabetes Care and Education dietetic practice group. *J. Am. Diet Assoc.* 1991; 91:1556.

Chapter 45
Galactosemia

Elizabeth Wenz

Classical galactosemia is an inherited metabolic disorder with low or absent activity of galactose-1-phosphate uridyl transferase and an elevated galactose-1-phosphate concentration in red blood cells.[1] The disorder is transmitted with an autosomal-recessive mode of inheritance. The incidence in North America is approximately 1 in 60,000 births.

The clinical symptoms are persistent vomiting, jaundice, weight loss, and hepatomegaly within the first few days of life after the infant has ingested breast milk or lactose-containing infant formulas.[2] Later, cataracts, cirrhosis of the liver, and retarded physical and intellectual development occur if the condition is not diagnosed and treated. If untreated, there is a high mortality rate in the affected infants, usually from sepsis.[3] The severity of the clinical picture has been reduced by routine screening of newborn infants or selective screening of sick infants in the first week of life.[4]

Galactose-1-phosphate concentrations in red blood cells are used to measure control of the condition.[2] The galactose-restricted diet is initiated when the galactose-1-phosphate level is 5 mg/dL or greater or in the presence of clinical symptoms, even in variant forms of galactosemia.[5]

Biochemical Abnormalities

The first step in galactose metabolism is the phosphorylation of galactose to galactose-1-phosphate by the enzyme galactokinase. Inactivity of this enzyme results in the accumulation of galactose and galactitol in the body. The second step in the metabolic pathway involves the enzyme galactose-1-phosphate uridyl transferase (transferase), which releases glucose-1-phosphate with the formation of uridine diphosphate galactose (UDP Gal). Inactivity of this enzyme results in a deficiency of uridine diphosphate galactose (UDP Gal) and an accumulation of galactose and galactose-1-phosphate in various tissues of the body (Fig. 45–1).[4] The accumulation of galactose and its metabolites, including galactitol, in the

liver, lens of the eye, brain, and kidney is the source of the serious clinical problems of untreated galactosemia.[6,7]

Gonadal dysfunction in girls with galactosemia is one of the late-onset complications of classical galactosemia.[8,9] Reproductive function in women with galactosemia is impaired; only 2 of the 26 women who were studied had normal ovarian function.[10] Two possible explanations are that accumulation of galactose-1-phosphate damages the ovary or that there is inadequate production of uridine diphosphate galactose (UDP Gal), the nucleotide sugar required for galactolipid, galactoprotein, and mucopolysaccharide synthesis.[11]

Variants of classical galactosemia have been identified by confirmation of the presumptive positive tests from newborn screening.[12,13] Patients with these variants who have even minimal transferase activity and have normal UDP Gal may have normal gonadal function.[11]

The classification of the forms of galactosemia according to the percentage of normal enzyme activity is shown in Table 45–1.

Factors to be Considered in Nutritional Evaluation

The treatment of galactosemia involves the restriction of dietary galactose to achieve and maintain blood galactose-1-phosphate in the acceptable range—1 to 4 mg/dL. Many of the clinical symptoms are resolved after a few weeks of dietary treatment. Lactose and galactose are the offending carbohydrates that must be eliminated. Milk and milk products, the principal dietary sources of lactose, therefore must be omitted from the infant's diet. The restriction of lactose is maintained throughout life.[2]

Incidental sources of lactose are found in ingredients in prepared foods and fillers (inert or excipient ingredients) in medicines and nutritional supplements. The manufacturers of foods should be contacted if the label information is unclear, and pharmaceutical companies should be contacted by a member of the health care team before the medication

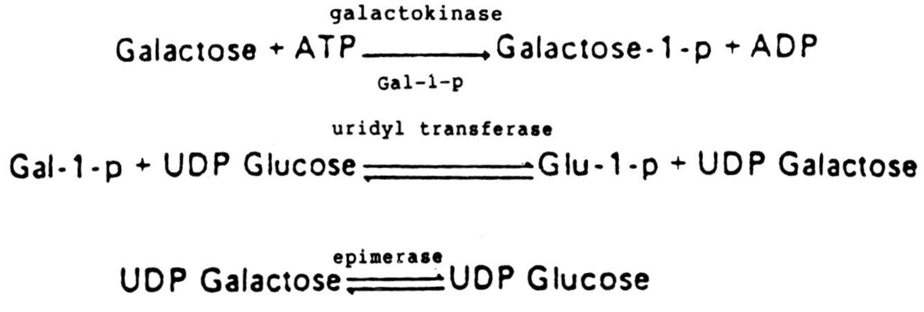

$$\text{Galactose} + \text{ATP} \xrightarrow{\text{galactokinase}} \text{Galactose-1-p} + \text{ADP}$$
Gal-1-p

$$\text{Gal-1-p} + \text{UDP Glucose} \underset{\text{uridyl transferase}}{\rightleftharpoons} \text{Glu-1-p} + \text{UDP Galactose}$$

$$\text{UDP Galactose} \underset{\text{epimerase}}{\rightleftharpoons} \text{UDP Glucose}$$

Fig. 45–1. The Leloir pathway of galactose metabolism.

Table 45–1. Percentage of Gal-1-P Transferase Activity

Type of Galactosemia	Designated Code	% of Normal Activity
Classical galactosemia		
Unaffected	NN	100
Carrier	GN	50
Homozygote	GG	0
Duarte variant/normal	DN	75
Duarte variant (homozygote)	DD	50
Duarte/galactosemia (double heterozygote)	DG	25

Adapted from Ng, W.G., Bergren, W.R., Donnell, G.N. A new variant of galactose-1-phosphate uridyltransferase in man. *Ann. Hum. Genet.* 1973; 37:1.

is prescribed. There are several references to help identify these substances so they can be eliminated.[14–19] In addition, some galactose is produced from glucose in a series of reversible reactions[20] (Fig. 45–1).

The content of complex carbohydrates, raffinose, and stachyose of foods is listed in the publication, *Sugar Content of Selected Foods*.[21] Although galactose has been isolated from these complex carbohydrates, there are no internal enzymes, alpha-galactosidases, to release galactose in human digestion. There is no clinical evidence that galactose-1-phosphate concentration in the blood of individuals with galactosemia increases after these complex carbohydrates are consumed.

Dietary Management

Adequacy of the diet

The diet can be adequate in all nutrients if soy protein isolate formula with added methionine is consumed as prescribed. In addition, the intake of calories should support an acceptable rate of growth. A ratio of protein to calories of 1.7 g protein to 100 calories, adjusted for protein quality,[22,23] is recommended.

Carnitine can be synthesized from lysine and methionine, but newborn infants lack that ability. Therefore, infants fed soy protein isolate formula without carnitine supplementation have low blood carnitine values and elevated plasma triglycerides and free fatty acid concentrations.[24] Carnitine has been added to infant soy formulas to improve metabolism of fatty acids for energy.[25,26]

Taurine can be synthesized from methionine, but is thought to be essential in the diet of newborn infants. It is present in human milk and is added to infant formulas.[25,26] Zinc may be deficient, as demonstrated by low serum zinc concentrations, despite adequate dietary intake due to residual phytate in soy protein.[27,28]

Analyses of diet records of formula and foods consumed by infants and children with galactosemia have been done by computer software.[29] These diet analyses are compared to the child's rate of growth, laboratory assessments of nutritional status, and the erythrocyte galactose-1-phosphate concentration. Comparison with the recommended dietary allowance for age indicated inadequate intakes of essential minerals, such as calcium, phosphorus, zinc, and magne-

sium, when insufficient amounts of food sources are consumed. Supplementation of minerals will contribute to nutrient needs if taken in a form that is well utilized by the body.

The galactose-restricted diet includes most protein-rich foods (other than milk or milk products), fruits, vegetables, grains, fats, and sugars (Table 45–2).

Food labels

The ingredient lists of labels of all processed foods must be read carefully for the presence of milk and milk products, such as dry milk solids, lactose, curds, or whey. These ingredients *must be avoided*. Labels do not specify the amounts of each ingredient, although food ingredients are given in descending order by weight.

The ingestion of casein as an incidental ingredient and caseinates *must be limited* because they are classified as milk proteins and contain approximately 0.4 to 1.2% lactose; therefore they contain some galactose.[16,30] If many foods or large amounts of any food that contain casein or caseinate are eaten, they may contribute significant amounts of galactose. The term, "hydrolyzed protein" can be used in place of the term "casein" on food labels.

Incidental inclusion of casein and whey may occur when milk-free products are produced in dairy-processing plants. Sodium caseinate may also be used and labeled only as "natural flavoring."[31]

Current guidelines for ingredient labeling now state that some foods containing food additives which are animal or plant derived must be labeled. Not all foods are regulated by the same government agency.[32] Careful reading of labels or contacting the manufacturer will prevent these accidental breaks in diet control. Alpha-lactalbumin and beta-lactoglobulin are two of the proteins in whey that may contain residual lactose. Most of the lactose in milk is contained in the whey portion, so these proteins may need to be limited.

Ripened cheeses contain 0.4 to 2 g lactose/100 g product[33] so quantities must be limited if allowed by the health care team and the galactose-1-phosphate concentrations are routinely monitored.

Vegetable gums are *permitted* because they do not contain free galactose and do not release galactose within the digestive system of humans. They are agar, acacia, gum arabic, carrageenan, locust bean gum (carob), guar gum, and tragacanth.[34]

The following products may be used because they do not contain lactose: lactate, lactic acid, lactylates, calcium compounds, and the animal fats, lard and suet. References are available that define the ingredients and give their function in foods; these are helpful to nutritionists and parents of children with galactosemia.[14–17]

Kosher designation of foods by symbols or such words as kosher, pareve, or parve can guide nutritionists and parents in selecting foods that are milk free. The designation is voluntary and is provided by the rabbinical organization at the expense of the manufacturer. Careful reading of labels is recommended, however, since manufacturing procedures vary in terms of the inclusion of milk and milk products in foods. Although the absence of the letter "D" (dairy) does not mean the food is milk-free, its presence does indicate reliably either that the food contains a dairy product or that

Table 45–2. The Galactose-Restricted Diet

Foods Permitted	Foods Not Permitted
Milk substitutes Soy milks fortified with methionine: Isomil, Prosobee, Nursoy, L-Soyalac Casein hydrolysates without added lactose: Nutramigen Nondairy cream substitutes made from soy protein	**Milk and milk products** Human milk All animal milks and milk products: buttermilk, cream, sour cream, yogurt, ice cream, ice milk, sherbet, butter, cheese, cottage cheese, cream cheese Casein, milk solids, lactose, whey, milk fat
Protein foods Plain meat, fish, poultry—without milk products All-meat frankfurters, sausage, cold cuts Eggs—without milk or milk products Nuts, nut butters Legumes (dried beans and peas)—kidney, pinto, navy etc.	**Protein foods** Organ meat: brains Seafood: mussels Processed meats with added milk products Fermented soy sauce, or soybean products in which enzyme processing is used
Fruits and vegetables Any fruits—fresh, frozen, canned, dried—unless processing with lactose or milk products Any vegetables—fresh, frozen, canned, dried—unless processed with lactose or milk products	**Fruits and vegetables** Fruits with milk, cream, or any milk products Vegetables with milk, cream, or any milk products
Grains and breads* Cooked and dry cereals without milk, lactose, or milk products added Breads, rolls, buns—without milk, milk products, or lactose added Crackers, Saltines, biscuits, cookies without lactose or other milk products added Flour or corn tortillas without milk or milk products Macaroni, noodles, spaghetti, rice	**Grains and breads*** Dry cereals with added whey, casein, or milk products Breads, rolls, buns, cakes, cookies, or any baked products with added milk or milk products
Fats† All vegetable oils—soybean, corn, olive, cottonseed, safflower, peanut, canola Margarine without milk or milk products Vegetable shortening, lard, suet	**Fats†** Butter, cream, sour cream, milk fat Margarines† with added milk or milk products
Miscellaneous Clear candies, gum drops, marshmallows, gum, fruit pectins Chocolate: dark, bitter, semi-sweet, cocoa, cocoa "butter" Sugar, corn syrup, molasses, honey; plain carob	**Miscellaneous** Milk chocolate, white "chocolate," caramels, carob with added milk—any with milk or lactose Cocoa mixes or syrups with milk products

*Prepare list of brand name of breads and baked goods in each geographic area if ingredient content on labels is incomplete.
†Prepare list of brand names of margarines in each geographic area if ingredient content on labels is incomplete.
From Children's Hospital of Los Angeles. Used with permission.

equipment had been used for a milk-containing food even though the food does not contain milk.

There is a need for consistent label information so consumers can interpret ingredient information and select appropriate foods.[35] Even though there are FDA standards of identity of foods,[17] approximately 18% of standardized foods do not have ingredient labels.[35] More accurate food labeling has been the subject of several recent articles.[36–38]

Diet during pregnancy

The woman who has galactosemia should remain on the galactose-restricted diet during pregnancy. Her infant will not be at risk for galactosemia unless the father has galactosemia or is a carrier for the galactosemia trait.[4] Known heterozygotes for galactosemia should be on a diet restricted in lactose and galactose during pregnancy and ideally before conception. During gestation, there is evidence that galac-tose and its metabolites, specifically galactitol, accumulate in affected fetuses. The elevated metabolites in amniotic fluid are evidence of this accumulation, which is thought to cause prenatal damage.[39] Cataract formation occurs in the lens of the eyes of the fetus. The affected newborn of an untreated pregnancy has elevated galactose-1-phosphate in cord blood due to the maternal ingestion of galactose and probably metabolites of galactose-containing compounds.[4,20,40] Even when the mother's diet is restricted during pregnancy, the cord blood Gal-1-P is elevated, but at a lower level than if the diet during pregnancy is unrestricted.[41]

Because the diet during pregnancy is restricted in milk and milk products, women need to be counseled regarding the nutrients that might be deficient when milk and milk products are omitted. The diet should be evaluated for nutritional adequacy during pregnancy, especially the status of such minerals as calcium, phosphorus, magnesium, and zinc. Mineral needs during pregnancy are described by Worthington-Roberts and Williams.[42]

Table 45–3. The Galactose-Restricted Diet: A Daily Guide for Children

Milk group	Protein group	Grains group
USE	USE	USE
24–32 oz (infants and adolescents)	4–6 cooked oz of meat, fish, poultry	4 servings (½ cup or 1 slice)
16–24 oz (young children)	Eggs, nuts, legumes (peas and beans)	Rice, oats, wheat, rye, corn, barley—in breads or cereals
Soy milk fortified with methionine	Peanut and other nut butters	
Casein hydrolysate without added lactose	Soybeans and soy products	
DO NOT USE	DO NOT USE	DO NOT USE
Cow's milk; any animal milks	Mussels (seafood)	Any made with milk or milk products
Butter, cream, milk fat	Brains (organ meat)	
Casein (hydrolyzed milk protein)	Creamed foods with sauce using milk, butter, cream	
Cheeses, fresh or aged	Fermented soy products	
Lactose		

Vegetable fruit group	Fats	Sugars
USE	USE	USE
4 servings (½ cup or 1 piece)	Recommended at least 1 Tbsp or as needed for calories	As needed for extra Calories
One citrus each day	Oil, shortening, lard	Sucrose (table sugar)
One deep green or yellow fruit or vegetable each day, as raw, cooked, dried or frozen	Milk-free margarines	Glucose, honey, syrup, molasses, sorghum
	Milk-free salad dressings	
DO NOT USE	DO NOT USE	DO NOT USE
Sauces with milk, butter, cream, or margarine with milk	Butter, cream, milk fat	Lactose
	Margarines with milk	
	Cream or cheese salad dressings	

From Children's Hospital of Los Angeles. Used with permission.

Follow-up and Standards of Care

The care of the child with galactosemia includes a complete assessment and monitoring at least every 6 months. Clinic visits may be more frequent for the young infant and less frequent for the older individual.

The periodic evaluation should include physical examination with palpation of the liver; growth measurements—height for age with percentiles of standards, weight for age with percentiles, weight for height; and head circumference until 3 years of age (other growth measurement continue indefinitely); and laboratory assessment of galactose-1-phosphate at each visit. An ophthamologic examination, including a slit-lamp examination for cataracts, is recommended each year. Psychological assessments and speech evaluations are part of good follow-up care. Written diet intake records should be obtained at every clinic visit to enable assessment of possible lactose ingestion and adequacy of all nutrients, including calories and minerals.

Clinical team

In addition to the health care professionals who perform and interpret the assessments described above, the parents of the child are important members of the treatment team. They are most responsible for management of the child's treatment as they interpret the guidelines from the health care providers. The interaction among team members and parents should provide education, motivation, and support when needed.

The nutritionist counsels the family members at each clinic visit, thereby providing ongoing education of the parents. He or she might need to obtain information on newly developed foods or to prepare recipes or to manage diet-related behavior problems. When instructing parents, the use of key words for milk products is important; for example, parents may not recognize that whey and casein are milk products.[43]

When the child begins school, meals away from home are planned to maintain the galactose-restricted diet. Taking lunch and snacks to school makes this planning easier at first. As the child gets older, choosing from the school lunch menus can be allowed when the schedule of meals and ingredients in all foods are known in advance. Tables 45–2 and 45–3 can serve as guides in selecting appropriate amounts of foods.

To help school personnel understand the galactose-restricted diet, parents can meet with the teacher before the school term begins to explain the diet limitations to everyone who will supervise the child. "A Teacher's Guide to Galactosemia"[44] is useful and gives creative activities for children in school.

In summary, early identification and treatment of galactosemia with the galactose-restricted diet continue to be the goals in managing this inherited metabolic disorder. The clinical team members work together with the parents to enhance the growth, intellectual performance, and nutritional status of the child with galactosemia.

References

1. Koch, R., Donnell, G.N., Fishler, K., Ng, W.G., Wenz, E. Galactosemia. In: Kelly, V.C., ed. *Practice of Pediatrics*. Philadelphia: Harper and Row; 1982.
2. Donnell, G.N., Koch, R., Fishler, K., Ng, W.G. Clinical aspects of galactosemia. In: Burman, D., Holton, J.B., Pennock, C.A., eds. *Inherited Disorders of Carbohydrate Metabolism*. Lancaster: MTP; 1980.
3. Levy, H.L., Sepe, S.J., Shih, V.E., Vawter, G.F., Klein, J.O. Sepsis due to E. Coli in neonates with galactosemia. *N. Engl. J. Med.* 1977; 297:823.
4. Komrower, G.M. Galactosemia—thirty years on. The experience of a generation. *J. Inher. Metab. Dis.* 1982; 5:96.
5. Treatment policy. Los Angeles: Childrens Hospital, 1987.
6. Schwarz, H.P., Zuppinger, K.A., Zimmerman, A., Dauwalder, H., Scherz, R., Bier, D.M. Galactose intolerance in individuals with double heterozygosity for Duarte variant and galactosemia. *J. Pediatr.* 1982; 100:704.
7. Schwarz, H.P., Schaefer, T., Bachmann, C. Galactose and galactitol in urine of children with compound heterozygosity for Duarte variant and classical galactosemia after an oral glucose load. *Clin. Chem.* 1985; 31:420.
8. Kaufman, F.R., Kogut, M.D., Donnell, G.M., Goebelsmann, U., March, C., Koch, R. Hypergonadotrophic hypogonadism in female patients with galactosemia. *N. Engl. J. Med.* 1981; 304:994.
9. Cramer, D.W., Harlow, B.L., Barbieri, R.L., Ng, W.G. Galactose-1-phosphate uridyl transferase activity associated with age at menopause and reproductive history. *Fertil. Steril.* 1989; 51:609.
10. Kaufman, F.R., Donnell, G.N., Roe, T.E., Kogut, M.D. Gonadal function in patients with galactosemia. *J. Inher. Metab. Dis.* 1986; 9:140.
11. Kaufman, F.R., Xu, Y.K., Ng, W.G., Donnell, G.N. Correlation of ovarian function with galactose-1-phosphate uridyl transferase levels in galactosemia. *J. Pediatr.* 1988; 112:754.
12. Ng, W.G., Kline, F., Lin, J., Koch, R., Donnell, G.N. Biochemical studies of a human low-activity galactose-1-phosphate uridyl transferase variant. *J. Inher. Metab. Dis.* 1978; 1:145.
13. Lee, J.E.S., Ng, W.G. Semi-micro techniques for the genotyping of galactokinase and galactose-1-phosphate uridyl transferase. *Clin. Chim. Acta.* 1982; 124:351.
14. Igoe, R.S., ed. *Dictionary of Food Ingredients*. 2nd ed. New York: Van Nostrand Reinhold; 1989.
15. Lewis, R.J., ed. *Food Additives Handbook*. New York: Van Nostrand Reinhold; 1989.
16. National Research Council. *Food Chemicals Codex*, 1981 and Supplements 1983 and 1986. Washington, DC: National Academy of Sciences; 1981, 1983, 1986.
17. *Code of Federal Regulations, Food and Drugs*, 21, parts 100–169 and 70–199. Washington, DC: U.S. Government Printing Office; 1988.
18. American Academy of Pediatrics Committee on Drugs. 'Inactive' ingredients in pharmaceutical products. *Pediatrics.* 1985; 76:635.
19. *Physician's Desk Reference and Physician's Desk Reference for Non-Prescription Drugs*. Oradell, New Jersey: Medical Economics; 1989.
20. Sardharwalla, L.B., Wraith, J.E. Galactosemia. *Nutr. Health.* 1987; 5:175.
21. Matthews, R.H., Pehrsson, P.R., Farhat-Sabet, M. *Sugar Content of Selected Foods*. Home Economics Research Report #48, Human Nutrition Information Service. Washington, DC: United States Department of Agriculture; 1987.
22. Beaton, G.H., Chery, A. Protein requirements of infants: a re-examination of concepts and approaches. *Am. J. Clin. Nutr.* 1988; 48:1403.
23. World Health Organization. *Energy and Protein Requirements*. Technical Report Series 724. Geneva: World Health Organization; 1985.
24. Olson, A.L., Nelson, S.E., Rebouche, C.J. Low carnitine intake and altered lipid metabolism in infants. *Am. J. Clin. Nutr.* 1989; 49:624.
25. *Ross Laboratories Product Handbook* G-124. Columbus, OH: Ross Laboratories; 1990.
26. *Mead Johnson Nutritionals Pediatric Product Handbook* L B 6 3–90. Evansville, IN: Mead Johnson/Bristol Myers; 1990.
27. Chan, G.M., Leeper, L., Book, L.S. Effects of soy formulas on mineral metabolism in term infants. *Am. J. Dis. Child.* 1987; 141:527.
28. Sandstrom, B., Cederblad, A., Lonnerdal, B. Zinc absorption from human milk, cow's milk and infant formulas. *Am. J. Dis. Child.* 1987; 141:527.
29. Kennedy, B., Anderson, K. *Amino Acid Analyzer Software*. Tallahassee, Nutrition Management Systems, 1987.
30. McBean, L.D. Food sensitivity and dairy products. *Dairy Council Digest.* 1989; 60:25.
31. Gern, J.E., Yang, E., Evrard, H.M., Sampson, H.A. Allergic reactions to milk–containing "nondairy products." *N. Engl. J. Med.* 1991; 324:976.
32. *Fed. Register* 1990; 55:7289, 9 CFR Parts 317 and 381.
33. Scrimshaw, N.S., Murray, E.B. The acceptance of milk and milk products in populations with a high prevalence of lactose intolerance. *Am. J. Clin. Nutr.* 1988; 48(S4):1083.
34. Bott, D.E., Hopley, P.J., Leach, R.H. Suspending agents in medications as possible sources of galactose to galactosemic child. *Arch. Dis. Child.* 1970; 45:436.
35. Kessler, D.A. The federal regulation of food labeling. *N. Engl. J. Med.* 1989; 321:717.
36. Little, L.V. Nutrition legislative update. *Nutr. Today.* 1989; 24:31.
37. Tillotson, J.E. The controversy over health claims on labels. *Food Tech.* 1988; 42:106.
38. Levine, A.S., Labuza, T.P., Morley, J.E. Food technology: a primer for physicians. *N. Engl. J. Med.* 1985; 312:628.
39. Allen, J.T., Gillett, M., Holton, J.B., King, G.S., Pettit, B.R. Evidence of galactosemia in utero. *Lancet.* 1980; 1:603.
40. Gitzelmann, R., Steinmann, B. Galactosemia: how does long term treatment change the outcome? *Enzyme.* 1984; 32:37.
41. Irons, M., Levy, H.L., Puschel, S., Castree, K. Accumulation of galactose-1-phosphate in the galactosemic fetus despite maternal milk avoidance. *J. Pediatr.* 1985; 107:261.
42. Worthington-Roberts, B., Williams, S.R. *Nutrition in Pregnancy and Lactation*. 4th ed. St. Louis: Times Mirror/Mosby College; 1989.
43. Leinhas, J.L. Food allergy challenges: guidelines and implications. *J. Am. Diet. Assoc.* 1987; 87:604.
44. Nardella, M. *A Teacher's Guide to Galactosemia*. Pheonix: Department of Health Services; 1986.

Chapter 46
Lactose Intolerance

Elizabeth Wenz

As a result of studies carried out within the last 10 years, lactose intolerance has been redefined and treatments for this carbohydrate disorder have been revised. Other commonly used names for the disorder are low lactase activity, lactase deficiency, lactase nonpersistence, and lactose sensitivity.[1,2] These terms refer to the gradual decrease in lactase activity that occurs in older children and adults in many populations. The term "lactose maldigestion" is preferred to lactose malabsorption, since lactose is split into galactose and glucose, rather than being absorbed as the disaccharide.[2,3]

The symptoms of lactose intolerance are rapid onset of nausea, bloating, flatulence, abdominal cramps, watery acidic stools, and, subsequently, dehydration. These symptoms can occur within 15 minutes to 2 hours after the consumption of lactose-containing foods.

Biochemical Abnormalities

Metabolism of lactose

Lactose is hydrolyzed to glucose and galactose in the brush border cells of the villi in the small intestine by the enzyme lactase, a beta-galactosidase.[4-6] Glucose and galactose are absorbed into the bloodstream by a common active transport system, and the galactose is then converted into glucose by the liver.

Lactase activity

Activity of intestinal lactase increases from the third month of fetal life to its peak, which occurs late in fetal life. Lactase decreases during infancy in most mammals and some humans. Studies indicate that 5% to 15% of Caucasian adults and 60% to 70% of non-Caucasian adults show low levels of lactase activity.[2,6] The decrease of lactase activity, which appears more frequently in certain racial groups, occurs rather early in children—from ages 1 to 5 years. It can be assumed that these individuals tolerated lactose in the first years of life, although in some exceptional cases, lactose sensitivity had already developed by 6 months of age.[2,3]

Congenital low lactase activity

This condition is extremely rare. Affected infants have deficient intestinal lactase activity from birth, and the enzyme defect lasts throughout life. Diarrhea is the main symptom, although severe vomiting and cramping may also occur. If the diarrhea persists, with subsequent loss of fluid, electrolytes, and lactose, malnutrition and failure to thrive can result.[5]

Primary low lactase activity

Primary lactase deficiency is a result of a genetically inherited decrease in lactase activity and is age related. Intestinal infections can exacerbate the clinical symptoms. Lactose-sensitive children with giardiasis were less tolerant of milk, suggesting that this condition may aggravate lactose sensitivity, since recurrent infections were common.[7]

The majority of adults, except for those of Northern European origin, have decreased tolerance for lactose in large amounts. Therefore, the condition is also described as lactase nonpersistence.[2,3]

In older adults, lactase production decreases, and lactose intolerance may present as gasiness and diarrhea. This condition can be more serious in frail elderly persons as all organs are compromised and because of the sudden loss of blood pressure associated with dehydration through colonic fluid loss.[1]

Secondary lactase deficiency

This condition occurs after prolonged illness, intestinal infections, diarrhea, or chronic malnutrition. It can also be caused by medications that alter the brush border cells of the gastrointestinal tract. The damage to the absorptive area in the small intestines may be transitory, and the intake of lactose as infant formulas or cow's milk can usually be resumed within 6 weeks.[8] Soy-based formulas or enteral products based on caseinate should be used to maintain nutritional adequacy. The nutrient content of these foods is described in product information from the manufacturer or on the product label.[9,10]

Factors to be Considered in Nutritional Evaluation

A diagnosis of low lactase activity requires a nutrition history and food intake record. Information on the amount of milk consumed, plain or flavored, taken alone or with other foods, and at what temperature will help interpret the clinical symptoms.[2,11]

The onset of symptoms and their severity in relation to the amount of milk consumed should be documented. The characteristics, volume, and frequency of the stools should be noted, as well as how soon they occur after the ingestion of milk.[5] Clinical symptoms can be a reliable measure of tolerance for lactose and can be helpful in the interpretation of laboratory tests.

Although there are commonly used screening tests for the diagnosis of lactose sensitivity, the breath hydrogen test has been used most often in recent years.[3,12] It is noninvasive and less painful than biopsy of the intestinal mucosa.[2,3] A baseline value is obtained from a fasting sample of expired air. After the administration of lactose, samples of breath are taken at intervals. An increase in breath hydrogen of greater than 10–20 ppm above the baseline value is considered abnormal and indicative of fermentation of nonabsorbed carbohydrate.[6,13]

Lactose loading studies indirectly measure the amount of lactase activity by measuring blood glucose. The lactose load is much greater than the normal intake of milk. It is comparable to an adult consuming 1 to 1.5 liters of milk in a short period of time.[6,14]

Dietary Management

Objectives of dietary management

The goal of nutritional management is the same as for all infants and older individuals: achieving adequacy of all major nutrients. Since milk and milk products provide well-utilized sources of calcium, phosphorus, protein, riboflavin, niacin, and vitamins A and D, other acceptable sources of these nutrients must be supplied when milk is omitted. Soy milk or casein hydrolysate-based products should be used in place of milk. In secondary lactose intolerance, aged cheeses are often tolerated.

Tolerance of milk products

In the manufacture of cheeses, whey is separated from casein, which removes most of the lactose. As they age, cheeses continue to decrease in lactose content, unless fresh milk is added to the finished product. The aged cheeses that have been analyzed contain 0.4% to 2% of lactose and are good sources of most of the nutrients in milk.[2,12,15]

Lactose-sensitive older children and adults can often tolerate some milk and milk products when they are offered in small amounts and with other foods.[16,17,18] Yogurt and fermented milk products are better tolerated in well-controlled studies.[19] Although yogurt contains lactose in laboratory analyses, the active yogurt cultures are beta-galactosidases and continue to function in the gastrointestinal tract. This is described as "auto-digestion" of yogurt, which can be as effective as lactose supplements.[20,21] The use of hydrolyzed-lactose milk or lactase tablets is also effective in reducing clinical symptoms in lactose-sensitive individuals.[22–24]

In a study of Gabonese children aged 5 to 14 years, the use of a spray-dried fermented milk, reconstituted as a formula, was better tolerated than was regular milk. The excretion of breath hydrogen was lower, and there was a decrease in clinical manifestations, such as flatulence. Because the dried fermented milk is more easily stored and utilized than fresh yogurt, it can be considered for feeding programs in countries where a high percentage of the population is lactase nonpersistent.[25]

Chocolate milk and cocoa appear to be better tolerated than plain milk, as seen by the reduction of the symptoms of lactose intolerance and breath hydrogen excretion in adults. One possible explanation is that the transit time of digestion is slower with chocolate milk than plain milk.[26]

When milk is reintroduced, whole fat milk is less likely to cause a return of the clinical symptoms than nonfat milk or low-fat milk. This is partially explained by the slower transit of fat through the intestinal tract.[2]

Lactose-restricted diet

Food labels. Labels of all processed foods include ingredients in descending order of quantity unless there is a FDA Standard of Identity.[27] Approximately 18% of these standardized foods do not have ingredient labels.[28]

Since ingredients in foods change frequently, all foods must be evaluated for their content of milk or milk products and labels should be reviewed before the food is consumed. Certain "key words" indicate the presence of milk in foods. Any product that contains *milk, dry milk solids, cream, lactose, or whey* should be avoided (Table 46–1). Other derivatives of these substances should be listed in educational materials for patient use.[29]

Imitation or substitute milks are defined as engineered foods that differ from the FDA Standards of Identity.[30] The lactose content is usually not reduced.[30] In addition, the nutritional content of these foods may not be equivalent to the foods they imitate.[30]

The use of casein and caseinates may need to be limited since they are derived from milk protein. The term "hydrolyzed protein" can be used in place of casein on food labels. These products typically contain less than 1% lactose, but may contain as much as 2%.[31] Their lactose content must be considered if many foods containing casein are consumed. Alpha-lactalbumin and beta-lactoglobulin are two whey proteins that may contain larger amounts of residual lactose.[32]

The following products *may be used* because they do not contain lactose: lactate, lactic acid, lactylates, suet and lard.

Food products that may contain lactose include the following:

- creamed foods, breaded foods, gravies, cream soups, chowders
- frozen breaded meats and fish or vegetable-meat casseroles
- meat, poultry, and fish entrees in fast-food restaurants
- prepared meats, such as sausage, cold cuts, or frankfurters
- commercial mixes for muffins, waffles, cakes, cookies, breads
- candies, such as milk chocolates, toffee, or caramels

In addition to Table 46–1, lists of commercially prepared foods for lactose-intolerant infants and older children can be developed. Manufacturers periodically issue ingredient information on baby and toddler foods.[33,34]

Consumers need consistent label information so they can interpret ingredient information and select appropriate foods.[35] The FDA has proposed new regulations on labeling that will require information on the percentage of major ingredients in food and more complete labeling of additives.[36] The presence and relative amounts of added sugars in processed foods should be noted in the ingredient lists on food labels to guide consumers.[37]

Medicines

Lactose is often used as a bulking agent in medications and dietary supplements. It may not be listed on the label because it is an inert ingredient or filler.[38–40] Several published references can be used as guides to lactose content.[41–43] However, health care professionals should contact the manufacturer for current information. A physician may rec-

Table 46–1. Lactose-Restricted Diet

Permitted	Not Permitted
Milk and Milk Products	
Soy milk, fortified with L-methionine for infants	Breast or human milk unless tolerated
Casein hydrolysate infant formulas or Enteral products for infants, children, and adults	Milk of any animal source, as whole, skim, dried, condensed, evaporated; whey, lactose
Cream substitutes, free of milk or milk derivatives, based on soy protein or casseinate	Most brands of filled or imitation milk
Yogurt with active yogurt cultures, if tolerated	
Lactose-reduced milk	
Protein Foods	
Plain meat, fish, or poultry	Creamed or breaded meats, fish, or poultry
Eggs prepared without milk or milk products	Sausage, frankfurters, or cold cuts that contain milk or milk products
Legumes, nuts, peanut butter	
Aged cheeses	
Breads and Cereals	
All may be included	
Fats	
Margarines without milk	Butter, unless tolerated
Oil, lard	Margarines with milk or milk products
Salad dressings without milk or cream	
Olives, nut butters	
Fruits and Vegetables	
All may be included unless prepared with milk and milk products—fresh, canned, frozen, dried, or as juice, when age appropriate	Breaded or creamed vegetables Fruits with milk or milk products
Soups	
Clear broths, consommes, vegetable soups	Cream soups, chowders, commercially prepared soups containing milk or milk products
Desserts	
Fruit ices, sorbets, water ices (popsicles)	Ice cream, sherbert
Fruit pies, cookies, cakes without milk	Custard, milk pudding
Soy-based frozen desserts without milk	Cream-filled pastries
Cocoa, baking chocolate, semi-sweet chocolate	Candies with milk or cream
	Milk chocolate
Miscellaneous	
Sucrose, honey, molasses	Seasoning mixes with lactose, whey, or other milk products
Carbonated beverages, fruit punch base	
Chewing gums	

ommend that a lactase enzyme table be taken with medications to improve the tolerance to the lactose contained in them.

Education and counseling

In addition to Table 46–1, parents need a listing of milk derivatives and ingredients that could be a source of lactose. There are several sources of information on food ingredients and additives.[27,44] Written materials, including sample labels and menus, can enhance nutritional counseling.[29] There are a number of recipe books that avoid milk or use soy milks, which can be used to add variety to meals.[45-50]

Follow-up

Lactase persistence or nonpersistence is age related and may change at times. Tolerance of milk and milk products may increase or decrease, so repeated diet and laboratory as-

sessments are recommended. Evaluation of low lactase activity for specific ages and ethnic groups is advisable, with a family pedigree to determine the familial intolerance of lactose.

In summary, the study of lactase sensitivity is a complex topic, and the evaluation by the clinical team should include laboratory assessments, diet history, and accurate intake records calculated for nutritional adequacy, as well as lactose content.

References

1. Solomons, N.W. An update on lactose intolerance. *Nutr. News.* 1986; 49:1.
2. Scrimshaw, N.S., Murray, E.B. The acceptability of milk and milk products in populations with a high prevalence of lactose intolerance. *Am. J. Clin. Nutr.* 1988; 48(suppl)4:1083.
3. Saavedra, J.M., Perman, J.A. Current concepts in lactose malabsorption and intolerance. *Annu. Rev. Nutr.* 1989; 9:475.
4. Prader, A., Auricchio, S. Defects of intestinal disaccharide absorption. *Annu. Rev. Med.* 1965; 16:345.

5. Montgomery, R.K., Jonas, M.M., Grand, R.J. Intestinal disaccharidases. In: *Carbohydrate Intolerance in Infancy*. New York: Marcel Dekker; 1982.

6. MacLean, W.C., Graham, G. Lactose intolerance and milk intolerance. In: *Pediatric Nutrition in Clinical Practice*. Menlo Park, CA: Addison-Wesley; 1982.

7. Tolboom, J.J.M. Milk intolerance due to lactose and giardiasis. *Am. J. Clin. Nutr.* 1989; 50:178.

8. *Meeting the Special Feeding Needs of Infants with Cows' Milk and Carbohydrate Intolerance*. Columbus, OH: Ross Laboratories; 1987. Publication F522.

9. *Product Handbook G-124*. Columbus, OH: Ross Laboratories; 1990.

10. *Product Handbook L-B63*. Evansville, IN: Mead Johnson Nutritionals; 1990.

11. Rosado, J.L., Allen, L.H., Solomons, N.W. Milk consumption, symptom response, and lactose digestion in milk intolerance. *Am. J. Clin. Nutr.* 1987; 45:1457.

12. McBean, L.D. Food sensitivity and dairy products. *Dairy Council Digest*. 1989; 60:25.

13. Lifschitz, C. Breath hydrogen testing in infants with diarrhea. In: *Carbohydrate Intolerance in Infancy*. New York: Marcel Dekker; 1982.

14. Lebenthal, E., Rossi, T.M. Correlation between lactase deficiency and lactose malabsorption to lactose intolerance. In: *Carbohydrate Intolerance in Infancy*. New York: Marcel Dekker; 1982.

15. Kirkpatrick, K.J., Fenwick, R.M. Manufacture and general properties of dairy ingredients. *Food Tech.* 1987; 41:58.

16. Solomons, N.W., et al. Dietary manipulation of postprandial colonic lactose fermentation. I. Effects of solid foods in a meal. *Am. J. Clin. Nutr.* 1985; 41:199.

17. Martini, M.C., Savaiano, D. Reduced intolerance symptoms for lactose consumed during a meal. *Am. J. Clin. Nutr.* 1988; 47:57.

18. Ladas, S.D., Katsiyiannaki-Latoufi, E., Raptis, S.A. Lactose maldigestion and milk intolerance in healthy Greek schoolchildren. *Am. J. Clin. Nutr.* 1991; 53:676.

19. American Academy of Pediatrics Committee on Nutrition. Practical significance of lactose in children: supplement. *Pediatrics*. 1990; 86:643.

20. Kolars, J.C., et al. Yogurt—an autodigesting source of lactose. *N. Engl. J. Med.* 1984; 310:1.

21. Kroger, M., Kurmann, J.A., Rasic, J.L. Fermented milks. *Food Tech.* 1989; 43:92.

22. Onwalata, C.I., Rao, D.R., Vankineni, P. Relative efficiency of yogurt, sweet acidopholus milk, hydrolyzed lactose milk, and commercial lactase tablet in alleviating lactose maldigestion. *Am. J. Clin. Nutr.* 1989; 49:1233.

23. Cultured and culture-containing dairy foods. *Dairy Council Digest*. 1984; 55:15.

24. Solomons, N.W., et al. Dietary manipulation of postprandial colonic lactose fermentation. II. Addition of exogenous microbial beta-galactosidases at mealtime. *Am. J. Clin. Nutr.* 1985; 41:209.

25. Gendrel, D., Dupont, C., Rickard-Lenable, D., Gendrel, C., Choussain, M. Feeding lactose-intolerant children with a powdered fermented milk. *J. Pediatr. Gastroenterol. Nutr.* 1990; 10:44.

26. Lee, C.M., Hardy, C.M. Cocoa feeding and human lactose intolerance. *Am. J. Clin. Nutr.* 1989; 49:840.

27. *Code of Federal Regulations, Food and Drugs 21*, Parts 100-169 and 170-199. Washington, DC: US Gov. Printing Office; 1988.

28. Levine, A., et al. Food technology: a primer for physicians. *N. Engl. J. Med.* 1985; 312:628.

29. Leinhas, J.L. Food allergy challenges: guidelines and implications. *J. Am. Diet. Assoc.* 1987; 87:604.

30. Imitation and substitute dairy products. *Dairy Council Digest*. 1983; 54:1.

31. National Research Council. *Food Chemicals Codex*. 1981 and supplements 1983 and 1986. Washington, DC: National Academy of Sciences; 1981, 1983, 1986.

32. Mulvihill, D.M., Kinsella, J.E. Gelation characteristics of whey proteins and beta-lactoglobulin. *Food Tech.* 1987; 41:102.

33. *Gerber Foods Ingredients*. Fremont, MI: Gerber Products Co.; 1988.

34. *Heinz Ingredients and Allergy Information*. Pittsburgh: H.J. Heinz Co.; 1984.

35. Kessler, D.A. The federal regulation of food labeling. *N. Engl. J. Med.* 1989; 321:717.

36. Legislative highlights. FDA announces examination of food labeling issues. *J. Am. Diet. Assoc.* 1989; 89:1594.

37. *The Surgeon General's Report on Nutrition and Health*. Washington, DC: US Government Printing Office; 1988. USDHHS publication 88-50211.

38. Brown, J.L. Incomplete labeling of pharmaceuticals: a list of inactive ingredients. *N. Engl. J. Med.* 1983; 309:439.

39. Brown, J.L. The health hazard of unlabeled ingredients in pharmaceuticals. *Pediatrics*. 1984; 73:402.

40. American Academy of Pediatrics Committee on Drugs. Inactive ingredients in pharmaceutical products. *Pediatrics*. 1985; 76:635.

41. *Physicians Desk Reference and Physicians Desk Reference for Non-Prescription Drugs*. Oradell, NJ: Medical Economics; 1989.

42. *Lactose Content Medications*. Pleasantville, NJ: Lactaid; 1990.

43. Bronson Pharmaceuticals. *Ingredient Listing*. La Canada, CA: 1986.

44. Igoe, R.S. *Dictionary of Food Ingredients*. New York: Van Nostrand Reinhold; 1989.

45. Bronson-Adatto, C., ed. *Food Sensitivity Series: Lactose Intolerance*. Chicago: American Dietetic Association; 1985.

46. Jones, J. *Mocha Mix Cookbook*. City of Industry, CA: Presto Food Products; 1986.

47. Borgwardt, B.N. *The No Milk Cookbook*. West Allis, WI: Parkway; 1982.

48. *Cooking with Isomil G-714*. Columbus, OH: Ross Laboratories; 1980.

49. *Meals without Milk*, L-F 17. Evansville, IN: Mead Johnson Nutritional Division; 1981.

50. *Nursoy Cookery* P426 R. Philadelphia, PA: Wyeth Laboratories; 1982.

Chapter 47
Adrenoleukodystrophy and Related Peroxisomal Disorders

Janet Borel

X-linked adrenoleukodystrophy (ALD) is a genetically determined disorder that affects the white matter of the nervous system and the adrenal gland. It can be manifested in several forms. The childhood form of the disease appears to be the most common. Clinically, the onset of progressive neurological degeneration and dementia occurs in affected boys at age 4–8 years after a period of normal growth and development. Within approximately 2 years from the onset of neurological symptoms, the child is in a vegetative state, is bedridden, and is unable to see, speak, or eat except by tube feeding. Subsequent survival ranges from 3 to 10 years.[1]

The adult form of the disorder, adrenomyeloneuropathy (AMN), is characterized by progressive spastic paraparesis, moderate sensory loss, and peripheral neuropathy, which often start at age 20 to 30 years and develop over a period of decades. Approximately 90% of patients of both phenotypes have adrenal insufficiency.[1]

Ten to 15% of female carriers of the disorder experience symptoms similar to men with AMN, although heterozygous women rarely have adrenal insufficiency. The average age of onset of symptoms in affected women is 43 ± 11 (SD) years.[1]

Biochemical Abnormalities

The key biochemical abnormality in X-linked ALD is the accumulation of saturated very long-chain fatty acids (VLCFA) in tissues and body fluids. This accumulation is caused by the deficient functioning of one enzyme in the series of steps necessary to oxidize, or degrade, VLCFA in the peroxisomes of cells. There is considerable evidence that the defective enzyme is lignoceroyl-CoA synthetase, the enzyme that catalyzes the formation of the coenzyme A derivative of VLCFA.[2] This defect results in an accumulation of unbranched saturated VLCFA, particularly hexacosanoic (C26:0), pentacosanoic (C25:0), and tetracosanoic (C24:0) acids. These fatty acids accumulate in all tissues and body fluids, but are particularly abundant in brain white matter and adrenal cortex. In X-linked ALD, the peroxisome structure is normal, as are all other metabolic functions of the peroxisomes.

VLCFA also accumulate in an entirely distinct group of disorders characterized by defects in peroxisome biogenesis such that peroxisomes are not formed or maintained in cells. In the absence of peroxisomes as the site of normal enzyme function, several peroxisomal enzyme systems are affected.[3] The biochemical abnormalities resulting from peroxisomes that are absent or reduced in number include accumulation of VLCFA, phytanic acid, L-pipecolic acid, and bile acid intermediates; decreased synthesis of plasmalogens; increased urinary excretion of dicarboxylic acids; and location of the enzyme catalase in the cytosol of cells, rather than in the peroxisome.[4–6] The disorders of peroxisomal biogenesis include Zellweger cerebrohepatorenal syndrome, neonatal ALD, and infantile Refsum disease. All of these are rare autosomal-recessive disorders and manifest the biochemical abnormalities listed above. They appear to vary in degree of biochemical abnormality and severity and range of symptoms, which can result in developmental delay and shortened life expectancy.[4]

Rhizomelic chondrodysplasia punctata (RCDP) is an autosomal-recessive disorder characterized by intact peroxisomes but a deficiency of more than one peroxisomal enzyme. The result is increased levels of phytanic acid and decreased plasmalogen synthesis, but normal levels of VLCFA, pipecolic acid, and bile acid intermediates.[7]

Refsum disease (heredopathia atactica polyneuritiformis) is an autosomal-recessive disorder characterized by a single enzyme defect in the oxidation of phytanic acid, which results in the accumulation of phytanic acid in blood and tissues.[8,9] Clinical symptoms include retinitis pigmentosa, peripheral neuropathy, hearing loss, and cerebellar ataxia. Onset of symptoms usually occurs before age 20 years, and without treatment there is a gradual deterioration of vision, hearing, and certain neurological functions. Peroxisome structure is normal, as are other peroxisomal functions,[10] and it is not clear whether Refsum disease is exclusively a peroxisomal disorder.[4] However, Refsum disease is included here for purposes of discussion of dietary treatment because the accumulation of phytanic acid is similar to that seen in disorders of peroxisomal biogenesis.

The biochemical abnormalities of these peroxisomal disorders are summarized in Table 47–1.

Factors to be Considered in Nutritional/ Biochemical Evaluation

Diagnosis of adrenoleukodystrophy and other peroxisomal disorders is based on clinical symptoms and measurement of abnormal levels of metabolic products in plasma, red blood cells, or fibroblasts (Table 47–1). The analysis of both phosphoethanolamine (PE) plasmalogen and impaired peroxisomal B oxidation due to a deficiency in acyl-COA oxidase are useful in prenatal diagnosis of these disorders.[11,12]

Dietary Management

X-linked adrenoleukodystrophy

The goal of dietary therapy of X-linked ALD and adrenomyeloneuropathy is to lower the levels of saturated VLCFA,

Table 47–1. Biochemical Abnormalities in Peroxisomal Disorders

	Disorders of Peroxisome Biogenesis*	Disorders of a Single Peroxisome Enzyme		Disorders of More Than One Peroxisome Enzyme
Peroxisomes	Absent or reduced in number	Normal (ALD & AMN)	Normal (Refsum)	Normal (RCDP†)
Metabolic products				
Plasma				
VLCFA‡	increased	increased	normal	normal
Bile acid intermediates	increased	normal	normal	normal
Pipecolic acid	increased	normal	normal	normal
Phytanic acid	increased	normal	increased	increased
Red blood cells				
Plasmalogens	decreased	normal	normal	decreased

*Zellweger syndrome, neonatal ALD, infantile Refsum disease.
†Rhizomelic chondrodysplasia punctata.
‡Very long-chain fatty acids.

particularly hexacosanoic acid (C26:0), as measured in the plasma. This goal is based upon the assumption, as yet unproven, that elimination of the "offending" metabolite will prove to be clinically beneficial. Experience with other disorders, such as PKU and Refsum disease, provides the rationale for this assumption.

The source of the VLCFA is the diet, as well as the endogenous elongation of shorter chain fatty acids, such as palmitic acid (C16:0) and stearic acid (C18:0).[13,14] Therefore, the dietary restriction of VLCFA intake alone is not effective in lowering plasma levels.[15] In vitro studies of cultured fibroblasts from ALD patients indicated that synthesis of saturated VLCFA was decreased in a medium that was high in oleic acid (C18:1).[16] A dietary regimen that combines restricted intake of the VLCFA and increased intake of oleic acid (to provide approximately 60% to 75% of fat calories) decreases plasma VLCFA levels by an average of 50%.[17,18] For most patients however, even after a 50% decrease in VLCFA, the level is still two to three times normal.

Normalization of saturated VLCFA appears to be possible with the addition to the diet of another monounsaturated fatty acid, erucic acid (C22:1).[19]

Restriction of VLCFA intake. Intake of saturated VLCFA, specifically C26:0, from a typical American diet is approximately 12–40 mg/day.[20] Dietary restriction of C26:0 intake to 3 mg or less per day is recommended,[17] although higher intakes of 5–10 mg/day are also reported to be effective in lowering plasma VLCFA when combined with high oleic acid intake.[18] For diets incorporating both oleic acid and erucic acid, dietary intake of VLCFA may not need to be as restrictive. It appears that a low-fat diet (20% of calories from fat) and avoidance of foods particularly high in VLCFA may be sufficient to normalize plasma VLCFA.[19]

The C26:0 content of various foods is listed in Table 47–2. The list is somewhat biased toward low-fat foods. Variations in C26:0 content due to processing, brand, methods of cooking, and geographical factors were not determined. Of note is the considerable difference in the C26:0 content of various

vegetable oils; peanut oil is particularly high with 208 mg C26:0 per 100 g oil. There is a significant difference in the C26:0 content of peeled versus unpeeled fruits and vegetables, reflecting the presence of VLCFA in the cutin of the waxy and leafy portions of some plants.[15]

Use of glycerol trioleate (GTO) oil. Oleic acid is provided in the form of glycerol trioleate (GTO) oil (manufactured by Karlshamns Lipid Specialties USA, 501 W. First Ave., Columbus, OH 43201). GTO oil is approximately 90% oleic acid. Oleic acid is present in more common food oils, such as corn oil (25%), sunflower seed oil (21%), or olive oil (70%).[21] Unlike these other oils, however, GTO oil has only trace amounts of VLCFA.

Use of glycerol trierucate (GTE). Erucic acid (C22:1) is a natural constituent of some marine oils and rapeseed oil, both of which are used as food oils in many parts of the world.[22] Concern about the safety of erucic acid is based on reports of cardiac lipidosis and focal cardiac necrosis in rats fed large amounts of C22:1.[23] However, adverse effects are not observed in normal human subjects,[22] and although ALD and AMN patients may not metabolize C22:1 at a normal rate, evidence suggests that ALD patients do not experience toxic effects from the dietary intake of erucic acid.[19]

For dietary therapy, erucic acid is isolated from high erucic acid rapeseed oil and made into glycerol trierucate (GTE) (Croda Universal Ltd, Hull, England). GTE is approximately 92% C22:1 and is free of VLCFA (Table 47–3). It is a white solid at room temperature.

For the diet, GTO oil and GTE are used to replace all other oils or fats, such as margarine, butter, mayonnaise, salad dressings, cooking oil, or shortening. It appears that a ratio of four parts GTO to one part GTE provides adequate GTE to normalize plasma VLCFA in ALD boys within 4 weeks.[19] The GTE can be melted and mixed with the GTO (the mixture is referred to as Lorenzo's oil and is also avail-

Table 47–2. C26:0 Content of Selected Foods (mg/100 g)

CEREALS

ALL BRAN, KELLOGGS	5.630
APPLE JACKS	1.565
CHEERIOS	3.100
CORN CHEX, RALSTON	0.087
CORN FLAKES, KELLOGGS	0.414
CREAM OF WHEAT, NABISCO, COOKED	1.700
CRISPEX, KELLOGGS	0.210
GRAPE NUTS, POST	0.889
GRITS, QUAKER INSTANT, COOKED	0.781
OAT BRAN	0.090
OATMEAL, REGULAR, DRY	3.349
OATMEAL, INSTANT, DRY	1.836
PUFFED RICE	1.020
RICE CHEX, RALSTON	0.277
RICE KRISPIES	1.067
SHREDDED WHEAT	2.014
SPECIAL K	0.219

BREADS

BAGEL, WATER BASED, LENDER'S	1.060
ENERGEN RYE CRISP	3.338
ENGLISH MUFFIN, THOMAS	0.934
FIBRE PLUS, WASA RYE KING (IRELAND)	6.419
ITALIAN BREAD, GIANT BRAND	1.066
ITALIAN BREAD, HOMEMADE	0.697
MATZO	2.990
PITA BREAD	23.474
POPCORN CAKES	0.535
PRETZELS, GOLDFISH, PEPPERIDGE FARMS	2.970
PRETZELS, SNYDERS	1.890
PRETZEL STICKS, THIN	0.964
RICE CAKES	0.003
RYE BREAD	1.018
SALTINES, NABISCO PREMIUM	3.530
TACO SHELL	0.987
WHITE BREAD, WITH CRUST	1.486
WHITE BREAD, NO CRUST	1.388

FRUIT

APPLESAUCE, MOTT'S	0.040
APRICOT, DRIED, STEWED	0.710
APPLE, GRANNY SMITH, PEELED	0.045
APPLE, GRANNY SMITH, UNPEELED	0.500
APPLE, DRIED, STEWED	0.042
BANANA	0.785
BLUEBERRY, FRESH	0.334
CANTALOUPE, FRESH	0.066
CHERRIES, FRESH, PEELED	0.077
FRUIT COCKTAIL, CANNED	0.077
GRAPES, GREEN SEEDLESS PEELED	0.314
GRAPES, GREEN SEEDLESS UNPEELED	0.643
MANGO, PEELED	0.121
MANGO, UNPEELED	0.303
PAPAYA, PEELED	0.701
PEAR, PEELED	0.042
PEAR, UNPEELED	0.292
PEACH, FRESH PEELED	0.043
PEACH, FRESH UNPEELED	0.091
PEACH, CANNED, LIBBY'S	0.028
PINEAPPLE	0.146
PLUM, PURPLE, FRESH, PEELED	0.060
PLUM, PURPLE, FRESH, WITH PEEL	0.104
RAISINS	3.800
STRAWBERRY, FRESH WITH SEEDS	0.094
WATERMELON	0.163

FRUIT JUICES

APPLE JUICE (MOTT'S)	0.014
GRAPE JUICE (MOTT'S)	0.014
GRAPEFRUIT JUICE, FRESH, STRAINED	
CRANBERRY JUICE, OCEAN SPRAY	0.010
ORANGE JUICE, FROM CONCENTRATE	0.941
ORANGE JUICE, FRESH, STRAINED	0.189
PRUNE JUICE, SUNSWEET	0.084

VEGETABLES

BEANS, STRING, FROZEN COOKED	0.245
BEANS, STRING, CANNED	1.483
BEET, CANNED	0.382
BROCOLLI, FROZEN, BOILED	0.449
BROCCOLI STEM, PEELED, STEAMED	
CABBAGE, FRESH, RAW	2.185
CARROTS, PEELED, COOKED	0.061
CELERY	0.257
CUCUMBER, DESEEDED, PEELED	0.098
EGGPLANT, FRESH, PEELED, COOKED	0.088
ENDIVE	0.070
FENNEL	0.113
LETTUCE HEARTS	0.372
MUSHROOMS, FRESH, BOILED	0.055
ONION, YELLOW, RAW	0.440
PEPPER, GREEN, FRESH	0.092
PICKLE, DILL, WITH SKIN	0.560
PICKLE, DILL, PEELED	0.410
SCALLION, GREEN	0.470
SCALLION, WHITE	0.716
SPINACH, FROZEN, COOKED	0.508
TOMATO, NO SKIN, NO SEEDS	0.071
TOMATO JUICE, CAMPBELL'S	0.051
TOMATO, WITH SKIN AND SEEDS	0.289
TURNIPS, FRESH, COOKED, PEELED	0.088
ZUCCHINI, FRESH, PEELED, COOKED	2.873

FATS AND OILS

APRICOT KERNEL OIL, HAINS	9.200
COCONUT OIL, HAINS	5.990
COD LIVER OIL	1.500
CORN OIL	31.300
COTTONSEED OIL	19.540
HALIBUT OIL	3.000
LARD (A&P)	3.400
LINSEED OIL	31.490
MAYONNAISE, HAINS IMITATION	5.250
MCT OIL	0.450
MICROLIPID	0.730
OLIVE OIL	19.900
PEANUT OIL	208.400
PUMPKINSEED OIL	13.940
PRIMROSE OIL	76.600
RAPESEED OIL	9.080
SAFFLOWER OIL	5.570
SESAME SEED OIL	23.130
SOY SOIL	12.640
SUNFLOWER OIL	8.810
WALNUT OIL	11.300
WHEAT GERM OIL	45.380

STARCHY VEGETABLES

CORN, NIBLET (A&P)	0.368
LIMA BEANS, SOAKED, COOKED WITH SKIN	0.176
LIMA BEANS, SOAKED, COOKED, NO SKIN	0.115
PINTO BEANS, FRESH, SOAKED, COOKED	0.588
PEAS, GREEN, FROZEN, COOKED	0.181
POP CORN, POPPED, PLAIN	0.353
POTATO, PEELED, BOILED	0.096
POTATO, FRENCH FRIES, FROZEN (A&P)	2.288
POTATO CHIPS	7.465
RICE, LONG GRAIN, COOKED	0.273
SQUASH, BUTTERNUT, FRESH, COOKED	0.191
SQUASH, ACORN, FRESH, COOKED	0.236
SQUASH, PUMPKIN, LIBBY'S CANNED	0.959
SWEET POTATO, BAKED	0.244

OTHER STARCHES

CORNMEAL FLOUR, YELLOW	2.290
FLOUR, BUCKWHEAT	1.815
FLOUR, WHITE (A&P)	0.320
FLOUR, PLAIN (BRITAIN)	1.831
FLOUR, WHOLE MEAL (BRITAIN)	3.409
FLOUR, SELF RISING (BRITAIN)	1.891
PASTA, COOKED SPAGHETTI, ST. GIORGIO	1.130
PASTA, SHELLS, ARTICHOKE FLOUR, DE BOLS	1.059
PASTA, HOMEMADE	0.344

MEATS

BEEF, GROUND ROUND, BROILED	0.120
BEEF, STEAK, FAT TRIMMED, BROILED	0.083
HAM, LEAN, FAT TRIMMED, BOILED	0.072
PORK CHOP, EXTRA LEAN, FAT TRIMMED	0.130

POULTRY

CHICKEN BREAST, SKINNED, BROILED	0.060
TURKEY BREAST, SKINNED, BROILED	0.220
CHICKEN FRANK, HOLLY FARMS	0.020

SEAFOOD

AMBER JACK FISH, BAKED	0.100
BASS, BAKED	1.120
CATFISH, FRESH, BAKED	0.055
CLAMS, WHOLE, FRESH	0.045

Table 47-2. (*Continued*)

COD, FRESH, BROILED	0.480	*OTHER*		MILK, NONFAT, DRY MIXED WITH WATER	0.020	SUSTACAL LIQUID MEAD JOHNSON	0.156
CRAB, FRESH, STEAMED	0.042	EGG WHITE	0.007	MILK, CHOCOLATE, LOWFAT	3.330	*MISCELLANEOUS*	
FLOUNDER, FRESH, BROILED	0.068	EGG BEATERS, FLEISHMANS	0.067	PUDDING, VANILLA, MADE W/SKIM		BOUILLON CUBE, BEEF OR CHICKEN	0.003
GROUPER, BAKED	0.038	PROTEIN IN POWDER, SHAKLEE	0.643	MILK, JELLO	0.011	BUTTER BUDS	0.556
HADDOCK, FRESH, POACHED	0.025	TOFU	0.850	INSTANT BREAKFAST, CARNATION,		CHOCOLATE, UNSWEETENED, BAKER'S	4.800
OCEAN PERCH, FROZEN, BAKED	0.070	*COMBINATION FOODS*		VANILLA MADE W/SKIM MILK	0.043	CHOCOLATE EXTRACT, McCORMICK	0.004
REDFISH, BAKED	0.235	SPAGHETTI SAUCE, PREGO	1.317	YOGURT, 2% FAT	0.470	COCOA POWDER, HERSHEY'S	3.649
SHRIMP, FRESH, BROILED, OR BOILED	0.760	SPAGHETTI & MEATBALLS, CHEF BOYARDEE	0.086	YOGURT, PLAIN, WHOLE MILK BASED	1.760	CATSUP	0.112
SWORDFISH, BAKED	0.687	SOUP, VEGETABLE, CAMPBELLS, MIXED		YOGURT, PLAIN, SKIM, COLUMBO	0.060	LECITHIN	5.150
TUNA, WATER PACKED, A&P	0.090	W/WATER	0.084	YOGURT, DANNON STRAWBERRY,		METAMUCIL	0.170
WALLEYE, BAKED	0.216	SOUP, TOMATO, CAMPBELLS, MIXED W/WATER	0.160	SKIM MILK BASED	0.471	MUSTARD, FRENCH'S YELLOW	0.830
				FORMULAS		MAPLE SYRUP	0.001
MEAT COMBINATIONS				ISOCAL, LIQUID, MEAD JOHNSON CO.	0.480	UNIFIBER, DIETARY FIBER POWDER	0.347
BOLOGNA, OSCAR MEYER	1.220	*DAIRY PRODUCTS*		NUTRAMIGEN, POWDER, MEAD JOHNSON	2.604	WORCESTERSHIRE SAUCE	0.150
FRANKFURTER, OSCAR MEYER, BEEF	1.226	COTTAGE CHEESE, 1% FAT	0.117	PORTAGEN, POWDER, MEAD		*BEVERAGES*	
POTTED MEAT, GIANT FOODS	0.160	COTTAGE CHEESE, DRY CURD	0.532	JOHNSON	0.550	BEER, MICHELOB	0.011
SALAMI	7.411	COUNT DOWN CHEESE	0.318	PREGESTIMIL, POWER, MEAD		COCA COLA	0.000
SAUSAGE, HOMEMADE, LEAN, GRILLED	0.840	MILK, SKIM	0.050	JOHNSON	2.500	COFFEE, BREWED	0.010
CHICKEN AND RICE, LEAN CUISINE	1.230	MILK, SKIM, EVAPORATED, CARNATION	0.100			TEA, INSTANT, LIPTON	0.007
						VODKA	0.002
						WINE, WHITE, ALMADEN	0.005

able in a commercial blend), or the two fats can be used separately.

A specific amount of GTO and GTE in a 4:1 ratio is prescribed, based on the individual's caloric requirements, to provide 20% of total calories. One tablespoon (15 mL) GTO oil weighs 13.2 grams and provides 116 calories (8.8 cal/g). When added to a low-fat diet of 15% to 20% of calories from other foods and fats, the result is a diet similar to the typical American diet in percent calories from fat (35% to 40%).

GTO oil is approximately 5% linoleic acid and thus provides about 1.25% of total calories from this essential fatty acid. Since intake of other fats and oils is restricted, it may

be necessary to supplement the diet with safflower oil to provide adequate essential fatty acid intake, especially for infants and young children. Safflower oil is recommended because it is approximately 74% linoleic acid[21] and is very low in C26:0 content (5.6 mg/100 g, Table 47-2).

GTO oil is an excellent cooking oil. Recipes for use of GTO oil in such products as mayonnaise and a margarine-like spread, as well as other recipes for the diet, are provided in the *ALD/AMN Diet Cookbook*.[24]

Using the foods determined to have low VLCFA content (Table 47-2), a food exchange list was developed to help patients and families with meal planning. Meals planned according to the C26:0 values of the exchange lists were found to be very close to the calculated and actual measured C26:0 content of the foods.[15] A sample meal pattern and one day's menu are shown in Table 47-4.

Related peroxisomal disorders

At present, of the several biochemical abnormalities observed in children with other peroxisomal disorders, dietary therapy has been applied successfully to reduce elevated levels of phytanic acid, as well as of VLCFA.[25,26] Efforts to lower levels of phytanic acid in children with peroxisomal disorders are based on experience with patients with Refsum disease, an autosomal-recessive disorder affecting adults and characterized by the accumulation of phytanic acid in blood and tissues.[8,9]

Phytanic acid is a 20-carbon branched-chain fatty acid that is normally present in human tissues in trace amounts. Plasma

Table 47-3. Fatty Acid Composition of Glycerol Trioleate (GTO) and Glycerol Trierucate (GTE)

		Percentage Present	
Fatty Acid		GTO	GTE
C12:0	Lauric	1.25	0
C16:0	Palmitic	1.07	0
C18:0	Stearic	3.02	0.5
C18:1	Oleic	87.45	0.5
C18:2	Linoleic	4.79	0.5
C18:3	Linolenic	0	0.5
C20:1	Eicosenoic	0	1.0-3.5
C22:1	Erucic	0	91.5-94.0
C24:0	Lignoceric	0	0
C24:1	Nervonic	0	1.0-3.5
C26:0	Hexacosanoic	trace	0

Table 47–4. Sample Diet Prescription and Menu

1500 CALORIES

GTO/GTE Prescription: 20% cal = 300 calories
= 2.5 Tbsp (37.5 mL) GTO/GTE mixture, in 4:1 ratio
= 7.5 mL (1.5 tsp) GTE plus
30.0 mL (2 Tbsp) GTO

SAMPLE MEAL PATTERN: 1500 cal

	Number of Exchanges	C26:0 (mg)
Protein	5	0.25
Starch	5	1.00
Fruit	2	0.20
Vegetables	2	0.20
Dairy products	2	0.20
Fat (GTO/GTE)	2.5 TBS	—
Desserts	1	0.10

SAMPLE DAY's MENU: 1500 cal

Breakfast	Exchange	C26:0 (mg)
Rice Krispies, 1 cup	1 Starch	0.20
Skim milk, 1 cup	1 Dairy	0.10
Apple juice, 4 oz	1 Fruit	0.10
Lunch		
Sandwich		
White bread, 2 slices	2 Starches	0.40
Ham, lean, 2 oz	2 Protein	0.10
Mustard	Free	—
GTO/GTE, 1 Tbsp		—
Lettuce	1 Vegetable	0.10
Peaches, canned, ½ cup	1 Fruit	0.10
Apple cake,* 1 slice	1 Dessert	0.10
Dinner		
Chicken breast, 3 oz	3 Protein	0.15
Potatoes, peeled, ½ cup	1 Starch	0.20
Carrots, cooked, ½ cup	1 Vegetable	0.10
GTO/GTE, 1.5 Tbsp		—
Skim milk, 1 cup	1 Dairy	0.10
Snack		
Popcorn, plain, 5 cups	1 Starch	0.20
	TOTAL	1.95 mg

*Use a low-fat recipe.

phytanic acid is normally 0.3 mg/dL or less than 0.5% of total plasma fatty acids.[27] In Refsum disease patients, phytanic acid can amount to 5% to 30% of plasma total fatty acids, a 10-to 60-fold increase above normal. Increased plasma phytanic acid levels are also observed in children with Zellweger syndrome, neonatal ALD, infantile Refsum disease, and RCDP[4] (Table 47–1).

Accumulation of phytanic acid is caused by the lack of the enzyme, phytanic acid oxidase, which is responsible for the alpha oxidation of phytanic acid.[6] The source of accumulated phytanic acid is exogenous, specifically from dietary phytanic acid. There is no evidence of endogenous synthesis of phytanic acid, although dietary-free phytol can be converted to phytanic acid.[28] However, phytol is normally bound to chlorophyll and, as such, is not well absorbed; thus, phytol is probably not a major source of phytanic acid.[6,29].

Data on the phytanic acid content of foods are limited,[8,30] and interpretation is complicated by the fact that the phytanic acid content of some foods is highly variable, depending on seasonal or regional differences in growth. Primary sources of phytanic acid are dairy products, ruminant fats, and ruminant meats.

Since green vegetables contain phytol bound to chlorophyll and phytol may be released during cooking,[8] several researchers have excluded green vegetables from the diet to lower phytanic acid levels.[31–33] However, as mentioned above, chlorophyll-bound phytol is not well absorbed, and it appears that phytol is not important as a source of phytanic acid in the diet. Nevertheless, it is probably best to restrict the intake of green vegetables until plasma phytanic acid levels decrease sufficiently. Then selected green vegetables can be added to the diet, one at a time, and the effect on plasma phytanic acid can be monitored.

The usual dietary intake of phytanic acid is approximately 0.1% of daily dietary fat intake or 100 mg or less per day.[8] Recommendations for the dietary therapy of Refsum disease have varied from restricting intake of phytanic acid to less than 3 mg/day to as much as 21 mg/day.[31-35] Plasmapheresis has been used to decrease plasma phytanic acid more rapidly, with subsequent maintenance of low levels by the dietary restriction of phytanic acid intake.[8,34] In patients in whom a change in diet has resulted in weight loss, plasma phytanic acid levels may increase, with concomitant worsening of clinical symptoms. It appears that phytanic acid is mobilized from adipose tissue and the liver during weight loss.[8,34]

In infants with disorders of peroxisomal biogenesis, phytanic acid may be elevated only moderately. This is probably because phytanic acid is exclusively of dietary origin, and accumulation occurs only after the child's diet begins to incorporate dairy products and meats.

Table 47-5 is a composite list of foods allowed and to be avoided to limit phytanic acid intake, as recommended by various researchers.[8,30-35] Children with disorders of peroxisomal biogenesis also have elevated plasma VLCFA and should combine the dietary treatment to lower VLCFA with restriction of phytanic acid intake. Fortunately, many aspects of both diets are the same, and combining the dietary recommendations does not further restrict food choices significantly.

It is important to note that for Zellweger and neonatal ALD patients, the diet to lower VLCFA should use GTO oil only. The use of GTE is not recommended since plasma monounsaturated VLCFA, including C22:1, are elevated in

these children, suggesting the impaired metabolism of these fats, as well as of saturated VLCFA.[3]

Pipecolic Acid. Children with Zellweger syndrome, infantile Refsum disease, and neonatal ALD also have elevated plasma levels of pipecolic acid, an amino acid involved in lysine metabolism. It may be possible to lower plasma levels of pipecolic acid by dietary restriction of foods known to be high in that substance,[36-38] but the clinical significance of such efforts is not known.

Potential nutritional problems

The diet to lower VLCFA can result in constipation, weight loss, and gastrointestinal upset. Constipation may be caused by the low dietary fiber content of the foods allowed, if skins and seeds of fruits and vegetables and whole grains are avoided due to their high C26:0 content. Avoidance of these high-fiber foods may not be as necessary with the use of GTE in addition to GTO if normalization of plasma VLCFA occurs. In addition to providing adequate fluid and exercise, patients should make a conscious effort to select higher fiber foods from those that are allowed on the diet. Constipation may also result from neurological impairment caused by the disease so that dietary measures may not be entirely effective in alleviating that problem.

Weight loss in adults and poor weight gain in children may result from lack of interest in eating because of the

Table 47-5. Diet to Restrict Phytanic Acid Intake

	Foods Allowed	Foods Forbidden

Dairy	Skim milk
	Nonfat yogurt
	Lean cheese
	  1% fat cottage cheese
	  Dry cottage cheese
	Eggs, egg white
		Whole milk
		All other cheeses
		Ice cream
		Butter

Meat	Chicken, turkey Lean fish—haddock, tuna in water All lean meats: veal, beef, pork, lamb	Fatty fish Fatty meats
Fat	Sunflower or safflower seed oil	Corn and vegetable oils Mayonnaise, salad dressing Lard, butter, animal fats
Breads/grains	Breads made without butter Pasta Rice White flour Cereals	
Other	Sugars, syrups, honey, jellies, jams	Nuts, chocolate, fresh green herbs

Vegetables	Beets, mushrooms, onions,
	  potatoes, carrots, parsnips,
	  swedes, corn, yellow squash
		All others

Fruits	Apricots, pears, pineapple, fruit
	  cocktail, oranges, peaches,
	  applesauce, grapefruit
		Bananas, grapes, rhubarb

Beverages	Tea, coffee, carbonated drinks, beer, fruit juices, wines, spirits	

limited food choices. C26:0 restriction to less than 3 mg/day may not meet caloric needs of adolescents and other individuals requiring more than approximately 2500 cal/day, without supplementation or liberalization of the C26:0 restriction. Calories can be supplemented with the use of foods that are "free" of C26:0.

Some patients report gastrointestinal upset, such as nausea or diarrhea, when changing to GTO oil and GTE as their primary fat sources. These fats are tolerated best when incorporated into foods, as is the case for most dietary fats. The daily dose of GTO and GTE should be divided throughout the day, taken at mealtimes, and incorporated into foods. GTO can be used for frying and baking and in recipes for mayonnaise and salad dressings.[24]

Even though the diet to lower VLCFA is restricted in the variety of foods allowed, with careful planning and inclusion of foods from all food groups, a nutritionally well-balanced diet is possible. However, because food choices are limited, a daily multivitamin and mineral supplement to provide the recommended dietary allowance for age and sex is recommended.

Follow-up

Plasma levels of VLCFA and of phytanic acid when applicable should be measured regularly to monitor the effect of diet. Using GTO oil only, plasma VLCFA levels may decrease significantly within 30–90 days and can be expected to decrease to 30% to 50% of baseline.[17,18] Despite the decrease, plasma levels of VLCFA may remain above the normal range. Normalization of plasma VLCFA occurs within 4 weeks of starting a diet with GTE and GTO.[19]

Essential fatty acid and vitamin E status should also be monitored periodically. Weight should be monitored to maintain appropriate weight in adults and adequate growth in children.

References

1. Moser, H.W., Naidu, S., Kumar, A.J., Rosenbaum, A.E. The adrenoleukodystrophies. *CRC Crit. Rev. Neurobiol.* 1987; 3:29.
2. Moser, H.W., Moser, A.B. Adrenoleukodystrophy (X-Linked). In: Scriver, C.R., Beaudet, A.L., Sly, W.S., Valle, D., eds. *The Metabolic Basis of Inherited Disease.* 6th ed. New York: McGraw-Hill; 1989.
3. Lazarow, P.B., Moser, H.W. Disorders of peroxisome biogenesis. In: Scriver, C.R., Beaudet, A.L., Sly, W.S., Valle, D., eds. *The Metabolic Basis of Inherited Disease.* 6th ed. New York: McGraw-Hill; 1989.
4. Moser, H.W. Peroxisomal diseases. In: *Advances in Pediatrics.* Chicago: Year Book Medical Publishers; 1989.
5. Sharp, P., Johnson, R., Poulos, A. Molecular species of phosphatidylcholine containing very long chain fatty acids in human brain: enrichment in x-linked adrenoleukodystrophy brain and diseases of peroxisome biogenesis brain. *J. Neurochem.* 1991; 56:30.
6. Singh, H., Usher, S., Johnson, D., Poulos, A. Metabolism of branched chain fatty acids in peroxisomal disorders. *J. Inher. Metab. Dis.* 1990; 13:387.
7. Hoefler, G., Hoefler, S., Watkins, P.A., Chen, W.W., Moser, A., Baldwin, V., McGillivary, B., Charrow, J., Friedman, M., Rutledge, L., Hashimoto, T., Moser, H.W. Biochemical abnormalities in rhizomelic chondrodysplasia punctata. *J. Pediatr.* 1988; 112:726.
8. Steinberg, D. Refsum disease. In: Scriver, C.R., Beaudet, A.L., Sly, W.S., Valle, D., eds. *The Metabolic Basis of Inherited Disease.* 6th ed. New York: McGraw-Hill; 1989.
9. Refsum, S. Heredopathia atactica polyneuritiformis (Refsum disease). In: Dyck, P.J., Thomas, P.K., Lambert, E.H., Bunge, R., eds. *Peripheral Neuropathy.* Philadelphia: W.B. Saunders; 1984.
10. Wanders, R.J.A., Heymans, H.S.A., Shutgens, R.B.H., Poll-The, B.T., Saudubray, J.M., Tager, J.M., Schrakamp, G., van den Bosch, H. Peroxisomal functions in classical Refsum's disease: comparison with the infantile form of Refsum's disease. *J. Neurol. Sci.* 1988; 84:147.
11. Wanders, R., Schelen, A., Feller, N., Schutgens, R., Stellaard, F., Jacobs, C., Mitulla, B., Leidlitz, G. First prenatal diagnosis of acyl-coa oxidase deficiency. *J. Inher. Metab. Dis.* 1990; 13:371.
12. Tanaka, K., Nishizawa, K., Yamamoto, H., Naruto, T., Izeki, E., Taga, T., Shimada, M., Saeki, Y. Analysis of very long-chain fatty acids and plasmalogen in the erythrocyte membrane: a simple method for detection of peroxisomal disorders and discrimination between adrenoleukodystrophy and Zellweger syndrome. *Neuropediatrics.* 1989; 21:119.
13. Moser, H.W., Pallante, S.L., Moser, A.B., Rizzo, W.B., Schulman, J.D., Fenelau, D. Adrenoleukodystrophy: origin of very long chain fatty acids and therapy. *Pediatr. Res.* 1983; 17:293A.
14. Kishimoto, Y., Moser, H.W., Kawamura, N., Platt, M., Pallante, S.L., Fenselau, C. Adrenoleukodystrophy: evidence that abnormal very long chain fatty acids of brain cholesterol esters are of exogenous origin. *Biochem. Biophys. Res. Comm.* 1980; 96:69.
15. Van Duyn, M., Moser, A.B., Brown, F.R., Sactor, N., Lui, A., Moser, H.W. The design of a diet restricted in saturated very long-chain fatty acids: therapeutic application in adrenoleukodystrophy. *Am. J. Clin. Nutr.* 1984; 40:277.
16. Rizzo, W.B., Watkins, P.A., Phillips, M.W., Cranin, D., Campbell, B., Avigan, J. Adrenoleukodystrophy: oleic acid lowers fibroblast saturated C22-26 fatty acids. *Neurology.* 1986; 36:357.
17. Moser, A.B., Borel, J.S., Odone, A., Naidu, S., Cornblath, D., Sanders, D.B., Moser, H.W. A new dietary therapy for adrenoleukodystrophy: biochemical and preliminary clinical results in 36 patients. *Ann. Neurol.* 1987; 21:240.
18. Rizzo, W.B., Phillips, M.W., Dammann, A.L., Leshner, R.T., Jennings, S.S., Avigan, J., Proud, V.K. Adrenoleukodystrophy: dietary oleic acid lowers hexacosanoate levels. *Ann. Neurol.* 1987; 21:232.
19. Rizzo, W.B., Leshner, R.T., Odone, A., Dammann, A.L., Craft, D.A., Jensen, M.E., Jennings, S.S., Davis, S., Jaitly, R., Sgro, J.A. Dietary erucic acid therapy for X-linked adrenoleukodystrophy. *Neurology.* 1989; 39:1415.
20. Brown, F.R., III, Van Duyn, M.A., Moser, A.B., Schulman, J.D., Rizzo, W.B., Snyder, R.D., Murphy, J.V., Kamoshita, S., Migeon, C.J., Moser, H.W. Adrenoleukodystrophy: effects of dietary restriction of very long chain fatty acids and administration of carnitine and clofibrate on clinical status and plasma fatty acids. *Johns Hopkins Med. J.* 1982; 15:164.
21. Agriculture Research Service, United States Department of Agriculture, *Handbook No.8-4, Fats and Oils.* Washington, DC: US Government Printing Office; 1979.
22. Kramer, J.K.G., Sauer, F.D., Pidgen, W.J., eds. *High and Low Eruic Acid Rapeseed Oils. Production, Usage, Chemistry and Toxicological Evaluation.* Toronto: Academic Press; 1983.
23. Roine, P., Uksila, E., Teir, H., Rapola, J. Histopathological changes in rats and pigs fed rapeseed oil. *Z. Ernahrungswiss.* 1960; 1:118.
24. Borel, J., Cohen, J., eds. *ALD/AMN Diet Cookbook.* Baltimore: Kennedy Institute and United Leukodystrophy Foundation, 1990.
25. Borel, J.S., Moser, A.B., Naidu, S., Moser, H.W. Dietary therapy for adrenoleukodystrophy and related peroxisomal disorders. *J. Am. Diet. Assoc.* Abstract in Outlooks for Tomorrow. 1987; 159.
26. Greenberg, C.R., Hajra, A.K., Moser, A.B. Triple therapy of a patient with a generalized peroxisomal disorder. *Am. J. Hum. Genet.* 1987; 41(suppl A):64.
27. Avigan, J. The presence of phytanic acid in normal human and animal plasma. *Biochim. Biophys. Acta.* 1966; 116:391.
28. Stoffel, W., Kablke, W. The transformation of phytol into 3,7,11,15-tetramethyhexadecanoic (phytanic) acid in heredo-

pathia atactica polyneuritiformis (Refsum's syndrome). *Biochem. Biophys. Res. Comm.* 1965; 19:33.

29. Baxter, J.H. Absorption of chlorophyll phytol in normal man and in patients with Refsum's disease. *J. Lipid Res.* 1968; 9:636.

30. Masters-Thomas, A., Bailes, J., Billimoria, J.D., Clemens, M.E., Gibberd, F.B., Page, N.G.R. Heredopathia atactica polyneuritiformis (Refsum's disease) 2. Estimation of phytanic acid in foods. *J. Hum. Nutr.* 1980; 34:251.

31. Masters-Thomas, A., Bailes, J., Billimoria, J.D., Clemens, M.E., Gibberd, F.B., Page, N.G.R. Heredopathia atactica polyneuritiformis (Refsum's disease) 1. Clinical features and dietary management. *J. Hum. Nutr.* 1980; 34:245.

32. Eldjarn, L., Try, K., Stokke, O., Munthe-Kaas, A.W., Refsum, S., Steinberg, D., Avigan, J., Mize, C. Dietary effects on serum-phytanic-acid levels and on clinical manifestations in hereopathia atactica polyneuritiformis. *Lancet.* 1966; 1:691.

33. Steinberg, D., Mize, C.E., Herndon, J.H., Fales, H.M., Engel, W.K., Vroom, F.Q. Phytanic acid in patients with Ref-

sum's syndrome and responses to dietary treatment. *Arch. Intern. Med.* 1970; 125:75.

34. Gibberd, F.B., Billimoria, J.D., Page, N.G.R., Retsas, S. Heredopathia atactica polyneuritiformis (Refsum's disease) treated by diet and plasma-exchange. *Lancet.* 1979; 1:575.

35. Eldjarn, L., Stokke, O., Try, K. Biochemical aspects of Refsum's disease and principles for the dietary treatment. In: Vinken, P.J., Bruyn, G.W., eds. *Handbook of Clinical Neurology. Metabolic and Deficiency Diseases of the Nervous System* New York: American-Elsevier, 1976.

36. Zacharius, R.M., Thompson, J.F., Steward, F.C. The detection, isolation and identification of L(−)pipecolic acid in the non-protein fraction of beans (Phaseolus vulgaris). *J. Am. Chem. Soc.* 1954; 76:2908.

37. Gatfield, P.D., Taller, R.T., Hinton, G.G., Wallace, A.C., Abdelnour, G.M., Haust, M.D. Hyperpipecolatemia: a new metabolic disorder associated with neuropathy and hepatomegaly: a case study. *Can. Med. Assoc. J.* 1968; 99:1215.

38. Burton, B.K., Reed, S.P., Remy, W.T. Hyperpipecolic acidemia: clinical and biochemical observations in two male siblings. *J. Pediatr.* 1981; 99:729.

Chapter 48
Broad Thumb-Hallux (Rubinstein-Taybi) Syndrome

Jack Rubinstein

In 1963, Dr. Taybi and the author published a report on a possible syndrome in seven children—two girls and five boys—with broad thumbs and great toes, as well as distinctive facial features, growth retardation, mental retardation, and cryptorchidism in boys.[1] Ten years after that publication, the author was informed[2] that in 1957 Michail et al.[3] published a single case report of a 7-year-old Greek boy with the same constellation of findings in a French orthopedic journal.[3]

Clinical Abnormalities

Common clinical findings in the broad thumb-hallux (BTHS; Rubinstein-Taybi) syndrome include stature below the 5th percentile; head circumference below the 2nd percentile; and mental, motor, language, and social retardation with intelligence often at a moderately retarded level.

Frequently noted facial findings produce a recognizable facial gestalt. These findings include prominent forehead, broad nasal bridge, beaked or straight nose with the nasal septum extending below the alae nasi, antimongoloid slant of palpebral fissures, clinical hypertelorism, strabismus, highly arched or heavy eyebrows, epicanthi, minimal abnormalities of external ears, mild retrognathia, grimacing smile, a high-arched palate, and dental irregularity and overcrowding (Fig. 48-1).

Broad, short thumbs, which may be radially angulated, and broad halluces, which may be duplicated by x-ray and/or angulated, are major findings. Broad terminal phalanges of other fingers and a stiff gait are often seen.

There usually is delayed or incomplete descent of testes in boys. Anomalies of kidneys and heart may occur, and hirsutism is common.

Factors to be Considered in Nutritional Evaluation

In individuals with BTHS, feeding difficulties in infancy were found in 77% of children in whom the presence or absence of the finding was mentioned.[4] In addition, neonatal distress and/or recurrent respiratory infection occurred in 78% of cases.[4] In at least some of the individuals with feeding difficulties, gastroesophageal reflux (GER) has been demonstrated.[5] The reflux may, in fact, have been responsible for some of the episodes of recurrent pneumonitis,[6] and some of the deaths in infants with BTHS may have been due to recurrent aspiration in conjunction with reflux. Two children with BTHS had sleep apnea, one of which was associated with GER. One child had an episode of apnea

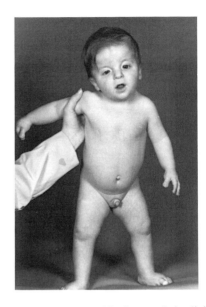

Fig. 48-1. A 1-year-old boy with characteristic clinical findings of BTHS. From the University Affiliated Cincinnati Center for Developmental Disorders. Used with permission.

with feeding. There may be an increased risk of aspiration in children with BTHS during anesthesia.[7] Significant GER may occur without vomiting.[8] GER may also cause esophagitis, esophageal stenosis, hematemesis, iron-deficiency anemia, irritability, epigastric pain, chronic cough, recurrent wheezing, and failure to thrive[9] (see Chapters 24 and 34).

There is considerable discussion in the literature about what constitutes significant GER and how best to confirm its presence in different age groups. A recent review[10] suggests that the main value of the radiologic barium swallow is to rule out structural abnormalities that may cause regurgitation and mimic GER. The barium swallow is associated with a false-positive rate of approximately 31% and a false-negative rate of 14% in children.[11] In infants with GER, an incidence of intestinal malrotation of around 50% was found on upper gastrointestinal barium contrast study.[12] Esophageal radionuclide scintiscan, which evaluates gastric emptying time and scans the lung fields, is also used, but it has a high percentage of false-negative and false-positive results.[10]

Esophageal manometry and endoscopy with or without biopsy may be used to document reduced lower esophageal sphincter pressure and the presence of esophagitis, respectively; however, they cannot confirm the diagnosis of GER.[10]

Of those patients with GER, 46% had normal mucosa at esophagoscopy, 3% had false-negative biopsies, and 13% had false-positive biopsies.[11]

Continuous monitoring of pH in the distal esophagus is used to confirm the presence of GER. When correctly used, it had approximately a 12% false-negative and 6% false-positive result.[11] If conducted as a part of polysomnographic studies, pH monitoring may demonstrate an association with apnea or other disturbances of physiological behavior.[10] Some authors have suggested that continuous 24-hour esophageal pH probing be used as the initial laboratory study for GER.[9]

Other gastrointestinal problems in BTHS include severe constipation in 54% of infants and young children[4] and, later in childhood and adolescence, obesity relative to the individuals' short stature.

Management

When GER is demonstrated, conservative measures are first used, including positioning the infant after feedings prone on a Herbst board with a 30° elevation.[13] The efficacy of thickened feedings has been disputed,[14] since this practice may be associated with occult GER of long duration. Bethanechol (Urecholine®) has been employed to control reflux.[15] If delayed gastric emptying is documented, a trial of metaclopromide (Reglan®) may be employed[6]; however, one study suggested that this regimen increased GER.[16] If esophagitis is documented, antacids (e.g., Maalox®)[17] and cimetidine may be considered.[6,18]

If medical measures have been exhausted and are not successful, a number of surgical procedures for GER may be attempted.[19] Nissen fundoplicaton with a feeding gastrostomy tube placement is often used. The gastrostomy tube also serves as a release valve to prevent distention (gas bloat) that may occur after the surgical procedure. The gastrostomy tube may be removed after several months if oral feedings are successful.

Follow-up

Complications of Nissen fundoplication for GER, which may require a reoperation, have included prolapse into the mediastinum of the fundoplication, intestinal obstruction, and esophageal stricture.[20] The incidence of postoperative complications was highest in children with mental retardation.[20] On long-term follow-up, complications included gas bloat,

inability to vomit, slow eating habits, and choking on solids[21] (see Chapter 24).

Severe constipation also has been a major challenge to overcome in infants and children with BTHS. The risk of relative obesity should be anticipated and prevented, if possible, or dealt with by weight reduction (see Chapters 19 and 35). Monitoring growth and weight is essential.

References

1. Rubinstein, J.H., Taybi, H. Broad thumbs and toes and facial abnormalities: a possible mental retardation syndrome. *Am. J. Dis. Child.* 1963; 105:588.
2. Matsoukas, J. Fatherhood of the so-called Rubinstein-Taybi syndrome. *Am. J. Dis. Child.* 1973; 126:860.
3. Michail, J., Matsoukas, J., Théodorou, S. Pouce bot arqué en forte abduction-extension et autres symptomes concomitants. *Rev. Chir. Orthop.* 1957; 43:142.
4. Rubinstein, J.H. Broad thumb-hallux (Rubinstein-Taybi) syndrome (1957–1988). *Am. J. Med. Genet.* 1990; 6:3.
5. Grunow, J.E. Case report: gastroesophageal reflux in Rubinstein-Taybi syndrome. *J. Pediatr. Gastroenterol. Nutr.* 1982; 1:273.
6. Orenstein, S.R., Orenstein, D.M. Gastroesophageal reflux and respiratory disease in children. *J. Pediatr.* 1988; 112:847.
7. Stirt, J.A. Anesthetic problems in Rubinstein-Taybi syndrome. *Anesth. Analg.* 1981; 60:534.
8. Paton, J.Y., Nanayakkhara, C.S., Simpson, H. Vomiting and gastro-oesophageal reflux. *Arch. Dis. Child.* 1988; 63:837.
9. Da Dalt, L., Mazzoleni, S., Montini, G., Donzelli, F., Zacchello, F. Diagnostic accuracy of pH monitoring in gastro-oesophageal reflux. *Arch. Dis. Child.* 1989; 64:1421.
10. Sondheimer, J.M. Gastroesophageal reflux: update on pathogenesis and diagnosis. *Pediatr. Clin. North Am.* 1988; 35:103.
11. Meyers, W.F., Roberts, C.C., Johnson, D.G., Herbst, J.J. Value of tests for evaluation of gastroesophageal reflux in children. *J. Pediatr. Surg.* 1985; 20:515.
12. Kumar, D., Brereton, R.J., Spitz, L., Hall, C.M. Gastro-oesophageal reflux and intestinal malrotation in children. *Br. J. Surg.* 1988; 75:533.
13. Meyers, W.F., Herbst, J.J. Effectiveness of positioning therapy for gastroesophageal reflux. *Pediatrics.* 1982; 69:768.
14. Vandenplas, Y., Sacré, L. Mild-thickening agents as a treatment for gastroesophageal reflux. *Clin. Pediatr.* 1987; 26:66.
15. Herbst, J.J. Gastroesophageal reflux. *J. Pediatr.* 1981; 98:859.
16. Machida, H.M., Forbes, D.A., Gall, D.G., Scott, R.B. Metoclopramide in gastroesophageal reflux of infancy. *J. Pediatr.* 1988; 112:483.
17. Sutphen, J.L., Dillard, V.L., Pipan, M.E. Antacid and formula effects on gastric acidity in infants with gastroesophageal reflux. *Pediatrics.* 1986; 78:55.
18. Cucchiara, S., Staiano, A., Romaniello, G., Capobianco, S., Auricchio, S. Antacids and cimetidine treatment for gastro-oesophageal reflux and peptic oesophagitis. *Arch. Dis. Child.* 1984; 59:842.
19. Johnson, D.G. Current thinking on the role of surgery in gastroesophageal reflux. *Pediatr. Clin. North Am.* 1985; 32:1165.
20. Spitz, L., Kirtane, J. Results and complications of surgery for gastro-oesophageal reflux. *Arch. Dis. Child.* 1985; 60:743.
21. Harnsberger, J.K., Corey, J.J., Johnson, D.G., Herbst, J.J. Long-term follow-up of surgery for gastroesophageal reflux in infants and children. *J. Pediatr.* 1983; 102:505.

Chapter 49
Celiac Disease

James Heubi and Deborah Gregg

Celiac disease or gluten-sensitive enteropathy was first described by Samuel Gee in 1888. Although presentation with signs and symptoms of disease most commonly occurs in the first 5 years of life, patients of all ages may present for evaluation. Symptoms in toddlers typically appear 4 months or more after introduction of gluten-containing products in the diet, including oats, wheat, rye, and barley. Diarrhea, poor weight gain or weight loss, abdominal pain, anorexia or excess appetite, and occasionally constipation are found in affected children. Clinical findings include abdominal distention, muscle wasting, growth (weight for height) impairment, and, less commonly, finger clubbing and long eyelashes. In older children, growth stunting and delayed pubertal development may be prominent clinical findings.

The incidence of celiac disease varies throughout the world. The highest incidence of 1 per 597 is found in Western Ireland, whereas in the United States and England, the incidence is approximately 1 in 3000. The incidence of celiac disease may be increasing as suggested by a Swedish study in which it was shown that the incidence was 0.31 cases per 1000 infants at age two years in 1970 versus 2.93 per 1000 in 1988.[1] Celiac disease commonly occurs in multiple family members. Intestinal biopsies may identify mucosal abnormalities in 5% to 10% of first-degree relatives. Histocompatibility antigen HLA-B8 is found in 60% to 90% of affected patients (versus 10% to 20% controls), whereas HLA-DR3 is found in 80% (20% to 30% controls). Between 1.5% and 3.5% of patients with type I diabetes mellitus also have celiac disease.[2-5]

Biochemical and Clinical Abnormalities

Only small intestinal biopsy can verify the diagnosis of celiac disease. In patients with untreated celiac disease, a small intestinal biopsy typically shows the loss of normal villus architecture, elongation of the crypts, shortening of the epithelial cell height, and a plasma cell and lymphocyte infiltration of the lamina propria. To confirm the diagnosis, the patient must have another biopsy after consuming a gluten-free diet for 6 months or longer. At that time, symptoms should have resolved, and there should be improved weight gain, reduced irritability, and resolution of diarrhea. Histological features of mucosal injury should be replaced by normal-appearing villus architecture, normalization of enterocyte height, and reduction in the lamina propria infiltrate. Some physicians recommend rechallenge with gluten to confirm the diagnosis, but others find rechallenge unnecessary and sometimes confusing since sensitivity to glu-

ten varies among individuals and years may be required before relapse can be documented (Fig. 49-1).

Screening tests may not be particularly effective in deciding who should undergo intestinal biopsy. Fecal fat measurements may be normal in as many as one-half of patients with celiac disease, and increased fat excretion is a nonspecific finding. Red blood cell folate concentration, anemia, and hypoalbuminemia are likewise nonspecific and do not improve identification of affected subjects. The D-xylose absorption test is considered to be the most sensitive screening test for celiac disease; however, false-negative tests are found in as many as 30% of subjects.[6] Tests measuring antigliadin and antiendomysial antibodies appear especially valuable for screening populations of suspected celiacs, including children with idiopathic short stature and diabetes mellitus.[7,8] Cacciari et al.[9] have found that 8.3% of 60 patients with idiopathic short stature without symptoms had celiac disease. In a similar population, Groll et al.[10] found celiac disease in 21% of 32 English children with short stature. Although there appear to be relatively few false-negative results, false-positive results are found in approximately 10% to 20% of patients with other gastrointestinal diseases.[10,11] In addition, measurement of antigliadin antibodies may be useful in assessing response to a gluten-free diet and gluten challenge.[12]

Etiology

Two theories have been proposed to explain the susceptibility of certain individuals to gluten-containing products: metabolic defect and immunological abnormality. Originally, it was believed that the absence of a specific detoxifying enzyme for gluten resulted in the accumulation of toxic material and ultimately destruction of the mucosal lining. Although peptidase deficiencies have been identified within the damaged mucosa, none has been found after resolution of histological injury. In recent years, the immunological theory of the disease has gained increasing support. A number of observations have given strong support to this theory: (1) antigliadin antibodies are found in the serum of untreated patients, but disappear with treatment, (2) circulating immune complexes with deposition in mucosa are found in celiac patients, (3) mucosa from celiacs produces macrophage-inhibition factor, and (4) organ cultures of celiac patients produce mucosa with active disease improves morphology and a rise in alkaline phosphatase. When the mucosa of patients in remission is incubated with gluten, no change is seen. When mucosa in remission and relapse are co-incubated, alkaline phosphatase activity does not rise in remission mucosa from celiac patients, and when cortisol is

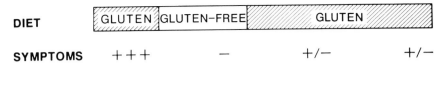

Fig. 49–1. The clinical and intestinal morphological response to a gluten-containing and gluten-free diet in a patient with celiac disease. Specific attention should be focused on the variable sensitivity to gluten as illustrated during rechallenge with gluten-containing foods.

added to the incubation media, the toxic effect of gluten is eliminated.

Factors to be Considered in Nutritional Evaluation

The disease affects the small bowel in the proximal-to-distal gradient, with most disease activity located where the mucosa has the most exposure to gluten-containing products. As a consequence of the mucosal injury, excess fluid and electrolytes may be lost. More importantly, excess protein loss and fat malabsorption are present in approximately 50% of patients. Secondary lactase deficiency may cause lactose malabsorption, and folate and iron levels may be reduced, resulting in mild-to-moderate anemia. Finally, fat-soluble vitamin deficiency may coexist, with the most serious acute consequence being hypoprothrombinemia and attendant bleeding risk.

Dietary Management

The mainstay of therapy is dietary. A strict gluten-free diet is essential for healing of the intestinal mucosa. Gluten is an elastic protein found in cereal grains that gives cohesiveness to dough. It is the gliadin fraction of gluten that is not tolerated by celiacs. Gliadin is found in wheat, barley, oats, and rye, and these grains must be eliminated from the diet (Table 49–1).

Initially lactose may need to be restricted until intestinal lactase activity increases. Milk and other dairy products may need to be limited during the first months after diagnosis. If fat malabsorption is a problem, a low-fat diet may be considered, which may help minimize stool fat loss. A fat-controlled diet emphasizes lean meats; low-fat milk; avoidance of fried foods, cream sauces, and gravies; and restriction of butter and margarine to 3 tsp/day. Since the absorptive lining of the intestine has been destroyed, the absorption of any nutrients, including iron, folic acid, and vitamins A, D, B_{12}, B_6, and K, have decreased, and thus, supplemental vitamins and minerals are recommended. Supplemental folate and iron may be necessary, and intramuscular vitamin K_1 should be administered if hypoprothrombinemia is present.

In most cases, the appetite improves with the initiation of a gluten-free diet, and weight gain occurs. It may take several months before good health is experienced, although irritability in children commonly improves within 1–2 weeks and diarrhea resolves in 4–6 weeks. The gluten-free diet must be followed strictly for the rest of the patient's life as celiac disease is a lifelong illness. It is important to remember that every patient has a different sensitivity to gluten, with affected children being more sensitive than adults. Even trace amounts of gliadin may destroy the villi every time the intestine is exposed. Regeneration of the villi will be more difficult with periodic gluten exposure, and normal absorption may not return completely in adults diagnosed later in life.[13]

In addition to food products made from wheat, barley, oats, and rye, gliadin-containing additives need to be avoided. These incidental ingredients include vegetable protein or hydrolyzed vegetable protein (HVP), malt or malt flavoring, modified starch, vegetable gum, and mono- and diglycerides. Soy sauce usually is made with wheat. Most commercial corn and rice cereals contain malt that is usually derived from barley or barley malt syrup. It is essential that all labels on prepared foods be carefully reviewed because many processed foods use cereal, flour, or gliadin-containing ingredients in their preparation. Also, all medications and over-the-counter drugs should be checked because they may contain wheat starch as a filler. Information can be obtained from pharmacists or drug companies. Thus, if any ingredient is questionable, the manufacturer should be contacted, and the product should be avoided until verification that it is gluten-free.

Several cookbooks and diet information sources are available for patients and/or parents:

- *What's Cooking with Cincinnati Celiacs Cookbook and Information Packet.* The Cincinnati Celiac Society, Clinical Research Center, Children's Hospital Medical Center, Cincinnati, OH 45229-2899.
- *Celiac Disease Needs a Diet for Life* and quarterly newsletters. Canadian Celiac Association National Office, 1087 Meyerside Drive, Suite #5, Mississauga, Ontario L5T 1M5, Canada.
- *Gluten-Free Diet.* CRC Dietitians, Clinical Research Center, University of Michigan Hospitals, University Hospital 7A118/0108, 1500 E. Medical Center Drive, Ann Arbor, MI 48109-0108.
- *Gluten-Intolerance Group Cookbook*, patient packet, diet instruction, fact sheet, and quarterly newsletters. The Gluten Intolerance Group of North America, P.O. Box 23053, Seattle, WA 98102-0353.

Table 49–1. Gluten-Free Diet*

Types of Foods and Amounts	Foods to Include	Foods to Avoid
Soups As desired	Homemade broth and unthickened vegetable soups; cream soups prepared with cornstarch, rice, potato, or soy bean flour	All canned, frozen, or dry soups containing gluten, noodle soups, canned soups,† bouillon, commercial thickened soup
Meat and meat substitutes 2–3 servings	Fresh meat, poultry, seafood; plain unbreaded frozen meats, fish, or poultry; canned fish in oil or water; natural or cream cheese; pure peanut butter; plain dried beans or peas; eggs	Prepared meats that contain wheat, rye, oats, or barley, such as sausage,† bologna,† luncheon meats,† chili,† meatloaf,† hamburger with cereal filler,† stews with noodles or dumplings, sandwich spreads;† pasteurized cheese spreads;† canned baked beans;† cottage cheese;† tuna in vegetable broth; fondue, creamed eggs, or souffles unless prepared with allowed flours
Potato and potato substitutes 1 or more servings	White or sweet potato; yams; white, brown or wild rice; hominy; Aproten® pasta and other brands	Creamed or escalloped potatoes unless prepared with allowed flours; macaroni, noodles, ravioli, spaghetti, lasagna, or vermicelli; commercial potato salad;† packaged rice and potato mixes;† dumplings; fritters
Vegetables 2 or more servings	All plain, fresh, frozen, canned (include a dark-green or deep-yellow vegetable daily for a source of vitamin A)	Breaded, creamed, or escalloped unless prepared with allowed flours; commercially prepared vegetables or salads†
Breads 3 or more servings	Breads or muffins made from rice flour, corn flour, tapioca flour, potato flour, soybean flour, and/or arrowroot flour; rice wafers or sticks (usually available at Oriental specialty stores); pure corn tortillas; gluten-free bread mixes; Ener-G Foods gluten-free breads	All bread, crackers, and products containing wheat, rye, barley, oats, bran, graham, wheat germ, quinoa, millet, malt, kasha, amaranth, pastry flour, durham flour, or bulgar; rye krisp, rusks, zwieback, pretzels; bread or cracker crumbs; wheat starch (contains protein fractions); communion wafers
Cereals 1 or more servings	ONLY puffed rice, pure corn meal, rice, hominy grits, hominy, cream of rice, puffed rice; Kellogg's Sugar Pops®; Post's Fruity and Cocoa Pebbles®; Health Valley's Golden Corn Lites®, Brown Rice Lites®, Brown Rice Fruit Lites™, and Golden Corn Fruit Lites™; General Mill's Cocoa Puffs®	Cereals made from wheat, rye, oats, or barley, such as cream of wheat, farina, Grape Nuts®, oatmeal, Ralston®, Wheatena®, pablum, wheat germ, granola, muesli.† Cereals with malt or malt flavoring, such as cornflakes, and Rice Krispies®
Fats As desired	Butter, cream, margarine, vegetable oils, animal fat, pure mayonnaise; homemade salad dressings and gravies prepared with allowed ingredients; bacon	Commercially prepared salad dressings, cream sauces, and gravies containing gluten stabilizers or thickened with gluten-containing flours;† shortenings†
Fruits 2 or more servings	Fresh, frozen, canned, or dried; fruit juices (include 1 serving citrus fruit or juice daily for a source of vitamin C)	Fruits prepared with wheat, rye, oats, or barley; commercially thickened fruits or pie fillings†
Desserts As desired	Homemade cakes, cookies, pastries, pies, puddings, prepared with allowed ingredients; gelatin desserts, meringues, custard, fruit ices and whips	Commercial cakes, cake decorations, cookies, pies, doughnuts, pastries, puddings, pie crust, ice cream cones; prepared mixes containing wheat, rye, oats, or barley; icing mixes. Ice cream and sherbet containing gluten stabilizers†
Milk 2 or more cups	Fresh, dry, evaporated, or condensed milk; sweet or sour cream; buttermilk	Malted milk, commercial chocolate drinks with cereal additives, instant milk drinks, cocoa mixes. Ovaltine®, nondairy creamers,† yogurt†
Beverages As desired	Sanka®, pure instant coffee, coffee, tea, carbonated beverages, fruit juices and drinks, cider, frozen lemonade concentrate; rum, tequila and other distilled liquors;† unfortified wine	Fruit punch powders; lager, ale, beer, stout, whiskey, gin, and vodka distilled from grain; Postum®, instant coffee, flavored coffees;† herbal teas with malted barley

Table 49–1. (*Continued*)

Miscellaneous As desired	Salt (iodized), sugar, marmalade, jam, honey, jelly, molasses, pure cocoa, carob, chocolate, coconut, olives, pure fruit syrup, herbs, flavoring extracts, artifical flavoring, food coloring; pure spices, such as cloves, ginger, nutmeg, and cinnamon; cornstarch, cider and wine vinegar, yeast, sodium bicarbonate, cream of tartar, nuts, unflavored popcorn, gluten-free potato and corn chips, dry mustard, monosodium glutamate. Gluten-free stabilizers: carrageenan, carob bean, locust bean, arabic, xanthan, tragacanth and guar gum, and lecithin	Chili seasoning mix,† gravy mixes,† meat sauces,† malt or malt flavoring, hydrolyzed vegetable protein (HVP), vinegar,† distilled or malt vinegar, chewing gum,† catsup,† mustard,† soy sauce,† curry powder,† chili powder,† pickles,† horseradish,† vegetable gum,† nuts with flour coating, modified food starch,† emulsifiers and stabilizers† may be derived from or may contain wheat, rye, oats, or barley

*When dining out, choose foods prepared simply, such as broiled or roasted meats, plain vegetables, and plain salads. Since flour and cereal products are quite often used in the preparation of foods, it is important to be aware of the methods of preparation used, as well as the foods themselves.
†These foods may or may not contain gluten. Check with the manufacturer to determine if food is gluten-free.
Adapted from Pemberton et al.,[14] Rawcliffe & Rolph,[15] Hartsook,[16] and Mercer et al.[17]

- *Delicious and Easy Rice Flour Recipes: A Sequel to Gourmet Food and Wheat-Free Diet, 1981.* Marion Wood, Charles C. Thomas, Publishers, 301 E. Lawrence Avenue, Springfield, IL 62717.
- *Good Food: Gluten-Free.* Hilda C. Hills, Keats Publishing, Inc., 27 Pine Street, Box 876, New Canaan, CT 06840; 1976.
- *Gluten-Intolerance: A Resource Including Recipes.* The Food Sensitivity Series, The American Dietetic Association, 208 South La Salle Street, Suite 1100, Chicago, IL 60604-1003; 1985.
- *Celiac Sprue Enteropathy: Basics for the Gluten-Free Diet, Gluten-Free Commercial Products Booklet, On the Celiac Condition: A Handbook for Celiacs and Their Families*, and quarterly newsletters. CSA/USA, Inc., P.O. Box 31700, Omaha, NE 68131-0700.
- *The Gluten-Free Diet Book.* Peter Rawcliffe, M.D., and Ruth Rolph, S.R.D., Arco Publishing, Inc., 215 Park Avenue South, NY, NY 10003; 1985.
- *Celiac Handbook*, food list, video: "The Celiac Condition." U.K. Holiday Guide, Society Recipe Books and Quarterly Magazine. Coeliac Society Office, P.O. Box 220, High Wycombe, Bucks HP11 2HY, Great Britain.

Commercial gluten-free products can be purchased in local stores or ordered by mail. The following is a list of companies who manufacture these special products and product selections:

- Bread, bread mixes, cookies, doughnuts, and pasta can be ordered from Ener-G Foods, Inc., 5960 First Avenue South, P.O. Box 84487, Seattle, WA 98124-5787; in Washington 1-800-325-9788 or out of state 1-800-331-5222.
- Noodles, bread, muffin, and cake mixes may be purchased from Dietary Specialties, P.O. Box 227, Rochester, NY 14601, 716-263-2787.
- Cereal, catsup, chips, and other snacks are available from Health Valley Foods, 700 Union Street, Montebello, CA 90640, 213-724-2211. These products may be found in grocery stores.
- Cybros Bakery, Inc., P.O. Box 851, Waukesha, Wisconsin 53187, 1-800-241-2360, ext. 292, has rice bread, rolls, and nuggets.

Oriental and specialty sections in grocery stores and health food stores sell gluten-free products, such as rice crackers or cakes, flours, bread mixes, rice products, and bread.

References

1. Ascher, H., Krantz, I., Kistiansson, B. Increasing incidence of coeliac disease in Sweden. *Arch. Dis. Child.* 1991; 66:870.
2. Anderson, C.M. *Paediatric Gastroenterology.* London: Blackwell; 1975.
3. Silverman, A., Roy, C.C. *Pediatric Clinical Gastroenterology.* 3rd ed. St. Louis: CV Mosby; 1983.
4. Thain, M.E., Hamilton, J.R., Ehrlich, R.M. Coexistence of diabetes mellitus and coeliac disease. *J. Pediatr.* 1974; 85:527.
5. Savilahti, E., Simell, O., Koshimies, S., Rilva, A., Akerblom, H.K. Celiac disease in insulin-dependent diabetes mellitus. *J. Pediatr.* 1986; 180:690.
6. Craig, R.M., Atkinson, A.J. Jr. D-xylose testing: a review. *Gastroenterology.* 1988; 95:223.
7. Rich, E.J., Christie, D.L. Anti-gliadin antibody panel and xylose absorption test in screening for celiac disease. *J. Pediatr. Gastroenterol. Nutr.* 1990; 10:174.
8. Rossi, T.M., Kumar, V., Lerner, A., Heitlinger, L.A., Tucker, N., Fisher, J. Relationship of endomysial antibodies to jejunal mucosal pathology: specificity towards both symptomatic and asymptomatic celiacs. *J. Pediatr. Gastroenterol. Nutr.* 1988; 7:858.
9. Cacciari, E., Salardi, S., Lazzazi, R., Collina, A., Pirazzoli, P., Tassoni, D., Biasco, G., Corazza, G.R., Cassio, A. A relationship to consider even in patients with no gastrointestinal tract symptoms. *J. Pediatr.* 1983; 103:708.
10. Groll, A., Candy, D.C.A., Preece, M.A., Tanner, J.M., Harries, J.T. Short stature as the primary manifestation of coeliac disease. *Lancet.* 1980; 2:1097.
11. Bürgin-Wolff, A., Bertele, R.M., Brger, R., Gaze, H., Harms, H.K., Just, M., Khanna, S., Schürmann, K., Signer, E., Tomovic, D. A reliable screening test for childhood celiac disease: fluorescent immunosorbent test for gliadin antibodies. A prospective multicenter study. *J. Pediatr.* 1983; 102:655.
12. Mayer, M., Greco, L., Troncone, R., Grimaldi, M., Pansa, G. Early prediction of relapse during gluten challenge in childhood celiac disease. *J. Pediatr. Gastroenterol. Nutr.* 1989; 8:474.
13. Trier, T.S., Falchuk, Z.M., Carey, M.C., Schreiber, D.S. Celiac sprue and refractory sprue. *Gastroenterology.* 1978; 75:307.
14. Pemberton, C.M., Moxness, K.E., German, M.J., Nelson, J.K., Gastineau, C.F. *Mayo Clinic Diet Manual.* 6th ed. Philadelphia: Decker; 1978.
15. Rawcliffe, P., Rolph, R. *The Gluten-Free Diet Book.* New York: Alco; 1985.
16. Hartsook, E.I. *Gluten-Restricted, Gliadin-Free Diet Instruction.* Seattle: Gluten Intolerance Group of North America; 1987.
17. Mercer, N., Kellogg, N., Hydrick Adair, C.R. *Gluten-Free Diet.* Ann Arbor: Clinical Research Center, University of Michigan Hospitals; 1982.

Chapter 50
Cystic Fibrosis

Melanie Hunt

Landsteiner in 1905 and Garrod and Hurtley in 1912[1] described conditions resembling cystic fibrosis. The disease was recognized as a distinct clinical entity in 1937 when Andersen[2] noted that many infants with a history of repeated chest infections and steatorrhea-like stools died at an early age and that the symptoms were often repeated in the same families. Few children lived beyond the preschool years before the advent of antibiotics and pancreatic enzyme replacements. Now, many patients reach adolescence or adulthood because of improved therapy. However, cystic fibrosis continues to be a lethal disorder of children, adolescents, and young adults.

Cystic fibrosis (CF) is an inherited disorder in which there is a generalized dysfunction of the exocrine glands, resulting in the production of abnormally viscous secretions. These secretions are difficult to clear from the lungs and ductules of other organs and lead to complications, including chronic pulmonary disease, pancreatic exocrine insufficiency, and high sweat electrolytes.[2] Severe liver involvement, heart failure, and cor pulmonale may follow.

Cystic fibrosis is transmitted as a Mendelian recessive trait. It occurs in all races, but is predominantly found in Caucasians of Northwest European descent. The incidence is 1 in 1600–2000 Caucasian live births, in 1 in 17,000 black live births,[3] and is rare in Orientals.[4] Although the specific etiology of CF is not known, the defective gene,[5] discovered in 1989, is located on the long arm of chromosome 7.[6] Significant advances in understanding the cellular defect of CF have been made during the 1980s so that reliable prenatal diagnosis is now possible and improved treatment based on molecular genetics may be anticipated.

Biochemical Abnormalities

The principal biochemical abnormalities are (1) a deficiency of the digestive enzymes—trypsin, lipase, and amylase—in the duodenal contents, (2) decreased bicarbonate in the duodenum, and (3) decreased duodenal bile acid concentrations.[7] Maldigestion and malabsorption occur, and secondary changes may include fat-soluble vitamin deficiency, essential fatty acid deficiency, inadequate production of cholesterol, depressed levels of albumin and urea nitrogen,[8] and lactosuria and sucrosuria.

The presence of increased amounts of albumin in meconium reflects a deficiency of proteolytic enzymes. This abnormality was the basis for a neonatal screening test for CF.[9] The observation that infants with CF have abnormally high levels of serum immunoreactive trypsin (IRT) led to screening studies using dried neonatal blood spots collected for the detection of other inborn errors of metabolism.[10,11] The most useful diagnostic test for CF is the quantitative pilocarpine iontophoretic test in which the amount of sodium and chloride in the sweat is measured. Elevation of sweat electrolytes is indicative of cystic fibrosis. Elevation of sweat chloride concentrations also occurs in adrenal insufficiency, hypothyroidism, some types of ectodermal dysplasia, and a few other rare conditions.

Factors to be Considered in Diagnosis

Individuals with CF can develop abdominal distress, chronic lower respiratory tract infection, wheezing, sinusitis, nasal polyps, unexplained heat prostration, and/or meconium ileus. The Schwachman and Kulczycki[12] clinical evaluation form or the one developed by the Cystic Fibrosis Clinic of the Children's Hospital Medical Center in Cincinnati (Table 50–1) can be used to assess an individual's condition. Physical activity, physical findings, nutritional status, and anthropometric measurements are areas that can be scored easily to determine the degree of involvement at a specific time.

Gastrointestinal involvement

Gastrointestinal symptoms involving the pancreas, liver, and intestines occur in more than 85% of the individuals who have CF.[13] The primary symptoms are distended abdomen; bulky, greasy, foul-smelling stools; cramps; lack of subcutaneous fat; voracious appetite; poor weight gain; poor rate of growth; occasionally, rectal prolapse; enlarged liver; poor muscle tone; jaundice; and edema.

The development and excess accumulation of thick, viscid secretions in the exocrine glands are thought to be responsible for these multiple problems. Obstruction of the pancreatic ducts by the viscous pancreatic secretions interrupts the flow of proenzymes from the pancreas, resulting in pancreatic enzyme deficiency. The inspissated pancreatic enzymes eventually digest part of the pancreas, causing progressive pancreatic fibrosis.

Steatorrhea and loss of nitrogen in stool reflect the disturbance of alimentary absorption. Proteins are usually better tolerated than fats, making nitrogen balance possible through increased dietary intake; however, fats should be used as tolerated. Utilization of carbohydrates is less impaired. The absorption of liposoluble vitamins varies, and deficiency of vitamins A, D, E, and K may occur. Retardation in physical growth secondary to malabsorption was suggested by Sproul and Huang,[14] even though in their study

Table 50–1. Clinical Evaluation Sheet

Name: _____ C.H. No. _____ Date: _____ Age: _____

A. 1. Height _____ Percentile _____ Ht., wt., above 25th %ile (3) 10–25th (2) Total Score _____

    2. Weight _____ Percentile _____   3–10th (1) below 3rd %ile (0)

    3. Pulse, resting   Normal (4) Sl. Elev. (3) Moderate elev. (2) Tachycardia (1)

    4. Respiration, resting   Normal (4) Sl. Elev. (3) Moderate elev. (2) Tachypnea (1)

    5. Muscle mass and tone   Good (4) Fair (3) Poor (2) Weak, flabby (1)

    6. Subcutaneous fat   Normal (5) Slight decrease (4) Moderate deficiency (3) Marked defic. (2) Absent (1)

    7. Posture

| Good (4) | Moderate rounding of shoulders (3) | Rounded shoulders, forward head (2) | Poor (1) |

    8. Clubbing   None (5) + to +1 (4) 1+–2+ (3) 2+–3+ (2) 3+–4+ (1)

    9. Lungs

| Clear (5) | Occasional harsh sounds (4) | Occasional rales, rhonchi (3) |

| Rales, rhonchi, wheezing usually present (2) | Generalized fine and course rales, rhonchi (1) |

   10. Sexual maturation   Normal (5) Sl. retarded (4) Definitely retarded (3) Failure (1)

   11. Abdominal status   Normal (5) Sl. distention (3) Moderate distension (2) Large, protuberant (1)

   12. Cyanosis   None (5) Usually (2) Always (1)

B. 1. Activity   Full (5) Slight limitation (4) Moderate limitation (2) Severe limitation (1)

    2. Exercise tolerance/endurance   Normal (4) Tires after exertion (3) Dyspneic after exertion (2)

Dyspnea and orthopnea (1)

    3. Motor development   Normal (5) Low normal (4) Slight retardation (3) Moderate retardation (2)

Marked retardation (1)

    4. Personality/disposition   Normal (4) Occasionally irritable (3) Fussy, irritable (2) Irritable or apathetic (1)

    5. School attendance   Good (4) Fair (3) Poor (2) Cannot attend (1)

    6. Cough   None (5) Occasional (4) Chronic in morning or after exertion (3)

| Chronic, repetitive frequent (2) | Severe, paroxysmal with vomiting or hemoptysis (1) |

    7. Appetite   Excellent (4) Normal (3) Fair (2) Poor (1)

    8. Stools

| Well formed, normal (5) | Frequent, slightly abnormal (4) | Abnormal, large, float but formed (3) |

| Bulky, poorly formed, foul (2) | Bulky, frequent, fatty, foul (1) |

C. Chest

    1. Overinflation   None (5) Minimal (4) Moderate (3) Marked (2) Severe (1)

    2. Marking increases   None (5) Mild (4) Moderate (3) Extensive (2) Severe (1)

    3. Infiltration or atelectasis   None (5) Occasional (3) Persistent (1)

Designed for the Cystic Fibrosis Clinic, Children's Hospital Medical Center, Cincinnati, OH.

there was a lack of correlation between the degree of growth retardation and degree of measurable pancreatic deficiency. Approximately 15% of affected individuals over 18 years of age have inflammation of the pancreas and develop diabetes mellitus.[15]

Intestinal malabsorption is associated with the accumulation of bulky and sticky intestinal contents, which can cause intestinal blockage, known during the neonatal period as "meconium ileus" or in the older patient as "meconium ileus equivalent." Meconium ileus occurs in 10% to 15% of the infants with CF, and the obstruction must be corrected promptly, usually by surgery. Problems that may occur at any age include intussusception due to fecal impaction, rectal prolapse due to malnutrition and mucosal abnormalities, and constipation because of intestinal dysmotility.

Hepatobiliary disease is another complication of CF. The pathogenesis is not understood, but inspissated bile that plugs the bile ductules is thought to be a contributory factor.[16] Depending on the type of disease, the condition can manifest in a variety of ways, i.e., bile acid deficiency, cholesterol gallstone formation, jaundice, and/or cirrhosis. Focal biliary cirrhosis is not unusual in older children or adolescents who have CF and is often asymptomatic. Portal hypertension with splenomegaly, ascites, lower extremity edema, and bleeding from esophogeal varices can be sequelae. Any of these problems compound those already associated with maldigestion and malabsorption.

Loss of sodium and chloride in sweat

CF subjects have excessive sweat salt loss, a process that is accentuated by fever, increased activity, or a warm environment. These characteristics of the disease allow for easy determination of sodium or chloride content of sweat by a quick procedure that causes minimal discomfort to the individual. Sweat is collected from an area of the skin that has been made to sweat profusely by pilocarpine iontophoresis. It is then analyzed for salt content. Levels of sodium and chloride above 60 mEq/L in eccrine sweat are consistent with the diagnosis of CF.

Pulmonary involvement

The respiratory system is usually the principal focus for medical treatment and research as pulmonary involvement is often extensive and the chronic lung disease is life threatening. The respiratory involvement is the result of airway obstruction caused by an accumulation of secretions and infection. This sets in motion a cycle of inflammation, more obstruction, and more inflammation, with long-term consequences of destructive changes in the airways, alveoli, and interstitium of the lung.[3] Pulmonary symptoms include increased respiratory rate, cough, increased sputum production, decreased activity, wheezing, cyanosis, digital clubbing, emphysema, and barrel chest deformity.

Factors to be Considered in Nutritional Evaluation

Cystic fibrosis is a multifaceted disease that confronts families with monumental financial obligations, frequent emotional stresses, and an inordinate amount of time and effort required to care for the individual who has CF. Treatment frequently includes aerosol therapy, postural drainage, chest physical therapy, supplemental vitamins, supplemental pancreatic enzymes, repetitive clinic visits, hospitalizations, and nocturnal feedings. All aspects of treatment must be considered when prescribing a diet for the child or adult with CF to avoid an atmosphere of guilt, anxiety, or antagonism. However, at least one investigator who studied the psychosocial functioning of malnourished CF patients and their families concluded "that the parents of children with CF function well, with little overt distress despite their many burdens."[17]

Supplemental nutrition

Most nutritionists, clinicians, and patients agree that supplemental nutrition is an important component of treating the individual with CF; determining at what point aggressive supplemental therapy should occur or at what point it should be discontinued is more difficult. Shepherd et al.[18] suggested that total body potassium (TBK), a noninvasive procedure for measuring functional tissue growth, may be a feasible and useful tool for deciding when aggressive therapy should be used. Another valuable clinical research technique is the measurement of total body nitrogen (TBN). Baur et al. discuss how this method can be used to "define the degree of protein depletion associated with malnutrition or to guide protein repletion during nutritional rehabilitation programs."[19] With an objective measure such as this, one may then be able to determine what kind of supplemental nutrition and how much would be most beneficial to the individual.

Formulas were developed during the 1970s, first in England and then in the United States, which modified specific nutrients and enhanced digestion and absorption. Allan et al.[20] recommended a formula of beef serum protein hydrolysate, medium-chain triglyceride (MCT), and modified starch, containing 4–6 glucose units, for CF patients to be used in addition to a regular diet. The diet and formula increased the growth and well-being of the children. Previously, MCT oil had been substituted for long-chain fats, but no significant increase in growth rate occurred.[21] In 1975, Berry et al.[8] reported on the use of a complete dietary supplement consisting of a beef serum hydrolysate, a glucose polymer, and MCT oil in 15 patients. The formula contained 55% to 70% of the calories as carbohydrates, 14% to 16% as amino acids, and 20% to 30% as fat. These ingredients were mixed with appropriate liquids and taken in 2 to 3 fluid ounce quantities, six to eight times daily, depending on the age of the patient. This formula was used in addition to the patient's regular diet. Patients who received the formula showed significant gain in weight, increased serum albumin, increased clinical score, and a significant drop in white blood cell count when compared to patients who did not take the supplement. Farrell et al.[22] also assessed the growth rates of CF patients fed different diets. They concluded that the regular use of a formula, such as Pregestimil, in infants promoted improved growth and permitted normalization of weight by 1 year of age.[22]

Essential fatty acids promote growth, are important in cell membrane structure, are converted into prostaglandins, and affect smooth muscle regulation.[23] Because of defective digestion and absorption of fat, linoleic acid deficiency is a common finding in CF patients, and correction of the deficiency may prevent some of the manifestations of the disease.[24] Hunt et al.[25] demonstrated that the use of an oral sonicated emulsion of safflower oil was an effective and inexpensive way to increase serum linoleic acid levels; Mischler et al.[26] made a similar observation.

The use of elemental, semi-elemental, or nonelemental (with supplemental pancreatic enzymes) formula increases the amount of protein and calories consumed by the patients. These formulas are usually taken as oral feedings during the day. However, if more calories and protein are needed than the individual can easily take while awake, the formula can be administered via nocturnal tube feeding. The type of tube used, whether nasogastric or jejunostomy, is a matter of individual preference.

Boland et al.[27] reported the successful use of nocturnal jejunostomy feeding of a nonelemental formula (Isocal® by Mead Johnson in Belleville, Canada or Ensure® by Ross Laboratories in Montreal, Canada), with added powdered pancreatic enzymes, in undernourished CF patients. All patients gained weight, had significant increase in weight for height, and had improved midarm muscle circumference. The approach by O'Loughlin and Forbes[28] was slightly different in that they recommended nocturnal use of a semi-synthetic formula (Vital® by Ross Laboratories in Montreal, Canada) via nasogastric tube. Their results were similar: weight gain was achieved in a majority of the patients and was associated with an increase in lean body mass, total body fat, and height velocity. Moore et al.[29] evaluated patients who had taken an elemental formula (Criticare HN® by Mead Johnson in Evansville, IN) as a nocturnal nasogastric feeding. This type of formula yielded an increase in energy intake, with concomitant increases in serum transferrin and retinol-binding protein and improved clinical scores.[29]

Perhaps Pelekanos et al.[30] summarize these conclusions best with their study, which analyzed protein turnover in CF individuals who were infused in random sequence with a semi-elemental formula (Criticare®, Mead Johnson, Evansville, IN), a nonelemental formula (Traumacal®, Mead Johnson) and a modified nonelemental formula (Modified Traumacal®, Mead Johnson). They found that the net protein deposition was greater in these subjects during the period when the nonelemental formula was used and concluded that the provision of calories was more important in protein accretion than the nature of the protein.[30]

As the CF individual becomes more debilitated with increased lung function deterioration, the ability to excrete the carbon dioxide load associated with eating is lost.[31] Michel and Mueller[32] recommend that food supplements that are rich in carbohydrate be limited once the patient reaches this stage of disease. However, one way to compensate for part of this phenomenon is to extend the feeding time by using an enterostomy tube.

Nocturnal tube feeding is an effective method for promoting growth. The patient is able to eat a regular diet during the day without the interference of nutritional supplements. Supplemental pancreatic enzymes are used with meals, but may not be necessary with some of the elemental or semi-elemental formulas. Weight gain and improved nu-

tritional status that have occurred during the period of nocturnal feedings may not be sustained if the night feedings are curtailed. Although pulmonary function may not be favorably altered, the use of nocturnal feedings is warranted if the patient gains weight, has improved sense of well-being, and has decreased frequency of illness.

Supplemental pancreatic enzymes

Two types of supplemental pancreatic enzymes are available: pancrelipase and pancreatin. Pancrelipase is derived from porcine pancreas. It contains not less than 24 USP units each of amylase and protease activity per milligram. Most of the supplemental pancreatic enzymes used in treating CF are pancrelipase. Pancreatin may be derived from either bovine or porcine pancreas. This supplement contains not less than 2 USP units of lipase activity and not less than 25 USP units each of amylase and protease activity per milligram.[33] Pancrelipase and pancreatin exert their primary effects of the duodenum and upper jejunum.

The purpose of the supplemental pancreatic enzymes is to aid digestion, and they should be given only with meals and formula. The amount of enzymes needed varies and is dependent upon the amounts of food eaten. Initially 1000 to 2000 IU's of lipase per 120 mL of formula (predigested formula, breast milk, or infant formula) may be recommended. The efficacy of supplemental pancreatic enzymes is not questioned. These products have evolved from a powder form, in which the enzyme activity was easily destroyed by moisture, heat, or gastric juices, to the current products, which are enteric-coated pH-sensitive microspheres. The enteric-coated microspheres, which dissolve in a pH over 5.5, do not completely correct the problem associated with malabsorption, but do improve the dyspeptic symptoms and decrease stool frequency.[35]

Supplemental vitamins and minerals

Vitamin and mineral deficiencies are rare in normal individuals but those with cystic fibrosis are at risk to develop one or more deficiencies because of maldigestion and malabsorption. For this reason, multivitamins in a water-miscible form are prescribed. The usual dosage for supplemental vitamins is twice the normal recommendations.

The fat-soluble vitamins are routinely prescribed for CF patients, usually as part of a multivitamin, and additional vitamin E may be given at 25 IU at 0–6 months to 200–400 IU after 10 years of age in a water soluble form.[34] Vitamin A helps the patient resist infection and should be given in a 5000 IU daily dosage.[34] Vitamin E protects vitamins A[36] and C and polyunsaturated fats from degradation. Vitamin K absorption from the intestine may be impaired because of abnormal bile production and altered intestinal flora caused by the daily use of antibiotics; however, supplemental vitamin K is only recommended if the individual has biliary cirrhosis, portal hypertension, or hemoptysis. If needed, Vitamin K supplementation is recommended at 2.5 mg/wk 0–12 months and 5.0 mg/wk after one year. Vitamin D should be given as a 400 IU daily dose (which is usually in the multivitamin).[34] Although an effort is made to prevent fat-soluble vitamin deficiencies, one must not forget that a fat-soluble vitamin toxicity might occur if massive pharmacological doses are used. Consequently, the patient's clinical status must be monitored closely when attempting to correct a deficiency state.[37]

Deficiencies of water-soluble vitamins are not a primary consideration in treating CF. However, vitamin C needs may be increased because of frequent pulmonary infection, and the supplemental pancreatic enzymes may decrease absorption of vitamin B_{12}. In 1986, Faraj et al.[38] conducted a study in which they demonstrated that pyridoxal-5'-phosphate (PLP) deficiency occurred in patients with CF. They found that good patient management and administration of a multivitamin did not ensure adequate levels of vitamin B_6 and concluded that the defect could be due either to an acquired or inherited defect in metabolism associated with cystic fibrosis.

Mineral deficiencies are seldom observed in CF patients. However, Ehrhardt et al.[39] observed that 32% of their study patients had low serum ferritin concentrations, which did not correlate with Schwachman score, Chrispin-Norman scores, or *Pseudomonas* infection. They concluded that the conflicting evidence about iron utilization, especially as it relates to bacterial infection and CF, necessitated iron supplementation for those who appear to be iron deficient. Most CF clinics routinely supplement the diet with iron.

Other supplemental minerals are not usually given, but several should be considered. Fluoride supplements are given to patients in geographic regions that do not have fluoride in the water. Zinc is essential for growth and wound healing and may be limited because supplemental pancreatic enzymes can inhibit absorption of this mineral. Selenium is not well absorbed by CF patients, but supplementation is not recommended because of toxicity.

Dietary Management

Alterations in diet can lessen digestive disturbance; improve the absorption of fat, protein, and carbohydrate; reduce the frequency and bulkiness of stools; decrease the risk of rectal prolapse; and improve linear growth and weight gain. Proper and adequate nutrition for patients with CF is essential, but one must keep in perspective the role of diet. The complexity of care often means that nutritional goals are difficult to attain.

Individuals who have CF require a diet that is both high in calories and high in protein to meet basic metabolic and energy needs as affected by activity, infections, and growth. Because of maldigestion and malabsorption, the recommended daily allowances may be inadequate for individuals with CF. Consequently, an energy intake about 150% of the RDA is recommended; however, many children with CF do well with a lower energy intake.[40] The Cystic Foundation[34] developed a concensus regarding assessment: if the current weight-height index is <85% of ideal weight, enteral supplementation is indicated, and if <75% of ideal weight enteral feedings or total parenteral nutrition are needed. The daily energy requirement can be calculated as:

$$\text{Daily energy requirements in joules} = \frac{\text{kcal/day}}{4.180} =$$

* basal metabolic rate (BMR)
$\times$ activity level (low 1.3 to high 1.7)
$+$ lung disease (mild 0.1 to severe 0.5)
$\times$ pancreatic sufficient coefficient of fat absorption (0.93)/coefficient of fat absorption as fraction of fat intake if collected or 0.85.
* see Table 4–9 (Chapter 4) to calculate body weight from BMR.

The problems associated with fat malabsorption have always been recognized for these patients, but of equal importance are the consequences of protein and carbohydrate malabsorption. Shohl et al.[41] demonstrated in 1943 that children with CF frequently excrete excess nitrogen in their stools if diets containing whole protein and fat were consumed, and disaccharide intolerance,[42,43] particularly of lactose, has been documented in these patients.

A satisfactory diet is one that provides a good selection of fruits, vegetables, meat, dairy products, and grains and is supplemented with a partially digested formula, such as Vital® or Pregestimil®. This combination of food will meet both psychological and nutritional requirements. However, some groups of food that have a high fat content, are concentrated sources of carbohydrate, or are heavily spiced may need to be limited or omitted from the diet. Part of the enigma of CF is the varying individual response to the foods. If a food is not well tolerated, there may be an increased frequency or bulkiness of bowel movements, abdominal cramping, or increased production of gas. Because foods that are tolerated vary greatly among individuals, new foods should be gradually introduced.

The CF patient with little hunger and a poor appetite is not unusual. In this situation, six to eight small feedings per day can be scheduled. This meal pattern enables the patient to consume more food without feeling too full and enhances the utilization of nutrients. Bizarre eating habits may develop, especially among toddlers and preschoolers, if the patient is allowed to circumvent his or her parents' good intentions. Singer et al.[44] describe how children may develop behavioral feeding disorder not only because of physiological factors but also because of parent-child interaction. Parental anxiety, coaxing and forced-feedings reinforce the child's avoidance to eating. Children who manipulate their parents with food are likely to do so with medications and treatments as well.

Pertinent considerations about the diet are summarized below.

- Broiled, roasted, or stewed meats; fish; and poultry are good sources of protein and calories. Corned beef, hot dogs, lunch-meat, sausage, oil-packed tuna fish, and similar foods may cause discomfort for some because of an increased amount of fat in these products.
- Eggs are an excellent source of protein and cholesterol and should be included in the diet.
- Vegetables and fruits provide fiber, and should be included in the diet each day. The dietary fiber may help decrease the possibility of intestinal impaction. Some vegetables, such as dried beans, dried peas, brussel sprouts, cabbage, cauliflower, corn, greens, and sauerkraut, can cause abdominal distention; use of these foods depends on individual tolerance.

• Homogenized milk is a good source of protein and provides essential fatty acids. Skim milk or 2% milk should be used only if there is obvious intolerance to homogenized milk. Dry skim milk powder (DSMP) is an easy way to increase protein and calories and blends easily with many foods. Four tablespoons of DSMP provides 109 calories and 10.9 g protein.

• High-fat or heavily spiced foods—gravy, peanut butter, margarine or butter, olives, salad dressing, canned fruits, candy, ice cream, rich desserts, potato chips, corn chips, tomato paste, pizzas, and spices similar to those in catsup, chili sauces, horseradish, and relishes—may result in generalized abdominal discomfort and an increased frequency of bowel movements.

Follow-up

The frequency of clinic visits is determined by the age of the child and the severity of disease. The Cystic Fibrosis Foundation[34] concensus recommends early intervention which involves complete anthropometry assessment every three months, nutritional and biochemical assessment at least yearly or more frequently as indicated (this is somewhat similar to the quality assurance criteria by the American Dietetic Association).[46] At each visit, height and weight measurements should be taken. A standard score devised by Sontag and Fels[45] may be calculated by subtracting the child's weight or height from the mean values for a child of the same sex and age and dividing the difference by the standard deviation for the age. This is a useful tool for research purposes as growth rates of children of different ages and sex can be compared on the same scale. Periodically, the physical examination should include an evaluation of criteria for nutrition quality assurance.[46,47] The survival of adolescent and young adult females with CF was significantly lower than of males (perhaps due to the males higher fat free body mass) in one study and may require special follow up care. Resting energy expendtiure also was significantly increased in CF patients when compared to anorexia nervosa and control patients.[48]

Dietary evaluation and suggestions for supplementation should be made frequently, as a lack of understanding or motivation may require innovative nutrition education techniques. Diet records are beneficial in assessing nutritional status; the kind and amount of supplemental pancreatic enzymes used should be noted on the diet records, as should any other kind of supplement. The person keeping the diet record should also note any sign of maldigestion. This data may then be considered with the biochemical and anthropometric data when assessing the nutritional status of these patients.

References

1. Schwachman, H., Barbero, G.J., di Sant'Agnese, P.A., Harrison, G.M., Matthews, L.W., Patterson, P.R. *Guide to Diagnosis and Management of Cystic Fibrosis.* Atlanta: Cystic Fibrosis Foundation; 1977.
2. Andersen, D.H. Cystic fibrosis of the pancreas. *J. Chron. Dis.* 1958; 7:58.
3. Hilman, B.C. Cystis fibrosis—a challenging masquerader. *Clin. Rev. Allerg.* 1983; 1:57.
4. di Sant'Agnese, P. Cystic fibrosis. In: Vaughan, C., III, McKay, J., Behrman, R.E., eds., *Nelson Textbook of Pediatrics.* 11th ed. Philadelphia: W.B. Saunders; 1979.
5. Rommens, J.M., Iannuzzi, M.C., Kerem, B.S., Drumm, M.L., Melmer, G., Dean, M., Rozmahel, R., Cole, J.L., Kennedy, D., Hidaka, N., Zsiga, M., Buchwald, M., Riordan, J.R., Tsui, L.C., Collins, F.S. Identification of the cystic fibrosis gene: chromosome walking and jumping. *Science.* 1989; 245:1059.
6. White, R., Woodward, S., Leppert, M., O'Connell, P., Hoff, M., Herbst, J., Lalouel, J.M., Dean, M., Woude, G.V. A closely linked genetic marker for cystic fibrosis. *Nature.* 1985; 318:381.
7. Sinaasappel, M., Bouquet, J., Neijens, H.J. Problems in the treatment of malabsorption in CF. *Acta Paediatr. Scand.* 1985; 317(suppl):22.
8. Berry, H., Kellogg, F., Hunt, M., Ingberg, R., Richter, L., Gutjahr, C. Dietary supplement and nutrition in children with cystic fibrosis. *Am. J. Dis. Child.* 1975; 129:165.
9. Berry, H.K., Kellogg, F.W., Lichstein, S.R., Ingberg, R.L. Elevated meconium lactase activity. *Am. J. Dis. Child.* 1980; 134:930.
10. Crossley, J.R., Elliott, R.B., Smith, P.A. Dried-blood spot screening for cystic fibrosis in the newborn. *Lancet.* 1979; 1:472.
11. Wilcken, B., Brown, A.R.D., Urwin, R., Brown, D.A. Cystic fibrosis screening by dried blood spot trypsin assay: results in 75,000 newborn infants. *J. Pediatr.* 1983; 102:383.
12. Schwachman, H., Kulczycki, L. Long term study of one hundred five patients with cystic fibrosis. *Am. J. Dis. Child.* 1958; 96:6.
13. Parsons, H.G., Shillabeer, G., Rademaker, A.W. Early onset of essential fatty acid deficiency in patients with cystic fibrosis receiving a semisynthetic diet. *J. Pediatr.* 1984; 105:958.
14. Sproul, A., Huang, N. Growth patterns in children with cystic fibrosis. *J. Pediatr.* 1964; 65:664.
15. Rodman, H.M., Doershuk, C.F., Roland, J.M. The interaction of 2 diseases: diabetes mellitus and cystic fibrosis. *Medicine.* 1986; 65:389.
16. Roy, C.C., Weber, A.M., Morin, C.L., Lepage, G., Brisson, G., Yousef, I., Lasalle, R. Hepatobiliary disease in cystic fibrosis: a survey of current issues and concepts. *J. Pediatr. Gastroenterol. Nutr.* 1982; 1:469.
17. Brennan, J.L., Todd, A.L., Jools, P.A., Gaskin, K.J. Malnutrition in cystic fibrosis: psychosocial functioning of patients and their families. *J. Paediatr. Child. Health.* 1990; 26:36.
18. Shepherd, R.W., Holt, T.L., Greer, R., Cleghorn, G.J., Thomas, B.J. Total body potassium in cystic fibrosis. *J. Pediatr. Gastroenterol. Nutr.* 1989; 9:200.
19. Baur, L.A., Waters, D.L., Allen, B.J., Glagojevic, N., Gaskin, K.J. Nitrogen deposition in malnourished children with cystic fibrosis. *Am. J. Clin. Nutr.* 1991; 53:503.
20. Allan, J.D., Milner, J., Moss, D. Therapeutic use of an artificial diet. *Lancet.* 1970; 1:785.
21. Gracey, M., Burke, V., Anderson, C.M. Assessment of medium-chain triglyceride feeding in infants with cystic fibrosis. *Arch. Dis. Child.* 1969; 44:401.
22. Farrell, P.M., Mischler, E.H., Sondel, S.A., Palta, M. Predigested formula for infants with cystic fibrosis. *J. Am. Diet. Assoc.* 1987; 87:1353.
23. Alfin Slater, R.B., Aftergood, L. Absorption, digestion, and metabolism of lipids. In: Wohl, M.G., Goodhart, R.S., eds. *Modern Nutrition in Health and Disease.* Philadelphia: Lea & Febiger; 1968.
24. Rivers, J.P.W., Hassan, A.G. Defective essential fatty-acid metabolism in cystic fibrosis. *Lancet.* 1975; 2:642.
25. Hunt, M.M., Berry, H.K., Kellogg, F.W. Sonicated emulsion of safflower oil (SESO) in treatment of essential fatty acid deficiency in cystic fibrosis. In: Lawson, D., ed. *Cystic Fibrosis:Horizons.* Proceedings of the 9th International Cystic Fibrosis Congress. Chichester, England: John Wiley and Sons; 1984.
26. Mischler, E.H., Parrell, S.W., Farrell, P.M., Raynor, W.J., Lemen, R.J. Correction of linoleic acid deficiency in cystic fibrosis. *Pediatr. Res.* 1986; 20:36.
27. Boland, M.P., MacDonald, N.E., Stoski, D.S., Soucy, P., Patrick, J. Chronic jejunostomy feeding with a non-elemental formula in undernourished patients with cystic fibrosis. *Lancet.* 1986; 1:232.
28. O'Loughlin, E., Forbes, D., et al. Nutritional rehabilitation of malnourished patients with cystic fibrosis. *Am. J. Clin. Nutr.* 1986; 43:732.
29. Moore, M.C., Greene, H.L., Donald, W.D., Dunn, G.D.

Enteral-tube feeding as adjunct therapy in malnourished patients with cystic fibrosis: a clinical study and literature review. *Am. J. Clin. Nutr.* 1986; 44:33.

30. Pelekanos, J.T., Holt, T.L., Ward, L.C., Cleghorn, G.J., Shepherd, R.W. Protein turnover in malnourished patients with cystic fibrosis: effects of elemental and nonelemental nutritional supplements. *J. Pediatr. Gastroenterol. Nutr.* 1990; 10:339.

31. Boland, M.P., Stoski, D.S., Patrick, J. Long-term nutritional rehabilitation in cystic fibrosis. *J. Pediatr.* 1986; 108:489. Letter.

32. Michel, S.H., Mueller, D.H. Practical approaches to nutrition care of patients with cystic fibrosis. *Top. Clin. Nutr.* 1987; 2:10.

33. Lewis, A.J., Gonzales, G.D. Winek, C.L., eds. *Modern Drug Encyclopedia and Therapeutic Index*, 16th ed. New York: Yorke Medical Books; 1981.

34. Ramsey, B., Farrell, P., Pencharz, P., and Concensus Committee. Nutritional Assessment and management in cystic fibrosis: a Consensus Report. *Am. J. Clin. Nutr.* 1992; 55:108.

35. Petersen, W., Heilmann, C., Garne, S. Pancreatic enzyme supplementation as acid-resistant microspheres versus enteric-coated granules in cystic fibrosis. *Acta Paediatr. Scand.* 1987; 76:66.

36. Ekvall, S., Mitchell, A. The effect of supplemental vitamin E on vitamin A serum levels in cystic fibrosis. *Int. J. Vit. Nutr. Res.* 1978; 48:325.

37. Eid, N.S., Shoemaker, L.R., Samiec, T.D. Vitamin A in cystic fibrosis: case report and review of the literature. *J. Pediatr. Gastroenterol. Nutr.* 1990; 10:265.

38. Faraj, B.A., Caplan, D.B., Camp, V., Pilzer, E., Kutner, M. Low levels of pyridoxal 5'-phosphate in patients with cystic fibrosis. *Pediatrics* 1986; 78:278.

39. Ehrhardt, P., Miller, M.G., Littlewood, J.M. Iron deficiency in cystic fibrosis. *Arch. Dis. Child.* 1987; 62:185.

40. Hubbard, V.S., Mangrum, P.J. Energy intake and nutrition counseling in cystic fibrosis. *J. Am. Diet. Assoc.* 1982; 80:127.

41. Shohl, A.T., May, C.D., Schwachman, H. Studies of nitrogen and fat metabolism on infants and children with pancreatic fibrosis. *J. Pediatr.* 1943; 23:267.

42. Francis, D.E.M. *Diets for Sick Children.* 3rd ed. London: Blackwell Scientific Publications; 1974.

43. Antonowicz, I., Reddy, V., Khaw, K.T., Schwachman, H. Lactase deficiency in patients with cystic fibrosis. *Pediatrics.* 1968; 42:492.

44. Singer, L.T., Nofer, J.A., Benson-Szekely, L.J., Brooks, L.J. Behavioral Assessment and Management of Food Refusal in Children with Cystic Fibrosis. *Dev. Beh. Pediatr.* 1991; 12:115.

45. Sontag, L.W, Reynolds, E.L. The Fels composite sheet. I. A practical method for analyzing growth progress. *J. Pediatr.* 1945; 26:327.

46. Wooldridge, N.H. Pulmonary diseases. In: Wooldridge, N.H., ed., *Quality Assurance Criteria for Pediatric Nutrition Conditions: A Model.* Chicago: American Dietetic Association; 1988.

47. Luder, E. Nutritional care of patients with cystic fibrosis. *Top. Clin. Nutr.* 1991; 6:39.

48. Vaisman, N., Clarke, R., Rossi, M., Goldberg, E., Zello, G., Pencharz, P. Protein turnover and resting energy expenditure in patients with undernutrition and chronic lung disease. *Am. J. Clin. Nutr.* 1992; 55:63.

Chapter 51
Diabetes Insipidus

Barbara Niedbala

Diabetes insipidus is characterized by polyuria and polydipsia resulting from an inability to concentrate urine. There are two forms of this disease: neurogenic diabetes insipidus, for which there is no diet therapy, and nephrogenic diabetes insipidus, in which diet therapy may play a major role. Although characterized by the same symptoms, the two forms of diabetes insipidus have differing etiologies and therefore differing treatments.

Neurogenic Diabetes Insipidus

Neurogenic diabetes insipidus, also termed central diabetes insipidus, results from a partial or total lack of arginine vasopressin (antidiuretic hormone; ADH). ADH is produced in the hypothalamus, stored in the posterior pituitary gland, and acts directly on the distal tubule and collecting ducts of the kidney to facilitate reabsorption of water. Disturbances of the neurohypophyseal unit, such as tumor growth, basal skull fracture, asphyxia, intraventricular hemorrhage, surgical procedures, or infectious lesions,[1,2] may induce diabetes insipidus. The induced diabetes insipidus may be either transient or permanent. Diabetes insipidus is hereditary in some persons.[3] In others, no known etiology is discovered, and it is termed idiopathic diabetes insipidus.[4] The incidence of idiopathic diabetes insipidus is approximately 9%.

Biochemical abnormality

Clinical manifestations of neurogenic diabetes inisipidus in infancy are rapid weight loss, vomiting, constipation, and hyperthermia. The infant may show a quieting response when given water, rather than formula. In the child, neurogenic diabetes insipidus may present as extreme thirst and constant urination, which make play, sleep, and learning difficult. The daily volume of urine is 4–10 liters and is diluted, with a specific gravity of 1.001–1.005 and an osmolality of 50–100 mOsm/kg H_2O.[3] Administration of vasopressin quickly raises urine osmolality.

Factors to be considered in nutritional evaluation

Nutrient needs are unchanged in an infant or child with neurogenic diabetes insipidus, with the exception of the need for water. It is imperative that free access to water be given and dehydration prevented. Repeated bouts of dehydration are associated with mental retardation.[5] When a child is unable to express thirst, as in cases of unconsciousness, delirium, and some forms of emotional or mental impair-

ment, life-threatening hypernatremia from water depletion may occur.

Medical treatment

If the disorder is mild, no treatment may be given other than free access to water. The inconvenience to the child and family usually depends on the degree of ADH deficiency. If therapy is warranted, chlorpropramide or desmopressin (1-desamino-8-D-arginine vasopressin; DDAVP) may be used. Apparently, when chlorpropramide is used to control urine-concentrating ability, secondary hypoglycemia is rare.[5] There are no observed drug-nutrient interactions with the long-term use of DDAVP. Also an antidiuretic effect of indapamide was observed with central diabetes insipidus and produced no adverse reactions.[6] Feeding problems are not inherent to the disease, but may present depending on its etiology.

A decreased ability to suck, chew, and swallow may occur after surgical procedures or brain injury. Nutritionally adequate liquid feedings with sufficient water may need to be provided by tube. Hydration status should be monitored frequently by laboratory data.

The prognosis for those with permanent neurogenic diabetes insipidus is generally good.[7] Possible long-term complications are bladder enlargement and hydronephrosis, resulting in decreased renal function later in life.

Nephrogenic Diabetes Insipidus

Nephrogenic diabetes insipidus (NDI) is a rare familial disease that is inherited either as a sex-linked recessive trait with variable penetrance in the female or as an autosomal-dominant trait with an X-linked gene.[8] The pathogenesis of NDI is still unclear, but it is known that the collecting ducts and renal tubules are unresponsive to both endogenous and exogenous vasopressin.

Biochemical and clinical abnormalities

The first symptoms of the disease occur soon after birth, or for the infant who is breastfed, symptoms are seen when the infant begins to receive a higher solute load diet from the addition of solid foods. Growth failure, polyuria, anorexia, constipation, vomiting, dehydration, and fever of unknown origin are all common symptoms.

Water intake and urine output are excessively high—7–10 L/day. Urine specific gravity is low (1.001–1.005), as is urine osmolality (50–100 mOsm/kg H_2O). The serum os-

Table 51–1. Sample Menu for Nephrogenic Diabetes Insipidus

Sample menu for 8-year-old child weighing 25 kg. Diet provides 2 g protein/kg/day and 2 mEq Na⁺/kg/day with approximately 1350 calories.

Exchanges used:	3 protein	4 starch	6 fruit
	4 milk	2 vegetable	4 fat

Breakfast
1/2 c whole milk
1 egg, fried in 1 tsp margarine
1 slice wheat toast, 1 tbsp jelly
1/2 c orange juice

Midafternoon Snack
8 oz grape juice
2 graham crackers

Evening Snack
1/2 banana
1/2 c whole milk

Lunch
1/2 c whole milk
1/2 sandwich, made with 1 oz chicken, 1 slice bread, 1 tsp mayonnaise, lettuce and tomato
1 apple

Dinner
1/2 c whole milk
1 oz roast beef
1/2 c mashed potatoes with 2 tsp margarine
1/2 green beans
1/2 c fruit cocktail

Sample menu for 1-year-old child weighing 10 kg. Diet provides 2 g protein/kg/day, 1.5 mEq Na⁺/kg/day, and approximately 95–100 cal/kg/day.

Exchanges used:	1 protein	2 starch	3 fruit
	0 milk	1 vegetable	3 fat

Breakfast
1/4 c iron-fortified infant cereal with 1 tsp salt-free margarine
2 oz orange juice
4 oz SMA® infant formula*

Lunch
1 oz chopped chicken
1/2 slice bread with 1 tsp salt-free margarine
1/4 c spinach
4 oz apple juice

Dinner
1/4 c mashed potatoes with 1 tsp salt-free margarine
1/4 c fruit cocktail
1/4 c green beans
4 oz grape juice

Midmorning snack
1/4 c Cheerios®†
4 oz SMA® infant formula

Midafternoon snack
4 oz SMA® infant formula

Nighttime Snack
4 oz SMA® infant formula

*SMA infant formula: 1/4 c Polycose® powder is added to 16 oz of SMA® formula each day to increase caloric content.
†Cheerios® may be measured in the morning and used throughout day as finger food.

molality is higher than normal (295 ± 6 mOsm/kg H₂O).[3] Since the presentation of nephrogenic diabetes insipidus is similar to that of neurogenic diabetes insipidus, a differential diagnosis must be made. This is done by performing a water deprivation test or by a trial of exogenous vasopressin with concurrent measurements of urine and serum osmolalities. NDI does not respond to vasopressin administration, whereas a greater urinary-concentrating ability is seen in the neurogenic form.

Factors to be considered in nutritional evaluation

Baseline anthropometric measurements of weight, length, and head circumference should be obtained upon diagnosis of nephrogenic diabetes insipidus. Infants with NDI usually present with severe delay or complete arrest of statural growth. Catch-up growth is observed with appropriate treatment.

Hypernatremia and volume contraction are thought to be the leading causes of growth retardation.[8,9] In addition, the vomiting and anorexia often observed result in a decreased nutrient intake that affects growth. There is also speculation whether growth retardation may be intrinsic to this inherited disease.[10,11] Growth measurements should be recorded routinely to follow the progression throughout childhood and adolescence.

A thorough dietary and feeding history should be completed and analyzed to determine the usual intake of nutrients. Emphasis should be placed on the amounts of calories, protein, sodium, and potassium as these nutrients are manipulated in the dietary treatment of NDI. The presence or absence of an intact thirst mechanism should be elicited, and the parent or caregiver should be taught an awareness of the infant's and young child's indicators of thirst. Accurate fluid intake and urine output records are helpful in measuring the efficacy of treatment when subsequent records are compared to baseline.

Dietary management

The usual treatment for nephrogenic diabetes insipidus is free access to water, a low-protein and low-sodium diet to lower the renal solute load, and diuretic therapy. The goal of treatment is to reduce the need for fluid intake.

Continued breastfeeding is ideal for infants with NDI because of the low solute load of breast milk. A low-solute infant formula (SMA®, S29®, Wyeth Laboratories or Similac PM 60/40®, Ross Laboratories) may be used, keeping protein restricted to 2 g/kg/day[8] (see Appendix 6). Sufficient calories are then provided through the use of additional carbohydrate (Polycose®, Ross Laboratories, or Sumacal®, Mead-Johnson) in the formula or through supplements of juice.

For older children, protein is restricted to 2 g/kg/day and sodium restricted to 1–2 mEq/kg/day.[8] Exchange lists for diabetes mellitus can be used. Sample menus are shown in Table 51–1. The planned diet should meet the calorie, vitamin, and mineral needs of the individual child and be revised periodically as the child grows. Because of the protein restriction, the dietary intake of calcium, iron, phosphorus, and vitamin D is inadequate, and supplements of these nutrients will be necessary. Carbohydrates and fats, if they are not moderate or high sources of sodium, will contribute the majority of calories in the diet. The caloric density of food may be increased by the addition of Polycose or Sumacal, and vegetable oil or low-sodium butter and margarine to allowed foods and liquids.

Because the amount of water needed daily may not be easily accepted by the infant, intravenous or gastric feedings may be necessary. In Niaudet's review[8] of 32 infants and children with NDI treated in a 25-year period, gastric feedings were used in infants as long as more than three drinks per night were necessary to maintain hydration. This situation often persisted until age 2 to 3.

In older children placed on diuretic therapy (hydrochlorothiazide), the sodium restriction of 1–2 mEq/kg/day should be maintained. The diet may be otherwise liberalized. Diuretic therapy reduces urinary volume by the induction of sodium depletion, which results in increased proximal tubular reabsorption of both sodium and water. Less water is then presented to the defective portion of the tubules, and the need for fluid is reduced. The effect of hydrochlorothiazide is not seen without dietary sodium restriction.[8,12] The well-known potassium-wasting effect of hydrochlorothiazide must be avoided, as potassium depletion in and of itself leads to an impairment of urinary-concentrating ability.[13] Dietary potassium should be increased, but more often potassium chloride supplements must be prescribed. To prevent the kaluresis seen with hydrochlorothiazide therapy, prostaglandins may be used in conjunction with hydrochlorothiazide and the low-sodium diet.[14–16]

Theoretically, dietary control alone may be used to achieve a reduction in polydipsia and polyuria. Dietary protein and sodium chloride are precursors of over half the urinary osmoles (urea and NaCl). Loss of urinary-concentrating ability causes the daily urine volume to become dependent upon the osmolar excretion. Decreasing urea and NaCl in the urine by controlling the dietary intake of protein and NaCl will therefore reduce water intake and urine volume. Blalock et al.[17] demonstrated this effect in their study of five subjects with diabetes insipidus. However, the protein and sodium restrictions used by these investigators in their study (1 g protein/kg/day and 8–10 mg sodium/kg/day for children under 13 years) are unrealistic for long-term compliance.

Follow-up

Nephrogenic diabetes insipidus is a chronic disease, but the prognosis is good when NDI is diagnosed early and treated appropriately. Mental retardation has been associated with NDI; the retardation is now recognized to be a result of secondary damage to the central nervous system through repeated episodes of hypernatremia, rather than being intrinsic to the disease itself.[7] Bladder enlargement with hydronephrosis leading to chronic renal failure is the primary cause of death in children with NDI.[9]

References

1. Greger, N.G., Kirkland, R.T., Clayton, G.W., Kirkland, J.L. Central diabetes insipidus. 22 years' experience. *Am. J. Dis. Child.* 1986; 140:551.
2. Weise, K., Zaritsky, A. Endocrine manifestations of critical illness in the child. *Pediatr. Clin. North Am.* 1987; 34:119.
3. Oliver, R.E., Jamison, R.L. Diabetes insipidus. A physiological approach to diagnosis. *Postgrad. Med.* 1980; 68:120.
4. Czernichow, P., Pomarede, R., Basmaciogullari, A., Brauner, R., Rappaport, R. Diabetes insipidus in children. III. Anterior pituitary dysfunction in idiopathic types. *J. Pediatr.* 1985; 106:41.
5. Ruess, A.L., Rosenthal, I.M. Intelligence in nephrogenic diabetes insipidus. *Am. J. Dis. Child.* 1963; 105:358.
6. Kocak, M., Karademir, B., Tetiker, A. Antidiuretic effect of indapamide in central diabetes insipidus. *Acta Endocrinol.*, 1990; 123:657.
7. Farrell, C.A., Staas, W.E. Diabetes insipidus in a quadriplegic patient. *Arch. Phys. Med. Rehabil.* 1986; 67:132.
8. Niaudet, P. Nephrogenic diabetes insipidus: clinical and pathophysiological aspects. *Adv. Nephrol.* 1984; 13:247.
9. Sprenger, K.J., Winship, W.S., Wittenberg, D.F. Nephrogenic diabetes insipidus presenting with infantile hypotonia. *S. Afr. Med. J.* 1986; 70:227.
10. Vest, M., Talbot, N.B., Crawford, J.D. Hypocaloric dwarfism and hydronephrosis in diabetes insipidus. *Am. J. Dis. Child.* 1963; 105:175.
11. Monn, E. Prostaglandin synthetase inhibitors in the treatment of nephrogenic diabetes insipidus. *Acta Paediatr. Scand.* 1981; 70:39.
12. Earley, L.E., Orloff, J. The mechanism of antidiuresis associated with administration of hydrochlorothiazide to patients with vasopressin-resistant diabetes insipidus. *J. Clin. Invest.* 1962; 41:1988.
13. Jamison, R.L., Oliver, R.E. Disorders of urinary concentration and diluation. *Am. J. Med.* 1982; 72:308.
14. Alon, U., Chan, J.C.M. Hydrochlorothiazide-amiloride in the treatment of congenital nephrogenic diabetes insipidus. *Am. J. Nephrol.* 1985; 5:9.
15. Anderson, O., Jacobsen, B.B. The renin-aldosterone system in nephrogenic diabetes insipidus and the influence of hydrochlorathiazide and indomethacin. *Acta Paediatr. Scand.* 1983; 72:717.
16. Hartenberg, M.A., Cory, M., Chan, J.C.M. Nephrogenic diabetes insipidus. Radiological and clinical features. *Int. J. Pediatr. Nephrol.* 1985; 6:281.
17. Blalock, T., Gerron, G., Quiter, E., Rudman, D. Role of diet in the management of vasopressin-responsive and -resistant diabetes insipidus. *Am. J. Clin. Nutr.* 1977; 30:1070.

Chapter 52
Fragile X Syndrome

Donna Runyan

Fragile X syndrome is the most common inherited form of mental retardation and the second most common chromosomal abnormality after Down's syndrome.[1] It was first described in 1969 by Lubs who found a marker on the X chromosome in several members of a family with mental retardation.[2] This marker was later characterized as a fragile site (Xq27.3) on the long arm of the X chromosome (Fig. 52–1). Laird hypothesized and Yu's et al.[3] data agree that four cis-acting alleles of Xq27 delay replication of this chromosome area, thus producing fragility.

Fragile X syndrome is seen in both sexes and all races.[1] It is generally viewed as a modified X-linked disorder, although the exact inheritance pattern is not clear since some individuals who carry the fragile X gene are unaffected.[4] It is more easily recognized in males since males have only one X chromosome. Approximately three-fourths of males with the fragile X gene show signs of the disorder.[5] The remainder are clinically unaffected, but will pass the gene to their daughters. In females, who have two X chromosomes, the normal X may suppress expression of the defective chromosome. Fifty percent of heterozygous females are affected to some degree.[1,5] Other females with the fragile X gene but no expression in the X chromosome are considered carriers. Females may or may not pass the gene to their offspring.

Genetic counseling is important for all family members at risk for carrying the fragile X gene. Prenatal diagnosis is available at experienced laboratories, but the degree of impairment of the affected fetus cannot be determined.[1,6]

Little was known about fragile X syndrome until the early 1980s when improved cytogenic techniques using folate-deficient media enabled researchers to detect the fragile site.[7] The percent of cells carrying the fragile X chromosome was found to vary from 1% to 50%.[8] The percentage of fragility appears to correlate with the degree of cognitive impairment of affected females.[9] In males, the comparable correlation is not as clear. Studies have shown, however, that fragile X males with normal intelligence have a very low percentage of defective cells.[10]

The incidence of fragile X syndrome is not easily determined since there is a wide variation in the degree of impairment of affected individuals. Current estimates put the incidence as high as 1 in 1000 because researchers believe that many individuals with this disorder have not yet been diagnosed.[1] More conservative estimates put the prevalence at 1 in 2000 males and 1 in 2500 females.[1,5] A carrier prevalence of 1 in 1000 females has been cited.[5]

Biochemical and Clinical Abnormalities

Diagnosis of the fragile X syndrome is based upon the results of cytogenetic assessment and direct DNA analysis.[11] Phenotypic expression of the defective chromosome results in characteristic physical features, which can aid in the diagnostic process. The classic triad in males is enlarged testes (macro-orchidism) following puberty (also evident in 20% to 40% of prepubertal males), large or prominent ears, and a long narrow face.[1,5,8] The precocious puberty may reflect an underlying disturbance of hypothalamic-pituitary-gonadal function in the fragile X syndrome.[12] Other common features are hyperextensible finger joints, ocular problems (myopia, strabismus), mitral valve prolapse, abnormal hand and foot creases, high-arched palate (8% cleft palate), and recurrent otitis media (Table 52–1).[5] It is felt that many of the physical features result from connective tissue dysplasia. Fragile X females with mental impairment frequently show subtle signs of the same characteristic facial features as affected males. Carrier females may not show any facial stigmata.[8]

There is wide variation in the cognitive functioning of affected individuals. The majority of fragile X males have some degree of intellectual dysfunction ranging from borderline to profound mental retardation. Retrospective studies have shown a decline in IQ over time, with mild mental retardation in childhood regressing to a moderate or severe level after puberty.[13] Fragile X males with normal IQ frequently have learning disabilities and attention problems.[1,8,14] The primary area of weakness is mathematics; strengths include reading and spelling. About 30% of affected females are mentally retarded, but they are usually higher functioning than their male counterparts.[1] An additional 20% have normal intelligence, but have significant

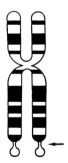

Fig. 52–1. The fragile X chromosome. Arrow points to the fragile site. From Hagerman, R.J., McBogg, P.M., eds. *The Fragile X Syndrome: Diagnosis, Biochemistry, and Intervention.* Dillon, CO, Spectra Publishing Co. Inc.; 1983. Used with permission.

Table 52–1. Clinical Features of the Fragile X Syndrome

Growth
    Slightly increased birth weight
    Average height in children
    Head circumference usually greater than
       75th percentile in children
Facies
    Long face
    Prominent large ears
    Prominent high forehead
    Mild coarsening of facial features
    High-arched palate
    Occasional brachycephaly
    Occasional prognathism in adults
    Epicanthic folds
    Dental crowding
    Occasional facial asymmetry
    Occasional strabismus
Genitalia
    Macro-orchidism in most adults, occasional in children
Musculoskeletal
    Hypotonia
    Hyperextensibility of fingers
    Pes planus
    Occasional scoliosis

Cardiovascular
    Mitral valve prolapse
    Occasional dilation of ascending aorta
Central nervous system
    Mild to profound mental retardation
       (occasional normal IQ with learning
       disabilities)
    Occasional seizures
Integument
    Fine velvety skin
    Callouses on hand from self-abuse
    Abnormal palmar creases
    Increased frequency of radial loops,
       whorls, and arches on third digits
Behavior
    Autistic features
    Shyness
    Stereotypical mannerisms
    Hyperactivity
    Hand flapping
    Hand biting
Speech
    Perseveration
    Echolalia
    Poor language content
    Cluttering

From Chudley & Hagerman,[5] with permission.

learning disabilities, again primarily in math. Most carrier females have normal intelligence. Recent studies, however, have also shown a characteristic academic weakness in mathematics among this group.[1,8]

Speech and language deficits are common among fragile X individuals.[8] Speech is poorly articulated, with frequent stuttering, perseveration, and echolalia.

Behavior problems among affected males vary from subtle inappropriateness to violent outbursts. Autistic-like behavior, especially poor eye contact and hand flapping, may be present. Some studies have shown a higher frequency of autism among male fragile X subjects than among mentally retarded controls, causing researchers to continue to look for an association between these two disabilities.[8] Most fragile X males, however, do not have the total lack of relatedness needed to meet the diagnostic criteria for infantile autism.[1] Affected females may be shy or withdrawn, but do not usually display more pronounced autistic-like behaviors. They tend to have psychosocial and emotional problems.

No metabolic abnormalities are associated with fragile X syndrome.[1,8] The majority of studies report normal gonadal and thyroid function in fragile X males despite enlarged testicles.[8] Since the fragile site on the X chromosome is visible only in a folate-deficient medium, some researchers have postulated an error in folate metabolism in fragile X subjects. Studies have shown, however, that the pathways of folic acid metabolism are intact and are, in fact, identical to those of normal controls.[15]

Factors to be Considered in Nutritional Evaluation

The growth pattern of fragile X children varies only slightly from normal.[16] The most striking feature is large head cir-

cumference (macrocephaly), which continues into adulthood. Height and weight are above normal during childhood, but normalize at maturity. This pattern differs from the low weight and small stature found in children with other chromosomal abnormalities.

Feeding difficulties may be present due to the high-arched palate and oral motor dysfunction characteristic of children with speech delays. Hypotonia, motor dysfunction, and mental retardation may delay the progression of feeding skills. Fragile X children should be monitored for constipation since oral motor dysfunction may limit the ingestion of high-fiber foods, and generalized hypotonia will reduce gastrointestinal motility (see Chapter 35).

If folic acid therapy is provided (see below), a multivitamin with B complex is recommended to counteract B vitamin deficiencies.[1] Hagerman et al.[17] found that three adults became deficient in vitamin B_6 while taking high doses of folic acid. Since folic acid may interfere with zinc absorption, serum zinc levels should also be monitored.[18]

Medications that interfere with folic acid metabolism should be used with caution in fragile X individuals.[19] Antibiotics containing trimethoprim, such as Bactrim, Trimpex (Roche), Proloprim, and Septra (Burroughs Welcome), lower folate levels through the inhibition of dihydrofolate reductase. This medication is commonly prescribed for acute otitis media, a condition frequently seen in fragile X children.[20]

Dietary Management

There is no cure for fragile X syndrome. Recent studies, however, have shown some promise in the use of folic acid for this condition.[17,21–27] Early anecdotal reports of greatly improved behavior of fragile X males given oral folic acid spurred researchers to conduct controlled, double-blind studies to investigate this phenomenon.[28,29] The results have been mixed.

A large, well-controlled study was conducted by Hagerman et al.,[17] who examined the effect of folic acid on 25 males, ages 1–31 (mean age, 16). Using a double-blind crossover design, 10 mg of folic acid or placebo (saline) was given orally for 6 months. Thirteen of the subjects showed mild or marked improvement in attention span, activity level, and frequency of tantrums. There was greater improvement in the prepubertal boys (75%) than in those who had passed puberty (41%). Intellectual performance (IQ) improved significantly in the younger boys. Two children, ages 3 and 6, had baseline IQs in the mentally retarded range. After folic acid treatment, their IQ increased to the normal range. The researchers related this change to improved behavior that affected the developmental testing. The younger children responded more clearly to the folic acid treatment than the adolescents and adults. Behavioral changes occurred within 2–4 weeks of folic acid therapy and carried over for a short time into the placebo period.

Similar results were found by Gillberg et al.,[21] who looked at four boys, ages 6–14, who had fragile X syndrome and infantile autism. Larger doses of folic acid were given (5 mg/kg/day) for 3 months in a double-blind ABA fashion. The older boy, who had gone through puberty, showed no change in behavior, but improvement was noted in the three younger subjects. Two of the boys were on seizure medications. No increase in seizure activity was evident during the treatment periods, despite large doses of folic acid.

Froster-Iskenius et al.[22] examined the effect of folic acid on eight females, ages 5–53, and ten males, ages 15–54. The only young child in the study group was a 5-year-old girl. She was given 5 mg of folic acid daily for 4 months; the others received 10 mg. No improvement was found in concentration, fine motor coordination, or comprehension in the adolescent or adult subjects. The 5-year-old girl, however, exhibited improved concentration after 2 months of folic acid treatment. No further improvement was noted after that time. Other studies have also shown positive results.[23-27]

However, there have been several negative reports in the literature.[30-32] In one study, Brown et al.[30] gave 250 mg folic acid to 5 males, ages 8–26, for two 3-month periods. No changes in IQ or behavior between the treatment and intervening placebo periods were found. However, this lack of change could be due to the high dosage given and the carryover effect since it takes 6–8 weeks for the folic acid level to normalize after therapy.

Summary and Follow-up

In summary, folic acid treatment in fragile X subjects remains controversial. It appears to be more effective in young children than in adolescents and adults. The primary improvements are seen in behavior, with possible benefits in cognitive function. The most commonly used dosage in the studies with positive results was 10 mg/day, often in divided doses. The treatment period should exceed 2 months (preferably 3–6 months) to allow sufficient time for behavioral

improvements. High doses of folic acid should be given only in a well-designed experimental study.[33] Until further research confirms the beneficial effects, folic acid is not recommended for general use in fragile X syndrome.

References

1. Hagerman, R.J. Fragile X syndrome. *Curr. Probl. Pediatr.* 1987; 17:621.
2. Lubs, H.A. A marker X chromosome. *Am. J. Hum. Genet.*, 1969; 21:231.
3. Yu, W-D., Wenger, S., Steele, M. X chromosome imprinting in fragile X syndrome. *Hum. Genet.* 1990; 85:590.
4. Shapiro, L.R. The fragile X syndrome: a peculiar pattern of inheritance. *N. Engl. J. Med.* 1991; 325:1736.
5. Chudley, A.E., Hagerman, R.J. Fragile X syndrome. *J. Pediatr.* 1987; 110:821.
6. Sutherland, G.R., Gedeon, A., Kornman, L., Donnelly, A., Byard, R.W., Mulley, J.C., Kremer, E., Lynch, M., Pritchard, M., Yu, S., Richards, R.I. Prenatal diagnosis of fragile X syndrome by direct detection of the unstable DNA sequence. *N. Engl. J. Med.* 1991; 325:1720.
7. McGavran, L., Maxwell, F. Cytogenetic aspects of the fragile X syndrome. In: Hagerman, R.J., McBogg, P.M., eds. *The Fragile X Syndrome: Diagnosis, Biochemistry, and Intervention.* Dillon, CO: Spectra; 1983.
8. Bregman, J.D., Dykens, E., Watson, M., Ort, S.I., Leckman, J.F. Fragile X syndrome: variability of phenotypic expression. *J. Am. Acad. Child. Adolesc. Psychiatr.* 1987; 26:463.
9. Kemper, M.B., Hagerman, R.J., Ahmad, R.S., Mariner, R. Cognitive profiles and the spectrum of clinical manifestations in heterozygous fragile X females. *Am. J. Med. Genet.*, 1986; 23:139.
10. Froster-Iskenius, U., McGillivray, B.C., Dill, F.J., Hall, J.G., Herbst, D.S. Normal male carriers in the fragile X form of X-linked mental retardation (Martin-Bell syndrome). *Am. J. Med. Genet.* 1986; 23:619.
11. Rousseau, F., Heitz, D., Biancalana, V., Blumenfeld, S., Kretz, C., Boué, J., Tommercup, N., Van Der Hagen, C., Delozier-Blanchet, C., Croquette, M., Gilgenkrantz, SD., Jalbert, P., Voelckel, M., Oberlé, I., Mandel, J. Direct diagnosis by DNA analysis of the fragile X syndrome of mental retardation. *N. Engl. J. Med.* 1991; 325:1673.
12. Moore, P., Chudley, A., Winter, J. True precocious puberty in a girl with fragile X syndrome. *Am. J. Med. Genet.* 1990; 37:265.
13. Lachiewicz, A.V., Gullion, C.M., Spiridigliozzi, G.A., Aylsworth, A.S. Declining IQ's of young males with the fragile X syndrome. *Am. J. Ment. Retard.* 1987; 92:272.
14. Hagerman, R.J., Kemper, M., Hudson, M. Learning disabilities and attentional problems in boys with the fragile X syndrome. *Am. J. Dis. Child.* 1985;139:674.
15. Wang, J.C., Erbe, R.W. Folate metabolism in cells from fragile X syndrome patients and carriers. *Am. J. Med. Genet.* 1984; 17:303.
16. Partington, M.W. The fragile X syndrome. II: Preliminary data on growth and development in males. *Am. J. Med. Genet.* 1984; 17:175.
17. Hagerman, R.J., Jackson, A.W., Levitas, A., Braden, M., McBogg, P., Kemper, M., McGavran, L., Berry, R., Matus, I., Hagerman, P.J. Oral folic acid versus placebo in the treatment of males with the fragile X syndrome. *Am. J. Med. Genet.* 1986; 23:241.
18. Milne, D.B. Canfield, W.K., Mahalko, J.R., Sandstead, H.H. Effect of oral folic acid supplements on zinc, copper and iron absorption and excretion. *Am. J. Clin. Nutr.* 1984; 39:535.
19. Hecht, F., Glover, T.W. Antibiotics containing trimethoprim and the fragile X chromosome. *N. Engl. J. Med.* 1983; 308:285. Letter.
20. Hagerman, R.J., Altshul-Stark, D., McBogg, P. Recurrent otitis media in the fragile X syndrome. *Am. J. Dis. Child.* 1987; 141:184.
21. Gillberg, C., Wahlstrom, J., Johansson, R., Tornblom, M., Albertsson-Wikland, K. Folic acid as an adjunct in the

treatment of children with the autism fragile X syndrome (AF-RAX). *Dev. Med. Child. Neurol.* 1986; 28:624.

22. Froster-Iskenius, U., Bodeker, K., Oepen, T., Matthes, R., Piper, U., Schwinger, E. Folic acid treatment in males and females with fragile X syndrome. *Am. J. Med. Genet.* 1986; 23:273.

23. Wells, T.E., Madison, L.S. Assessment of behavior change in a fragile X syndrome male treated with folic acid. *Am. J. Med. Genet.* 1986; 23:291.

24. Gustavson, K.H., Dahlbom, K., Flood, A., Holmgren, G., Blomquist, H.K., Sanner, G. Effect of folic acid treatment in the fragile X syndrome. *Clin. Genet.* 1985; 27:463.

25. Lejeune, J., Rethore, M.O., deBlois, M.C., Ravel, A. Trial of folic acid treatment in fragile X syndrome. *Ann. Genet.* (Paris) 1984; 27:230.

26. Brown, W.T., Jenkins, E.C., Friedman, E., Brooks, J., Cohen, I.L., Duncan, C., Hill, A.L., Malik, M.N., Morris, V., Wolf, E. Folic acid therapy in the fragile X syndrome. *Am. J. Med. Genet.* 1984; 17:289.

27. Carpenter, N.J., Barber, D.H., Jones, M., Lindley, W., Carr, C. Controlled six-month study of oral folic acid therapy in boys with fragile X-linked mental retardation. Abstract 243. *Am. J. Hum. Genet.* 1983; 35(suppl 82A).

28. Lejeune, J. Is the fragile X syndrome amenable to treatment? *Lancet.* 1982; 1:273. Letter.

29. Harpey, J.P. Treatment of fragile X. *Pediatrics.* 1982; 69:670. Letter.

30. Brown, W.T., Cohen, I.L., Fisch, G.S., Wolf-Schein, E.G., Jenkins, V.A. Malik, M.N., Jenkins, E.C. High dose folic acid treatment of fragile X males. *Am. J. Med. Genet.* 1986; 23:263.

31. Madison, L.S., Wells, T.E., Fristo, T.E., Benesch, C.G. A controlled study of folic acid treatment on three fragile X syndrome males. *J. Dev. Behav. Pediatr.* 1986; 7:253.

32. Rosenblatt, D.S. Duschenes, E.A., Hellstrom, F.V., Golick, M.S., Vekemans, M.J., Zeesman, S.F., Andermann, E. Folic acid blinded trial in identical twins with fragile X syndrome. *Am. J. Hum. Genet.* 1985; 37:543.

33. Nussbaum, R.L., Ledbetter, D.H. The fragile X syndrome. In: Scriver, C.R., Beaudet, A.L., Sly, W.S., Valle, D., eds. *The Metabolic Basis of Inherited Disease*, 6th ed. Vol. 1. New York: McGraw-Hill; 1989.

Chapter 53
Hyperuricemias (Lesch-Nyhan Syndrome)

R. Jean Hine

Purine nucleotide biosynthesis is achieved via both a de novo synthetic pathway and a salvage pathway. The cytoplasmic enzyme, hypoxanthine-guanine phosphoribosyl transferase (HGPRT), catalyzes the reutilization of preformed purine bases (hypoxanthine and guanine) in the purine nucleotide salvage pathway. Human HGPRT is encoded by a single structural gene; its amino acid sequence has been characterized.[1] The importance of an efficient purine nucleotide salvage pathway is underscored by the clinical manifestations of inherited disorders of purine metabolism.

The Lesch-Nyhan syndrome (LN) results from a total lack of HGPRT. LN is an X-linked, recessive disorder that was first described in 1964.[2] This disorder is characterized by excessive uric acid synthesis with consequent development of uric acid nephrolithiasis, choreoathetosis, spasticity, growth failure, and mental retardation. A compulsive pattern of self-mutilation associated with LN involves biting of the fingers, lips, and buccal mucosa (Fig. 53–1). Males with LN typically have a reduced life-span, living to between 20 and 30 years of age. Death is frequently caused by renal failure or infection.

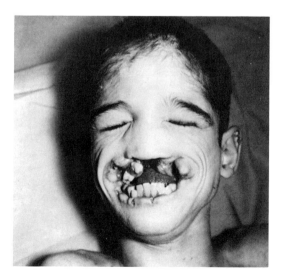

Fig. 53–1. A 14-year-old boy illustrating an extreme degree of mutilation around the face. From Nyhan, W.L., Sahati, N.O. *Diagnostic Recognition of Genetic Disease.* Philadelphia: Lea & Febiger; 1987. Used with permission.

Most subjects with partial HGPRT deficiency escape the serious neurological and behavioral abnormalities that accompany LN, but they usually suffer from severe gouty arthritis or uric acid nephrolithiasis as adults. Twenty percent of patients with partial enzyme deficiency have mild neurological problems, but they do not exhibit the dramatic self-mutilation observed in LN patients. Also in contrast with LN patients, those with partial HGPRT deficiency have a normal life expectancy.

Biochemical Abnormalities

A virtually complete lack of HGPRT was originally observed in the red cells and fibroblasts of patients with LN. The enzyme defect was later confirmed in other tissues, including the liver and brain of patients with both complete and partial HGPRT deficiency.

LN is somewhat confusing in a metabolic sense. Purine nucleotides are synthesized in two ways.[3] In the de novo pathway, the purine ring structure is completed in a stepwise fashion. The salvage pathway reassembles purine nucleotides from 5-phosphoribosyl-1-pyrophosphate (PRPP) and free purines, including guanine and hypoxanthine. The salvage of hypoxanthine and xanthine regulates purine biosynthesis. In the salvage pathway, HGPRT catalyzes the transfer of the phosphoribosyl moiety of PRPP to hypoxanthine and guanine to form inosinic acid (IMP) or guanosine 5' monophosphate (GMP), respectively. The HGPRT deficiency affects the purine nucleotide salvage pathway with resultant excessive production of purine nucleotides. Yet, hyperuricemia in patients with HGPRT deficiency is a consequence of an increased rate of de novo purine synthesis. This is probably because of decreased feedback inhibition by nucleotide end products in combination with a loss of hypoxanthine from cells.

There are reports in the literature of megaloblastic changes in the bone marrow and red blood cells of LN patients. Low plasma folic acid levels were also observed in these patients.[4,5] These problems with folic acid status could occur because of an increased demand for the vitamin, which acts as a co-factor in two steps of purine biosynthesis.

The mechanism responsible for the neurological problems associated with LN is unclear. However, excess uric acid production does not appear to be related to development of neurological problems. This conclusion is supported by the finding of normal uric acid levels in the cerebrospinal fluid (CSF) of all patients in whom it has been measured and by the failure of pharmacological treatment of hyperuricemia to alleviate neurological symptoms in LN patients.[6]

However, hypoxanthine is found in CSF in amounts four times that of control individuals. Neurotransmitters have been implicated in the behavioral features of the disease.[7]

Factors to be Considered in Diagnosis/Evaluation

There appear to be no pronounced differences in the occurrence of LN among ethnic or racial groups. The incidence of LN is estimated to be 1 in 10,000 males.[8] Wilson et al.[9] evaluated 24 unrelated patients with varying degrees of HGPRT deficiency and found evidence of marked genetic heterogeneity in disorders of HGPRT.

Primary clinical symptoms of HGPRT deficiency occur only in males, with transmission through female carriers. Although males with LN syndrome are sterile, those with partial deficiency of HGPRT do reproduce. No male-to-male transmission of the disorder has been observed, which is consistent with an X-linked mode of transmission. Several reports in the literature suggest that heterozygotes for HGPRT deficiency exhibit subtle abnormalities of purine metabolism, although they are generally asymptomatic clinically. The carrier state can be detected using in vitro methods.[10,11] Prenatal diagnosis of LN can be achieved by directly measuring HGPRT levels in cells obtained from chorionic villus sampling during the first trimester of pregnancy.

Two groups of investigators published results of their longitudinal experience in treating LN in the United States and Japan.[12,13] Their data supplied much needed insights into the clinical course of the disorder. Infants with LN usually appear to be normal at birth. Sometimes, hypotonia, recurrent vomiting, and other feeding problems are seen in the first 3 months of life. Delayed motor development is observed as early as 4 months of age. Before 1 year, extrapyramidal signs develop, including fine, athetoid movements of the extremities, chorea, and dystonia. Pyramidal tract involvement is also apparent by 1 year. The diagnosis of cerebral palsy is sometimes given before a patient is identified as having LN. Neurological involvement is such that patients with LN are nonambulatory. Approximately half the LN patients reported in the literature had seizure disorders. The pathogenesis of neural dysfunction is poorly understood.

The diagnosis of LN is not usually made until families become concerned about the self-mutilation behavior. Between 2 and 16 years of age, boys with LN develop compulsive self-injurious and aggressive behavior. Christie et al.[12] found that 26 months was the average age of onset of self-mutilation in the 19 subjects studied. The self-mutilation often includes biting the buccal mucosa, lips, and fingers. Head banging is common as well, but it is sometimes difficult to distinguish from accidental head injury resulting from involuntary movements. Although the seriousness of the self-mutilation and aggression is variable, measures, such as restraints and extraction of the teeth, may be necessary to prevent self-mutilation.

Most males with LN are mentally retarded, with IQs between 40–60. However there have been reports of boys with near-normal intelligence.[12] LN patients' performance on standardized intelligence tests is limited by dysarthria, choreoathetosis, and by the arm restraints that may be necessary to prevent self-injury.

Patients with LN produce and excrete large amounts of uric acid. The serum urate is elevated, ranging from 7–18 mg/dL. The excretion of uric acid ranges from 25–143 mg/kg/day (the upper limit for normal children is 18 mg/kg/day). This increased quantity of urinary uric acid results in uric acid crystal formation. Orange uric acid crystals in a wet diaper can be the first sign of the disorder. Untreated patients develop uric acid nephrolithiasis, subsequent obstructive uropathy, and early death. Three-quarters of those with partial HGPRT deficiency have had uric acid nephrolithiasis, and half of these individuals develop gout.

Bacterial infections are a significant problem in patients with LN. Death may be caused by pneumonia or complications associated with urinary tract infections. There is, however, no consistent evidence of compromised immunity among those with LN or partial HGPRT deficiency.

Most patients with LN have bilaterally dislocated hips. Some delay in bone age is seen among patients with LN, but it is not as marked as the growth retardation seen in these individuals. One group of researchers suggests that the growth retardation may reflect a nutritional deficit, rather than a primary manifestation of the disorder.[13]

Management

The treatment of HGPRT deficiency focuses on reducing the excessive synthesis of uric acid and the amelioration of neurological problems. Allopurinol inhibits xanthine oxidase and can thereby limit the accumulation of uric acid in body fluids. The enzyme, xanthine oxidase, is responsible for the conversion of hypoxanthine to xanthine and of xanthine to uric acid, the end product of purine biosynthesis. Allopurinol administration prevents uric acid stone formation, urate nephropathy, gouty arthritis, and the development of tophi. Christie et al.[12] recommend an initial daily dose of 15–20 mg/kg, with monitoring of uric acid blood levels until they fall to 3 mg/dL or below. Stout and Caskey[8] suggest a low initial dose of 10 mg/kg/day, with a maximum dose of 800 mg/day. The formation of uric acid and xanthine stones is minimized by monitoring urinary levels of uric acid, xanthine, and hypoxanthine. There is no effective drug therapy for the neurological problems associated with LN.

Prevention of the genetic defect responsible for LN is preferable to its symptomatic treatment. Therefore, this disease has become a prototype for gene replacement therapy.[1]

Nutritional care

Nutritional care of LN patients is a component of their overall therapeutic management. As recommended by Thompson and Smith,[14] it is important to assess the nutritional status of patients with handicapping conditions. Longitudinal measurement of height and weight can be used to document growth rate. Height and weight measurements of older LN patients may be complicated by their nonambulatory status or aggressive behavior. Often, arm circumference and skinfold measurements can supply useful information about body composition.

Clinical examination of patients should be done to screen for overt physical signs of nutrient deficiencies. The nutritionist should briefly review medical records to obtain a history of such problems as anemia, recurrent infections, or food allergies.

Laboratory assessment of nutritional status should be performed to determine the biochemical correlates of nutritional status. If undernutrition is suspected, plasma proteins should be measured. In patients with LN, it may be helpful to measure plasma or red cell folate levels or at least to assess red blood cells for any macrocytic changes. Abnormal indices of folate status may be caused by an increased requirement of folic acid for purine synthesis or may result from anticonvulsant drug therapy. Descriptive information about food intake, dietary patterns, feeding skills, and use of nutritional supplements is necessary to help the clinician develop a realistic nutritional care plan.

Christie et al.[12] found that 58% of the LN patients they studied had feeding problems. Feeding skill development is delayed in boys with LN because of athetosis and is sometimes further hindered by the presence of arm restraints to prevent self-mutilation. Parents may spend large amounts of time feeding a child with LN. If teeth have been extracted to prevent self-injury, the diet texture needs to be modified accordingly. A delay in feeding skill acquisition would not be anticipated among children with partial HGPRT deficiency.

Several recommendations have been made regarding dietary intake of patients with LN or partial HGPRT deficiency. Some assert that growth retardation is a phenotypic manifestation of LN,[15] whereas others suggest that energy supplements enhance the growth of LN patients. At least some growth deficits seen in LN syndrome are secondary to low energy intake. Dietary purines, which are found in protein-rich foods, such as meat (particularly high in organ meats), poultry, fish, dried beans and lentils, meat soups, and stews, are thought to be of little consequence in HGPRT deficiency.[16] Bran, wheat germ, peas, asparagus, and mushrooms are also high in purines. Because there is no evidence that restriction of dietary purines improves LN, it is not recommended unless renal function is very poor or control of hyperuricemia is unsatisfactory.[16] (A sample purine-free diet is shown in a table in *The Metabolic Basis of Inherited Diseases*.[16] Since the elevated urinary excretion of uric acid results from excessive purine production, fluid intake should be promoted to increase urinary volume.

The question of folic acid status and a possible need for folic acid supplementation is controversial. At least one patient was resistant to B$_{12}$ and folinic acid therapy. Unfortunately, investigators did not state the levels of either nutrient or other specific information about the supplementation trial.[4] Depending on the folate status of the patient, clinicians may wish to counsel families about regular inclusion of folate-rich foods in the diet.

Follow-up and Summary

A nutrition care plan with follow-up should be an integral part of an individualized family service plan (IFSP) for boys with LN syndrome according to the requirement of PL 99-457. As recommended by the American Public Health Association Maternal and Child Health Section's Committee on Children with Special Health Care Needs, respite care should also be a part of the ISFP because it can periodically relieve parents from the responsibilities of continuous supervision, care, and feeding of children with LN.[17]

References

1. Stout, J.T., Caskey, C.T. Hypoxanthine phosphoribosyl-transferase deficiency: the Lesch-Nyhan syndrome and gouty arthritis. In: Scriver, C.R., Beaudet, A.L., Sly, W.S., Valle, D., eds. *The Metabolic Basis of Inherited Disease*. 6th ed. Vol. I. New York: McGraw-Hill; 1989.
2. Lesch, M., Nyhan, W.L. A familial disorder of uric acid metabolism and central nervous system function. *Am. J. Med.* 1964; 36:561.
3. Lehninger, A.L., Anderson, S., Fox, J., eds. Biosynthesis of amino acids and nucleotides. In: *Principles of Biochemistry*. New York: Worth; 1984.
4. Van Der Zee, S.P.M., Schretlen, E.D.A.M., Monnens, L.A.H. Megaloblastic anemia in the Lesch-Nyhan syndrome. *Lancet.* 1968; 1:1427.
5. Hernandez-Nieto, L., Brito-Barraso, M.C., Nyhan, W.L. Megaloblastic anemia in Lesch-Nyhan syndrome. *Sangre.* 1988; 29:175.
6. Sweetman, L. Urinary and cerebrospinal oxypurine levels and allopurinol metabolism in the Lesch-Nyhan syndrome. *Fed. Proc.* 1968; 27:1055.
7. Castells, S., Chakrabarti, C., Winsberg, B.G., Hurwic, M., Perel, J.M., Nyhan, W.L. Effects of 5-hydroxytryptophan in the Lesch-Nyhan syndrome. *J. Autism Dev. Disord.* 1979; 9:95.
8. Stout, J.T., Caskey, C.T. The Lesch-Nyhan syndrome: clinical, molecular and genetic aspects. *Trends Genet.* 1988; 4:175.
9. Wilson, J.M., Stout, J.T., Palella, T.D., Davidson, B.L., Kelly, W.V., Caskey, C.T. A molecular survey of hypoxanthine-guanine phosphoribosyltransferase deficiency in man. *J. Clin. Invest.* 1986; 77:188.
10. Kamatani, N., Yamanaka, H., Nishioka, K., Nishida, Y., Mikanagi, K. Diagnosis of Lesch-Nyhan heterozygotes in peripheral blood. *Adv. Exp. Med. Biol.* 1986; 195:157.
11. Gibbs, D.A. Advances in the study of inherited metabolic disease. *J. Inher. Metab. Dis.* 1989; 12:240.
12. Christie, R., Bay, C., Kaufman, I., Bakay, B., Borden, M., Nyhan, W.L. Lesch-Nyhan disease: clinical experience with nineteen patients. *Dev. Med. Child. Neurol.* 1982; 24:293.
13. Mizuno, T. Long-term follow-up of ten patients with Lesch-Nyhan syndrome. *Neuropediatrics.* 1986; 17:158.
14. Thompson, M.L., Smith, M.A.H. *1987 Update Guidelines for Nutrition Training in University Affiliated Programs.* Memphis: University of Tennessee Child Development Center; 1987.
15. Thompson, G., Pacy, P., Watts, W., Hallidy, D. Protein metabolism in phylketonuria and Lesch-Nyhan syndrome. *Pediatr. Res.* 1990; 28:240.
16. Palella, T.D., Fox, I.H. Hyperuricemia and gout. In: Scriver, C., Beaudet, A., Sly, W., Valle, D., eds. *Metabolic Basis of Inherited Diseases.* 6th ed. Vol. I. New York: McGraw-Hill; 1989.
17. American Public Health Association, Maternal and Child Health Section. *Committee Statement on Children with Special Health Care Needs.* Washington, D.C.; 1989.

Chapter 54
Hyperlipidemias in Children

Ellen Gerber Illig

Lipids are fats that are present in blood and body tissues and serve as a concentrated and efficient form of energy storage. Clinical and experimental evidence suggests that a relationship exists between elevated levels of lipids (hyperlipidemia), especially cholesterol and saturated fat, and the development of atherosclerosis.[1]

Cholesterol is a waxy type of lipid found in all animal tissues. The cholesterol level in the blood is affected by the cholesterol produced by the body (blood cholesterol) and the saturated fat and cholesterol in the diet (dietary cholesterol). Although cholesterol is essential for many of the body's chemical processes, including the manufacture of hormones, bile acid, and vitamin D, too much in the blood can lead to heart and blood vessel disease.

Cholesterol is carried in the blood bound to proteins called lipoproteins. The lipoproteins are classified according to their density. The three most significant lipoproteins are high-density lipoprotein cholesterol (HDL-C), low-density lipoprotein cholesterol (LDL-C), and very low-density lipoprotein cholesterol (VLDL-C)[2] (Table 54–1).

- *High-Density Lipoprotein Cholesterol (HDL-C)*: The high-density lipoproteins remove cholesterol from the blood and blood vessels and transport it to the liver where it is converted to bile acids for excretion from the body. This is a "good" cholesterol; the higher the level, the lower the risk.
- *Low-Density Lipoprotein Cholesterol (LDL-C)*: The low-density lipoproteins carry most of the cholesterol and deposit it in the blood vessels, contributing to atherosclerosis (hardening of the arteries). This is the "bad" cholesterol; the higher the level, the higher the risk of heart disease.
- *Very Low-Density Lipoprotein Cholesterol (VLDL-C)*: The very low-density lipoproteins carry some cholesterol, but primarily carry the triglycerides in the blood.
- *Triglycerides (TG) are another type of fat in the blood*: They can be manufactured in the body from simple sugars and alcohol or obtained from fats in the diet. High levels can lead to heart disease.

Hyperlipidemias include elevated cholesterol levels (hypercholesterolemia), depressed levels of HDL-C, elevated LDL-C, elevated triglyceride levels, or a combination of these. Dietary treatment varies depending on the specific lipoprotein abnormality.

Development of atherosclerosis begins in childhood. The severity of the atherosclerosis in the aorta and coronary arteries of children is related to the concentration of serum LDL-C and total cholesterol.[3] Total cholesterol measurements in childhood also are predictors of adult total and LDL-C levels, with 25% to 50% of adult cholesterol variability explained by childhood levels.[4] A change of eating habits in early childhood may delay or prevent cardiovascular disease development.[5,6]

Children at "high risk" are defined as those with hypercholesterolemia or coronary heart disease in a parent or grandparent before the age of 55. Their family histories should be carefully obtained and should include parents, grandparents, and all first-degree relatives. Physicians should obtain at least two and preferably three blood cholesterol determinations.

Biochemical Abnormalities

A normal cholesterol level for an infant or child is ≤ 165 mg/dL (50th percentile). Infants at high risk should have an appropriate blood test conducted once before age 2. If the level is normal, a repeat check every 5–7 years during childhood (age 2–19) seems prudent.[7]

In infants or children with abnormally high cholesterol levels, a plasma total cholesterol (TC), triglyceride (TG), and HDL-C should be measured, with calculation of LDL-C

Table 54–1. Lipid and Lipoprotein Values for Children

	Percentiles						
	5	10	25	50	75	90	95
Plasma total cholesterol (mg/dL)	115	125	140	155	170	185	200
Plasma triglyceride (mg/dL)	35	40	45	55	70	90	110
Plasma LDL-cholesterol (mg/dL)	65	70	80	95	110	125	135
Plasma HDL-cholesterol (mg/dL)	35	40	45	55	60	70	75

Modified from Goldman et al.,[8] with permission.

[TC − HDL-C − (TG < 400 mg/dL ÷ 5)] to determine if the child has high levels of LDL cholesterol or low levels of HDL cholesterol (Table 54–1).[8] It is also important to make sure that the hypercholesterolemia is not due to other diseases or drugs.

Factors to be Considered in Nutritional Evaluation

Most children with high total and LDL cholesterol levels have an excessive intake of saturated fat and cholesterol, rather than familial hypercholesterolemia. Therefore, children with blood cholesterol levels between the 75th and 90th percentile (170–185 mg/dL) should be counseled regarding diet and other cardiovascular risk factors and followed at 1-year intervals. Those above the 90th percentile (>185 mg/dL) require special dietary instruction and close supervision with the evaluation of other risk factors. A child with a blood cholesterol level above the 95th percentile (200 mg/dL) and LDL-C level above 130 to 135 mg/dL on two occasions is in a special category and may have one of the hereditary hypercholesterolemias.[8] Strict dietary intervention is indicated and usually is sufficient to reduce LDL-C levels approximately 5% to 15%. Nonresponders over 10 years of age should be considered for treatment with a lipid lowering medication.[7,9,10] Fatty acids of marine origin (n-3) lowered systolic blood pressure and triglycerides, but raised LDL cholesterol compared with fatty acids from plants (n-3 and n-6).[11]

Physician agreement with cholesterol treatment goals is an important component of a successful program to reduce cholesterol levels.[12] The American Academy of Pediatrics, as well as the National Cholesterol Education Program have established recommendations to reduce cardiovascular risk factors in children, including setting guidelines for cholesterol screening and reduction (Fig. 54–1).[13,14]

Dietary Management

During the first 2 years of life, infants and toddlers should not be given low-fat or nonfat foods, such as skim milk, because they need the extra fat and calories for development of the nervous system and proper growth. If fat is restricted before age 2, growth can be temporarily slowed. Human milk or prepared formula, supplemented with infant foods after 4–6 months of age, is appropriate for infants at risk of developing atherosclerosis, as well as for infants not at risk. After 1 year of age, a varied diet including foods from each of the major food groups is the best assurance of nutrition adequacy. At age 2 years, the serum lipid patterns begin to reflect the dietary intake. Children at high risk are 2.7 times more likely to have serum cholesterol values greater than the 95th percentile than are children in the general population.[15]

Whether the hyperlipidemia is familial or not, it is beneficial and practical for the whole family to follow the dietary recommendations. It is important that the child not feel deprived of all preferred foods and treats. Recipes can be developed or altered to include acceptable substituted items, and many of the child's customary foods can be eaten. Fat reductions to lower the risk of cardiovascular disease can also cause weight loss. For an overweight child, this can be an incentive to follow the diet.[16]

Hypercholesterolemia

The diet for treating simple hypercholesterolemia is called a type IIa diet (NIH nomenclature). It corresponds to the American Heart Association prudent diet (Table 54–2) which is the most highly recommended treatment for moderately elevated cholesterol levels (75th to 90th percentile). This diet recommends that 30% of total calories come from fat, with less than 10% of total calories as saturated fat and the remaining 20% from polyunsaturated or monounsaturated fat. Fewer than 300 mg of cholesterol should be eaten per day. These recommendations are similar for both children and adults; quantities and kinds of foods can vary. Preschool children should have about 1 ounce of meat, fish, or poultry for each year of age.[17]

Dietary cholesterol

Cholesterol is found in animal products only, which includes red meats, fish, poultry, eggs, and high fat dairy products. Vegetables, vegetable oils, grains, and fruits contain no cholesterol. Egg yolks and organ meats are major sources of dietary cholesterol. Children should be discouraged from eating more than two egg yolks per week, although egg whites and yolkless egg substitutes can be consumed freely. Organ meats, including liver, should be limited to less than 3 oz/month. Meat, fish, and poultry intake needs to be limited, but peanut butter can be used occasionally as a good cholesterol-free source of protein.

There are an increasing number of vegetable protein meat substitutes, such as tofu, which are made primarily from soybean protein. These products although cholesterol-free and low in saturated fats, are high in sodium content.

Turkey can be used in place of some high-fat meats for bologna, salami, sausage, and other lunchmeats or cold cuts. Although lower in saturated fat, turkey is an animal food containing cholesterol and still needs to be limited.

Saturated fats

Saturated fat causes the body to produce more cholesterol, which can raise both total and LDL cholesterol levels. According to the American Heart Association, restricting saturated fat has been shown to be twice as effective in lowering cholesterol levels, gram for gram, as increasing polyunsaturated fat.[10]

Saturated fat can come from either animal or vegetable sources. The primary sources are meat fat, whole-milk dairy products, solid vegetable shortening, and cocoa butter (chocolate). The hypercholesterolemic patient should use very lean meats with little marbling. Fat should be trimmed from all meat before cooking, when possible, or before being eaten. Poultry skin should be removed, preferably before cooking. Lard, bacon fat, chicken fat, and other meat fats should not be used for frying, baking, seasoning, or gravies. Usual meat-containing entrees, such as spaghetti sauce, chili, stew, or lasagna, can be made and enjoyed without meat.

The consumption of low-fat dairy products should be encouraged. Milk should be skim or low fat (0–1%). Cheese with 6 grams of fat per ounce or less, 0–1% fat cottage cheese, and low-fat (1%) or nonfat plain yogurt are acceptable choices. Mixing the yogurt with fresh fruit makes a good meal or snack. Ice cream should be discouraged

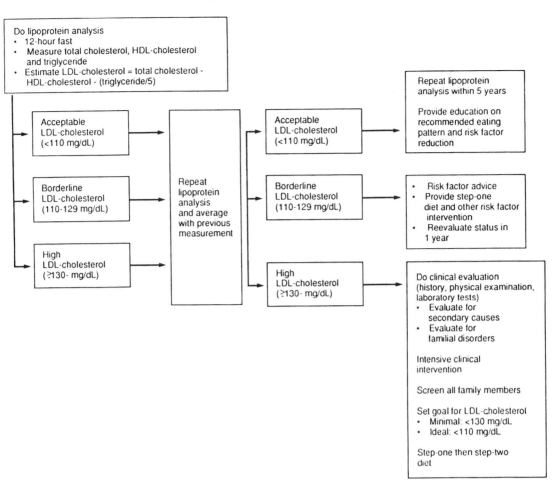

Fig. 54–1. Classification, education and follow-up of children and adolescents based on LDL-cholesterol levels. Step one diet removes obvious sources of saturated fatty acids and cholesterol in the diet. Step two diet requires planning with a registered dietitian to insure adequate nutrients, minerals and vitamins. From National Cholesterol Education Program. *Report of the Expert Panel on Blood Cholesterol Levels in Children and Adolescents.* Bethesda, MD: U.S. Department of Health and Human Services, Public Health Service, National Institute of Health, National Heart, Lung, Blood Institute, 1991.

because of its high saturated fat content. Although ice milk, sherbet, and frozen yogurt seem to be good alternatives, many contain cream, whole milk, and/or egg yolk solids, so ingredient labels must be read carefully. Fruit ice, sorbet, and nonfat egg-free frozen yogurts are better choices. Butter, cream cheese, sour cream, and products made from them should be eliminated. "Lite" or "diet" products often are still too high in fat or contain the wrong kind of fat and should be used sparingly.

The most widely used vegetable sources of saturated fats are coconut, palm, and palm kernel oils. These are the major ingredients in many commercial products, such as nondairy whipped topping, artificial sour cream, coffee whiteners (both powder and liquid), granola cereal and candy, dry pudding mixes, pudding pops, and commercial cookies and cakes. Any product containing one or more of these fats should be avoided. Just because a label says "vegetable oil" or "vegetable shortening" does not preclude the use of coconut or palm oil.

Any baked good containing meat fat—lard, beef fat, chicken fat, or butter—should be avoided. Cookies, cakes, and pie crusts can all be made at home using polyunsaturated oil or margarine. Two egg whites or one-fourth cup of egg substitute can be used in place of one whole egg in recipes.

The cocoa butter in chocolate is highly saturated and should be discouraged. Baked goods and puddings can be prepared using pure cocoa or cocoa syrup (which is cocoa + sucrose + water) instead of chocolate. Oil or margarine can be added to the cocoa as a replacement for the cocoa butter fraction. Carob chips, although made from vegetable oil instead of cocoa butter, are not a good substitute for chocolate chips as they are made from coconut or palm oil.

Polyunsaturated fats

Polyunsaturated fats, which generally come from vegetable sources, help lower total and LDL cholesterol levels. Safflower, sunflower, corn, soybean, sesame, and cottonseed oils are predominantly polyunsaturated fat. These oils are available to the consumer in the form of cooking oil, margarine, mayonnaise, and salad dressing. In general, the more liquid a fat is at room temperature, the higher the ratio of polyunsaturated to saturated fat (P/S ratio). A product should contain at least twice as much polyunsaturated fat as saturated fat to be most beneficial in changing lipid levels.

The desired P/S ratio of a child's total diet is in the range of 1.0 to 1.5. Generally, this ratio can be achieved by eating

Table 54–2. Basic Guidelines for a Cholesterol-Lowering Diet

Food	Amount to be eaten
MEATS	
Meat, fish, poultry	6 oz/day or less
Red meat	1–3 servings/week
Meatless, low-meat entrees	3+ servings/week
Egg yolks	1–2/week
Shrimp, liver, organ meat	3 oz/month or less
High-fat lunch meat	AVOID
DAIRY	
Skim milk (0–1.0% milk fat) cottage cheese (0–1.0%), low-fat (1.0% milk fat) or nonfat yogurt	1/2–1 cup, 2–4 servings/day
Low-fat cheese (2–6 g of fat/ounce)	1 oz as substitute for 1 oz meat, fish, poultry
Whole milk, whole milk products	AVOID
FATS/OILS	
Polyunsaturated and/or monounsaturated fat	6 tsp/day
Saturated fats (coconut oil, palm oil, fully hydrogenated vegetable oil, lard, solid vegetable shortening, etc.	AVOID
FRUITS/VEGETABLES	
Most fruits and vegetables	6+ servings/day
Coconut, avocado	AVOID
BREADS	
Bread, pasta, potato, rice cereal (hot or cold)	4+ servings/day
Breads containing >2 g fat/ serving and/or saturated fat	AVOID

From The Cholesterol Center at The Jewish Hospital, Cincinnati, OH, 1987. Used with permission.

one teaspoon of polyunsaturated fat (P/S ≥ 2) for every ounce of animal sources of protein consumed. For example, if a child eats 4–5 oz/day of meat, fish, or poultry, the child needs 4–5 teaspoons of polyunsaturated fat.

Commercial products are often labeled "partially hydrogenated." This means that hydrogen has been added to a fat to saturate the chemical bonds, which hardens the fat. If the fat began as safflower, sunflower, corn, soybean, or cottonseed oil and then was partially hydrogenated, it becomes a monounsaturated fat (P/S 1:1). This is still an acceptable product, as monounsaturated fat has been shown to lower total cholesterol and LDL cholesterol without lowering the protective HDL cholesterol. Partially hydrogenated coconut or palm oils, as well as fats that are fully hydrogenated, are unacceptable.

Hypertriglyceridemia

The dietary treatment for hypertriglyceridemia (type IV diet) is similar to the diet for hypercholesterolemia, but with the addition of controlled simple sugars. The therapeutic treatment of choice is weight loss to approximately ideal body weight. The great majority of children with familial hypertriglyceridemia who exhibit the hypertriglyceridemic phenotype before age 21 are usually 30% or more above ideal body weight. Weight loss toward ideal body weight almost always results in normal triglyceride levels and helps HDL cholesterol move into the normal range. Modest weight loss can be achieved by using a diet that provides 80% of the calories needed to maintain weight.

Approximately 45% of the diet should be made up of carbohydrates, especially complex carbohydrates. Complex carbohydrates, such as whole-grain breads and cereals and dried beans with high fiber content, and fruits and vegetables with many antioxidant vitamins should be encouraged. Products containing simple sugars, such as sugar-sweetened soft drinks, carbonated and noncarbonated fruit drinks, syrups, jellies and jams, honey, molasses, presweetened cereals, candy, cookies, cakes, and pies, should be avoided or severely restricted.

Artificial sweeteners and artificially sweetened beverages can be used with parental discretion. Fruit and 100% unsweetened fruit juice can be used for "sweetening" cereals, as snacks or desserts, in baking, or for popsicles, instead of sugar or other sweetened flavoring agents.

Fad diets and severely restricted diets are *not* recommended for children. Skipping meals or fasting to lose weight should be discouraged. A child on any restricted diet should be carefully monitored by the physician, dietitian, and parents for any symptoms of an eating or behavioral disorder, including anorexia nervosa or bulimia.[10]

If a child has severe hypertriglyceridemia (> 1000 mg/dL), the child is classified as type V. Total calories need reduction, and fat should be restricted to 20% to 25% of these calories because of the possibility of developing pancreatitis. Cholesterol intake is moderately restricted, and alcoholic beverages should be avoided. An exercise program also is important.

Exercise

Studies have shown that long-term supervised aerobic exercise programs are beneficial for obese children and result in significant weight reduction and improvement in lipoprotein metabolism.[18,19] Aerobic exercise maintains or increases lean body mass while reducing "fatness." It can include 20–30 minutes of brisk walking, indoor or outdoor bicycle riding (10–12 mph), jogging, dancing, rope-skipping, cross-country skiing, swimming, handball, racquetball, skating, running, basketball, or soccer and should be done at least three to four times per week. Aerobic exercise has also been shown to reduce triglyceride levels and elevate the protective HDL cholesterol.

Fiber

Dietary fiber can be grouped into two categories, water soluble and water insoluble. Insoluble fiber is found in wheat bran (the type of bran in most cereals), some vegetables, and most grain fibers. Water-soluble fiber is found in dried beans and peas, some fresh vegetables (peas, carrots, zucchini, sweet potatoes, cauliflower, and green beans), oats, barley, apples, and other high-pectin fruits (oranges, grapefruit, plums, and strawberries). Insoluble fiber promotes regularity and may help reduce the incidence of colon cancer. It has little or no effect on lowering cholesterol. Water-soluble fiber has a hypocholesterolemic effect and less of an impact on regularity. An important recent finding is that water-soluble fiber has been shown to slow glucose absorption and lower serum cholesterol. Some researchers theorize that soluble fiber binds with bile acids and accelerates the clearance of LDL cholesterol from the blood. It also tends to raise HDL cholesterol.

Oat bran is one of the best sources of water-soluble fiber. It is rich in oat gum, a glucan. Animal studies suggest that oat gum is the ingredient active in lowering serum cholesterol. Oat bran can be used as a hot or cold cereal, made into muffins or bread, sprinkled on foods, or used as a filler or food coating.

The recommended amount of dietary fiber to assure an adequate intake of both water-soluble and insoluble fiber in adult diets is 20–35/g/1000 cal.[20–23] Breads are 2.0 g,

cooked legumes are 5.0 g, cereal and pasta are 4.0 g, vegetables are 2.0 g, and fruit and nuts are 2.5 g. The recommended daily allowance for children has not been established.

Fiber should be added to the diet gradually to minimize intestinal discomfort. Excessive fiber intake can cause bloating and diarrhea, as well as the loss of some trace minerals (zinc, calcium, copper, iron and magnesium) due to binding by the fiber.

Although high-carbohydrate, low-fiber diets often raise fasting plasma triglyceride levels, high-carbohydrate, high-fiber diets maintain or lower triglycerides in individuals with normal values, and lower triglycerides significantly in individuals with elevated levels.[18–24]

Several studies have been conducted to test the effect of lecithin on serum cholesterol, but most of these studies were poorly designed. Lecithin is a phospholipid found primarily in soybeans. The combined results of the four appropriately controlled trials suggest that dietary lecithin does not lower serum cholesterol.[25]

Guar gum, a gel-forming dietary fiber, has been shown to be effective in reducing serum cholesterol levels,[26] but there are still many questions concerning the effectiveness of long-term guar gum therapy.[27]

Pectins are a group of high molecular weight polysaccharides found primarily in apples, citrus fruits, and strawberries. When ingested, pectin can lower serum cholesterol levels in some people.[28,29] It has been suggested that pectin lowers serum cholesterol only in the presence of dietary cholesterol. If a prudent diet is followed that reduces the intake of dietary cholesterol, the addition of pectin has little or no cholesterol-lowering effect.[30]

Dining out

A child cannot be expected to eat all meals at home. Snacking and eating at friends' homes, restaurants, snack bars, and parties are all part of today's busy lifestyles. The child can, however, be instructed in good food choices, which may include turkey, ham, grilled chicken (no breading, not fried), baked fish, or well-trimmed roast beef. Sandwiches should not be topped with cheese or bacon, but a mayonnaise-type dressing is acceptable. Hamburgers that are broiled or charcoal-grilled are more acceptable than those that are fried, and cheese should not be added because of its high fat content. If fried chicken is selected; much of the fat can be eliminated by removing and discarding the breading and skin. A fruit cup, tossed salad, corn-on-the-cob, cole slaw, and applesauce would be good accompaniments, rather than french fries, onion rings, or other fried items.

Pizza made with part skim mozzarella cheese is a good choice, but only if it is plain or topped with vegetables. Sausage, pepperoni, and hamburger add too much fat and cholesterol and should be avoided.[10]

Follow-up

The aim of any dietary restriction for the child with hyperlipidemia is lifelong adherence.[31] It is therefore important that the diet not be too rigid or unappealing. The diet regimen recommended for children is not as strict as that suggested by the American Heart Association for adults. A moderately restricted diet that is followed on a long-term basis is more successful in reducing cardiovascular disease than an extremely rigid diet followed only for a short time. Whether following a diet to lower cholesterol or triglyceride levels, children still need to meet the recommended dietary allowances established by the American Dietetic Association for their age group.

In general, diet and lifestyle intervention should be tried at least 6 months before resorting to drug treatment to normalize lipid levels. If drug treatment is necessary, it is important that the patient remain on the prescribed diet to achieve the best results.

References

1. Palmer, S., Esterman, P. Preventable nutritional problems in infancy. In: Palmer, S., Ekvall, S., eds. *Pediatric Nutrition in Developmental Disorders*. Springfield, IL: Charles C. Thomas; 1978.
2. *Blood Cholesterols*. Cincinnati: The Cholesterol Center of The Jewish Hospital; 1987.
3. Nicklas, T.A., Farris, R.P., Frank, G.C., Webber, L.S., Cresanta, J.L., Berenson, G.S. Cardiovascular disease risk factors from birth to seven years of age: Bogalusa heart study, dietary intakes. *Pediatrics*. 1987; 805(suppl):767.
4. Lauer, R.M., Lee, J., Clarke, W.R. Factors affecting the relationship between childhood and adult cholesterol levels: the Muscatine study. *Pediatrics*. 1988; 82:309.
5. Farris, R.P., Cresanta, J.L., Webber, L.S., Berenson, G.S. Macronutrient intakes of 10-year-old children, 1973 to 1982. *J. Am. Diet. Assoc*. 1986; 86:765.
6. Cresanta, J.L., Farris, R.P., Croft, J.B., Frank, G.C., Berenson, G.S. Trends in fatty acid intakes of 10-year old children, 1973 to 1982. *J. Am. Diet. Assoc*. 1988; 88:178.
7. Consensus Conference. Lowering blood cholesterol to prevent heart disease. *JAMA*. 1985; 253:2080.
8. Goldman, S., Illig, E., Mellies, M., Glueck, C.J. Nutrition and hyperlipidemia. In: Grand, R.J., Sutphen, J.L., Dietz, W.H., eds. *Pediatric Nutrition Theory and Practice*. Boston: Butterworth Publishers; 1987.
9. Glueck, C.J. Pediatric primary prevention of atherosclerosis. *N. Engl. J. Med*. 1986; 314:175.
10. Snetselaar, L., Lauer, R. Childhood, diet and atherosclerotic process. *Nutr. Today* 1992; 27:22.
11. Kestin, M., Clifton, P., Belling, G., Nestel, P. n-3 Fatty acids of marine origin lower systolic pressure and triglycerides but raise LDL cholesterol compared with n-3 and n-6 fatty acids from plants. *Am. J. Clin. Nutr*. 1990; 51:1028.
12. Superko, H.R., Desmond, D.A., deSantos, P.A., Vranizan, K.M., Farquhar, J.W. Blood cholesterol treatment attitudes of community physicians: A major problem. *Am. Heart J.* 1988; 113:849.
13. National Cholesterol Education Program, 1991. Report of the Expert Panel on Blood Cholesterol Levels in Children and Adults. Bethesda, MD: U.S. Department of Health and Human Services, National Institute of Health, National Heart, Lung, Blood Institute.
14. American Academy of Pediatrics Committee on Nutrition. Indications for cholesterol testing. *Pediatrics*. 1989; 83:141.
15. American Academy of Pediatrics Committee on Nutrition. Toward a prudent diet for children. *Pediatrics*. 1983; 71:78.
16. Taras, H.L., Sallis, J.F., Rupp, J.W. Early childhood diet: recommendations of pediatric health care providers. *J. Am. Diet. Assoc*. 1988; 88:1417.
17. *The American Heart Association Diet: An Eating Plan for Healthy Americans*. Dallas: The American Heart Association; 1985.
18. Sasaki, J., Shindo, M., Tanaka, H., Ando, J., Arakawa, K. A long-term aerobic exercise program decreases the obesity index and increases the high density lipoprotein cholesterol concentration in obese children. *Int. J. Obes*. 1987; 11:339.
19. Anderson, J.W., Tietyen-Clark, J. Dietary fiber: hyperlipidemia, hypertension and coronary heart disease. *Am. J. Gastroenterol*. 1986; 81:907.
20. Anderson, J.W., Bridges, S.R., Tietyen, J., Gustafson, N.J. Dietary fiber content of a simulated American diet and selected research diets. *Am. J. Clin. Nutr*. 1989; 49:352.
21. Anderson, J.W., Bridges, S.R. Dietary fiber content of selected foods. *Am. J. Clin. Nutr*. 1988; 47:440.
22. *Back to Fiber*. Minneapolis: General Mills; 1986.
23. *The High Fiber Diet*. Cincinnati: Procter and Gamble; 1985.
24. Anderson, J.W., Gustafson, N.J., Bryant, C.A., Tietyen-Clark, J. Dietary fiber and diabetes: a comprehensive review and practical application. *J. Am. Diet. Assoc*. 1987; 87:1189.
25. Knuiman, J.T., Beynen, A.C., Katan, M.B. Lecithin intake and serum cholesterol. *Am. J. Clin. Nutr*. 1989; 49:266.
26. Uusitupa, M., Siitonen, O., Savolainen, K., Silvasti, M. Penttila, I. Metabolic and nutritional effects of long-term use of guar gum in the treatment of noninsulin-dependent diabetes of poor metabolic control. *Am. J. Clin. Nutr*. 1989; 49:345.
27. Superko, H.R., Haskell, W.L., Sawrey-Kubicek, L., Farquhar, J. Effects of solid and liquid guar gum on plasma cholesterol and triglyceride concentrations in moderate hypercholesterolemia. *Am. J. Cardiol*. 1988; 65:51.
28. Siragusa, R.J., Cerda, J.J., Baig, M.M., Burgin, C.W., Robbins, F.L. Methanol production from the degradation of pectin by human colonic bacteria. *Am. J. Clin. Nutr*. 1988; 47:848.
29. Slavin, J.L. Dietary fiber: classification, chemical analysis, and food sources. *J. Am. Diet. Assoc*. 1987; 87:1164.
30. Kay, R.M., Truswell, A.S. Effect of citrus pectin on blood lipids and fecal steroid excretion in man. *Am. J. Clin. Nutr*. 1977; 30:171.
31. Copperman, N., Schebendach, J., Arden, M., Jacobson, M. Practical management of pediatric hyperlipidemia. *Top. Clin. Nutr*. 1991; 6:51.

Chapter 55
Lowe's Syndrome

Marietta Llenado and Shirley Walberg Ekvall

Lowe's syndrome is a congenital hereditary disorder that was originally described in 1952 by Lowe et al.[1] The terms "oculocerebrorenal syndrome" and "Lowe's syndrome" have been used interchangeably because of the triad of congenital ocular abnormalities, cerebral dysfunction, and renal abnormalities.[2-4]

Patients with Lowe's syndrome are characterized by growth retardation, hypotonia, mild or severe metabolic acidosis, generalized hyperaminoaciduria, proteinuria, rickets, and characteristic eye changes.[5] Prominent opthalmological features include congenital cataracts, glaucoma, corneal degeneration, and strabismus[4] (Fig. 55–1). Muscles are abnormally weak and hypotonic, resulting in a "floppy" appearance.

The natural history of Lowe's syndrome has been divided into three stages.[2] In the first stage, there may be only proteinuria and ocular abnormalities in the neonatal period. During the first year of life, the second stage may appear with aminoaciduria, organic aciduria, and metabolic acidosis. Seizures may be seen in this stage. Rickets, phosphaturia, and hypophosphatemia follow unless there is adequate prophylaxis with vitamin D, phosphate, and alkali. The final phase is characterized by the reduction of metabolic disturbances; the patient remains retarded mentally and physically, with a significant visual handicap and chronic renal failure.[6]

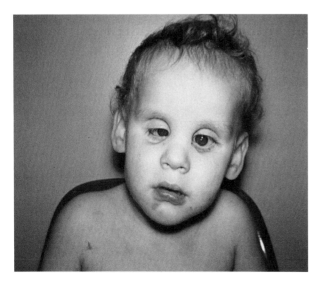

Fig. 55–1. Ocular defects (bilateral dense nuclear cataracts) in Lowe's syndrome. From University Affiliated Cincinnati Center for Developmental Disorders. Used with permission.

Lowe's syndrome is considered to be a rare disease. Estimates of the number of persons with Lowe's syndrome range from several hundred to a few thousand throughout the world.[4] Deaths at all ages have been reported from kidney failure, dehydration, and pneumonia. However, children can be expected to live at least to their twenties and thirties if no complications occur.[4]

There is abundant evidence of familial occurrence of the syndrome. The disease is believed to be X-linked recessive and affects young males more than females, with few female cases reported.[4,5,7,8] At present, the etiology of the disease is not well understood, and there is no specific diagnostic test available. Not all affected children will have every characteristic feature at all ages. Typically, the diagnosis is made in the first year of life and is based upon the physical examination, laboratory findings, and family history.

Biochemical Abnormalities

A review of the literature suggests that the exact metabolic defect in Lowe's syndrome is not yet fully understood. Metabolic disturbances, such as proteinuria, sialic aciduria, and the excretion of undersulfated chrondroitin sulfate A, that occur in this syndrome are also found in a variety of inborn errors of metabolism. Laboratory findings that could warrant recognition of Lowe's syndrome include persistent metabolic acidosis with normal plasma amino acid concentration; serum calcium level varying from low to normal, with reduced serum inorganic phosphate concentrations and increased serum alkaline phosphatase[9]; and hypokalemia with potassium values varying between 2.3 and 3.5 mEq/L.[10]

The renal involvement in Lowe's syndrome is related to the tubular dysfunction, which is characterized by impaired reabsorption of bicarbonate, glucose, phosphate, potassium, amino acids, and uric acid.[11]

Some progress in research has been made in recent years in clarifying the underlying biochemical defect of the oculocerebrorenal syndrome (OCRS). Wisnewski et al.[11] reported that the clinical stigmata of OCRS may be related to a defect in glycosaminoglycans (GAG) metabolism. Urinary excretion of GAG was four to five times greater in OCRS patients than in normal controls. During behavioral agitation, one patient showed a tenfold increase in urinary GAG excretion. Yoshida et al.[12] demonstrated that nucleotide pyrophosphatase activity was markedly elevated in cultured skin fibroblasts from OCRS patients. It was suggested that this increase in breakdown of sugar nucleotides and active sulfate would disturb GAG metabolism. In a similar study using cultured fibroblasts obtained from OCRS patients, it was reported that an excessive synthesis of under-sulfated chrondroitin-4-sulfate is the consequence of elevated nucleotide pyrophosphatase activity.[13] Yokoi et al.,[14] in their study of synthesis of intracellular glycosaminoglycans in cultured cells from patients with Lowe's syndrome, found no evidence of a defect in sulfation of heparan sulfate, but rather an impairment of synthesis. Palmieri et al.[15] extended the studies on cultured fibroblasts to include an examination of collagen formation. They observed that cultured fibroblasts originating from patients with Lowe's syndrome consistently accumulated more intracellular proline, suggesting a possible abnormality in the intracellular fate of this amino acid. Although the mechanism of this increased proline entry has not been established, it is possible that the difference in proline uptake may be used to characterize fibroblasts from fetuses suspected of having Lowe's syndrome. Therefore, this biochemical tool possibly could be used for prenatal diagnosis.[16]

Careful orthopedic evaluation of OCRS patients disclosed musculoskeletal deformities that are commonly seen in other known connective tissue disorders, particularly the mucopolysaccharidoses (MPS).[17] Clinical findings of scoliosis, kyphosis, platyspondylia, dislocated and/or subluxed hips, and cervical spine abnormalities were reported in six patients.[3] These findings were never reported previously. The investigators in this study used oral doses of 0.25–0.50 ug/day of a synthetic vitamin D_3 analog, 1 α, 25 dihydroxycholecalciferol (Rocaltrol®). Some form of alkali supplementation had been given to facilitate resolution of the bone disease. Porosis and reduced bone age and muscle mass were consistent with a clinical diagnosis of the syndrome. Bone changes related to renal defects have been treated with vitamin D from 1000 to 2000 IU/day in conjunction with alkali of 50 to 100 mEq/day.[18,19]

Pronounced hypotonia and retarded motor development are generally associated with Lowe's syndrome. Patients may be partially or totally blind. Feeding problems, such as poor sucking ability and active tongue thrusting without direction, are often observed. The level of feeding skills development may vary according to the extent of the abnormality and other combinations of problems that are present in each case (see Chapter 24 for specific feeding facilitation techniques). The general syndrome of hypotonia can cause constipation (atonic type), which should be an important aspect of nutrition evaluation.

Reported cases of pulmonary infections should be investigated if the patient is in a poor nutritional state[10] (see Chapter 28).

Factors to be Considered in Nutritional Evaluation and Dietary Management

There is no specific dietary management for Lowe's syndrome. A study by Fogelson and Berry[17] investigating a galactose-restricted diet with three infant boys having OCRS found that the diet decreased aminoaciduria. Although the diet did not improve the problems of mental retardation, cataracts, glaucoma, and hypotonia, the patients were reported to be happier, easier to care for, more agile, and had no episodes of dehydration.

Dietary treatment is individualized according to the evaluation of the patient's existing problems. Generally, the diet should be high in calories, fiber, and fluid, and there should be small frequent feedings. Although birth weight in Lowe's syndrome is normal, patients are reported to feed poorly during the first few days of life.[10,18] Weight and stature are usually retarded and can fall to the 3rd percentile after a few months.

Because frequent vomiting and unexplained fever with dehydration are common, provision should be made for a high calorie and fluid intake. Constipation caused by the general syndrome of hypotonia should be treated similarly to atonic constipation with increased fiber and fluid intake (see Chapter 35).

Follow-up

A medical examination every 6 to 8 months is suggested for the purpose of evaluating renal, ocular, and neurological functions. Anthropometric measurements—fatfold, height, weight, and head circumference—are useful parameters for assessing physical growth and development and should be evaluated at each visit. Dietary intake and feeding abilities also should be evaluated to determine the adequacy of nutrition for normal growth and development.

References

1. Lowe, C. V., Terry, M., MacLachlan, E. A. Organic aciduria, decreased ammonia production, hydrophthalmus and mental retardation. A clinical entity. *Am. J. Dis. Child.* 1952; 84:164.
2. Curtis, J.A., Goel, K.M. Oculo-cerebro-renal syndrome (Lowe's syndrome)—a report of three cases. *Practitioner.* 1982; 226:1159.
3. Holtgrewe, J.L., Kalen, V. Orthopedic manifestations of the Lowe (oculocerebrorenal) syndrome. *J. Pediatr. Orthop.* 1986; 6:165.
4. *Living with Lowe's Syndrome, A Guide for Families, Friends, and Professionals.* Lowe's Syndrome Association; 1987.
5. Yamashina, I., Fuqui, S., Funakoshi, I. Biochemical studies on Lowe's syndrome. *Mol. Cell. Biochem.* 1983; 52:107.
6. Harris, L.S., Gitter, K.A., Galin, M.A., Plechaty, G.P. Oculo-cerebro-renal syndrome. Report of a case in a baby girl. *Br. J. Opthalmol.* 1970; 54:278.
7. Hodgson, S.V., Heckmatt, J.Z., Hughes, E., Crolla, J.A., Dubowitz, V., Bobrow, M. A balanced de novo X/autosome translocation in a girl with manifestations of Lowe's syndrome. *Am. J. Med. Genet.* 1986; 23:837.
8. O'Brien, D. Rare inborn errors of metabolism. In: *Children with Disorders of Amino Acid Metabolism.* Washington, DC: US Government Printing Office; 1970. US DHEW publication no. 2049.
9. Cyvin, K.B., Weideman, J., Bathen, J. Lowe's syndrome. *Acta Paediatr. Scand.* 1973; 62:309.
10. Baluarte, H.J. Renal abnormalities in Lowe's syndrome. *Lowe's Synd. Fam. Newsl. (On the Beam)* 1983; 1:7.
11. Wisnewski, K., Kierras, F., French, J., Houck, G., Ramos, P. Ultrastructural, neurological, and glycosaminoglycan abnormalities in Lowe's syndrome. *Ann. Neurol.* 1984; 16:40.
12. Yoshida, H., Fukui, S., Yamashina, I., Tanaka, T., Sakano, T., Usui, T., Shimotsuji, T., Yabuuchi, H., Owada, M., Kitagawa, T. Elevation of nucleotide pyrophosphatase activity in skin fibroblasts from patients with Lowe's syndrome. *Biochem. Biophys. Res. Comm.*, 1982; 107:1144.
13. Fukui, S., Yoshida, H., Tanaka, T., Sakano, T., Usui, T., Yamashina, I.: Glycosaminoglycan synthesis by cultured skin fibroblasts from a patient with Lowe's syndrome. *J. Biol. Chem.* 1981; 256:10313.
14. Yokoi, T., Taniguchi, N., Ikawa, K. Impaired synthesis of intracellular heparin sulfate in skin fibroblasts of Lowe's syndrome. *J. Lab. Clin. Med.* 1982; 100:461.

15. Palmieri, M., O'Hara, J., States, B., Segal, S. Decreased pre-collagen production in cultured fibroblasts from patients with Lowe's syndrome. *J. Inher. Metab. Dis.* 1985; 8:187.

16. States, B., Palmieri, M.J., Segal, S. Uptake of proline in cultured cells from patients with Lowe's syndrome. *Biochem. Biophys. Res. Comm.*, 1982; 109:428.

17. Fogelson, M., Berry, H. Nutritional investigation in the ocu-locerebrorenal syndrome of Lowe. *Birth Defects*. 1974; 10:149.

18. Michelbergeron, M., Gougoux, A. In: Scriver, C., Beaudet, A., Sly, W., Valle, D., eds. *The Metabolic Basis of Inherited Diseases*. 6th ed. Vol. 1. New York: McGraw-Hill; 1989.

19. Loughead, J., Mimouni, F., Schilling, S., Feingold, M. Lowe's syndrome. *Am. J. Dis. Child.* 1991; 145:113.

Chapter 56
Williams Syndrome

Lusia Hornstein

Williams syndrome is a complex condition of unknown etiology, involving multiple organ systems and with a characteristic facies. It is associated with mental retardation, usually of a mild degree.

In 1951, Fanconi[1] and Butler[2] reported almost simultaneously observations of infants with failure to thrive, elfin-like facies, and hypercalcemia. Williams et al.[3] described in 1961 four young children with a peculiar facies, supravalvular aortic stenosis (SVAS), and mental retardation. Beuren et al.[4] in 1962 added three more patients with the same findings noted by Williams and questioned whether the association of SVAS, mental retardation, and facial characteristics constituted a syndrome. It was Black and Bonham Carter[5] who noted in 1963 that the facies of children with SVAS described by Williams and co-workers and those with idiopathic hypercalcemia described by Fanconi were quite similar and suggested that these children had different manifestations of the same condition. With time and through efforts of many workers, it became obvious that the facial appearances, SVAS, occasional infantile hypercalcemia, and other characteristics are part of the same syndrome, which came to be referred to as "infantile hypercalcemia-supravalvular aortic stenosis" or "Williams syndrome." Jones and Smith pointed out in 1975[6] that not all children have SVAS and hypercalcemia. Of the 19 individuals with Williams syndrome studied, 8 of whom had serum calcium determinations in the first year of life, none had hypercalcemia.

Clinically, pregnancy is usually reported to be normal, and birth weight, although on the lower end, tends to be within the normal range. At birth an unusual facial appearance may be noted. In many infants, feeding difficulties occur almost from the first days of life. Vomiting is frequent, and failure to gain weight is noted, particularly during the first few months of life. Occasionally, a high serum calcium level is documented during this period. Many of the infants are described as extremely irritable and refusing to eat. Constipation is a frequent occurrence and hernias—umbilical, inguinal, and epigastric—are not uncommon. As time progresses, the feeding difficulties and failure to thrive lessen, but delays in motor, mental, and language development; poor motor coordination; and in some a deep husky voice become more apparent. Parents may report hyperacusis and fear of heights, such as descending stairs, sitting in a highchair, etc., which may continue into adulthood.[7,8]

Physical characteristics include mild microcephaly with bitemporal depressions, flat nasal bridge, anteverted nares, full cheeks particularly in the lower portion, long philtrum, full lips with frequent sagging of the lower lip, epicanthic folds, periorbital fullness, frequently blue irides with stellate pattern, strabismus that is prominent at times, low-set ears, micrognathia, and high-arched palate. These facial characteristics have led to the description "elfin like" or "pixy like." As the children grow, their body build may also be quite characteristic. Many of the children continue to be small and thin. The neck and the torso may be long, and pectus excavatum occurs frequently. The shoulders tend to be narrow and sloping. Clinodactyly of the fifth fingers, hallux valgus, and abnormal palmar creases may be noted. Teeth may be small, irregularly spaced, and with enamel hypoplasia and bite abnormalities (Fig. 56–1).

Of particular importance are cardiac and vascular anomalies. The most frequently encountered lesion is SVAS, but there may be other associated lesions, such as pulmonary artery stenosis, aortic hypoplasia, septal defects, and others. Narrowing of other vessels of the body may be seen, and systemic hypertension, at times secondary to renal artery stenosis, may be present.[9,10]

Renal anomalies have been described, as well as urinary bladder diverticula. A mild neurological dysfunction may be present. The deep tendon reflexes are characteristically hyperactive. Hypotonia may be present, particularly during infancy and childhood. Decreased flexion in the ankle joints and limitation of joint movements may occur. Some older individuals may become obese.[10]

Individuals with Williams syndrome usually are mildly retarded (IQ, 50–80) with poor visuomotor coordination and with particular strength in vocabulary and language. Socially, most are outgoing, friendly, and very talkative. However, some may become upset easily, are stubborn and hyperactive, and show behavior problems.

Williams syndrome occurs sporadically in about 1 in 20,000 births. The etiology is unknown. Chromosomal abnormalities have been found infrequently, but these have been inconsistent, involving different chromosomes. In most instances, chromosomes have been normal.

Biochemical Abnormalities

Hypercalcemia is found in some children with Williams syndrome during infancy. It appears to be present only during the first few months of life, and unless the diagnosis of Williams syndrome is made during this period, in most cases it cannot be documented later. The vomiting, constipation, irritability, and failure to thrive frequently seen during infancy in children with Williams syndrome may be related to hypercalcemia, but not all children with these symptoms have a high serum calcium level.

The etiology of the hypercalcemia is not yet understood, despite numerous clinical and animal studies. In the early

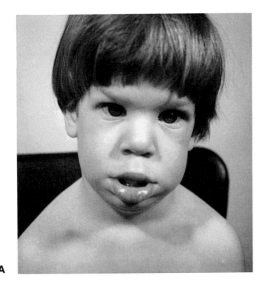

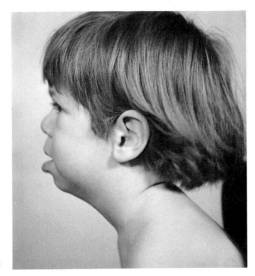

Fig. 56–1. *A*, Front view and *B*, profile of 1-year-old child with Williams syndrome. From University Affiliated Cincinnati Center for Developmental Disorders. Used with permission.

post-World War II years a large number of cases of infantile hypercalcemia and SVAS were identified in the United Kingdom and in Germany. During those years infants were ingesting large amounts of vitamin D, approximately 4000 units per day; milk, cereals, and other products were fortified with large doses of vitamin D in an attempt to eliminate rickets. In Germany, it was customary to give infants prophylactical injections of vitamin D containing as much as 400,000–600,000 units several times during the first year of life.[11] Mothers may have also been exposed to large amounts of vitamin D during pregnancy. After a drastic reduction in vitamin D supplementation, the incidence of idiopathic hypercalcemia syndrome in the United Kingdom was reduced dramatically.

Vitamin D has three classic forms. The dietary form and the form produced in the skin, calciferol, are converted in the liver to 25-hydroxycholecalciferol. This form is converted in the kidneys to the very potent 1,25-dihydroxycholecalciferol, which maintains the serum calcium level through absorption from the intestine. Some authors believe there may be hypersensitivity to vitamin D either in the infant or pregnant mother. How this possible hypersensitivity affects the vitamin D regulation of calcium metabolism is unknown. Another hypothesis involves a possible disturbance in the homeostasis of calcium in utero. Friedman and Mills[12] gave pregnant rabbits very large doses of vitamin D and were able to produce lesions in the aorta and some of the craniofacial stigmata seen in Williams syndrome in their offspring.

Martin et al.[13] measured metabolites of vitamin D in 83 patients with idiopathic infantile hypercalcemia (Williams syndrome) who at the time of the study had normal calcium levels and could not demonstrate any abnormality of vitamin D metabolism. Garabedian et al.[14] measured plasma concentrations of 1,25-dihydroxycalciferol in four young infants with Williams syndrome with hypercalcemia. These levels were elevated between 5 and 9 months of age. They were higher than those in three children with the syndrome but without hypercalcemia and in eight children with hypercalcemia but no dysmorphic features. The authors concluded that the hypercalcemia in these four infants may be secondary to the abnormal degradation of 1,25-dihydroxycholecalciferol.

Most recently, calcitonin has been implicated as a possible cause of the hypercalcemia. Calcitonin, a hormone produced by the parafollicular cells of the thyroid gland, helps clear calcium from blood. Culler et al.[15] studied the effects of provocative infusions of calcium and parathyroid hormone in five children with Williams syndrome and found delayed clearance of calcium after intravenous calcium loading. They concluded that individuals with Williams syndrome have a defect in the synthesis or release of calcitonin.

Factors to be Considered in Nutritional Evaluation

Not all children with Williams syndrome have a history of feeding problems, vomiting, and failure to thrive. However, these difficulties, together with the extreme irritability, constitute the main reason for morbidity during the first year of life. Even later, some of the children tend to be "picky eaters."

In Williams syndrome, therapy goals have to be directed toward feeding difficulties, failure to thrive, hypercalcemia, constipation, and, in later years, occasionally obesity.

Dietary Management

Providing dietary advice during infancy is very important to ensure that the infant receives adequate amount of calories, fluid, and nutrients for growth and to compensate for the vomiting. In severe cases of vomiting, a nasogastric tube supplementation may be utilized during the night. Offering reassurance to parents is essential during this period. The infants are very difficult to feed, and mothers frequently feel guilty and sometimes are made to feel responsible for their infant's failure to thrive, particularly in yet undiagnosed cases.

Some believe that the irritability, feeding difficulties, vomiting, and constipation occur primarily in children whose calcium level is higher than the normal range. Therefore, lowering of the calcium level may result in an improvement in symptomatology. Martin et al.[16] suggest that plasma calcium levels be investigated in children with profuse vomiting and failure to thrive in association with a heart murmur. In their survey, children were treated with a low-calcium and vitamin-D-restricted diet. In addition, some received a course of corticosteroids for 1 to 4 weeks. Noted adverse effects were hypocalcemia in 21% and iatrogenic rickets in 9%. Even on the diet, feeding problems continued, but there was some lessening of vomiting and a slow weight gain. The authors recommend that the therapy should not be continued longer than 6 to 12 months.

Constipation is seen frequently in children with Williams syndrome. In young infants it is felt to be related to hypercalcemia. A diet high in fiber and fluid probably is useful in the older child. Foods high in fiber, such as fruits, vegetables, and whole-grain cereals and breads, are recommended (see Chapter 35).

Follow-up

Although most children with Williams syndrome are thin or have normal weight, some tend to become somewhat obese during adolescence. These individuals should be under dietary supervision to prevent obesity (see Chapter 19). Anthropometric measures, dietary history (particularly related to adequate growth, fiber, and fluids), feeding history, and appropriate serum levels should be performed each visit.

References

1. Fanconi, G. Uber Chronische Storungen des Calcium and Phosphatstoffwechsels im Kindesalter. *Schweiz. Med. Wochenschr.* 1951; 81:908.
2. Butler, N.R. Generalized retardation with renal impairment, hypercalcemia and osteosclerosis of skull. *Proc. Roy. Soc. Med.*, 1951; 44:296.
3. Williams, J.C.P., Barratt-Boyes, B.G., Lowe, J.B. Supravalvular aortic stenosis. *Circulation.* 1961; 24:1311.
4. Beuren, A.J., Apitz, J., Harmjan, D. Supravalvular aortic stenosis in association with mental retardation and certain facial appearance. *Circulation.* 1962; 26:1235.
5. Black, J.A., Bonham Carter, R.E. Association between aortic stenosis and facies of severe infantile hypercalcemia. *Lancet.* 1963; 2:745.
6. Jones, K.L., Smith, D.W. The Williams elfin facies syndrome. *J. Pediatr.* 1975; 86:718.
7. Udwin, O. A survey of adults with Williams syndrome and idiopathic infantile hypercalcemia. *Dev. Med. Child. Neurol.* 1990; 32:129.
8. Klein, A.J., Armstrong, B.L., Greer, M.K., Brown, F.R. Hyperacusis and otitis media in individuals with Williams syndrome. *J. Speech Hear. Disord.* 1990; 55:339.
9. Daniels, S.R., Loggie, J.M.H., Schwartz, D.C., Strife, J.L., Kaplan, S. Systemic hypertension secondary to peripheral vascular anomalies in patients with Williams syndrome. *J. Pediatr.* 1985; 102:249.
10. Morris, C.A., Demsey, S.A., Leonard, C.O., Dilts, C., Blackburn, B.L. Natural history of Williams syndrome: physical characteristics. *J. Pediatr.* 1988; 114:318.
11. Tsang, R.C., Noguchi, A., Steichen, J.J. Pediatric parathyroid disorders. *Pediatr. Clin. North Am.* 1979; 26:223.
12. Friedman, W.F., Mills, L.F. The relationship between vitamin D and the craniofacial dental anomalies of the supravalvular aortic stenosis syndrome. *Pediatrics.* 1969; 43:12.
13. Martin, N.D.T., Snodgrass, G.J.A.I., Cohen, R.D., Porteous, C.E., Coldwell, R.D., Porteous, Trafford, D.J.H., Makin, H.L.J. Vitamin D metabolites in idiopathic infantile hypercalcemia. *Arch. Dis. Child.* 1985; 60:1140.
14. Garabedian, M., Jacoz, E., Guillozo, H., Grimberg, R., Guillot, M., Gagnadoux, M., Broyer, M., Lenoir, G., Balsan, S. Elevated plasma 1,25-dihydroxyvitamin D concentration in infants with hypercalcemia and an elfin facies. *N. Engl. J. Med.* 1985; 312:948.
15. Culler, F.L., Jones, K.J., Deftos, L.N. Impaired calcitonin secretion in patients with Williams syndrome. *J. Pediatr.* 1985; 107:720.
16. Martin, N.D., Snodgrass, G.J.A.I., Cohen, R.D. Idiopathic infantile hypercalcemia—a continuing enigma. *Arch. Dis. Child.* 1984; 59:605.

Chapter 57
Wilson's Disease

Florence Stevens

Wilson's disease (WD), inherited as an autosomal-recessive condition, is caused by the abnormal transport or storage of copper, which results in damage to the liver, kidney, brain, and cornea. Chronic copper poisoning occurs with hepatolenticular degeneration. The prevalence of WD is 30 per 1,000,000.[1] Though copper is toxic in WD, it is also essential for life. Chromosome 13 and Exterase-D have been mapped for WD. Genetic screening is important in terms of diagnosis. Chromosome 13 is close to the retinoblastoma locus. To identify gene carriers, a retinoblastoma probe is used in the diagram of siblings and relatives.[2] The gene affects the synthesis and processing rather than the regulation of ceruloplasmin. Affected children are identified between the age of 6 and the early teens. For most children, the initial presentation is hepatic. If the liver biopsy of a sibling indicates WD, the diagnosis of WD in infants should be delayed 6 months because of low ceruloplasmin levels. The disease onset is neurological or psychiatric between the second and fourth decade of life.[3]

Some observable characteristics indicating the onset of WD are deterioration of handwriting, weakness, deterioration of general school performance (decreased coordination, decreased fine motor ability, increased behavioral problems, decreased mental function) rigidity, dysphagia, dysarthria, deterioration in self-help skills, or spasticity.[1] In the advanced stage of WD, cirrhosis of the liver, a Kayser-Fleischer ring in the cornea, choreathetosis, dystonia, reduced serum ceruloplasmin, increased copper excretion, increased liver copper content, a "wing-beating" tremor, and open-mouth grimace are frequently seen.[4] Pancreatitis also may be associated with WD.[5]

Biochemical Abnormalities

WD is confirmed by low serum copper concentrations (<80 ug/100 dL), decreased serum ceruloplasmin levels (<20 ug/100 mL), increased excretion of copper (100 mcg/24 hr),[6] and urine zinc. Serum phosphatase and serum uric acid levels are decreased. Testing should include routine liver function tests, computerized axial tomography scan, and determination of radiocopper incorporation into ceruloplasmin. As toxicity progresses, liver cells are destroyed and replaced by fibrous tissue. In liver biopsy, hepatic copper is greater than 100 ug per gram of dry weight. A renal Fanconi syndrome presents with generalized aminoaciduria and increased glucose, uric acid, calcium, and phosphate in urine.[7] Heterozygous carriers have decreased ceruloplasmin and increased liver copper levels, even though they are symptom-free.

Penicillamine is the chelating agent used for most WD patients. When penicillamine is begun, functioning levels decrease before improvement is seen. For those who are allergic to the medication, trientine has been effective in cases of penicillamine-induced neutropenia, thrombocytopenia, systemic lupus erythematosis, and nephrosis. Seizures have occurred in a minority of patients utilizing drug therapy. Zinc acetate has been developed as an effective and nontoxic therapy for WD. Without drug intervention, the progress of the toxicity and its effects increase. Noncompliance is devastating, and in severe cases recovery takes years.

Factors to be Considered in Nutritional Evaluation

Nutritional assessment is required to establish nutritional needs and identify feeding problems. Obesity may be a factor when there is limited mobility. Motor coordination and swallowing problems make self-feeding and normal mastication of food difficult. Requirements for adaptive equipment and alterations in food textures and calories are required in advanced stages or relapse. Penicillamine drug-nutrient interaction causes the increased excretion of zinc, iron, copper, manganese, and pyridoxine, with possible anemias, iron deficiency, drug-induced peripheral neuropathy, and reduced white blood cells and platelets. Supplements are needed. Other side effects are unpleasant taste, decreased taste for salt and sweet, and anorexia perhaps due to lowered zinc levels.[8] When zinc acetate alone is used, it blocks copper absorption. Patients with neurological disease often worsen initially on penicillamine. Zinc also acts slower than desired. Without neurological disease, a period of treatment is required to induce intestinal cell metallotheonein, which interacts with copper with a high affinity and prevents its serosal transfer. It is excellent for maintenance therapy and the treatment of the presymptomatic patient.

The decreased ability to perform daily functions is a result of copper intoxication. (Biochemical information is diagnostic.) A 24-hour dietary recall and frequency cross-check should be taken to evaluate the copper, calorie, and protein content of the diet.

Drooling and loss of fluids due to feeding problems require a fluid intake assessment. The presence of copper plumbing and copper cooking utensils contributes to copper ingestion. If water contains more than 0.1 mg Cu/L, distilled water should be used. Copper cooking utensils should be used as copper can be leached from food being cooked.

Table 57–1. Copper Content of Foods

Foods	(mg/100 g)	Foods	(mg/100 g)
	Foods High in Copper (>1 mg/100 g)		
Oysters, all varieties	17.14	Lobster	1.69
Calves' liver	7.90	Crab, canned, all variety	1.52
Beef liver	2.80	Molasses	1.42
Wheat germ	2.39	High protein, dry baby cereal	1.20
Sunflower seeds	1.77		
	Foods Intermediate in Copper (0.05 to 1.00 mg/100 g)		
Meat, Fish, Eggs		Vegetable and Vegetable Products	
Beef ground	.08	Tomato sauce	.10
Pork cured, ham	.09	Mushrooms	.26
Pork chop	.19	Onion rings, breaded	.10
Veal cutlet	.10	French fries, commercial	.14
Chicken breasts, fried	.05	Potato chips, commercial	.35
Bologna	.06	Peas	.10
Fish sticks	.07		
Tuna	.05	Fruit and Dried Fruit	
Eggs, soft	.06	Raisins	.31
		Prunes	.29
Nuts and Nut Products		Avocado	.19
Peanuts, dry roasted	.67		
Peanut butter, cream	.61	Desserts	
		Ice cream, chocolate	.14
Legumes		Chocolate cake	.23
Navy beans	.28	Chocolate chip cookies	.23
Cowpeas	.27	Chocolate cookies	.32
		Milk chocolate	.45
Grains and Grain Products		Cocoa	.76
Whole-wheat bread	.25		
Pancakes	.07		
Macaroni	.08		
Shredded wheat cereal	.47		
Raisin bran	.48		
Granola	.34		
	Foods Low in Copper (<0.05 mg/100 g)		
Milk and Milk Products		Fruits	
Whole milk	.003	Apples, raw	.02
Cheese, American	.045	Apple juice, canned	.01
Yogurt	.004	Orange, raw	.04
		Orange juice, frozen reconstituted	.02
Vegetables		Watermelon	.02
Coleslaw	.017		
Lettuce, raw	.028	Beverages	
Tomato	.05	Tea	.006
Potatoes, mashed	.05	Coffee	.001
Corn, boiled, fresh	.04		

Adapted from Pennington et al.[13]

Dietary Management

The goals of dietary management are related to the medical management of WD. These goals are to inhibit the absorption of copper from the intestinal tract, remove copper from tissues and prevent its reaccumulation, maintain normal levels of copper necessary for copper balance, and monitor caloric intake, eating and feeding problems, and changes in gag reflex or dysphagia as needed.[9]

The chelating agent penicillamine, which mobilizes copper from tissues and promotes its excretion, is taken 2 hours before or 2 hours after meals. Potassium sulfide supplements also are given during meals to absorb dietary copper and prevent its absorption in intestinal tract. A daily pyridoxine supplement is necessary to prevent pyridoxine deficiency as a result of penicillamine administration. When penicillamine is not tolerated, trientine hydrochloride is utilized to increase the urinary excretion of copper. Ammonium tetrathiomolybdate has been used successfully as an initial therapy when acute neurological symptoms of WD have presented.[10] Pediatric patients have been treated with oral zinc and have maintained a negative or zero copper balance with no side effects or complications. Oral zinc given every 4 hours during the day and at bedtime or zinc sulfate given three times a day can be used as an adjunctive therapy. Zinc acetate alone, given in doses of 50 mg three times daily 1 hour before eating, safely blocks the uptake of copper. Zinc supplementation prevents zinc deficiency caused by the chelation therapy or reduces the amount of penicillamine chelation therapy required.[10] When zinc acetate alone is used, it controls abnormal positive copper balance, blocks the uptake of orally administered ^{64}Cu, controls urine and plasma copper, prevents the reaccumulation of hepatic copper, and prevents the development or progression of copper toxicity in WD.

Dietary levels of copper must be determined. Foods in the low range and a limited amount from the moderate range of copper can be consumed (Table 57–1). With school-aged children, it is important to maintain a low-copper diet and adequate fluid intake at school. Food textures and calories require monitoring to ensure adequate intake. The school should be advised of dietary therapy and the necessity for rigid compliance with the medication/mealtime sequence. Biochemical monitoring of red, white, and platelet cells is necessary every 2 weeks during the first 6 months of penicillamine administration.[12,13]

Follow-up

Nutritional care should coincide with medical check-ups. Height, weight, skinfold, and heat circumference (if the child is under age 3), along with biochemical profiles, are required for children every 3 months. A 24-hour recall and frequency cross-check or 3-day diet diary should be used to evaluate dietary copper intake, calories, and protein. Supplements should be added when required. Management of eating and medication to be consumed in the school setting is essential. Feeding skills relate to the level of progression of the disease and require continuous re-evaluation.

When dysphagia related to difficulty in swallowing or chewing, decreased gag reflex, drooling of saliva, spasticity, tremors, or anorexia occur, several approaches are required:

provide an appropriate texture of food, offer milkshakes (low in copper, high in calories), check the gag reflex and swallowing ability before feeding, massage the face and neck muscles before eating, readjust to an upright position during meals, feed slowly, and take weekly calorie counts and weights. For constipation and drooling, one should increase fluid intake (see Chapter 35). Adaptive equipment should be provided whenever necessary to enhance self-feeding skills. (see Chapter 24).

References

1. Mandell, A., Issacs-Glaberman, K., Scheinberg, H. Neuropsychological impairment in Wilson's Disease. *Arch. Neurol.* 1988; 45:502.
2. Brewer, G., Yuzbasiyan-Gurban, V., Lee, D. Use of zinc-copper metabolic interactions in the treatment of Wilson's disease. *J. Am. Coll. Nutr.* 1990; 9:487.
3. Grossman, D. Wilson's disease: a genetic disorder of copper metabolism. *J. Neurosci. Nurs.* 1987; 19:216.
4. Fahn, S. Differential diagnosis of tremors. *Med. Clin. North Am.* 1972; 56:1363.
5. Weizman, Z., Picard, E., Barki, Y., Moses, S. Wilson's disease associated with pancreatitis. *J. Pediatr. Gastroenterol. Nutr.* 1988; 7:931.
6. Sheinberg, I.H., Sternlieb, I. *Wilson's Disease.* Philadelphia: W.B. Saunders; 1984.
7. Carpenter, T.O., Pendrak, M.L., Anast, C.S. Metabolism of 25-hydroxyvitamin D in copper-laden rat: a model of Wilson's disease. *Am. J. Physiol.* 1988; 254:150.
8. Powers, D.E., Moore, A.D. *Food and Medication Interactions,* 6th ed. Phoenix: Food Medication Interactions; 1988.
9. Escott-Stump, S., ed. *Nutrition and Diagnosis-Related Care.* Philadelphia: Lea & Febiger; 1988.
10. Brewer, G., Dick, R., Yuzbasiyan-Gurkin, V., Tankanow, R., Young, A., Kluin, K. Initial therapy of patients with Wilson's Disease with tetrathiomolybdate. *Arch. Neurol.* 1991; 48:42.
11. Van Ness, M., Hall, L. Wilson's disease: a treatable form of liver disease. *Consult.* 1986; 8,143.
12. Pennington, J., Calloway, D. Copper content of foods. *J. Am. Diet. Assoc.* 1973; 63:143.
13. Pennington, J.A.T., Young, B.E., Wilson, D.B., Johnson, R.D., Vanderveen, J.E. Mineral content of foods and total diets: the selected minerals in food survey, 1982 to 1984. *J. Am. Diet. Assoc.* 1986; 86:876.

Appendix 1
Recommended Dietary Allowances
and U.S. RDI

1–1 Food and Nutrition Board, National Academy of Sciences (U.S. RDA), 1989

Designed for the maintenance of good nutrition of practically all healthy people in the United States

Category	Age (years) or Condition	Weight (kg)	Weight (lb)	Height (cm)	Height (in)	Protein (g)	Fat-Soluble Vitamins				Water-Soluble Vitamins							Minerals						
							Vitamin A (μg RE)	Vitamin D (μg)	Vitamin E (mg α-TE)	Vitamin K (μg)	Vitamin C (mg)	Thiamin (mg)	Riboflavin (mg)	Niacin (mg NE)	Vitamin B6 (mg)	Folate (μg)	Vitamin B12 (μg)	Calcium (mg)	Phosphorus (mg)	Magnesium (mg)	Iron (mg)	Zinc (mg)	Iodine (μg)	Selenium (μg)
Infants	0.0–0.5	6	13	60	24	13	375	7.5	3	5	30	0.3	0.4	5	0.3	25	0.3	400	300	40	6	5	40	10
	0.5–1.0	9	20	71	28	14	375	10	4	10	35	0.4	0.5	6	0.6	35	0.5	600	500	60	10	5	50	15
Children	1–3	13	29	90	35	16	400	10	6	15	40	0.7	0.8	9	1.0	50	0.7	800	800	80	10	10	70	20
	4–6	20	44	112	44	24	500	10	7	20	45	0.9	1.1	12	1.1	75	1.0	800	800	120	10	10	90	20
	7–10	28	62	132	52	28	700	10	7	30	45	1.0	1.2	13	1.4	100	1.4	800	800	170	10	10	120	30
Males	11–14	45	99	157	62	45	1,000	10	10	45	50	1.3	1.5	17	1.7	150	2.0	1,200	1,200	270	12	15	150	40
	15–18	66	145	176	69	59	1,000	10	10	65	60	1.5	1.8	20	2.0	200	2.0	1,200	1,200	400	12	15	150	50
	19–24	72	160	177	70	58	1,000	10	10	70	60	1.5	1.7	19	2.0	200	2.0	1,200	1,200	350	10	15	150	70
	25–50	79	174	176	70	63	1,000	5	10	80	60	1.5	1.7	19	2.0	200	2.0	800	800	350	10	15	150	70
	51+	77	170	173	68	63	1,000	5	10	80	60	1.2	1.4	15	2.0	200	2.0	800	800	350	10	15	150	70
Females	11–14	46	101	157	62	46	800	10	8	45	50	1.1	1.3	15	1.4	150	2.0	1,200	1,200	280	15	12	150	45
	15–18	55	120	163	64	44	800	10	8	55	60	1.1	1.3	15	1.5	180	2.0	1,200	1,200	300	15	12	150	50
	19–24	58	128	164	65	46	800	10	8	60	60	1.1	1.3	15	1.6	180	2.0	1,200	1,200	280	15	12	150	55
	25–50	63	138	163	64	50	800	5	8	65	60	1.1	1.3	15	1.6	180	2.0	800	800	280	15	12	150	55
	51+	65	143	160	63	50	800	5	8	65	60	1.0	1.2	13	1.6	180	2.0	800	800	280	10	12	150	55
Pregnant						60	800	10	10	65	70	1.5	1.6	17	2.2	400	2.2	1,200	1,200	320	30	15	175	65
Lactating	1st 6 months					65	1,300	10	12	65	95	1.6	1.8	20	2.1	280	2.6	1,200	1,200	355	15	19	200	75
	2nd 6 months					62	1,200	10	11	65	90	1.6	1.7	20	2.1	260	2.6	1,200	1,200	340	15	16	200	75

[a] The allowances, expressed as average daily intakes over time, are intended to provide for individual variations among most normal persons as they live in the United States under usual environmental stresses. Diets should be based on a variety of common foods in order to provide other nutrients for which human requirements have been less well defined. See text for detailed discussion of allowances and of nutrients not tabulated.

[b] Weights and heights of Reference Adults are actual medians for the U.S. population of the designated age, as reported by NHANES II. The median weights and heights of those under 19 years of age were taken from Hamill et al. (1979) (see pages 16–17). The use of these figures does not imply that the height-to-weight ratios are ideal.

[c] Retinol equivalents. 1 retinol equivalent = 1 μg retinol or 6 μg β-carotene. See text for calculation of vitamin A activity of diets as retinol equivalents.

[d] As cholecalciferol. 10 μg cholecalciferol = 400 IU of vitamin D.

[e] α-Tocopherol equivalents. 1 mg d-α tocopherol = 1 α-TE. See text for variation in allowances and calculation of vitamin E activity of the diet as α-tocopherol equivalents.

[f] 1 NE (niacin equivalent) is equal to 1 mg of niacin or 60 mg of dietary tryptophan.

1–2 Nutrients, Weights, Heights, and Energy Intake (U.S. RDA), 1989

Estimated Safe and Adequate Daily Dietary Intakes of Selected Vitamins and Minerals[a]

Category	Age (years)	Vitamins	
		Biotin (µg)	Pantothenic Acid (mg)
Infants	0–0.5	10	2
	0.5–1	15	3
Children and adolescents	1–3	20	3
	4–6	25	3–4
	7–10	30	4–5
	11+	30–100	4–7
Adults		30–100	4–7

Category	Age (years)	Trace Elements[b]				
		Copper (mg)	Manganese (mg)	Fluoride (mg)	Chromium (µg)	Molybdenum (µg)
Infants	0–0.5	0.4–0.6	0.3–0.6	0.1–0.5	10–40	15–30
	0.5–1	0.6–0.7	0.6–1.0	0.2–1.0	20–60	20–40
Children and adolescents	1–3	0.7–1.0	1.0–1.5	0.5–1.5	20–80	25–50
	4–6	1.0–1.5	1.5–2.0	1.0–2.5	30–120	30–75
	7–10	1.0–2.0	2.0–3.0	1.5–2.5	50–200	50–150
	11+	1.5–2.5	2.0–5.0	1.5–2.5	50–200	75–250
Adults		1.5–3.0	2.0–5.0	1.5–4.0	50–200	75–250

[a] Because there is less information on which to base allowances, these figures are not given in the main table of RDA and are provided here in the form of ranges of recommended intakes.

[b] Since the toxic levels for many trace elements may be only several times usual intakes, the upper levels for the trace elements given in this table should not be habitually exceeded.

Median Heights and Weights and Recommended Energy Intake

Category	Age (years) or Condition	Weight		Height		REE[a] (kcal/day)	Average Energy Allowance (kcal)[b]		
		(kg)	(lb)	(cm)	(in)		Multiples of REE	Per kg	Per day[c]
Infants	0.0–0.5	6	13	60	24	320		108	650
	0.5–1.0	9	20	71	28	500		98	850
Children	1–3	13	29	90	35	740		102	1,300
	4–6	20	44	112	44	950		90	1,800
	7–10	28	62	132	52	1,130		70	2,000
Males	11–14	45	99	157	62	1,440	1.70	55	2,500
	15–18	66	145	176	69	1,760	1.67	45	3,000
	19–24	72	160	177	70	1,780	1.67	40	2,900
	25–50	79	174	176	70	1,800	1.60	37	2,900
	51+	77	170	173	68	1,530	1.50	30	2,300
Females	11–14	46	101	157	62	1,310	1.67	47	2,200
	15–18	55	120	163	64	1,370	1.60	40	2,200
	19–24	58	128	164	65	1,350	1.60	38	2,200
	25–50	63	138	163	64	1,380	1.55	36	2,200
	51+	65	143	160	63	1,280	1.50	30	1,900
Pregnant	1st trimester								+0
	2nd trimester								+300
	3rd trimester								+300
Lactating	1st 6 months								+500
	2nd 6 months								+500

[a] Calculation based on FAO equations (Table 3-1), then rounded.

[b] In the range of light to moderate activity, the coefficient of variation is ±20%.

[c] Figure is rounded.

1–3   Recommended Dietary Intakes (U.S. RDI), 1989

Nutrient	Unit of Measurement	Adults and children 4 or more years of age	Children less than 4 years of age	Infants	Pregnant women	Lactating women
Vitamin A	Retinol equivalents	875	400	375	800	1,300
Vitamin C	Milligrams	60	40	33	70	95
Calcium	.....do......	900	800	500	1,200	1,200
Iron	.....do......	12	10	8.0	30	15
Vitamin D	Micrograms	6.5	10	9.0	10	10
Vitamin E	a-Tocopherol equivalents	9.0	6.0	3.5	10	12
Vitamin K	Micrograms	65	15	7.5	65	65
Thiamin	Milligrams	1.2	0.7	0.4	1.5	1.6
Riboflavin	......do......	1.4	0.8	0.5	1.6	1.8
Niacin	Niacin equivalents	16	9.0	5.5	17	20
Vitamin B_6	Milligrams	1.5	1.0	0.5	2.2	2.1
Folate	Micrograms	180	50	30	400	280
Vitamin B_{12}	.....do......	2.0	0.7	0.4	2.2	2.6
Biotin	.....do......	60	20	13	65	65
Pantothenic acid	Milligrams	5.5	3.0	2.5	5.5	5.5
Phosphorus	.....do......	900	800	400	1,200	1,200
Magnesium	.....do......	300	80	50	320	355
Zinc	.....do......	13	10	5.0	15	19
Iodine	Micrograms	150	70	45	175	200
Selenium	.....do......	55	20	13	65	75
Copper	Milligrams	2.0	0.9	0.6	2.5	2.5
Manganese	.....do......	3.5	1.3	0.6	3.5	3.5
Fluoride	.....do......	2.5	1.0	0.5	3.0	3.0
Chromium	Micrograms	120	50	33	130	130
Molybdenum	.....do......	150	38	26	160	160
Chloride	Milligrams	3,150	1,000	650	3,400	3,400

Adapted from the Federal Register, Washington, D.C., November 27, 1991: Volume 56, No. 229, 60390.
For more specifics regarding recommended dietary intakes according to age group see: Liu, J. and Guthrie, H.:
Nutrient labeling – a tool for nutrition education.   Part 1: nutrient units of protein, vitamins and minerals.
Nutrition Today, 1992; 27:2.

1-4 Recommended Nutrient Intakes (Canadian)

Age	Sex	Weight kg	Protein g	Vit A RE[a]	Vit D µg	Vit E mg	Vit C mg	Folate µg	Vit B12 µg	Calcium mg	Phosphorus mg	Magnesium mg	Iron mg	Iodine µg	Zinc mg	Energy kcal	Thiamin mg	Riboflavin mg	Niacin NE[b]	n-3 PUFA[a] g	n-6 PUFA g
Months																					
0-4	Both	6.0	12[b]	400	10	3	20	50	0.3	250f	150	20	0.3d	30	2d	600	0.3	0.3	4	0.5	3
5-12	Both	9.0	12	400	10	3	20	50	0.3	400	200	32	7	40	3	900	0.4	0.5	7	0.5	3
Years																					
1	Both	11	19	400	10	3	20	65	0.3	500	300	40	6	55	4	1100	0.5	0.6	8	0.6	4
2-3	Both	14	22	400	5	4	20	80	0.4	550	350	50	6	65	4	1300	0.6	0.7	9	0.7	4
4-6	Both	18	26	500	5	5	25	90	0.5	600	400	65	8	85	5	1800	0.7	0.9	13	1.0	6
7-9	M	25	30	700	2.5	7	25	125	0.8	700	500	100	8	110	7	2200	0.9	1.1	16	1.2	7
	F	25	30	700	2.5	6	25	125	0.8	700	500	100	8	95	7	1900	0.8	1.0	14	1.0	6
10-12	M	34	38	800	2.5	8	25	170	1.0	900	700	130	8	125	9	2500	1.0	1.3	18	1.4	8
	F	36	40	800	5	7	25	180	1.0	1100	800	135	8	110	9	2200	0.9	1.1	16	1.1	7
13-15	M	50	50	900	5	9	30	150	1.5	1100	900	185	10	160	12	2800	1.1	1.4	20	1.4	9
	F	48	42	800	5	7	30	145	1.5	1000	850	180	13	160	9	2200	0.9	1.1	16	1.2	7
16-18	M	62	55	1000	5	10	40e	185	1.9	900	1000	230	10	160	12	3200	1.3	1.6	23	1.8	11
	F	53	43	800	2.5	7	30e	160	1.9	700	850	200	12	160	9	2100	0.8	1.1	15	1.2	7
19-24	M	71	58	1000	2.5	10	40e	210	2.0	800	1000	240	9	160	12	3000	1.2	1.5	22	1.6	10
	F	58	43	800	2.5	7	30e	175	2.0	700	850	200	13	160	9	2100	0.8	1.1	15	1.2	7
25-49	M	74	61	1000	2.5	9	40e	220	2.0	800	1000	250	9	160	12	2700	1.1	1.4	19	1.5	9
	F	59	44	800	2.5	6	30e	175	2.0	700	850	200	13	160	9	2000	0.8	1.0	14	1.1	7
50-74	M	73	60	1000	5	7	40e	220	2.0	800	1000	250	9	160	12	2300	0.9	1.3	16	1.3	8
	F	63	47	800	5	6	30e	190	2.0	800	850	210	8	160	9	1800	0.8c	1.0c	14c	1.1c	7c
75+	M	69	57	1000	5	6	40e	205	2.0	800	1000	230	9	160	12	2000	0.8	1.0	14	1.0	7
	F	64	47	800	2.5	5	30e	190	2.0	800	850	210	8	160	9	1700	0.8c	1.0c	14c	1.1c	7c
Pregnancy(additional)																					
1st Trimester			5	100	2.5	2	0	300	1.0	500	200	15	0	25	6	100	0.1	0.1	0.1	0.05	0.3
2nd Trimester			20	100	2.5	2	10	300	1.0	500	200	45	5	25	6	300	0.1	0.3	0.2	0.16	0.9
3rd Trimester			24	100	2.5	2	10	300	1.0	500	200	45	10	25	6	300	0.1	0.3	0.2	0.16	0.9
Lactation (additional)			20	400	2.5	3	25	100	0.5	500	200	65	0	50	6	450	0.2	0.4	0.3	0.25	1.5

a. Retinol Equivalents
b. Protein is assumed to be from breast milk and must be adjusted for infant formula.
c. Infant formula with high phosphorus should contain 375 mg calcium
d. Breast milk is assumed to be the source of the mineral.
e. Smokers should increase vitamin C by 50%.

a. PUFA, polyunsaturated fatty acids
b. Niacin Equivalents
c. Level below which intake should not fall
d. Assumes moderate physical activity

From: Health and Welfare Canada, 1990. *Nutrition Recommendations*. Ottawa: Canadian Government Publishing Centre. Reproduced with permission of the Minister of Supply and Services Canada.

Appendix 2
Growth Grids for Special Conditions

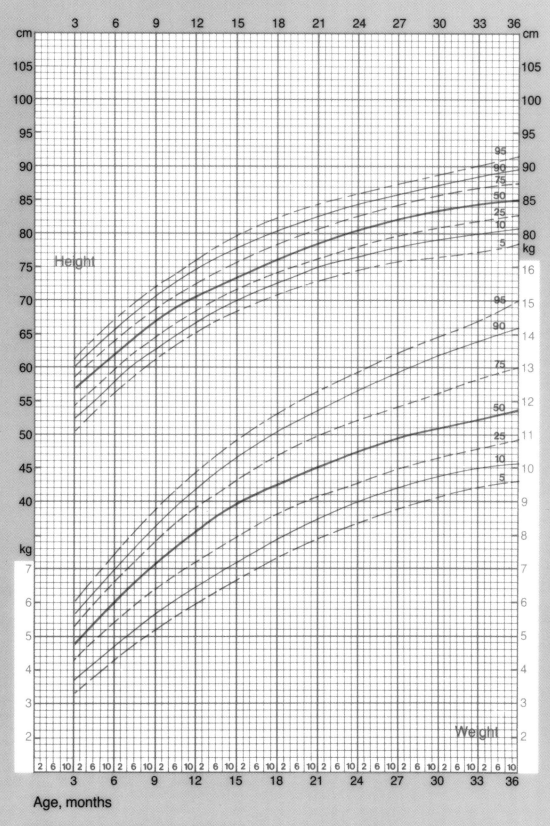

2-18 years on reverse (comparison with Tanner-Whitehouse standards)
CRONK, CROCKER, PUESCHEL, SHEA, ZACKAI, PICKENS, REED
(Reproduced with permission. *Pediatrics* Vol. 81 p102 ©1988)

Height

Weight

Age, months

Data collection supported by The March of Dimes, grant number (6-449)

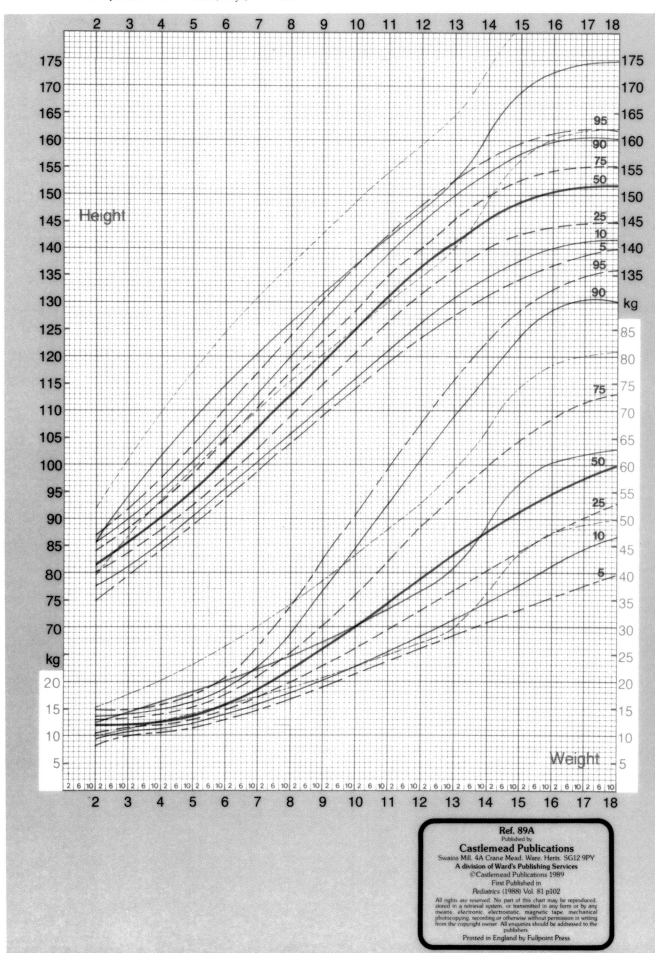

Ref. 89A
Published by
Castlemead Publications
Swains Mill. 4A Crane Mead. Ware. Herts. SG12 9PY
A division of Ward's Publishing Services
©Castlemead Publications 1989
First Published in
Pediatrics (1988) Vol. 81 p102

Printed in England by Fullpoint Press

2-18 years on reverse (comparison with Tanner-Whitehouse standards)

CRONK, CROCKER, PUESCHEL, SHEA, ZACKAI, PICKENS, REED
(Reproduced with permission. *Pediatrics* Vol. 81 p102 ©1988)

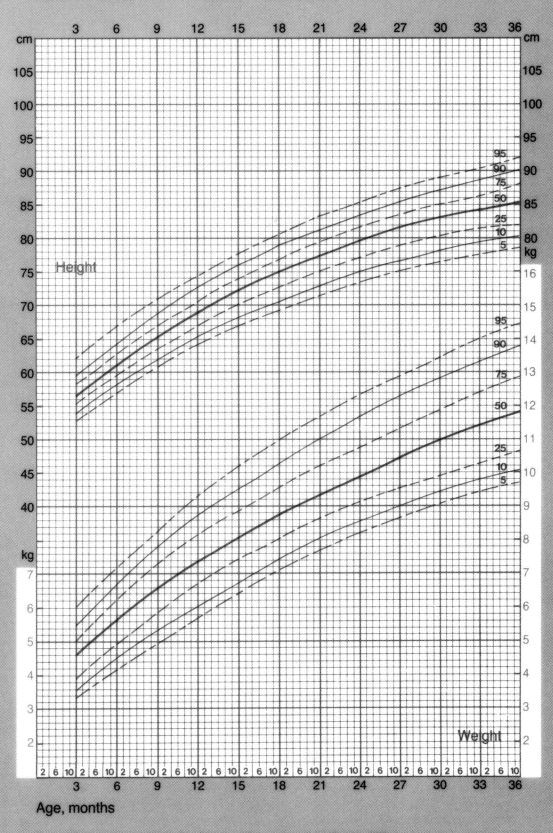

Age, months

Data collection supported by The March of Dimes, grant number (6-449)

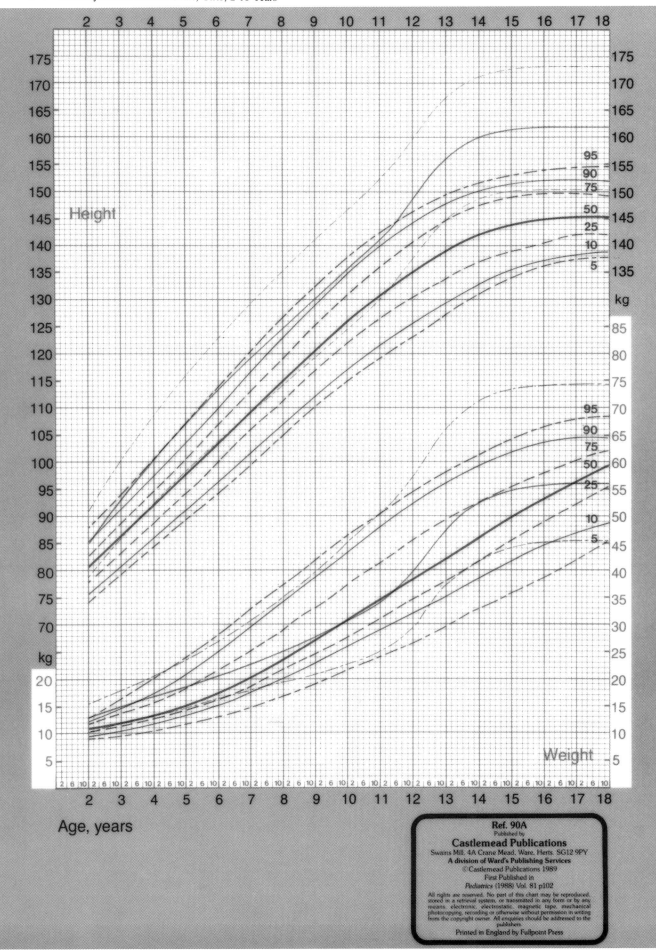

Age, years

Ref. 90A
Published by
Castlemead Publications
Swains Mill, 4A Crane Mead, Ware, Herts. SG12 9PY
A division of Ward's Publishing Services
© Castlemead Publications 1989
First Published in
Pediatrics (1988) Vol. 81 p102

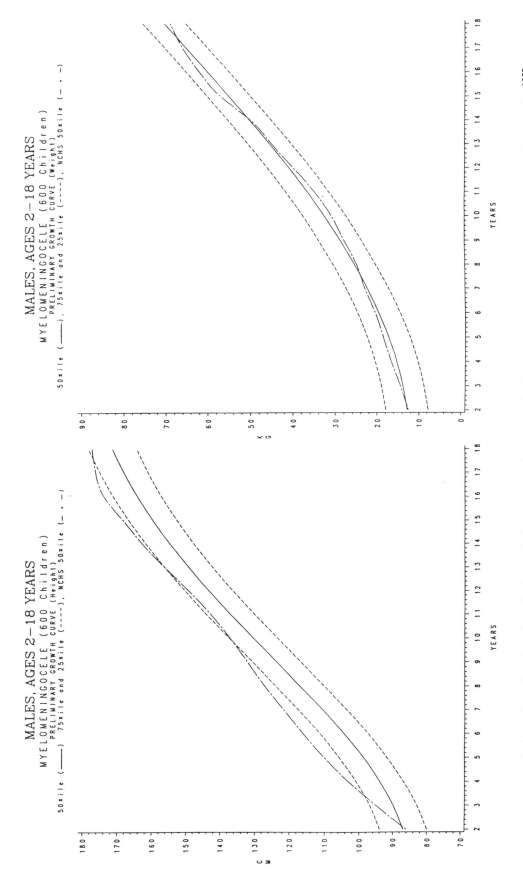

2-5 Myelomeningocele Growth Chart, Boys, 2-18 Years

Preliminary growth charts for myelomeningocele with NCHS standard growth curve developed by Ekvall, S., Schwiegeraht, L., Bigley, B., Beck, C. and Leonti, G., 1992.

2–6 Myelomeningocele Growth Chart, Girls, 2-18 Years

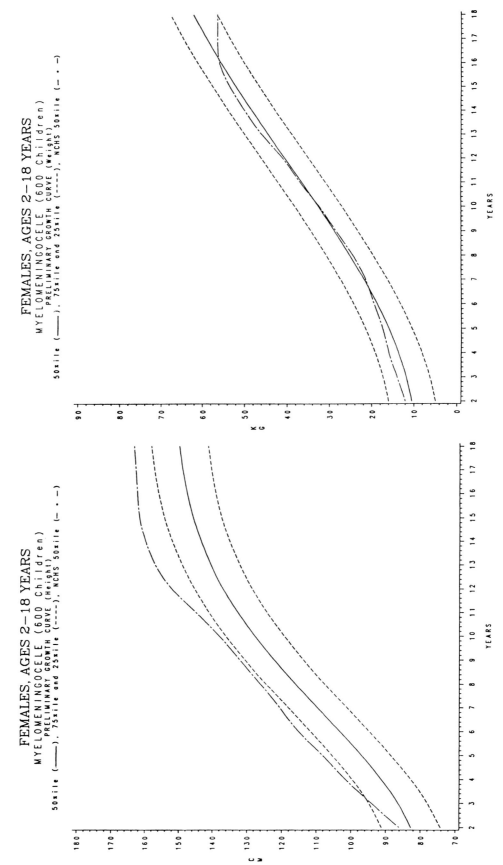

FEMALES, AGES 2–18 YEARS
MYELOMENINGOCELE (600 Children)
PRELIMINARY GROWTH CURVE (Height)
50xile (———), 75xile and 25xile (-----), NCHS 50xile (— • —)

FEMALES, AGES 2–18 YEARS
MYELOMENINGOCELE (600 Children)
PRELIMINARY GROWTH CURVE (Weight)
50xile (———), 75xile and 25xile (-----), NCHS 50xile (— • —)

Preliminary growth charts for myelomeningocele with NCHS standard growth curve developed by Ekvall, S., Schwiegeraht, L., Bigley, B., Beck, C. and Leonti, G., 1992.

2-7 Prader-Willi Growth Chart, Males, 3-25 Years

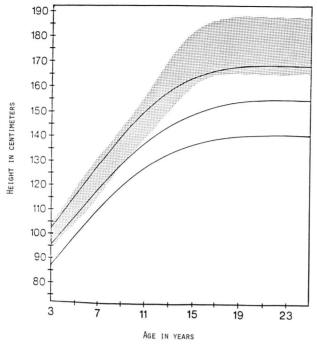

Holm, V. A.: Appendix A: Growth charts for Prader-Willi syndrome. In
Greensway, L. R. and Alexander, P. C. (Eds.): Management of Prader-Willi
Syndrome, New York, Springer Verlag Pub, 1988.

2-8 Prader-Willi Growth Chart, Females, 3-25 Years

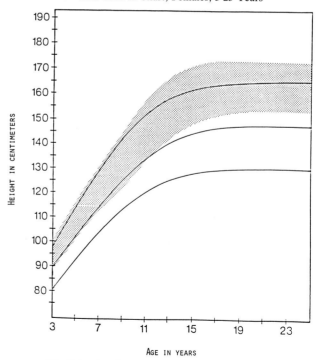

Holm, V. A.: Appendix A: Growth charts for Prader-Willi syndrome. In
Greensway, L. R. and Alexander, P. C. (Eds.): Management of Prader-Willi
Syndrome, New York, Springer Verlag Pub, 1988.

2–9   Sickle Cell Anemia Growth Chart, a Male, 2-18 Years

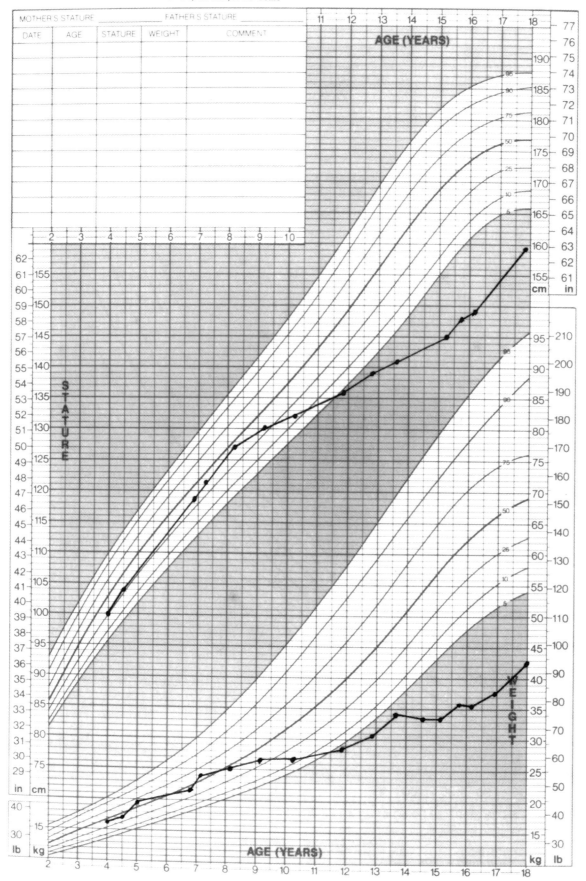

2–10 Sickle Cell Anemia Growth Chart, a Female, 2-18 Years

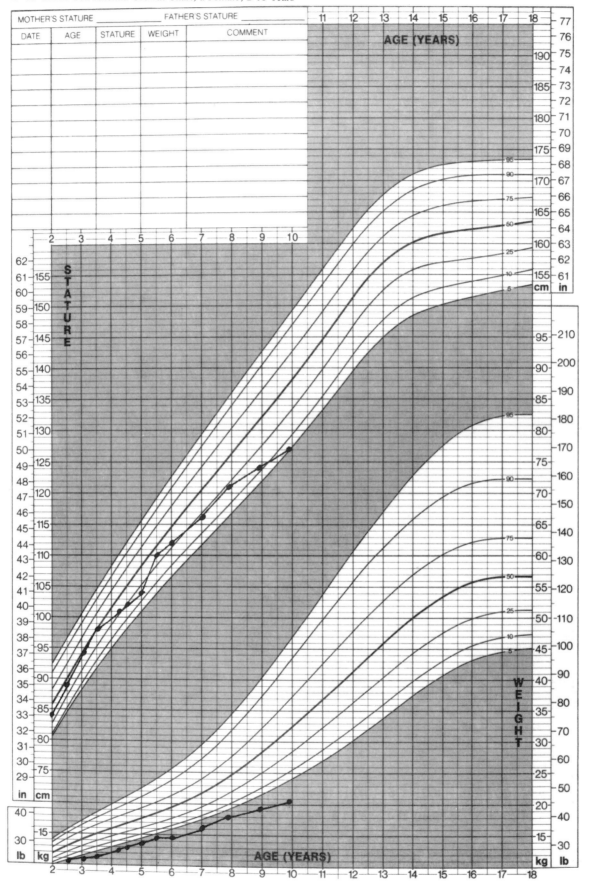

2–11 Sickle Cell Anemia, Velocity Curve Chart, a Male, 2-18 Years

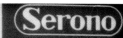

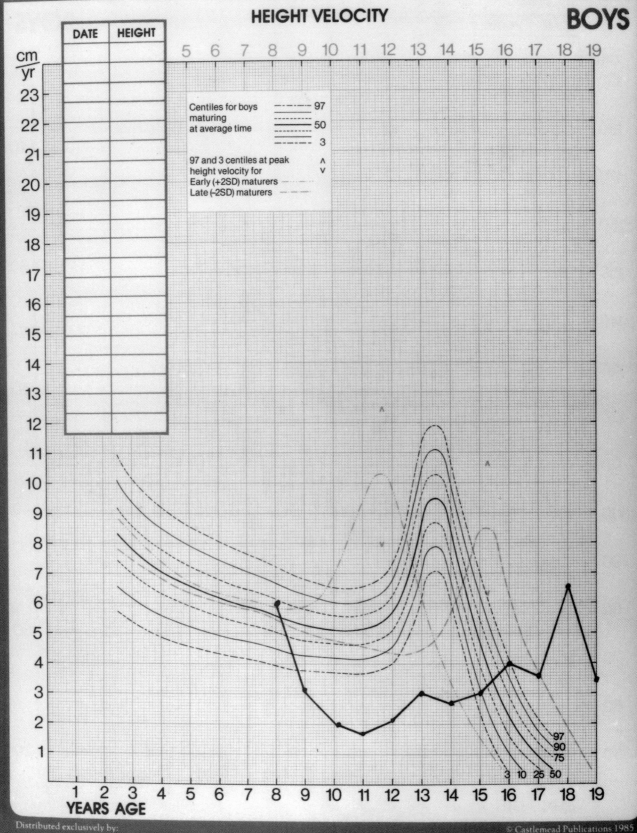

Tanner JM, Davis PSW. Journal of Pediatrics 1985; 107

NAME _____ RECORD # _____

■ ▦ NORMAL GIRLS*
■ UNTREATED TURNER PATIENTS**

*Percentiles derived from National Center for Health Statistics
**Turner Percentiles from Lyon, A.J., Preece, M.A., and Grant, D.B.
Growth curve for girls with Turner Syndrome. Archives of Disease in Childhood 60: 932-935 (1985).

AGE (YEARS)

DATE	HEIGHT	GROWTH RATE

STATURE

STATURE

AGE (YEARS)

Appendix 3
Growth Grids—NCHS for General Pediatric Population

3–1 Weight and Height of Males and Females to Age 18 in U.S., 1989

	Males, by percentile							Females, by percentile						
	Weight, kg (lb)			Height, cm (in)			Weight, kg (lb)			Height, cm (in)			
Age	5th	50th	95th	5th	50th	95th	5th	50th	95th	5th	50th	95th
Months												
1	3.16	4.29 (9.4)	5.38	50.4	54.6 (21.5)	58.6	2.97	3.98 (8.8)	4.92	49.2	53.5 (21.1)	56.9
3	4.43	5.98 (13.2)	7.37	56.7	61.1 (24.1)	65.4	4.18	5.40 (11.9)	6.74	55.4	59.5 (23.4)	63.4
6	6.20	7.85 (17.3)	9.46	63.4	67.8 (26.7)	72.3	5.79	7.21 (15.9)	8.73	61.8	65.9 (25.9)	70.2
9	7.52	9.18 (20.2)	10.93	68.0	72.3 (28.5)	77.1	7.00	8.56 (18.8)	10.17	66.1	70.4 (27.7)	75.0
12	8.43	10.15 (22.3)	11.99	71.7	76.1 (30.0)	81.2	7.84	9.53 (21.0)	11.24	69.8	74.3 (29.3)	79.1
18	9.59	11.47 (25.2)	13.44	77.5	82.4 (32.4)	88.1	8.92	10.82 (23.8)	12.76	76.0	80.9 (31.9)	86.1
Years												
2	10.49	12.34 (27.1)	15.50	82.5	86.8 (34.2)	94.4	9.95	11.80 (26.0)	14.15	81.6	86.8 (34.2)	93.6
3	12.05	14.62 (32.2)	17.77	89.0	94.9 (37.4)	102.0	11.61	14.10 (31.0)	17.22	88.3	94.1 (37.0)	100.6
4	13.64	16.69 (36.7)	20.27	95.8	102.9 (40.5)	109.9	13.11	15.96 (35.1)	19.91	95.0	101.6 (40.0)	108.3
5	15.27	18.67 (41.1)	23.09	102.0	109.9 (43.3)	117.0	14.55	17.66 (38.9)	22.62	101.1	108.4 (42.7)	115.6
6	16.93	20.69 (45.5)	26.34	107.7	116.1 (45.7)	123.5	16.05	19.52 (42.9)	25.75	106.6	114.6 (45.1)	122.7
7	18.64	22.85 (50.3)	30.12	113.0	121.7 (47.9)	129.7	17.71	21.84 (48.0)	29.68	111.8	120.6 (47.5)	129.5
8	20.40	25.30 (55.7)	34.51	118.1	127.0 (50.0)	135.7	19.62	24.84 (54.6)	34.71	116.9	126.4 (49.8)	136.2
9	22.25	28.13 (61.9)	39.58	122.9	132.2 (52.0)	141.8	21.82	28.46 (62.6)	40.64	122.1	132.2 (52.0)	142.9
10	24.33	31.44 (69.2)	45.27	127.7	137.5 (54.1)	148.1	24.36	32.55 (71.6)	47.17	127.5	138.3 (54.4)	149.5
11	26.80	35.30 (77.7)	51.47	132.6	143.3 (56.4)	154.9	27.24	36.95 (81.3)	54.00	133.5	144.8 (57.0)	156.2
12	29.85	39.78 (87.5)	58.09	137.6	149.7 (58.9)	162.3	30.52	41.53 (91.4)	60.81	139.8	151.5 (59.6)	162.7
13	33.64	44.95 (98.9)	65.02	142.9	156.5 (61.6)	169.8	34.14	46.10 (101.4)	67.30	145.2	157.1 (61.9)	168.1
14	38.22	50.77 (111.7)	72.13	148.8	163.1 (64.2)	176.7	37.76	50.28 (110.6)	73.08	148.7	160.4 (63.1)	171.3
15	43.11	56.71 (124.8)	79.12	155.2	169.0 (66.5)	181.9	40.99	53.68 (118.1)	77.78	150.5	161.8 (63.7)	172.8
16	47.74	62.10 (136.6)	85.62	161.1	173.5 (68.3)	185.4	43.41	55.89 (123.0)	80.99	151.6	162.4 (63.9)	173.3
17	51.50	66.31 (145.9)	91.31	164.9	176.2 (69.4)	187.3	44.74	56.69 (124.7)	82.46	152.7	163.1 (64.2)	173.5
18	53.97	68.88 (151.5)	95.76	165.7	176.8 (69.6)	187.6	45.26	56.62 (124.6)	82.47	153.6	163.7 (64.4)	173.6

SOURCE: Adapted from Hamill et al. (1979).

Data in this table have been used to derive weight and height reference points in the present report. It is not intended that they necessarily be considered standards of normal growth and development. Data pertaining to infants 2 to 18 months of age are taken from longitudinal growth studies at Fels Research Institute. Ages are exact, and infants were measured in the recumbent position. The measurements were based on some 867 children followed longitudinally at the institute between 1929 and 1975. Data pertaining to children between 2 and 18 years of age were collected between 1962 and 1974 by the National Center for Health Statistics and involve some 20,000 individuals comprising nationally representative samples in three studies conducted between 1960 and 1974. In these studies, children were measured in the standing position with no upward pressure exerted on the mastoid processes. In the ninth edition of this report, data for children up to 6 years of age were taken from longitudinal growth studies in Iowa and Boston, where children were measured in the recumbent position. This explains the systematically smaller heights for 2- to 5-year-old children in this current table compared with those represented in previous editions. In this table, actual age is represented.

3–2   NCHS Percentile Growth Chart, Boys, 0-36 Months

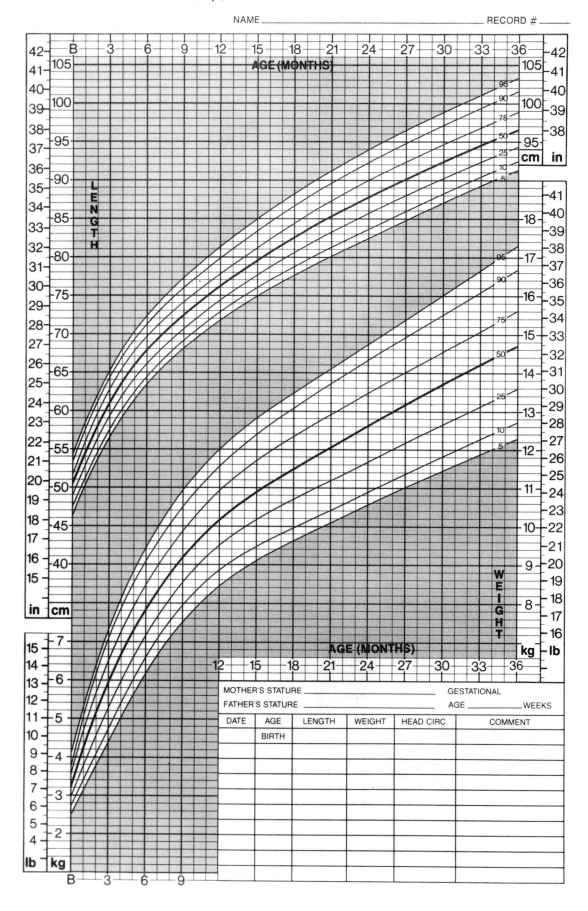

3–3 NCHS Head Circumference, Weight for Length, Boys, 0-36 Months

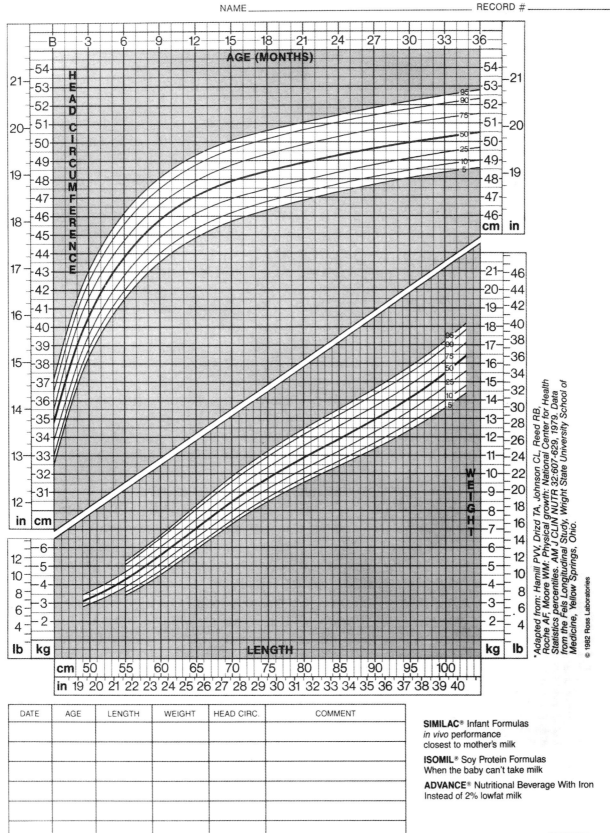

*Adapted from: Hamill PVV, Drizd TA, Johnson CL, Reed RB, Roche AF, Moore WM: Physical growth: National Center for Health Statistics percentiles. AM J CLIN NUTR 32:607-629, 1979. Data from the Fels Longitudinal Study, Wright State University School of Medicine, Yellow Springs, Ohio.

© 1982 Ross Laboratories

DATE	AGE	LENGTH	WEIGHT	HEAD CIRC.	COMMENT

3–4   NCHS Percentile Growth Chart, Girls, 0-36 Months

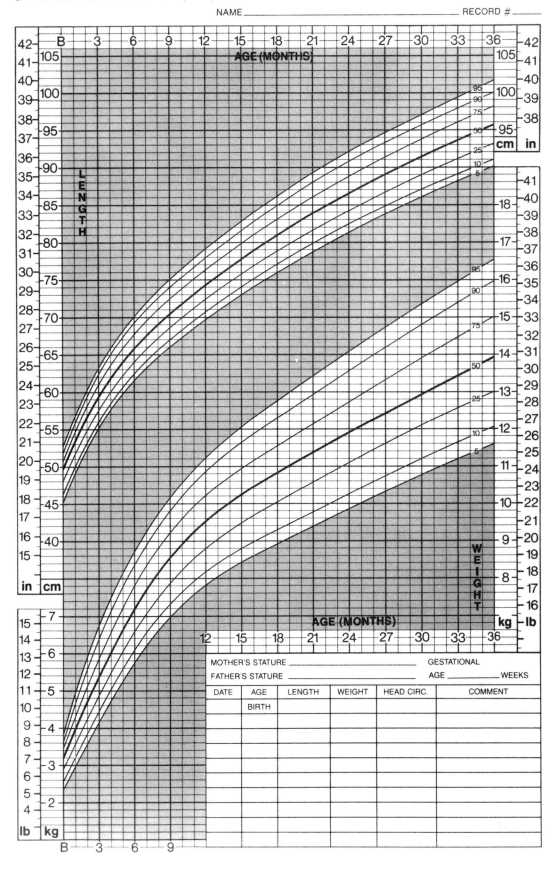

3–5 NCHS Head Circumference, Weight for Length, Girls, 0-36 Months

NAME _____   RECORD # _____

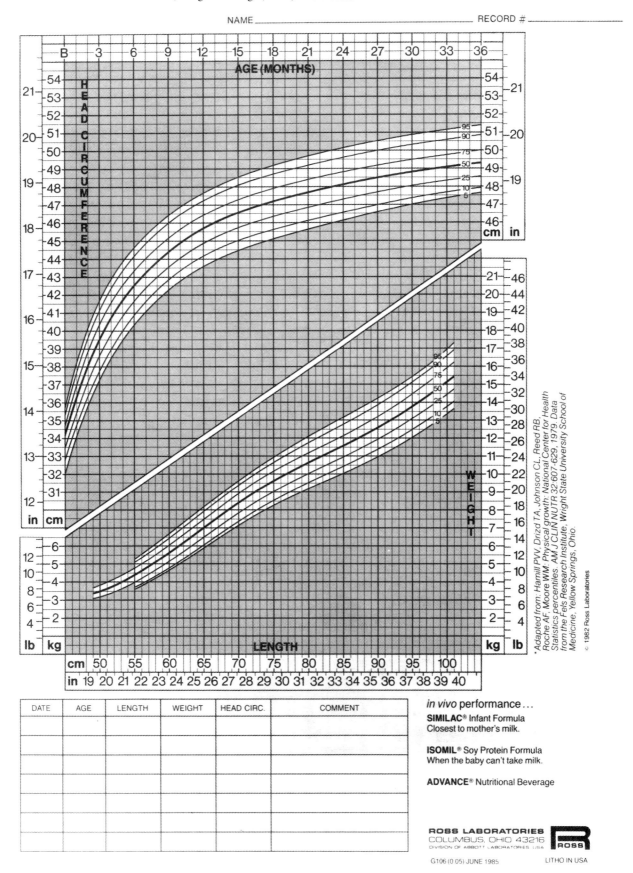

DATE	AGE	LENGTH	WEIGHT	HEAD CIRC.	COMMENT

*Adapted from: Hamill PVV, Drizd TA, Johnson CL, Reed RB, Roche AF, Moore WM: Physical growth: National Center for Health Statistics percentiles. AM J CLIN NUTR 32:607-629, 1979. Data from the Fels Research Institute, Wright State University School of Medicine, Yellow Springs, Ohio.

© 1982 Ross Laboratories

3–6 NCHS Growth Chart, Boys, 2-18 Years

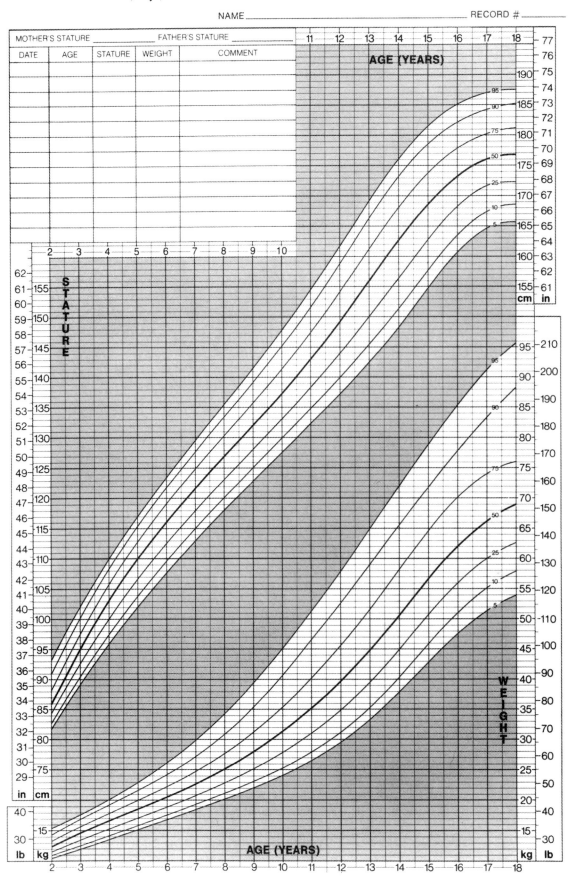

3–7 NCHS Weight for Stature, Boys

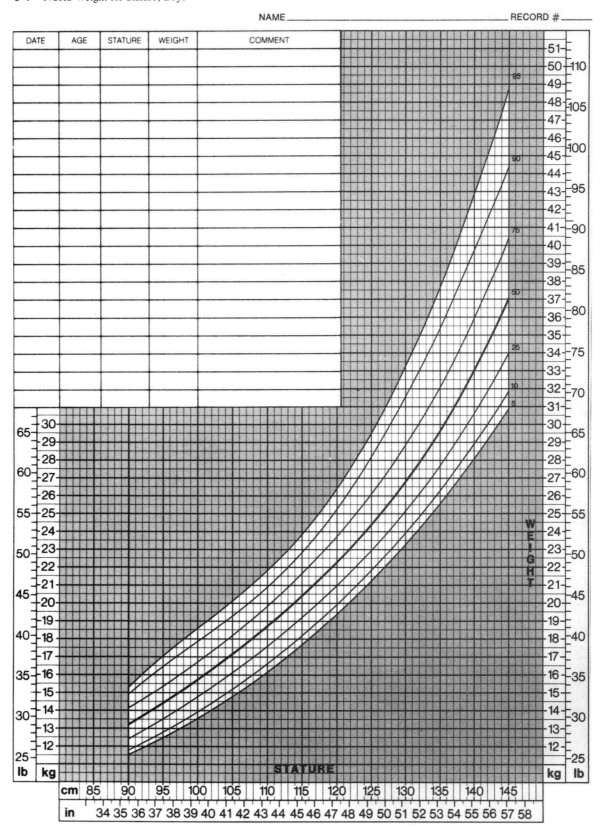

3–8   NCHS Growth Chart, Girls, 2-18 Years

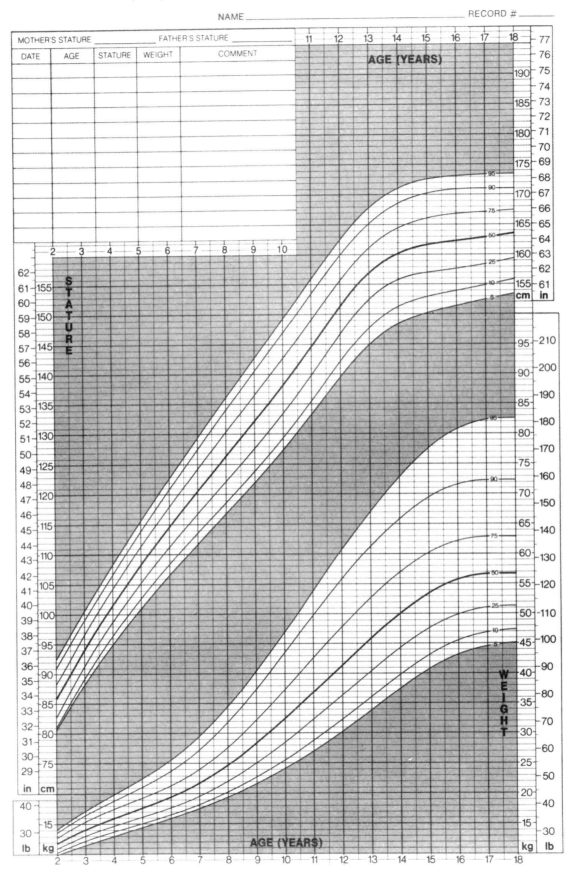

3–9 NCHS Weight for Stature, Girls

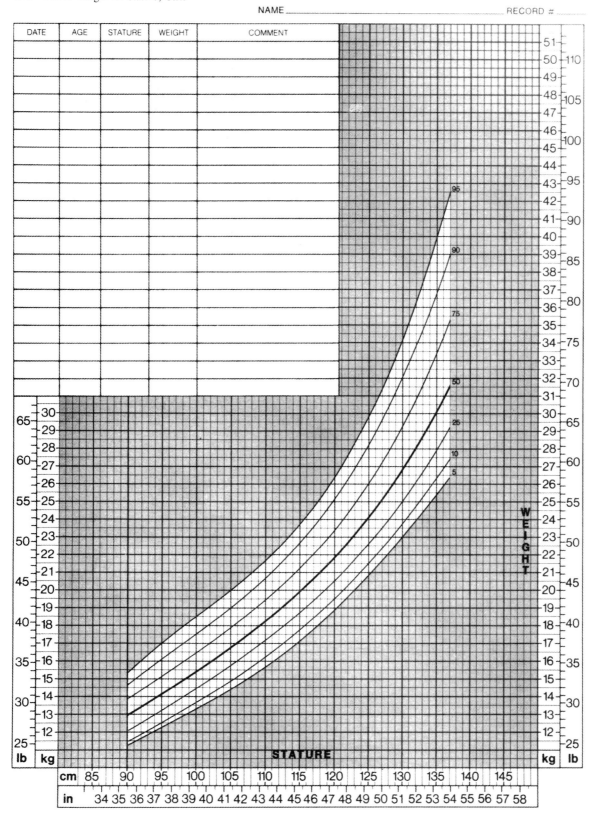

Appendix 4
Nutrition Assessment Records, University Affiliated Cincinnati Center for Developmental Disorders, Children's Hospital Medical Center

4–1 Nutrition Indepth Assessment Record, UACCDD, CHMC

NAME:
BIRTHDATE:
AGE: _____ SEX: _____ RACE: _____
BIRTH WEIGHT:
DATE SEEN:

ADDRESS:
TELEPHONE:
INFORMANT:
EVAL. COORDINATOR:
Interviewer:
Press. Nutr. Prob.

BACKGROUND INFORMATION:

	Mother	Father	Siblings
Height:			
Weight:			
Age:			
Parents:			

Med. Diagnosis:
IQ. _____ A.B. _____

ANTHROPOMETRIC MEASUREMENTS:
Ht. cm. _____ %ile   Upper Arm Segment cm. _____   MAMC cm. _____
Wt. kg. _____ %ile   Upper Arm Circum. cm. _____   Bone Ag/Den. _____
Wt/Ht. Index _____ / _____ %ile   Fatfold Tricep mm. _____   Blood Pressure _____
Avg. _____   Head Circumference cm. _____

CHEMISTRY:
Hb. _____ Serum Fe _____
Hct. _____ Other _____
Vit/Mineral Supp. (Doctor's orders Y/N)
(frequency/type)
Meds:
Nutrient/Drug Interaction Discussed:
Yes _____ No _____ NA _____
Caretaker knowledge demonstrated Y/N

INTERDISCIPLINARY FINDINGS:
Gross Motor:
Speech:

DENTAL CARE:
Daily Source of Fluoride? Y/N
Brushes teeth regularly? Y/N
Sees dentist regularly? Y/N
Caries-causing foods named

MEDICAL:
Hx. of hospitalizations
Hx. Infections:

SOCIO-ECONOMIC:
Income: $ _____ Weekly/Monthly
Food: $ _____
No. of family members:
Using Food Stamp Program or Supplemental
Food Program Yes _____ No _____ NA _____

PRENATAL DIETARY CARE:

NEONATAL FEEDING HISTORY:
Period Breast Fed
Period Formula Fed
Type Tolerated
Feeding Problems: Sucking, Swallowing,
Colic, Vomiting, Diarrhea,
Constipation, Weight Gain Abnormal

ORDER OF INFANT FOOD ADDED:

Age	Amts	How Taken

(Solid food should not be given before four months of age)

SUPPLEMENTS:
AGE BEGAN: _____ TIME CONTINUED: _____

AGE: Weaned from bottle _____ Liquid from cup _____ Unassisted _____
Age: Finger Fed _____ Used Spoon _____ Unassisted _____
Bottle night feeding (other than water) Yes _____ No _____

PRESENT FEEDING ABILITIES:
Table Foods _____ Chopped Foods _____ Jr. Foods _____ Strained _____
Normal Feeding Period: _____ Behavioral Problems _____ Reward System _____
(Circle): Choking, Swallowing, Chewing, Tongue Thrust, Constipation, Anorexia, Pica,
(Clay, Starch, Plaster, Ashes, Bugs, Crayons) — How much? _____

DIETARY EVALUATION

FOOD INTAKE (24 Hr. Recall)*

Name: _____

Patterns:
	Breakfast	Amt.
Time	Fruit	
	Meat	
	Egg	
Where	Bread	
	Fat	
With Whom	Cereal	
	Beverage	
Who Prepared	Other	

	Lunch	
Time	Meat	
	Veg.	
Where	Bread	
	Fruit	
With Whom	Beverage	
	Other	
Who Prepared		

	Dinner	
Time	Soup	
	Meat or subst.	
Where	Potato	
	Vegetable: Cooked	
With Whom	Raw	
	Salad	
Who Prepared	Bread	
	Fat	
	Desert	
	Beverage	
	Other	

	Between Meals	
Time:		

FOOD SUMMARY

GROUP	Amt. per day	Amt. per week	Possible points or daily serv.	**Actual Points
Dairy Products:			3	
Milk				
Cheese				
Cottage Cheese				
Yogurt				
Other				
Meat or Alternatives: ***Fat & Chol.			2	
***Meat, Eggs				
Fish, Poultry				
Dr. Beans/ peas				
Peanut Butter				
Vegetables: (No Vit. A/C-1/2 cr)			3	
Vit A Veg.				
Vit C Veg.				
Other				
Fruits:			2	
Vit C Fruit				
Other Fruits				
Whole Grains/Starches: (No w/grains-1/2 cr)			6	
Cereal				
Bread				
Pasta, Rice				
Other				
TOTAL			16	
Others:				
Candy/Sugar			If daily-1	
Chips/t. salt			If daily-1	
Soft Drinks			If daily-1	
Desserts			None daily-1	
Water				
***Fats & Chol.				
Fiber			3 ser. d.-1 None daily-1	
TOTAL				

Frequency/wk. of eating outside the home:
Food allergies:
Foods regularly omitted: _____ Why: _____

Favorite Foods:
Impression of diet:
Validity of record:
Activity Score:

Are you using iodized salt? _____ Cooking: _____ Table: _____ Using vitamin D fortified mix? Yes/No
Caretaker knowledge/fiber & fluid Yes/No   Can plan Basic 4 diet Yes/No

*If dietary recall, anthropometric measures, or clinical assessment abnormal, obtain 3 day food intake record and 3 day physical activity record for evaluation.
**When the number of servings eaten exceeds the number possible, those servings are not counted. Score below 10 requires follow-up visit, score 10–12 is borderline nutritionally.
***Group with possible high fat and cholesterol.

Fig. 4–1 (Continued)

NUTRITIONAL CLINICAL EVALUATION
Code: 0 = absent; 1 = present; 2 = does not apply

Code Doubtful   Code Doubtful   Code Doubtful

Hair:
all
neg.
— dry
— dispigmented
— easily pluckable
— abnormal texture

Eyes:
all
neg.
— cloudy
— reddened
— dry

Lips:
all
neg.
— angular lesions
— angular scars

Gums:
all
neg.
— swelling
— redness
— hypertrophy
— bleeding

Teeth:
all
neg.
— visible caries
— missing teeth
— calculus
— mottling
— striated discoloration
— malocclusion

Tongue:
all
neg.
— glossy
— fissures
— magenta
— geographic

Nails:
all
neg.
— clubbed
— ridged
— spooned
— blue
— combinations

Face & Neck:
all
neg.
— thyroid enlarged
— facial stigmata of syndrome

Skin:
all
neg.
— folicular hyperkeratosis
— hyperpigmentation
— dry and scaling
— cold
— dispigmentation

Skeletal or Muscular:
all
neg.
— proturberant abdomen
— bowed legs
— knocked-knees
— beading of ribs
— enlargement of wrist
— winged scapula
— scoliosis
— muscle wasting

Lower Extremities:
all
neg.
— pretibial edema

General Appearance: Circle if appropriate
skinny   ambulatory
fat   nonambulatory
well proportioned   no speech
alert   unintelligible speech
apathetic   intelligible speech
irritable   poor feeding behavior
uncooperative   very active

Parent-Child Interaction
___ Appropriate   ___ Slight
___ Moderate   ___ None

PHYSICAL ACTIVITY RECORDS
Estimation of Caloric Needs

WEIGHT: _____ kg. _____ (lbs.) _____ %ile _____ Caloric Input _____

HEIGHT: _____ cm. _____ (in.) _____ %ile _____ Caloric Input _____

RDA caloric average for ages _____ to _____ = _____

RDA range for age _____ – _____

A. Record the following activities as accurately as possible:

	Activity	Time in Hours		Calories/ lb./hr.		Total per lb.
1.	Sleeping		× 0.4	=		
2.	Sitting at rest (watching TV, reading, etc.)		× 0.7	=		
3.	Sitting (Hand activities, i.e., playing with toys)		× 1.0	=		
4.	Walking with crutches		× 1.5	=		
5.	Walking with crutches, total self care		× 2.0	=		
6.	Walking doing light exercise (playground walking, sandbox playing, swinging)		× 2.0	=		
7.	Moderate exercise (active games, i.e., playing ball, stair climbing dancing)		× 2.7	=		
8.	Strenuous exercise (running, swimming, bicycle riding, etc.)		× 4.3	=		
		Total 24				TOTAL

Calorie Output (total per lb. × weight in lbs.): _____

Optional:

B. Recommended kcal. per cm height: _____ × height (cm) = _____ kcal/day
(use only for children with motor dysfunction, ages 5–12.)
(ambulatory, motor dysfunction, 13.9 cal/cm.)
(nonambulatory, severe motor dysfunction, 11.1 cal/cm.)

Caretaker demonstrates knowledge of relationship of calories to physical activity: YES/NO

Fig. 4–1 (Continued)

FEEDING SKILL DEVELOPMENT

Birth	Total Body response	28 Weeks	Sits with some support	1 Year	Importance of mouth as primary sensory organ diminishing
	Rooting reflex		Takes solids well		
	Sucking reflex		Feet to mouth – *36 Weeks		Grasps cup with both hands
	Swallowing				Drinks from cup
	Tearless hunger cry		Grasps spoon, nipple, cup rim	15 Months	Bottle Discarded
	Retrussion reflex				Grasp inhibition
4 Weeks	Face brightens on satiety	32 Weeks	Bites, chews toys *18 months		Uses spoon, upside down
	Looks at Mother's face		Acquire sitting balance		Releases finger food into cup
	Tonic necks reflex position of head		Guides Mother's hand during feeding		Casts toy or finger food
	2 night feedings – *8 weeks	36 Weeks	Holds feeding bottle		Grasps cup with both hands
	Tongue projects after spoon is removed		Feeds self cracker well		Sucks through straw
8 Weeks	1 night feeding – *28 weeks	40 Weeks	Sits well, creeps	18 Months	Feeds self in part spills – *36 months
12–16 Weeks	Choking response to solids		Combines 2 toys, utensils		Hands empty dish to Mother
16 Weeks	Head erect but set forward		Chooses pellet, finger food		Finger feeds with pieces of food
	Anticipates on sight of food	44 Weeks	Tries to feed self	21 Months	Handles cup well
	Arms activate at toys or food		Drinks from cup in part		Verbalizes "Fat," "All Gone" asks for food
	Mouth poises for nipple		Tries to use spoon		Spoon to mouth right side up
20 Weeks	Pats bottle or breast *36 weeks	48 Weeks	Net pincer grasp	2 Years	Uses spoon well
	Closes in on bottle with both hands		Cessation of drooling except when talking		Feeds doll
	Scratches table top or flat surface				Fond of ritual
24 Weeks	Brings hand to mouth			3 Years	Spills little
	Sits in chair when securely supported				Pours well from small pitcher
					Feeds self well using utensils

FEEDING SKILL ASSESSMENT CHART

	Number of Observations									
	1	2	3	4	5	6	7	8	9	10
Breathes through mouth										
Sits with good head control										
Grasp response follows a tactile stimulus										
Lip closure occurs										
Can protrude tongue										
Can lateralize tongue (from side to side moves easily)										
Can elevate tongue										
Removes food from spoon with lips										
Control of drooling										
Drinks from cup (in part)										
Holds own cup (spills easily)										
Holds own cup (few spills)										
Holds own cup by handles, drinks well										
Has hand to mouth movements										
Finger feeds (cracker)										
Removes food from spoon with lips, not teeth										
Uses spoon (spills frequently)										
Uses spoon (few spills)										
Fills spoon, brings to mouth, and eats										
Uses fork										
Uses knife										
Feeds self using utensils										
Shows independence in eating and talking well										
Eats rapidly										
Can straw suck										
Pours from pitcher										
Can serve self										
Can set table										

Key: X adequate / attempt + with help − unable to do 0 not tested

Food Guide Pyramid
A Guide to Daily Food Choices

KEY
☐ Fat (naturally occurring and added) ☐ Sugars (added)

These symbols show fats, oils, and added sugars in foods.

Fats, Oils, & Sweets
USE SPARINGLY

Milk, Yogurt, & Cheese Group
2-3 SERVINGS

Meat, Poultry, Fish, Dry Beans, Eggs, & Nuts Group
2-3 SERVINGS

Vegetable Group
3-5 SERVINGS

Fruit Group
2-4 SERVINGS

Bread, Cereal, Rice, & Pasta Group
6-11 SERVINGS

FOOD GUIDE

What is your score?

Group	High Score	Add Your Score
Milk		
1 pint or more for an adult	3	
3 to 4 cups for children	3	
1 quart or more for teen-agers	3	
1 quart or more for women during pregnancy and nursing (pregnant and nursing teens 5 cups or more)	3	
Fruits (vitamin C source)		
2 servings or more of citrus fruit, tomato, broccoli, raw cabbage, peppers, melon, or berries	2	
Vegetables (vitamin A source)		
2 servings or more of dark-green or deep yellow vegetables or fruits	2	
1 or more servings of other vegetables and fruits, including potatoes	1 / 3	
Meat/Meat Alternatives		
2 or more servings of meat, poultry fish, eggs (3 servings if pregnant)	1	
(If one serving of above foods, and one of dry beans, dry peas, lentils, nuts, peanuts, or peanut butter)	1 / 2	
Whole Grains		
6 or more servings of whole grain cereals, breads, pasta, rice, and other grain products	6	
6 or more servings enriched or restored	3	
	6 / 16	

COMPARISON SCORE

16	14	12	10	8	6	4	2
100	90	80	70	60	50	40	30

Adapted from the University of California Agricultural Extension Service

---

Fig. 4–1 (Continued)

MUELLER PRESPEECH AND FEEDING EVALUATION

Name: _____ Date: _____

	N	Abn	Nt*
1. *Facial Expression*			
2. *Feeding Reflexes*			
Rooting Reflex			
Suck/Swallow Reflex			
Bite Reflex			
Gag Reflex			
3. *Feeding Behavior*			
Sucking/Drinking			
Swallowing			
Chewing – Rotary?			
4. *Response to Digital Stimulation*			
Outside mouth			
Inside mouth			
5. *Dental Development*			
Bite			
Teeth			
Gums			
6. *Jaws*			
At rest			
In motion			
7. *Lips*			
At rest			
In motion			
8. *Tongue*			
At rest			
In motion			
9. *Breathing*			
At rest			
In motion			
10. *Voice*			
Pitch, Range			
Loudness			
Rate			
Intonation			

*Could not be tested

SUMMARY

PROCEDURE RECOMMENDED

Fig. 4–1. (Continued)

CHILD
Nutritional Assessment (Case Workup) Evaluation

I DEMOGRAPHIC DATA – 100 POINTS TOTAL Points

   A. Chart reviewed for pertinent data from other evaluations and parental
      questionnaire pertaining to nutrition. 10
   B. Anthropometric data completed with accurate calculations and
      percentiles. 10
   C. Prenatal, newborn and pertinent family data recorded. 10
   D. Laboratory data compiled. 10
   E. Twenty four hour recall and food summary evaluated. 20
   F. Physical Activity Record 10
   G. Clinical Evaluation 10
   H. Feeding Skill and Assessment 20

II NUTRITION RECORD SUMMARY – 100 POINTS TOTAL Evaluation

   A. Pertinent Nutritional History 18
      —prenatal
      —newborn food intake
      —infant food
      —supplements
      —feeding milestones development
      —diet history of infancy and early childhood

   B. Evaluation of Current Nutritional Status 12
      —behavior patterns during feeding/reward system
      —present dietary pattern/fiber/fluid, caloric intake and expenditure
      —associated problems
      —caretaker knowledge

   C. Anthropometric Data 8
      —growth grid completed and curve plotted
      —current measurements and percentiles/weight-height ratio and status to
        ideal weight and age

   D. Biochemical Data 4
      —medications
      —drug/food interactions/caretaker knowledge
      —laboratory values
      —supplements

   E. Clinical Observations 16
      —physical signs and symptoms
      —current feeding abilities – a, b, and c
      —observation of behavior during interview
      —interaction with parents

   F. Presenting Nutritional Problem 6

   G. Impressions 20
      —overall nutritional status
      —weight/height ratio, number of pounds over or under ideal weight
      —adequacy of diet expressed in foods and nutrients/medication
        interaction; % of RDA, if a 3DDD
      —physical activity/relationship to caloric intake/expenditure
      —feeding skills level

   H. Recommendations: Care Plan 16
      —recommendations made during interview/caretaker knowledge
      —translate low or excessive nutrients into appropriate food sources/plus
        adequate fiber and fluids
      —food budgeting, selection, and preparation
      —special techniques to improve feeding skills
      —physical activities beneficial to client
      —referral to other programs
      —type of counseling, treatment needed from Nutrition Department
      —pertinent, practical and realistic planning goals/timetable/how
        measured
      —format of written report

4–2   Nutrition Mid-level Clinical Assessment Record (Infant to Toddler), UACCDD, CHMC

INFANT–TODDLER NUTRITION FORM
(High Risk and Myelomeningocele Clinics)

Name: \
Birthdate: Age: Parents Name \
Date: Address: \
Pediatrician: \
Diagnosis: Siblings:

Height: (____ cm.) \
Weight: (____ kg.) \
Ht/Wt Ratio ____ / ____ \
Head Circumf. ____ \
Skinfold ____

Hct ____ %   low/normal \
Hgb ____ %   low/normal \
Hx of infections: YES/NO \
Allergies: YES/NO

Growth since last clinic visits: Ht. ____ Wt. ____ Plot growth curve \
Clinical Evaluation: NEG/POS (area) \
Physical Limitations (Scale 1–8, 8 high)/Dx: \
Vitamins/Minerals: YES/NO TYPE: \
Medications: YES/NO Nutrient Interaction: \
Fluoride Source: YES/NO \
WIC YES/NO

Appetite \
Diet/Eating Concerns \
Feeding Problems: sucking/chewing/choking/drooling/swallowing/colic/spitting/ \
     tongue thrust/pica

DIET

*Breast fed \
*Formula (type) \
Amount per day \
Infant Foods: How taken \
   Age started \
YES/NO: Table Salt ___ Table sugar ___ \
   Pop ___ \
*Water: Amt. per day

Constipation: YES/NO \
Diarrhea: YES/NO \
*Food Allergies: YES/NO \
*Nursing Bottle Syndrome: YES/NO \
*Solid foods should not be given \
   before 4 months of age. \
Review Quantity of Food, Sample Menu: \
YES/NO

Caretaker knowledge demonstrated: \
   caloric expenditure   YES/NO \
   nutrition   YES/NO \
   fiber & fluid   YES/NO \
   dental health   YES/NO \
   food & drug interaction YES/NO

Time	24 HOUR RECALL	Amount	Score
	B. Fruit		
	Meat/Egg		
	Bread		
	Fat		
	Cereal		
	Beverage		
	L. Meat		
	Veg.		
	Bread		
	Fruit		
	Beverage		
	D. Meat		
	Veg.		
	Salad		
	Bread		
	Fat		
	Dessert		
	Beverage		

Time	BETWEEN MEALS

Developmental Assessment

Feeding: SPOON -- Grasps YES/NO, unable, palmer, pincer (assisted) (unassisted) \
(Fine   <u>Control</u>: beginning, fair, good \
Motor)   CUP   -- Grasps YES/NO, both hands, one hand (assisted) (unassisted) \
            <u>Control</u>: beginning, fair, good

     BOTTLE – YES/NO \
     INFA-FEEDER – YES/NO \
     FINGER FEEDING – YES/NO

<u>Gross Motor</u>   sitting ____ (with or without support) \
       hand to mouth control ____ \
       chewing ____ \
       creeping ____ \
       crawling ____

     pullup ____ \
     stand alone ____ \
     cruising ____ \
     walking ____ \
     run ____

Manner Fed: high chair   pumpkin seat   held

Transition to table foods/Reward System

Overall Feeding Skills Assessment: age appropriate   delayed

Caloric intake ____ or ____ kcal/kg.   LOW/ACCEPTABLE/ABOVE RDA

*RDA range kcal   0 – 6 mos   kg x 115 kcal = ____   (range) \
             6 mo – 1 yr   kg x 105 = ____   (95–145) \
             1 – 3   3000 (900–1800)   (80–135)

*RDA protein   0 – 6 mos   kg x 2.5 gm = ____ \
            6 mo – 1 yr   kg x 2.0 = ____ \
            1 – 3 yr   23 gm

Water needs

Overall Diet Adequacy: ACCEPTABLE/NOT ACCEPTABLE

<u>ADDITIONAL COMMENTS</u>

<u>SOAP NUTRITION CARE PLAN/RECOMMENDATIONS/FOLLOW UP</u> \
Goals/Timetable/How measured

_____ Nutritionist

6/84 Prepared by J. Wessel, E. Grace, M. Schmidt, S. Ekvall

4–3 Nutrition Mid-level Clinical Assessment Record (Above Toddler Age), UACCDD, CHMC

```
          UNIVERSITY AFFILIATED CINCINNATI CENTER FOR DEVELOPMENTAL DISORDERS
                      Myelomeningocele and Cerebral Palsy Clinic
                            Nutrition Evaluation Form
                                 (>Toddler Age)
     Name:                                  Address:
     Birthdate:
     Date:                                  Age:
     Height: _____(_____cm)_____%           Hct_____low/normal Hgb_____low/normal
     Weight: _____(_____kg)_____%           (from CCDD/CHMC record)
     Ht/Wt Ratio:_____%, if under 10 yrs.   Hx of infections_____ Allergies: YES/NO
     Brace Wt_____                      Constipatin YES/NO - Method: _____
     Head Circumf. ____cm.                  Diet Restrictions: YES/NO - Type:_____
     Upper Arm Circumf._____(__cm)____%     Vitamins/Minerals: YES/NO - Type:_____
     Tricep___mm (Median for age__is__mm)   Nutrients affected:_____
     Arm Muscle Circumf._____cm_____%       Feeding skills assesment:NORMAL/DELAYED
     Arm Muscle Area_____cm             Behavioral problems____ Reward system__
     Thorax_____mm Abdomen_____mm           Caretaker knowledge demonstrated:YES/NO
     Waist Circumf._____inches            ___caloric expenditure ___dental health
     Nutrition Clinical Eval.: NEG/POS      ___nutrition      ___food & drug
     Physical Limitations: wheelchair -     ___fiber & fluid    interaction    =YES
       braces - walker - self-ambulator
     Physical Activity Score (1-8): ___     Food Stamps: YES/NO
     Diet History: YES/NO  Nutrient deficits:_____
     Food Summary Score: _____ Estimated caloric intake: _____ Expenditure: _____
```

```
          24 HOUR RECALL                          FOOD SUMMARY
                          Amt.                Amt.   Amt.  Possible
     Breakfast                                per    per   points or  **Actual
          Fruit    _____  _____             day    week  daily serv. Points
          Meat     _____  _____     GROUP
          Egg      _____  _____     Dairy Products:              3
          Bread    _____  _____       Milk       ____  ____  ____     ____
          Fat      _____  _____       Cheese     ____  ____  ____     ____
          Cereal   _____  _____       Cottage Cheese ___  ___  ___    ____
          Beverage _____  _____       Yogurt     ____  ____  ____     ____
          Other    _____  _____       Other      ____  ____  ____     ____
     Lunch                            Meat or Alternates:*** Fat & Chol.2
          Meat     _____  _____     ***Meat, Eggs ____  ____  ____     ____
          Veg.     _____  _____       Fish, Poultry ___  ___  ___     ____
          Bread    _____  _____       Dr. Beans/peas ___ ___  ___     ____
          Fruit    _____  _____       Peanut Butter ___  ___  ___     ____
          Beverage _____  _____     Vegetables: (No Vit. A/C-1/2 cr)  3
          Other    _____  _____       Vit A Veg. ____  ____  ____     ____
     Dinner                             Vit C Veg. ____  ____  ____     ____
          Soup     _____  _____       Other      ____  ____  ____     ____
          Meat or Subst. ____  _____   Fruits:                    2
          Potato   _____  _____       Vit C Fruit ___  ____  ____     ____
          Veg.: Cooked      _____       Other Fruits ___  ____  ____     ____
                 Raw        _____     Whole Grains/Starches: (No w/grains-1/2 cr)
          Salad    _____  _____                                 6
          Bread    _____  _____       Cereal     ____  ____  ____     ____
          Fat      _____  _____       Bread      ____  ____  ____     ____
          Dessert  _____  _____       Pasta, Rice ___  ____  ____     ____
          Beverage _____  _____       Other      ____  ____  ____     ____
          Other    _____  _____                        TOTAL  16      ____
                                      Others:
     Time Between Meals                 Candy/Sugar ___  ____  If daily-1 ____
                                        Chips/t. salt ___ ___  If daily-1 ____
     ____  _____  _____             Soft Drinks ___  ____  If daily-1 ____
     ____  _____  _____             Desserts   ____  ____  If daily-1 ____
     ____  _____  _____             Water      ____  ____  None daily-1 ___
                                        ***Fats & Chol. ___ ___ 3 ser. d.-1 ____
     Water flouridated: Yes/No          Fiber      ____  ____  None daily-1 ___
                                                         TOTAL            ____
```

(>Toddler Age) Form - Page 2

NUTRITION ASSESSMENT REPORT AND SOAP NUTRITION CARE PLAN

Recommendations/Follow Up/Goals/Timetable/How Measured

```
                          _____
                            Team Nutritionist
     3/91 Revised by Nutrition Staff-UACCDD
```

4–4   Nutrition Mini-level, Clinical Assessment Record, UACCDD, CHMC

<u>NUTRITION SCREENING/MINI EVALUATION</u>
Community Outreach – Developmental Consultation Team (DCT)

<u>Teacher</u>/<u>Nurse</u> Observation Checklist for Nutritional evaluation:

	Yes	No
Disproportionate weight for height	___	___
Frequent absenteeism	___	___
Falls asleep in class	___	___
Lacks ambition	___	___
Behaves clumsily or falls easily	___	___
Delayed healing of minor injuries	___	___
Bites nails	___	___
Signs of hyperactivity	___	___
Many food dislikes (if known)	___	___
Balanced lunch including protein food, fruit and milk	___	___

_____

	Yes	No
Frequent colds or respiratory infections	___	___
Good appetite	___	___
Frequent headaches	___	___
Frequent digestive disturbances	___	___
Allergies (if known)	___	___

Additional Health of nutritional information of importance not included in above_____

_____

_____

Checklist for Screening to be completed by <u>Nutritionist</u>:

Height_____   Percentile_____
Weight_____   Percentile_____
Head Circumference_____   Percentile_____

Physical Appearance:

	Satisfactory	If Unsatisfactory, Describe
Hair	_____	_____
Skin	_____	_____
Nails	_____	_____
Eyes	_____	_____
Teeth	_____	_____
Gums	_____	_____
Lips	_____	_____
Tongue	_____	_____
Posture	_____	_____
Abdomen	_____	_____
Skeletal development	_____	_____

Other Comments_____

The <u>Social Worker</u> Inteview with parents:

Questions on family food practices, such as feeding history (feeding difficulties) and dietary history (food purchasing, food preparation, eating habits)_____

*Prepared by Catherine Grogan, M.Ed., R.D., and Patricia Lierman, R.D., M.Ed., DCT Staff Nutritionists
From <u>Clinical Instruction Techniques In An Interdisciplinary Setting</u>, S. Ekvall

4–5 Nutrition 3 Day Diet Diary and Physical Activity Record, UACCDD, CHMC

NAME: _____ AGE: _____ WT: _____ HT: _____

SEX: _____

DATES: From _____ to _____

INSTRUCTION SHEET FOR RECORDING OF DIETARY INTAKE

1. Record what the child has eaten immediately after each meal or snack. Do not trust your memory at the end of the day!

2. Date each sheet – have consecutive days (unless illness intervenes).

3. Be exact as to amounts, i.e. report in terms of level tablespoons, cups, dimensions of slices of meat, size of fruit, etc. "Bowlfuls", "glasses", and "servings" do not indicate accurate measures of food contained therein!

4. Describe accurately the kind of food recorded:

   a. State brand name whenever possible.
   b. Type of milk used: whole, powdered, evaporated, etc. Mention whenever butter, milk or sugar are used in cream sauce, etc.
   c. Differentiate between ice milk and ice cream.
   d. Type of bread or cereal used: whole wheat, white, rye, cornflakes, oatmeal, etc.
   e. Method of cooking: boiled, fried, creamed, roasted, etc., give entire recipes (list of ingredients) of mixed dishes.
   f. State whether canned, dried, fresh, or frozen product.

5. Be sure to record everything eaten:

   a. Vitamin preparations and medicines.
   b. "Hidden foods", – sugar on cereal or fruit, butter, oleo, or mayonnaise on bread, vegetables, popcorn, crumb or cheese topping, etc.
   c. Candy, pop, potato chips, state kind and amount.

6. At the end of this period, please complete the following.

   a. Was this a typical week (does child usually eat these foods and these amounts?

   b. If not, how was it different? _____

   c. Was there any illness during this period?

MEAL PATTERN	KIND OF FOOD	AMOUNT	CALORIES	DAY
BREAKFAST Time _____ Where _____ With Whom _____				
Mid-Morning Snacks				
LUNCH Time _____ Where _____ With Whom _____				
Afternoon Snacks				
DINNER Time _____ Where _____ With Whom _____				
Evening Snacks				
Water				
Vitamins or Minerals				
Appetite				
		TOTAL		

PHYSICAL ACTIVITY RECORD

Record below all activities during the day from time of waking up until going to bed in the evening and falling asleep.

Example:	Time		Kind of Activity	Where
	from	until		
	11:00	11:30	Played Ball	Outdoors

TIME From Until	KIND OF ACTIVITY	WHERE

Appendix 5
Nutritional Assessment Records, Developmental Evaluation Center, Boston Children's Hospital Medical Center Other Nutritional Assessment Forms

5–1 Indepth Nutrition Assessment Record, Developmental Evaluation Center, Boston Children's Hospital Medical Center

Child's Name _____ Date _____

Child's Birth Date _____ Age _____

Person Completing Form _____

Relationship to child _____

Early Feeding Problems

	Never	0-6 Months	6-12 Months	1-3 Years	3-6 Years
Sucking					
Swallowing					
Chewing					
Tongue Control					
Lip Control					
Color Change with Feeding					
Gagging					
Colic					
Spitting-up					
Vomiting					
Appetite					
Food Intolerances					
Diarrhea					
Constipation					
Anemia					
Dehydration					
Underweight					
Overweight					
Poor Growth					
Gastrostomy					
Nasogastric					
Hyperalimentation					
Intravenous					

What are your child's feeding problems?

1.

2.

3.

4.

5.

How much did your child weigh at birth?

What was your child's length at birth?

Was your child a full term baby?

How long did your child stay in hospital at birth?

Has your child had any hospitalizations since birth?

Has your child ever been treated with a special diet?

Circle the answer that applies

Weight gain from birth has been: satisfactory   slow   fluctuating

Weight gain recently has been: satisfactory   slow   fluctuating

How does this child compare to siblings at the same age? larger   same   smaller

How much does mother weigh?

How tall is mother?

How much does father weigh?

How tall is father?

Has your child ever been treated with a special diet?

5-1 (Continued)

How Often Does Your Child Eat These Foods?

	Daily	Occasionally	Seldom
Milk			
Cheese, ice cream			
Cold or hot cereal			
Sweet rolls or donuts			
Sandwiches			
Soup			
Fruit or fruit juice			
Peanut butter or nuts			
Dried peas or beans			
Meat in casseroles			
Red meat, fish or poultry			
Cooked or raw vegetable			
Potato, rice or noodles			
Cookies or crackers			
Pie, cake or brownies			
Potato chips or corn chips			
Candy			
Soft drinks or kool-aid			

Feeding Development

	0-3 Months	4-6 Months	7-9 Months	10-12 Months	13-15 Months	16-18 Months	19-21 Months	22-24 Months	2-2½ Years	2½-3 Years	Not Yet
Baby Food Introduction											
Junior Foods											
Finger Feeding											
Cup Drinking											
Weaning											
Whole Table Foods											
Use of Spoon											
Independent Feeding											
Self Preparation of Food											

Present Feeding

What is the hungriest time of the day for your child?   a.m.   noon   p.m.

Does your child ever crave or eat non-food items?   yes   no

Please Record the Usual Daily Food Intake:

Time of meal or snack	Food eaten	Amount

Is your child on a vitamin-mineral supplement?   yes   no   name _____

List the medications taken by your child

     Past _____

     Now _____

What is your child's position during feeding?   held   in seat   sits independently

How long does a feeding take?   15 minutes or less   ½ hour   ½ hour or more

Who usually feeds your child?   mother   father   other

Describe the texture of your child's food.   strained   ground   cut   regular

How is your child fed?   bottle   cup   spoon   gastrostomy   nasogastric

Describe your child's appetite: excellent   fair   poor

Does your child bring toys or fingers to his or her mouth?   yes   no

Describe your child's level of independence.   totally independent   partially independent   dependent

Does your child close his or hands around a bottle?   yes   no

Does your child finger feed?   yes   no

Does your child attempt to grasp the spoon as you feed?   yes   no

Is your child sipping from a cup?   yes   no

Does your child: Drink independently from a cup?
     raises cup
     drinks
     replaces

Does your child eat independently with a spoon?
     - grasps spoon
     - dips in dish
     - fills spoon
     - brings spoon to mouth
     - replaces spoon

Does your child use a fork?   yes   no

5-1 (Continued)

NUTRITION ASSESSMENT

DEVELOPMENTAL EVALUATION CLINIC

NAME:------------------- PARENTS:-------------------
D.O.B.:------- AGE:------ ADDRESS:-------------------
D.O.E.:-------
EVALUATOR:------------- TELEPHONE:-----------------
DIAGNOSIS:-----------------

ANTHROPOMETRICS

HEIGHT:------/------IN./CM ------% ------%(DS)
WEIGHT:------/------LBS./KG ------% ------%(DS)
WT/HT RELATIONSHIP:------% HEAD CIRCUMFERENCE:------IN/CM----%
HEIGHT AGE:------ WEIGHT AGE:------ IDEAL BODY WEIGHT:------%
SKIN FOLD:------MM/------% ARM CIRCUMFERENCE:------MM/------%
MAMC:------CM/------%

ACTIVITY LEVEL AND MUSCLE TONE

------AMBULATORY ------WHEELCHAIR BOUND ------INVOLUNTARY
MOVEMENTS ------NORMAL TONE ----HYPERTONIA ------HYPOTONIA
------VARIABLE TONE ----SIT WITH /WITHOUT SUPPORT
------STAND WITH/WITHOUT SUPPORT.

PRENATAL AND INFANT HISTORY:

GESTATIONAL LENGTH:------ PRENATAL WEIGHT GAIN:------
BIRTH COMPLICATIONS:------
BIRTH WEIGHT:------ BIRTH LENGTH:------
BREAST FED:------ BOTTLE FED:------ FORMULA:------
AGE SOLID FOODS WERE STARTED:------
DIFFICULTIES:------

BIOCHEMICAL DATA:

SERUM ALBUMIN:------(GM/DL) SERUM TOTAL PROTEIN:------(GM/DL)
HEMOGLOBIN:------(GM/DL) HCT:------(%) SERUM TRANSFERRIN(MG/DL)
------ OTHER:------

NUTRITIONAL HISTORY:

FEEDING SKILLS:

------NO SELF-FEEDING SKILLS ----ABLE TO FEED SELF WITH
ASSISTANCE ------HOLDS BOTTLE ----FINGER FEEDS ----WEANED FROM
BOTTLE
INDEPENDENT WITH ----SPOON ------FORK ----STRAW

DIET TEXTURE:

------STRAINED BABY FOODS ------JUNIOR BABY FOODS
------BLENDERIZED/MASHED TABLE FOODS ------GROUND ------CHOPPED
FINE ------REGULAR

24-HOUR RECALL(TYPICAL DAY):

BREAKFAST   LUNCH   DINNER   SNACKS

TOTAL CALORIES:------   KCAL/KG:------
PROTEIN(GMS)/KG:------   FLUID INTAKE:------(OZ/CC)
ESTIMATED NEEDS:
CALORIES:------ KCAL/DAY, ------KCAL/KG
PROTEIN:------ GM/DAY, ------GM/KG
FLUID: ------CC/DAY

NUTRITIONAL RELATED CONCERNS:

ORAL MOTOR------ BEHAVIORAL------ POSITIONING------
FOOD TOLERANCES------ VOMITING/GAGGING------
CONSTIPATION/DIARRHEA------ DENTAL PROBLEMS:------
MEDICATIONS:------
VITAMIN/MINERAL SUPPLEMENTS:------
OTHER CONCERNS:------

NUTRITIONAL IMPRESSIONS:

RECOMMENDATIONS:

1.------
2.------
3.------
4.------

8/88

5-2   WIC Nutrition Education/Care Plan, Ohio

Date _____

Participant's Name _____

Participant's Age _____

Location of Program Application: _____

Circle type of encounter: Initial   Recent

Follow-up: Date _____
     Ind   Grp   HR   Tel

S Participant comments/statements:
U
B Health professional comments/observations:
J
E
C
T Location of medical chart:
I Other clinical/medical data:
V
E Language Barrier?   Yes   No

O
B Ht: ___ in ___ %ile
J Wt: ___ lb ___ oz ___ %ile
E Hct/Hgb:
C See: ___ Growth chart
T ___ Certification form
I Location of medical chart:
V Other clinical/medical data:
E

Minimum Requirements for Nutrition Education

Required at initial certification. Restate needed thereafter.

( ) Information Covered.
___ 1. Explanation of nutritional need condition.
___ 2. Explanation that foods are for recipient and not entire family.
___ 3. Information regarding what constitutes an adequate diet for the participant.
___ 4. Explanation that the WIC foods are supplemental.
___ 5. Information regarding possible uses of the WIC foods.
___ 6. Information regarding the nutritional value of the WIC foods.
___ 7. Explanation of the importance of health care.
___ 8. Explanation of breastfeeding (pregnant women only).

Parental heights: Mother _____ Father _____
Weight gain/loss: _____ lb at _____ weeks gestation
Wrist Measurement: _____ in Frame size _____
EDC (Date) _____

	WIC CODE	PRIORITY	COMMENTS
A Anthropometric			
S Weight/Growth: WNL O U	11, 12, 13, 14, 15	1,6	
S Height: WNL Low Stature	51, 52, 53, 54	1,3	
E Hematological			
S WNL LOW N/A	20	1, 3, 6	
S Nutritional			
M 24 hour recall:			
E WNL Inadequate			
N Food Frequency:	30, 62	4, 5, 6	
T WNL Inadequate			

Other Risk Assessments
Age   40, 41   1, 3
Breastfeeding   70, 71, 72   1, 2, 4
Infants   61, 64   2
Medical Condition   44   1, 3
Previous/Current OB
   History   42, 43, 45   1, 4
Prevention of Regression   63   1, 3, 6
Substance Abuse   46, 47, 48   1
Transfers   80, 81   1, 2, 3, 4, 6
Other Assessment Information
Receptive to counseling?   Yes   No
Objectives met?   Yes   No

High risk _____ Reason:
Ineligible _____ Reason:

	COUNSELING		HANDOUTS
P	___ Basic Nutrition		___ Daily Food Guide
L	___ Breastfeeding		___ Breastfeeding: Baby's Best Start
A	___ Dental/Baby Bottle Tooth Decay		___ Food For the Preschooler: I II III
N	___ Infant Feeding/Solids		___ Feeding Your Baby
	___ Iron		___ Eating Right For Your Baby
	___ Postpartum Nutrition		___ Relief From Common Problems
	___ Prenatal Nutrition		___ ABC's of Smart Snacking
	___ Snacking		___ Food For Red Blood
	___ Vitamins/Minerals		___ Counting Your Calories
	___ Weight Control		___ Your Baby's Weight
	___ Other:		___ Your Child's Weight
			___ Other:

Objectives set:

High Risk Plan:

Referrals:
___ Well Child Clinic   ___ Headstart
___ Immunizations   ___ Physician
___ HEALTHCHEK   ___ Dentist
___ Prenatal Clinic   ___ Food Stamps
___ Family Planning   ___ Childbirth Class
___ Breastfeeding   ___ Other:
   Support
___ Human Services/Medicaid

Health Professional's Signature _____

Follow-up Contact (Date): _____

From: Ohio Department of Health, Division of Women, Infants, and Children. Used with Permission.

Name: _____ Date: _____

What did you eat for:	HOW MUCH? (Amount of each food)	Milk	Meat & Alternatives	Fruit & Vegetables	Grain	Other
Morning						
Between Meals						
Noon						
Between Meals						
Evening						
In Evening Before Bedtime						
	Totals					

5–2 (Continued)

FOOD FREQUENCY FOR WOMEN

Name: _____ Today's Date: _____

DIRECTIONS: For each GROUP of foods, write in the number of times PER DAY or WEEK the woman eats any of them and CIRCLE the serving size that is closest to what she USUALLY eats.

Foods	Frequency	Your Usual Serving Size 1/2	1	2	Tally + or -
Milk, Yogurt, Pudding, Custard, Creamed Soup		4 oz or 1/2 C	8 oz or 1 C	12-16 oz or 1-1/2 C	
Cheese			1/2-1 slice	1-1/2 slices 2-3 slices	
Cottage Cheese, Ice Cream, Milk Shake		1/2-1 C	2 C	3-4 C	
Meat, Poultry, Fish, Eggs		1 oz or 1 egg	2 oz or 1 egg	4 oz or 1 egg	
Dried Beans (Pinto, Kidney, etc.), Dried Peas (Split Peas)		1/4 C cooked	3/4 C cooked	1-1/2 C cooked	
Nuts, Seeds, Peanut Butter		1/2 oz or 1 T	1 oz or 2 T	2 oz or 4 T	
Vit C - Citrus Fruit or Juice, Tomato, Broccoli, Brussels Sprouts, Strawberries enriched Apple Juice, Green Peppers, Greens		1/4 C cooked or juice or 1/2 C raw	1/2 C cooked or juice or 1 C raw	1 C cooked or juice or 1-1/2 C raw	
Vit A - Spinach, Cantaloupe, Apricots Peaches, Sweet Potato, Yams, Carrots		1/4 C fresh 1/2 piece	1/2 C fresh 1 piece	1 C fresh 2 pieces	
White Potato, Peas, Corn, Lettuce, Zucchini, Green or Yellow Beans, Beets, Celery, Cucumber		1/4 C cooked or 1/2 C raw	1/2 C cooked or 1 C raw	1 C cooked or 2 C raw	
Apples, Banana, Plums, Pears, Grapes		1/4 C or 1/2 piece	1/2 C or 1 piece	1 C or 2 pieces	
Enriched or Whole Grain Breads, Muffins, Biscuits, Pancakes, Waffles, Crackers		1/2 slice	1 slice	2 slices	
Cereal (hot) and Rice, Pasta, Grits		1/4 C	1/2-3/4 C	1-1 1/2 C	
Cereals, Ready-to-Eat		1/2 C	1 C	2 C	
Sweet Roll, Donut, Cake, Pie, Cookies		1/2 piece	1 piece	2 pieces	
French Fries, Potato Chips, Corn Chips Cheese Curls, Pretzels, etc.		1 oz bag	1 C	2 C	
Pot Pies, TV Dinners, Canned or Packaged Spaghetti, Ravioli, Macaroni and Cheese, Beefaroni, or Canned Soup		1/2 C	1 C	2 C	
Coffee (regular), Tea		1/2 C	1 C	2 C	
Soda Pop, Hi-C, Kool-Aid, Cocoa, Fruit Drinks		6 oz	12 oz	16 oz	
Sugar, Honey, Maple Syrup		1 T	2 T	4 T	

List any other foods you usually eat and how often: _____

From: Ohio Dept. of Health, Division of WIC. Used with permission.

5–3   Nutritional Assessment, Perinatal, California

Perinatal *

Name:_____ Date of HV:_____

Address:_____ City:_____

Birth Date:_____ Age:_____ Phone #:_____

Race: ☐ White ☐ Asian ☐ Indochinese ☐ Phillipino   Language Spoken _____

☐ Black ☐ Amer. Indian ☐ Pacific Islander ☐ Hispanic   Head of Household, Family Name _____

Evaluator_____

Program ☐☐☐   Signature _____

I. ANTHROPOMETRIC

	DATA	A	AG/I
0 Height			
1 Current Weight			
Post Partum (PP)			
2 Recommended Body Weight (RBW)			
◇ 3 Percent RBW			
◇ 4 Weight Change			
Ante Partum (AP)			
6 Pregravid Weight			
7 Pregravid RBW			
8 Pregravid Percent RBW			
9 Prenatal Weight Change			
GOAL			O
PP - Client at RBW			
AP - Adequate weight gain rate			

III. DIETARY

	DATA	A	AG/I
30 Adequate Food Groups			
◇ 31 Vitamin-mineral supplements			
◇ 33 Fad Diet			
◇ 34 Pica			
◇ 35 Food allergy/intolerance/dislikes			
36 Change in appetite			
38 Fat intake			
39 Sugar intake			
40 Alcohol intake			
41 Salt intake			
42 Caffeine intake			
43 Fluid intake			
44 Exercise			
45 Financial resources			
46 Food preparation/storage facilities			
47 Food preparation ability			
48 Breastfeeding			
◇ 49 Special diet			
GOAL			O
59 DIETARY is WNL			

*page 2 - weight grid, summary and referral

II. BIOCHEMICAL

	DATA	A	AG/I
◇ 20 Hemoglobin			
◇ 21 Hematocrit			
◇ 22 Blood glucose			
23 Urinalysis — protein			
24 glucose			
25 ketones			
GOAL			O
29 BIOCHEM is WNL			

IV. MEDICAL

	DATA	A	AG/I
◇ 60 Blood pressure			
◇ 61 Days of hospitalization			
62 Chewing ability			
◇ 64 Malnutrition			
◇ 65 Nutrient-drug interactions			
◇ 66 Nausea/vomiting			
◇ 67 Heartburn			
◇ 68 Constipation			
◇ 69 Diarrhea			
◇ 70 Frequent conception			
◇ 71 Age			
72 Gravida/Para			
73 Multiple births			
74 Smoking			
◇ 76 Dental caries			

HYPERMETABOLIC CONDITIONS

	*	AG/I
◇ 80 Major surgery		
81 Minor surgery		
82 Burns		
83 Long bone fracture		
84 Other		

PREVIOUS OBSTETRICAL COMPLICATIONS

		AG/I
◇ 90 Birthweight < 5 lbs 8 oz or > 8 lbs 13 oz		
◇ 91 Glucose intolerance in pregnancy		
92 Congenital anomalies		
93 Fetal or neonatal deaths		
◇ 94 Pre-eclampsia/Toxemia		
◇ 95 Anemia		
◇ 96 Weight gain < 20 or > 40 lbs		

CHRONIC DISEASE

	AG/I
101 Cardiovascular disease	
◇ 102 —anemia	
◇ 105 —G6PD	
◇ 106 —hyperlipidemia	
◇ 107 —hypertension	
◇ 108 —sickle cell	
109 Endocrine disorder	
◇ 110 —diabetes	
112 Gastrointestinal disease	
118 Infectious disease	
120 Kidney disease	
125 Liver and Biliary disease	
◇ 127 —cholecystitis	
129 Metabolic disease	
132 Neurological disease	
138 Orthopedic disease	
142 Psychological dysfunction	
◇ 143 —alcoholism	
◇ 144 —depression	
◇ 145 —eating disorder	
◇ 146 —substance abuse	
147 Respiratory disease	
149 Other	
GOAL	O
150 MEDICAL is WNL	

LEGEND
AG = Anticipatory Guidance
T = Teach
D = Demonstrate
L = Literature
R = Refer
S = Supervise
C = Contract
K = Counsel

◇ = Refer to nutritionist/RD
A = Assessment
␥ = WNL
P = Problem
+ = Optimal Problem Management
— = Not appropriate
Y = Yes, condition is present
N = No, condition is not present
I = Intervention

O = Outcome
1 = Goal Met
= Goal Not Met
2a = Still working towards goal
2b = Lost to follow up
2c = Refused
2d = Client failed to follow through
2e = Referred to another District or Co.
3 = Continue on appropriate flow sheet

County of San Bernardino — Department of Public Health   341.003.H41

Clay, G., Bouchard, C., and Hemphill, K.: A comprehensive nutrition case management system. J Am Diet Assoc 88 (2);197, 1988. Used with permission.

5-4 Mental Health Institution Nutrition Assessment, Ohio

Living Area/Ward	Sex	Age	Height	Weight	Ideal Weight		Amount of Foods Eaten Daily					
							Milk	Meat	Eggs	Vegetables	Fruit Juices	Desserts
Weight History	Mid Arm Circ.	Triceps Skinfold			Mid Arm Musc. Circ.		Bread	Cereal	Potato, Pasta	Fats	Sugar, Candy	Snack Foods

Admitting Diagnosis

Family History (diabetes, mental deficiency, obesity, etc.)

Pertinent Medical History

Diet Order

Assessment

Medications

Pertinent Lab Values (date and result)

| HGB | HCT | Alb | FBS |
| BUN | Chol | Other | |

Motor Development (dexterity, coordination)

Sensory Skills

Speech/Communication | Vision | Hearing

Habits Related to Foods

Occupation/Daily Activity

Sleep Patterns

Total Hours: Exercise: ☐ Continuous ☐ Interrupted   ☐ Restrictive ☐ Inactive ☐ Moderate ☐ Excessive

Tobacco (kind, amount)   Alcohol (kind, amount)   Drugs (kind, amount)

Elimination: ☐ Regular ☐ Diarrhea ☐ Constipation ☐ Laxatives   Appetite: ☐ Excessive ☐ Good ☐ Fair ☐ Poor

Food Likes   Food Dislikes

Allergies, Intolerances, Religious Restrictions

Nutritional Care Plan

Goals

Objectives   Strategies

Special Problems Affecting Eating

Dentition: ☐ Own Teeth ☐ Dentures ☐ No Teeth ☐ Swallowing

Feeding: ☐ Feeds Self ☐ Needs Assistance ☐ Adaptive Equipment (specify)

Ambulation: ☐ Ambulatory ☐ Mobil Nonambulatory ☐ Nonambulatory

Comments:

Source of Information (if other than patient)

Signature of Interviewer (if other than Dietitian)   Date   Signature of Dietitian   Date

DMH-0021   Rev. 8/82   **DIETARY HISTORY** DMH-MedR-1017 ⊜   DMH-MedR-1017 ⊜

From: Department of Mental Health, Ohio. Used with permission.

5–5 Nutrition Screening Questionnaire, Health Department, New Mexico

CHILD_____BIRTHDATE_____TODAY'S DATE_____

HOME PHONE_____

HOW IS YOUR CHILD EATING AND GROWING?

(Please circle yes or no in response to the following questions)

(7)	yes	no	1.	Is it easy to tell when your child is hungry or thirsty?
(10)	yes	no	2.	Do you have any concerns about his/her eating or growing?
(5B)	yes	no	3.	Is your child on a special diet? If yes, what? _____
(5D)	yes	no	4.	Does he/she take vitamins and minerals? If yes, what? _____
(5E)	yes	no	5.	Does he/she take medications? If yes, what?_____
(5C)	yes	no	6.	Does your child eat anything that is not food, such as paint or dirt?
(5A)	yes	no	7.	Do you have trouble buying or making your child's food?
	yes	no	8.	Does your child participate in the WIC Program? If yes, where?_____

WHAT DOES YOUR CHILD EAT AND DRINK?

(5A) 9. How many meals and snacks does he/she eat most days? _____Meals _____Snacks

(8E) 10. How long does it take him/her to finish a meal or feeding? _____ Minutes

(6) 11. Please check the choice(s) that best describe(s) what your child eats.

____Breastmilk   ____Baby Cereal   ____Ground Meats/Finely Ground Table Foods

____Formula   ____Strained Baby Foods   ____Cut Up Meats/Soft Table Foods

____Cow's Milk   ____Junior Foods   ____Finger Foods

(5A) 12. Circle any of the following food groups that you feel your child is not eating enough of.

1. Milk & Milk Products   2. Meat, Beans, Eggs   3. Fruits & Vegetables   4. Breads & Cereals

(5A) 13. Fill in the amount (cups or ounces) your child usually drinks in one day (24 hours).

Water_____   Sweet Drinks_____   Juice_____   Cow's Milk_____

Baby Formula_____   What kind of formula?_____

How do you make formula?   _____

(8) ARE ANY OF THESE A PROBLEM FOR YOUR CHILD? IF YES, PLEASE CHECK.

___Vomiting	___Eating too slowly	___Holding up his/her head
___Diarrhea	___Refusing to eat	___Sitting up alone
___Constipation	___Spitting out food	___Sucking on nipple
___Food Allergies	___Gagging & Choking	___Chewing
___Bad Teeth/Sore Mouth	___Getting upset at meals	___Swallowing
		___Drooling

==

STAFF USE ONLY

(9) DX _____

(1,2) Height_____Weight_____ %tiles : Ht/Age_____ Wt/Age_____ Wt/Ht_____

(3)(4) Birthweight (birth to 2 years) _____ Hematocrit _____ % Hemoglobin _____ gm/dl

Comments:_____

_____

_____

Name_____Agency_____Phone_____

Nutrition Bureau, Public Health Division, New Mexico Health & Environment Department
Adapted from Child Nutrition Questionnaire, Colorado Department of Health
Used with permission.

Appendix 6
Intensive Care Nursery Protocol
Formula Composition and Preventive Nutrition

6-1   Medical Nutrition Formula Composition, Alabama

FORMULA (Distributor) kcal/cc	Pro. g/cc	Pro. Source	CHO g/cc	CHO Source	Fat g/cc	Fat Source	Na mEq/cc	K mEq/cc	Ca mg/cc	P mg/cc	Mg mg/cc	Zn mg/cc	Fe mg/cc	Osmolality mOsm/kgH₂O	Renal Solute Load mOsm/L
Sustacal 1.00 (Mead Johnson)	0.061	calcium caseinate soy protein isolate sodium caseinate	0.140	sucrose corn syrup	0.023	partially hydrogenated soy	0.041	0.054	1.010	0.930	0.380	0.014	0.017	650	360
Carnation Instant Breakfast 1.00	0.058	milk casein soy protein	0.140	sucrose lactose corn syrup	0.031	whole milk	0.041	0.070	—	—	—	—	0.019	—	—
Ensure Plus 1.50 (Ross)	0.055	sodium & calcium caseinates soy protein isolate	0.200	corn syrup sucrose	0.053	corn	0.049	0.053	0.700	0.700	0.279	0.016	0.013	690	473
Magnacal 2.00 (Sherwood)	0.070	sodium & calcium caseinates	0.250	maltodextrin sucrose	0.080	partially hydrogenated soy	0.044	0.032	1.000	0.000	0.400	0.030	0.018	590	382
Amin Aid 2.00 (McGaw)	0.019	crystalline essential amino acids	0.366	maltodextrin sucrose	0.046	soy lecithin mono, diglycerides	0.014	0.005	—	—	—	—	—	1095	90
Hepatic Aid 1.10 (McGaw)	0.044	crystalline amino acids branched chain a.a.	0.169	sucrose	0.036	maltodextrin mono, diglycerides soy lecithin	0.014	0.055	—	—	—	—	—	560	—
Jevity 1.00 (Ross)	0.042	partially hydrolyzed whey, meat and soy free amino acids	0.185	hydrolyzed cornstarch sucrose	0.011	safflower MCT 45%	0.020	3.034	0.666	.0666	0.266	0.015		500	317
Reabilan 1.00 (O'Brien)	0.031	small peptides	0.131	maltodextrin tapioca starch	0.038	MCT soy	0.030	0.032	0.499	0.499	0.250	0.010	0.010	350	248
Tolerex 1.00 (was Vivonex) (Sandoz)	0.021	free amino acids	0.231	oligosaccharides glucose	0.001	safflower	0.020	0.030	0.500	0.500	0.222	0.008	0.010	550	244
Vital 1.06 3.4g fiber 240cc (Ross)	0.045	casein	0.152	hydrolyzed cornstarch	0.037	MCT 505 corn oil	0.041	0.040	0.910	0.760	0.300	0.017	0.012	300	260
Enrich 1.10 3.4gm dietary fiber/240cc (Ross)	0.040	sodium & calcium caseinates soy	0.162	hydrolized corn starch sucrose soy, polysaccharide	0.037	corn	0.036	0.040	0.710	0.710	0.280	0.016	0.013	480	344
Ensure 1.06 (Ross)	0.037	sodium & calcium caseinates soy protein isolate	0.145	corn syrup sucrose	0.037	corn	0.036	0.040	0.521	0.521	0.208	0.012	0.009	470	329

6–1 (Continued)

FORMULA (Distributor)	Pro. g/cc kcal/cc	Pro. Source	CHO g/cc Pro. Source	Fat g/cc CHO Source	Na Fat Source	K mEq/cc	Ca mg/cc	P mg/cc	Mg mg/cc	Zn mg/cc	Fe mg/cc	Osmolality mOsm/kgH$_2$O	Renal Solute Load mOsm/L
Pediasure 1.00 (Ross)	0.030	low lactose whey protein sodium carbinate 18.82 blend	0.110 corn syrup sucrose	0.049 safflower soy MCT 205	0.016	0.033	0.910	0.800	0.200	0.011	0.013	325	198
Portagen 0.67 (Mead Johnson)	0.023	casein lactose, sucrose	0.077 glucose polymers corn	0.032 MCT 85%	0.014	0.021	0.626	0.4671	0.140	0.006	0.013	220	150
Pedialyte 0.10 (Ross)	—		0.025 dextrose	—	0.045	0.020	—	—	—	—	—	250	100
Rehydralyte 0.10 (Ross)	—		0.025 dextrose	—	0.075	0.020	—	—	—	—	—	305	85
Osmolite 1.06 (Ross)	0.037	sodium & calcium caseinates soy protein isolate	0.145 glucose polymers	0.037 MCT 50% corn, soy	0.027	0.026	0.521	0.521	0.208	0.012	0.009	300	289
Isocal 1.06 (Mead Johnson)	0.034	caseinates soy protein isolate	0.133 sodium & calcium	0.044 maltodextrin	0.023 soy, MCT 20%	0.034	0.634	0.528	0.211	0.011	0.010	300	210
Precision Isotonic Diet 1.00	0.029	egg white solids sodium caseinate	0.144 maltodextrin sucrose	0.030 partially hydrogenated soy	0.034	0.025	0.025	0.641	0.256	0.010	0.010	300	210
Isosource 1.25 (Sandoz)	0.043	casein	0.175 maltodextrin	0.042 MCT, corn oil	0.032	0.043	0.660	0.660	0.260	0.016	0.012	300	280
Isotein HN 1.20 (Sandoz)	0.068	delactosed lactalbumin sodium caseinate	0.156 fructose	0.034 maltodextrin hydrogenated soy MCT	0.0265 partially	0.0274	0.056	0.056	0.226	0.008	0.010	300	354

Formula	Indications
S-14 (Wyeth)	Leucine sensitive hypoglycemia
S-29 (Wyeth)	Very low renal solute load:
S-44 (Wyeth)	Diabetes Insipidus, Renal disease, Cardiac disease Hypercalcemia
RCF (Ross)	Carbohydrate intolerance CHO Free, Soy protein base, must add CHO
Modular Core (8501) (Ross)	CHO intolerance; contains calcium caseinate, fat Must add CHO

Other formulas for inborn errors of metabolism can be found in individual chapters.

Prepared by H. Cloud, Sparks Center for Developmental and Learning Disorders, University of Alabama at Birmingham, Birmingham, Alabama

6-2 University Hospital Neonatal Intensive Care Unit Protocol, Cincinnati

POLICY: ENTERAL VITAMIN AND IRON SUPPLEMENTATION

POPULATION: All infants admitted to the neonatal intensive care unit.

A. PRETERM INFANTS

1. Vitamin Supplementation: When an infant is tolerating full feeding volume, vitamin supplementation should be started. Neonatal nutritionists may individualize vitamin recommendations when the following guidelines do not meet infant needs.

FEEDING TYPE	SUPPLEMENT
Human Milk	0.5 cc Polyvisol
	0.5 cc Aquasol E (first 4 weeks of full enteral feeding)
Human Milk plus fortifier	0.5 cc Aquasol E (first 4 weeks of full enteral feeding)
Preterm Formula	0.5 cc Aquasol E (first 4 weeks of full enteral feeding)
Term Formula	0.5 cc Polyvisol
	0.5 cc Aquasol E (first 4 weeks of full enteral feeding)

2. Iron Supplementation: A dose of 2 mg elemental iron/kg/d should be begun in preterm infants between 1 and 2 months of age. The dose should be adjusted for weight until a maximum dose of 15 mg/d is achieved. Iron supplementation should be continued for the first year of life. Iron supplementation can be provided by Fer-in-sol drops (25 mg/cc) or iron fortified preterm formula (~ 1.8 mg/100 kcal)or term formula (~ 1.8 mg/100 kcal).

B. TERM INFANTS

1. Multivitamin Supplementation: Neonatal nutritionists may individualize vitamin recommendations when the following guidelines do not meet an infant's needs.

FEEDING TYPE	SUPPLEMENT
Human Milk	1.0 cc Tri-Vi-Flor
Term Formula	no supplement

2. Iron Supplementation: In full term infants receiving own mother's milk, a dietary or supplementary source of iron should be provided by the time the infant is 6 months old.

Iron fortified formulas are the feedings of choice for formula-fed full term infants.

Written by: Susan Krug-Wispe, Barbette Tohline, Jacqueline Wessel
Reviewed by:

Donald Houchins, R.N., M.S.N.   POL:26B   Uma R. Kotagal, M.D.
Head Nurse - NICU   Director of Nurseries
Written: 4/1/90

6-2 (Continued)

POLICY: NUTRITION

    ENTERAL FEEDING GUIDELINES

POPULATION: All infants less than 2000 grams and larger infants that have primary illnesses which have delayed the
    introduction of enteral feeding.

A. **ENERGY/FLUID GOALS**

	Preterm Infants	Term Infants
Energy	120 kcal/kg	110 kcal/kg
Fluid needed to meet energy goal with:		
— 20 kcal/oz	180 cc/kg	165 cc/kg
— 22 kcal/oz	165 cc/kg	
— 24 kcal/oz	150 cc/kg	135 cc/kg

Actual weight is used to calculate enteral feeding intakes and prescriptions with the following exceptions:

    a. birth weight may be used during the first 10 days of life
    b. estimated "dry weight" may be used in edematous infants

Once feedings are established, fluid and energy goals should be individualized to achieve a rate of growth that
maintains or, for those where catch up growth is desired, improves the infants position on the growth curve.

B. **STARTING HUMAN MILK FEEDINGS**

Strength: Full strength human milk from infant's mother.

Starting Volume: 15 to 35 cc/kg/24 hr
(approximately 10% - 20% of full feeding volume)

Rate/Frequency of feeding: Divided into 8 or 12 bolus
feedings, or an hourly rate if continuous feeding to be
used.

> **Example:** Recommended starting intake range for 1500 gm
> infant.
> 24 hr volume: 15 cc/kg/24 hr X 1.5 kg = 22.5 cc/24 hr
>
>   35 cc/kg/24 hr X 1.5 kg = 52.5 cc/24 hr
>
>   24 hr intake range = 22.5 to 52.5 cc
>
> Feeding volume: 22.5 cc/24 hr ÷ 12 fdg/24 hr = 1.9 cc/fdg
>   round off to 2 cc/fdg
>
>   52.5 cc/24 hr ÷ 12 fdg/24 hr = 4.4 cc/fdg
>   round off to 4 cc/fdg
>
>   Feeding volume range = 2 to 4 cc/fdg every 2 hr

Increasing Volume: Incremental increases up to a
maximum of 35 cc/kg/24 hr until full feeding is achieved.

NOTE: Each increase in feeding volume should be based
on the infant's demonstrated tolerance.

> **Example:** 1500 gram infant receiving 4 cc human milk
> every 2 hr.
>
> Maximum daily advance: 35 cc/kg/24 hr X 1.5 kg = 52.5
>   cc/24 hr
>
> Maximum increase per fdg: 52.5 cc/24 hr ÷ 12 fdg/24 hr =
>   4.4 cc/fdg
>   round off to 4 cc/fdg
>
> A schedule that advances the infant's feedings by 2 cc
> every 12 hours would provide the maximum allowance after
> the first 48 hours.

Fortification: In preterm infants with birth weights < 1500 grams, fortification with either Enfamil Human Milk
        Fortifier or Similac Natural Care should be started when intakes of human milk equal to 135-150 cc/kg
        are tolerated. DO NOT INCREASE VOLUME OF FEEDING on the day fortifier is started. Establish tolerance
        first, then continue feeding increases until full feeding established.

Human milk fortifiers increase the calorie density of human milk as follows (assuming human milk to be 20 kcal/oz):

Enfamil Human Milk Fortifier: (powder)	1 pkt / 50 cc human milk results in 22 kcal/oz
	1 pkt / 25 cc human milk results in 24 kcal/oz
Similac Natural Care (SNC):	50 : 50 mix, SNC : human milk results in 22 kcal/oz

6–2 (Continued)

C. STARTING FORMULA FEEDINGS

Strength: 1/2 strength x 3 days
            advance to <u>full strength on 4th day</u> of feeding.

Starting Formula: <u>Preterm infant formula (Similac Special Care)</u> for infants with birth weights < 2000 grams. Standard infant formula for infants with birth weights > 2000 grams.

Starting Volume: <u>35 cc/kg/24 hr</u>
(approximately 20% of full feeding volume).

Starting Frequency: Divided into 8 or 12 bolus feedings, or an hourly rate if continuous feeding to be used.

Daily Advances: <u>Incremental increases of 35 cc/kg/24 hr</u> are recommended while using 1/2 str. formula. DO NOT INCREASE FEEDING VOLUME ON DAY 4 when a transition to full str. formula is made. Once full str. formula is tolerated, incremental increases up to a maximum of 35 cc/kg/24 hr are continued until full volume is achieved.

> **Example:** Recommended starting intake for 1500 gram infant
>
> 24 hour volume: 35 cc/kg/24 hr X 1.5 kg = 52.5 cc/24 hr
>
> Feeding volume: 52.5 cc/24 hr ÷ 12 fdg/24 hr = 4.4 cc/fdg
>   round off to 4 cc/fdg

> **Example:** 1500 gram infant receiving 4 cc 1/2 str Similac Special Care 20 every 2 hr.
>
> | Day of Feeding | Strength | Final Feeding Volume |
> |---|---|---|
> | 2 | 1/2 | 6 cc every 2 hr x 12 hr
8 cc every 2 hr x 12 hr |
> | 3 | 1/2 | 10 cc every 2 hr x 12 hr
12 cc every 2 hr x 12 hr |
> | 4 | 3/4
full | 12 cc every 2 hr x 12 hr
12 cc every 2 hr x 12 hr |
> | 5 | full | 14 cc every 2 hr x 12 hr
16 cc every 2 hr x 12 hr |
>
> Increases continued until full feeding volume of 180 cc/kg is achieved based on current weight.

D. TOLERANCE

Infants need to be closely monitored for feeding tolerance. Physicians should routinely assess tolerance prior to advancing rate of feeding. Nursing should notify the resident physician of clinical and laboratory findings that reflect a change in the infants feeding tolerance (aspirates, abdominal distention, emesis, guaiac + or clinitest + stools, feeding associated apnea and bradycardia).

Aspirates: The resident should be notified when an infant who previously tolerated feedings develops an aspirate equal to or greater than 10% of the previous feeding volume. Some infants consistently have small aspirates. For these infants, the resident should be notified when the aspirate is greater than usual (a physician's order clarifying volume for notification is recommended).

E. ROUTINE FEEDING ASSESSMENT

The feeding prescription should be evaluated at least <u>twice weekly</u> (e.g. Monday and Thursday) for adequacy. Once full feedings have been established and weight gain achieved, the volume and/or calorie density of the feeding should be regularly adjusted to maintain a rate of growth that maintains or improves the infant's position on the growth curve.

To accurately assess growth, the infant's weight, length and head circumference should regularly be measured and plotted on the standard growth chart included in the bedside notebook for each infant. Preterm infants' growth measurements should be plotted according to post-conceptional age.

F. STOPPING HUMAN MILK FORTIFICATION

Human milk fortification is automatically weaned as the frequency and volume of milk provided by breastfeeding increases. Fortification of bottle/gavage human milk feedings is discontinued one week prior to home discharge or when the infant achieves a weight of 3500 grams -- whichever comes first.

G. STOPPING PRETERM FORMULA

Formula fed preterm infants are changed from preterm formula to iron fortified term formula when the infant is one week prior to home discharge or achieves a weight of 3500 grams—whichever comes first.

Written by: Reviewed by: Director of Nurseries
Head Nurse—NICU   POL:25B
Written:
Revised:

6–3 Naturally Occurring Toxins and Syndromes They Produce in Humans

TYPE OF TOXIN	EFFECTS IN HUMANS
Protease inhibitors*	IgE antibodies to the Kunitz soybean trypsin inhibitor produce angioedema and anaphylaxis
Hemagglutinins/lectins	Diarrhea and poor growth
Glucosinolates/thioglucosides	Goitrogenic syndromes of theoretical concern only
Cyanogens*	Tropical ataxic syndrome from chronic ingestion. Acute poisoning is similar to that from inorganic cyanide
Saponins/glycosides	No obvious effects
Gossypol polyphenolic pigments	Anorexia, cachexia, and infertility
Lathyrogens*	Neurolathyrism (osteolathyrism does not occur in humans)
Pyrimidine analogues*	Favism—acute hemolytic anemia in patients with deficiency of glucose 6 phosphate dehydrogenase
Non-physiologic amino acids*	L-canavanine can induce or exacerbate the lupus syndrome
Allergens*	Target of allergies may be the skin, lungs, gastrointestinal tract, musculoskeletal or nervous system
Carcinogens and mutagens*	Aflatoxins are probably etiologic in the pathogenesis of some malignancies
Anti-vitamin factors*	Pellagra is endemic in India because of an antiniacin factor on jowar, a plant with a high content of leucine (which interferes with the metabolism of tryptophan and nicotinic acid)
Estrogenic products of plants	None described
Hallucinogens*	Acute or chronic hallucinosis, drug dependence, or both
Pressor amines*	High levels in some fruits, cheeses, beans, and nuts increase blood pressure
Hypoglycemic agents*	Intake of unripe ackee fruit in Jamaica and Nigeria has been associated with hypoglycemia and depression of the central nervous system
Antienzymes*	Solanine, an anticholinestrase present in sprouts and skin of "night-shade plants," can act as a poison
Other toxins	Purple mint plant has a ketone substitutedfuran and can cause pulmonary emphysema in several species of animals. Rose in humans is unknown

*Clinically significant.

From: Corman, L.C. The relationship between nutrition, infection and immunity. *Med Clin N Am*, 69(3):519, 1985. Used with permission.

PLANT SOURCES

Grain Family
- corn
  - corn starch
  - corn oil
  - corn sugar
  - corn syrup
  - cerulose
  - dextrose
  - glucose
- barley
  - malt
- oats
- rice
- rye
- sorghum
- wheat
  - graham flour
  - gluten flour
  - bran
  - wheat germ
- wild rice

Arrowroot Family
- arrowroot

Arum Family
- taro
  - poi
- cane
  - cane sugar
  - molasses

Spurge Family
- tapioca

Buckwheat Family
- buckwheat
- rhubarb

Composite Family
- leaf lettuce
- head lettuce
- endive
- escarole
- artichoke
- dandelion
- oyster plant
- chicory

Goosefoot Family
- beet
  - beet sugar
- spinach
- swiss chard

Gourd Family
- pumpkin
- squash
- cucumber
- cantaloupe
- muskmelon
- honeydew
- persian melon
- casaba
- watermelon

Legume Family
- navy bean
- kidney bean
- lima bean
- string bean
- soybean
  - soybean oil
- lentil
- black-eyed pea
- pea
- peanut
  - peanut oil
- licorice
- anacia
- senna

Lily Family
- asparagus
- onion
- garlic
- leek
- chive
- aloes

Morning Glory Family
- sweet potato
- yam

Mustard Family
- mustard
- cabbage
- cauliflower
- broccoli
- brussel sprouts
- turnip
- rutabaga
- kale
- collard
- celery cabbage
- kohlrabi
- radish
- horseradish
- watercress

Parsley Family
- parsley
- parsnip
- carrot
- celery
- celeriac
- caraway
- anise
- dill
- coriander
- fennel

Pomegranate Family
- pomegranate

Potato Family
- potato
- tomato
- eggplant
- red pepper
- cayenne
- green pepper
- chili

Sunflower Family*
- jerusalem artichoke
- sunflower seed oil

Apple Family
- apple
  - cider
  - vinegar
  - apple pectin
- pear
- quince
  - quince seed

Banana Family
- banana
- plantain

Citrus Family
- orange
- grapefruit
- lemon
- lime
- tangerine
- kumquat

Ebony Family
- persimmon

Gooseberry Family
- gooseberry
- currant

Grape Family
- grape
- raisin
- cream of tartar

Heath Family
- cranberry
- blueberry

Honeysuckle Family
- eldberry

Laurel Family
- avocado
- cinnamon
- bay leaves

Olive Family
- green olive
- ripe olive
- olive oil

Pawpaw Family
- papaya

Pineapple Family
- pineapple

Plum Family
- plum
  - prune
- cherry
- peach
- apricot
- nectarine
- almond

Rose Family
- raspberry
- blackberry
- loganberry
- youngberry
- dewberry
- strawberry

Beech Family
- beechnut
- chestnut

Birch Family
- filbert
- hazelnut
- oil of birch
  - (wintergreen)

Cashew Family
- cashew
- pistachio
- mango

Fungi Family
- mushroom
- yeast

Ginger Family
- ginger
- turmeric
- cadamon

Legythis Family
- brazil nut

Madder Family
- coffee

Mallow Family
- okra (gumbo)
- cottonseed

Maple Family
- maple syrup
- maple sugar

Mint Family
- mint
- peppermint
- spearmint
- thyme
- sage
- marjoram
- savory

Miscellaneous
- honey

Mulberry Family
- mulberry
- fig
- hop
- breadfruit

Myrtle Family
- allspice
- cloves
- pimento
- guava

Nutmeg Family
- nutmeg

Orchid Family
- vanilla

Palm Family
- coconut
- date
- sago

Pedalium Family
- sesame oil

Pepper Family
- black pepper

Pine Family
- juniper

Poppy Family
- poppy seed

Stercula Family
- cocoa
- chocolate

Tea Family
- tea

Walnut Family
- english walnut
- black walnut
- butternut
- hickory nut
- pecan

ANIMAL SOURCES

Amphibians
- frog

Crustaceans
- crab
- lobster
- shrimp
- squid*

Fish
- sturgeon
  - caviar
- anchovy
- sardine
- herring
- smelt
- trout
- salmon
- whitefish
- chub
- shad
- eel
- carp
- sucker
- buffalo
- catfish
- bullhead
- pike
- pickerel
- muskellunge
- mullet
- barracuda
- mackerel
- tuna
- pompano
- bluefish
- butterfish
- harverstfish
- swordfish
- sunfish
- bass
- perch
- snapper
- croaker
- weakfish
- drum
- scup
- porgy
- flounder
- sole
- halibut
- rosefish
- codfish
- scrod
- haddock
- hake
- pollack
- cusk

Mollusks
- abalone
- mussel
- oyster
- scallop
- clam

Reptiles
- turtle

Birds
- chicken
  - chicken eggs
- duck
  - duck eggs
- goose
  - goose eggs
- turkey
- guinea hen
- pheasant
- partridge
- grouse

Mammals
- beef
- veal
- cow's milk
- butter
- cheese
- goat
  - goat's milk
  - cheese
- mutton
- lamb
- pork
- ham
- bacon
- venison
- horse meat
- rabbit
- squirrel

*Sometimes place in composite family. Modified from Sheldon, J.M., Lovell, R.G. and Mathews, K.P.(Eds.): Food and Gastrointestinal Allergy. In A Manual of Clinical Allergy, Philadelphia, Saunders, 1967. Used with permission.

6–5 Factors in Cancer Causation and Prevention

Disease	Risk factors	Mechanism	Protective elements	Mechanism
Lung cancer	Cigarette smoking	Complex mixture of genotoxic carcinogens, polycyclic aromatic hydrocarbons and tobacco specific nitrosamines and risk-determining enhancing, promoting agents. Asbestos, air pollutants have strong cocarcinogenic effect	Yellow-green vegetables	Retinoids, β-carotene inhibit development of early lesions through strengthening patency of gap junctions
	Occupational	Polycyclic hydrocarbons coal gas work, bis(chloromethyl)ether, bis(chloroethyl)sulfide, arsenic, nickel, and chromate ores		
Oral cancer	Smoking; tobacco chewing; betel chewing; smoking and alcohol	Carcinogens in tobacco (mainly tobacco-specific nitrosamines), betel nut; hydroxy radicals	Yellow-green vegetables	Retinoids, β-carotene
Kidney cancer	Smoking; other factors unknown	Carcinogens from tobacco, unknown mechanisms	?	?
	Obesity	Endocrines; fat cells produce estrogens acting as carcinogens?	Weight control/loss	Lowers excessive nonphysiologic estrogen levels
Nasopharyngeal cancer	Salted, pickled fish	Contains specific nitrosamine?	?	?
	Viral factors	Can increase cell cycling	Vaccination?	
	Occupational	Wood and leather workers		
Esophageal cancer	Salted, pickled food?	Specific nitrosamine	Yellow-green vegetables	Role of vegetables unknown if risk factor present in food
	Alcohol intake + smoking	Alcohol modifies esophageal metabolism of tobacco-specific carcinogens	Yellow-green vegetables	(β-carotene, protective element)
	Tobacco chewing	Tobacco-specific carcinogens and promoters?	Vegetables	β-Carotene, retinoids
Gastric cancer (intestinal)	Salted, pickled food	Nitrosoindoles, phenolic diazotates	Green-yellow vegetables	Role of vegetables unknown if risk factor present in food, but may assist in differentiation
	Geochemical nitrate and salt	Formation of gastric carcinogens, above, in stomach	Green-yellow vegetables, fruits, vitamins C and E	Prevent formation of carcinogen; cellular tissue defenses
Bladder cancer	Bilharzia: schistosomiasis	Carcinogens unknown; increased cell proliferation enhances risk	Yellow-green vegetables	?
	Smoking	Unknown	Yellow-green vegetables	Retinoids
	Occupational	Arylamines	—	—
Endocrine-related cancers; prostate, breast, ovary	Total dietary fat (saturated + ω-6 polyunsaturated lipids)	Complex multieffector elements; hormonal balances, membrane and intracellular effectors	Monounsaturated oil (olive); ω-3 polyunsaturated oils	Neutral or protective action on hormone metabolism
			Medium-chain triglycerides	Caloric equivalent to carbohydrate
			Cereal fiber and pectin; yellow-green vegetables	Affects enteroheptic cycling of hormones
Endometrium	Same as above; excessive body weight	Same as above; fat cells generate estrogen	Same as above; weight control/loss	Same as above; lowers excessive nonphysiologic estrogen levels
Pancreas	Same as endocrine;	Fat affects physiology	Low-fat diets	Protects function
	Cigarette smoking	Tobacco-specific nitrosamines	?	?
Colon cancer Proximal	?	?	?	?
Distal	Same as endocrine related cancers	Biosynthesis of cholesterol, thence bile acids, and colon cancer promotion including higher cell cycling	Cereal fiber	Increases stool bulk; dilutes promoters; lower intestinal pH
Rectal cancer	Alcoholic beverages, especially beer	Increases cell cycling in rectum	Cereal fiber?	Dilutes effectors by increasing stool bulk
Liver cancer	Mold contaminated foods	Mycotoxins	Avoid moldy, pickled foods, improve nutrition, more protein, fruits and vegetables	Lower carcinogen intake
	Some plants	Pyrrolizidine alkaloids		
	Pickled foods	Nitrosamines		
	Chronic virus	Hepatitis B	Vaccination	
	High level of specific alcoholic beverages	Damages liver, risk of cirrhosis potentiates effect of carcinogens	Decrease intake of alcohol	May lower cell duplication rates
	Occupational	Vinyl chloride	Lower exposure	
	Iatrogenic	Some oral contraceptives (infrequent occurrence)		

From: Weisburger, J.H.: Nutritional approach to cancer prevention with emphasis on vitamins, antioxidants and carotenoids. Am J Clin Nut, 53(1):227S, 1991. Used with permission.

Appendix 7
Quality Assurance Standards

7–1 Nutrition Quality Assurance Criteria, Developmental Disorders

Target Population: Patients With Developmental Disabilities (Generic)
Variables: Age 0 to 18 Years, Ambulatory Care, Nonacute

Criteria*	Critical time	Accepted level of performance	Exceptions	References	Audit data source
(P) 1. Nutrition screening completed, including the following minimal elements: a. Diagnosis b. Review of health history† c. Weight/height (or length) d. Rate of growth e. Dietary intake f. Ambulation	Each clinic visit		Clinic visit for nutrition assessment or routine therapy		Medical record
(P) 2. Nutrition assessment completed, including the following minimal elements: a. Height (or length) and weight b. Triceps and subscapular skin-fold measurements c. Iron status d. Dietary e. Clinical/dental f. Feeding skills/behaviors g. Elimination patterns h. Nutrient-drug interaction i. Nutrient supplementation j. Frequent infections k. Physical activity/ambulation l. Maturation	Initial evaluation period and as indicated in nutrition care plan Nutrient-drug interactions evaluated with each medication change Maturation evaluated during preadolescence and adolescence			1, 2	Medical record
(P) 3. Nutrition care plan developed jointly by patient/caregiver and nutritionist according to established guidelines for documentation.	At or within 2 wk of completion of nutrition assessment				Medical record
(P) 4. Nutrition care plan implemented as written or revised.	Duration of treatment or according to timetable identified in nutrition care plan				Medical record
(P) 5. Patient/caregiver given food and fluid information appropriate to patient's age, development, and condition.	Initial clinic visit and as indicated in nutrition care plan			3, 4	Medical record
(O) 6. Patient/caregiver reports patient consumes (or progresses toward) diet as specified in nutrition care plan.	Following initial instruction and with each change in diet				Medical record
(O) 7. Solid or supplemental foods introduced no earlier than age 4 mo.	First 4 mo of life		Solid or supplemental foods introduced to patient prior to initial clinic visit	5	Medical record
(O) 8. Patient's texture progression of food appropriate for developmental status.	Until mature eating pattern achieved		Team assessment identifies that patient's maximum potential achieved but is below mature eating pattern	3, 6	Medical record
(O) 9. Patient progresses toward or achieves mature feeding skills.	Until mature feeding skills achieved		Team assessment identifies that patient's maximum potential achieved but is below mature feeding skills	6	Medical record
(O) 10. Patient with prescribed diet modification and/or caregiver can devise 1-day meal plan with number of servings, portion sizes, and kinds of foods specified in diet pattern agreed upon with nutritionist.	Clinic visit following initial counseling, or as specified in nutrition care plan		Precluded by functioning level of patient and/or caregiver		Medical record
(O) 11. Patient/caregiver can identify diet and activity as factors contributing to patient's weight status.	Clinic visit following initial counseling, or as specified in nutrition care plan		Precluded by functioning level of patient and/or caregiver; patient's weight is appropriate and unlikely to be affected adversely by condition	7, 8	Medical record
(O) 12. Patient/caregiver can identify fluid and dietary fiber intake and exercise as important factors in prevention of constipation.	Clinic visit following initial counseling, or as specified in nutrition care plan		Precluded by functioning level of patient and/or caregiver; constipation not usual manifestation of clinical condition	9, 10	Medical record

7–1 (Continued)

(O) 13. Patient/caregiver reports appropriate use of rewards (reinforcers).	Clinic visit following initial counseling, or as specified in nutrition care plan		3, 8	Medical record
(P) 14. Patient/caregiver counseled on relationship between diet and dental/oral health.	Initial evaluation period and/or as indicated in nutrition care plan		8, 11	Medical record
(O) 15. Patient/caregiver can identify inappropriate bottle feeding.	Clinic visit following initial counseling, or as indicated in nutrition care plan	Patient no longer using bottle	11	Medical record
(O) 16. Patient maintains, progresses toward, or achieves weight/height between the 10th and 90th percentiles according to National Center for Health Statistics (NCHS) growth chart, and/or triceps and subscapular skin-fold measurements between 10th and 90th percentiles of most appropriate reference data available.‡	Each clinic visit following initial visit, or as indicated in nutrition care plan	Growth potential compromised by nonnutritional factors	12-15	Medical record
(O) 17. Patient/caregiver can identify nutrition risk related to nutrient-drug interactions.	Clinic visit following initial counseling, or as indicated in nutrition care plan	Precluded by functioning level of patient and/or caregiver; patient is not receiving drugs that affect nutrition	16, 17	Medical record

§

* P, process; O, outcome.

‡ These percentiles are used because of the importance of detecting a potential growth problem early, as growth problems are often found in this population.

§ This criteria set was one of the first to be developed. It does not include a specific criterion regarding referral of the client to food and/or nutrition resources. Practitioners are encouraged to add such a criterion when using this criteria set.

† Iron status, feeding skills/behaviors, elimination patterns, nutrient supplementation, nutrient-drug interaction, frequent infections.

References

1. Smith MAH, et al: Developmental feeding tool, in: *Feeding Management of a Child With a Handicap: A Guide for Professionals*. Memphis, University of Tennessee Center for the Health Sciences Child Development Center, 1982.

2. Smith MAH (ed): *Guides for Nutritional Assessment of the Mentally Retarded and Developmentally Disabled*. Memphis, University of Tennessee Center for the Health Sciences Child Development Center, 1976.

3. Pipes PL, Carmen P: Nutrition and feeding of children with developmental delays and related problems, in Pipes PL and Carman P (eds): *Nutrition in Infancy and Childhood*. St. Louis, Times Mirror/Mosby Co, 1985.

4. Rickard K, Brady MS, Gresham EL: Nutrition in the chronically ill child. Congenital heart disease and myelomeningocele. *Pediatr Clin North Am* 24:157, 1977.

5. American Academy of Pediatrics Committee on Nutrition: On the feeding of supplemental foods to infants. *Pediatrics* 65:1178, 1980.

6. Smith MAH, et al: Normal feeding development chart, in: *Feeding Management of a Child With a Handicap: A Guide for Professionals*. Memphis, University of Tennessee Center for the Health Sciences Child Development Center, 1982.

7. Heins JN: Obesity in children, in Palmer S, Ekvall S (eds): *Pediatric Nutrition Developmental Disorders*. Springfield, IL, Charles C Thomas, 1978.

8. Howard RB, Harbold NH: *Nutrition in Clinical Care*. New York, McGraw-Hill, 1982.

9. Infant and child nutrition: Concerns regarding the developmentally disabled. *J Am Diet Assoc* 78:443, 1981.

10. Frequently reported nutrition problems and factors contributing to high nutritional risk of children with handicapping conditions, in Baer MT (ed): *Nutrition Services for Children With Handicaps. A Manual for State Title V Programs*. Los Angeles, University Affiliated Training Program, Center for Child Development Disorders, 1982.

11. Nizel AE: Nutritional support for optimizing children's dental health, in Suskind R (ed): *Textbook of Pediatric Nutrition*. New York, Raven Press, 1981.

12. National Center for Health Statistics: *NCHS Growth Curves for Children 0-18 Years, US*. Vital and Health Statistics, series 11, no. 165. Health Resources Administration, US Government Printing Office, 1977.

13. National Center for Health Statistics: *Height and Weight of Youths 12-17 Years, US*. Vital and Health Statistics, series 11, no. 124. Health Services and Mental Health Administration, US Government Printing Office, 1973.

14. National Center for Health Statistics: *Basic Data on Anthropometric Measurements and Angular Measurement of the Hip and Knee Joints for Selected Age Groups, 1-74 Years of Age, US 1971-1975*. Vital and Health Statistics, series 11, no. 219. US Government Printing Office, 1981.

15. Cronk CE: Growth of children with Down's syndrome: Birth to age 3 years. *Pediatrics* 61:564, 1978.

16. Springer NS, Fricke NL: Endogenous malnutrition following drug therapy, in Palmer S, Ekvall S (eds): *Pediatric Nutrition in Developmental Disorders*. Springfield, IL, Charles C Thomas, 1978.

17. Springer NS: Drug-nutrient interactions, in: *Nutrition Casebook on Developmental Disabilities*. Syracuse, NY, Syracuse University Press, 1982.

Developmental Disabilities Quality Assurance Committee

Among those involved in the development and/or field testing of these criteria were:

Mariel Caldwell, MS, MPH, RD, chairperson
Marion Baer, PhD, RD
Elaine Blyler, MS, RD
Harriet Cloud, MS, RD
Sandra Eardley, PhD, RD
Shirley M. Ekvall, PhD, RD
Sheila Farnan, MPH, RD
Barbara Free, MS, RD
Kate Hohenbrink, MS, RD
Betty Kozlowski, PhD
Jackie Krick, MS, RD
Judith Oliver, MS, RD
Peggy Pipes, MPH, RD

Field-test Sites:

Southern Illinois University School of Medicine
Springfield, Illinois

Sparks Center for Developmental and Learning Disorders
University of Alabama at Birmingham
Birmingham, Alabama

University Affiliated Cincinnati Center for Developmental Disorders
University of Cincinnati
Cincinnati, Ohio

7–2 Nutrition Quality Assurance Criteria, Myelomeningocele

Target Population: Patients With Myelodysplasia
Variables: Age 0-18 Years, Ambulatory Care, Nonacute

Criteria*	Critical time	Accepted level of performance	Exceptions	References	Audit data source
(P) 1. Nutrition screening completed, including the following minimal elements: a. Review of health history† b. Weight/height (or length) and/or skin-fold	Each clinic visit or as indicated in nutrition care plan		Clinic visit for nutrition assessment		Medical record
(P) 2. Nutrition assessment completed, including the following minimal elements: a. Height (or length) b. Weight and/or skin-fold c. Iron status d. Dietary intake e. Clinical/medical history f. Feeding skills	Initial clinic visit and as indicated in nutrition care plan			1	Medical record
(P) 3. Nutrition care plan developed jointly by patient/caregiver and nutritionist according to established guidelines for documentation.	At or within 2 wk of completion of nutrition assessment				Medical record
(P) 4. Nutrition care plan implemented as written or revised.	According to timetable identified in nutrition care plan				Medical record
(P) 5. Patient maintains, progresses toward, or achieves: a. Body weight/height between the 10th and 75th percentiles according to National Center for Health Statistics (NCHS) growth chart (for patients aged 2-10 yr) and/or	Duration of treatment		Patient is not aged 2-10 yr	2-5	Medical record
b. Body weight/height between the 10th and 90th percentiles according to Health and Nutrition Examination Survey (HANES) data (for patients aged 12-17 yr) and/or			Patient is not aged 12-17 yr		
c. A triceps or subscapular skin-fold between the 10th and 90th percentiles for age and sex according to HANES data (for patients aged 1-18 yr)‡			Patient is not aged 1-18 yr		
(O) 6. Patient/caregiver given the following information related to patient's age, development, and condition (each element evaluated separately): a. Appropriate food and fluid intake b. Avoidance of high-calorie, low-nutrient foods c. Nursing bottle syndrome	Each clinic visit or as indicated in nutrition care plan		Patient is no longer using bottle	2	Medical record
(O) 7. Patient/caregiver reports patient consumes or progresses toward diet as specified in nutrition care plan.	Following initial diet instruction and as indicated by nutrition care plan				Medical record
(O) 8. Solid or supplemental foods introduced no earlier than age 4 mo.	First 4 mo of life		Solid or supplemental foods introduced to patient prior to intial clinic visit	6	Medical record
(O) 9. Patient/caregiver reports texture progression of food appropriate for developmental readiness.	Until mature feeding skills achieved		Team assessment identifies that patient's maximum potential is achieved, but is below mature eating pattern	7	Medical record
(O) 10. Patient progresses toward or achieves mature feeding skills appropriate for developmental or chronologic age.	Until mature feeding skills achieved		Team assessment identifies that patient's maximum potential is achieved, but is below mature feeding skills	8	Medical record
(O) 11. Patient/caregiver correctly identifies low-nutrient, high-calorie foods in patient's diet history.	Clinic visit following initial counseling, or as specified in nutrition care plan		Patient has diagnosis of failure to thrive; patient is below 5th percentile as measured in criterion 5	2, 9	Medical record

7–2 (Continued)

Criterion	Time frame	Exceptions		Data source
(O) 12. Patient with prescribed diet modification and/or caregiver can devise 1-day meal with recommended number of servings, portion sizes, and kinds of foods consistent with those specified in diet pattern agreed upon with nutrition counselor.	Clinic visit following initial instruciton or as specified in nutrition care plan	Patient does not have prescribed diet modification		Medical record
(O) 13. Patient/caregiver can identify that patient's specific diet and activity factors contribute to weight control.	Clinic visit following initial instruction or as specified in nutrition care plan		10	Medical record
(O) 14. Patient/caregiver can identify fluid and dietary fiber intake and exercise as important factors in prevention of constipation.	Clinic visit following initial instruction or as specified in nutrition care plan		11	Medical record
(O) 15. Patient/caregiver reports use of only nonfood items as rewards.	Clinic visit following initial instruction or as specified in nutrition care plan			Medical record
(O) 16. Patient's drug/medical intake evaluated for effect on nutrient utilization.	At initial clinic visit and following each drug/medication change		12	Medical record

§

* P, process; O, outcome.

§ This criteria set was one of the first to be developed. It does not include a specific criterion regarding referral of the client to food and/or nutrition resources. Practitioners are encouraged to add such a criterion when using this criteria set.

‡ These percentiles are used because of the importance of detecting a potential growth problem early, as growth problems are often found in this population.

References

1. Christakis G (ed): Nutrition assessment in health programs. *Am J Public Health* 63:38, 1973.
2. Rickard K, Brady MS, Gresham EL: Nutritional management of the chronically ill child: Congenital heart disease and myelomeningocele, in Neumann CG, Jelliffe DB (eds): *Pediatric Clinics of North America.* Philadelphia, W.B. Saunders Co, 1977.
3. National Center for Health Statistics: *NCHS Growth Curves for Children 0-18 Years, US.* Vital and Health Statistics, series 11, no. 165. Health Resources Administration, US Government Printing Office, 1977.
4. National Center for Health Statistics: *Height and Weight of Youths 12-17 Years, US.* Vital and Health Statistics, series 11, no. 124. Health Services and Mental Health Administration, US Government Printing Office, 1973.
5. National Center for Health Statistics: *Basic Data on Anthropometric Measurements and Angular Measurement of the Hip and Knee Joints for Selected Age Groups, 1-74 Years of Age, US, 1971-1975.* Vital and Health Statistics, series 11, no. 219. US Government Printing Office, 1981.
6. American Academy of Pediatrics Committee on Nutrition: On the feeding of supplemental foods to infants. *Pediatrics* 65:1178, 1980.
7. Pipes PL (ed): *Nutrition in Infancy and Childhood.* St. Louis, C.V. Mosby, 1981.
8. Smith MAH, et al: Normal feeding development chart, in: *Feeding Management of a Child With a Handicap: A Guide for Professionals.* Memphis, University of Tennessee Center for the Health Sciences Child Development Center, 1982.
9. *Nutritive Value of Foods.* Home and Garden Bulletin no. 72. Department of Agriculture, 1981.
10. Heins JN: Obesity in children, in Palmer S, Ekvall S (eds): *Pediatric Nutrition in Developmental Disorders.* Springfield, IL, Charles C Thomas, 1978.
11. Infant and child nutrition: Concerns regarding the developmentally disabled. *J Am Diet Assoc* 78:443, 1981.
12. Springer NS, Fricke NL: Endogenous malnutrition following drug therapy, in Palmer S, Ekvall S (eds): *Pediatric Nutrition in Developmental Disorders.* Springfield, IL, Charles C. Thomas, 1978.

Myelodysplasia Quality Assurance Committee

Among those involved in the development and/or field testing of these criteria were:

Mariel Caldwell, MS, MPH, RD, chairperson
Mary Sue Brady, RD, DMSc
Shirley M. Ekvall, PhD, RD
Sheila Farnan, MPH, RD
Barbara Free, MS, RD
Betty Krauss, RD
Anne Nalepp, RD
Jill Reynolds, MPH, RD
Karyl Rickard, RD, PhD
Alice Smith, MS, RD

Field-test Sites

Children's Hospital of Michigan
Detroit, Michigan

Children's Memorial Hospital
Chicago, Illinois

James Whitcomb Riley Hospital for Children
Indiana University Medical Center
Indianapolis, Indiana

Mary Freebed Hospital
Grand Rapids, Michigan

University Affiliated Cincinnati Center for Developmental Disorders
University of Cincinnati
Cincinnati, Ohio

Appendix 8
Skinfold Grids—Children
Other Anthropometry Standards

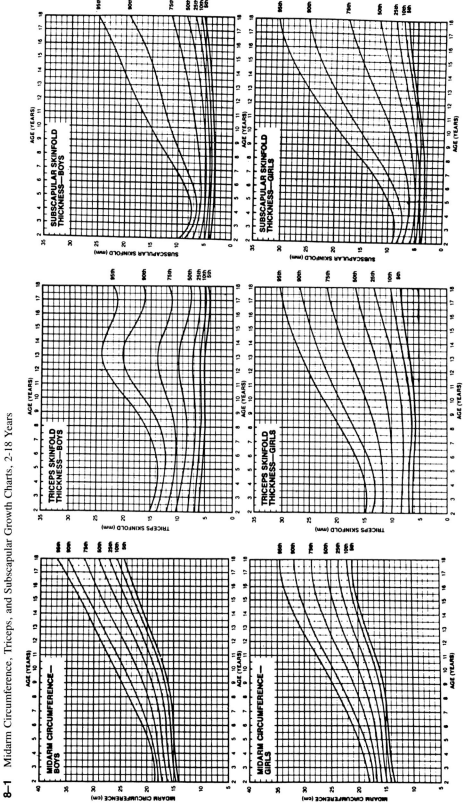

8–1   Midarm Circumference, Triceps, and Subscapular Growth Charts, 2-18 Years

Figures adapted from Johnson, C. L., Fulwood, R., Abraham, S., et al: Basic data on anthropometric measurements and angular measurements of the hip and knee joints for selected age groups, 1-74 years of age, United States, 1971-1975. Vital and Health Statistics Series 11, No. 219. DHHS Publication No. (PHS) 81-1669, 1981.

8-2 Upper Arm Circumference and Upper Arm Muscle Area Percentiles, 1-75 Years

Upper Arm Circumference

Males

Age (yrs)	5	10	15	25	50	75	85	90	95
1.0-1.9	14.2	14.7	14.9	15.2	16.0	16.9	17.4	17.7	18.2
2.0-2.9	14.3	14.8	15.1	15.5	16.3	17.1	17.6	17.9	18.6
3.0-3.9	15.0	15.3	15.5	16.0	16.8	17.6	18.1	18.4	19.0
4.0-4.9	15.1	15.5	15.8	16.2	17.1	18.0	18.5	18.7	19.3
5.0-5.9	15.5	16.0	16.1	16.6	17.5	18.5	19.1	19.5	20.5
6.0-6.9	15.8	16.1	16.5	17.0	18.0	19.1	19.8	20.7	22.8
7.0-7.9	16.1	16.8	17.0	17.6	18.7	20.0	21.0	21.8	22.9
8.0-8.9	16.5	17.2	17.5	18.1	19.2	20.5	21.6	22.6	24.0
9.0-9.9	17.5	18.0	18.4	19.1	20.1	21.8	23.2	24.5	26.0
10.0-10.9	18.1	18.6	19.1	19.7	21.1	23.1	24.8	26.0	27.9
11.0-11.9	18.5	19.3	19.8	20.6	22.1	24.5	26.1	27.6	29.4
12.0-12.9	19.3	20.1	20.7	21.5	23.1	25.4	27.1	28.5	30.3
13.0-13.9	20.0	20.8	21.6	22.5	24.5	26.6	28.2	29.0	30.8
14.0-14.9	21.6	22.5	23.2	23.8	25.7	28.1	29.1	30.0	32.3
15.0-15.9	22.5	23.4	24.0	25.1	27.2	29.0	30.3	31.2	32.7
16.0-16.9	24.1	25.0	25.7	26.7	28.3	30.6	32.1	32.7	34.7
17.0-17.9	24.3	25.1	25.9	26.8	28.6	30.8	32.2	33.3	34.7
18.0-24.9	26.0	27.1	27.7	28.7	30.7	33.0	34.4	35.4	37.2
25.0-29.9	27.0	28.0	28.7	29.8	31.8	34.2	35.5	36.6	38.3
30.0-34.9	27.7	28.7	29.3	30.5	32.5	34.9	36.2	36.7	38.2
35.0-39.9	27.4	28.6	29.5	30.7	32.9	35.1	36.1	36.9	38.2
40.0-44.9	27.8	28.9	29.7	31.0	32.8	34.9	36.1	36.9	38.1
45.0-49.9	27.2	28.6	29.4	30.6	32.6	34.5	36.1	36.9	38.3
50.0-54.9	27.1	28.3	29.1	30.2	32.3	34.3	35.8	36.8	37.8
55.0-59.9	26.8	28.1	28.6	30.4	32.3	34.0	35.5	36.6	37.5
60.0-64.9	26.6	27.8	28.6	29.7	32.0	34.0	35.1	36.0	36.6
65.0-69.9	25.4	26.7	27.7	29.0	31.1	33.2	34.5	35.3	38.5
70.0-74.9	25.1	26.2	27.1	28.5	30.7	32.6	33.7	34.8	37.5

Females

Age (yrs)	5	10	15	25	50	75	85	90	95
1.0-1.9	13.6	14.1	14.4	14.8	15.7	16.4	17.0	17.2	17.8
2.0-2.9	14.2	14.6	15.0	15.4	16.1	17.0	17.4	18.0	18.5
3.0-3.9	14.4	15.0	15.2	15.7	16.6	17.4	18.0	18.4	19.0
4.0-4.9	14.8	15.3	15.7	16.1	17.0	18.0	18.5	19.0	19.5
5.0-5.9	15.2	15.7	16.1	16.5	17.5	18.5	19.4	20.0	21.0
6.0-6.9	15.7	16.2	16.5	17.0	17.8	19.0	19.9	20.5	22.0
7.0-7.9	16.4	16.7	17.0	17.5	18.6	20.1	20.9	21.6	23.3
8.0-8.9	16.7	17.2	17.6	18.2	19.5	21.2	22.2	23.2	25.1
9.0-9.9	17.6	18.1	18.6	19.1	20.6	22.2	23.8	25.0	26.7
10.0-10.9	17.8	18.4	18.9	19.5	21.2	23.4	25.0	26.1	27.3
11.0-11.9	18.8	19.6	20.0	20.6	22.2	25.1	26.5	27.9	30.0
12.0-12.9	19.2	20.0	20.5	21.5	23.7	25.8	27.6	28.3	30.2
13.0-13.9	20.1	21.0	21.5	22.5	24.3	26.7	28.3	30.1	32.7
14.0-14.9	21.2	21.8	22.5	23.5	25.1	27.4	29.5	30.9	32.9
15.0-15.9	21.6	22.2	22.9	24.4	25.2	27.7	28.8	30.0	33.5
16.0-16.9	22.3	23.2	23.5	24.5	26.1	28.5	29.9	31.6	35.4
17.0-17.9	22.0	23.1	23.6	24.8	26.6	29.0	30.7	32.8	35.2
18.0-24.9	22.4	24.0	24.0	25.5	26.8	29.2	31.2	32.4	37.1
25.0-29.9	23.1	24.7	24.5	26.4	27.6	30.6	34.1	34.3	38.5
30.0-34.9	23.8	25.2	25.4	26.8	28.6	32.0	35.0	36.0	39.0
35.0-39.9	24.1	25.4	25.8	27.2	29.4	32.6	35.5	36.8	38.8
40.0-44.9	24.3	25.5	26.2	27.4	29.7	33.2	35.6	37.2	40.0
45.0-49.9	24.2	26.0	26.3	27.8	30.1	33.5	35.9	37.5	39.3
50.0-54.9	24.8	26.1	26.8	28.0	30.6	33.8	36.7	38.0	40.0
55.0-59.9	24.8	26.1	27.0	28.2	30.9	34.3	37.3	38.0	39.3
60.0-64.9	25.0	26.1	27.1	28.4	30.8	34.3	36.7	37.3	39.6
65.0-69.9	24.3	25.7	26.7	28.0	30.5	33.4	35.7	36.5	38.5
70.0-74.9	23.8	25.3	26.3	27.6	30.3	33.1	34.7	35.8	37.5

Percentiles

Upper Arm Muscle Area

Males

Age (yrs)	5	10	15	25	50	75	85	90	95
1.0-1.9	9.7	10.4	10.8	11.6	13.0	14.6	15.4	16.3	17.2
2.0-2.9	10.1	10.9	11.3	12.4	13.9	15.6	16.4	16.9	18.4
3.0-3.9	11.2	12.0	12.6	13.5	15.0	16.4	17.4	18.3	19.5
4.0-4.9	12.0	12.9	13.5	14.5	16.2	17.9	18.8	19.8	20.9
5.0-5.9	13.2	14.2	14.7	15.7	17.6	19.5	20.7	21.7	23.2
6.0-6.9	14.4	15.3	15.8	16.8	18.7	21.3	22.9	23.8	25.7
7.0-7.9	15.1	16.2	17.0	18.5	20.6	22.6	24.5	25.2	28.6
8.0-8.9	16.3	17.8	18.5	19.5	21.6	24.0	25.5	26.6	29.0
9.0-9.9	18.2	19.3	20.3	21.7	23.5	26.7	28.7	30.4	32.9
10.0-10.9	19.6	20.7	21.6	23.0	25.7	29.0	32.2	34.0	37.1
11.0-11.9	21.0	22.0	23.0	24.8	27.7	31.6	33.6	36.1	40.3
12.0-12.9	22.6	24.1	25.3	26.9	30.4	35.9	39.3	40.9	44.9
13.0-13.9	24.5	26.7	28.1	30.4	35.7	41.3	45.3	48.1	52.5
14.0-14.9	28.3	31.3	33.1	36.1	41.9	47.4	51.3	54.0	57.5
15.0-15.9	31.9	34.9	36.9	40.3	46.3	53.1	56.3	57.7	63.0
16.0-16.9	37.0	40.9	42.4	45.9	51.9	57.8	63.6	66.2	70.5
17.0-17.9	39.6	42.6	44.8	48.0	53.4	60.4	64.3	67.9	73.1
18.0-24.9	34.2	37.3	39.6	42.7	49.4	57.1	61.8	65.0	72.0
25.0-29.9	36.6	39.9	42.4	46.0	53.0	61.4	66.1	68.9	74.5
30.0-34.9	37.9	40.9	43.4	47.3	54.4	63.2	67.6	70.8	76.1
35.0-39.9	38.5	42.6	44.6	47.9	55.3	64.0	69.1	72.7	77.0
40.0-44.9	38.4	42.1	45.1	48.7	56.0	64.0	68.5	71.6	77.0
45.0-49.9	37.7	41.3	43.7	47.9	55.2	63.3	67.6	72.2	76.2
50.0-54.9	36.0	40.0	42.7	46.6	54.0	62.7	67.0	70.4	75.1
55.0-59.9	36.5	40.8	42.7	46.7	54.3	61.9	66.4	69.6	71.6
60.0-64.9	34.5	38.7	41.2	44.9	52.1	60.0	64.8	67.5	69.4
65.0-69.9	31.4	35.8	38.4	42.3	49.1	57.3	61.2	64.3	69.4
70.0-74.9	29.7	33.8	36.1	40.2	47.0	54.6	59.1	62.1	67.3

Females

Age (yrs)	5	10	15	25	50	75	85	90	95
1.0-1.9	8.9	9.7	10.1	10.8	12.3	13.8	14.6	15.3	16.2
2.0-2.9	10.1	10.6	10.9	11.8	13.2	14.7	15.6	16.4	17.3
3.0-3.9	10.8	11.4	11.8	12.6	14.3	15.8	16.7	17.4	18.8
4.0-4.9	11.2	12.2	12.7	13.6	15.3	17.0	18.0	18.6	19.8
5.0-5.9	12.4	13.2	13.9	14.8	16.4	18.3	19.4	20.6	22.1
6.0-6.9	13.5	14.1	14.6	15.6	17.4	19.5	21.0	22.0	24.2
7.0-7.9	14.4	15.2	15.8	16.7	18.9	21.2	22.6	23.9	25.3
8.0-8.9	15.2	16.0	16.8	18.2	20.8	23.2	24.6	26.5	28.0
9.0-9.9	17.0	17.9	18.7	19.8	21.9	25.4	27.2	28.3	31.1
10.0-10.9	17.6	18.5	19.3	20.9	23.8	27.0	29.1	31.0	33.1
11.0-11.9	19.5	21.0	21.7	23.2	26.4	30.7	33.5	35.7	39.2
12.0-12.9	20.4	21.8	23.1	25.5	29.0	33.2	36.3	37.8	40.5
13.0-13.9	22.8	24.5	25.4	27.1	30.8	35.3	38.1	39.6	43.7
14.0-14.9	24.0	26.2	27.1	29.0	32.8	36.9	39.8	41.7	47.5
15.0-15.9	24.4	25.8	28.2	29.2	33.0	37.3	40.2	41.7	45.9
16.0-16.9	25.2	26.8	28.8	30.0	33.6	38.0	43.4	46.2	48.3
17.0-17.9	25.9	27.5	28.9	30.7	34.3	39.6	45.6	50.8	50.8
18.0-24.9	19.5	21.5	22.8	24.5	28.3	33.1	34.3	39.0	44.2
25.0-29.9	20.5	21.9	23.1	25.2	29.4	34.9	36.4	39.6	47.8
30.0-34.9	21.1	23.0	24.2	26.3	30.9	36.8	38.5	41.9	50.8
35.0-39.9	21.1	23.4	24.7	27.3	31.8	36.7	41.2	46.1	51.3
40.0-44.9	21.3	23.4	25.5	27.5	32.3	39.8	43.1	47.8	54.2
45.0-49.9	21.6	23.1	24.8	27.4	32.5	39.5	45.8	49.5	55.8
50.0-54.9	22.2	24.6	25.7	28.3	33.4	40.4	44.7	48.4	56.1
55.0-59.9	22.8	24.8	26.5	28.7	34.7	42.3	47.3	52.1	58.8
60.0-64.9	22.4	24.5	26.3	29.2	34.5	41.1	45.6	49.1	55.1
65.0-69.9	21.9	24.5	26.2	28.9	34.6	41.6	46.3	49.6	56.5
70.0-74.9	22.2	24.4	26.0	28.8	34.3	41.8	46.4	49.2	54.6

Modified from Frisancho, A. R.: Anthropometric Standards for the Assessment of Growth and Nutritional Status. Ann Arbor, The University of Michigan Press, 1990.

8-3   Triceps and Subscapular Skinfold Percentiles, 1–75 Years

Triceps Skinfold

Age (yrs)	5	10	15	25	50	75	85	90	95
Males									
1.0–1.9	6.5	7.0	7.5	8.0	10.0	12.0	13.0	14.0	15.5
2.0–2.9	6.0	6.5	7.0	8.0	10.0	12.0	13.0	14.0	15.0
3.0–3.9	6.0	7.0	7.0	8.0	9.5	11.5	12.5	13.5	15.0
4.0–4.9	5.5	6.5	7.0	7.5	9.0	11.0	12.0	12.5	14.0
5.0–5.9	5.0	6.0	6.0	7.0	8.0	10.0	11.5	13.0	14.5
6.0–6.9	5.0	5.5	6.0	6.5	8.0	10.0	12.0	13.0	16.0
7.0–7.9	4.5	5.5	6.0	6.0	8.0	10.5	13.0	14.0	16.0
8.0–8.9	5.0	5.5	6.0	7.0	8.5	11.0	13.0	16.0	19.0
9.0–9.9	5.0	5.5	6.0	6.5	9.0	12.5	15.5	17.0	20.0
10.0–10.9	5.0	6.0	6.0	7.5	10.0	14.0	17.0	20.0	24.0
11.0–11.9	5.0	6.0	6.0	7.5	10.0	16.0	19.5	23.0	27.0
12.0–12.9	4.5	6.0	6.5	7.5	10.5	14.5	18.0	22.5	27.5
13.0–13.9	4.5	5.5	5.5	7.0	9.0	13.0	17.0	20.5	25.0
14.0–14.9	4.0	5.0	5.0	6.0	8.5	12.5	15.0	18.0	23.5
15.0–15.9	5.0	5.0	5.1	6.0	7.5	11.0	15.0	18.0	23.5
16.0–16.9	4.0	5.0	5.5	6.0	8.0	12.0	14.0	17.0	23.0
17.0–17.9	4.0	5.0	5.0	6.0	7.0	11.0	13.5	16.0	19.5
18.0–24.9	4.0	5.0	5.5	6.5	10.0	14.5	17.5	20.0	23.5
25.0–29.9	4.5	5.0	6.0	7.0	11.0	15.5	19.0	21.5	25.0
30.0–34.9	4.5	6.0	6.5	8.0	12.0	16.5	20.0	22.0	25.0
35.0–39.9	5.0	6.0	7.0	8.0	12.0	16.0	18.5	20.5	24.5
40.0–44.9	5.0	6.0	6.9	8.0	12.0	16.0	19.0	21.5	26.0
45.0–49.9	5.0	6.0	7.0	8.0	12.0	16.0	19.0	21.0	25.0
50.0–54.9	5.0	6.0	7.0	8.0	11.5	15.0	18.5	20.8	25.0
55.0–59.9	5.0	6.0	6.5	8.0	11.5	15.5	18.0	20.5	25.0
60.0–64.9	5.0	6.0	7.0	8.0	11.5	15.5	18.5	20.5	24.0
65.0–69.9	4.5	5.0	6.5	8.0	11.0	15.0	18.0	20.0	23.5
70.0–74.9	4.5	6.0	6.5	8.0	11.0	15.0	17.0	19.0	23.0
Females									
1.0–1.9	6.0	7.0	7.0	8.0	10.0	12.0	13.0	14.0	16.0
2.0–2.9	6.0	7.0	7.5	8.5	10.0	12.0	13.5	14.5	16.0
3.0–3.9	6.0	7.0	7.0	8.5	10.0	12.0	13.0	14.0	16.0
4.0–4.9	6.0	7.0	7.5	8.0	10.0	12.0	13.0	14.0	15.5
5.0–5.9	5.5	7.0	7.0	8.0	10.0	12.0	13.5	15.0	17.0
6.0–6.9	6.0	6.5	7.0	8.0	10.0	12.0	13.0	15.0	17.0
7.0–7.9	6.0	7.0	7.0	8.5	10.5	12.5	15.0	16.0	19.0
8.0–8.9	6.0	7.0	7.5	9.0	11.0	14.5	17.0	18.0	22.5
9.0–9.9	6.5	7.0	8.0	9.0	12.0	16.0	19.0	21.0	25.0
10.0–10.9	7.0	8.0	8.0	10.0	12.5	17.5	20.0	22.5	27.0
11.0–11.9	7.0	8.0	8.5	10.0	13.0	18.0	21.5	24.0	29.0
12.0–12.9	7.0	8.0	9.0	11.0	14.0	18.5	21.5	24.0	27.5
13.0–13.9	7.0	8.0	9.0	11.0	15.0	20.0	24.0	25.0	30.0
14.0–14.9	8.0	9.0	9.0	11.5	16.0	21.0	23.5	26.5	32.0
15.0–15.9	8.0	9.5	10.5	12.0	16.5	20.5	23.0	26.0	32.5
16.0–16.9	10.5	11.5	12.0	14.0	18.0	23.0	26.5	29.0	34.5
17.0–17.9	9.0	11.0	12.0	13.0	18.0	24.0	28.5	29.0	36.0
18.0–24.9	9.0	11.0	12.0	14.0	18.5	24.5	31.0	34.0	36.0
25.0–29.9	10.0	12.0	13.0	15.0	20.0	26.5	33.0	35.5	38.0
30.0–34.9	10.5	13.0	15.0	17.0	22.5	29.5	35.0	37.0	41.5
35.0–39.9	11.0	13.0	15.5	18.0	23.5	30.0	35.0	38.5	41.0
40.0–44.9	12.0	14.5	16.5	19.0	24.5	30.5	35.5	39.0	42.5
45.0–49.9	12.0	15.0	17.0	19.5	25.5	32.0	36.0	38.0	42.0
50.0–54.9	12.5	15.0	17.5	20.5	25.5	32.0	36.0	38.5	42.5
55.0–59.9	12.0	16.0	17.0	20.5	26.0	32.0	35.5	39.0	42.5
60.0–64.9	12.0	16.0	17.5	20.5	26.0	32.0	36.0	38.0	42.5
65.0–69.9	12.0	14.5	16.0	19.0	25.0	30.0	33.5	36.0	40.0
70.0–74.9	11.0	13.5	15.5	18.0	24.0	29.5	32.0	35.0	38.5

Subscapular Skinfold

Age (yrs)	5	10	15	25	50	75	85	90	95
Males									
1.0–1.9	4.0	4.0	4.5	5.0	6.0	7.0	8.0	8.5	10.0
2.0–2.9	3.5	4.0	4.0	4.5	5.5	7.0	7.5	8.5	10.0
3.0–3.9	3.5	4.0	4.0	4.5	5.0	6.0	7.0	7.0	9.0
4.0–4.9	3.0	3.5	4.0	4.0	5.0	6.0	6.5	7.0	8.0
5.0–5.9	3.0	3.5	4.0	4.0	5.0	5.5	6.5	7.0	8.0
6.0–6.9	3.0	3.5	3.5	4.0	4.5	5.5	6.5	8.0	13.0
7.0–7.9	3.0	3.5	4.0	4.0	5.0	6.0	7.0	8.0	12.0
8.0–8.9	3.5	3.5	4.0	4.0	5.0	6.0	7.5	9.0	12.5
9.0–9.9	3.0	3.5	4.0	4.0	5.0	7.0	9.5	12.0	14.5
10.0–10.9	3.5	4.0	4.0	4.5	6.0	8.0	11.0	14.0	19.5
11.0–11.9	4.0	4.0	4.5	5.0	6.0	9.0	15.0	18.5	26.0
12.0–12.9	4.0	4.0	4.5	5.0	6.0	9.5	15.0	19.0	24.0
13.0–13.9	4.0	4.0	5.0	5.0	6.5	9.0	13.0	17.0	25.0
14.0–14.9	4.0	5.0	5.0	5.5	7.0	9.0	12.0	15.5	22.5
15.0–15.9	5.0	5.0	5.5	6.0	7.0	10.0	13.0	16.0	22.0
16.0–16.9	4.0	6.0	6.0	7.0	8.0	11.0	14.0	16.0	22.0
17.0–17.9	5.0	6.0	6.0	7.0	8.0	11.0	14.0	17.0	21.5
18.0–24.9	5.0	7.0	8.0	8.0	11.0	16.0	20.0	24.0	30.0
25.0–29.9	6.0	7.0	9.0	11.0	13.0	20.0	24.5	26.5	31.0
30.0–34.9	6.0	8.0	9.5	11.0	15.5	22.0	25.5	29.0	33.0
35.0–39.9	7.0	8.0	9.0	11.5	16.0	22.5	25.5	28.0	33.0
40.0–44.9	7.0	8.0	9.0	11.5	16.0	22.0	25.5	29.5	34.5
45.0–49.9	7.0	8.0	9.5	11.5	17.0	23.5	27.0	30.0	34.0
50.0–54.9	7.0	8.0	9.5	11.5	16.0	22.5	26.5	29.5	34.0
55.0–59.9	6.5	8.0	9.5	11.5	16.5	23.0	26.0	28.5	32.0
60.0–64.9	7.0	8.0	10.0	12.0	17.0	23.0	26.0	29.0	34.0
65.0–69.9	6.0	7.5	8.5	10.5	15.0	21.5	25.0	28.0	32.5
70.0–74.9	6.5	7.0	8.0	10.3	15.0	21.0	25.0	27.5	31.0
Females									
1.0–1.9	4.0	4.0	4.5	5.0	6.0	7.5	8.5	9.0	10.0
2.0–2.9	4.0	4.0	4.5	5.0	6.0	7.0	8.0	9.0	10.5
3.0–3.9	3.5	4.0	4.0	5.0	5.5	7.0	7.5	8.5	10.0
4.0–4.9	3.5	3.5	4.0	4.5	5.5	7.0	8.0	8.5	10.5
5.0–5.9	3.5	4.0	4.0	4.5	5.5	7.0	8.0	9.0	12.0
6.0–6.9	3.5	4.0	4.0	4.5	6.0	7.5	8.0	10.0	11.5
7.0–7.9	3.5	4.0	4.5	5.0	6.0	8.0	9.5	11.0	13.0
8.0–8.9	4.0	4.5	5.0	5.5	6.5	9.5	11.5	14.5	21.0
9.0–9.9	4.0	4.5	5.0	5.5	7.0	11.5	13.0	18.0	24.0
10.0–10.9	4.0	4.5	5.0	6.0	8.0	12.0	16.0	19.5	24.0
11.0–11.9	4.5	5.0	5.0	6.5	9.0	13.0	16.0	20.0	28.5
12.0–12.9	5.0	5.5	6.0	7.0	10.0	15.5	17.0	22.0	30.0
13.0–13.9	5.0	6.0	6.0	7.0	10.0	15.5	19.0	23.0	26.5
14.0–14.9	6.0	6.0	7.0	7.5	10.0	16.0	20.5	25.0	30.0
15.0–15.9	7.0	7.5	8.0	8.0	10.0	15.0	20.0	23.0	28.0
16.0–16.9	6.0	7.0	8.0	9.0	11.5	16.5	24.0	26.0	34.0
17.0–17.9	7.0	7.5	8.0	9.0	12.5	19.0	24.5	28.0	34.0
18.0–24.9	6.5	7.0	8.0	9.0	13.0	20.0	25.5	29.0	36.0
25.0–29.9	6.5	7.5	8.0	10.0	14.0	23.0	29.0	33.0	38.5
30.0–34.9	7.0	7.5	8.5	10.5	18.0	26.5	32.5	37.0	43.0
35.0–39.9	7.0	8.0	9.0	11.0	18.0	28.5	34.0	36.5	43.0
40.0–44.9	6.5	8.0	9.0	11.5	19.0	28.5	34.0	37.0	42.0
45.0–49.9	7.0	8.5	10.0	12.5	20.0	29.5	34.0	37.5	43.5
50.0–54.9	7.0	9.0	11.0	14.0	21.9	30.0	35.0	39.0	43.5
55.0–59.9	7.0	9.0	11.0	13.5	22.0	31.0	35.0	38.0	45.0
60.0–64.9	7.5	9.0	11.0	14.0	21.5	30.5	35.0	38.0	43.0
65.0–69.9	7.0	8.0	10.0	13.0	20.0	28.0	33.0	36.0	41.0
70.0–74.9	6.5	8.5	10.0	12.0	19.5	27.0	32.0	35.0	38.5

Modified from Fisancho, A. R.: Anthropometric Standards for the Assessment of Growth and Nutritional Status, Ann Arbor, The University of Michigan Press, 1990.

8—4   Acromial Radiale (Upper Arm) Length and Knee Height Growth Chart, 2–18 Years

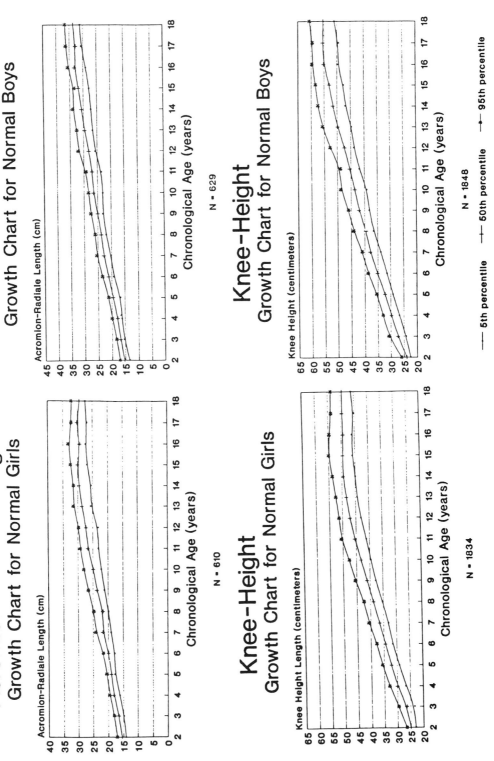

Acromion-Radiale Length
Growth Chart for Normal Boys

Acromion-Radiale Length (cm)

Chronological Age (years)

N = 629

Acromion-Radiale Length
Growth Chart for Normal Girls

Acromion-Radiale Length (cm)

Chronological Age (years)

N = 610

Knee-Height
Growth Chart for Normal Boys

Knee Height (centimeters)

Chronological Age (years)

N = 1848

Knee-Height
Growth Chart for Normal Girls

Knee Height Length (centimeters)

Chronological Age (years)

N = 1834

—— 5th percentile   —+— 50th percentile   —✱— 95th percentile

From charts developed by T. K. White and S. W. Ekvall, 1992 as adapted from data by Snyder, R. G., Highway Safety Research Institute, University of Michigan, 1977.

8–5   Directions for Ross Knee Height Caliper Measurement

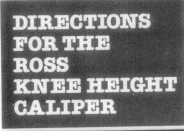

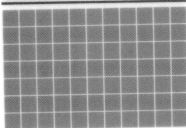

Stature can be estimated from knee height when standing height cannot be measured. Estimated stature can be used in nutritional assessment parameters, including reference weights for height, energy expenditure equations, body surface area equations, and the creatinine-height and body mass indices. Knee height may also be used with midarm circumference to predict weight in individuals who cannot be weighed by conventional methods.

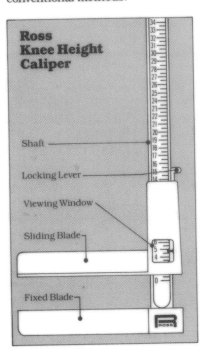

KNEE HEIGHT MEASUREMENTS

1. With the subject lying on his or her back, bend both the left knee and left ankle to a 90° angle (Fig 1). Check the angles using the triangle (Fig 2).

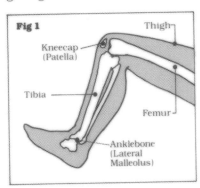

2. Open the caliper and place the fixed blade under the heel. Press the sliding blade down against the thigh about 2 in. behind the kneecap (patella) (Fig 3). The shaft of

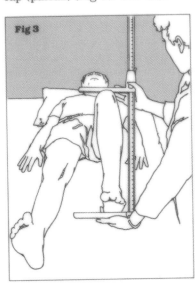

the caliper should be in line with the large bone in the lower leg (tibia) and be over the ankle bone (lateral malleolus) (Fig 4).

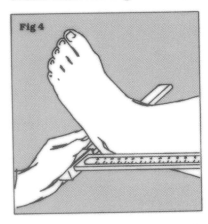

3. To hold the measurement, push the locking lever away from the blades (Fig 5). Read the measurement through the viewing window to the nearest 0.1 cm (Fig 6).

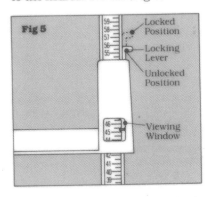

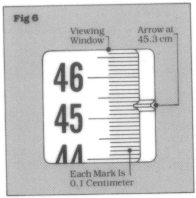

4. Release the locking lever by pushing it toward the caliper blades. Repeat the process to take a second measurement. Both measurements should be within 0.5 cm of each other.

8–6 Estimations of Stature and Weight from Knee Height

Stature may be estimated from knee height for children, adults, and the elderly using age-, gender-, and race-specific equations. Equations have been developed from national surveys of healthy, normal individuals and reflect normal patterns of growth and development.

1. Average the two knee height measurements, rounding the result to the nearest 0.1 cm.

2. Use the appropriate equation to determine height.

3. To convert the estimated stature from centimeters to inches, use the following:

$$\text{Stature in inches} = \frac{\text{Stature in cm}}{2.54}$$

MALES 6 TO 18 YEARS		NOTE: Estimated stature should be within…
White Males	Stature (cm) = [Knee Height (cm) × 2.22] + 40.54	± 8.42 cm of actual stature for 95% of white boys.
Black Males	Stature (cm) = [Knee Height (cm) × 2.18] + 39.60	± 9.16 cm of actual stature for 95% of black boys.
MALES 19 TO 59 YEARS		
White Males	Stature (cm) = [Knee Height (cm) × 1.88] + 71.85	± 7.94 cm of actual stature for 95% of white men.
Black Males	Stature (cm) = [Knee Height (cm) × 1.79] + 73.42	± 7.20 cm of actual stature for 95% of black men.
MALES 60 TO 80 YEARS		
White Males	Stature (cm) = [Knee Height (cm) × 2.08] + 59.01	± 7.84 cm of actual stature for 95% of white men.
Black Males	Stature (cm) = [Knee Height (cm) × 1.37] + 95.79	± 8.44 cm of actual stature for 95% of black men.
FEMALES 6 TO 18 YEARS		
White Females	Stature (cm) = [Knee Height (cm) × 2.15] + 43.21	± 7.79 cm of actual stature for 95% of white girls.
Black Females	Stature (cm) = [Knee Height (cm) × 2.02] + 46.59	± 8.77 cm of actual stature for 95% of black girls.
FEMALES 19 TO 59 YEARS		
White Females	Stature (cm) = [Knee Height (cm) × 1.86] − [Age (years) × 0.05] + 70.25	± 7.20 cm of actual stature for 95% of white women.
Black Females	Stature (cm) = [Knee Height (cm) × 1.86] − [Age (years) × 0.06] + 68.10	± 7.60 cm of actual stature for 95% of black women.
FEMALES 60 TO 80 YEARS		
White Females	Stature (cm) = [Knee Height (cm) × 1.91] − [Age (years) × 0.17] + 75.00	± 8.82 cm of actual stature for 95% of white women.
Black Females	Stature (cm) = [Knee Height (cm) × 1.96] + 58.72	± 8.26 cm of actual stature for 95% of black women.

ESTIMATING WEIGHT FROM KNEE HEIGHT

Weight can be estimated using age-, gender-, and race-specific equations. Measurements of midarm circumference (MAC) are also needed. Equations have been developed from national surveys of healthy, normal individuals and reflect normal patterns of growth and development.

1. Average the two knee height and midarm circumference measurements, rounding the results to the nearest 0.1 cm.

2. Use the appropriate equation to determine weight.

3. To convert weight in kilograms to pounds, use the following:

$$\text{Weight (lbs)} = [\text{Weight (kg)} \times 2.2]$$

MALES 6 TO 18 YEARS		NOTE: Estimated weight should be within…
White Males	Weight (kg) = [Knee Height (cm) × 0.68] + [MAC (cm) × 2.64] − 50.08	± 7.82 kg of actual weight for 95% of white boys.
Black Males	Weight (kg) = [Knee Height (cm) × 0.59] + [MAC (cm) × 2.73] − 48.32	± 7.50 kg of actual weight for 95% of black boys.
MALES 19 TO 59 YEARS		
White Males	Weight (kg) = [Knee Height (cm) × 1.19] + [MAC (cm) × 3.21] − 86.82	± 11.42 kg of actual weight for 95% of white men.
Black Males	Weight (kg) = [Knee Height (cm) × 1.09] + [MAC (cm) × 3.14] − 83.72	± 11.30 kg of actual weight for 95% of black men.
MALES 60 TO 80 YEARS		
White Males	Weight (kg) = [Knee Height (cm) × 1.10] + [MAC (cm) × 3.07] − 75.81	± 11.46 kg of actual weight for 95% of white men.
Black Males	Weight (kg) = [Knee Height (cm) × 0.44] + [MAC (cm) × 2.86] − 39.21	± 7.04 kg of actual weight for 95% of black men.
FEMALES 6 TO 18 YEARS		
White Females	Weight (kg) = [Knee Height (cm) × 0.77] + [MAC (cm) × 2.47] − 50.16	± 7.20 kg of actual weight for 95% of white girls.
Black Females	Weight (kg) = [Knee Height (cm) × 0.71] + [MAC (cm) × 2.59] − 50.43	± 7.65 kg of actual weight for 95% of black girls.
FEMALES 19 TO 59 YEARS		
White Females	Weight (kg) = [Knee Height (cm) × 1.01] + [MAC (cm) × 2.81] − 66.04	± 10.60 kg of actual weight for 95% of white women.
Black Females	Weight (kg) = [Knee Height (cm) × 1.24] + [MAC (cm) × 2.97] − 82.48	± 11.98 kg of actual weight for 95% of black women.
FEMALES 60 TO 80 YEARS		
White Females	Weight (kg) = [Knee Height (cm) × 1.09] + [MAC (cm) × 2.68] − 65.51	± 11.42 kg of actual weight for 95% of white women.
Black Females	Weight (kg) = [Knee Height (cm) × 1.50] + [MAC (cm) × 2.58] − 84.22	± 14.52 kg of actual weight for 95% of black women.

8-7 Sitting Height Percentiles, 2-75 Years, Body Mass Index and Two Skinfolds and Anthropometry Nutritional Assessment, Boy, 8 Years

Age, years	BMI 50th M	BMI 50th F	BMI 85th M	BMI 85th F	BMI 95th M	BMI 95th F	Sum of Two Skinfolds 50th M	50th F	85th M	85th F	95th M	95th F
6	15.4	15.2	16.8	17.1	18.2	18.5	12	14	16	19	20	27
7	15.6	15.4	17.1	17.6	18.9	19.6	12	15	17	22	24	28
8	16.0	15.9	18.1	18.6	20.2	21.1	13	16	19	25	28	36
9	16.2	16.3	19.0	19.5	22.4	22.9	14	17	23	29	34	41
10	16.5	16.9	19.2	20.6	21.8	23.6	14	18	24	32	33	43
11	17.2	17.5	20.9	20.9	24.2	24.8	15	19	28	31	39	43
12	17.8	18.6	21.4	22.6	24.1	26.2	15	20	24	34	44	47
13	18.7	19.4	22.6	23.4	26.6	26.8	15	21	28	39	46	52
14	19.6	20.7	23.2	24.7	26.7	26.5	14	24	27	37	39	53
15	20.4	20.7	24.0	24.7	27.8	29.4	14	25	25	41	40	56
16	20.8	20.9	24.0	24.9	26.9	29.6	14	26	24	42	39	58
17	21.5	21.0	24.9	24.3	28.5	29.3	15	27	26	42	41	59

From Lohman, T: *Advances in Body Composition Assessment*. Champaign, Human Kinetics, 1992.

Characteristics	Computation	Variable
Child's stature (CS)	N.A.	123.0 cm
Father's stature	N.A.	187.0 cm
Mother's stature	N.A.	165.0 cm
Midparent stature (MPS)	(187 + 165)/2	176.0 cm
Adjusted for midparent stature	123 - 4.27	118.7 cm
Weight	N.A.	31.0 kg
Sitting Height	N.A.	69.0 cm
Sitting Height Index	(69/123) x 100	56.0%
Triceps Skinfold	11/10 = 1.1 cm	11.0 mm
Subscapular Skinfold	N.A.	5.0 mm
Sum of Skinfold Thicknesses	N.A.	16.0 mm
Upper Arm Circumference	N.A.	22.0 cm
Total Upper Arm Fat Area (TUA)	$22^2/12.57$	38.5 cm²
Upper Arm Muscle Area (UMA)	$[(22.0 - 1.1) \times 3.1416]^2/12.57$	27.4 cm²
Upper Arm Fat Area (UFA)	38.5 - 27.4	11.1 mm²
Arm Fat Index (AFI)	(11.1/38.5) x 100	28.8%

Growth and Nutritional Status Evaluation

Reference	Z-score	Category	Percentile	Category
Stature by Age	-1.08	Below Ave.	>5th but <15	Below Ave.
Adj. midparent stature	-1.87	Short	< 5th	Short
Wt. by Age	N.A.	N.A.	>15th but <85th	Average
Wt. by Ht.	N.A.	N.A.	>95th	High Wt.
Sitting Ht. Index	0.76	Average	>95th	Large Trunk
UMA by Age	1.26	Above Ave.	>85th but <95th	Above Ave.
UMA by Ht.	2.19	Above Ave.	>85th but <95th	Above Ave.
Sum of Skinfolds	N.A.	N.A.	>15th but <85th	Average
Arm Fat Index	N.A.	N.A.	>15th but <85th	Average

Interpretation. The subject is short for his age and, considering his parents' height, he should have been taller than he is now. In other words, he seems to be below his genetic potential as far as his height is concerned. However, the subject is heavy for his age. As judged by the measurements of body composition, the excess weight is not due to an excess of fat but to the subjects' high muscularity and short legs (which is indicated by the high sitting height index).

Sitting Height Percentiles

Age (yrs)	5	10	15	25	50	75	85	90	95
Males									
2.0-2.9	50.0	51.0	51.3	52.0	54.0	56.0	57.0	57.0	58.0
3.0-3.9	52.1	54.0	54.0	55.0	57.0	58.8	59.6	60.0	61.0
4.0-4.9	55.0	56.0	57.0	60.0	60.0	61.7	63.0	63.0	64.3
5.0-5.9	57.9	59.0	59.3	63.0	62.3	64.0	65.0	66.0	67.0
6.0-6.9	59.5	61.0	62.0	63.0	65.0	67.0	68.0	69.0	69.4
7.0-7.9	62.0	63.2	64.0	65.3	67.2	69.2	70.0	71.0	72.0
8.0-8.9	64.1	65.4	66.0	67.5	69.0	71.4	72.6	73.0	74.6
9.0-9.9	66.0	67.5	68.0	69.0	71.4	74.0	75.0	75.6	76.7
10.0-10.9	68.0	69.0	70.0	71.6	73.8	76.0	77.0	78.0	79.4
11.0-11.9	69.3	71.0	71.9	73.0	76.0	78.0	79.6	80.4	82.0
12.0-12.9	71.7	72.9	74.0	75.1	78.0	81.0	82.3	84.2	86.0
13.0-13.9	74.0	75.0	76.0	78.0	81.7	85.3	87.2	88.5	90.5
14.0-14.9	76.7	79.3	80.5	82.5	86.0	88.9	90.5	91.5	92.9
15.0-15.9	80.4	82.0	83.5	85.4	88.1	91.1	92.6	93.8	95.0
16.0-16.9	84.1	85.2	86.1	87.6	90.5	93.4	94.5	95.1	96.5
17.0-17.9	84.3	86.0	87.0	88.4	91.1	93.5	94.7	95.9	97.3
18.0-24.9	86.2	87.6	88.5	90.0	92.4	95.2	96.3	97.2	98.5
25.0-29.9	86.5	88.0	89.0	90.3	92.9	95.2	96.7	97.6	98.8
30.0-34.9	86.7	87.9	88.8	90.3	92.7	95.1	96.4	97.4	98.7
35.0-39.9	86.4	87.6	88.6	90.0	92.5	95.1	96.4	97.0	98.3
40.0-44.9	86.3	87.8	88.8	90.1	92.4	94.5	96.0	96.9	98.2
45.0-49.9	85.5	87.2	88.3	89.6	92.1	94.2	95.6	96.4	97.8
50.0-54.9	85.3	86.8	87.6	89.2	91.6	93.8	95.1	96.0	97.3
55.0-59.9	84.8	86.2	87.3	88.6	91.1	93.5	94.6	95.4	96.6
60.0-64.9	84.8	86.1	86.8	88.0	90.5	92.9	94.1	94.8	96.1
65.0-69.9	83.3	84.5	85.5	86.7	89.4	91.7	93.3	94.1	95.2
70.0-74.9	81.9	83.6	84.8	86.2	88.7	91.0	92.4	93.5	94.4
Females									
2.0-2.9	49.0	49.8	50.0	51.0	53.0	54.4	55.0	56.0	56.7
3.0-3.9	51.0	52.3	53.0	54.0	55.7	57.2	58.3	59.0	60.0
4.0-4.9	54.0	55.0	56.0	57.0	58.8	60.7	61.3	62.0	63.0
5.0-5.9	56.6	58.0	58.9	60.0	61.6	63.1	64.2	65.0	66.0
6.0-6.9	59.2	60.0	61.0	62.0	64.0	66.0	67.0	68.0	69.0
7.0-7.9	62.0	62.8	63.1	64.5	68.4	71.0	72.0	73.0	74.1
8.0-8.9	64.0	64.7	65.9	67.0	69.0	71.6	72.0	73.0	77.2
9.0-9.9	65.5	66.7	67.8	69.2	71.0	73.5	75.0	76.0	81.0
10.0-10.9	68.0	69.2	70.1	71.4	73.5	75.8	77.3	78.9	83.9
11.0-11.9	70.0	71.6	72.2	74.0	76.6	80.0	81.2	82.3	84.6
12.0-12.9	70.0	74.0	75.1	77.2	80.5	83.1	84.6	85.5	86.4
13.0-13.9	76.2	77.7	78.7	80.1	82.7	85.0	86.3	86.9	87.8
14.0-14.9	78.1	79.1	80.4	81.7	84.3	86.9	87.8	88.6	89.5
15.0-15.9	79.8	81.1	82.2	83.3	85.3	87.5	88.5	89.9	91.5
16.0-16.9	79.3	81.0	81.9	83.5	85.8	88.0	88.8	89.8	91.5
17.0-17.9	80.0	81.1	82.4	83.8	86.0	88.1	89.4	90.3	92.0
18.0-24.9	80.4	81.9	82.8	84.4	86.4	88.5	89.9	90.6	91.9
25.0-29.9	80.9	82.2	83.1	84.4	86.5	88.7	89.9	90.6	92.0
30.0-34.9	81.0	82.3	83.1	84.4	86.5	89.0	90.1	91.1	92.3
35.0-39.9	81.0	82.1	83.1	84.5	86.7	88.8	90.2	91.0	92.3
40.0-44.9	80.6	82.0	82.8	84.1	86.3	88.4	89.7	90.5	91.7
45.0-49.9	80.5	82.0	83.0	84.2	86.4	88.3	89.4	90.3	91.6
50.0-54.9	80.5	81.6	82.4	83.4	85.5	88.3	89.4	89.7	90.7
55.0-59.9	78.9	80.5	81.5	82.6	85.0	87.1	88.3	88.8	90.0
60.0-64.9	78.6	80.0	80.9	82.1	84.4	86.5	87.7	88.4	89.7
65.0-69.9	77.4	78.8	79.7	81.0	83.3	85.5	86.7	87.4	88.6
70.0-74.9	76.5	77.9	78.7	80.0	82.4	84.4	85.7	86.5	87.6

Modified from Frisancho, A.R.: *Anthropometric Standards for the Assessment of Growth and Nutritional Status*, Ann Arbor, The University of Michigan Press, 1990.

8–8 Percentage Body Fat from Triceps plus Subscapular Skinfolds, Equations and Chart, Children

For Triceps and Subscapular

Prepubescent White Males: PFDWB = 1.21 (triceps + subscapular) - .008 (triceps + subscapular)^2 - 1.7

Prepubsecent Black Males: PFDWB = 1.21 (triceps + subscapular) - .008 (triceps + subscapular)^2 - 3.2

Pubescent White Males: PFDWB = 1.21 (triceps + subscapular) - .008 (triceps + subscapular)^2 - 3.4

Pubescent Black Males: PFDWB = 1.21 (triceps + subscapular) - .008 (triceps + subscapular)^2 - 5.2

Postpubescent White Males: PFDWB = 1.21 (triceps + subscapular) - .008 (triceps + subscapular)^2 - 5.5

Postpubescent Black Males: PFDWB = 1.21 (triceps + subscapular) - .008 (triceps + subscapular)^2 - 6.8

All Females: PFDWB = 1.33 (triceps + subscapular) - .013 (triceps + subscapular)^2 - 2.5

For a sum of tricep and subscapular greater than 35 mm, the following equation should be applied.

All Males PFDWB = .783 (triceps + subscapular) + 1.6

All Females PFDWB = .546 (triceps + subscapular) + 9.7

From Slaughter, M. H. Lohman, T. G., Boileau, R. A., Horswill, C. A., Stillman, R. J., Van Loan, M.D. and Bemben, D. A.: Skinfold equations for estimation of body fatness in children and youth. Human Biol, 60:709, 1988. Used with permission.

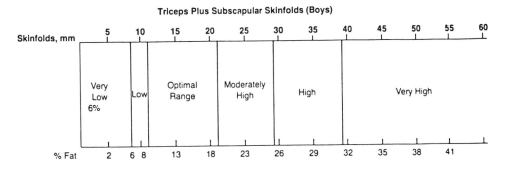

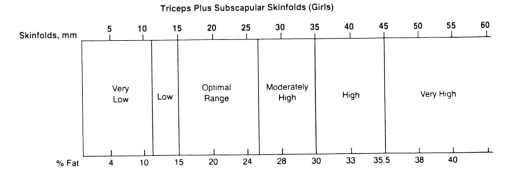

Figure 1.

Lohman, T. G.: The use of skinfold to estimate body fatness on children and youth. J Phy Ed Rec, 58:98, 1987.

8–9   Percentage Body Fat from Triceps plus Calf Skinfolds, Equations and Chart, Children

<u>For Triceps and Calf</u>
Males:PFDWB = .735 (triceps + calf) + 1.0
Females:PFDWB = .610 (triceps + calf) + 5.1

From Slaughter, M. H. Lohman, T. G., Boileau, R. A., Horswill, C. A., Stillman,
R. J., Van Loan, M.D. and Bemben, D. A.: Skinfold equations for estimation of
body fatness in children and youth. <u>Human Biol</u>, 60:709, 1988. Used with
permission.

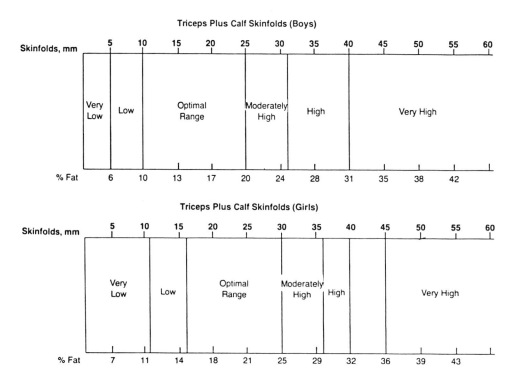

Figure 1.

Lohman, T. G.: The use of skinfold to estimate body fatness on children and
youth. <u>J Phy Ed Rec</u>, 58:98, 1987.

8–10 Free Amino Acids in Serum

micromol per liter

| | Children Birth-6 yrs | Normal Adults Mean (S.D) | |
		MALE	FEMALE
Taurine	110 (40)	86 (28)	80 (25)
Aspartic Acid	33 (14)	28 (11)	21 (10)
Hydroxyproline	31 (14)	15 (6)	13 (5)
Threonine	157 (47)	150 (26)	147 (47)
Serine	194 (54)	192 (45)	177 (58)
Asparagine	71 (18)	63 (21)	60 (21)
Glutamic Acid	113 (43)	103 (41)	88 (32)
Glutamine	647 (116)	599 (61)	562 (98)
Proline	223 (58)	210 (64)	173 (58)
Glycine	367 (95)	298 (52)	303 (84)
Alanine	417 (107)	376 (96)	354 (99)
Citrulline	22 (8)	34 (8)	31 (8)
Aminobutyric	10) 6)	21 (12)	17 (11)
Valine	213 (53)	271 (48)	214 (36)
Cystine	36 (10)	44 (18)	39 (12)
Methionine	34 (11)	24 (4)	20 (4)
Isoleucine	66 (21)	70 (14)	54 (12)
Leucine	122 (32)	143 (24)	112 (20)
Tyrosine	81 (28)	61 (15)	57 (17)
Phenylalanine	72 (17)	76 (18)	61 (15)
Tryptophan	40 (13)	42 (12)	40 (13)
Ornithine	95 (38)	115 (23)	103 (33)
Lysine	169 (41)	199 (37)	172 (38)
Histidine	90 (16)	98 (18)	90 (18)
Arginine	95 (29)	54 (9)	54 (22)

From the Metabolic Disease Center, Children's Hospital Medical Center, Cincinnati, OH, 45229 (unpublished data). Data for children respresent the 10th to 90th percentiles of values from 440 consecutive amino acid analyses on a Beckman 6300 Amino Acid Analyzer (Beckman Instruments, Fullerton, CA) using operating settings and reagents recommended by the manufacturer for analysis of physiological fluids. Adult values represent two specimens each from 10 men and 18 women.

8-11 Laboratory Evaluation Data

Nutrient & Units	Age of Subject (years)	Criteria of Status Deficient	Marginal	Acceptable
Hemoglobin (g/dl)	1 week			13-20
	1 month			>14
	6-23 months	<9.0	9.0-9.9	10.0+
	2-5	<10.0	10.0-10.9	11.0+
	6-12	<10.0	10.0-11.4	11.5+
	13-16M	<12.0	12.0-12.9	13.0+
	13-16F	<10.0	10.0-11.4	11.5+
	16+M	<12.0	12.0-13.9	14.0+
	16+F	<10.0	10.0-11.9	12.0+
	Pregnant 2nd trimester	<9.5	9.5-10.9	11.0+
	3rd trimester	<9.0	9.0-10.5	10.5+
Hematocrit (packed cell volume in %)	1 week			43-66
	1 month			>50
	3 months			>35
	6 months-5 years			>38
	6-12	<30	30-35	36+
	13-16M	<37	37-39	40+
	13-16F	<31	31-35	36+
	16+M	<37	37-43	44+
	16+F	<31	31-37	33+
	Pregnant	<30	30-32	33+
Mean corpuscular volume (μm^3)	All ages			80-94
Mean corpuscular hemoglobin (μg)	All ages			27-35
Mean corpuscular hemoglobin concentration (%)	All ages			32-36
Serum iron (μg/dl)	<2	<30		30+
	2-5	<40		40+
	6-12	<50		50+
	12+M	<60		60+
	12+F or pregnant	<40	40	40+
Transferrin saturation (%)	<2	<15.0		15.0+
	2-12	<20.0		20.0+
	12+M	<20.0		20.0+
	12+F or pregnant	<15.0	15	15.0+
Serum ascorbic acid (mg/dl)	All ages	<0.1	0.1-0.19	0.2+
Plasma vitamin A (μg/dl)	All ages	<10	10-19	20+
Plasma carotene (μ/dl)	All ages	<20	20-39	40+
	pregnant		40-79	80+

Nutrient & Units	Age of Subject (years)	Criteria of Status Deficient	Marginal	Acceptable
Serum folic acid (ng/ml)	All ages; pregnant	<2.0	2.1-5.9	6.0+
Serum vitamin B$_{12}$ (pg/ml)	All ages; pregnant	<100	100	100+
Thiamine in urine (μg/g of creatinine)	1-3	<120	120-175	175+
	4-5	<85	85-120	120+
	6-9	<70	70-180	180+
	10-15	<55	55-150	150+
	16+	<27	27-65	65+
	Pregnant	<21	21-49	50+
Riboflavin in urine (μg/g of creatinine)	1-3	<150	150-499	500+
	4-5	<100	100-299	300+
	6-9	<85	85-269	270+
	10-16	<80	70-199	200+
	16+	<27	27-79	80+
	Pregnant	<30	30-89	90+
Tryptophan load (mg xanthurenic acid excreted) Adults (Dose: 100 mg/kg body weight)	6 hr	25+		<25
	24 hr	75+		<75
Urinary pyridoxine (μg/g of creatinine)	1-3	<90		90+
	4-6	<80		80+
	7-9	<60		60+
	10-12	<40		40+
	13-15	<30		30+
	16+	<20		20+
Urinary N'methyl nicotinamide (mg/g of creatinine)	All ages	<0.2	0.2-5.59	0.6+
	Pregnant	<0.8	0.8-2.49	2.5+
Urinary pantothenic acid (μg)	All ages	<200		200+
Vitamine E (serum tocopherol)(mg/dl)	Birth			0.22
	2 mos.			0.33
	2-12 yr.			0.72
	Adults			0.85
Transaminase index (ratio) EGOT	Adult	2.0+		<2.0
EGPT	Adult	1.25+		<1.25

Modified from: Zeman, F. J.: Clinical Nutrition and Dietetics. New York, Macmillan, 1991. M=male subjects; F=female subjects; EGOT=erythrocyte glutamic oxaloacetic transaminase; EGPT=erythrocyte glutamic pyruvic transaminase.

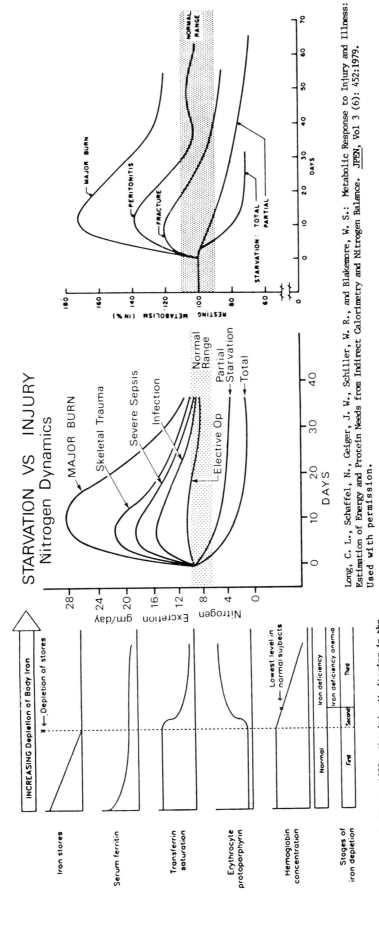

8–12 Depletion of Body Iron, Increases in Urinary Nitrogen Excretion, and Changes in Resting Metabolism Over Time

Long, C. L., Schaffel, N., Geiger, J. W., Schiller, W. R., and Blakemore, W. S.: Metabolic Response to Injury and Illness: Estimation of Energy and Protein Needs from Indirect Calorimetry and Nitrogen Balance. JPEN, Vol 3 (6): 452:1979. Used with permission.

From: LSRO, FASEB. 1989. Nutrition Monitoring in the United States: An Update Report on Nutrition Monitoring Washington, D.C.: U.S. Government Printing Office, Figure 6.1, page 131.

Appendix 9
Adolescent Maturational Charts & Psychological Tests

Typical Progression of Male Pubertal Development

Pubertal development in size of male genitalia.

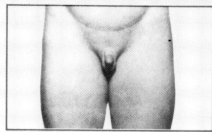

Stage 1. The penis, testes, and scrotum are of childhood size.

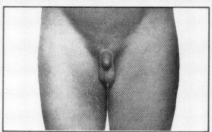

Stage 2. There is enlargement of the scrotum and testes, but the penis usually does not enlarge. The scrotal skin reddens.

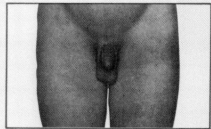

Stage 3. There is further growth of the testes and scrotum and enlargement of the penis, mainly in length.

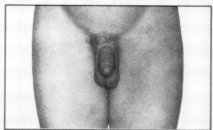

Stage 4. There is still further growth of the testes and scrotum and increased size of the penis, especially in breadth.

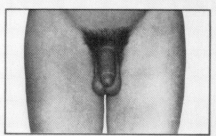

Stage 5. The genitalia are adult in size and shape.

Pubertal development of male pubic hair.

Stage 1. There is no pubic hair.

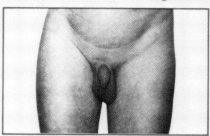

Stage 2. There is sparse growth of long, slightly pigmented, downy hair, straight or only slightly curled, primarily at the base of the penis.

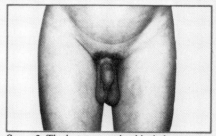

Stage 3. The hair is considerably darker, coarser, and more curled. The hair spreads sparsely over the junction of the pubes.

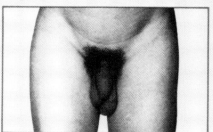

Stage 4. The hair, now adult in type, covers a smaller area than in the adult and does not extend onto the thighs.

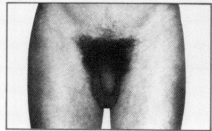

Stage 5. The hair is adult in quantity and type, with extension onto the thighs.

Sequence of Pubertal Events—
Average American Male

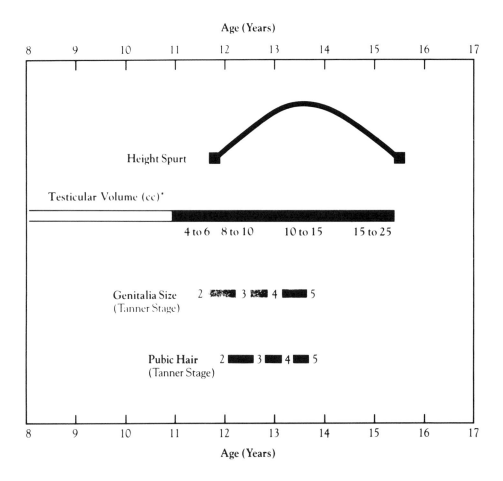

Adapted from Brookman RR, Rauh JL, Morrison JA, et al:
The Princeton Maturation Study, 1976, unpublished data for
adolescents in Cincinnati, Ohio.

*Testicular volume less than 4 cc using orchidometer (Prader Beads)
represents prepubertal stage.

Prader Beads may be obtained from M. Benesch,
Secretary to Professor Prader, Universitats-Kinderklinik,
Steinwiesstrasse 75, CH-8032, Zurich, Switzerland.
Enclose check for 70 Swiss francs and allow 4 to 5 months
for delivery.

Typical Progression of Female Pubertal Development

Pubertal development in size of female breasts.

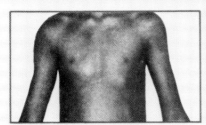

Stage 1. The breasts are preadolescent. There is elevation of the papilla only.

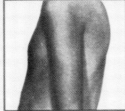
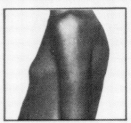

Stage 2. Breast bud stage. A small mound is formed by the elevation of the breast and papilla. The areolar diameter enlarges.

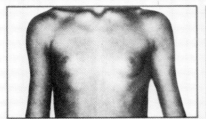
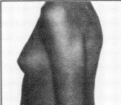

Stage 3. There is further enlargement of breasts and areola with no separation of their contours.

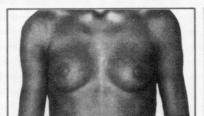
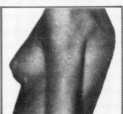

Stage 4. There is a projection of the areola and papilla to form a secondary mound above the level of the breast.

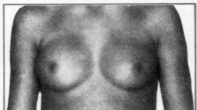
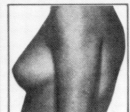

Stage 5. The breasts resemble those of a mature female as the areola has recessed to the general contour of the breast.

Pubertal development of female pubic hair.

Stage 1. There is no pubic hair.

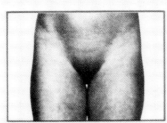
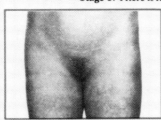
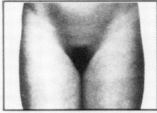
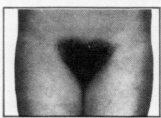

Stage 2. There is sparse growth of long, slightly pigmented, downy hair, straight or only slightly curled, primarily along the labia.

Stage 3. The hair is considerably darker, coarser, and more curled. The hair spreads sparsely over the junction of the pubes.

Stage 4. The hair, now adult in type, covers a smaller area than in the adult and does not extend onto the thighs.

Stage 5. The hair is adult in quantity and type, with extension onto the thighs.

Sequence of Pubertal Events— Average American Female

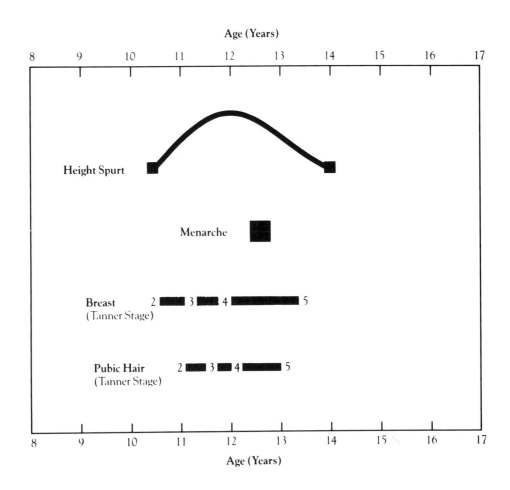

Adapted from Brookman RR, Rauh JL, Morrison JA, et al:
The Princeton Maturation Study, 1976, unpublished data for
adolescents in Cincinnati, Ohio.

	MATURATIONAL STAGE					
	I	II	III	IV	V	Adult
Follicle–stimulating hormone (mIU/ml) [*]						
Male mean – 21 Range 16–21	4.5	5.9	8.1	8.5	8.0	range 5.0–20.0
Female mean – 21	4.2	5.5	8.0	8.0	12.3	range 4.0–20.0
Luteinizing hormone (mIU/ml) [*]						
Male mean – 21 Range 16–21	3.9	6.8	8.5	9.5	11.5	range 5.0–20.0
Female mean – 21	2.9	3.9	8.4	11.3	18.9	range 4.0–25.0
Follicle–stimulating hormone (mIU/ml) [**]						
Male mean – 24	3.8	3.9	6.8	7.4	6.4	
Luteinzing hormone (mIU/ml) [**]						
Male mean – 24	5.4	5.6	7.5	9.1	9.3	
Follicle stimulating hormone (IU) [++]						
Male mean – 22	1.6	3.2	3.7	4.7	2.8	
Female mean – 22	1.5	4.0	6.0	3.8	2.3	
Luteinizing hormone (IU) [++]						
Male mean – 22	2.0	5.9	13.5	17.0	21.6	
Female mean – 22	1.9	5.0	13.7	14.9	16.6	
Prolactin (mIU/ml) [**]						
Male mean –	3.6–10.3	2.4–18.9	3.0–15.2	4.3–18.1	3.1–15.7	
Female mean – 20	3.8–13.5	3.1–11.7	3.8–19.2	4.2–16.8	5.0–18.0	
Estrone (ng/dl) [*]						
Male mean – 16	2.0	3.0	3.0	4.0	3.0	range 2.0– 6.0
Female mean – 16	4.0	5.0	7.0	12.0	3.0	range 2.0–18.2
Estradiol (ng/dl) [*]						
Male mean – 16	2.0	1.0	2.0	4.0	3.0	range 1.5– 5.0
Female mean – 16	2.0	3.0	13.0	16.0	8.0	range 1.5–40.0
Progesterone (ng/dl) [*]						
Male mean – 21	30.0	36.0	40.0	40.0	35.0	range 16– 60
Female mean – 21	10–13	16.0	16–23	30–161	29–75 (follicular)	range 20–2000
17-hydroxyprogesterone (ng/dl) [*]						
Male mean – 21	30–60	34–40	52–62	78–93	97.0	range 38–200
Female mean – 21	32–38	38–52	55–69	101–127	11–80	range
Testosterone (ng/dl) [*]						
Male mean – 16	10	18	52	170	350	range 300–800
Female mean – 16	11	19	28	48	38	range 15– 85
Dehydrotestosterone (ng/dl) [*]						
Male mean – 16	3	4	13	26	16	range 30–80
Female mean – 21	2–16	3–24	9–25	9–32		range 10–32
Androstenedione (nd/dl) [*]						
Male mean – 16	54	49	85	69	90	range 100–180
Female mean – 16	35	72	103	176	141	range 40–300
Dehydroepiandrosterone (ng/dl) [*]						
Male mean – 16	192	300	396	396	450	range 200–700
Female mean – 16	133	326	427	498	741	range 200–1500
Dehydroepiandrosterone sulfate (mg/dl) [*]						
Male mean – 33	42	63	73	103	123	range 125–300
Female mean – 33	43	49	71	86	120	range 125–300
Testosterone (ng/dl) [*]						
Male mean – 24	31	132	368	423	490	

[*] plasma   [**] serum   [++] 24 hour urine collection

9-6 Body Composition of Reference Adolescents

Body Composition of Reference Adolescents.

Age (years)	Height (cm)	Weight (kg)	Fat (kg)	Fat (%)	FFBM (kg)	Protein	Components of Fat-Free Body Mass (FFBM) (% of body weight)						FFBM Density (g/cm³)
							Water			Minerals		Carbohydrate	
							Total Body	Extracellular	Cellular	OM	NOM		
Males													
10.5	140.3	33.30	5.34	16.0	27.96	16.2	63.1	27.2	36.0	3.3	0.9	0.6	1.086
11.5	146.4	37.46	6.46	17.2	31.00	16.1	62.2	26.5	35.7	3.2	0.8	0.6	1.086
12.5	153.0	42.27	6.90	16.3	35.37	16.4	62.7	26.4	36.4	3.2	0.9	0.6	1.086
13.5	159.9	47.81	7.05	14.8	40.76	16.8	63.7	26.4	37.3	3.4	0.9	0.6	1.087
14.5	166.2	53.76	7.32	13.6	46.44	17.1	64.4	26.2	38.2	3.5	0.9	0.6	1.088
15.5	171.5	59.51	7.73	13.0	51.78	17.4	64.6	25.8	38.8	3.6	0.9	0.6	1.090
16.5	175.2	64.39	8.22	12.8	56.17	17.6	64.5	25.4	39.1	3.8	0.9	0.6	1.091
17.5	176.7	67.78	8.61	12.7	59.17	17.7	64.4	25.0	39.4	3.8	0.9	0.7	1.092
18.5	177.0	69.88	9.01	12.9	60.87	17.7	64.1	24.7	39.4	3.9	0.9	0.7	1.093
Females													
10.5	141.5	34.72	8.14	23.5	26.58	15.0	57.3	25.3	32.0	3.0	0.8	0.5	1.087
11.5	148.2	39.23	8.90	22.7	30.33	15.2	57.7	25.4	32.3	3.2	0.8	0.5	1.088
12.5	154.6	43.84	9.41	21.5	34.43	15.4	58.5	25.6	32.9	3.4	0.8	0.5	1.090
13.5	159.0	48.26	10.53	21.8	37.73	15.4	58.0	25.2	32.8	3.6	0.8	0.5	1.092
14.5	161.2	52.10	12.09	23.2	40.01	15.1	56.8	24.4	32.4	3.6	0.8	0.5	1.093
15.5	162.1	54.96	13.59	24.7	41.37	14.9	55.5	23.7	31.8	3.7	0.8	0.5	1.094
16.5	162.7	56.44	14.34	25.4	42.10	14.8	54.9	23.4	31.6	3.7	0.7	0.4	1.095
17.5	163.4	56.71	14.28	25.2	42.43	14.8	55.1	23.4	31.7	3.7	0.7	0.4	1.095
18.5	164.0	56.97	14.24	25.0	42.77	14.9	55.2	23.5	31.7	3.7	0.7	0.4	1.096

OM = osseous minerals, NOM = norosseous minerals

From Haschke, F.: Body Composition During Adolescence. In Klish, W. J. and Kretchmer, N. (Eds.): Body Composition Measurements in Infants and Children, Report of the Ninety-Eighth Ross Conference on Pediatric Research, Columbus, Ohio, Ross Laboratories, 1989, p. 78. Used with permission.

9-7   Multidimensional Eating Disorder Inventory

DRIVE FOR THINNESS: Subscale Items
I eat sweets and carbohydrates without feeling nervous.
I think about dieting.
I feel extremely guilty after overeating.
I am terrified of gaining weight
I exaggerate or magnify the importance of weight.
I am preoccupied with the desire to be thinner.
If I gain a pound, I worry that I will keep gaining.

INTEROCEPTIVE AWARENESS: Subscale Items
I get frightened when my feelings are too strong.
I get confused about what emotion I am feeling.
I can clearly identify what emotion I am feeling.
I don't know what's going on inside me.
I get confused as to whether or not I am hungry.
I worry that my feelings will get out of control.
I feel bloated after eating a small meal.
When I am upset, I don't know if I am sad, frightened
or angry.
I have feelings I can't quite identify.
When I am upset, I worry that I will start eating.

BULIMIA: Subscale Items
I eat when I am upset.
I stuff myself with food.
I have gone on eating binges where I have felt that I
could not stop.
I thing about bingeing (overeating).
I eat moderately in front of others and stuff myself
when they're gone.
I have the thought of trying to vomit in order to lose
weight.
I eat or drink in secrecy.

BODY DISSATISFACTION: Subscale Item
I think that my stomach is too big.
I think that my thighs are too large.
I think that my stomach is just the right size.
I feel satisfied with the shape of my body.
I like the shape of my buttocks.
I think my hips are too big.
I think that my thighs are just the right size.
I think my buttocks are too large.
I think that my hips are just the right size.

INEFFECTIVENESS: Subscale Items
I feel ineffective as a person.
I feel alone in the world.
I feel generally in control of things in my life.
I wish I were someone else.
I feel inadequate.
I feel secure about myself.
I have a low opinion of myself.
I feel that I can achieve my standards.
I feel that I am a worthwhile person.
I feel empty inside (emotionally).

MATURITY FEARS: Subscale Items
I wish that I could return to the security of childhood.
I wish that I could be younger.
The happiest time in life is when you are a child.
I would rather be an adult than a child.
The demands of adulthood are too great.
I feel happy that I am not a child anymore.
I feel that people are happiest when they are children.
The best years of your life are when you become an adult.

PERFECTIONISM: Subscale Items
Only outstanding performance is good enough in
my family.
As a child, I tried very hard to avoid disappointing
my parents and teachers.
I hate being less than best at things.
My parents have expected excellence of me.
I feel that I must do things perfectly or not do them
at all.
I have extremely high goals.

INTERPERSONAL DISTRUST: Subscale Items
I am open about my feelings.
I trust others.
I can communicate with others easily.
I have close relationships.
I have trouble expressing my emotions to others.
I need to keep people at a certain distance (feel
uncomfortable if someone tries to get too close).
I can talk about personal thoughts or feelings.

Adapted from: Garner, D. M., Olmstead, M. P., and Polivy, J.: Development and validation of a multidimensional eating disorder inventory for anorexia nervosa and bulimia. Int'l J Eating Disorders, 2(2):15, 1989.

9-8 Eating Attitudes Test

SELF

1. Am terrified about being overweight.
2. Avoid eating when I am hungry.
3. Find myself preoccupied with food.
4. Have gone on eating binges where I feel that I may not be able to stop.
5. Cut my food into small pieces.
6. Am aware of the calorie content of foods that I eat.
7. Particularly avoid foods with a high carbohydrate content (e.g. bread, rice, potatoes, etc.).
8. Feel that others would prefer if I ate more.
9. Vomit after I eat.
10. Feel extremely guilty after eating.
11. Am preoccupied with a desire to be thinner.
12. Think about burning calories when I exercise.
13. Other people think that I am too thin.
14. Am preoccupied with the thought of having fat on my body.
15. Take longer than others to eat my meals.
16. Avoid foods with sugar in them.
17. Eat diet foods.
18. Feel that food controls my life.
19. Display self-control around food.
20. Feel that others pressure me to eat.
21. Give too much time and thought to food.
22. Feel uncomfortable after eating sweets.
23. Engage in dieting behavior.
24. Like my stomach to be empty.
25. Enjoy trying new rich foods.
26. Have the impulse to vomit after meals.
27. Exercise to prevent weight gain.
28. Use laxatives or diuretics to prevent weight gain.

PARENT

1. Is terrified about being overweight.
2. Avoids eating when she is hungry.
3. Is preoccupied with food.
4. Has gone on eating binges where she is not able to stop.
5. Cuts her food into small pieces.
6. Is aware of the calorie content of foods that she eats.
7. Particularly avoids foods with a high carbohydrate content (e.g. bread, rice, potatoes, etc).
8. Feels that others would prefer if she ate more.
9. Vomits after she eats.
10. Feels extremely guilty after eating.
11. Is preoccupied with a desire to be thinner.
12. Thinks about burning up calories when she exercises.
13. Feels other eople think she is too thin.
14. Is preoccupied with the thought of having fat on her body.
15. Takes longer than others to eat her meals.
16. Avoids foods with sugar in them.
17. Eats diet foods.
18. Feels that food controls her life.
19. Displays self-control around food.
20. Feels that others pressure her to eat.
21. Gives too much time and thought to food.
22. Feels uncomfortable after eating sweets.
23. Engages in dieting behavior.
24. Likes her stomach to be empty.
25. Enjoys trying new rich foods.
26. Has the impulse to vomit after meals.
27. Exercises to prevent weight gain.
28. Uses laxatives or diuretics to prevent weight gain.

0 = Never   1 = Rarely   2 = Sometimes   3 = Often   4 = Usually   5 = Always

Adapted from: Kagan, D. M. and Squires, R. L.: Eating disorders among adolescents: patterns and prevalence. Adolesc, 19(73):15, 1984. Kagan, D. M. and Squires, R. L.: Dieting, compulsive eating and feelings of failure among adolescents. Int'l J Eating Disorders, 3(1):15, 1983.

9-9 Depression Inventory (Symptoms, Attitude, Categories)

A (Mood)
0 I do not feel sad
1 I feel blue or sad
2a I am blue or sad all the time and I can't snap out of it
2b I am so sad or unhappy that it is very painful
3 I am so sad or unhappy that I can't stand it

B (Pessimism)
0 I am not particularly pessimistic or discouraged about the future
1a I feel discouraged about the future
2a I feel I have nothing to look forward to
2b I feel that I won't ever get over my troubles
3 I feel that the future is hopeless and that things cannot improve

C (Sense of Failure)
0 I do not feel like a failure
1 I feel I have failed more than the average person
2a I feel I have accomplished very little that is worthwhile or that means anything
2b As I look back on my life all I can see is a lot of failures
3 I feel I am a complete failure as a person (parent, husband, wife)

D (Lack of Satisfaction)
0 I am not particularly dissatisfied
1a I feel bored most of the time
1b I don't enjoy things the way I used to
2 I don't get satisfaction out of anything any more
3 I am dissatisfied with everything

E (Guilty Feeling)
0 I don't feel particularly guilty
1 I feel bad or unworthy a good part of the time
2a I feel quite guilty
2b I feel bad or unworthy practically all the time now
3 I feel as though I am very bad or worthless

F (Sense of Punishment)
0 I don't feel I am being punished
1 I feel that something bad may happen to me
2 I feel I am being punished or will be punished
3a I feel I deserve to be punished
3b I want to be punished

G (Self Hate)
0 I don't feel disappointed in myself
1a I am disappointed in myself
1b I don't like myself
2 I am disgusted with myself
3 I hate myself

H (Self Accusations)
0 I don't feel I am any worse than anybody else
1 I am very critical of myself for my weaknesses or mistakes
2a I blame myself for everything that goes wrong

I (Self-Punitive Thoughts)
0 I don't have any thought of harming myself
1 I have thoughts of harming myself but I would not carry them out
2a I feel I would be better off dead
2b I have definite plans about committing suicide
2c I feel my family would be better off if I were dead
3 I would kill myself if I could

J (Crying Spells)
0 I don't cry any more than usual
1 I cry more now than I used to
2 I cry all the time now. I can't stop it
3 I used to be able to cry but now I can't cry at all even though I want to

K (Irritability)
0 I am no more irritated now that I ever am
1 I get annoyed or irritated more easily than I used to
2 I feel irritated all the time now
3 I don't get irritated at all the things that used to irritate me

L (Social Withdrawal)
0 I have not lost interest in other people
1 I am less interested in other people now than I used to be
2 I have lost all my interest in other people and have little feeling for them
3 I have lost all my interest in other people and don't care about them at all

M (Indecisiveness)
0 I make decisions about as well as ever
1 I am less sure of myself now try to put off making decisions
2 I can't make decisions at all without help
3 I can't make any decisions at all any more

N (Body Image)
0 I don't feel I look any worse than I used to
1 I am worried that I am looking old or unattractive
2 I feel that there are permanent changes in my appearance and they make me look unattractive
3 I feel that I am ugly or repulsive looking

O (Work Inhibition)
0 I can work about as well as before
1a It takes extra effort to get started at doing something
1b I don't work as well as I used to
2 I have to push myself very hard to do anything
3 I can't do any work at all

P (Sleep Disturbance)
0 I can sleep as well as usual
1 I wake up more tired in the morning than I used to
2 I wake up 1–2 hours earlier than usual and find it hard to get back to sleep
3 I wake up early every day and can't get more than 5 hours sleep

Q (Fatigability)
0 I don't get any more tired than usual
1 I get tired more easily than I used to
2 I get tired from doing anything
3 I get too tired to do anything

R (Loss of Appetite)
0 My appetite is no worse than usual
1 My appetite is not as good as it used to be
2 My appetite is much worse now
3 I have no appetite at all any more

S (Weight Loss)
0 I haven't lost much weight, if any, lately
1 I have lost more than 5 pounds
2 I have lost more than 10 pounds
3 I have lost more than 15 pounds

T (Somatic Preoccupation)
1 I am no more concerned about my health than usual
1 I am concerned about aches and pains or upset stomach or constipation or other unpleasant feelings in my body
2 I am so concerned with how I feel or what I feel that it's hard to think of much else
3 I am completely absorbed in what I feel

U (Loss of Libido)
0 I have not noticed any recent change in my interest in sex
1 I am less interested in sex than I used to be
2 I am much less interested in sex now
3 I have lost interest in sex completely

*Scoring: None, mild, moderate, severe
Adapted from: Beck, A.T., Ward, C.H., Mendelson, M., Mock, J., and Erbaugh, J.: An inventory for measuring depression. Arch Gen Psychiatry 4:53, 1961.

9–10 Twelve Step Approach for Eating Disorders and Questionnaire on Health and Nutrition for the Homeless

TWELVE STEP APPROACH FOR EATING DISORDERS

1. Admit being powerless over food

2. Request power within self to restore self to sanity.

3. Make decisions to turn life over to God.

4. Make searching and fearless inventory of self.

5. Confess to God, self, and another person that eating habits are bad.

6. Be entirely ready to ask God to remove all defects of character.

7. Humbly ask God to remove all shortcomings.

8. Make a list of all people harmed and make willing amends.

9. Make direct amends.

10. Continue to take personal inventory, and admit any wrong doings.

11. Seek through prayer and meditation a conscience which is content with God.

12. Having had a spiritual awakening, try to carry this message to other people with eating disorders and practice these principles in all affairs.

From: Devlin, C. L., Twelve Step Approach Intervention in Compulsive Eating. *J Am Diet Assoc*, 1991:A186.

Percentage of 96 homeless persons answering "yes" to questions on a health and nutrition questionnaire.

Question	Yes %
1. Do you have enough to eat?	90
2. Do you have a good appetite?	73
3. Are there cooking facilities available to you?	43
4. How many meals do you prepare for yourself per day?	
0 meals	57
1 meal	16
2–3 meals	27
5. Do you have any money to buy food? How much per week?	
0 dollars	15
20 dollars	31
21–50 dollars	38
51 dollars or more	16
6. Have you been told by an M.D. that you should or should not eat particular foods?	52
7. If yes, are you able to follow this diet?	48
8. Do you smoke cigarettes?	65
9. Do you drink alcohol?	32
10. Do you use street drugs?	5
11. Do you use vitamin supplements?	47
12. Has your weight changed over the past year?	58
If yes, did it go up?	47
Or, did it go down?	53
13. Do you have any medical conditions?	89
If yes, are you taking medications for these conditions?	98

From: Luder, E., Cupens-Okado, E., Karen-Roth, A., Martinez-Weber, C. Health and nutrition survey in a group of urban homeless adults. *J Am Diet Assoc*, 1990, 90:1387.

Appendix 10
Adult Nutrition Records and Nutrition Values

10–1 Nutrition Assessment Summary, Adult

NUTRITION TODAY

By _____

Individual Patient
Nutritional Assessment Summary © *

PATIENT _____

INSTITUTION _____

DATE _____

Triceps Skin-fold	% of standard	——
Mid Upper Arm Circum.	% of standard	——

Mid Upper Arm Muscle Circumference
(Mid Arm Circum. cm-πx Triceps Skinfold
cm) (N adult male 25.3, female

23.2 cm)	% of standard	——
Albumin	% of standard	——

Height/Creatinine mg/24 hrs/cm Height
(See tables on reverse side for normal values for males
and females of ideal weight for their height, of urinary
creatinine/cm body height.)

Height/Creatinine	% of standard	——

Total Lymphocyte Count
(Should be 1,500/mm³)   ——   /mm³

Total Lymphocyte Count   % of standard   ——

Transferrin
(or TIBC level)   % of standard   ——

Cellular Immunity Skin Testing

	Reactive	Unre-active
PPD (0.1 mg, 5 Tuberculin units)	——	——
Candida (Hollister-Stier)	——	——
DNCB	——	——

Assessment of CMI—adequate .... Impaired ....

SUMMARY (CHECK)

STANDARD PARAMETERS	>90%	60-90%	<60%
Weight/Height			
Triceps Skinfold			
Mid Arm Circumference			
Mid Arm Muscle Circum.			
Albumin			
Height/Creatinine			
Lymphocyte Count			
Transferrin			
Cellular Immunity			

Other Risk Factors: Absent   Present

Vitamin Deficiency
a. Clinical Signs
b. Laboratory Evidence

Mineral or Electrolyte
Imbalance
a. Clinical Signs
b. Laboratory Evidence

Drug-Nutrient-Hormone
Interaction

General Assessment
(Socio-Economic, Habits,
Behavior, Underlying
Diagnosis, etc.)

Types of Protein-Calorie Malnutrition   (Check):

Acute Visceral Attrition ("Kwashiorkor-like")
(Wt/Ht, TSF, MUAC, MUAMC, Ht/Creat, Preserved;
alb and transferrin acutely depressed)   ☐

Chronic Depletion of Parietal Muscle & Fat
("Adult Marasmus")
(Wt/Ht, TSF, MUAC, MUAMC, Ht/Creat, depressed;
Alb and Transferrin preserved until late)   ☐

**Acute Visceral Attrition Superimposed on Chronic
Depletion of Muscle & Fat**
(Advanced PCM:)
(Wt/Ht, TSF, MUAC, MUAMC, Ht/Creat, Alb, Trans-
ferrin, Lymphocytes, Immunity, all depressed)   ☐

Other Nutritional Disorders   (Check):
Vitamin Deficiency   ☐
Specify Predominant Syndromes,
Or if multiple, so state
Mineral or Electrolyte Imbalance   ☐
(e.g. Iron, Calcium, Magnesium, Phosphorus, Zinc,
Sodium, Potassium, etc.)
Specify

PRIMARY DIAGNOSIS

*From "Hospital Malnutrition and Nutritional Assessment," Nutrition Today
10:8 (March/April) '75. This form is copyrighted by Nutrition Today, Inc., 101
Ridgely Ave., Annapolis, Md. 21404. Available in pads of 100 sheets each at
$4.00 a pad, postpaid. Nutrition Today Society members entitled to 10
percent discount. Payment must accompany order.

10-2 Adult Indepth Nutrition Record, UACCDD, CHMC

NAME: _____ ADDRESS: _____
BIRTHDATE: _____ TELEPHONE: _____
AGE: _____ WORK HOURS: _____
MARITAL STATUS: _____ DATE SEEN: _____
OCCUPATION: _____

BACKGROUND INFORMATION: Current Diagnosis: _____
PARENTS: DIED FROM AT AGE Sex: ___ Race: ___
  Mother _____ Interviewer: _____
  Father _____
SIBLINGS:
  Brother/s _____
  Sister/s _____

ANTHROPOMETRIC MEASUREMENTS:
          Present   Ideal
Ht. cm _____
Wt. kg _____
Wt. loss or gain (circle one) in 6 mo. _____
Amt. (kg.) _____

$\frac{\text{Usual weight} - \text{Current Weight}}{\text{Usual Weight}} \times 100 = $ ___ % wt. loss

Upper arm circ. ___ cm Pulse rate ___
Fatfold tricep ___ mm B.P. ___
Muscle mass ___ cm
Bone Age ___ Bone density ___

CHEMISTRY:
Hb. ___ Hct. ___ CBC ___
Transferin ___ Urinalysis ___
TG ___ Serum Albumin ___
Chol. ___ Blood Sugar ___
Kidney ___ Chest ___ Stomach ___
Eyes ___ Hearing ___

CLINICAL/PHYSICAL DATA (check if appropriate)
Chronic Diseases
Cancer ___
Chronic Liver Disease ___
Chronic Renal Disease ___
Coronary Artery Disease ___
Diabetes Mellitus ___
Hypertension ___

INTERDISCIPLINARY FINDINGS:
Dental: ___
Gross Motor: ___
Speech: ___
Hx. Infections: ___

Recent Major Surgery or Illness ___
Type of Surgery Performed ___
Increased Metabolic Needs:
  burns ___
  fever ___
  infection ___
  trauma ___

Increased Losses:
  burns ___
  draining abscesses ___
  draining fistulas ___
  open wounds ___

Gastrointestinal Function:
Dysgeusian ___ Dysphasia ___
Enteric Fistula ___
Head/neck cancer-radiation or trauma ___
Inflammatory bowel disease ___
Mechanical Obstruction of GI tract ___
Persistent diarrhea ___ or vomiting ___

PRESENT FEEDING ABILITIES:
Table foods ___ Chpd. foods ___ Jr. Foods ___ Strained ___
Length of Normal Feeding Period ___
Circle: Choking, Swallowing, Chewing, Tongue Thrust, Constipation, Anorexia

---

Name: _____

DIETARY EVALUATION

FOOD INTAKE (24 Hr. Recall)

Patterns:

	Breakfast	Amt.
Time	Fruit	
	Meat	
	Egg	
	Bread	
	Fat	
Where	Cereal	
With Whom	Beverage	
	Other	
Who Prepared		

	Lunch	
Time	Meat	
	Veg.	
Where	Bread	
	Fruit	
With Whom	Beverage	
	Other	
Who Prepared		

	Dinner	
Time	Soup	
	Meat or subst.	
Where	Potato	
With Whom	Vegetable: Cooked / Raw	
	Salad	
Who Prepared	Bread	
	Fat	
	Dessert	
	Beverage	
	Other	

Between Meals
Time: _____

Alcohol ___ Smoking ___
How much salt is used at each meal ___
Vit. & Mineral Supp. ___
Drugs: ___
Income ___ Spent on Food ___ /wk.mo.

Are you using iodized salt? ___ Are you using vitamin D fortified milk? ___
Are you on food stamp or supplemental food program? ___
Favorite Foods ___ What foods do you believe are good for you? ___
(religion, region, nationality, illness, special diet, allergies, etc.)
affecting the diet? ___ Foods regularly omitted ___

FOOD SUMMARY

GROUP	Amt. per day	Amt. per week	Possible points or daily serv.	**Actual Points
Dairy Products:				
Milk			3	
Cheese				
Cottage Cheese				
Yogurt				
Other				
Meat or Alternates:*** Fat & Chol.2				
***Meat, Eggs				
Fish, Poultry				
Dr. Beans/peas				
Peanut Butter				
Vegetables: (No Vit. A/C-1/2 cr)			3	
Vit A Veg.				
Vit C Veg.				
Other				
Fruits:			2	
Vit C Fruit				
Other Fruits				
Whole Grains/Starches: (No w/grains-1/2 cr)			6	
Cereal				
Bread				
Pasta, Rice				
Other		TOTAL	16	
Others:				
Candy/Sugar			If daily-1	
Chips/t. salt			If daily-1	
Soft Drinks			If daily-1	
Desserts			If daily-1	
Water			None daily-1	
***Fats & Chol.			3 ser. d.-1	
Fiber			None daily-1	
			TOTAL	

Frequency/wk. of eating outside the home: _____
Food allergies: _____
Foods regularly ommitted: _____ Why: _____

Favorite Foods: _____
Impression of diet: _____
Validity of record: _____
Activity Score: _____

Fig. 10-2. (Continued)

NUTRITIONAL CLINICAL EVALUATION

Code: 0 = absent; 1 = present; 2 = does not apply
Code Doubtful
Code Doubtful

Hair:
all — dry
neg. — dispigmented
— easily pluckable
— abnormal texture

Eyes:
all — cloudy
neg. — reddened
— dry

Lips:
all — angular lesions
neg. — angular scars

Gums:
all — swelling
neg. — redness
— hypertrophy
— bleeding

Teeth:
all — visible caries
neg. — missing teeth
— calculus
— mottling
— striated discoloration
— malocclusion

Tongue:
all — glossy
neg. — fissures
— magenta
— geographic

Nails:
all — clubbed
neg. — ridged
— spooned
— blue
— combinations

Face & Neck:
all — thyroid enlarged
neg. — facial stigmata
— of syndrome

Skin:
all — follicular
neg. — hyperkeratosis
— hyperpigmentation
— dry and scaling
— cold
— dispigmentation

Skeletal or Muscular:
all — protuberant
neg. — abdomen
— bowed legs
— knocked-knees
— beading of ribs
— enlargement of
— wrist
— winged scapula
— scoliosis
— muscle wasting

Lower Extremities:
all — pretibial edema
neg.

General Appearance: Circle if appropriate
skinny — ambulatory
fat — nonambulatory
well proportioned — no speech
alert — unintelligible speech
apathetic — intelligible speech
irritable — poor feeding behavior
uncooperative — very active

Parent-Child Interaction
— Appropriate — Slight
— Moderate — None

PHYSICAL ACTIVITY RECORDS
Estimation of Caloric Needs

WEIGHT: kg. _____ (lbs.) _____ %ile _____ Caloric Input _____

HEIGHT: cm. _____ (in.) _____ %ile _____ Caloric Output _____

RDA calorie average for ages _____ to _____ = _____

RDA range for age _____ - _____

A. Record the following activities as accurately as possible:

Activity	Time in Hours	Calories/ lb./hr.	Total per lb.
1. Sleeping		x 0.4 =	
2. Sitting at rest (watching TV, reading, etc.)		x 0.7 =	
3. Sitting (Hand activities, i.e., playing with toys)		x 1.0 =	
4. Walking with crutches		x 1.5 =	
5. Walking with crutches, total self care		x 2.0 =	
6. Walking doing light exercise (playground walking, sandbox playing, swinging)		x 2.0 =	
7. Moderate exercise (active games, i.e., playing ball, stair climbing dancing)		x 2.7 =	
8. Strenuous exercise (running, swimming, bicycle riding, etc.)		x 4.3 =	
	Total 24		TOTAL

Calorie Output (total per lb. x weight in lbs.): _____
Optional:

B. Recommended kcal. per cm. height: _____ x height (cm) = _____ kcal/day
(use only for children with motor dysfunction, ages 5-12.)
(ambulatory, motor dysfunction, 13.9 cal/cm.)
(nonambulatory, severe motor dysfunction, 11.1 cal/cm.)
Caretaker demonstrates knowledge of relationship of calories to physical activity: YES/NO

Fig. 10-2. (Continued)

ADULT
Nutritional Assessment (Case Workup) Evaluation
Nutrition Record Summary

Evaluation

Demographic Data
  anthropometric data   9
  family data
  lab data

Pertinent Nutritional History   6
  medication and disease history
  diet history

Current Nutritional and Feeding Status   27
  present dietary pattern
  any neurological impairment that affects feeding
  physical activity
  socioeconomic problems
  presenting nutrition problem
  anthropometric - height, weight, skinfold, circumference

Biochemical   16
  medications, drug interaction, nutrition supplements lab data

Clinical Observations   12
  physical signs and symptoms/overt signs of poor nutrition
  feeding skill evaluation
  behavioral problems
  interaction with people

Impressions   12
  1. Height and weight, percentiles and statements to reflect
     nutritional status such as thin or overweight, etc.
  2. Adequacy of diet expressed in nutrients.
  3. Feeding skills level.

Recommendations   18
  1. Good nutrition-translation of low or excessive nutrients into
     appropriate food sources.
  2. Food planning, purchasing and preparation suggestions.
  3. Social interaction - suggestions in eating or techniques in feeding.
  4. Physical activity suggestions.
  5. Follow up or disposition of case.

10-3 Weight for Height—Males and Females, 18-74 Years

Weight (lbs.) For Height (in.), Males

Height in inches	Percentile	18-24	25-34	35-44	45-54	55-64	65-74
62 inches	50	130	141	143	147	143	143
	15	102	109	115	118	113	116
	5	85	91	98	100	96	100
63 inches	50	135	145	148	152	147	147
	15	107	113	120	123	117	120
	5	90	95	103	105	100	104
64 inches	50	140	150	153	156	153	151
	15	112	118	125	127	123	124
	5	95	100	108	109	106	108
65 inches	50	145	156	158	160	158	156
	15	117	124	130	131	128	129
	5	100	106	113	113	111	113
66 inches	50	150	160	163	164	163	160
	15	122	128	135	135	133	133
	5	105	110	118	117	116	117
67 inches	50	154	165	169	169	168	164
	15	126	133	141	140	138	137
	5	109	115	124	122	121	121
68 inches	50	159	170	174	173	173	169
	15	131	138	146	144	143	142
	5	114	120	129	126	126	126
69 inches	50	164	174	179	177	178	173
	15	136	142	151	148	148	146
	5	119	124	134	130	131	130
70 inches	50	168	179	184	182	183	177
	15	140	147	156	153	153	150
	5	123	129	139	135	136	134
71 inches	50	173	184	190	187	189	182
	15	145	152	162	158	159	155
	5	128	134	145	140	142	139
72 inches	50	178	189	194	191	193	186
	15	150	157	166	162	163	159
	5	133	139	149	144	146	143
73 inches	50	183	194	200	196	197	190
	15	155	162	172	167	167	163
	5	138	144	155	149	150	147
74 inches	50	188	199	205	200	203	194
	15	160	167	177	171	173	167
	5	143	149	160	153	156	150

Weight (lbs.) For Height (in.), Females

Height in inches	Percentile	18-24	25-34	35-44	45-54	55-64	65-74
57 inches	50	114	118	125	129	132	130
	15	85	85	89	94	97	100
	5	68	65	67	73	77	82
58 inches	50	117	121	129	133	136	134
	15	88	88	93	98	101	104
	5	71	68	71	77	81	86
59 inches	50	120	125	133	136	140	137
	15	91	92	97	101	105	107
	5	74	72	75	80	85	89
60 inches	50	123	128	137	140	143	140
	15	94	95	101	105	108	110
	5	77	75	79	84	88	92
61 inches	50	126	132	141	143	147	144
	15	97	99	105	108	112	114
	5	80	79	83	87	92	96
62 inches	50	129	136	144	147	150	147
	15	100	103	108	112	115	117
	5	83	83	86	91	95	99
63 inches	50	132	139	148	150	153	151
	15	103	106	112	115	118	121
	5	86	86	90	94	98	103
64 inches	50	135	142	152	154	157	154
	15	106	109	116	119	122	124
	5	89	89	94	98	102	106
65 inches	50	138	146	156	158	160	158
	15	109	113	120	123	125	128
	5	92	93	98	102	105	110
66 inches	50	141	150	159	161	164	161
	15	112	117	123	126	129	131
	5	95	97	101	105	109	113
67 inches	50	144	153	163	165	167	165
	15	115	120	127	130	132	135
	5	98	100	105	109	112	117
68 inches	50	147	157	167	168	171	169
	15	118	124	131	133	136	139
	5	101	104	109	112	116	121

From: **Weight by Height and Age for Adults 18-74 Years: U. S. 1971-74, National Health Survey. Vital Health Statistics Series 11, No. 208, U. S. Dept. Health, Education, and Welfare, P.H.S., 1979** and 15th percentile Bishop, C. W., Bowen, P. E., Ritchey, S. J.: Norms for nutritional anthropometry of Americans and adults by upper arm anthropometry. _Am J Clin Nutr_, 34:2530, 1981. Used with permission.

10—4 Elbow Breadth/Percentiles 1-75 Years, and Elbow Breadth/Stature Index for Frame Size, 18-75 Years

Age (yrs)	Percentiles								
	5	10	15	25	50	75	85	90	95
Males									
1.0–1.9	36.0	37.0	37.0	39.0	40.0	42.0	43.0	44.0	45.0
2.0–2.9	38.0	39.0	40.0	41.0	42.0	44.0	45.0	46.0	47.0
3.0–3.9	40.0	41.0	42.0	43.0	44.0	46.0	47.0	48.0	50.0
4.0–4.9	42.0	43.0	43.0	44.0	46.0	48.0	49.0	50.0	52.0
5.0–5.9	43.0	44.0	45.0	46.0	48.0	50.0	51.0	52.0	53.0
6.0–6.9	45.0	46.0	47.0	48.0	50.0	52.0	54.0	55.0	56.0
7.0–7.9	47.0	48.0	49.0	49.0	52.0	54.0	55.0	56.0	57.0
8.0–8.9	48.0	49.0	50.0	51.0	54.0	56.0	57.0	58.0	60.0
9.0–9.9	50.0	51.0	52.0	53.0	56.0	58.0	60.0	61.0	63.0
10.0–10.9	51.0	53.0	54.0	56.0	58.0	60.0	62.0	63.0	65.0
11.0–11.9	53.0	54.0	56.0	57.0	60.0	62.0	64.0	65.0	67.0
12.0–12.9	55.0	57.0	58.0	60.0	63.0	66.0	68.0	68.0	72.0
13.0–13.9	59.0	61.0	61.0	63.0	66.0	69.0	71.0	72.0	74.0
14.0–14.9	62.0	64.0	64.0	66.0	69.0	71.0	73.0	74.0	75.0
15.0–15.9	63.0	64.0	65.0	67.0	70.0	72.0	74.0	75.0	77.0
16.0–16.9	64.0	66.0	66.0	68.0	70.0	73.0	74.0	76.0	77.0
17.0–17.9	64.0	66.0	67.0	68.0	71.0	73.0	75.0	76.0	77.0
18.0–24.9	65.0	66.0	67.0	69.0	71.0	74.0	76.0	76.0	78.0
25.0–29.9	65.0	67.0	68.0	69.0	72.0	74.0	76.0	77.0	78.0
30.0–34.9	65.0	67.0	68.0	70.0	72.0	75.0	77.0	77.0	79.0
35.0–39.9	66.0	67.0	69.0	70.0	73.0	76.0	77.0	78.0	80.0
40.0–44.9	67.0	68.0	69.0	70.0	73.0	76.0	78.0	78.0	80.0
45.0–49.9	66.0	68.0	69.0	71.0	73.0	76.0	77.0	78.0	80.0
50.0–54.9	67.0	68.0	70.0	71.0	73.0	76.0	78.0	78.0	81.0
55.0–59.9	67.0	68.0	69.0	71.0	73.0	77.0	78.0	80.0	81.0
60.0–64.9	67.0	68.0	69.0	71.0	73.0	76.0	78.0	79.0	81.0
65.0–69.9	66.0	68.0	69.0	71.0	73.0	76.0	78.0	79.0	81.0
70.0–74.9	67.0	68.0	69.0	71.0	73.0	76.0	78.0	79.0	81.0
Females									
1.0–1.9	34.0	35.0	36.0	37.0	39.0	41.0	42.0	42.0	43.0
2.0–2.9	36.0	37.0	38.0	39.0	41.0	42.0	44.0	44.0	45.0
3.0–3.9	38.0	39.0	40.0	41.0	43.0	44.0	45.0	46.0	47.0
4.0–4.9	40.0	41.0	41.0	42.0	44.0	46.0	47.0	48.0	49.0
5.0–5.9	42.0	43.0	43.0	44.0	46.0	48.0	49.0	50.0	51.0
6.0–6.9	43.0	44.0	45.0	46.0	48.0	50.0	51.0	52.0	53.0
7.0–7.9	44.0	45.0	46.0	48.0	50.0	52.0	53.0	54.0	55.0
8.0–8.9	46.0	47.0	48.0	49.0	51.0	54.0	55.0	56.0	58.0
9.0–9.9	48.0	50.0	50.0	51.0	54.0	56.0	57.0	59.0	60.0
10.0–10.9	50.0	51.0	51.0	53.0	55.0	58.0	60.0	61.0	62.0
11.0–11.9	52.0	53.0	53.0	55.0	58.0	61.0	63.0	63.0	64.0
12.0–12.9	54.0	55.0	55.0	57.0	59.0	61.0	62.0	64.0	65.0
13.0–13.9	54.0	55.0	56.0	57.0	60.0	62.0	63.0	64.0	66.0
14.0–14.9	55.0	56.0	57.0	58.0	60.0	62.0	64.0	65.0	66.0
15.0–15.9	54.0	56.0	57.0	58.0	61.0	63.0	65.0	66.0	66.0
16.0–16.9	55.0	56.0	57.0	58.0	61.0	63.0	65.0	66.0	67.0
17.0–17.9	54.0	56.0	57.0	59.0	61.0	64.0	64.0	66.0	67.0
18.0–24.9	55.0	56.0	57.0	59.0	61.0	63.0	65.0	66.0	68.0
25.0–29.9	55.0	57.0	57.0	59.0	62.0	64.0	65.0	66.0	69.0
30.0–34.9	56.0	57.0	58.0	60.0	62.0	65.0	66.0	67.0	69.0
35.0–39.9	56.0	58.0	59.0	60.0	63.0	65.0	66.0	68.0	70.0
40.0–44.9	57.0	58.0	59.0	61.0	63.0	66.0	67.0	68.0	70.0
45.0–49.9	57.0	59.0	60.0	61.0	63.0	66.0	68.0	69.0	71.0
50.0–54.9	57.0	59.0	60.0	61.0	64.0	67.0	68.0	69.0	71.0
55.0–59.9	58.0	59.0	60.0	62.0	64.0	67.0	69.0	70.0	72.0
60.0–64.9	58.0	60.0	61.0	62.0	64.0	67.0	69.0	70.0	72.0
65.0–69.9	58.0	59.0	60.0	61.0	64.0	67.0	69.0	70.0	72.0
70.0–74.9	58.0	60.0	60.0	62.0	64.0	67.0	69.0	71.0	72.0

Categories of frame size derived with reference to Frame Index 2 [[elbow breadth (mm) / stature (cm)] x 100], by age and by height

Frame Index 2 = [elbow breadth (mm) / stature (cm)] x 100

Frame Index 1: elbow breadth (mm)

Age (yrs.)	Male			Female		
	Small	Medium	Large	Small	Medium	Large
18.0–24.9	<38.4	38.4 to 41.6	>41.6	<35.2	35.2 to 38.6	>38.6
25.0–29.9	<38.6	38.6 to 41.8	>41.8	<35.7	35.7 to 38.7	>38.7
30.0–34.9	<38.6	38.6 to 42.1	>42.1	<35.7	35.7 to 39.0	>39.0
35.0–39.9	<39.1	39.1 to 42.4	>42.4	<36.2	36.2 to 39.8	>39.8
40.0–44.9	<39.3	39.3 to 42.5	>42.5	<36.7	36.7 to 40.2	>40.2
45.0–45.9	<39.6	39.6 to 43.0	>43.0	<36.7	37.2 to 40.7	>40.7
50.0–54.9	<39.9	39.9 to 43.3	>43.3	<37.2	37.2 to 41.6	>41.6
55.0–59.9	<40.2	40.2 to 43.8	>43.8	<37.8	37.8 to 41.9	>41.9
60.0–64.9	<40.2	40.2 to 43.6	>43.6	<38.2	38.2 to 41.8	>41.8
65.0–69.9	<40.2	40.2 to 43.6	>43.6	<38.2	38.2 to 41.8	>41.8
70.0–74.9	<40.2	40.2 to 43.6	>43.6	<38.2	38.2 to 41.8	>41.8

Frame Index 2: Elbow breadth by height

Height (cm)	Male			Female		
	Small	Medium	Large	Small	Medium	Large
141–146	—	—	—	<56	56 to 61	>61
147–152	—	—	—	<57	57 to 62	>62
153–158	<66	66 to 70	>70	<60	60 to 63	>63
159–164	<66	66 to 71	>71	<61	61 to 65	>65
165–170	<68	68 to 72	>72	<61	61 to 65	>65
171–176	<70	70 to 73	>73	<62	62 to 65	>65
177–182	<71	71 to 75	>75	<62	62 to 66	>66
183–188	<71	71 to 76	>76	—	—	—
189–194	<73	73 to 76	>76	—	—	—

Modified from Frisancho, A.R.: Anthropometric Standards for the Assessment of Growth and Nutritional Status, Ann Arbor, The University of Michigan Press, 1990.

10–5 Percentile Weight by Frame Size, Adults

Males

Age (yrs)	5	10	15	25	50	75	85	90	95
Males with small frames									
18.0–24.9	54.5	57.4	59.8	63.2	69.3	76.4	81.0	83.9	89.6
25.0–29.9	57.9	60.9	62.1	66.1	73.1	81.6	85.8	88.3	97.9
30.0–34.9	59.6	63.0	65.1	68.4	75.4	83.3	87.0	91.5	97.6
35.0–39.9	56.6	61.7	63.3	67.9	76.5	83.9	88.6	91.6	96.0
40.0–44.9	62.3	64.6	68.8	71.9	77.6	87.4	93.0	96.8	101.3
45.0–49.9	58.8	62.3	63.8	68.3	76.8	84.1	89.4	92.6	96.4
50.0–54.9	57.3	62.8	65.2	67.5	75.4	83.0	88.2	90.5	99.4
55.0–59.9	54.0	58.2	61.8	66.4	75.1	81.5	87.2	90.9	94.7
60.0–64.9	56.4	60.2	62.5	65.8	73.6	80.8	85.7	88.4	93.3
65.0–69.9	51.1	56.0	59.0	62.9	71.4	79.9	84.1	86.8	91.8
70.0–74.9	50.1	54.5	58.7	62.6	70.5	78.1	82.6	84.9	92.2
Males with medium frames									
18.0–24.9	57.9	60.8	62.4	65.9	72.3	81.0	87.0	93.1	100.5
25.0–29.9	59.5	63.0	65.2	69.3	76.7	84.6	88.9	93.2	100.7
30.0–34.9	60.0	63.4	66.2	69.7	78.1	85.7	91.6	94.0	99.1
35.0–39.9	60.9	66.3	69.8	73.7	80.6	87.1	91.5	94.6	101.6
40.0–44.9	61.2	65.3	68.4	72.5	79.9	88.4	93.4	97.8	102.6
45.0–49.9	60.1	65.2	67.3	72.1	79.8	88.6	93.3	96.7	101.3
50.0–54.9	58.6	63.4	66.4	70.9	78.5	86.4	91.7	96.7	102.2
55.0–59.9	60.2	65.8	67.1	71.2	78.0	85.4	91.1	95.4	100.9
60.0–64.9	58.4	61.8	65.3	69.2	76.9	84.5	88.6	91.5	97.8
65.0–69.9	56.7	60.7	63.4	67.9	75.1	83.2	87.0	90.8	96.7
70.0–74.9	55.2	59.1	62.9	66.6	73.7	81.8	86.6	90.3	93.9
Males with large frames									
18.0–24.9	58.4	61.5	62.7	67.6	75.0	85.4	91.2	95.0	103.3
25.0–29.9	61.2	66.0	68.3	72.8	82.0	90.9	99.3	102.1	113.5
30.0–34.9	64.6	69.1	70.9	76.3	86.0	94.0	101.0	104.3	115.5
35.0–39.9	59.6	67.4	71.4	75.4	83.6	92.6	98.4	104.1	115.3
40.0–44.9	63.6	67.4	68.7	73.4	81.8	92.2	100.3	107.4	113.8
45.0–49.9	64.2	67.3	69.4	75.3	83.9	92.5	97.9	103.2	113.2
50.0–54.9	64.3	66.6	68.8	73.0	82.4	92.5	100.9	102.8	110.2
55.0–59.9	64.8	68.1	71.5	75.1	84.5	92.8	100.0	102.6	116.3
60.0–64.9	62.7	66.7	69.5	73.1	80.1	89.4	94.5	98.9	107.3
65.0–69.9	58.2	62.0	66.3	71.0	78.9	87.5	92.2	95.7	103.9
70.0–74.9	55.8	61.6	64.8	68.4	76.9	83.2	90.5	94.7	99.6

Females

Age (yrs)	5	10	15	25	50	75	85	90	95
Females with small frames									
18.0–24.9	44.0	46.7	48.5	50.6	54.9	60.9	64.5	66.9	71.5
25.0–29.9	44.4	47.3	48.5	51.3	55.9	60.9	63.7	66.1	72.6
30.0–34.9	46.1	48.3	50.0	52.6	57.0	62.5	66.8	68.8	77.1
35.0–39.9	45.9	48.2	50.0	53.4	59.4	66.2	71.0	74.7	78.4
40.0–44.9	48.0	50.3	51.8	54.5	58.8	65.2	69.3	72.5	78.1
45.0–49.9	46.5	48.8	50.9	53.5	60.1	66.3	70.5	73.1	79.7
50.0–54.9	46.8	49.3	51.5	54.4	59.2	66.7	70.4	72.9	76.5
55.0–59.9	45.4	48.5	51.6	54.2	60.7	64.9	69.6	72.3	79.1
60.0–64.9	46.6	48.5	50.6	53.5	60.0	67.9	71.4	73.9	79.8
65.0–69.9	45.1	48.4	51.1	53.5	60.0	67.3	70.8	73.5	79.0
70.0–74.9	42.6	45.9	48.5	51.5	59.6	66.4	72.0	74.2	79.3
Females with medium frames									
18.0–24.9	46.6	48.8	50.2	52.6	57.9	64.1	68.1	71.9	77.8
25.0–29.9	46.9	49.1	50.2	52.7	58.1	66.1	72.2	76.0	81.6
30.0–34.9	47.2	50.0	51.7	54.2	60.1	68.3	73.7	78.6	83.6
35.0–39.9	49.2	51.7	53.0	55.9	60.8	67.6	72.8	76.7	83.5
40.0–44.9	49.0	51.0	53.2	56.1	61.6	68.8	75.4	80.1	90.6
45.0–49.9	47.7	50.9	53.0	55.9	62.8	71.2	76.9	81.9	89.0
50.0–54.9	48.8	52.4	54.5	57.3	63.6	72.3	78.0	81.6	89.6
55.0–59.9	48.2	50.6	53.6	57.3	64.2	73.3	78.4	84.1	89.2
60.0–64.9	49.1	51.7	53.3	57.3	64.2	72.7	77.6	81.1	87.2
65.0–69.9	48.5	51.3	53.3	56.3	64.4	72.7	78.1	81.1	87.8
70.0–74.9	47.1	50.6	52.5	56.6	62.5	70.2	75.9	79.1	83.9
Females with large frames									
18.0–24.9	48.6	50.8	52.7	55.3	62.1	74.3	81.9	86.4	102.1
25.0–29.9	49.8	52.7	55.1	57.8	66.0	79.7	87.7	96.3	104.0
30.0–34.9	50.5	53.6	56.8	60.1	69.3	87.2	95.6	101.3	109.4
35.0–39.9	52.3	55.0	56.7	61.5	71.8	86.1	94.5	98.9	108.9
40.0–44.9	52.3	56.8	59.9	64.0	73.5	86.8	94.9	100.6	110.8
45.0–49.9	56.0	60.3	63.2	65.8	76.0	86.1	97.6	102.2	112.5
50.0–54.9	50.6	58.7	61.2	65.5	73.0	85.5	93.1	98.5	106.7
55.0–59.9	55.9	59.8	61.9	66.1	70.4	88.2	92.9	99.1	105.6
60.0–64.9	56.0	58.5	61.3	65.7	75.8	84.7	91.3	98.8	104.2
65.0–69.9	54.8	58.4	60.8	63.8	73.8	82.5	90.8	97.2	105.7
70.0–74.9	53.9	57.6	60.7	65.7	74.4	81.9	87.0	90.0	93.9

Modified from Frisancho, A. R.: Anthropometric Standards for the Assessment of Growth and Nutritional Status, Ann Arbor, The University of Michigan Press, 1990.

10–6 Percentiles of Percent Body Fat by Age, and Nomograms for Conversion of Skinfolds to Percent Body Fat, Adults

Age (yrs)	Percentiles								
	5	10	15	25	50	75	85	90	95
Males									
18.0–24.9	8.0	9.0	10.0	12.0	16.0	20.0	23.0	25.0	28.0
25.0–29.9	9.0	10.0	11.0	13.0	18.0	23.0	25.0	26.0	29.0
30.0–34.9	16.0	17.0	18.0	20.0	23.0	26.0	27.0	28.0	30.0
35.0–39.9	15.0	17.0	18.0	20.0	23.0	25.0	27.0	27.0	29.0
40.0–44.9	14.0	16.0	18.0	21.0	26.0	30.0	32.0	34.0	36.0
45.0–49.9	15.0	17.0	19.0	21.0	26.0	30.0	32.0	34.0	36.0
50.0–54.9	15.0	17.0	19.0	22.0	27.0	31.0	33.0	35.0	37.0
55.0–59.9	15.0	18.0	20.0	22.0	27.0	31.0	33.0	35.0	37.0
60.0–64.9	16.0	18.0	20.0	22.0	27.0	31.0	33.0	35.0	37.0
65.0–69.9	13.0	16.0	18.0	21.0	26.0	30.0	33.0	35.0	37.0
70.0–74.9	13.0	16.0	18.0	21.0	26.0	30.0	33.0	34.0	36.0
Females									
18.0–24.9	17.0	19.0	21.0	23.0	27.0	33.0	35.0	37.0	40.0
25.0–29.9	18.0	20.0	21.0	24.0	29.0	34.0	37.0	39.0	41.0
30.0–34.9	21.0	23.0	25.0	27.0	31.0	36.0	38.0	40.0	42.0
35.0–39.9	22.0	24.0	25.0	28.0	32.0	37.0	39.0	40.0	42.0
40.0–44.9	25.0	28.0	29.0	31.0	35.0	39.0	41.0	42.0	43.0
45.0–49.9	26.0	28.0	29.0	32.0	36.0	39.0	41.0	42.0	44.0
50.0–54.9	27.0	30.0	32.0	35.0	39.0	43.0	46.0	47.0	48.0
55.0–59.9	27.0	30.0	32.0	35.0	39.0	44.0	45.0	47.0	49.0
60.0–64.9	28.0	31.0	32.0	35.0	40.0	43.0	45.0	46.0	48.0
65.0–69.9	27.0	30.0	32.0	34.0	38.0	42.0	44.0	46.0	47.0
70.0–74.9	26.0	29.0	31.0	34.0	38.0	42.0	44.0	45.0	47.0

Sum of Three Skinfolds* (mm)

♂ ♀

Percent Body Fat

Age in Years

* ♂ Chest, Abdomen, Thigh
  ♀ Triceps, Thigh, Suprailium

Modified from Frisancho, A.R.: Anthropometric Standards for the Assessment of Growth and Nutrition Status, Ann Arbor, The University of Michigan Press, 1990.

From: The Research Quarterly for Exercise and Sport, 1981, 52:380. Used with permission.

10-7 Sum of Skinfold to Determine Body Fat in Adults by Jackson and Pollock, 3 Sites

Percent Fat: Men, Sum of three sites:
1. Abdomen
2. Ilium
3. Tricep

$$\text{Percent fat} = .39287\,(\Sigma 3) - .00105\,(\Sigma 3^2) + .15772\,(\text{AGE}) + 5.18845$$

R = .893   SE = 3.63% fat

Percent Fat Estimates for Three Sites — Men

Sum of 3 skinfolds	| Age to Last Year								
	18-22	23-27	28-32	33-37	38-42	43-47	48-52	53-57	>58
8-12	1.8	2.6	3.4	4.2	4.9	5.7	6.5	7.3	8.1
13-17	3.6	4.4	5.2	6.0	6.8	7.6	8.4	9.1	9.9
18-22	5.4	6.2	7.0	7.8	8.6	9.3	10.1	10.9	11.7
23-27	7.1	7.9	8.7	9.5	10.3	11.1	11.9	12.6	13.4
28-32	8.8	9.6	10.4	11.2	12.0	12.8	13.5	14.3	15.1
33-37	10.4	11.2	12.0	12.8	13.6	14.4	15.2	15.9	16.7
38-42	12.0	12.8	13.6	14.4	15.2	15.9	16.7	17.5	18.3
43-47	13.5	14.3	15.1	15.9	16.7	17.5	18.3	19.0	19.8
48-52	15.0	15.8	16.6	17.4	18.1	18.9	19.7	20.5	21.3
53-57	16.4	17.2	18.0	18.8	19.6	20.3	21.1	21.9	22.7
58-62	17.8	18.5	19.3	20.1	20.9	21.7	22.5	23.3	24.1
63-67	19.1	19.9	20.6	21.4	22.2	23.0	23.8	24.6	25.4
68-72	20.3	21.1	21.9	22.7	23.5	24.3	25.1	25.8	26.6
73-77	21.5	22.3	23.1	23.9	24.7	25.5	26.3	27.0	27.8
78-82	22.7	23.5	24.3	25.0	25.8	26.6	27.4	28.2	29.0
83-87	23.8	24.6	25.3	26.1	26.9	27.7	28.5	29.3	30.1
88-92	24.8	25.6	26.4	27.2	28.0	28.8	29.6	30.3	31.1
93-97	25.8	26.6	27.4	28.2	29.0	29.8	30.5	31.3	32.1
98-102	26.7	27.5	28.3	29.1	29.9	30.7	31.5	32.3	33.1
103-107	27.6	28.4	29.2	30.0	30.8	31.6	32.4	33.2	33.9
108-112	28.5	29.3	30.1	30.8	31.6	32.4	33.2	34.0	34.8
113-117	29.3	30.0	30.8	31.6	32.4	33.2	34.0	34.8	35.6
118-122	30.0	30.8	31.6	32.4	33.1	33.9	34.7	35.5	36.3
123-127	30.7	31.5	32.3	33.0	33.8	34.6	35.4	36.2	37.0
128-132	31.3	32.1	32.9	33.7	34.4	35.2	36.0	36.8	37.6
133-137	31.9	32.7	33.4	34.2	35.0	35.8	36.6	37.4	38.2
138-142	32.4	33.2	34.0	34.8	35.5	36.3	37.1	37.9	38.7
143-147	32.9	33.6	34.4	35.2	36.0	36.8	37.6	38.4	39.2
148-152	33.3	34.1	34.8	35.6	36.4	37.2	38.0	38.8	39.6
153-157	33.6	34.4	35.2	36.0	36.8	37.6	38.4	39.2	39.9
158-162	33.9	34.7	35.5	36.3	37.1	37.9	38.7	39.5	40.3
163-167	34.2	35.0	35.8	36.6	37.4	38.1	38.9	39.7	40.5
168-172	34.4	35.2	36.0	36.8	37.6	38.4	39.1	39.9	40.7
173-177	34.6	35.3	36.1	36.9	37.7	38.5	39.3	40.1	40.9
178-182	34.7	35.4	36.2	37.0	37.8	38.6	39.4	40.2	41.0

Percent Fat: Women, Sum of three sites:
1. Abdomen
2. Ilium
3. Tricep

$$\text{Percent fat} = .41563\,(\Sigma 3) - .00112\,(\Sigma 3^2) + .03661\,(\text{AGE}) + 4.03653$$

R = .825   SE = 3.98% fat

Percent Fat Estimates for Three Sites — Women

Sum of 3 skinfolds	| Age to Last Year								
	18-22	23-27	28-32	33-37	38-42	43-47	48-52	53-57	>58
8-12	8.8	9.0	9.2	9.4	9.5	9.7	9.9	10.1	10.3
13-17	10.8	10.9	11.1	11.3	11.5	11.7	11.8	12.0	12.2
18-22	12.6	12.8	13.0	13.2	13.4	13.5	13.7	13.9	14.1
23-27	14.5	14.6	14.8	15.0	15.2	15.4	15.6	15.7	15.9
28-32	16.2	16.4	16.6	16.8	17.0	17.1	17.3	17.5	17.7
33-37	17.9	18.1	18.3	18.5	18.7	18.9	19.0	19.2	19.4
38-42	19.6	19.8	20.0	20.2	20.3	20.5	20.7	20.9	21.1
43-47	21.2	21.4	21.6	21.8	21.9	22.1	22.3	22.5	22.7
48-52	22.8	22.9	23.1	23.3	23.5	23.7	23.8	24.0	24.2
53-57	24.4	24.4	24.6	24.8	25.0	25.2	25.3	25.5	25.7
58-62	25.7	25.9	26.0	26.2	26.4	26.6	26.8	27.0	27.1
63-67	27.1	27.2	27.4	27.6	27.8	28.0	28.2	28.3	28.5
68-72	28.4	28.6	28.7	28.9	29.1	29.3	29.5	29.7	29.8
73-77	29.6	29.8	30.0	30.2	30.4	30.6	30.7	30.9	31.1
78-82	30.9	31.1	31.2	31.4	31.6	31.8	32.0	32.1	32.3
83-87	32.0	32.2	32.4	32.6	32.7	32.9	33.1	33.3	33.5
88-92	33.1	33.3	33.5	33.7	33.8	34.0	34.2	34.4	34.6
93-97	34.1	34.3	34.5	34.7	34.9	35.1	35.2	35.4	35.6
98-102	35.1	35.3	35.5	35.7	35.8	36.0	36.2	36.4	36.6
103-107	36.1	36.2	36.4	36.6	36.8	37.0	37.1	37.3	37.5
108-112	36.9	37.1	37.3	37.5	37.7	37.9	38.0	38.2	38.4
113-117	37.8	38.0	38.1	38.3	38.5	38.7	38.9	39.1	39.5
118-122	38.5	38.7	38.9	39.1	39.2	39.4	39.6	39.8	40.0
123-127	39.2	39.4	39.6	39.8	39.9	40.1	40.3	40.5	40.7
128-132	39.9	40.1	40.2	40.4	40.6	40.8	41.0	41.2	41.3
133-137	40.5	40.7	40.8	41.0	41.2	41.4	41.6	41.7	41.9
138-142	41.0	41.2	41.4	41.6	41.7	41.9	42.1	42.3	42.5
143-147	41.5	41.7	41.9	42.0	42.2	42.4	42.6	42.8	43.0
148-152	41.9	42.1	42.3	42.5	42.6	42.8	43.0	43.2	43.4
153-157	42.3	42.5	42.8	52.8	43.1	43.4	43.6	43.7	43.7
158-162	42.6	42.9	43.0	43.1	43.3	43.5	43.8	44.0	44.1
163-167	42.9	43.1	43.2	43.4	43.6	43.8	44.0	44.1	44.3
168-172	43.1	43.2	43.4	43.6	43.8	43.9	44.2	44.3	44.5
173-177	43.2	43.3	43.5	43.6	43.9	44.0	44.3	44.5	44.7
178-182	43.3	43.5	43.7	43.8	44.0	44.2	44.4	44.6	44.8

Equations and tables based on Jackson, A.S. and Pollock, M.L.: Generalized equations for predicting body density of man. Br J Nutr, 40:497, 1978. From Golding, L.A., Myers, C.R., and Sinning, W.E.: Y's Way to Physical Fitness, Champaign, IL., Human Kinetics, 1989. Used with permission.

10-8 Sum of Skinfold to Determine Body Fat in Adults by Jackson and Pollock, 4 Sites

Percent Fat: Men - Sum of four sites:
  1. Abdomen   3. Tricep
  2. Ilium   4. Thigh
Percent fat = .29288 (Σ4)-.0005 (Σ4²)+.15845 (AGE)-5.76377
  R = .901   SE = 3.49% fat

Percent Fat Estimates for Four Sites - Men

Sum of 4 skinfolds	Age to Last Year								
	18-22	23-27	28-32	33-37	38-42	43-47	48-52	53-57	>58
13-17	1.7	2.5	3.3	4.1	4.9	5.6	6.4	7.2	8.0
18-22	3.1	3.9	4.6	5.4	6.2	7.0	7.8	8.6	9.4
23-27	4.4	5.2	6.0	6.8	7.6	8.4	9.2	10.0	10.7
28-32	5.7	6.5	7.3	8.1	8.9	9.7	10.5	11.3	12.1
33-37	7.0	7.8	8.6	9.4	10.2	11.0	11.8	12.6	13.4
38-42	8.3	9.1	9.9	10.7	11.5	12.3	13.1	13.9	14.6
43-47	9.6	10.3	11.1	11.9	12.7	13.5	14.3	15.1	15.9
48-52	10.8	11.6	12.4	13.2	13.9	14.7	15.5	16.3	17.1
53-57	12.0	12.8	13.6	14.4	15.1	15.9	16.7	17.5	18.3
58-62	13.1	13.9	14.7	15.5	16.3	17.1	17.9	18.7	19.5
63-67	14.3	15.1	15.9	16.7	17.5	18.2	19.0	19.8	20.6
68-72	15.4	16.2	17.0	17.8	18.6	19.4	20.2	21.0	21.8
73-77	16.5	17.3	18.1	18.9	19.7	20.5	21.3	22.1	22.8
78-82	17.6	18.4	19.2	20.0	20.7	21.5	22.3	23.1	23.9
83-87	18.6	19.4	20.2	21.0	21.8	22.6	23.4	24.2	25.0
88-92	19.6	20.4	21.2	22.0	22.8	23.6	24.4	25.2	26.0
93-97	20.6	21.4	22.2	23.0	23.8	24.6	25.4	26.2	27.0
98-102	21.6	22.4	23.2	24.0	24.8	25.6	26.4	27.1	27.9
103-107	22.5	23.3	24.1	24.9	25.7	26.5	27.3	28.1	28.9
108-112	23.5	24.3	25.1	25.9	26.7	27.4	28.2	29.0	29.8
113-117	24.4	25.2	26.0	26.7	27.5	28.3	29.1	29.9	30.7
118-122	25.2	26.0	26.8	27.6	28.4	29.2	30.0	30.8	31.6
123-127	26.0	26.8	27.6	28.4	29.2	30.0	30.8	31.6	32.4
128-132	26.9	27.7	28.4	29.2	30.0	30.8	31.6	32.4	33.2
133-137	27.7	28.4	29.2	30.0	30.8	31.6	32.4	33.2	34.0
138-142	28.4	29.2	30.0	30.8	31.6	32.4	33.2	34.0	34.8
143-147	29.2	29.9	30.7	31.5	32.3	33.1	33.9	34.7	35.5
148-152	29.9	30.7	31.5	32.2	33.0	33.8	34.6	35.4	36.2
153-157	30.6	31.3	32.1	32.9	33.7	34.5	35.3	36.1	36.9
158-162	31.2	32.0	32.8	33.6	34.4	35.2	36.0	36.8	37.6
163-167	31.8	32.6	33.4	34.2	35.0	35.8	36.6	37.4	38.2
168-172	32.5	33.3	34.1	34.9	35.6	36.4	37.2	38.0	38.8
173-177	33.0	33.8	34.6	35.4	36.2	37.0	37.8	38.6	39.4
178-182	33.6	34.4	35.2	36.0	36.8	37.6	38.4	39.2	39.9
183-187	34.1	34.9	35.7	36.5	37.3	38.1	38.9	39.7	40.5

Percent Fat: Women, Sum of four sites:
  1. Abdomen   3. Tricep
  2. Ilium   4. Thigh
Percent fat = .29669 (Σ4)-.00043 (Σ4²)+.02963 (AGE)+1.4072
  R = .846   SE = 3.89% fat

Percent Fat Estimates for Four Sites - Women

Sum of 4 skinfolds	Age to Last Year								
	18-22	23-27	28-32	33-37	38-42	43-47	48-52	53-57	>58
23-27	8.6	9.3	9.4	9.6	9.7	9.9	10.0	10.2	10.3
28-32	10.0	10.7	10.8	11.0	11.0	11.3	11.4	11.6	11.7
33-37	11.3	12.0	12.2	12.3	12.4	12.6	12.7	12.9	13.0
38-42	12.6	13.3	13.5	13.6	13.7	13.9	14.1	14.2	14.4
43-47	13.9	14.6	14.8	14.9	15.0	15.2	15.4	15.5	15.7
48-52	15.2	15.9	16.1	16.2	16.3	16.5	16.7	16.8	17.0
53-57	16.5	17.2	17.3	17.5	17.5	17.8	17.9	18.1	18.2
58-62	17.7	18.4	18.6	18.7	18.8	19.0	19.1	19.3	19.4
63-67	18.9	19.6	19.8	19.9	20.0	20.2	20.4	20.5	20.7
68-72	20.1	20.8	21.0	21.1	21.2	21.4	21.6	21.7	21.9
73-77	21.3	22.0	22.1	22.3	22.3	22.6	22.7	22.9	23.0
78-82	22.5	23.1	23.3	23.4	23.5	23.7	23.9	24.0	24.2
83-87	23.6	24.3	24.4	24.6	24.6	24.9	25.0	25.2	25.3
88-92	24.7	25.4	25.5	25.7	25.7	26.0	26.1	26.3	26.4
93-97	25.8	26.5	26.6	26.8	26.8	27.1	27.2	27.4	27.5
98-102	26.8	27.5	27.7	27.8	27.9	28.1	28.3	28.4	28.6
103-107	27.9	28.6	28.7	28.9	28.9	29.2	29.3	29.5	29.6
108-112	28.9	29.6	29.7	29.9	30.0	30.2	30.3	30.5	30.6
113-117	29.9	30.6	30.7	30.9	31.0	31.2	31.3	31.5	31.6
118-122	30.9	31.6	31.7	31.9	31.9	32.2	32.3	32.5	32.6
123-127	31.9	32.5	32.7	32.8	32.9	33.1	33.3	33.4	33.6
128-132	32.8	33.5	33.6	33.8	33.8	34.1	34.2	34.4	34.5
133-137	33.7	34.4	34.5	34.7	34.7	35.0	35.1	35.3	35.4
138-142	34.6	35.3	35.4	35.6	35.6	35.9	36.0	36.2	36.3
143-147	35.5	36.2	36.3	36.5	36.5	36.7	36.9	37.0	37.2
148-152	36.3	37.0	37.2	37.3	37.4	37.6	37.8	37.9	38.0
153-157	37.2	37.8	38.0	38.1	38.2	38.4	38.6	38.7	38.9
158-162	38.0	38.6	38.8	38.9	39.0	39.2	39.4	39.5	39.7
163-167	38.8	39.4	39.6	39.7	39.8	40.0	40.2	40.3	40.5
168-172	39.5	40.2	40.3	40.5	40.6	40.8	40.9	41.1	41.2
173-177	40.3	40.9	41.1	41.2	41.3	41.5	41.7	41.8	42.0
178-182	41.0	41.7	41.8	42.0	42.0	42.3	42.4	42.6	42.7
183-187	41.7	42.4	42.5	42.7	42.7	43.0	43.1	43.3	43.4
188-192	42.4	43.0	43.2	43.3	43.4	43.6	43.8	43.9	44.1
193-197	43.0	43.7	43.9	44.0	44.1	44.3	44.4	44.6	44.7
198-202	43.7	44.3	44.5	44.6	44.7	44.9	45.1	45.2	45.4

Equations and tables based on Jackson, A.S. and Pollock, M.L.: Generalized equations for predicting body density of man. Br J Nutr, 40:497, 1978. From Golding, L.A., Myers, C.R., and Sinning, W.E.: Y's Way to Physical Fitness, Champaign, IL., Human Kinetics, 1989. Used with permission.

10–9   Sample Adult Body Composition and Body Fat Classification for Athletes and Non Athletes

Men	Women
Age = 20-24	Age = 20-24
Height = 68.5 in.	Height = 64.5 in.
Weight = 154 lb.	Weight = 125 lb.
Total fat = 23.1 lb. (15.0%)	Total fat = 3.8 lb. (27.0%)
Storage fat = 18.5 lb. (12.0%)	Storage fat = 18.8 lb. (15.0%)
Essential fat = 4.6 lb. (3.0%)	Essential fat = 15.0 lb. (12.0%)
Muscle = 69 lb. (44.8%)	Muscle = 45 lb. (36.0%)
Bone = 23 lb. (14.9%)	Bone = 15 lb. (12.0%)
Remainder = 38.9 lb. (25.3%)	Remainder = 31.2 lb. (25.0%)
Lean body weight = 136 lb.	Minimal weight = 107 lb.

Gross body composition of a reference man and woman.

Adapted from McArdle, W.D., Katch, F.I., and Katch, V.L.: Exercise Physiology, Lea & Febiger, 1983.

BODY FAT VALUES in ATHLETES and VO₂ max

Athletic Group or Sport	MALE %fat	MALE VO$_2$ max ml/kg/min	FEMALE %fat	FEMALE VO$_2$max ml/kg/min
Baseball	12-15	48-56		
Basketball	7-12	45-55	18-27	40-44
Canoeing	10-14	55-67		
Football:				
Defensive backs	9-12	48-55		
Offensive backs	9-12	48-55		
Linebackers	13	48-55		
Offensive linemen	19	46-52		
Defensive linemen	19	42-48		
Quarterback, kickers	14	48-55		
Gymnastics	3- 6	52-58	8-18	37-44
Ice hockey	12-16	50-63		
Jockeys	6-14	50-60		
Skiing:				
Alpine	10-17	57-68	20-28	48-60
Cross-country	7-13	65-90	18-24	60-75
Ski jumping	12-16	58-63		
Soccer	7-12	54-64	16-22	45-55
Swimming	4-10	50-70	14-25	40-55
Track and field:				
Runners				
Distance,elite	5-12	60-80	10-18	60-75
Distance			15-20	50-60
Sprint	5-12	55-65	15-20	50-60
Discus	12-18	42-52	22-28	
Jumpers and hurdlers	6-13	50-60	12-22	48-60
Shot put	14-20	40-46	23-30	35-42
Tennis	12-16		15-22	
Volleyball	10-15		20-23	
Weight lifting	6-16			
Wrestling	6-12			

BODY FAT CLASSIFICATIONS for NON-ATHLETES

		Male	Female
Very low fat	skinny	7- 9.9	14 -16.9
Low fat	trim	10 -12.9	17 -19.9
Average fat	normal	13 -16.9	20 - 26.9
Above normal	plump	17 - 24.9	27 - 30.9
Very high fat	fat	25+	31+

From: Tufts University and United States Department of Agriculture, Human Nutrition Research Center on Aging.

10–10 Pathophysiology of Obesity, Waist to Hip Ratio, and Blood Pressure Classification, Male and Female, Adults

PATHOPHYSIOLOGY OF OBESITY

CLASSIFICATION OF BLOOD PRESSURE# IN ADULTS AGE 18 YEARS OR OLDER

Range, mm Hg	Category*
Diastolic	
< 85	Normal Blood Pressure
85-89	High normal blood pressure
90-104	Mild Hypertension
105-114	Moderate hypertension
≥ 115	Severe Hypertension

Systolic, when diastolic blood pressure is <90

< 140	Normal blood pressure
140-159	Borderline isolated systolic hypertension
≥ 160	Isolated systolic hypertension

#classification based on the average of two or more readings on two or more occasions.

*A classification of borderline isolated systolic hypertension (SBP 140 to 159 mm Hg) or isolated systolic hypertension (SBP ≥ 160 mm Hg) takes precedence over high normal blood pressure (diastolic blood pressure, 85 to 89 mm Hg) when both occur in the same person. High normal blood pressure (DBP 85 to 39 mm Hg) take precedence over a classification of normal blood pressure (SBP < 140 mm Hg) when both occur in the same person.

From: The 1988 Report of the Joint National Committee on Detection, Evaluation, and Treatment of High Blood Pressure, U.S. Dept. of Health and Human Services, Public Health Services, National Institute of Health.

Waist Hip Ratio by Age and Sex*

Risk	20-29	30-39	40-49	50-59	60-69
Very High	0.95(0.82)	0.96(0.85)	1.00(0.87)	1.20(0.88)	1.39(0.91)
Moderate	0.87(0.78)	0.92(0.79)	0.94(0.80)	0.95(0.82)	0.97(0.85)
Low	0.83(0.71)	0.84(0.73)	0.88(0.75)	0.90(0.76)	0.91(0.78)

*Female values in parenthesis.
Adapted from: Bray, G., Pathophysiology of obesity. Am J Clin Nutr, 1992: 55, 4885.

BODY MASS INDEX NOMOGRAM

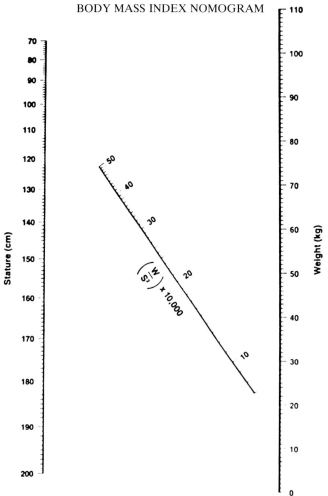

From: *Am J Clin Nutr*, 34, 2831, 1981. © *Am J Clin Nutr*, American Society for Clinical Nutrition. Used with permission.

BODY FAT NOMOGRAM

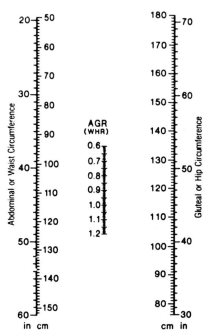

From: Bray, G. A., and D. S. Gray. Obesity. Part I: pathogenesis. *Western Medical Journal*, 1988, 149:429. Used with permission.

10-12 Nomogram for Adults and Upper Arm Anthropometry

Triceps Skinfold (mm), Males

Age (years)	Percentile		
	50th	15th	5th
18-24	9.5	6.0	4.0
25-34	12.0	6.0	4.5
35-44	12.0	7.0	5.0
45-54	11.0	7.0	5.0
55-64	11.0	6.5	5.0
65-74	11.0	6.5	4.5

Triceps Skinfold (mm), Females

Age (years)	Percentile		
	50th	15th	5th
18-24	18.0	12.0	9.4
25-34	21.0	13.5	10.5
35-44	23.0	16.0	12.0
45-54	25.0	17.0	13.0
55-64	25.0	16.0	11.0
65-74	23.0	16.0	11.5

Midarm Muscle Circumference (cm), Males

Age (years)	Percentile		
	50th	15th*	5th
18-24	27.2	25.0	23.5
25-34	28.0	25.8	24.2
35-44	28.7	26.2	25.0
45-54	28.1	25.6	24.0
55-64	27.9	25.4	22.8
65-74	26.9	24.3	22.5

Midarm Muscle Circumference (cm), Females

Age (years)	Percentile		
	50th	15th*	5th
18-24	20.6	18.8	17.7
25-34	21.4	19.3	18.3
35-44	22.0	19.7	18.5
45-54	22.2	19.9	18.8
55-64	22.6	20.1	18.6
65-74	22.5	20.0	18.6

Midarm Circumference (cm), Males

Age (years)	Percentile		
	50th	15th	5th
18-24	30.7	27.6	25.7
25-34	32.0	28.9	27.0
35-44	32.7	29.5	27.8
45-54	32.0	28.9	26.7
55-64	31.7	28.2	25.6
65-74	30.7	27.3	25.3

Midarm Circumference (cm), Females

Age (years)	Percentile		
	50th	15th	5th
18-24	26.4	23.5	22.1
25-34	27.8	24.8	23.3
35-44	29.2	25.8	24.1
45-54	30.3	26.6	24.3
55-64	30.2	26.1	23.9
65-74	29.9	26.2	23.8

*Values provided by investigator, Charles W. Bishop, PhD, University of Wisconsin From Bishop, C.W., Bowen, P. D., Ritchey, S.J.: Norms for nutritional assessment of American adults by upper arm anthropometry, Am J Clin Nutr 34:2530, 1981. Used with permission.

ARM ANTHROPOMETRY NOMOGRAM FOR ADULTS

*Reproduced with permission from: Gurney, J. and Jelliffe, D.: Arm anthropometry in nutritional assessments: nomogram for rapid calculation of muscle circumference and cross-sectional muscle and fat areas. Am J Clin Nutr, 26:912, 1973.

TRICEPS FATFOLD (mm); ARM MUSCLE AREA (cm²); ARM MUSCLE CIRCUMFERENCE (cm); ARM AREA (cm²); ARM CIRCUMFERENCE (cm)

10–13 Target Weight by Percent Body Fat, Women and Men

Target Weight – Women (23% Fat)

	Body Weight (lb)																		
%fat	105	110	115	120	125	130	135	140	145	150	155	160	165	170	175	180	185	190	195
24	104	109	114	118	123	128	133	138	143	148	153	158	163	168	173	178	183	188	192
25	102	107	112	117	122	127	131	136	141	146	151	156	161	166	170	175	180	185	190
26	101	106	111	115	120	125	130	135	139	144	149	154	159	163	168	173	178	183	187
27	100	104	109	114	119	123	128	133	137	142	147	152	156	161	166	171	175	180	185
28	98	103	108	112	117	122	126	131	136	140	145	150	154	159	164	168	173	178	182
29	97	101	106	111	115	120	124	129	134	138	143	148	152	157	161	166	171	175	180
30	95	100	105	109	114	118	123	127	132	136	141	145	150	155	159	164	168	173	177
31	94	99	103	108	112	116	121	125	130	134	139	144	149	152	157	161	166	170	175
32	93	97	102	106	110	115	119	124	129	132	137	141	146	150	155	159	163	168	172
33	91	96	100	104	109	113	117	122	126	131	135	139	144	148	152	157	161	165	170
34	90	94	99	103	107	111	116	120	124	129	133	137	141	146	150	154	159	163	167
35	89	93	97	101	106	110	114	118	122	127	131	135	139	144	148	152	156	160	165
36	87	91	96	100	104	108	112	116	121	125	129	133	137	141	145	150	154	158	162
37	86	90	94	98	102	106	110	115	119	123	127	131	135	139	143	147	151	155	160
38	85	89	93	97	101	105	109	113	117	121	125	129	133	137	141	145	149	153	157
39	83	87	91	95	99	103	107	111	115	119	123	127	131	135	139	143	147	151	154
40	82	86	90	94	97	101	105	109	113	117	121	125	129	132	136	140	144	148	152

Target Weight – Men (16% Fat)

	Body Weight (lb)																							
%Fat	120	125	130	135	140	145	150	155	160	165	170	175	180	185	190	195	200	205	210	215	220	225	230	235	240
17	119	123	129	133	138	143	148	153	158	163	168	173	179	183	188	193	198	203	208	212	217	222	227	232	237
18	117	122	127	132	137	142	146	151	156	161	166	171	176	181	186	190	195	200	205	210	215	220	225	229	234
19	116	121	125	130	135	140	145	149	154	159	164	169	174	178	183	188	193	198	203	207	212	217	222	225	231
20	114	119	124	129	133	138	143	148	152	157	162	167	171	176	181	186	190	195	200	205	210	214	219	224	229
21	113	118	122	127	132	136	141	146	150	155	160	165	169	174	179	183	188	193	198	202	207	212	216	221	226
22	111	116	121	125	130	135	139	144	149	153	158	162	167	172	176	181	186	190	195	200	204	209	214	218	223
23	110	115	119	123	128	133	138	142	147	151	156	160	165	170	174	179	183	188	193	197	202	206	211	215	220
24	109	113	118	122	127	131	136	140	145	149	154	158	163	167	172	176	181	186	190	195	199	204	208	213	217
25	107	112	116	121	125	129	134	138	143	147	152	156	161	165	170	174	179	183	188	192	196	201	205	210	214
26	106	110	115	119	123	128	132	137	141	145	150	154	158	163	167	172	176	181	185	189	194	198	203	207	211
27	104	109	113	117	122	126	130	135	139	143	148	152	156	161	165	169	174	178	183	187	191	196	200	204	209
28	103	107	111	116	120	124	129	133	137	141	146	150	154	159	163	167	171	176	180	184	189	193	197	201	208
29	102	106	110	114	118	123	127	131	135	139	144	148	152	156	161	165	169	173	178	182	186	190	194	199	203
30	100	104	108	113	117	121	125	129	133	137	142	146	150	154	158	162	167	171	175	179	183	188	192	196	200
31	99	103	107	111	115	119	123	127	131	136	140	144	149	152	156	160	164	168	173	177	181	185	189	193	197
32	97	101	105	109	113	117	121	125	130	134	138	142	146	150	154	158	162	166	170	174	178	182	186	190	194
33	96	100	104	108	112	116	120	124	128	132	136	140	144	148	152	156	160	164	168	171	175	179	183	187	191
34	94	98	102	106	110	114	118	122	126	130	134	137	141	145	149	153	157	161	165	169	173	177	181	185	189
35	93	97	101	104	108	112	116	120	124	128	132	135	139	143	147	151	155	159	163	166	170	174	178	182	186
36	91	95	99	103	107	110	114	118	122	126	130	133	137	141	145	149	152	156	160	164	168	171	175	179	183
37	90	94	98	101	105	109	113	116	120	124	128	131	135	139	143	146	150	154	158	161	165	169	173	176	180
38	89	92	96	100	103	107	111	114	118	122	125	129	133	137	140	144	148	151	155	159	162	166	170	174	177
39	87	91	94	98	102	105	109	112	116	120	123	127	131	134	138	142	145	149	153	156	160	163	167	171	174
40	86	89	93	96	100	104	107	111	114	118	121	125	129	132	136	139	143	146	150	154	157	161	164	168	173

NOTE: To use, find the subject's present weight at the top of the table, then descend vertically to the horizontal row corresponding to the estimated percent fat.

From Golding, L.A., Myers, C.R., and Sinning, W.E.: Y's Way to Fitness, Champaign, IL., Human Kinetics, 1989. Used with permission.

10–14 Percentiles of Anthropometry, Older Adults

Subscapular Skinfold Thickness

Age (years)	Men 95%	Men 50%	Men 5%	Age (years)	Women 95%	Women 50%	Women 5%
65	35.7	20.0	11.2	65	33.1	16.4	8.5
70	34.0	18.2	9.4	70	32.5	15.8	7.9
75	32.2	16.4	7.7	75	31.9	15.2	7.3
80	30.4	14.7	5.9	80	31.3	14.6	6.7
85	28.7	12.9	4.1	85	30.7	14.0	6.1
90	26.9	11.2	2.4	90	30.1	13.5	5.5

Midarm Muscle Area

Age (years)	Men 95%	Men 50%	Men 5%	Age (years)	Women 95%	Women 50%	Women 5%
65	77.1	59.4	43.2	65	66.4	44.5	33.5
70	75.3	57.7	41.4	70	65.9	44.1	33.0
75	73.5	55.9	39.6	75	65.5	43.6	32.6
80	71.7	54.1	37.8	80	65.1	43.2	32.2
85	69.9	52.3	36.0	85	64.7	42.8	31.8
90	68.2	50.5	34.3	90	64.2	42.4	31.3

Midarm Circumference

Age (years)	Men 95%	Men 50%	Men 5%	Age (years)	Women 95%	Women 50%	Women 5%
65	37.8	31.9	26.7	65	37.0	30.5	25.3
70	37.2	31.3	26.0	70	36.6	30.2	24.9
75	36.6	30.7	25.4	75	36.3	29.8	24.6
80	36.0	30.1	24.8	80	35.9	29.5	24.2
85	35.3	29.4	24.2	85	35.6	29.1	23.9
90	34.7	28.8	23.5	90	35.2	28.9	23.5

Weight

Age (years)	Men 95%	Men 50%	Men 5%	Age (years)	Women 95%	Women 50%	Women 5%
65	102.0 (224.9)	79.5 (175.0)	62.6 (138.0)	65	87.1 (192.0)	66.8 (147.3)	51.2 (112.9)
70	99.1 (218.5)	76.5 (168.7)	59.7 (131.6)	70	84.9 (187.2)	64.6 (142.4)	49.0 (108.0)
75	96.3 (212.3)	73.6 (162.3)	56.8 (125.2)	75	82.8 (182.5)	62.4 (137.6)	46.8 (103.2)
80	93.4 (205.9)	70.7 (155.9)	53.9 (118.8)	80	80.6 (177.7)	60.2 (132.7)	44.7 (98.5)
85	90.5 (199.5)	67.8 (149.5)	51.0 (112.4)	85	78.4 (172.8)	58.0 (127.9)	42.5 (93.7)
90	87.6 (193.1)	64.9 (142.8)	48.1 (106.0)	90	76.2 (168.0)	55.9 (123.2)	40.3 (88.8)

Stature

Age (years)	Men 95%	Men 50%	Men 5%	Age (years)	Women 95%	Women 50%	Women 5%
65	181.6 (71.5)	170.3 (67.0)	159.1 (62.6)	65	171.6 (67.6)	161.0 (63.4)	153.1 (60.3)
70	181.6 (71.5)	169.9 (66.9)	158.7 (62.5)	70	169.8 (66.9)	159.1 (62.6)	151.3 (59.6)
75	181.2 (71.3)	169.5 (66.7)	158.4 (62.4)	75	167.9 (66.1)	157.3 (61.9)	149.4 (58.8)
80	180.9 (71.2)	169.1 (66.6)	158.0 (62.2)	80	166.1 (65.4)	155.4 (61.2)	147.6 (58.1)
85	180.5 (71.1)	168.8 (66.5)	157.7 (62.1)	85	164.2 (64.6)	153.6 (60.5)	145.7 (57.4)
90	180.2 (70.9)	168.5 (66.3)	157.3 (61.9)	90	162.4 (63.9)	151.7 (59.7)	143.9 (56.6)

Triceps Skinfold Thickness

Age (years)	Men 95%	Men 50%	Men 5%	Age (years)	Women 95%	Women 50%	Women 5%
65	27.0	13.8	8.6	65	33.0	21.6	13.5
70	26.1	12.9	7.7	70	32.0	20.6	12.5
75	25.2	12.0	6.8	75	31.0	19.6	11.5
80	24.3	11.2	6.0	80	30.0	18.6	10.5
85	23.4	10.3	5.1	85	29.0	17.6	9.5
90	22.6	9.4	4.2	90	28.0	16.6	8.5

From: Nutritional Assessment of the Elderly through Anthropometry. Chumlea W.C., Roches, A.F., and Mukherjee, D., Fels Research Institute, Yellow Springs Ross Laboratories, Columbus, Ohio. Used with permission.

Stroke Risk Factor Prediction Chart

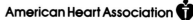
American Heart Association

1. Find Points For Each Risk Factor

Men

Age	SBP	HYP RX	Diabetes	Cigs	CVD	AF	LVH
54–56 = 0	95–105 = 0	No = 0	No = 0	No = 0	No = 0	No = 0	No = 0
57–59 = 1	106–116 = 1	Yes = 2	Yes = 2	Yes = 3	Yes = 3	Yes = 4	Yes = 6
60–62 = 2	117–126 = 2						
63–65 = 3	127–137 = 3						
66–68 = 4	138–148 = 4						
69–71 = 5	149–159 = 5						
72–74 = 6	160–170 = 6						
75–77 = 7	171–181 = 7						
78–80 = 8	182–191 = 8						
81–83 = 9	192–202 = 9						
84–86 = 10	203–213 = 10						

Women

Age	SBP	HYP RX	Diabetes	Cigs	CVD	AF	LVH
54–56 = 0	95–104 = 0	No = 0	No = 0	No = 0	No = 0	No = 0	No = 0
57–59 = 1	105–114 = 1	If Yes see below	Yes = 3	Yes = 3	Yes = 2	Yes = 6	Yes = 4
60–62 = 2	115–124 = 2						
63–65 = 3	125–134 = 3						
66–68 = 4	135–144 = 4						
69–71 = 5	145–154 = 5						
72–74 = 6	155–164 = 6						
75–77 = 7	165–174 = 7						
78–80 = 8	175–184 = 8						
81–83 = 9	185–194 = 9						
84–86 = 10	196–204 = 10						

If Currently Under Anti-Hypertensive Therapy Add The Following Points Depending On SBP Level

SBP	95–104	105–114	115–124	125–134	135–144	145–154
Points	6	5	5	4	3	3

SBP	155–164	165–174	175–184	185–194	195–204
Points	2	1	1	0	0

2. Sum Points For All Risk Factors

_____ + _____ + _____ + _____ + _____ + _____ + _____ + _____ = _____

Age   SBP   HYP RX   Diabetes   CIGS   CVD   AF   LVH   Point Total

3. Look Up Risk Corresponding To Point Total

Men 10 Yr.

Pts.	Prob.	Pts.	Prob.	Pts.	Prob.
1	2.6%	11	11.2%	21	41.7%
2	3.0%	12	12.9%	22	46.6%
3	3.5%	13	14.8%	23	51.8%
4	4.0%	14	17.0%	24	57.3%
5	4.7%	15	19.5%	25	62.8%
6	5.4%	16	22.4%	26	68.4%
7	6.3%	17	25.5%	27	73.8%
8	7.3%	18	29.0%	28	79.0%
9	8.4%	19	32.9%	29	83.7%
10	9.7%	20	37.1%	30	87.9%

Women 10 Yr.

Pts.	Prob.	Pts.	Prob.	Pts.	Prob.
1	1.1%	11	7.6%	21	43.4%
2	1.3%	12	9.2%	22	50.0%
3	1.6%	13	11.1%	23	57.0%
4	2.0%	14	13.3%	24	64.2%
5	2.4%	15	16.0%	25	71.4%
6	2.9%	16	19.1%	26	78.2%
7	3.5%	17	22.8%	27	84.4%
8	4.3%	18	27.0%		
9	5.2%	19	31.9%		
10	6.3%	20	37.3%		

4. Compare To Average 10-Year Risk

Avg. 10 Yr. Prob. By Age

	Men		Women
55–59	5.9%	55–59	3.0%
60–64	7.8%	60–64	4.7%
65–69	11.0%	65–69	7.2%
70–74	13.7%	70–74	10.9%
75–79	18.0%	75–79	15.5%
80–84	22.3%	80–84	23.9%

Key For Symbols:

SBP — Systolic blood pressure
HYP RX — Under anti-hypertensive therapy?
DIABETES — History of diabetes?
CIGS — Smokes cigarettes?

CVD — History of myocardial infarction, angina pectoris, coronary insuffiency, intermittent claudication or congestive heart failure?
AF — History of atrial fibrillation?
LVH — Left ventricular hypertrophy on ECG?

Coronary Heart Disease Risk Factor Prediction Chart

1. Find Points For Each Risk Factor

Age (If Female)				Age (If Male)				HDL-Cholesterol		Total-Cholesterol		Systolic Blood Pressure		Other	
Age	Pts.	Age	Pts.	Age	Pts.	Age	Pts.	HDL-C	Pts.	Total-C	Pts.	SBP	Pts.	Other	Pts.
30	−12	47–48	5	30	−2	57–59	13	25–26	7	139–151	−3	98–104	−2	Cigarettes	4
31	−11	49–50	6	31	−1	60–61	14	27–29	6	152–166	−2	105–112	−1	Diabetic-male	3
32	−9	51–52	7	32–33	0	62–64	15	30–32	5	167–182	−1	113–120	0	Diabetic-female	6
33	−8	53–55	8	34	1	65–67	16	33–35	4	183–199	0	121–129	1	ECG-LVH	9
34	−6	56–60	9	35–36	2	68–70	17	36–38	3	200–219	1	130–139	2		
35	−5	61–67	10	37–38	3	71–73	18	39–42	2	220–239	2	140–149	3	0 pts for each NO	
36	−4	68–74	11	39	4	74	19	43–46	1	240–262	3	150–160	4		
37	−3			40–41	5			47–50	0	263–288	4	161–172	5		
38	−2			42–43	6			51–55	−1	289–315	5	173–185	6		
39	−1			44–45	7			56–60	−2	316–330	6				
40	0			46–47	8			61–66	−3						
41	1			48–49	9			67–73	−4						
42–43	2			50–51	10			74–80	−5						
44	3			52–54	11			81–87	−6						
45–46	4			55–56	12			88–96	−7						

2. Sum Points For All Risk Factors

_____ + _____ + _____ + _____ + _____ + _____ + _____ = _____

Age   HDL-C   Total-C   SBP   Smoker   Diabetes   ECG-LVH   Point Total

NOTE: *Minus Points Subtract From Total.*

3. Look Up Risk Corresponding To Point Total

Pts.	5 Yr.	10 Yr.	Pts.	5 Yr.	10 Yr.	Pts.	5 Yr.	10 Yr.	Pts.	5 Yr.	10 Yr.
≤1	<1%	<2%	10	2%	6%	19	8%	16%	28	19%	33%
2	1%	2%	11	3%	6%	20	8%	18%	29	20%	36%
3	1%	2%	12	3%	7%	21	9%	19%	30	22%	38%
4	1%	2%	13	3%	8%	22	11%	21%	31	24%	40%
5	1%	3%	14	4%	9%	23	12%	23%	32	25%	42%
6	1%	3%	15	5%	10%	24	13%	25%			
7	1%	4%	16	5%	12%	25	14%	27%			
8	2%	4%	17	6%	13%	26	16%	29%			
9	2%	5%	18	7%	14%	27	17%	31%			

4. Compare To Average 10 Year Risk

Probability

Age	Women	Men
30–34	<1%	3%
35–39	<1%	5%
40–44	2%	6%
45–49	5%	10%
50–54	8%	14%
55–59	12%	16%
60–64	13%	21%
65–69	9%	30%
70–74	12%	24%

These charts were prepared with the help of William B. Kannel, M.D., Professor of Medicine and Public Health and Ralph D'Agostino, Ph.D., Head, Department of Mathematics, both at Boston University; Keaven Anderson, Ph.D., Statistician, NHLBI, Framingham Study; Daniel McGee, Ph.D., Associate Professor, University of Arizona.

Framingham Heart Study

Index

Note: Page numbers followed by f refer to illustrations, page numbers followed by t refer to tables, and page numbers followed by A refer to Appendices.